Supplements and New Media

For Instructors

Instructor's Resource Manual
ISBN: 0-13-143234-6

This manual contains a wealth of material to help faculty plan and manage the medical-surgical nursing course. It includes chapter overviews, detailed lecture suggestions and outlines, learning objectives, a complete test bank, answers to the textbook critical thinking exercises, teaching tips, and more for each chapter. The IRM also guides faculty on how to assign and use the text-specific Companion Website, www.prenhall.com/lemone, and the free student CD-ROM that accompany the textbook, as well as Prentice Hall's Research Navigator online.

Instructor's Resource CD-ROM
ISBN: 0-13-045581-4

This cross-platform CD-ROM provides discussion points and illustrations in PowerPoint from the new Third Edition of this textbook for use in classroom lectures. It also contains an electronic test bank, answers to the textbook critical thinking exercises, and animations from the Student CD-ROM. This supplement is available to faculty free upon adoption of the textbook.

Companion Website Syllabus Manager
www.prenhall.com/lemone

Faculty adopting this textbook have free access to the online Syllabus Manager on the Companion Website, www.prenhall.com/lemone. Syllabus Manager offers a whole host of features that facilitate the students' use of the Companion Website, and allows faculty to post syllabi and course information online for their students. For more information or a demonstration of Syllabus Manager, please contact a Prentice Hall Sales Representative.

Online Course Management Systems

Also available are online companions available for schools using course management systems. The online course management solutions feature interactive modules, electronic test bank, PowerPoint images, animations, assessment activities, and more. For more information about adopting an online course management system to accompany Medical-Surgical Nursing, please contact your Prentice Hall Health Sales Representative or go online to the appropriate website below and select "Courses," then "Nursing."

WebCT: http://cms.prenhall.com/webct/index.html/
BlackBoard: http://cms.prenhall.com/blackboard/index.html/
CourseCompass: http://cms.prenhall.com/coursecompass/

D1372484

Brief Contents

MEDICAL-SURGICAL NURSING

Critical Thinking in Client Care

VOLUME ONE
THIRD EDITION

PRISCILLA LEMONE, RN, DSN
University of Missouri–Columbia, Columbia, Missouri

KAREN BURKE, RN, MS
Clatsop Community College, Astoria, Oregon

PEARSON

Prentice
Hall

Upper Saddle River, NJ 07458

Cover art from "Kaleidoscope XVIII: Chai," by Paula Nadelstern, reproduced from *Kaleidoscope Artistry,* by Cozy Baker, published by C&T Publishing, Inc.

Taken from:

Medical Surgical Nursing: Critical Thinking in Client Care, Third Edition
by Priscilla LeMone and Karen Burke
Copyright © 2004 by Pearson Education, Inc.
Published by Prentice Hall, Inc.
Upper Saddle River, New Jersey 07458

This special edition published in cooperation with Pearson Custom Publishing.

Printed in the United States of America

10 9 8 7 6 5 4 3 2 1

ISBN 0-13-114768-4

BA 998419

JC

Please visit our web site at *www.pearsoned.com*

PEARSON CUSTOM PUBLISHING
75 Arlington Street, Suite 300, Boston, MA 02116
A Pearson Education Company

I dedicate this book to the people I love.
    Priscilla LeMone

To my husband and best friend, Steve, who never waivers in his love and support; our daughter, Kristin, who makes me unbelievably proud and awestruck; and our son, Nathan, whose spirit, humor, and incredible courage will always be with us.
    Karen Burke

DETAILED CONTENTS

PART 3
ELIMINATION PATTERNS   609

Unit 6
Responses to Altered Bowel Elimination   611

Chapter 23
Assessing Clients with Bowel Elimination Disorders   612

Chapter 24
Nursing Care of Clients with Bowel Disorders   617

Unit 7
Responses to Altered Urinary Elimination   693

Unit 9
Responses to Altered Peripheral Tissue Perfusion   917

Chapter 31
Assessing Clients with Hematologic, Peripheral Vascular, and Lymphatic Disorders   918

Chapter 32
Nursing Care of Clients with Hematologic Disorders   931

PART 5
COGNITIVE AND PERCEPTUAL PATTERNS 1287

Unit 12
Responses to Altered Neurologic Function 1289

Chapter 49
Nursing Care of Clients with Sexually Transmitted Infections 1598

At no other time in recent history has there been a greater need for nurses. In fact, the need for new nurses is projected to be at or greater than 1 million by 2010. Registered nurses are the largest group of health care professionals in the United States, numbering over 2.6 million. However, various forces are in effect that may decrease their numbers or challenge their ability to meet client needs. As our currently employed nurses age and retire, the population will also become older. As the population ages, more people will develop chronic illnesses and disabilities that require skilled nursing care. This means that your knowledge and skills will be in demand to meet health care needs well into the future.

Students are expected to build on a knowledge foundation of basic sciences, social sciences, and fundamentals of nursing to synthesize and critically analyze new knowledge necessary to provide holistic care that addresses the individualized human responses to potential or actual alterations in health. The third edition of *Medical-Surgical Nursing: Critical Thinking in Client Care* has been completely revised to provide you with that knowledge and the skills needed to care for clients to promote health, facilitate recovery from illness and injury, and provide support when coping with disability or grieving.

The kaleidoscope cover image is a strong reflection of health care today. The meditative aspect of focusing on the images in the kaleidoscope calms and helps to integrate the mind, spirit, and body. As with nursing care, healing benefits are discovered through various complementary and alternative therapy methods. Nursing care, like the kaleidoscope, is the integration of mind-body-spirit.

GOALS FOR THIS TEXTBOOK

Although the information has been totally updated, we continue to believe that students learn best within a nursing model of care with consistent organization and understandable text. From the first edition, we have held fast to our vision that this textbook will:

- Provide the most current information possible about the art and science of nursing.

- Provide clear explanations of the pathophysiologic processes of human illnesses and injury, integrating that information as a vital component of treatment and nursing care.

- Emphasize the nurse's role as an essential member of the health care team.

- Prioritize nursing diagnoses and interventions specific to altered responses to illness.

- Provide case studies for each major illness or injury so students can envision the client as a person requiring care.

- Foster critical thinking and decision-making skills in clinical practice.

NEW TO THIS EDITION

The third edition of this textbook includes new content on cultural diversity that is integrated throughout the narrative as well as incorporated into the following feature boxes: Focus on Diversity, Nursing Care of the Older Adult, Meeting Individualized Needs, Nursing Research, and Multisystem Effects. Additionally, new content covers health promotion, gerontology, complementary and alternative therapies, genetics, and diseases specific to bioterrorism. The new health-promotion heads can be found in the nursing care section in every disorder chapter. Complementary and alternative therapies are integrated throughout the textbook where appropriate. Genetics as a risk factor or that increases incidence of a disease is included with the disorders, such as Huntington's chorea, Von Willebrand's disease, sickle cell disease, and hemophilia. Diseases are included if more prevalent as the result of inheritance (such as diabetes). Genetic counseling is included in nursing care as appropriate. Information about infections that may be caused by bioterrorism is included in Chapter 8. Based on reviewer feedback, two new chapters have been added: Chapter 12 concerns care of clients with substance abuse and Chapter 39 deals with care of clients with musculoskeletal disorders (two separate chapters in the previous edition). This combined chapter is more consistent and easier for students to follow.

ORGANIZATION

The book has six major parts, organized by functional health patterns. Each part opens with a concept map illustrating the relationship of each functional health pattern to possible nursing diagnoses. The parts are then divided into units based on alterations in human structure and function. Each unit with a focus on altered health states opens with an assessment chapter that provides a review of normal anatomy and physiology, questions for a health history, and assessment techniques with possible abnormal findings. Students will find a detailed health history questionnaire, using functional health patterns as a guide, on the Companion Website. Also on the CD, students will find a comprehensive review of anatomy and physiology complete with animations, three-dimensional structures, and exercises. This draws upon the student's prerequisite knowledge, and serves to reinforce basic principles of anatomy and physiology as applied to physical assessment.

Following the assessment chapter in each unit, information about major conditions and diseases follows a consistent chapter format. Key components of the clinical chapters include the following:

PATHOPHYSIOLOGY. The discussion of each major illness or condition begins with an overview of pathophysiology, followed by manifestations and complications. In the new edition, we have increased coverage of pathophysiology and highlighted it as a section within the disease. A new feature, Focus on Diversity, is included with some disorders to demonstrate, for example, how race, age, and gender affect differences in incidence, prevalence, and mortality.

COLLABORATIVE CARE. Collaborative care considers the treatment of the illness or condition by the health care team. Information in this section includes, as appropriate, diagnostic tests, medications, surgery and treatments, fluid management, dietary management, and complementary therapies.

NURSING CARE. Because the prevention of illness is a critical factor in health care today, this section begins with health-promotion information. A brief section on assessment provides a focused health history interview and physical examination guides, as well as information about assessment of the older adult. Nursing care is discussed within a context of priority nursing diagnoses and interventions, with rationales provided for each intervention. As care is increasingly provided in the home, nursing care is followed by a list of topics and resources for teaching about home care. Lastly, for each major disorder or condition, a narrative Nursing Care Plan is provided. Each plan begins with a brief case study, followed by the steps of the nursing process in action. Critical thinking questions specific to the care plan conclude this part, with a section called Evaluate Your Response that provides additional guidance for critical thinking. Suggested guidelines are found in Appendix C.

CHAPTER REVIEW. This new section at the end of each chapter concludes with five multiple-choice review questions, to reinforce comprehension of the chapter content. The student will also find the section entitled EXPLORE MediaLink, which encourages students to use the CD-ROM and the Companion Website to apply what they have learned from the textbook in case studies, to practice NCLEX questions, and to use additional resources such as animation tutorials and more.

HALLMARK FEATURES

Thoughtful attention was given to existing features that students and faculty liked in the previous edition. We give them more emphasis in the new edition.

- **Manifestations** boxes reinforce understanding of the effects of illness or injury, and guide assessments and interventions.
- **Pathophysiology Illustrated** and **Multisystem Effects** features provide visual illustrations of the causes and consequences of pathophysiology.
- **Nursing Implications** boxes provide students with nursing implications that they need to be aware of when their client is undergoing a particular diagnostic test. These boxes address nursing care and client/family teaching.
- **Meeting Individualized Needs** boxes contain information specific to altered health, age, gender, race, and culture.

- **Procedure** boxes describe common or important procedures in detail.
- **Nursing Care of the Client** boxes describe nursing care for various medical or surgical procedures.

NEW FEATURES

In addition to the hallmark features that have made this textbook so popular with students and faculty, we provide new items that help students learn the concepts in this textbook, apply them in clinical settings, and hone their clinical judgment skills. These include the following:

- **MediaLink,** at the beginning of each chapter, lists specific content, animations, anatomy and physiology review, NCLEX review questions, tools, and other interactive exercises that appear on the accompanying student CD-ROM and the Companion Website. Special MediaLink tabs appear throughout the chapter in the margins, encouraging the students to use the media supplements for specific activities, applications, and resources. The purpose of the MediaLink feature is to further enhance the student experience, build on knowledge gained from the textbook, prepare students for NCLEX, and foster critical thinking.
- **Medication Administration** boxes provide examples of drugs commonly prescribed for specific illnesses, followed by nursing responsibilities and client/family teaching. The medication boxes reflect the role of nurses, who administer medications.
- **Focus on Diversity** boxes list incidence, prevalence, etiology, and more for a particular disorder as effected by race or ethnicity.
- **Nursing Care of the Older Adult** boxes are found throughout the text, as well as in the assessment sections for disorders. As the population continues to age, this is critical information for nursing care in any setting, and provides guidelines for assessing and teaching in home care for the elderly.
- **Nursing Care Plans** throughout the text help students approach care from a nursing process perspective. The care plan is followed by critical thinking questions for students to apply their knowledge to a plan of care for a specific client. Suggested responses to the critical thinking questions can be found in Appendix C. Additional care plan activities can be found on the Companion Website at www.prenhall.com/lemone. These activities provide students with client scenarios so they can write comprehensive care plans and email them to instructors as homework assignments.
- **NANDA, NIC, and NOC** charts illustrate the most up-to-date information on nursing language, and demonstrate how these items are related for specific disorders.
- **Nursing Research: Evidence-Based Practice** boxes are included to show how nursing research is used to provide rationales for nursing care.
- **Practice Alerts** are integrated into nursing care purposefully to help students consider all aspects of nursing even

though they may be focusing on only one aspect of client needs.

- **End of Chapter Review Section** provides students with an opportunity to evaluate their comprehension of the chapter. The student-friendly section includes:
- **Test Yourself**—Review questions at the end of every chapter.
- **EXPLORE MediaLink**—at the end of every chapter, encourages students to use the CD-ROM and Companion Website to apply their knowledge of the chapter through additional case studies, practice NCLEX questions, A&P review, animation tutorials, and additional resources.

COMPREHENSIVE TEACHING-LEARNING PACKAGE

Clinical Handbook ISBN: 0-13-048397-4

Serves as a portable, quick reference to medical-surgical nursing. Organized alphabetizing provides a succinct review of common disorders and conditions, including pathophysiology, nursing diagnoses, interventions, client teaching, and home care. This handbook will allow students to bring the information they learn from class into any clinical setting.

Study Guide ISBN: 0-13-113666-6

Provides anatomy and physiology review, study tips, review exercises, case studies, care plan activities, NCLEX review, and more. MediaLinks refer students to activities on the CD-ROM and Companion Website.

Student CD-ROM

Packaged *free* with the textbook, the student CD-ROM provides an interactive study program that allows students to practice answering NCLEX-style questions with rationales for right and wrong answers. It also contains an audio glossary, animations, anatomy and physiology review, and a link to the Companion Website (an Internet connection is required).

Companion Website

A *free* online study guide is designed to help students apply the concepts presented in the book. Each chapter-specific module features objectives, audio glossary, chapter summary for lecture notes, NCLEX review questions, case studies, care plan activities, MediaLink applications, WebLinks, and nursing tools, such as functional health pattern concept maps, assessment guides, and more.

SUPPLEMENTS AND NEW MEDIA FOR INSTRUCTORS

Instructor's Resource Manual ISBN: 0-13-143234-6

This manual contains a wealth of material to help faculty plan and manage the medical-surgical nursing course. It includes chapter overviews, detailed lecture suggestions and outlines, learning objectives, a complete test bank, answers to the textbook critical thinking exercises, teaching tips, and more for each chapter. The IRM also guides faculty how to assign and use the text-specific Companion Website, www.prenhall.com/lemone, and the free student CD-ROM that accompany the textbook.

Instructor's Resource CD-ROM ISBN: 0-13-045581-4

This cross-platform CD-ROM provides illustrations in PowerPoint from the new third edition of this textbook for use in classroom lectures. It also contains an electronic test bank, answers to the textbook critical thinking exercises, and animations from the student CD-ROM. This supplement is available to faculty free upon adoption of the textbook.

Companion Website Syllabus Manager

www.prenhall.com/lemone

Faculty adopting this textbook has *free* access to the online Syllabus Manager on the Companion Website, www.prenhall.com/lemone. Syllabus Manager offers a whole host of features that facilitate the students' use of the Companion Website, and allows faculty to post syllabi and course information online for students. For more information or a demonstration of Syllabus Manager, please contact a Prentice Hall sales representative.

Online Course Management Systems

Also available are online companions for schools using course management systems. The online course management solutions feature interactive modules, electronic test bank, PowerPoint images, animations, assessment activities, and more. For more information about adopting an online course management system to accompany *Medical-Surgical Nursing*, please contact your Prentice Hall Health sales representative or go online to one of the following websites and select "courses."

WebCT: http://cms.prenhall.com/webct/index.html/

Blackboard: http://cms.prenhall.com/blackboard/index.html/

CourseCompass: http://cms.prenhall.com/coursecompass/

CONTRIBUTORS

Text Contributors

Jane Bostick, PhD, RN
Sinclair School of Nursing
University of Missouri-Columbia
  Columbia, MO

Chapter 12: Nursing Care of Clients
  with Problems of Substance Abuse

Roxanne W. McDaniel, PhD, RN
Sinclair School of Nursing
University of Missouri-Columbia
  Columbia, MO

Chapter 10: Nursing Care of Clients with
  Cancer

Elaine Mohn-Brown, RN, EdD
Chemeketa Community College
Salem, OR

Chapter 8: Nursing Care of Clients with
  Infection

Chapter 9: Nursing Care of Clients with
  Altered Immunity

Chapter 45: Nursing Care of Clients with
  Eye and Ear Disorders

Margorie Whitman, RN, MSN, AOCN
Sinclair School of Nursing
University of Missouri-Columbia
  Columbia, MO

Chapter 7: Nursing Care of Clients Having
  Surgery

SUPPLEMENT AND MEDIA WRITERS
Student CD-ROM

Joseann DeWitt, RN, MSN, BC, CLNC
Alcorn State University School of Nursing
Department of Baccalaureate Nursing
Natchez, MS

Rebecca Gesler, RN, MSN
Nursing Professor
Saint Catharine College
St. Catharine, KY

Laurie Kaudewitz, RNC, BSN, MSN
Assistant Professor
East Tennessee State University
Johnson City, TN

**Douglas Turner, PhD(C), RN, MSN, CNS,
  CRNA**
Lead Instructor
Forsyth Technical Community College
Winston-Salem, NC

Linda White, PhD(C), MSN, CNS, RN
Lead Instructor
Forsyth Technical Community College
Winston-Salem, NC

Companion Website

Joseann DeWitt, RN, MSN, BC, CLNC
Alcorn State University School of Nursing
Department of Baccalaureate Nursing
Natches, MS

Peggy Ellis, PhD, RNCS, ANP
University of Missouri
Barnes College of Nursing
St. Louis, MO

Lynne Bryant, PhD, RN, MSN
Associate Professor, Nursing Technology
Broward Community College
Davie, FL

Rebecca Gesler, RN, MSN
Nursing Professor
Saint Catherine College
St. Catherine, KY

Vincent Salyers, RN, EdD
Associate Professor
Palomar College
San Marcos, CA
Adjunct Professor
University of Phoenix
San Diego, CA

Study Guide

Jacqueline B. Brinkman, RN, BSN, CPN
College of the Redwoods
Eureka, CA

Joseann DeWitt, RN, MSN, BC, CLNC
Alcorn State University School of Nursing
Department of Baccalaureate Nursing
Natchez, MS

Golden Tradewell, PhD, RN, MSN, MA
Associate Professor
McNeese State University
College of Nursing
Lake Charles, LA

Instructor's Resource Manual

Joyce Hammer, RN, MSN
Lourdes College
Sylvania, OH

Edna Hull, RN, MSN, CPN
Assistant Professor
Delgado Community College–Charity
  School of Nursing
New Orleans, LA

REVIEWERS

Marianne Adam, MSN, RN, CRNP
Assistant Professor
Moravian College—St. Luke's School of
　　Nursing
Bethlehem, PA

Ellise D. Adams, CNM, MSN, CD, ICCE
Nursing Faculty
Calhoun Community College
Decatur, AL

Martha Baker, PhD, RN, CS, CCRN
Associate Professor
Missouri Southern State College
Joplin, MO

Claudia P. Barone, EdD, RN, LNC, CPC
Clinical Assistant Professor, Dean for the
　　Master's Program,
Chairperson Department of Nursing Practice
University of Arkansas for Medical Sciences
Little Rock, AR

Gail Bolling, MS, RN, CCRN
Associate Professor
Montgomery College
Takoma Park, MD

Joanne Bonesteel, MS, RN
Nursing Faculty
Excelsior College
Albany, NY

Tara Brenner, MS, RN, CS
Assistant Professor
SUNY Brockport
Brockport, NY

Polly Cameron Haigler, PhD, RN
Clinical Assistant Professor
University of South Carolina
Columbia, SC

Candice Cherrington, PhD, RN
Assistant Professor
Wright State University
Dayton, OH

Betty Christeson, BSNE, MN, EdD
Adjunct Faculty
Greenville Technical College
Greenville, SC

Patty Clark, RN, MSN
Associate Professor
Abraham Baldwin College
Tifton, GA

Janet M. Clifton, MS
Instructor
Danville Area Community College
Danville, IL

Maureen Cochran, RN, PhD
Nursing Faculty
Suffolk University
Boston, MA

Ruth F. Craven, EdD, RN, BC, FAAN
Professor and Associate Dean
University of Washington
Seattle, WA

Janice A. Cullen, EdD, RN
Associate Professor
University of South Carolina-Aiken
Aiken, SC

Cynthia L. Dakin, RN, PHD
Clinical Specialist
Northeastern University
Boston, MA

Ann Denney, RN, MSN
Assistant Professor
Thomas More College
Crestview Hills, KY

Nancy Dentlinger, AS, BS, MS
Assistant Director
Redlands Community College
El Reno, OK

Susan DeSanto-Madeya, RN, DNSc
Assistant Professor
Moravian College—St. Luke's School of
　　Nursing
Bethlehem, PA

Susan Dipert-Scott, RN, MS
Adjunct Faculty
Wright State University
Dayton, OH

Mary Jo Distel, MS
Assistant Professor
Midwestern State University
Wichita Falls, TX

Jean Forsha, MSN, RN
Nursing Faculty
Westchester University
Westchester, PA

Rebecca Gesler, RN, MSN
Director
Saint Catherine College
St. Catherine, KY

Paula Gilbert, BS, RN, ANP
Nursing Instructor
Arnot Ogden Medical Center
Elmira, NY

LaVerne Grant, MS, RN
Assistant Professor
University of Mississippi Medical Center
Jackson, MS

**Corinne Grimes, RN, MSN, DNSc,
AOCN**
Assistant Professor
Texas Women's University
Dallas, TX

Barbara F. Harrah, RN, MSN
Assistant Professor
Kent State University
East Liverpool, OH

Anne Helm, RN, BSN, MSN
Associate Professor
Owens Community College
Toledo, OH

Mary Ann Helm, MSN, MRE, RN
Assistant Professor
Nursing Faculty
Tennessee State University
Nashville, TN

Beverly K. Hogan, MSN, RN, CS
Nursing Faculty
University of Alabama-Birmingham
Birmingham, AL

Susan P. Holmes, MSN, CRNP
Nursing Faculty
Auburn University
Auburn, AL

**Karen C. Johnson-Brennam, EdD,
RN, MSN**
Professor and Associate Director
San Francisco State University
San Francisco, CA

Paula R. Klemm, DNSc, RN, OCN
Associate Professor
University of Delaware
Newark, DE

Wilma La Cava, RNC, MSN
Assistant Professor
Riverside Community College
Riverside, CA

Kristine M. Lecuyer, RN, MSN
Adjunct Assistant Professor
Saint Louis University
St. Louis, MO

Camille Little, MS, RN, CS
Assistant Professor
Illinois State University
Normal, IL

Karen Martin, RN, MS
Assistant Professor
Pikeville College
Paintsville, KY

Arlene McGrory, DNSc, RN
Associate Professor
University of Massachusetts-Lowell
Lowell, MA

Shirley McIntosh, RNC, MSN, LNC
Clinical Instructor
Kent State University
Kent, OH

Donna Nayduch, RN, MSN, ACNP
Regional Trauma Director
Benner Health System
Greeley, CO

Dula F. Pacquiao, EdD, RN, CTN
Professor and Director
Kean University
Union, NJ

Lily Paull, SDN, BSN, MAE
Clinical Instructor
University of Washington
Seattle, WA

Dianne Reed, APRN, BC
Associate Professor
Texarkana College
Texarkana, TX

Renee S. Schnieder, MSN, RN
Faculty Advisor
Southeast Community College
Lincoln, NE

Beth Scott, MS, RN
Nursing Faculty
Redlands Community College
El Reno, OK

Nancy Severance, MS, RNCS
Instructor
Boise State University
Boise, ID

Audrey Stephan, EdD, RN, CCRN
Associate Professor
Bergen Community College
Paramus, NJ

Jean Stroud, RN, MS
Professor
Imperial Valley College
Imperial, CA

Scott Thigpen, RN, MSN, CCRN
Assistant Professor
South Georgia College
Douglas, GA

Marie Thonis Colucci, RN, MN, EdD
Associate Professor
Riverside Community College
Riverside, CA

Rosemary Valentine, MSN, RN
Associate Professor, Associate Degree
    Department Chair
University of Charleston
Charleston, WV

Evelyn Wills, RN, PhD
Associate Professor
University of Louisiana-Lafayette
Lafayette, LA

Janet M. Witucki-Brown, PhD, RN
Assistant Professor
University of Tennessee
Knoxville, TN

Cynthia Wolfer, RN, MSN
Clinical Assistant Professor
Pacific Lutheran University
Tacoma, WA

Eden Zabat, RN, DNSC
Faculty Instructor
Westchester University
Westchester, PA

Dolores M. Zygmont, PhD, RN
Assistant Professor
Temple University
Philadelphia, PA

PRISCILLA LEMONE, RN, DSN, FAAN

Priscilla LeMone has spent most of her career as a nurse educator, teaching medical-surgical nursing and patho-physiology at all levels from diploma to doctoral students. She has a diploma in nursing from Deaconess College of Nursing (St. Louis, Missouri), baccalaureate and master's degrees from Southeast Missouri State University, and a doctorate in nursing from the University of Alabama-Birmingham. She is currently an Associate Professor and Director of Undergraduate Studies, Sinclair School of Nursing, University of Missouri-Columbia.

Dr. LeMone has had numerous awards for scholarship and teaching during her over 30 years as a nurse educator. She is most honored for receiving the Kemper Fellowship for Teaching Excellence from the University of Missouri-Columbia, the Unique Contribution Award from the North American Nursing Diagnosis Association, and for being selected as a Fellow in the American Academy of Nursing.

She believes that her education gave her solid and everlasting roots in nursing. Her work with students has given her the wings that allow her love of nursing and teaching to continue through the years.

A widow, Dr. LeMone lives with her dog and shares time with her two children and her granddaughter. When she has time, she enjoys growing flowers and reading fiction.

KAREN M. BURKE, RN, MS

Karen Burke has practiced nursing in acute intensive and coronary care, in community-based settings, and in nursing education. As an educator, she has taught nursing skills, fundamentals, pathophysiology, and basic to advanced medical-surgical nursing. Ms. Burke has a diploma in nursing from Emanuel Hospital School of Nursing in Portland, Oregon, later completing baccalaureate studies at Oregon Health & Science University, and a master's degree at University of Portland.

Ms. Burke has been part of the nursing faculty at Clatsop Community College in Astoria, Oregon, since the inception of the Associate Degree Nursing program in 1983, most recently serving as Director of Health Occupations and Nursing. In this role, she is known as a leader and an innovator. She led the nursing faculty in developing an online program to deliver basic nursing education to a distant rural community. This program continues, serving as a model for other community college nursing programs to reach out to geographically isolated communities. Ms. Burke is actively involved in nursing education and developing strategies to address the nursing shortage in Oregon. She is a member of the Oregon Council of Associate Degree Nursing Programs (OCAP) and the Oregon Nursing Leadership Council (ONLC), currently serving as chair of the ONLC Education Committee. She is coauthor of several other texts: *Medical-Surgical Nursing Care,* with Priscilla LeMone and Elaine Mohn-Brown; *Fundamentals of Nursing: Concepts, Process, and Practice* (6th edition), with Barbara Kozier, Glenora Erb, and Audrey Berman; and a clinical handbook to accompany this text.

Ms. Burke sees herself as a nurse first, then a nurse educator and educational administrator. She strongly values the nursing profession and the importance of providing a solid education in the art and science of nursing for all students entering the profession.

When possible, Ms. Burke and her husband Steve spend time with their extended family and traveling. She enjoys a passion for quilting, and, when the weather allows, gardening.

Guide to
MEDICAL-SURGICAL NURSING

PART **II**

NUTRITION AND METABOLIC PATTERNS

Unit 3
Responses to Altered Integumentary
Structure and Function
Unit 4
Responses to Al_____ction

CHAPTER 3

Community-Based
and Home Care
of the Adult Client

MediaLink

www.prenhall.com/lemone
Additional resources for this chapter
can be found on the Student CD-ROM
accompanying this textbook, and on
the Companion Website at
www.prenhall.com/lemone. Click on
Chapter 3 to select the activities for
this chapter.

CD-ROM
• Audio Glossary
• NCLEX Review

Companion Website
• More NCLEX Review
• Case Study
   Home Health Nursing
• Care Plan Activity
   Home Health Assessment
• MediaLink Applications
   Hospice: Purpose and Benefits

After completing this chapter, you will be able to:
• Define community-based nursing care.
• Discuss factors affecting health status in the community.
• Describe community-based health care services.
• Describe home health nursing and the roles of the home
   health nurse.
• Describe the components of the home health care system,
   including agencies, clients, referrals, physicians, reimburse-
   ment, and legal considerations.
• Discuss the effect of the home setting on nursing practice.
• Apply the nursing process to care of the client in the home.

LEARNING OUTCOMES

Functional Health Patterns with Related Nursing Diagnoses

HEALTH PERCEPTION HEALTH MANAGEMENT
• Perceived health status
• Perceived health management
• Health care behaviors: health
  promotion and illness prevention
  activities, medical treatments,
  follow-up care

VALUE-BELIEF
• Values, goals, or beliefs (including
  spirituality) that guide choices or
  decisions
• Perceived conflicts in values, beliefs,
  or expectations that are health
  related

COPING-STRESS-TOLERANCE
• Capacity to resist challenges to
  self-integrity
• Methods of handling stress
• Support systems
• Perceived ability to control and
  manage situations

NUTRITIONAL-METABOLIC
• Daily consumption of food and fluids
• Favorite foods
• Use of dietary supplements
• Skin lesions and ability to heal
• Condition of the integument
• Weight, height, temperature

**Part 2
Nutrition and Metabolic Patterns
NANDA Nursing Diagnoses**
• Risk for Aspiration
• Risk for Imbalanced Body
  Temperature
• Impaired Dentition
• Feeding Self-Care Deficit
• Fluid Volume Deficit
• Fluid Volume Excess
• Risk for Deficient Fluid Volume
• Hyperthermia
• Hypothermia
• Risk for Infection
• Impaired Oral Mucous Membranes
• Nausea
• Imbalanced Nutrition: Less than
  Body Requirements
• Imbalanced Nutrition: More than
  Body Requirements
• Impaired Skin Integrity
• Risk for Impaired Skin Integrity
• Impaired Swallowing
• Ineffective Thermoregulation
• Impaired Tissue Integrity
• Risk For Trauma
• Adult Failure to Thrive

SEXUALITY-REPRODUCTIVE
• Satisfaction with sexuality or sexual
  relationships
• Reproductive pattern
• Female menstrual and perimeno-
  pausal history

ELIMINATION
• Patterns of bowel and urinary
  excretion
• Perceived regularity or irregularity of
  elimination
• Use of laxatives or routines
• Changes in time, modes, quality or
  quantity of excretions
• Use of devices for control

ROLE-RELATIONSHIP
• Perception of major roles,
  relationships, and responsibilities in
  current life situation
• Satisfaction with or disturbances in
  roles and relationships

ACTIVITY-EXERCISE
• Patterns of personally relevant
  exercise, activity, leisure, and
  recreation
• ADLs which require energy
  expenditure
• Factors that interfere with the desired
  pattern (e.g., illness or injury)

SELF-PERCEPTION-SELF-CONCEPT
• Attitudes about self
• Perceived abilities, worth, self-image,
  emotions
• Body posture and movement, eye
  contact, voice and speech patterns

SLEEP-REST
• Patterns of sleep and rest-/relaxation
  in a 24-hr period
• Perceptions of quality and quantity
  of sleep and rest
• Use of sleep aids or routines

COGNITIVE-PERCEPTUAL
• Adequacy of vision, hearing, taste,
  touch, smell
• Pain perception and management
• Language, judgment, memory,
  decisions

Part Openers

Each Part Opener is followed by a
Functional Health Pattern Concept Map.
These concept maps relate nursing diagnoses
to specific patterns covered in that part.

MediaLink introduces each chapter of the
text and lists additional specific content,
animations, NCLEX Review, tools, and
other interactive exercises, which appear on
the accompanying Student CD-ROM and
the Companion Website.

Learning Outcomes appear at the start
of each chapter, identifying important concepts students should know by the end of the
chapter.

CONTINUOUS CARDIAC MONITORING. Continuous monitoring of the cardiac rhythm is provided by bedside and central monitoring stations. Electrodes placed on the client's chest attach to cables connected to a monitor. The heart rate and rhythm is visually displayed on a bedside monitor connected to a central monitoring station. The central station allows simultaneous monitoring of multiple clients within a nursing unit. Alarms on both bedside and central monitors warn of potential problems such as very rapid or very slow heart rates. Alarm limits are preset by the nurse for the individual client. Procedure 29–1 describes how to place a client on cardiac monitoring.

Telemetry may be used in acute care settings when the client is ambulatory. Chest electrodes are connected to a portable transmitter worn around the neck or waist; the ECG is trans-mitted electronically to a central monitoring station for continuous monitoring.

HOME MONITORING. Clients often complain of palpitations or other heart symptoms but are asymptomatic during evaluation in a hospital or community-based setting. Ambulatory or Holter monitoring may be used to identify intermittent dysrhythmias, to detect silent ischemia, to assess pacemaker or automatic cardioverter-defibrillator function. Electrodes are applied and the leads attached to the portable telemetry monitor that records and stores all electrical activity. Clients are instructed to leave the electrode pads in place during monitoring, record any cardiac symptoms or events in a journal (such as chest pain, palpitations, syncope), and are told when to return to the clinic. After the prescribed period, usu-

Procedure 29–1

Initiating Cardiac Monitoring

SUPPLIES

- Bedside monitor and cable or telemetry unit with fresh battery
- Electrodes—self-adherent, pregelled, disposable
- Lead wires
- Washcloth, soap, and towel
- Alcohol prep pads
- Dry gauze pads or ECG prep pads

4. Clean sites with soap and water, and dry thoroughly. Alcohol may be used to remove skin oils; allow the skin to dry for 60 seconds after use.
5. Gently rub the site with a dry gauze pad or ECG prep pad to remove dead skin oils, debris, and residue.
6. Open the electrode package; peel the backing from the electrode, and check to ensure that the center of the pad is moist with conductive gel.
7. Apply electrode pads, pressing firmly to ensure contact (see figure).
8. Attach leads and position cable with sufficient slack for comfort. Place the telemetry unit (if used) in gown pouch or pocket.
9. Assess ECG tracing on the monitor, adjusting settings as needed.

10. Set monitor alarm limits typically at 20 BPM higher and lower than the client's baseline rate. Turn alarms on, and leave on at all times. Assess immediately if an alarm is triggered.
11. Time and date pads with every change.

BEFORE THE PROCEDURE

Explain the reason for ECG monitoring. Reassure client that changes in heart rhythm can be noted and immediately treated if necessary. Explain that loose or disconnected lead wires, poor electrode contact, excessive movement, electrical interference, or equipment malfunction may trigger alarms and alert the staff, allowing correction of the problem. Reassure that movement allowed, within activity restrictions, while on the monitor. Explain skin preparation procedure. Provide for privacy, and drape appropriately.

PROCEDURE

1. Follow standard precautions.
2. Check equipment for damage (i.e., fraying, bent, or broken wires). Connect lead wires to cable, and secure connections.
3. Select electrode sites on the chest wall, avoiding areas of excessive movement, joints, skin creases, scar tissue, or other lesions.

AFTER THE PROCEDURE

Monitor periodically for comfort. Assess electrode and lead wire connections as needed. Remove and apply new pads every 24 to 48 hours or whenever the pad becomes dislodged or nonadherent. Clean gel residue from previous site, and document skin condition under the pads. Choose an alternative site if the skin appears irritated or blistered. Document ECG strips according to unit policy and/or physician's order, as well as when the cardiac rhythm or the client's condition changes (especially with complaints of chest pain, decreased level of consciousness or changes in vital signs). Note the date, time, client identification, monitor lead, duration of PR and QT intervals, and rhythm interpretation on each ECG strip.

Procedures explain common nursing skills in a step-by-step manner.

- Physical assessment: Height/weight ratio; tion) of extremities, peripheral pulses, skin and mucous membranes (hair loss, appearance, lesions, rash, itching, vaginal discharge)

Nursing Diagnoses and Interventions

Although many different nursing diagnoses are appropriate for the person with diabetes, those discussed in this section address problems with skin integrity, infection, injury, sexuality, coping, and health maintenance. The goals of care are to maintain function, prevent complications, and teach self-management.

Risk for Impaired Skin Integrity

The person with diabetes is at increased risk for altered skin integrity as a result of decreased or absent sensation from neuropathies, decreased tissue perfusion from cardiovascular complications, and infection. In addition, poor vision increases the risk of trauma, and an open lesion is more prone to infection and delayed healing. Impaired skin and tissue integrity, with resultant gangrene, is especially common in the feet and lower extremities.

- Conduct baseline and ongoing assessments of the feet, including:
  - Musculoskeletal assessment that includes foot and ankle joint range of motion, bone abnormalities (bunions, hammertoes, overlapping digits), gait patterns, use of assistive devices for walking, and abnormal wear patterns on shoes.
  - Neurologic assessment that includes sensations of touch and position, pain, and temperature.

warts, ingr... sure points, blisters... People with diabetes are at sign... gangrene. Peripheral neuropathies may result in alterations in the perception of pain, loss of deep tendon reflexes, loss of cutaneous pressure and position sensation, foot drop, changes in the shape of the foot, and changes in bones and joints. Peripheral vascular disease may cause intermittent claudication, absent pulses, delayed venous filling on elevation, dependent rubor, and gangrene. Injuries, lesions, and changes in skin hydration potentiate infections, delayed healing, and tissue loss in the person with diabetes mellitus.

- Teach foot hygiene. Wash the feet daily with lukewarm water and mild hand soap; pat dry, and dry well between water toes. Apply a very thin coat of lubricating cream if dryness is present (but not between the toes). Proper hygiene decreases the chance of infection. Temperature receptors may be impaired, so the water should always be tested before use.

PRACTICE ALERT Teach the person with diabetes to always test the water temperature in the shower or bath before stepping in. ■

- Discuss the importance of not smoking if client smokes. *Nicotine in tobacco causes vasoconstriction, further decreasing the blood supply to the feet.*

Practice Alerts appear throughout the text as helpful hints for clinical practice.

Diabetes me... adults. Howev... of the client... greatly. Consi...

- Cheryl Dra... oped diabet... severe panc... ful about tak... ing regularly... sion is getti... her legs, esp... Cheryl says... her more th...

- Tom Chang... nosed with type 2 diabetes. Although Tom was taught about the disease and the importance of taking his oral medications, following his diet plan, and getting exercise, he rarely did more than take the medication. Five years ago, he was hospitalized for hyperglycemia and started taking insulin. Last year Tom had a stroke, leaving him unable to walk. He has now been admitted to the hospital for treatment of gangrene of the large toe on his left foot.

- Grace Staples is an independent 82-year-old woman who lives alone and happily takes care of her two cats. She is slightly overweight. Last year, during Grace's annual eye examination, eye changes typical for diabetes were found. She was referred to her family doctor, who diagnosed type 2 diabetes and started her on oral medications. Grace sticks to her diet, walks a mile every day, and plans to live to be 100.

As illustrated in these examples, diabetes mellitus is not a single disorder but a group of chronic disorders of the endocrine pancreas, all categorized under a broad diagnostic label. The condition is characterized by inappropriate hyperglycemia caused by a relative or absolute deficiency of insulin, or by a cellular resistance to the action of insulin. Of the several classifications of diabetes, this chapter will focus on the two major types, type 1 and type 2. **Type 1 DM** is the result of pancreatic islet cell destruction and a total deficit of circulating insulin; **type 2 DM** results from insulin resistance with a defect in compensatory insulin secretion.

Diabetes mellitus has been recognized as a disease for centuries. Diabetes derives from a Greek word meaning "to siphon," referring to the increased output of urine. Mellitus derives from a Latin word meaning "sweet." The two words together identify the disease as an outpouring of sweet urine. It was not until 1921 that techniques were developed for extracting insulin from pancreatic tissue and for measuring blood glucose. At the same time, researchers discovered that insulin, when injected, produces a dramatic drop in blood glucose. This meant that diabetes could now be controlled. Since that time, oral hyperglycemic drugs, human insulin products, insulin pumps, home blood glucose monitoring, and transplantation of the pancreas or of pancreatic islet or beta cells have advanced the treatment and care of people with diabetes.

Diabetes is the sixth leading cause of death by disease in the United States, primarily because of the widespread cardiovascular effects that result in atherosclerosis, coronary artery disease, and stroke. People with diabetes are 2 to 4 times more likely to have heart disease, and 2 to 6 times more likely to have a stroke than people who do not have diabetes. Diabetes is the leading cause of end-stage renal disease (kidney failure), and the major cause of newly diagnosed blindness in people ages 20 to 74. Diabetes also is the most frequent cause of nontraumatic amputations.

Americans with diabetes use a disproportionate share of the nation's health care services. They visit outpatient services and physicians' offices more often than people who do not have the disease, and they require more frequent hospitalizations with longer days of in-hospital treatment. The cost of illness and resulting loss of productivity for people with diabetes exceeds $98 billion per year, according to an estimate by the National Institute for Diabetes and Kidney Disease.

Focus on Diversity

RISK AND INCIDENCE OF DIABETES MELLITUS

- 11.4 million (7.8%) of all non-Hispanic whites have diabetes.
- 2.8 million (13%) of all non-Hispanic African Americans have diabetes, and are 2 times as likely to have diabetes as non-Hispanic whites of similar age. African Americans with type 2 diabetes have higher rates of coronary heart disease, CVA, and end-stage renal disease than do Caucasians with the disease.
- 1.2 million (10.2%) of all Mexican Americans have diabetes, and are 1.9 times as likely to have diabetes as non-Hispanic whites of similar age.
- On average, Hispanic/Latino Americans are about 2 times more likely to have diabetes as non-Hispanic whites of similar age.
- Native Americans are 2.8 times more likely to have diabetes than non-Hispanic whites, and diabetes is especially prevalent in middle-aged and older American Indians. According to the World Health Organization, 50% of the Pima tribe have diabetes, and 90% are diagnosed by age 65 (Burke, 2001).

Focus on Diversity boxes list incidence, prevalence, etiology, and more for a particular disorder as affected by race or ethnicity.

Pathophysiology Illustrated are three-dimensional illustrations that help students to visualize the pathophysiological process of a particular disorder. Additional animations can be found on the Student CD-ROM.

Nursing Care Plan

Throughout the text, nursing care plans help students approach care from a nursing process perspective. The care plan is followed by critical thinking questions for students to apply their knowledge to plan the care for a specific client. Suggested responses to the critical thinking questions can be found in Appendix C. Additional Care Plan activities can be found on the Companion Website.

Multisystem Effects are labeled illustrations that point out the effects a disorder has on various body systems.

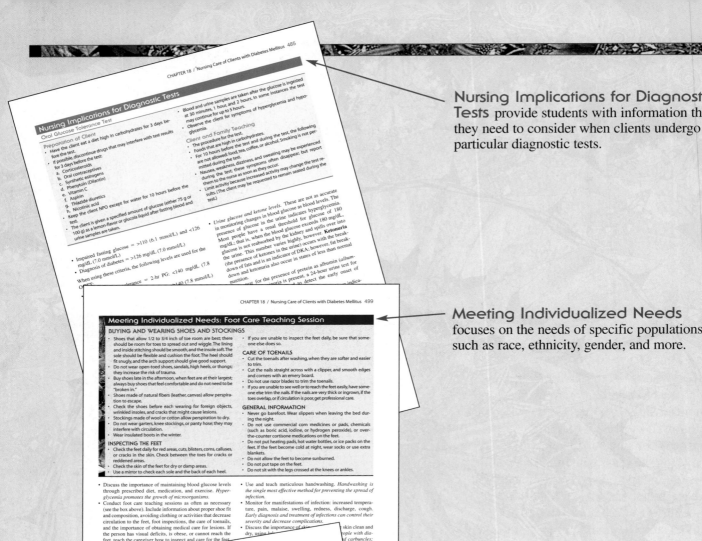

Nursing Implications for Diagnostic Tests
Oral Glucose Tolerance Test

Preparation of Client
- Have the client eat a diet high in carbohydrates for 3 days before the test.
- If possible, discontinue drugs that may interfere with test results for 3 days before the test:
  a. Corticosteroids
  b. Oral contraceptives
  c. Synthetic estrogens
  d. Phenytoin (Dilantin)
  e. Vitamin C
  f. Aspirin
  g. Thiazide diuretics
  h. Nicotinic acid
- Keep the client NPO except for water for 10 hours before the test.
- The client is given a specified amount of glucose (either 75 g or 100 g) as a lemon-flavor or glucola liquid after fasting blood and urine samples are taken.

- Blood and urine samples are taken after the glucose is ingested at 30 minutes, 1 hour, and 2 hours. In some instances the test may continue for up to 5 hours.
- Observe the client for symptoms of hyperglycemia and hypoglycemia.

Client and Family Teaching
- The procedure for the test.
- Foods that are high in carbohydrates.
- For 10 hours before the test and during the test, the following are not allowed: food, tea, coffee, or alcohol. Smoking is not permitted during the test.
- Nausea, weakness, dizziness, and sweating may be experienced during the test; these symptoms often disappear, but report them to the nurse as soon as they occur.
- Limit activity because increased activity may change the test results. (The client may be requested to remain seated during the test.)

- Impaired fasting glucose = >110 (6.1 mmol/L) and <126 mg/dL (7.0 mmol/L)
- Diagnosis of diabetes = >126 mg/dL (7.0 mmol/L)

When using these criteria, the following levels are used for the OGTT:
- Glucose tolerance = 2-hr PG: <140 mg/dL (7.8 ... >140 (7.8 mmol/L)

Urine glucose and ketone levels. These are not as accurate in monitoring changes in blood glucose as blood levels. The presence of glucose in the urine indicates hyperglycemia. Most people have a renal threshold for glucose of 180 mg/dL; that is, when the blood glucose exceeds 180 mg/dL, glucose is not reabsorbed by the kidney and spills over into the urine. This number varies highly, however. **Ketonuria** (the presence of ketones in the urine) occurs with the breakdown of fats and is an indicator of DKA; however, fat breakdown and ketonuria also occur in states of less than normal nutrition.

Meeting Individualized Needs: Foot Care Teaching Session

BUYING AND WEARING SHOES AND STOCKINGS
- Shoes that allow 1/2 to 3/4 inch of toe room are best; there should be room for toes to spread out and wiggle. The lining and inside stitching should be smooth, and the insole soft. The sole should be flexible and cushion the foot. The heel should fit snugly, and the arch support should give good support.
- Do not wear open-toed shoes, sandals, high heels, or thongs; they increase the risk of trauma.
- Buy shoes late in the afternoon, when feet are at their largest; always buy shoes that feel comfortable and do not need to be "broken in."
- Shoes made of natural fibers (leather, canvas) allow perspiration to escape.
- Check the shoes before each wearing for foreign objects, wrinkled insoles, and cracks that might cause lesions.
- Stockings made of wool or cotton allow perspiration to dry.
- Do not wear garters, knee stockings, or panty hose; they may interfere with circulation.
- Wear insulated boots in the winter.

INSPECTING THE FEET
- Check the feet daily for red areas, cuts, blisters, corns, calluses, or cracks in the skin. Check between the toes for cracks or reddened areas.
- Check the skin of the feet for dry or damp areas.
- Use a mirror to check each sole and the back of each heel.

- If you are unable to inspect the feet daily, be sure that someone else does so.

CARE OF TOENAILS
- Cut the toenails after washing, when they are softer and easier to trim.
- Cut the nails straight across with a clipper, and smooth edges and corners with an emery board.
- Do not use razor blades to trim the toenails.
- If you are unable to see well or to reach the feet easily, have someone else trim the nails. If the nails are very thick or ingrown, if the toes overlap, or if circulation is poor, get professional care.

GENERAL INFORMATION
- Never go barefoot. Wear slippers when leaving the bed during the night.
- Do not use commercial corn medicines or pads, chemicals (such as boric acid, iodine, or hydrogen peroxide), or over-the-counter cortisone medications on the feet.
- Do not put heating pads, hot water bottles, or ice packs on the feet. If the feet become cold at night, wear socks or use extra blankets.
- Do not allow the feet to become sunburned.
- Do not put tape on the feet.
- Do not sit with the legs crossed at the knees or ankles.

- Discuss the importance of maintaining blood glucose levels through prescribed diet, medication, and exercise. *Hyperglycemia promotes the growth of microorganisms.*
- Conduct foot care teaching sessions as often as necessary (see the box above). Include information about proper shoe fit and composition, avoiding clothing or activities that decrease circulation to the feet, foot inspections, the care of toenails, and the importance of obtaining medical care for lesions. If the person has visual deficits, is obese, or cannot reach the feet, teach the caregiver how to inspect and care for the feet. Feet should be inspected daily. *Foot care is ...*

- Use and teach meticulous handwashing. *Handwashing is the single most effective method for preventing the spread of infection.*
- Monitor for manifestations of infection: increased temperature, pain, malaise, swelling, redness, discharge, cough. *Early diagnosis and treatment of infections can control their severity and decrease complications.*
- Discuss the importance of skin ...

Nursing Care of the Older Adult

CARDIAC DYSRHYTHMIAS
Aging affects the heart and the cardiac conduction system, increasing the incidence of dysrhythmias and conduction defects. Older adults may experience dysrhythmias even when no evidence of heart disease is found.

Older adults have a higher incidence of both ventricular and supraventricular dysrhythmias without detrimental effects than younger people. Ectopic beats, including short runs of ventricular tachycardia, occur more commonly during exercise in older adults. These dysrhythmias do not affect cardiac morbidity or mortality. Fibrosis of the bundle branches can lead to atrioventricular blocks; a prolonged PR interval is common in clients over the age of 65. Older adults also have a higher incidence of diseases that may affect heart rhythm. An elderly client with hyperthyroidism, for example, may present with atrial fibrillation, syncope, and confusion instead of the usual manifestations of goiter, tremor, and exophthalmos.

ASSESSING FOR HOME CARE
Assessing older adults for problems related to cardiac dysrhythmias focuses on the effect of the dysrhythmia on functional health status.
- Ask about a history of cardiovascular disease and current medications.
- Ask about symptoms such as episodes of dizziness, lightheadedness, fainting, palpitations, chest pain, or shortness of breath.

- Ask about relationship of symptoms such as palpitations to intake of certain foods and caffeine-containing beverages.
- Evaluate for other contributing factors such as smoking or alcohol intake.
- Inquire about a history of falls, particularly those occurring without apparent reason.

TEACHING FOR HOME CARE
Teach measures to reduce the risk of cardiac dysrhythmias and potential adverse consequences of dysrhythmias.
- Emphasize the importance of taking medications as prescribed. Discuss possible effects of over-the-counter medications on the heart.
- Encourage reducing or eliminating caffeine intake. Caffeine increases the risk of ectopic beats and rapid heart rates.
- Encourage participation in a smoking cessation program and reduce or eliminate alcohol intake if appropriate.
- Encourage engaging in regular exercise. Discuss the beneficial effects of exercise to maintain muscle mass, including cardiac muscle, and cardiovascular health.
- Instruct to contact primary care provider for evaluation of symptoms such as dizziness, fainting, frequent palpitations, shortness of breath, unexplained falls, or chest pain.

- *Automaticity* is the ability of pacemaker cells to spontaneously initiate an electrical impulse. The SA node, the dominant pacemaker, normally generates impulses at the fastest rate, 60 to 100 times a minute. Myocardial muscle cells do not possess this ability.
- *Excitability* is the ability of myocardial cells to respond to stimuli generated by pacemaker cells.
- *Conductivity* is the ability to transmit an impulse from cell to cell. When one cell is stimulated, the impulse rapidly spreads throughout the heart muscle.
- *Contractility* is the ability of myocardial fibers to shorten in response to a stimulus. Heart muscle responds in an *all-or-nothing* manner: Stimulation of one muscle fiber causes the entire muscle mass to contract to its fullest extent as one unit.

The Action Potential
Movement of ions across cell membranes causes the electrical impulse that stimulates muscle contraction. This electrical activity, called the *action potential*, produces the waveforms represented on ECG strips.

In the resting state, positive and negative ions align on either side of the cell membrane, producing a relatively negative charge within the cell and a positive extracellular charge (Figure 29–9 ■). The cell is said to be *polarized*. The negative resting membrane potential is maintained at about − 90 millivolts (mV) by the sodium–potassium pump in the cell membrane.

When the resting cell is stimulated by an electrical charge from a neighboring cell or by a spontaneous event, its cell membrane permeability changes. Sodium ions enter the cell rapidly through openings called *fast sodium channels*. Slow *calcium–sodium channels* also open, allowing calcium into the cell. The membrane becomes less permeable to potassium ions. Addition of these positively charged ions to intracellular fluid changes the membrane potential from negative to slightly positive at − 20 to + 30 mV. This change in the electrical charge across the cell membrane is called **depolarization.**

As the cell becomes more positive, it reaches a point called the *threshold potential.* When the threshold potential is reached, an action potential is generated. The action potential causes a chemical reaction of calcium within the cell. This, in turn, causes actin and myosin filaments to slide together, producing cardiac muscle contraction. The action potential spreads to surrounding cells, causing a coordinated muscle contraction. As soon as the myocardium is completely depolarized, repolarization begins.

Repolarization returns the cell to its resting, polarized state. During *rapid repolarization*, fast sodium channels close abruptly, and the cell begins to regain its negative charge. During the *plateau phase*, muscle contraction is prolonged as slow calcium–sodium channels remain open. When these channels close, the sodium–potassium pump restores ion concentration to normal resting levels. The cell membrane is then polarized, ready for the cycle to start again. Each heartbeat represents one

---

Nursing Implications for Diagnostic Tests provide students with information that they need to consider when clients undergo particular diagnostic tests.

Meeting Individualized Needs focuses on the needs of specific populations, such as race, ethnicity, gender, and more.

Nursing Care of the Older Adult is found throughout the text, as well as in the assessment sections for disorders. As the population continues to age, this is critical information for nursing care in any setting, and provides guidelines for assessing and teaching in home care.

Medication Administration boxes help students learn the implications of certain medications the client is taking. Nursing responsibilities and client and family teaching practices are included.

NANDA, NIC, and NOC charts relate NANDA nursing diagnoses to NIC interventions and NOC outcomes for specific disorders.

Nursing Research: Evidence-Based Practice highlights nursing research and evidence-based practice as it applies to particular disorders or procedures, and provides critical thinking questions for students to apply that research.

Nursing Care of the Client

describes nursing care for various medical or surgical procedures.

EXPLORE MediaLink

Found at the end of every chapter, EXPLORE MediaLink encourages students to use the CD-ROM and the Companion Website to apply what they have learned from the text in case studies, practice NCLEX questions, and use additional resources.

Test Yourself allows students to test their knowledge of the chapter.

ADDITIONAL MEDIA RESOURCES:

Animation and Video Tutorials—On the Student CD-ROM, the student will find animations illustrating difficult concepts or reinforcing content in the text.

NCLEX Reviews—Both the Student CD-ROM and the free Companion Website offer the student an abundance of NCLEX review questions for each chapter of the book. The questions provide comprehensive rationales, as well as identify how the questions correlate to the NCLEX test plan.

Care Plan Activities—Each clinical chapter on the Companion Website provides the student with a case

scenario and asks the student to develop a care plan for the client. Students can e-mail these care plans to instructors as homework assignments.

Case Studies—For each clinical chapter on the Companion Website, the student can review a client scenario and answer critical thinking questions related to that client's care. Students can e-mail their responses to the case studies to instructors as homework assignments.

MediaLink Applications—Students are asked to go to websites to research the questions that are presented here.

SPECIAL FEATURES

 Nursing Care Plans

NANDA, NIC, and NOC Linkages

Focus on Diversity

 Meeting Individualized Needs

Procedures

Multisystem Effects of ...

Pathophysiology Illustrated

Medication Administration

Manifestations of ...

MEDICAL-SURGICAL NURSING PRACTICE

Unit 1

Dimensions of Medical-Surgical Nursing

Unit 2

Alterations in Patterns of Health

Functional Health Patterns with Related Nursing Diagnoses

HEALTH PERCEPTION HEALTH MANAGEMENT
- Perceived health status
- Perceived health management
- Health care behaviors: health promotion and illness prevention activities, medical treatments, follow-up care

VALUE-BELIEF
- Values, goals, or beliefs (including spirituality) that guide choices or decisions
- Perceived conflicts in values, beliefs, or expectations that are health related

COPING-STRESS-TOLERANCE
- Capacity to resist challenges to self-integrity
- Methods of handling stress
- Support systems
- Perceived ability to control and manage situations

NUTRITIONAL-METABOLIC
- Daily consumption of food and fluids
- Favorite foods
- Use of dietary supplements
- Skin lesions and ability to heal
- Condition of the integument
- Weight, height, temperature

Part 1
Medical-Surgical Nursing Practice NANDA Nursing Diagnoses

- Latex Allergy Response
- Caregiver Role Strain
- Chronic Sorrow
- Compromised Family Coping
- Death Anxiety
- Anxiety
- Decisional Conflict
- Disturbed Body Image
- Fatigue
- Fear
- Deficient Fluid Volume
- Excess Fluid Volume
- Ineffective Health Maintenance
- Health-Seeking Behaviors
- Risk for Infection
- Deficient Knowledge
- Nausea
- Acute Pain
- Chronic Pain
- Risk for Injury
- Powerlessness
- Disturbed Personal Identity
- Ineffective Protection
- Delayed Surgical Recovery
- Self-Care Deficit
- Low Self-Esteem
- Disturbed Sleep Pattern
- Ineffective Therapeutic Regimen Management
- Disturbed Thought Process
- Risk for Violence

SEXUALITY-REPRODUCTIVE
- Satisfaction with sexuality or sexual relationships
- Reproductive pattern
- Female menstrual and perimenopausal history

ELIMINATION
- Patterns of bowel and urinary excretion
- Perceived regularity or irregularity of elimination
- Use of laxatives or routines
- Changes in time, modes, quality or quantity of excretions
- Use of devices for control

ROLE-RELATIONSHIP
- Perception of major roles, relationships, and responsibilities in current life situation
- Satisfaction with or disturbances in roles and relationships

ACTIVITY-EXERCISE
- Patterns of personally relevant exercise, activity, leisure, and recreation
- ADLs which require energy expenditure
- Factors that interfere with the desired pattern (e.g., illness or injury)

SELF-PERCEPTION–SELF-CONCEPT
- Attitudes about self
- Perceived abilities, worth, self-image, emotions
- Body posture and movement, eye contact, voice and speech patterns

SLEEP-REST
- Patterns of sleep and rest-/relaxation in a 24-hr period
- Perceptions of quality and quantity of sleep and rest
- Use of sleep aids and routines

COGNITIVE-PERCEPTUAL
- Adequacy of vision, hearing, taste, touch, smell
- Pain perception and management
- Language, judgment, memory, decisions

DIMENSIONS OF MEDICAL-SURGICAL NURSING

The Medical-Surgical Nurse

MediaLink

www.prenhall.com/lemone

Additional resources for this chapter can be found on the Student CD-ROM accompanying this textbook, and on the Companion Website at www.prenhall.com/lemone. Click on Chapter 1 to select the activities for this chapter.

CD-ROM
- Audio Glossary
- NCLEX Review

Companion Website
- More NCLEX Review
- Case Study
    Advance Directive
- Care Plan Activity
    Nursing Process

After completing this chapter, you will be able to:

- Describe the activities and characteristics of the nurse as caregiver, educator, advocate, leader and manager, and researcher.

- Discuss the attitudes, mental habits, and skills necessary for critical thinking.

- Discuss the relationship between critical thinking and the nursing process in client care.

- Describe the importance of nursing codes and standards as guidelines for medical-surgical nursing care.

- Discuss the effect of legal and ethical dilemmas on nursing care.

- Discuss selected trends and issues in health care that affect medical-surgical nursing care.

Medical-surgical nursing is the health promotion, health care, and illness care of adults, based on knowledge derived from the arts and sciences and shaped by knowledge (the science) of nursing. Medical-surgical nursing focuses on the adult client's response to actual or potential alterations in health. In this textbook, discussions of those human responses are structured within the framework of functional health patterns, and nursing care is presented within the context of nursing diagnoses.

Medical-surgical nursing encompasses many interrelated components. The adult client—the person with whom and for whom nursing care is designed and implemented—ranges in age from the late teens to the early 100s. The human responses that nurses must consider when planning and implementing care result from changes in the structure and/or function of all body systems, as well as the interrelated effects of those changes on the psychosocial, cultural, spiritual, economic, and personal life of the client. The wide range of ages and the variety of health care needs specific to individual clients make medical-surgical nursing an ever-changing and challenging area of nursing practice.

ROLES OF THE NURSE IN MEDICAL-SURGICAL NURSING PRACTICE

Health care today is a vast and complex system. It reflects changes in society, changes in the populations requiring nursing care, and a philosophical shift toward health promotion rather than illness care. Roles of the medical-surgical nurse have broadened and expanded in response to these changes. Medical-surgical nurses are not only caregivers but also educators, advocates, leaders and managers, and researchers. The nurse assumes these various roles to promote and maintain health, to prevent illness, and to facilitate coping with disability or death for the adult **client** (a person requiring health care services) in any setting.

The Nurse as Caregiver

Nurses have always been caregivers. However, the activities carried out within the caregiver role have changed tremen-

Figure 1–1 ■ In the role of caregiver, the nurse provides comprehensive, individualized care to the adult client.

dously in the 21st century. From 1900 to the 1960s, the nurse was almost always female and was regarded primarily as the person who gave personal care and carried out physicians' orders. This dependent role has changed as a result of the increased education of nurses, research in and the development of nursing knowledge, and the recognition that nurses are autonomous and informed professionals.

The caregiver role for the nurse today is both independent and collaborative. Nurses independently make assessments and plan and implement client care based on nursing knowledge and skills (Figure 1–1 ■). Nurses also collaborate with other members of the health care team to implement and evaluate care.

As a caregiver, the nurse is a practitioner of nursing both as a science and as an art. Using **critical thinking** in the nursing process as the framework for care, the nurse provides interventions to meet not only the physical needs but also the psychosocial, cultural, spiritual, and environmental needs of clients and families. (Box 1–1 discusses culturally competent nursing care.) Considering all aspects of the client ensures a holistic approach to nursing. **Holistic nursing care** is based on a philosophical view that interacting wholes are greater than the sum of their parts. A holistic approach also emphasizes the uniqueness of the individual.

In providing comprehensive, individualized care, the nurse uses critical thinking skills to analyze and synthesize knowledge from the arts, the sciences, and nursing research and theory. The science (knowledge base) of nursing is translated into the art of nursing through caring. Caring is the means by which the nurse is connected with and concerned for the client (Benner & Wrubel, 1989). Thus, the nurse as caregiver is knowledgeable, skilled, empathic, and caring.

The Nurse as Educator

The nurse's role as educator is becoming increasingly important for several reasons. Health care providers and consumers as well as local, state, and federal governments are placing greater emphasis on health promotion and illness prevention; hospital stays are becoming shorter; and the number of chronically ill in our society is increasing. All these factors make the educator role essential to maintaining the health and well-being of clients.

The framework for the role of educator is the teaching-learning process. Within this framework, the nurse assesses learning needs, plans and implements teaching methods to meet those needs, and evaluates the effectiveness of the teaching. To be an effective educator, the nurse must have effective interpersonal skills and be familiar with adult learning principles (Figure 1–2 ■).

A major component of the educator role today is discharge planning. **Discharge planning,** which begins on admission to a health care setting, is a systematic method of preparing the client and family for exit from the health care agency and for maintaining continuity of care after the client leaves the setting. Discharge planning also involves making referrals, identifying community and personal resources, and arranging for necessary equipment and supplies for home care.

BOX 1–1 ■ Culturally Sensitive Nursing

The primary focus of nursing care is the client as the client relates to the environment and experiences events or situations related to health or illness. These experiences are given shape and personal meaning by culture—the socially inherited characteristics of a human group. These characteristics include the beliefs, practices, habits, likes, dislikes, customs, and rituals people learn from their families and pass on to their children. Cultural background is an essential component of a person's ethnic identity. A person's ethnic identity includes belonging to a social group within a culture and a social system and sharing a common religion, language, ancestry, and physical characteristics.

The health care system encompasses clients who are culturally diverse. This diversity includes differences in country of origin, health beliefs, sexual orientation, race, socioeconomic level, and age. Despite increasing diversity, nursing has been slow to address the need for culturally sensitive care. Many different factors account for this inattention, including ethnocentrism (people's belief that their own cultural group's beliefs and values are the only acceptable ones) and prejudice. The health care system is itself a culture, primarily, of white middle-class people, and it often serves as a barrier to culturally sensitive care.

The 1992 American Academy of Nursing Expert Panel on Culturally Competent Nursing Care identified several reasons why it has become increasingly important that nurses plan culturally sensitive care:

- The demographic and ethnic composition of the population of the world in general, and the United States in particular, has changed markedly, and there is a lack of ethnic representation in health care professionals in the health care system. Information on and knowledge about values, beliefs, experiences, and health care needs of various populations is limited.
- There is a growing awareness and acceptance of diversity and an increased willingness to maintain and support ethnic and cultural heritage.

- People of color and immigrants are facing increasing unemployment, decreasing opportunity, and limited access to health care. These conditions may contribute to the establishment of new minorities, such as the homeless.
- The international focus on providing health care for all people (within the context of inequity, barriers, and lack of access) may have raised the consciousness of health care professionals to some of the inequities inherent in health care systems in both developing countries and developed countries.
- Nurses comprise the largest force in the delivery of health care and therefore have the potential to contribute to the changing inequities in and inaccessibility to health care.
- Consumers are becoming increasingly aware of what is competent and sensitive health care.

This same panel of experts proposed general principles for nurses for becoming sensitive to cultural diversity and providing culturally sensitive care. For example:

- Nurses must learn to appreciate intergroup and intragroup cultural diversity and commonalties in racial/ethnic minority populations.
- Nurses must understand how social structure factors shape health behaviors and practices among members of racial/ethnic minorities.
- Nurses must confront their own ethnocentrism and racism.
- Nurses must begin rehearsing, practicing, and evaluating services provided to cross-cultural populations.

People of every culture have the right to have their cultural values known, respected, and addressed appropriately in nursing and other health care services (Leininger, 1991). To provide nursing care that is culturally sensitive, nurses must develop a sensitivity to personal fundamental values about health and illness; must accept the existence of differing values; and must be respectful of, interested in, and understanding of other cultures without being judgmental.

The Nurse as Advocate

The client entering the health care system is often unprepared to make independent decisions. The nurse as client advocate actively promotes the client's rights to autonomy and free choice. The nurse as advocate speaks for the patient, mediates between the patient and other persons, and/or protects the patient's right to self-determination (Ellis & Hartley, 1998). The goals of the nurse as advocate are to:

- Assess the need for advocacy.
- Communicate with other health care team members.
- Provide client and family teaching.
- Assist and support client decision making.
- Serve as a change agent in the health care system.
- Participate in health policy formulation.

The nurse must practice advocacy based on the belief that clients have the right to choose treatment options, based on information about the results of accepting or rejecting the treatment, without coercion. The nurse must also accept and respect the decision of the client, even though it may differ from the decision the nurse would make.

Figure 1–2 ■ The nurse's role as educator is an essential component of care. As part of the discharge planning process, the nurse provides teaching for self-care at home.

The Nurse as Leader and Manager

All nurses are leaders and managers. They practice leadership and they manage time, people, resources, and the environment in which they provide care. Nurses carry out these roles by directing, delegating, and coordinating nursing activities. Nurses also evaluate the quality of care provided.

Models of Care Delivery

Nurses are leaders and managers of client care within a variety of models of care delivery. Examples are primary nursing, team nursing, and case management.

PRIMARY NURSING. **Primary nursing** allows the nurse to provide individualized direct care to a small number of clients during their entire inpatient stay. This model was developed to reduce the fragmentation of care experienced by the client and to facilitate family-centered continuity of care. In primary nursing, the nurse provides care; communicates with clients, families, and other health care providers; and carries out discharge planning.

TEAM NURSING. **Team nursing** is practiced by teams of variously educated health care providers. For example, a team may consist of a registered nurse, a licensed practical nurse, and two unlicensed assistive personnel. The registered nurse is the team leader. The team leader is responsible for making assignments and has overall responsibility for patient care by team members. All team members work together, each performing the activities for which he or she is best prepared.

CASE MANAGEMENT. **Case management** focuses on management of a caseload (group) of clients and the members of the health care team caring for those clients. The purpose of case management is to maximize positive outcomes and contain costs. The nurse who is case manager is usually a clinical specialist, and the caseload consists of clients with similar health care needs. As case manager, the nurse makes appropriate referrals to other health care providers and manages the quality of care provided, including accuracy, timeliness, and cost. The case manager also is in contact with clients after discharge, ensuring continuity of care and health maintenance.

Delegation

Delegation is carried out when the nurse assigns appropriate and effective work activities to other members of the health care team. When the nurse delegates nursing care activities to another person, that person is authorized to act in the place of the nurse, while the nurse retains the accountability for the activities performed. Delegation skills are becoming increasingly important in health care as agencies restructure and implement cost containment measures. More categories of health care workers with often minimal nursing education and experience are being hired to assist the registered nurse as *nurse extenders*. Guidelines for delegation (Ellis & Hartley, 1998) include the following:

- Know the level of competence of each member of the health care team, the complexity of the task to be assigned, and the amount of time available to supervise the tasks.

- Know the level of nursing judgment and evaluation required for the task.
- Consider the potential harm and difficulty of performing the task.
- Know the state's nurse practice act and any practice limitations that may exist.
- Know the job descriptions for each category of worker.
- Assign the right job to the right person. Tasks that are routine and standard are the best to assign to others.
- Give clear and complete directions for assignments. Ask questions to be sure directions have been understood.
- Give the team member the authority to complete the task.
- Monitor the outcomes of the care provided and give constructive evaluation if necessary.

Evaluating Outcomes of Nursing Care

CRITICAL PATHWAYS. A **critical pathway** is a health care plan designed to provide care with a multidisciplinary, managed action focus. Critical pathways, also called critical paths, are one model for this approach to health care. Such pathways are generally developed for specific diagnoses—usually high volume, high risk, and high cost case types—with the collaboration of members of the health care team. This client care management tool describes how resources will be used to achieve predetermined outcomes. It also establishes the sequence of multidisciplinary interventions, including education, discharge planning, consultations, medication administration, diagnostics, therapeutics, and treatments. Figure 1–3 ■ shows a sample critical pathway.

The goals of critical pathways are to:

- Achieve realistic, expected client and family outcomes.
- Promote professional and collaborative practice and care.
- Ensure continuity of care.
- Guarantee appropriate use of resources.
- Reduce costs and length of stay.
- Provide the framework for continuous improvement.

Critical pathways are often used in conjunction with case management models and/or quality improvement efforts. The overall goal is to design pathways that facilitate a reproducible standard of care for specific client populations and improve the quality and proficiency of that care.

The agency determines the process for developing a critical pathway. Information imperative to the development of any critical pathway includes literature reviews, chart reviews, expert opinion, and insurance reimbursements for the designated case type. A typical approach is to first identify high cost, high volume, and high risk case types for the agency. Next, a multidisciplinary team, including physicians, develops a consensus around the management of the case type and a critical pathway. The pathway is then piloted with a designated group of clients, and revisions are based on the number and types of variances. The goal is to develop a pathway that best meets the needs of clients in the particular practice setting.

When clients do not achieve expected outcomes, variances (deviations from the established plan) from the critical pathways are recorded and studied by the multidisciplinary team. In many agencies, critical pathways are designed so that

	Date _____ Preoperative	Date _____ 1st 24 hours following surgery
	Expected length of stay: less than 24 hours	
Daily outcomes	Client will • Verbalize understanding of preoperative teaching, including turning, coughing, deep breathing, mobilization, and pain management. • Demonstrate ability to cope.	Client will • Be afebrile. • Have a dry, clean dressing. • Have nasal packing, splint/cast, and mustache dressing intact and in place. • Manage pain with nonpharmacologic measures or oral medications. • Be independent in self-care. • Be fully ambulatory. • Verbalize/demonstrate home care instructions. • Tolerate usual diet. • Demonstrate ability to cope with ongoing stressors.
Tests and treatments	CBC Urinalysis Baseline physical assessment with a focus on respiratory status Anesthesia consultation	Vital signs and O_2 saturation, neurovascular assessment, dressing, edema, and wound drainage assessment q15min × 4, q30min × 4, q1h × 4, and then q4h if stable. Assess for posterior nasal bleeding. Assess lung sounds q4h and prn. Assess voiding—if unable to void, try suggestive voiding techniques or catheterize q8h or prn if unable to void. Cool compresses to nose, eyes, or face to reduce swelling and prevent excessive discoloration.
Knowledge deficit	Orient to room and surroundings. Include family in teaching. Provide simple, brief instructions. Review preoperative preparation, including hospital and surgical routines. Reinforce preoperative teaching regarding specific postoperative care: turning, coughing, deep breathing, mobilization, and pain management. Assess understanding of teaching.	Reorient to room and postoperative routine. Include family in teaching. Review plan of care and importance of early mobilization, as well as any activity restrictions. Complete discharge teaching regarding splint/cast care/dressing change, follow-up care, signs and symptoms to report, medications, and diet. Instruct the client to avoid activities that might result in a blow or pressure on the nose and procedures to follow if bleeding occurs. Instruct client to avoid the Valsalva's maneuver and to avoid aspirin and other nonsteroidal medications. Assess understanding of teaching.
Psychosocial	Assess anxiety related to pending surgery. Assess fears of the unknown and surgery. Encourage verbalization of concerns. Provide emotional support to client and family. Provide information regarding surgery. Minimize stimuli (e.g., noise, movement).	Assess level of anxiety. Encourage verbalization of concerns. Provide emotional support to client and family. Provide information and ongoing support and encouragement.
Diet	NPO	Advance to clear liquids. If tolerated, advance to full liquids/soft diet following surgery.
Activity	OOB ad lib until premedicated for surgery.	Provide safety precautions. Place in semi-Fowler's position. Allow bathroom privileges with assistance on evening after surgery. Begin progressive ambulation to tolerance the morning following surgery until fully ambulatory.
Medications	NPO except ordered medications.	IM or PO analgesics. Antibiotics if ordered. IV fluids until adequate PO intake then intermittent IV. Discontinue prior to discharge.
Transfer/ discharge plans	Assess discharge plans and support system.	Probable discharge within 24 hours of surgery. Complete discharge home care teaching when client is fully awake and oriented and before discharge. Provide a written copy of discharge instructions.

Figure 1–3 ■ Critical pathway for a client following a rhinoplasty.

interventions and variances can be easily documented. Most documentation systems require a checkoff when interventions are performed or variances occur.

In many agencies, critical pathways are replacing traditional nursing care plans. The advantages of critical pathways are that they are outcome driven and provide a time line to achieve specified goals. Additionally, critical pathways provide opportunities for health care workers to collaborate and establish dynamic plans of care that consider all of the clients' needs. Although initially developed for acute hospitalizations, critical pathways are now developed to manage clients in home health, outpatient, and long-term settings.

QUALITY ASSURANCE. As a leader and manager, the nurse is responsible for the quality of client care through a process called **quality assurance.** It consists of the quality control activities that evaluate, monitor, or regulate the standard of services provided to the consumer. Clients are assured of quality care through professional and technical licensure of individual care providers; accreditation of hospitals (e.g., by the Joint Commission on Accreditation of Healthcare Organizations [JCAHO]); licensure of hospitals, pharmacies, and nursing homes; and certification in specialty areas.

Quality assurance methods also are used to evaluate client care. They commonly evaluate actual care against an established set of standards of care. Nurses and other health care providers make this evaluation by reviewing documentation, by conducting client surveys and nurse interviews, and/or by direct observation of nurse or client performance. The data are then used to identify differences between actual practice and established standards and to develop a plan of action to resolve the differences. The actions are then assessed through internal peer review or by an external medical review organization, called a utilization and quality control peer review organization (PRO), to determine whether they were effective in improving practice. These reviews have resulted in such health care changes as an increase in outpatient surgeries with a resultant decrease in the number of inpatient surgeries.

The Nurse as Researcher

Nurses have always identified problems in client care. Although they have developed interventions to meet specific needs, the activities often have not been conducted within a scientific framework or communicated to other nurses through nursing literature. To develop the science of nursing, nursing knowledge must be established through clinical research and then published, so that the findings can be used by all nurses to provide evidence-based client care.

To be relevant, nursing research must have a goal to improve the care that nurses provide clients. This means that all nurses must consider the researcher role to be integral to nursing practice. Summaries of relevant nursing research are included in almost all the nursing care chapters of this textbook. After the summary and discussion of each study, a critical thinking section specifically related to the findings of the study encourages the student to apply the findings to the clinical setting.

FRAMEWORK FOR PRACTICE: CRITICAL THINKING IN THE NURSING PROCESS

The **nursing process** is the series of critical thinking activities nurses use as they provide care to clients. These activities define a nursing model of care, differentiating nursing from other helping professions. The nursing process can be used in any setting. The purpose of care may be to promote wellness, maintain health, restore health, or facilitate coping with disability or death. Regardless of the purpose of care, the planned process of nursing allows for the inclusion of specific, individualized, and holistic activities.

Critical Thinking

Critical thinking is, most basically, thinking about one's own thinking. It is self-directed thinking that is focused on what to believe or do in a specific situation. It involves attitudes and skills. Critical thinking occurs when the nurse uses knowledge to consider a client care situation and uses the nursing process to make judgments and decisions about what to do in that situation. As you practice critical thinking, you must consider:

- The purpose of the thinking (e.g., is it to collect more data or is it to report the data to someone else?).
- Your level of acquired knowledge.
- Prejudices that may influence thinking (e.g., believing that all people in poverty are dirty or that the aged are incapable of learning how to care for themselves, or letting emotions affect decision making).
- Information that is needed from other sources such as faculty members, a skilled clinical nurse, a textbook or journal article, or the policies of the health care agency.
- The ability to identify other possible options, evaluate the alternatives, and reach a conclusion.
- Personal values and beliefs.

Critical thinking takes practice so that it becomes an integral component of the nurse's attitudes and skills. Critical thinking exercises are included throughout this book to provide that practice.

Attitudes and Mental Habits Necessary for Critical Thinking

Thinking critically involves more than just cognitive (knowledge) skills. It is strongly influenced by one's attitudes and mental habits. To think critically, you must focus your attention on your attitudes and how they affect your thinking. These attitudes and mental habits are:

- Being able to *think independently* so that you make clinical decisions based on sound thinking and judgment. This means, for example, you are not influenced by negative comments from other health care providers about a client.
- Being willing to listen to and be fair in your evaluation of others' ideas and beliefs by having *intellectual courage.* This involves listening carefully to other ideas and thoughts, and making a decision based on what you learn instead of how you feel.
- Having *intellectual empathy* by being able to put yourself in the place of another to better understand that other person.

For example, if you put yourself in the place of the person with severe pain, you are better able to understand why he or she is so upset when pain medications are late.

- Being fair-minded and considering all viewpoints before making a decision through an *intellectual sense of justice* and being *intellectually humble*. This means you consider the viewpoints of others that may be different from yours before reaching a conclusion. You also realize that you are constantly learning from others. You are not afraid to say, "I don't know the answer to that question, but I will find out and let you know."
- Being *disciplined* so that you do not stop at easy answers, but continue to consider alternatives.
- Being *creative* and *self-confident*. Nurses often need to consider different ways of providing care and constantly look for better, more cost-effective methods. Confidence in one's decisions is gained through critical thinking.

Critical Thinking Skills

Critical thinking skills are the mental abilities that are used. Major critical thinking skills are as follows:

- *Divergent thinking* is having the ability to weigh the importance of information. This means that when you collect data from a client, you can sort out the data that are relevant for the care of your client from the data that are not relevant and explore alternatives to draw a conclusion. Abnormal data are usually considered relevant; normal data are helpful but may not change the care you provide.
- *Reasoning* is having the ability to discriminate between facts and guesses. By using known facts, problems are solved and decisions are made in a systematic, logical way. For example, when you take a pulse you must know the facts of normal pulse rate for a person of this age, types of medications the client is taking that may alter the pulse rate, and the emotional and physical state of the client. Based on these facts, you are able to decide if the pulse rate is normal or abnormal.
- *Clarifying* is defining terms and noting similarities and differences. For example, when caring for a client with chronic pain, you must know the definition of chronic pain and the similarities and differences between acute pain and chronic pain.
- *Reflection* occurs when you take time to think about something. It cannot take place in an emergency situation. As you reflect on your experiences in nursing, many of those experiences may in turn become alternatives when caring for a different client.

Critical thinking is an expected ability of all nurses. Using critical thinking to provide care that is structured by the nursing process allows the nurse to provide safe, effective, holistic, and individualized care. See Table 1–1.

The Nursing Process

The five steps or phases in the nursing process are assessment, diagnosis, planning, implementation, and evaluation. These steps are interrelated and interdependent. The steps are most often used cyclically, as illustrated in Figure 1–4 ■. The steps have been legitimized by the American Nurses Association (ANA) Standards of Practice, state nursing practice acts, and licensing examinations that are structured on a nursing model of care based on the nursing process.

This textbook assumes that the student already has a basic understanding of the nursing process and is now ready to expand and apply that knowledge to adult clients with medical-surgical health problems. The following discussion is intended to serve only as a review; for more information, consult books specifically focused on the use of the nursing process, and read the case studies in the nursing care chapters throughout this textbook.

Assessment

Assessment is usually listed as the first step of the nursing process, but in actuality it is a critical element in each of the steps. It begins with the client's first encounter with the health care system and continues as long as the client requires care. During assessment, data (pieces of information) about health status are collected, validated, organized, clustered into patterns, and communicated either verbally or in written form. Assessment serves as the basis for deriving accurate nursing diagnoses, for planning and implementing both initial and ongoing individualized care, and for evaluating care.

The data that the nurse collects must be holistic; that is, the nurse must carefully consider all dimensions of an individual. The data collected are both objective and subjective. Information that the nurse perceives by the senses is **objective data;** it is seen, heard, touched, or smelled, and can be verified by another person (e.g., blood pressure, temperature, pulse, or the presence of infected drainage). Information that is perceived only by the person experiencing it (e.g., pain, dizziness, or anxiety) is **subjective data.**

Nurses assess clients in two ways: through an initial assessment and through focused assessments. The **initial assessment** of the client, conducted through a nursing history and physical assessment, is necessary to:

- Accumulate comprehensive data about health responses.
- Identify specific factors that contribute to these responses in a specific individual.
- Facilitate mutually established goals and outcomes of care. (Iyer, Taptich, & Bernocchi-Losey, 1994)

Focused assessments are ongoing and continuous, occurring whenever the nurse interacts with the client. They enable the nurse to evaluate nursing actions and make decisions about whether to continue or change interventions to meet outcomes. They also provide structure for documenting nursing care. In addition, focused assessments enable the nurse to identify responses to a disease process or treatment modality not present during the initial assessment, or to monitor the status of an actual or potential problem previously identified (Alfaro, 1998).

To make accurate and holistic assessments, nurses must have and use a wide variety of knowledge and skills. The ability to assess the physical status of the client is essential, as is the ability to use effective communication techniques. Nurses must be knowledgeable in pathophysiology and pharmacology and be able to identify abnormal laboratory and diagnostic test data. Finally, nurses must have a solid foundation of nursing knowledge and skill that will enable them to interpret assessment data and to use that interpretation as the basis for individualized care.

MediaLink | NURSING CARE PLAN

TABLE 1–1   Using Critical Thinking in the Nursing Process

Nursing Process Step	Critical Thinking Skills	Questions to Check Your Thinking
Assessment	Making reliable observations Distinguishing relevant from irrelevant data Distinguishing important from unimportant data Validating data Organizing data Categorizing data according to a framework Recognizing assumptions	What assumptions am I making about the patient? Is my data correct and accurate? How reliable are my sources? What data is important? Relevant? What biases do I have that might cause me to miss important information? Am I listening carefully to get the patient's and family's perspective? Do I have all the facts? What other data might I need?
Diagnosis	Finding patterns and relationships among cues Identifying gaps in the data Making inferences Suspending judgment when lacking data Making interdisciplinary connections Stating the problem Examining assumptions Comparing patterns with norms Identifying factors contributing to the problem	Do I know what is within normal limits for the data? Do I have enough data to make a valid inference? What biases might I have that could affect how I see the patient's problems? Do I have enough data to make a nursing diagnosis or should I make a "possible" diagnosis? What other problems might this data suggest other than the one that seems most obvious to me?
Planning	Forming valid generalizations Transferring knowledge from one situation to another Developing evaluative criteria Hypothesizing Making interdisciplinary connections Prioritizing client problems Generalizing principles from other sciences	Do I need help to plan interventions, or am I qualified to do it? Did I remember to give high priority to the problems the patient and family identified as important? What are the most important problems we need to solve? What interventions worked in similar situations? Is this situation similar enough to merit using them with this patient? Are there other plans that might be more agreeable to the patient, and therefore more likely to work? Why do I expect these interventions to be effective? Based on what knowledge?
Implementation	Applying knowledge to perform interventions Using interventions to test hypotheses	Has the patient's condition changed since the plan was made? Have I overlooked any new developments? What is the patient's initial response to the intervention? Are there any safety issues I have overlooked?
Evaluation	Deciding whether hypotheses are correct Making criterion-based evaluations	What are the patient reponses after the interventions? Have I overlooked anything? Does the data indicate that goals were met? Does the patient feel the goals were met? Does the patient trust me enough to give honest answers? Am I sure the problem is really resolved? What might we have done that would have been more effective? What nursing care is still needed, if any?

Note. From Nursing Process and Critical Thinking (3rd ed.) by J. M. Wilkinson, 2001. Reprinted by permission of Pearson Education, Inc., Upper Saddle River, NJ.

Diagnosis

The ANA defines nursing as "the diagnosis and treatment of human responses to actual or potential health problems" (1980, p. 9). The nurse labels each response with a **nursing diagnosis,** defined by the North American Nursing Diagnosis Association (NANDA) as "a clinical judgment about individual, family, or community responses to actual or potential health problems/life processes. Nursing diagnoses provide the basis for selection of nursing interventions to achieve outcomes for which the nurse is accountable" (NANDA, 2001,

p. 245). Nurses develop and implement a plan of care for actual responses; they also plan interventions to support health concerns and prevent illness concerns for potential human responses.

The nurse analyzes data collected during the assessment step to support appropriate nursing diagnoses. During analysis, the nurse clusters data into categories of information that can be used to identify actual or potential alterations in health. Data can be organized within a variety of frameworks and methods for identifying patterns of human behavior

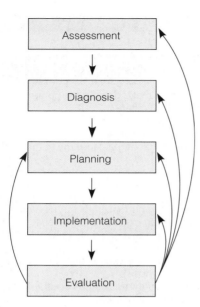

Figure 1–4 ■ Steps of the nursing process. Notice that the steps are interrelated and interdependent. For example, evaluation of the client might reveal the need for further assessment, additional nursing diagnoses, and/or a revision of the plan of care.

(Wilkinson, 2000). Methods commonly used are basic human needs (Maslow, 1970), body systems, human response patterns, and functional health patterns (Gordon, 1982). The broad organizational structure used to categorize information in this book is based on Gordon's (1994) functional health patterns, outlined in Box 1–2.

Making a diagnosis is a complex process that always involves uncertainty. Therefore, the nurse uses diagnostic reasoning to choose nursing diagnoses that best define the individual client's health problems. Diagnostic reasoning is a form of clinical judgment (Radwin, 1990) used to make decisions about which label (or diagnosis) best describes the patterns of data. Radwin's review of research about diagnostic reasoning

in nursing found that elements of the clinical judgment process include data gathering and validation, data categorization, intuition, and prior clinical experience.

Although there is no universal list of diagnoses used in nursing, the work of NANDA is widely accepted. The diagnoses are classified by a taxonomy; that is, they are grouped into classes and subclasses based on patterns and relationships. Work on both the nursing diagnoses and the taxonomy is ongoing. The NANDA system was accepted in 1988 by the ANA as the official system of diagnosis for the United States. Nursing diagnoses within the NANDA taxonomy are used in this book.

A diagnosis is written in two parts joined by the phrase "related to." The first part of the statement is the particular human response that has been identified from the analysis of data. It identifies what needs to change in a specific client as a result of nursing interventions, and it also identifies the client outcomes that measure the change. The part of the statement that follows the "related to" phrase identifies the physical, psychosocial, cultural, spiritual, and/or environmental factors (etiologies) that cause or contribute to the occurrence of the response.

Many nurses write nursing diagnoses using a method known as PES (Gordon, 1994). Diagnoses written with this method have three components:

1. The problem (P), which is the NANDA label.
2. The etiology (E) of the problem, which names the related factors and is indicated by the phrase "related to."
3. The signs and symptoms (S), which are the defining characteristics and are indicated by the phrase "as manifested by."

Examples of nursing diagnoses written with the PES method are as follows:

- *Anxiety* related to hospitalization as manifested by statements of nervousness and by crying
- *Bowel incontinence* related to loss of sphincter control as manifested by involuntary passage of stool

---

BOX 1–2 ■ Functional Health Patterns

1. *Health-perception–health-management pattern.* Describes client's perceived pattern of health and well-being and how health is managed.
2. *Nutritional-metabolic pattern.* Describes pattern of food and fluid consumption relative to metabolic need and pattern indicators of local nutrient supply.
3. *Elimination pattern.* Describes pattern of excretory function (bowel, bladder, and skin).
4. *Activity-exercise pattern.* Describes pattern of exercise, activity, leisure, and recreation.
5. *Cognitive-perceptual pattern.* Describes sensory-perceptual and cognitive patterns.
6. *Sleep-rest pattern.* Describes patterns of sleep, rest, and relaxation.

7. *Self-perception–self-concept pattern.* Describes self-concept pattern and perceptions of self (e.g., body comfort, body image, feeling state).
8. *Role-relationship pattern.* Describes patterns of role-engagements and relationships.
9. *Sexuality-reproductive pattern.* Describes client's patterns of satisfaction and dissatisfaction with sexuality; describes reproductive patterns.
10. *Coping–stress-tolerance pattern.* Describes general coping pattern and effectiveness of the pattern in terms of stress tolerance.
11. *Value-belief pattern.* Describes patterns of values, beliefs (including spiritual), or goals that guide choices or decisions.

Note. Adapted from Nursing Diagnosis: Process and Application *(3rd ed.) by M. Gordon, 1994, St. Louis: Mosby-Year Book.*

- *Fatigue* related to the side effects of chemotherapy as manifested by the inability to carry out normal daily routines and statements of overwhelming exhaustion

Planning

During the **planning** step, the nurse develops a list of nursing interventions (actions) and client outcomes to promote healthy responses and to prevent, reverse, or decrease unhealthy responses. **Outcomes,** which are mutually established by the client and nurse, identify what the client will be able to do as a result of the nursing interventions. Both outcomes and nursing interventions are documented in a written plan of care that directs nursing activities and documentation and provides a tool for evaluation (Alfaro, 1998). The plan of care may be documented in a variety of formats.

Nurses plan interventions for two types of client problems: those that require nursing management, stated as nursing diagnoses; and those that require collaborative management, which may be referred to as collaborative or clinical problems. Nursing diagnoses provide the basis for selecting nurse-initiated interventions to achieve outcomes for which the nurse is accountable. Collaborative problems are pathophysiologic, treatment-related, personal, environmental, and maturational situations which nurses monitor for detection of onset or changes in status. Both physician-initiated and nurse-initiated interventions minimize the complications of collaborative problems (Carpenito, 1999).

Outcome criteria for nursing diagnoses are client centered, time specific, and measurable. They are classified into three domains: cognitive (knowing), affective (feeling), and psychomotor (doing). The nurse considers all three domains to ensure holistic care.

Outcome criteria for collaborative problems are nursing goals, usually written as statements that begin with "to detect and report early signs and symptoms of potential complications of . . . " and "to implement preventive and corrective nursing interventions ordered by . . . " (Alfaro, 1998). In many instances, these goals are not written as part of the plan of care. Preventive and corrective nursing interventions for collaborative problems may be ordered by the physician or by institutional policy, procedures, protocols, or standards.

The nursing interventions planned must be specific and individualized. If, for example, the nurse identifies that a client is at risk for fluid volume deficit, it is not enough that the nurse simply encourage the client to drink increased amounts of fluid. The nurse and the client together must identify those liquids the client prefers, the times that will be best for drinking them, and the amount of fluid (in ounces or milliliters); this information must be documented as a nursing order on the written care plan. Only then does care truly become a part of the plan of care.

Implementation

The **implementation** step is the action or "doing" phase of the nursing process, during which the nurse carries out planned interventions. Ongoing assessment of the client before, during, and after the intervention is an essential component of implementation. Although the plan may be appropriate, many variables can modify or negate any planned intervention, making a change in the plan necessary. For example, the nurse would not be able to force fluids if the client were nauseated or vomiting.

When implementing the planned interventions, the nurse follows several important principles:

- Set daily priorities, based on initial assessments and on the client's condition as reported during the change of shift report and/or documented in the client's chart. Ensure that critical assessments (such as status of invasive lines, fluids infusing, or changes in health status during the preceding shift) take first priority.
- Be aware of the interrelated nature of nursing interventions. For example, while giving a bath the nurse can also assess physical and psychologic status, use therapeutic communication, teach the client, do range-of-motion exercises, and provide skin care.
- Determine the most appropriate interventions for each client, based on health status and illness treatment. Examples of appropriate interventions include:
  - Directly performing the activity for the client.
  - Assisting the client to perform the activity.
  - Supervising the client/family while they are performing the activity.
  - Teaching the client/family about health care.
  - Monitoring the client at risk for potential complications or problems.
- Use available resources to provide interventions that are realistic for the situation and practical in terms of equipment available, financial status of the client, and resources available (including staff, agency, family, and community resources).

Documenting interventions is the final component of implementation, and it is a legal requirement. There are many different ways of documenting care. The traditional narrative source-oriented and problem-oriented charting methods are used, as are newer methods such as focused charting, charting by exception, and computer-assisted documentation.

Evaluation

The **evaluation** step allows the nurse to determine whether the plan was effective and either to continue the plan, to revise the plan, or to terminate the plan. The outcome criteria that were established during the planning step provide the basis for evaluation. Although evaluation is listed as the last part of the nursing process, it takes place continuously throughout client care.

To evaluate a plan, the nurse collects data from the client and reviews the chart. The nurse then compares the status of the client with the written outcomes. If the outcomes have been accomplished, the nurse may either continue or terminate the plan. If the outcomes have not been accomplished, the nurse must modify the nursing diagnoses, outcomes, or plan.

Benefits of the Nursing Process

The nursing process benefits nurses who provide care, clients who receive care, and settings where care is provided. As nurses gain increasing autonomy in their practice, the use of the nursing process helps them identify their independent practice domain. The nursing process also provides a common reference system and a common terminology to serve as a base for improving

BOX 1–3	■ The International Council of Nurses Code for Nurses

The fundamental responsibility of the nurse is fourfold: to promote health, to prevent illness, to restore health, and to alleviate suffering. The need for nursing is universal. Inherent in nursing is respect for life, dignity, and the rights of man. It is unrestricted by considerations of nationality, race, creed, color, age, sex, politics, or social status. Nurses render health services to the individual, the family, and the community and coordinate their services with those of related groups.

NURSES AND PEOPLE

The nurse's primary responsibility is to those people who require nursing care. The nurse, in providing care, promotes an environment in which the values, customs, and spiritual beliefs of the individual are respected. The nurse holds in confidence personal information and uses judgment in sharing this information.

NURSES AND PRACTICE

The nurse carries responsibility for nursing practice and for maintaining competence by continual learning. The nurse maintains the highest standards of nursing care possible within the reality of a specific situation. The nurse uses judgment in relation to individual competence when accepting and delegating responsibilities. The nurse when acting in a professional capacity should at all times maintain standards of personal conduct that reflect credit upon the profession.

NURSES AND SOCIETY

The nurse shares with other citizens the responsibility for initiating and supporting action to meet the health and social needs of the public.

NURSES AND COWORKERS

The nurse sustains a cooperative relationship with coworkers in nursing and other fields. The nurse takes appropriate action to safeguard the individual when his or her care is endangered by a coworker or any other person.

NURSES AND THE PROFESSION

The nurse plays the major role in determining and implementing desirable standards of nursing practice and nursing education. The nurse is active in developing a core of professional knowledge. The nurse, acting through the professional organization, participates in establishing and maintaining equitable social and economic working conditions in nursing.

Note. From ICN Code for Nurses: Ethical Concepts Applied to Nursing by International Council of Nurses, 1973, Geneva: Imprimeries Populaires. Copyright © 1973 by ICN. Reprinted by permission.

clinical practice through research. In addition, the nursing process can serve as a framework for the evaluation of quality care.

The nursing process also benefits the client receiving care and the agency or institution providing that care. The client receives planned, individualized interventions; participates in all steps of the process; and is assured continuity of care through the written care plan. The nursing process benefits the health care institution through better resource utilization, increased client satisfaction, and improved documentation of care.

The Nursing Process in Clinical Practice

With experience, the nurse does not consciously stop and consider each step. Rather, using the process as a framework, the nurse provides care based on the client's specific, individualized needs. For example, when caring for a client who is hemorrhaging, the nurse uses all five steps simultaneously to meet critical, life-threatening needs. In contrast, when considering long-term needs for a client with a chronic illness or disability, the nurse makes in-depth assessments, mutually determines goals with the client, and provides documentation through a written plan of care that can be developed and revised as necessary by all nurses providing care. As a nurse becomes an expert practitioner, the nursing process becomes so much a part of the nurse that he or she may not even consciously consider it while providing care; the practice is the process (Benner, 1984).

GUIDELINES FOR NURSING PRACTICE

Nursing practice is structured by codes of ethics and standards that guide nursing practice and protect the public. These guidelines are especially important because nurses encounter legal and ethical problems almost daily. A discussion of representative issues also is included.

Codes for Nurses

An established code of ethics is one criterion that defines a profession. **Ethics** are principles of conduct. **Ethical behavior** is concerned with moral duty, values, obligations, and the distinction between right and wrong. Codes of ethics for nurses provide a frame of reference for "professionally valued and ideal nursing behaviors that are congruent with the principles expressed in the Code for Nurses" (Ketefian, 1987, p. 13).

The large number of ethical issues facing nurses in clinical practice makes the established codes for nurses critical to moral and ethical decision making. The codes also help to define the roles of nurses. The codes of ethics presented here were developed by and for members of the International Council of Nurses (ICN) and the ANA.

The ICN Code

The ICN Code for Nurses (Box 1–3) helps guide nurses in setting priorities, making judgments, and taking action when they face ethical dilemmas in clinical practice.

The ANA Code

The ANA Code for Nurses (Box 1–4) states principles of ethical concern, which guides the behavior of nurses and also defines nursing for the general public.

Standards of Nursing Practice

A **standard** is a statement or criterion that can be used by a profession and by the general public to measure quality of practice. Established standards of nursing practice make each individual nurse accountable for practice. This means that each nurse providing care has the responsibility or obligation to account for his or her own behaviors within that role. Professional nursing

BOX 1–4	■ The American Nurses Association Code of Ethics for Nurses

■ The nurse, in all professional relationships, practices with compassion and respect for the inherent dignity, worth, and uniqueness of every individual, unrestricted by considerations of social or economic status, personal attributes, or the nature of health problems.

■ The nurse's primary commitment is to the patient, whether an individual, family, group, or community.

■ The nurse promotes, advocates for, and strives to protect the health, safety, and rights of the patient.

■ The nurse is responsible and accountable for individual nursing practice and determines the appropriate delegation of tasks consistent with the nurse's obligation to provide optimum patient care.

■ The nurse owes the same duties to self as to others, including the responsibility to preserve integrity and safety, to maintain competence, and to continue personal and professional growth.

■ The nurse participates in establishing, maintaining, and improving health care environments and conditions of employment conducive to the provision of quality health care and consistent with the values of the profession through individual and collective action.

■ The nurse participates in the advancement of the profession through contributions in practice, education, administration, and knowledge development.

■ The nurse collaborates with other health professionals and the public in promoting community, national, and international efforts to meet health needs.

■ The profession of nursing, as represented by associations and their members, is responsible for articulating nursing values, for maintaining the integrity of the profession and its practice, and for shaping social policy.

Note. Reprinted with permission from American Nurses Association, Code of Ethics for Nurses with Interpretive Statements, © 2001, American Nurses Publishing. American Nurses Foundation/American Nurses Association, Washington, DC.

organizations develop and implement standards of practice to identify clearly the nurse's responsibilities to society.

The ANA standards of clinical nursing practice (1998) are outlined in Box 1–5. These standards allow objective evaluation of nursing licensure and certification, institutional accreditation, quality assurance, and public policy.

LEGAL AND ETHICAL DILEMMAS AND ISSUES IN NURSING

A **dilemma** is a choice between two unpleasant, ethically troubling alternatives. Nurses who provide medical-surgical nursing care face dilemmas almost daily—so many that a complete discussion of them is impossible here. However, many commonly experienced dilemmas involve caring for the client with acquired immune deficiency syndrome (AIDS), client rights, and issues of dying and death. The nurse must use ethical and legal guidelines to make decisions about moral actions when providing care in these and in many other situations.

Nurses respect the right to confidentiality of client information found in the client's record or secured during interviews. (In most instances, state nursing practice acts legally require nurses to uphold this right.) Rights of the client as an individual, however, can result in dilemmas for the nurse in the clinical setting. For example, the right to privacy and confidentiality creates a dilemma when it conflicts with the nurse's right to information that may affect personal safety. The may happen when the nurse does not know a client's HIV status. The current

BOX 1–5	■ The American Nurses Association Standards of Clinical Nursing Practice

STANDARDS OF CARE

Assessment: The nurse collects patient health data.

Diagnosis: The nurse analyzes the assessment data in determining diagnoses.

Outcome Identification: The nurse identifies expected outcomes individualized to the patient.

Planning: The nurse develops a plan of care that prescribes interventions to attain expected outcomes.

Implementation: The nurse implements the interventions identified in the plan of care.

Evaluation: The nurse evaluates the patient's progress toward attainment of outcomes.

STANDARDS OF PROFESSIONAL PERFORMANCE

Quality of Care: The nurse systematically evaluates the quality and effectiveness of nursing practice.

Performance Appraisal: The nurse evaluates one's own nursing practice in relation to professional practice standards and relevant statues and regulations.

Education: The nurse acquires and maintains current knowledge and competency in nursing practice.

Collegiality: The nurse interacts with and contributes to the professional development of peers and other health care providers as colleagues.

Ethics: The nurse's decisions and actions on behalf of patients are determined in an ethical manner.

Collaboration: The nurse collaborates with the patient, family, and other health care providers in providing patient care.

Research: The nurse uses research findings in practice.

Resource Utilization: The nurse considers factors related to safety, effectiveness, and cost in planning and delivering patient care.

Note. Reprinted with permission from American Nurses Association, Code of Ethics for Nurses with Interpretive Statements, © 2001, American Nurses Publishing. American Nurses Foundation/American Nurses Association, Washington, DC.

law in most states mandates that HIV test results can be given to another person only if the client provides written consent for the release of that information. Many health care providers believe that this law violates their own right to personal safety and are actively working to change the law.

The right to refuse treatment (including surgery, medication, medical therapy, and nourishment) is another client right that raises nursing dilemmas. The nurse, as client advocate, must first establish that the client is competent. If the client is competent, the situation, the alternatives, and the potential harm from refusal must be carefully explained. By law, the client must establish an advance directive on admission to a health care agency stating the client's choice about preserving or prolonging life. An **advance directive,** or **living will,** is a document in which a client formally states preferences for health care in the event that he or she later becomes mentally incapacitated. The client also names a person who has durable power of attorney to serve as a substitute decision maker to implement the client's stated preferences. This document becomes a part of the client's hospital record and is honored even if the client becomes incompetent during the period of treatment. The dilemma arises when the client's preferences conflict with the law. For example, the client may indicate that there is to be no food or fluids given during end-of-life care. However, several states assert that artificial feeding is not a procedure that may be rejected under living will statutes. The nurse is faced with the dilemma of carrying out the client's wishes or following the law.

Questions about who lives, who dies, and who decides often arise in the health care setting. The issues surrounding dying and death have become increasingly pressing as advances in technology extend the lives of people with chronic debilitating illness and major trauma. These changes have altered concepts of living and dying, resulting in ethical conflicts regarding quality of life and death with dignity versus technologic methods of preserving life in any form.

Even if the client is competent and requests that no heroic measures be used to maintain life, many questions arise in nursing care. What constitutes an heroic measure? Should nursing interventions to provide comfort include administering narcotics at a level known to depress respirations? Should a feeding tube be placed in the client who is terminally ill? These and other questions are being debated not only within the health care system but also in the courts.

TRENDS AND ISSUES IN MEDICAL-SURGICAL NURSING

Health care is a vast and complicated system, affected by, and reflecting changes in, society. The trends and issues facing medical-surgical nurses will shape both the philosophy and the provision of care in the 21st century. Following are some of the many trends and issues affecting nursing care today.

- The population over the age of 65 is increasing more rapidly than any other age group. Older adults have more chronic illnesses and recover less rapidly from acute illnesses than young and middle-aged adults. Treatment of illness requires a large number of hospital beds; the possibility exists that hospitals will become intensive care settings for older adults. Older adults also require more long-term care, community services, and home care. As a result, nursing care will be increasingly geared toward meeting the needs of the older adult in health and illness. The older adult is discussed in Chapter 2. ⨪

- HIV infection is no longer ranked as a leading cause of death for all people in the United States. However, it still ranks as the fifth cause of death among 25 to 44 year olds, and is the leading cause of death for black men of this age. HIV infection is discussed in Chapter 9. ⨪

- Persons who are medically indigent—those without any type of public or private insurance and who cannot pay for health care out of pocket—put increasing demands on state and federal health care budgets. Many clients who are medically indigent either do not seek preventive and restorative health care interventions or receive them too late to avoid serious illness.

- The findings of the Human Genome Project may dramatically affect the way disease is diagnosed and treated. Scientists have identified at least 36 proteins that may be markers for ovarian, breast, and colon cancer; and may also indicate depression, bipolar disorder, and schizophrenia. Pharmaceutical companies are using data from the project in research to develop medications that may, for example, eliminate the beta amyloid tangles responsible for Alzheimer's disease.

- Health problems in the homeless population include both physical and mental alterations. People who are homeless are more prone to injuries and to acute illnesses such as respiratory infections, food poisoning, and skin infestations. Chronic problems affecting the homeless include high blood pressure, chronic respiratory problems (including tuberculosis), heart and peripheral vascular disorders, and malnutrition. Mental health problems that contribute significantly to physical alterations are schizophrenia, depression, and substance abuse. Most care is provided by community health nurses (Figure 1–5 ■).

Figure 1–5 ■ Care for the homeless is often provided by nurses working in the community setting.

EXPLORE MediaLink

NCLEX review questions, case studies, care plan activities, MediaLink applications, and other interactive resources for this chapter can be found on the Companion Website at www.prenhall.com/lemone.

Click on Chapter 1 to select the activities for this chapter. For animations, video clips, more NCLEX review questions, and an audio glossary, access the Student CD-ROM accompanying this textbook.

TEST YOURSELF

1. Which of the following is a collaborative nursing activity?
   a. Taking a health history on a newly admitted client
   b. Assessing changes in heart rate
   c. Teaching a client with diabetes how to give insulin
   d. Administering prescribed medications

2. What goal is a component of the nurse's role as advocate?
   a. Assisting and supporting client decision making
   b. Conducting research about the effects of exercise
   c. Delegating responsibilities for client care to others
   d. Performing range-of-motion exercises

3. A method of establishing a standard of care and evaluating outcomes of that standard involves:
   a. Writing a dress code policy for a health care agency
   b. Creating a critical pathway for a specific type of surgical client
   c. Establishing quality assurance regulations
   d. Implementing a new procedure to change dressings

4. Which one of the following statements is most true of assessment in the nursing process?
   a. Assessment is the first step in the nursing process
   b. Assessment is the last step in the nursing process
   c. Assessment is a component of all steps of the nursing process
   d. Assessment is rarely used as a step in the nursing process

5. A client tells you that he wants no treatment for his cancer. What must the nurse do first?
   a. Ask the client's family members if they agree
   b. Report the information to the legal department
   c. Establish that the client is competent
   d. Ignore the statement

See Test Yourself answers in Appendix C.

BIBLIOGRAPHY

Alfaro, R. (1998). *Applying nursing diagnoses and nursing process: A step-by-step guide* (4th ed.). Philadelphia: Lippincott.

American Association of Retired Persons. (2002). *Profile of older Americans.* Washington, DC: Resource Services Group.

American Nurses Association. (1980). Nursing: A social policy statement. Kansas City, MO: ANA.

———. (1988). *Ethics in nursing: Position statement and guidelines.* Kansas City, MO: ANA.

———. (1991). *Nursing's agenda for health care reform.* Kansas City, MO: ANA.

———. (1995). *Nursing's social policy statement.* Washington, DC: American Nurses Publishing.

———. (1996). *Position statement on cultural diversity in nursing practice.* Washington, DC: ANA.

———. (1998). *Standards of clinical nursing practice.* Washington, DC: ANA.

———. (2001). *Code of ethics for nurses.* Washington, DC: ANA.

Anderson, C. A. (1999). Social change and its impact on nursing. *Nursing Outlook, 47*(2), 53–54.

Andrews, M., & Boyle, J. (1997). Competence in transcultural nursing care. *American Journal of Nursing, 97*(8), 16–20.

Benner, P. (1984). *From novice to expert: Excellence and power in clinical nursing practice.* Redwood City, CA: Addison-Wesley Nursing.

Benner, P., & Wrubel, J. (1989). *The primacy of caring: Stress and coping in clinical nursing practice.* Redwood City, CA: Addison-Wesley Nursing.

Carpenito, L. (1999). *Nursing care plans and documentation* (3rd ed.). Philadelphia: Lippincott.

———. (2000). *Nursing diagnoses: Application to clinical practice* (8th ed.). Philadelphia: Lippincott.

Centers for Disease Control, National Center for Health Statistics. (2002). *Deaths/mortality.* Hyattsville, MD: U.S. Department of Health and Human Services.

Chitty, K. (2001). *Professional nursing: Concepts & challenges* (3rd ed.). Philadelphia: Saunders.

Clemen-Stone, S., McGuire, S., & Eigsti, D. (1998). *Comprehensive community health nursing* (5th ed.). St. Louis: Mosby.

Ebert, J. (2000). Utilizing the nursing "team model" to enhance the role of case manager. *Nursing Case Management, 5*(5), 199–201.

Ellis, J., & Hartley, C. (1998). *Nursing in today's world: Challenges, issues, and trends* (6th ed.). Philadelphia: Lippincott.

Finkelman, A. W. (2001). *Managed care: A nursing perspective.* Upper Saddle River, NJ: Prentice Hall.

Flynn, L. (1997). The health practices of homeless women: A causal model. *Nursing Research, 46*(2), 72–77.

Gordon, M. (1982). *Nursing diagnosis: Process and application.* New York: McGraw-Hill.

———. (1987). *Nursing diagnosis: Process and application.* (2nd ed.) New York: McGraw-Hill.

———. (1994). *Nursing diagnosis: Process and application* (3rd ed.). St. Louis: Mosby.

Green, C. (2000). *Critical thinking in nursing: Case studies across the curriculum.* Upper Saddle River, NJ: Prentice Hall.

Hanshett, M., & OpNeal, J. (2001). Improving client education with the patient pathway. *Hospital Case Management, 9*(3), 39–42, 48.

International Council of Nurses. (1973). *ICN code for nurses: Ethical concept applied to nursing.* Geneva: Imprimeries Populaires.

Iyer, P., Taptich, B., & Bernocchi-Losey, D. (1994). *Nursing process and care planning* (2nd ed.). Philadelphia: Saunders.

Ketefian, S. (1987). Moral behavior in nursing. *Advances in Nursing Science, 9*(1), 10–19.

Klenner, S. (2000). Mapping out a clinical pathway. *RN, 63*(6), 33–36.

Leininger, M. (1991). Transcultural care principles, human rights, and ethical considerations. *Journal of Transcultural Nursing, 3*(1), 21–23.

Lipson, J., Dibble, S., & Minarik, P. (1996). *Culture & nursing care: A pocket guide.* San Francisco: UCSF Nursing Press.

Madigan, E. (2001). Home healthcare nurses can be leaders in evidence-based practice. *Home Healthcare Nurse, 19*(2), 120.

Maslow, A. (1970). *Motivation and personality.* New York: Harper & Row.

North American Nursing Diagnosis Association. (2001). *Nursing diagnoses: Definitions & classification 2001–2002.* Philadelphia: NANDA.

Radwin, L. (1990). Research on diagnostic reasoning in nursing. *Nursing Diagnosis, 1*(2), 70–77.

Roberts, S., & Cleary, V. (2000). Sustaining care delivery—team nursing with intensive care assistants. *Nursing in Critical Care, 5*(2), 68–71.

Rossi, P. (1999). *Case management in healthcare. A practical guide.* Philadelphia: Saunders.

Rosswurm, M. A., & Larrabee, J. H. (1999). A model for change to evidence-based practice.

Image: Journal of Nursing Scholarship, 31(4), 317–322.

Spector, R. (2000). *Cultural diversity in health and illness* (5th ed.). Norwalk, CT: Appleton & Lange.

Understanding differences can improve education: Examine own biases before teaching other cultures. (2001). *Patient Education Management, 8*(5), 57–58, 60.

Wilkinson, J. (2000). *Nursing process in action: A critical thinking approach.* Upper Saddle River, NJ: Prentice Hall.

The Adult Client in Health and Illness

MediaLink

www.prenhall.com/lemone

Additional resources for this chapter can be found on the Student CD-ROM accompanying this textbook, and on the Companion Website at www.prenhall.com/lemone. Click on Chapter 2 to select the activities for this chapter.

CD-ROM
• Audio Glossary
• NCLEX Review

Companion Website
• More NCLEX Review
• Case Study
    Developing Teaching Programs
• Care Plan Activity
    The Family and Chronic Illness
• MediaLink Application
    The Older Adult and Preventive Health

LEARNING OUTCOMES

After completing this chapter, you will be able to:

- Compare and contrast the physical status, risks for alterations in health, assessment guidelines, and healthy behaviors of the young adult, middle adult, and older adult.

- Discuss the definitions, functions, and developmental stages and tasks of the family.

- Define health, incorporating the health-illness continuum and the concept of high-level wellness.

- Identify factors affecting health status.

- Discuss the nurse's role in health promotion.

- Describe the primary, secondary, and tertiary levels of illness prevention.

- Compare and contrast illness and disease.

- Describe illness behaviors and needs of the client with acute illness and chronic illness.

- Discuss the role of the nurse in providing care as a part of rehabilitation.

Gordon Hight, a 21-year-old college student, is admitted to the emergency room with multiple injuries and head trauma following a motorcycle accident. Mary Green, a 38-year-old homemaker, arrives at same-day surgery for biopsy of a tumor in her left breast. Sam Rosengarten, a 55-year-old attorney, is in the intensive care unit for treatment of a myocardial infarction. Margarite Schlefer, age 82, is receiving home health care following a fall that fractured her right hip. These examples demonstrate the striking variety among adult clients—the focus of care in medical-surgical nursing.

THE ADULT CLIENT

The adult years commonly are divided into three stages: the young adult (age 18 to 40), the middle adult (age 40 to 65), and the older adult (over age 65). Although developmental markers are not as clearly delineated in the adult as in the infant or child, specific changes do occur with aging in intellectual, psychosocial, and spiritual development, as well as in physical structures and functions.

The developmental theories specific to the adult, with related stages and tasks, are listed in Table 2–1. Applying a vari-

TABLE 2–1   Theories of Adult Development

	Theorist	Age	Task
Psychosocial Development	Erikson	18–25	Identity versus role confusion • Establishing an intimate relationship with another person • Committing oneself to work and to relationships
		25–65	Generativity versus stagnation • Accepting one's own life as creative and productive • Having concern for others
		65–death	Integrity versus despair • Accepting worth of one's own life • Accepting inevitability of death
Spiritual Development	Fowler	After 18 After 30	• Having a high degree of self-consciousness • Constructing one's own spiritual system • Being aware of truth from a variety of viewpoints
	Westerhoff	Young adult	Searching Faith • Acquiring a cognitive and an affective faith through questioning one's own faith
		Middle–older adult	Owned Faith • Putting faith into action and standing up for beliefs
Moral Development	Kohlberg	Adult	Post-Conventional Level Social contract/legalistic orientation • Defining morality in terms of personal principles • Adhering to laws that protect the welfare and rights of others
			Universal-Ethical Principles • Internalizing universal moral principles • Respecting others; believing that relationships are based on mutual trust
Developmental Tasks	Havighurst	18–35	• Selecting and learning to live with a mate • Starting a family and rearing children • Managing a home • Starting an occupation • Taking on civic responsibility • Finding a congenial social group
		35–60	• Achieving civic and social responsibility • Establishing and maintaining an economic standard of living • Assisting teenage children in becoming responsible and happy adults • Developing leisure-time activities • Relating to one's spouse as a person • Accepting and adjusting to the physiologic changes of middle age • Adjusting to aging parents
		60 and over	• Meeting civic and social obligations • Establishing an affiliation with one's own age group • Establishing satisfactory physical living arrangements • Adjusting to decreasing physical strength, health, retirement, reduced income, death of spouse

Note. Adapted from Childhood and Society (2nd ed.) by E. Erickson, 1963, New York: Norton; Stages of Faith: The Psychology of Human Development and the Quest for Meaning by J. W. Fowler, 1981, New York: Harper & Row; Human Development and Education (3rd ed.) by R. J. Havighurst, 1972, New York: Longman; The Meaning and Measurement of Moral Development by L. Kohlberg, 1979, New York: Clark University; and Will Our Children Have Faith? by J. Westerhoff, 1976, New York: Seabury Press.

ety of developmental theories is important to the holistic care of the adult client as nurses perform assessments, implement care, and provide teaching.

THE YOUNG ADULT

From age 18 to 25, the healthy young adult is at the peak of physical development. All body systems are functioning at maximum efficiency. Then, during the 30s, some normal physiologic changes begin to occur. A comparison of physical status for young adults during their 20s and 30s is shown in Table 2–2.

Risks for Alterations in Health

The young adult is at risk for alterations in health from accidents, sexually transmitted diseases, substance abuse, and physical or psychosocial stressors. These risk factors may be interrelated.

Accidents

Accidents are the leading cause of injury and death in people between ages 15 and 24 (Centers for Disease Control and Prevention [CDC], 1999b). Most injuries and fatalities occur as the result of motor vehicle accidents; but injuries and death also result from drowning, fire, guns, occupational accidents, and exposure to environmental hazards. Accidental injury or death is often associated with the use of alcohol or other chemical substances, or with psychologic stress.

Sexually Transmitted Diseases

Sexually transmitted diseases include genital herpes, chlamydia, gonorrhea, syphilis, and HIV/AIDS. The young adult who is sexually active with a variety of partners and who does not use condoms is at greatest risk for development of these diseases.

Substance Abuse

Substance abuse is a major cause for concern in the young adult population. Although alcohol abuse occurs at all ages, it is greater in the 20s than during any other decade of the life span. Alcohol contributes to motor vehicle accidents and physical violence, and it is damaging to the developing fetus in pregnant women. It can also cause liver disease and nutritional deficits.

Other substances that are commonly abused include nicotine, marijuana, amphetamines, cocaine, and crack. Smoking increases the risk of respiratory and cardiovascular diseases. Cocaine and crack can cause death from cardiovascular effects (increased heart rate and ventricular dysrhythmias), and can lead to addiction and health problems in the baby born to an addicted mother.

Physical and Psychosocial Stressors

Physical stressors that increase the risk of illness include environmental pollutants and work-related risks (e.g., electrical hazards, mechanical injuries, or exposure to toxins or infectious agents). Other physical stressors include exposure to the sun, ingestion of chemical substances (e.g., caffeine, alcohol, nicotine), and pregnancy.

Many different and individualized psychosocial stressors may affect the young adult. Choices must be made about education, occupation, relationships, independence, and lifestyle. The young adult without adequate education or job skills may face unemployment, poverty, homelessness, and limited access to health care. Divorces in the United States are increasing. Three of every five marriages end in divorce, and this number is even higher among young adults (Edelman & Mandle, 2002). Divorce often results in loneliness, feelings of failure, financial difficulties, domestic violence, and child abuse. The inability of the young adult to cope with these stressors may result in suicide, which ranks next to accidents as a major cause of death in this age group. Although difficult to prove, it is believed that some accidental deaths, especially when associated with substance abuse, are actually suicides.

Assessment Guidelines

The following guidelines are useful in assessing the achievement of significant developmental tasks in the young adult. Does the young adult:

- Feel independent from parents?
- Have a realistic self-concept?
- Like oneself and the direction in which life is going?
- Interact well with family?
- Cope with the stresses of constant change and growth?
- Have well-established bonds with significant others, such as marriage partners or close friends?
- Have a meaningful social life?

MediaLink | NATIONAL HEALTH STATISTICS

TABLE 2–2	Physical Status and Changes in the Young Adult Years	
Assessment	**Status During the 20s**	**Status During the 30s**
Skin	Smooth, even temperature	Wrinkles begin to appear
Hair	Slightly oily, shiny Balding may begin	Graying may begin Balding may begin
Vision	Snellen 20/20	Some loss of visual acuity and accommodation
Musculoskeletal	Strong, coordinated	Some loss of strength and muscle mass
Cardiovascular	Maximum cardiac output 60–90 beats/min Mean BP: 120/80	Slight decline in cardiac output 60–90 beats/min Mean BP: 120/80
Respiratory	Rate: 12–20 Full vital capacity	Rate: 12–20 Decline in vital capacity

- Have a career or occupation?
- Demonstrate emotional, social, and economic responsibility for own life?
- Have a set of values that guide behavior?
- Have a healthy lifestyle? (Kozier, Erb, Berman, & Burke, 2000)

Physical assessment of the young adult includes height and weight, blood pressure, and vision. During the health history, the nurse should ask specific questions about substance use, sexual activity and concerns, exercise, eating habits, menstrual history and patterns, coping mechanisms, any familial chronic illnesses, and family changes.

Promoting Healthy Behaviors in the Young Adult

The nurse promotes health in the young adult by teaching the behaviors listed in Box 2–1. Health information for the young adult is primarily provided in community settings. Examples are as follows:

- Health-related courses and seminars at colleges and universities include information on the use of sports and exercise facilities, alcohol and drug abuse, smoking cessation, mental health, and sexual health.
- Workplace programs include blood pressure monitoring, exercise, smoking cessation, cafeteria nutrition guidelines, and stress-reduction activities.
- Community programs include media information, health fairs, support groups, and information about risk factors for disease and injury.

THE MIDDLE ADULT

The middle adult, age 40 to 65, has physical status and function similar to that of the young adult. However, many changes take place between ages 40 and 65. Table 2–3 lists the physical changes that normally occur in the middle years.

Risks for Alterations in Health

The middle adult is at risk for alterations in health from obesity, cardiovascular disease, cancer, substance abuse, and physical and psychosocial stressors. These factors may be interrelated.

Obesity

The middle adult often has a problem maintaining a healthy weight. Weight gain in middle adulthood is usually the result of continuing to consume the same number of calories while decreasing physical activity and experiencing a decrease in basal metabolic rate. Obesity affects all the major organ systems of the body, increasing the risk of atherosclerosis, hypertension, elevated cholesterol and triglyceride levels, and diabetes. Obesity is also associated with heart disease, osteoarthritis, and gallbladder disease.

Cardiovascular Disease

The major risk factors, especially for coronary artery disease, include age, male gender, physical inactivity, cigarette smoking, hypertension, elevated blood cholesterol levels, and diabetes. Other contributing factors include obesity, stress, and lack of exercise. The middle adult is at risk for disorders of peripheral vascular, cerebrovascular, and cardiovascular disease.

Cancer

Cancer is the third leading cause of death in adults between ages 25 and 64 in the United States, with one-third of cases occurring between ages 35 and 64. Cancers of the breast, colon, lung, and reproductive system are common in the middle years. The middle adult is at risk for cancer as a result of increased length of exposure to environmental carcinogens, as well as alcohol and nicotine use.

Substance Abuse

Although the middle adult may abuse a variety of substances, the most commonly abused are alcohol, nicotine, and prescription drugs. Excess alcohol use in the middle adult contributes

---

BOX 2–1	■ Healthy Behaviors in the Young Adult

- Choose foods from all food groups, and eat a variety of foods.
- Choose a diet low in fat (30% or less of total calories), saturated fat (less than 10% of calories), and cholesterol (less than 300 mg daily).
- Choose a diet that each day includes at least three servings of vegetables, two servings of fruits, and six servings of grains.
- Use sugar, salt, and sodium in moderation.
- For females, increase to or maintain 18 mg of iron daily in the diet, and 400 mg of folic acid per day through diet or supplements.
- Make exercise a regular part of life, carrying out activities that increase the heart rate to a set target, and maintain that rate for 30–60 minutes three or four times a week.
- Include exercise as part of any weight-reduction program.

- Have regular physical examinations, including assessment for cancer of the thyroid, ovaries, lymph nodes, and skin (every 3 years).
- Have a vision examination every 2–4 years.
- Have an annual dental checkup.
- For females between age 20 and 39 have a CBE* by a health care professional every 3 years.
- For females, have Pap tests as recommended by a physician: annually until three or more consecutive normal results, and then at physician's discretion.
- For males, have testicular and prostate examinations every 5 years.
- Conduct BSE* or testicular self-examination monthly.
- Maintain immunizations.

*CBE = clinical breast examination
BSE = breast self-examination

MediaLink | TEACHING PROGRAM CASE STUDY

TABLE 2-3	Physical Changes in the Middle Adult Years
Assessment	**Changes**
Skin	• Decreased turgor, moisture, and subcutaneous fat result in wrinkles. • Fat is deposited in the abdominal and hip areas.
Hair	• Loss of melanin in hair shaft causes graying. • Hairline recedes in males.
Sensory	• Visual acuity for near vision decreases (presbyopia) during the 40s. • Auditory acuity for high-frequency sounds decreases (presbycusis); more common in men. • Sense of taste diminishes.
Musculoskeletal	• Skeletal muscle mass decreases by about age 60. • Thinning of intervertebral discs results in loss of height (about 1 inch [2.5 cm]). • Postmenopausal women may have loss of calcium and develop osteoporosis.
Cardiovascular	• Blood vessels lose elasticity. • Systolic blood pressure may increase.
Respiratory	• Loss of vital capacity (about 1 L from age 20 to 60) occurs.
Gastrointestinal	• Large intestine gradually loses muscle tone; constipation may result. • Gastric secretions are decreased.
Genitourinary	• Hormonal changes occur: menopause, women (↓ estrogen); andropause, men (↓ testosterone).
Endocrine	• Gradual decrease in glucose tolerance occurs.

to an increased risk of liver cancer, cirrhosis, pancreatitis, hyperlipidemia, and anemia. Alcoholism also increases the risk of accidental injury or death and disrupts careers and relationships. Cigarette smoking increases the risk of cancer of the larynx, lung, mouth, pharynx, bladder, pancreas, esophagus, and kidney; of chronic obstructive pulmonary disorders; and of cardiovascular disorders.

Physical and Psychosocial Stressors

The middle adult years are ones of change and transition, frequently resulting in stress. Both men and women must adapt to changes in physical appearance and function and accept their own mortality. Children may leave home or choose to remain at home longer than they are welcome. Parents are aging, with illness probable and death inevitable. The middle adult thus becomes part of what has been called "the sandwich generation," caught between the need to care for both children and aging parents. Both men and women may make career changes, and approaching retirement becomes a reality. Divorce in the middle years is a major emotional, social, and financial stressor.

Assessment Guidelines

The following guidelines are useful in assessing the achievement of significant developmental tasks in the middle adult. Does the middle adult:

• Accept the aging body?
• Feel comfortable with and respect oneself?
• Enjoy some new freedom to be independent?
• Accept changes in family roles?
• Enjoy success and satisfaction from work and/or family roles?
• Interact well and share companionable activities with a partner?

• Expand or renew previous interests?
• Pursue charitable and altruistic activities?
• Consider plans for retirement?
• Have a meaningful philosophy of life?
• Follow preventive health care practices? (Kozier et al., 2000)

Physical assessment of the middle adult includes all body systems, including blood pressure, vision, and hearing. Monitoring for risks and onset of cancer symptoms is essential. During the health history, the nurse should ask specific questions about food intake and exercise habits, substance abuse, sexual concerns, changes in the reproductive system, and coping mechanisms.

Promoting Healthy Behaviors in the Middle Adult

The nurse promotes health in the middle adult by teaching the behaviors listed in Box 2–2. Information about health for the middle adult may be provided in a variety of community settings, including outpatient clinics, occupational health clinics, and private practice. Examples are as follows:

• Specific programs emphasize accepting responsibility for one's own health. This type of teaching can be in a seminar or on a one-to-one basis, and includes information specific to a group of individuals with an identified need, such as smokers, women who have just entered the workforce, or men nearing retirement.
• The community and industries provide information about safety hazards in the home and workplace, as well as during leisure activities.
• Literature about community resources is available for health promotion, including programs offered at alcohol/drug abuse

---

BOX 2–2 ■ **Healthy Behaviors in the Middle Adult**

- Choose foods from all food groups, and eat a variety of foods.
- Choose a diet low in fat (30% or less of total calories), saturated fat (less than 10% of calories), and cholesterol (less than 300 mg daily). Adjust daily calorie intake to maintain healthy weight.
- Choose a diet that each day includes at least three servings of vegetables, two servings of fruits, and six servings of grains.
- Use sugar, salt, and sodium in moderation.
- Increase calcium intake (in perimenopausal women) to 1200 mg daily.
- Consume high-fiber foods.
- Make exercise a part of life, carrying out regular exercise that is moderately strenuous, is consistent, and avoids overexertion; exercise for 30 minutes at least three times a week.
- Include exercise as part of any weight-reduction program.
- Have an annual vision examination.
- Have an annual dental checkup.

- Have a physical examination annually, including assessment for cancer of the thyroid, testes, prostate, mouth, ovaries, skin, colon, and lymph nodes.
- For females, have a mammogram every year from age 40 on. Have a CBE* annually.
- For females, have a Pap test as recommended for the young adult (see Box 2–1).
- Have an annual stool blood test; a digital rectal examination and a flexible sigmoidoscopy every 5 years; and a colonoscopy and digital rectal examination every 10 years or a double-contrast barium enema and a digital examination every 5–10 years.
- For males, have testicular and prostate examinations annually, including a PSA,* after age 50.
- Conduct BSE* or testicular self-examination every month. (The perimenopausal woman should set a specific date each month for the exam, as menstrual periods may be irregular or absent.)

*BSE = breast self-examination
CBE = clinical breast examination
PSA = prostate-specific antigen blood test

---

treatment centers, clinics and health centers, counseling services, crisis intervention centers, spouse abuse programs, and health education and promotion agencies (e.g., American Red Cross, American Cancer Society, American Heart Association, YWCA, YMCA).

THE OLDER ADULT

The older adult period begins at age 65, but it can be further divided into three periods: the young-old (age 65 to 74), the middle-old (age 75 to 84), and the old-old (age 85 and over). With increasing age, a number of normal physiologic changes occur, as listed in Table 2–4.

The older adult population is increasing more rapidly than any other age group. In the last century, the number of adults in the United States living to age 65 or older increased from 4% in 1900 to 12.8% in 1999. There will be 70 million older adults by the year 2030, more than twice the number in 1999. The life expectancy in the United States is 73.6 years for men and 79.4 years for women (American Association of Retired Persons [AARP], 2001; CDC, 1999).

The increase in numbers of older adults has important implications for nursing. Clients needing health care in all settings will be older, requiring nursing interventions and teaching specifically designed to meet needs that differ from those of young and middle adults. Although **gerontologic nursing** (care of the older adult) is a nursing specialty area, it is also an integral component of medical-surgical nursing (Figure 2–1 ■).

Risks for Alterations in Health

The older adult is at risk for alterations in health from a variety of causes. Approximately 40% of all older adults report having a limitation caused by a chronic illness, and more than 50% report having at least one disability (AARP, 2001). The most frequently occurring conditions in the older adult are arthritis, hypertension, hearing impairments, cardiovascular diseases, cataracts, sinusitis, orthopedic disorders, visual impairments, and diabetes. The leading causes of death are heart disease, cancer, and stroke.

Like the middle adult, the older adult is at risk for alterations in health from obesity, cardiovascular disease, and cancer. Other risk factors specific to this age group include injuries, pharmacologic effects, and physical and psychosocial stress.

Injuries

Injuries in the older adult cause many different problems: illness, financial burdens, hospitalization, self-care deficits, loss of independence, and even death. The risk of injury is increased by normal physiologic changes that accompany aging, pathophysiologic alterations in health, environmental hazards, and lack of support systems. The three major causes of injury in the older adult are falls, fires, and motor vehicle accidents. Of these, falls with resultant hip fractures are the most significant in terms of long-term disability and death.

Pharmacologic Effects

A number of risk factors predispose the older adult to experiencing drug toxicity. Age-related changes in tissue and organ structure and function alter the absorption of both oral and parenteral medications. Low nutritional levels and decreased liver function may alter drug metabolism. The aging kidney may not excrete drugs at the normal clearance rate. Self-administration of both prescribed and over-the-counter medications presents risks for error resulting from confusion, forgetfulness, or misreading the directions. In addition, the older adult may take several drugs at once, and it is difficult to know how drugs interact with each other (Weitzel, 2001).

Physical and Psychosocial Stressors

The older adult is exposed to the same environmental hazards as the young and middle adult, but the accumulation of years of

TABLE 2–4	Physical Changes in the Older Adult Years
Assessment	**Changes**
Skin	• Decreased turgor and sebaceous gland activity result in dry, wrinkled skin. Melanocytes cluster, causing "age spots" or "liver spots."
Hair and nails	• Scalp, axillary, and pubic hair thins; nose and ear hair thickens. Women may develop facial hair. • Nails grow more slowly; may become thick and brittle.
Sensory	• Visual field narrows, and depth perception is distorted. • Pupils are smaller, reducing night vision. • Lenses yellow and become opaque, resulting in distortion of green, blue, and violet tones and increased sensitivity to glare. • Production of tears decreases. • Sense of smell decreases. • Age-related hearing loss progresses, involving middle- and low-frequency sounds. • Threshold for pain and touch increases. • Alterations in proprioception (sense of physical position) may occur.
Musculoskeletal	• Loss of overall mass, strength, and movement of muscles occurs; tremors may occur. • Loss of bone structure and deterioration of cartilage in joints results in increased risk of fractures and in limitation of range of motion.
Cardiovascular	• Systolic blood pressure rises. • Cardiac output decreases. • Peripheral resistance increases, and capillary walls thicken.
Respiratory	• Continued loss of vital capacity occurs as the lungs become less elastic and more rigid. • Anteroposterior chest diameter increases; kyphosis. • Although blood carbon dioxide levels remain relatively constant, blood oxygen levels decrease by 10% to 15%.
Gastrointestinal	• Production of saliva decreases, and decreased number of taste buds decrease accurate receptors for salt and sweet. • Gag reflex is decreased, and stomach motility and emptying are reduced. • Both large and small intestines have some atrophy, with decreased peristalsis. • The liver decreases in weight and storage capacity; gallstones increase; pancreatic enzymes decrease.

Genitourinary	• Kidneys lose mass, and the glomerular filtration rate is reduced (by nearly 50% from young adulthood to old age).
	• Bladder capacity decreases, and the micturition reflex is delayed. Urinary retention is more common.
	• Women may have stress incontinence; men may have an enlarged prostate gland.
	• Reproductive changes in men occur:
	  — Testosterone decreases.
	  — Sperm count decreases.
	  — Testes become smaller.
	  — Length of time to achieve an erection increases; erection is less full.
	• Reproductive changes in women occur:
	  — Estrogen levels decrease.
	  — Breast tissue decreases.
	  — Vagina, uterus, ovaries, and urethra atrophy.
	  — Vaginal lubrication decreases.
	  — Vaginal secretions become alkaline.

Endocrine	• Pituitary gland loses weight and vascularity. • Thyroid gland becomes more fibrous, and plasma T_3 decreases. • Pancreas releases insulin more slowly; increased blood glucose levels are common. • Adrenal glands produce less cortisol.

exposure may now appear. For example, exposure to the sun in earlier years may be manifested by skin cancer, and the long-term effects of exposure to noise pollution can result in impaired hearing. The older adult (especially the older male) is at increased risk for respiratory disorders as a result of years of smoking, or from such pollutants as coal or asbestos dust. Living conditions and economic constraints may prevent the older adult from having necessary heating and cooling, contributing to thermal-related illness and even death. Elder abuse and neglect further increase the risk of injury or illness.

Psychosocial stressors for the older adult include the illness or death of a spouse, decreased or limited income, retirement, isolation from friends and family because of lack of transportation or distance, return to the home of a child, or relocation to

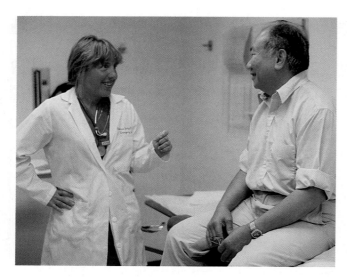

Figure 2–1 ■ The older adult population is increasing more rapidly than any other age group, making gerontologic nursing an integral component of medical-surgical nursing practice.

a long-term health care facility. A further stressor may be role loss or reversal—for example, when the wife becomes the caretaker of her chronically ill husband.

Assessment Guidelines

The following guidelines are useful in assessing the achievement of significant developmental tasks in the older adult. Does the older adult:

- Adjust to the physiologic changes related to aging?
- Manage retirement years in a satisfying manner?
- Have satisfactory living arrangements and income to meet changing needs?
- Participate in social and leisure activities?
- Have a social network of friends and support persons?
- View life as worthwhile?
- Have high self-esteem?
- Have the abilities to care for self or to secure appropriate help?
- Gain support from a value system or spiritual philosophy?
- Adapt lifestyle to diminishing energy and ability?
- Accept and adjust to the death of significant others? (Kozier et al., 2000)

Physical assessment of the older adult includes a careful examination of all body systems. During the health history, the nurse should ask specific questions about usual dietary patterns; elimination; exercise and rest; use of alcohol, nicotine, over-the-counter medications, and prescription drugs; sexual concerns; financial concerns; and support systems.

Promoting Healthy Behaviors in the Older Adult

The nurse promotes health in the older adult by teaching the behaviors listed in Box 2–3. Older adults get the same benefits from health teaching as young adults and middle adults; they should never be viewed as being "too old" for healthy living

practices. However, nurses should structure teaching activities to meet age-related physiologic changes, such as using charts and literature with large print. Health education for the older adult is provided in hospitals, long-term care facilities, retirement centers, outpatient clinics, senior citizen centers, and other community settings. Examples are as follows:

- Educational seminars teach about accident prevention in the home, in automobiles, and when taking public transportation.
- Health screenings and information in health fairs can specifically aid the older adult.
- Community programs provide immunization for influenza and pneumonia.
- Literature is available about financial assistance for health care, crisis hot lines, community services and resources (as described earlier for the middle adult), transportation, and nutrition (such as the Meals-on-Wheels program).

THE FAMILY OF THE ADULT CLIENT

Although some clients are totally alone in the world, most have one or more people who are significant in their lives. These significant others may be related or bonded to the client by birth, adoption, marriage, or friendship. Although not always meeting traditional definitions, people (or even pets) significant to the client are the client's family. The nurse includes the family as an integral component of care in all health care settings.

Definitions and Functions of the Family

What is a **family?** The definitions of a family are changing as society changes. According to one definition, a family is a unit of people related by marriage, birth, or adoption (Duvall, 1977). An expanded definition states that "a family is composed of two or more people who are emotionally involved with each other and live in close geographical proximity" (Freidman, 1981, p. 8). In a global society, it may not be possible for family members to live in close proximity, but they do remain emotionally involved.

Although every family is unique, all families have certain structural and functional features in common. **Family structure** (family roles and relationships) and **family function** (interactions among family members and with the community) provide the following:

- *Interdependence.* The behaviors and level of development of individual family members constantly influence and are influenced by the behaviors and level of development of all other members of the family.
- *Maintaining boundaries.* The family creates boundaries that guide its members, providing a distinct and unique family culture. This culture, in turn, provides values.
- *Adapting to change.* The family changes as new members are added, current members leave, and the development of each member progresses.
- *Performing family tasks.* Essential tasks maintain the stability and continuity of the family. These tasks include physical maintenance of the home and the people in the home, the production and socialization of family members, and the maintenance of the psychologic well-being of members.

BOX 2–3	■ Healthy Behaviors in the Older Adult

■ Choose foods from all food groups, and eat a variety of foods. Include some high-quality protein at each meal, such as low-fat milk and cheese, peanut butter, meat, fish, or poultry.

■ Choose a diet low in fat (30% or less of total calories), saturated fat (less than 10% of calories), and cholesterol (less than 300 mg daily). Adjust daily caloric intake to balance energy expenditure and maintain healthy weight. A daily caloric intake of 1200 kcal is recommended, but it may vary according to body build and activity level.

■ Choose a diet that each day includes at least three servings of vegetables, two servings of fruits, and six servings of grains. Increased amounts of high-fiber foods may be necessary; if so, fluid intake should also be increased.

■ Use sugar, salt, and sodium in moderation.

■ Increase calcium intake to at least 800 mg per day (1000–1500 mg per day may be recommended).

■ Make exercise a part of life, following a regular program of moderate exercise, such as walking or swimming. Avoid overexertion.

■ Have an annual vision examination.

■ Have an annual dental checkup.

■ Have an annual physical examination that includes urinalysis and assessment for cancer of the thyroid, testes, prostate, mouth, ovaries, skin, colon, and lymph nodes.

■ For females, have a CBE* and a mammogram annually.

■ For females, have Pap tests as recommended by health care provider.

■ For males, have an annual testicular and prostate examination including a PSA.*

■ Have a digital rectal examination and stool blood test annually. Have examinations as recommended for the middle adult (see Box 2–2).

■ Conduct BSE* or testicular self-examination every month.

■ Maintain immunizations for diphtheria and tetanus by having boosters every 10 years.

■ Obtain annual immunizations against influenza, especially with a history of chronic cardiovascular or respiratory illness.

■ Obtain pneumococcal pneumonia immunization.

■ Practice the following to avoid injury:

  a. Have adequate lighting in all rooms of the house including stairs, basement, and bedrooms.

  b. Avoid sitting or standing rapidly; if dizziness occurs, remain in one position until dizziness is gone.

  c. Have handrails installed by the toilet and in the shower or bathtub.

  d. Do not use throw rugs.

  e. Install smoke alarms.

  f. Never step into a tub or shower without checking the temperature of the water.

  g. Always wear corrective lenses and/or hearing aids when driving.

  h. Do not drive a car after taking medications that cause drowsiness or dizziness.

*BSE = breast self-examination
CBE = clinical breast examination
PSA = prostate-specific antigen blood test

Family Developmental Stages and Tasks

The family, like the individual, has developmental stages and tasks. Each stage brings change, requiring adaptation; each new stage also brings family-related risk factors for alterations in health. The nurse must consider the needs of the client both at a specific developmental stage and within a family with specific developmental tasks. Family developmental stages and developmental tasks are described next; related risk factors and health problems for each stage are listed in Table 2–5.

Couple

Two people, living together with or without being married, are in a period of establishing themselves as a couple. The developmental tasks of the couple include adjusting to living together as a couple, establishing a mutually satisfying relationship, relating to kin, and deciding whether to have children.

Family with Infants and Preschoolers

The family with infants or preschoolers must adjust to having and supporting the needs of more than two members. Other developmental tasks of the family at this stage are developing an attachment between parents and children, adjusting to the economic costs of having more members, coping with energy depletion and lack of privacy, and carrying out activities that enhance growth and development of the children.

Family with School-Age Children

The family with school-age children has the developmental tasks of adjusting to the expanded world of children in school and encouraging educational achievement. A further task is promoting joint decision making between children and parents.

Family with Adolescents and Young Adults

The developmental tasks of the family with adolescents and young adults focus on transition. While providing a supportive home base and maintaining open communications, parents must balance freedom with responsibility and release adult children as they seek independence.

Family with Middle Adults

The family with middle adults (in which the parents are middle-aged and children are no longer at home) has the developmental tasks of maintaining ties with older and younger generations and planning for retirement. If the family consists of just the middle-aged couple, they have the developmental task of reestablishing the relationship and (if necessary) acquiring the role of grandparents.

Family with Older Adults

The older adult family has the developmental tasks of adjusting to retirement, adjusting to aging, and coping with the loss of a spouse. If a spouse dies, further tasks include adjusting to living alone or closing the family home.

TABLE 2–5 Family-Related Risk Factors for Alterations in Health

Stage	Risk Factors	Health Problems
Couple, or Family with Infants and Preschoolers	• Lack of knowledge about family planning, contraception, sexual and marital roles • Inadequate prenatal care • Altered nutrition: inadequate nutrition, overweight, underweight • Smoking, alcohol/drug abuse • First pregnancy before age 16 or after age 35 • Low socioeconomic status • Lack of knowledge about child health and safety • Rubella, syphilis, gonorrhea, AIDS	Premature pregnancy Low-birth-weight infant Birth defects Injury to infant or child Accidents
Family with School-Age Children	• Unsafe home environment • Working parents with inappropriate or inadequate resources for child care • Low socioeconomic status • Child abuse or neglect • Multiple, closely spaced children • Repeated infections, accidents, and hospitalizations • Unrecognized and unattended health problems • Poor or inappropriate nutrition • Toxic substances in the home • Immature, dependent parents • Generational pattern of using social agencies as a way of life	Behavior problems Speech and vision problems Learning disabilities Communicable diseases Physical abuse Cancer Developmental delay Obesity, underweight
Family with Adolescents and Young Adults	• Family values of aggressiveness and competition • Racial and ethnic family origin • Socioeconomic factors contributing to peer relationships • Lifestyle and behavior leading to chronic illness (substance abuse, inadequate diet) • Lack of problem-solving skills • Conflicts between parent and children	Violent death and injury Alcohol/drug abuse Unwanted pregnancy Suicide Sexually transmitted diseases Domestic abuse
Family with Middle Adults	• High-cholesterol diet • Overweight • Hypertension • Smoking, alcohol abuse • Physical inactivity • Genetic predisposition, heredity • Personality patterns related to stress • Habits: low-fiber and high-cholesterol diet; charcoal grilling • Exposure to environment: sunlight, radiation, asbestos, water or air pollution • Depression • Gingivitis	Cardiovascular disease (coronary artery disease and cerebral vascular disease) Cancer Accidents Suicide Mental illness Periodontal disease, loss of teeth
Family with Older Adults	• Age • Depression • Drug interactions • Metabolic and endocrine disorders • Chronic illness • Death of spouse • Reduced income • Poor nutrition • Lack of exercise • Past environment and lifestyle	Impaired vision and hearing Hypertension Acute illness Chronic illness Infectious diseases (influenza, pneumonia) Injuries from burns and falls Depression Alcohol abuse

Note. Adapted from Healthy People: The Surgeon General's Report on Health Promotion and Disease Prevention, *Health and Human Services Pub. No. 79-55071, 1992, Washington, DC: US Government Printing Office, and* Healthy People 2001: National Health Promotion and Disease Prevention Objectives (Summary), *American Public Health Association, 2000, Washington, DC: US Government Printing Office.*

HEALTH AND ILLNESS IN THE ADULT CLIENT
Health

The World Health Organization (WHO) defines **health** as "a state of complete physical, mental, and social well-being, and not merely the absence of disease or infirmity" (WHO, 1974, p. 1). However, this definition does not take into account the various levels of health a person may experience, or that a person may be clinically described as ill and still define oneself as well. These additional factors, which greatly influence nursing care, include the health-illness continuum and high-level wellness.

The Health-Illness Continuum and High-Level Wellness

The **health-illness continuum** represents health as a dynamic process, with high-level wellness at one extreme of the continuum and death at the opposite extreme (Figure 2–2 ■). Individuals place themselves at different locations on the continuum at specific points in time.

Dunn (1959) expanded the concept of a continuum of health and illness in his description of **high-level wellness.** Dunn conceptualized wellness as an active process influenced by the environment. He differentiated good health from wellness:

> Good health can exist as a relatively passive state of freedom from illness in which the individual is at peace with his environment. . . . Wellness is an integrated method of functioning, which is oriented toward maximizing the potential of which the individual is capable, within the environment where he is functioning. (1959, p. 4)

A variety of factors influence wellness, including self-concept, environment, culture, and spiritual values. Providing care based on a framework of wellness facilitates active involvement by both the nurse and the client in promoting, maintaining, or restoring health. It also supports the philosophy of holistic health care, in which all aspects of a person (physical, psychosocial, cultural, spiritual, and intellectual) are considered as essential components of individualized care.

Factors Affecting Health

Many different factors affect a person's health or level of wellness. These factors often interact to promote health or to become risk factors for alterations in health. The factors affecting health are described next.

GENETIC MAKEUP. Each person's genetic makeup influences health status throughout life. Genetic makeup affects personality, temperament, body structure, intellectual potential, and susceptibility to the development of hereditary alterations in health. Examples of chronic illnesses that are associated with genetic makeup include sickle cell disease, hemophilia, diabetes mellitus, and cancer.

COGNITIVE ABILITIES AND EDUCATIONAL LEVEL. Although cognitive abilities are determined prior to adulthood, the level of cognitive development affects whether people view themselves as healthy or ill; cognitive levels also may affect health practices. Injuries to and illnesses affecting the brain may alter cognitive abilities. Educational level affects the ability to understand and follow guidelines for health. For example, if an individual is functionally illiterate, written information about healthy behaviors and health resources is worthless.

RACE, ETHNICITY, AND CULTURAL BACKGROUND. Certain diseases occur at a higher rate of incidence in some races and ethnic groups than in others. For example, in the United States, hypertension is more common in African Americans, tuberculosis and diabetes mellitus are among the leading causes of illness in Native Americans, and eye disorders are more prevalent in Chinese Americans. The ethnic and cultural background of an individual also influences health values and behaviors, lifestyle, and illness behaviors. Every culture defines health and illness in a way that is unique; in addition, each culture has its own health beliefs and illness treatment practices.

AGE, GENDER, AND DEVELOPMENTAL LEVEL. Age, gender, and developmental level are factors in health and illness. Cardiovascular disorders are uncommon in young adults, but the incidence increases after the age of 40. Myocardial infarctions are more common in men than women until women are past menopause. Some diseases occur only in one gender or the other (e.g., prostate cancer in men and cervical cancer in women). The older adult has increased incidence of chronic illness and increased potential for serious illness or death from infectious illnesses such as influenza and pneumonia.

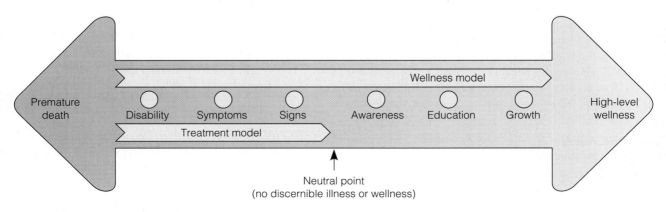

Figure 2–2 ■ The health/illness continuum.

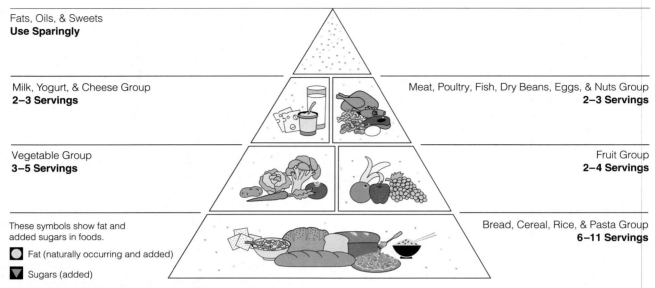

Fats, Oils, & Sweets
Use Sparingly

Milk, Yogurt, & Cheese Group
2–3 Servings

Meat, Poultry, Fish, Dry Beans, Eggs, & Nuts Group
2–3 Servings

Vegetable Group
3–5 Servings

Fruit Group
2–4 Servings

These symbols show fat and
added sugars in foods.

◯ Fat (naturally occurring and added)

▽ Sugars (added)

Bread, Cereal, Rice, & Pasta Group
6–11 Servings

Figure 2–3 ■ The food guide pyramid is designed to be used as a guide when buying foods and preparing meals.

Source: U.S. Department of Agriculture and U.S. Department of Health and Human Services.

LIFESTYLE AND ENVIRONMENT. The components of a person's lifestyle that affect health status include patterns of eating, use of chemical substances (alcohol, nicotine, caffeine, legal and illegal drugs), exercise and rest patterns, and coping methods. Examples of altered responses are the relationship of obesity to hypertension, cigarette smoking to chronic obstructive pulmonary disease, a sedentary lifestyle to heart disease, and a high-stress career to alcoholism. The environment has a major influence on health. Occupational exposure to toxic substances (such as asbestos and coal dust) increases the risk of pulmonary disorders. Air, water, and food pollution increase the risk of respiratory disorders, infectious diseases, and cancer. Environmental temperature variations can result in hypothermia or hyperthermia, especially in the older adult.

SOCIOECONOMIC BACKGROUND.   Both lifestyle and environmental influences are affected by one's income level. The culture of poverty, which crosses all racial and ethnic boundaries, negatively influences health status. Living at or below the poverty level often results in crowded, unsanitary living conditions or homelessness. Housing often is overcrowded, lacks adequate heating or cooling, and is infested with insects and rats. Crowded living conditions increase the risk of transferring communicable diseases. Other problems include lack of infant and child care, lack of medical care for injuries or illness, inadequate nutrition, use of addictive substances, and violence.

GEOGRAPHIC AREA.   The geographic area in which one lives influences health status. Such illnesses as malaria are more common in tropical areas of North America, whereas multiple sclerosis occurs with greater frequency in the northern United States and Canada. Other geographic influences are seen in the number of skin cancers in people living in sunny, hot areas and sinus infections in people living in areas of high humidity.

Health Promotion and Maintenance

For many years, the emphasis in nursing was on care of the acutely ill client in the hospital setting. With changes in society and in health care, this emphasis is shifting toward preventive, community-based care. Although the focus of this textbook is not community health nursing, the importance of teaching health maintenance and providing continuity of care as a client moves among health care settings is an essential component of medical-surgical nursing.

HEALTHY LIVING.   Practices that are known to promote health and wellness are:

- Eating three balanced meals a day and including foods according to the food guide pyramid (Figure 2–3 ■).
- Eating moderately to maintain a healthy weight.
- Exercising moderately, following a regular routine.
- Sleeping 7 to 8 hours each day.
- Limiting alcohol consumption to a moderate amount.
- Eliminating smoking.
- Keeping sun exposure to a minimum.

The nurse promotes health by teaching the activities that maintain wellness, by providing information about the characteristics and consequences of diseases when risk factors have been identified, and by supplying specific information about decreasing risk factors (Pender, Parsons, & Murdaugh, 2002). The nurse also promotes health by following healthy practices and serving as a role model.

NATIONAL HEALTH PROMOTION.   The U.S. Department of Health and Human Services (2000) published national health objectives for the year 2010. Goals and leading health indicators are described in Box 2–4.

ILLNESS PREVENTION.   Activities to prevent illness include any measures that limit the progression of an illness at any point of its course. Three levels of illness prevention have been

BOX 2–4	■ Goals and Leading Health Indicators: Healthy People 2010

Healthy People 2010 has two major goals: to increase the quality and years of healthy life and to eliminate health disparities.

The major goals are divided into 28 focus areas, with each area having a specific goal. For example, for cancer, the goal is to reduce the number of new cancer cases as well as the illness, disability, and death caused by cancer.

The leading indicators used to measure the expected goals are as follows:

■ Physical activity
■ Overweight and obesity
■ Tobacco use
■ Substance abuse
■ Responsible sexual behavior
■ Mental health
■ Injury and violence
■ Environmental quality
■ Immunization
■ Access to health care

Note. Adapted from Healthy People 2010 *by US Department of Health and Human Services, 2000, Washington, DC: USDHHS.*

defined (Leavell & Clark, 1965). Each level of prevention occurs at a distinct point in the development of a disease process and requires specific nursing interventions (Edelman & Mandle, 2002). The levels are as follows:

1. Primary level of prevention includes generalized health-promotion activities as well as specific actions that prevent or delay the occurrence of a disease. Following are examples of primary prevention activities:
   • Protecting oneself against environmental risks, such as air and water pollution
   • Eating nutritious foods
   • Protecting oneself against industrial hazards
   • Obeying seat belt and helmet laws
   • Obtaining sex counseling and practicing safe sex
   • Obtaining immunizations
   • Undergoing genetic screenings
   • Eliminating the use of alcohol and cigarettes
2. Secondary level of prevention involves activities that emphasize early diagnosis and treatment of an illness that is already present, to stop the pathologic process and enable the person to return to his or her former state of health as soon as possible. Following are examples of secondary prevention activities:
   • Having screenings for diseases such as hypertension, diabetes mellitus, and glaucoma
   • Obtaining physical examinations and diagnostic tests for cancer
   • Performing self-examination for breast and/or testicular cancer
   • Obtaining tuberculosis skin tests

   • Obtaining specific treatment of illness (e.g., the treatment of streptococcal infections of the throat will prevent secondary infections involving the heart and/or kidneys)
3. Tertiary level of prevention focuses on stopping the disease process and returning the affected individual to a useful place in society within the constraints of any disability. The activities primarily revolve around rehabilitation. Following are examples of tertiary prevention measures:
   • Obtaining medical or surgical treatment for an illness
   • Enrolling in specific rehabilitation programs for cardiovascular problems, head injuries, and strokes
   • Joining work training programs following illness or injury
   • Educating the public to employ rehabilitated people to the fullest possible extent

Disease and Illness

Disease and *illness* are terms that are often used interchangeably, but in fact they have different meanings. In general, nursing is concerned with illness, whereas medicine is concerned with disease.

Disease

Disease (literally meaning "without ease") is a medical term describing alterations in structure and function of the body or mind. Diseases may have mechanical, biologic, or normative causes. Mechanical causes of disease result in damage to the structure of the body and are the result of trauma or extremes of temperature. Biologic causes of disease affect body function and are the result of genetic defects, the effects of aging, infestation and infection, alterations in the immune system, and alterations in normal organ secretions. Normative causes are psychologic but involve a mind-body interaction, so that physical manifestations occur in response to the psychologic disturbance.

The cause of many diseases is still unknown. The following are generally accepted as common causes of disease:

• Genetic defects
• Developmental defects resulting from exposure to viruses, chemicals, or drugs that affect the developing fetus
• Biologic agents or toxins (including viruses, bacteria, rickettsia, fungi, protozoa, and helminths)
• Physical agents such as temperature extremes, radiation, and electricity
• Chemical agents such as alcohol, drugs, strong acids or bases, and heavy metals
• Generalized response of tissues to injury or irritation
• Alterations in the production of antibodies, resulting in allergies or hypersensitivities
• Faulty metabolic processes (e.g., a production of hormones or enzymes above or below normal)
• Continued, unabated stress

Diseases may be classified as acute or chronic, communicable, congenital, degenerative, functional, malignant, psychosomatic, idiopathic, or iatrogenic. These classifications are defined in Table 2–6. In all types of disease, alterations in structure or function cause signs and symptoms (**manifestations**) that

TABLE 2–6	Disease Classifications and Definitions
Classification	**Definition**
Acute	A disease that has a rapid onset, lasts a relatively short time, and is self-limiting
Chronic	A disease that has one or more of these characteristics: (1) is permanent, (2) leaves permanent disability, (3) causes nonreversible pathophysiology, (4) requires special training of the client for rehabilitation, (5) requires a long period of care
Communicable	A disease that can spread from one person to another
Congenital	A disease or disorder that exists at or before birth
Degenerative	A disease that results from deterioration or impairment of organs or tissues
Functional	A disease that affects function or performance but does not have manifestations of organic illness
Malignant	A disease that tends to become worse and cause death
Psychosomatic	A psychologic disease that is manifested by physiologic symptoms
Idiopathic	A disease that has an unknown cause
Iatrogenic	A disease that is caused by medical therapy

prompt a person to seek treatment from a physician or traditional healer. Although both subjective symptoms and objective signs commonly appear with disease, objective signs often predominate. Examples include bleeding, vomiting, diarrhea, limitation of movement, swelling, visual disturbances, and changes in elimination. However, pain (a subjective symptom) is often the primary reason that prompts a person to seek health care.

Illness

Illness is the response a person has to a disease. This response is highly individualized, as the person responds not only to his or her own perceptions of the disease but also to the perceptions of others. Illness integrates pathophysiologic alterations; psychologic effects of those alterations; effects on roles, relationships, and values; and cultural and spiritual beliefs. A person may have a disease and not categorize himself or herself as ill, or may validate feelings of illness through the comments of others ("You don't look as though you feel well today").

ACUTE ILLNESS. An **acute illness** occurs rapidly, lasts for a relatively short time, and is self-limiting. The condition responds to self-treatment or to medical-surgical intervention. Clients with uncomplicated acute illnesses usually have full recovery and return to normal pre-illness functioning.

Illness behaviors are the way people cope with the alterations in health and function caused by a disease. Illness behaviors are highly individualized and are influenced by age, gender, family values, economic status, culture, educational level, and mental status. Following is a sequence of illness behaviors (Suchman, 1972):

1. *Experiencing symptoms.* In the first stage of an acute illness, a person experiences one or more manifestations that serve as cues for an awareness that a change in normal health is occurring. The most significant manifestation is pain. Examples of other symptoms that signal an illness are bleeding, swelling, fever, or difficulty with breathing.

If the manifestations are mild or are familiar (such as symptoms of the common cold or influenza), the person usually uses over-the-counter medications or a traditional remedy for self-treatment. If the symptoms are relieved, no further action is taken; however, if the symptoms are severe or become worse, the person moves to the next stage.

2. *Assuming the sick role.* In the second stage of the sequence, the person assumes the sick role. This role assumption signals acceptance of the symptoms as proof that an illness is present. The person usually validates this belief with others and seeks support for the need to have professional treatment or to stay at home from school or work. Self-preoccupation is characteristic of this stage, and the person focuses on alterations in function resulting from the illness. If the illness is resolved, the person validates a return to health with others and resumes normal activities; however, if manifestations remain or increase in severity and others agree that no improvement has occurred, the person moves to the next stage by seeking medical care.

3. *Seeking medical care.* In our society, a physician or other health care provider most often provides validation of illness. People who believe themselves to be ill (and who are encouraged by others to contact a health care provider) make the medical contact for diagnosis, prognosis, and treatment of the illness. If the medical diagnosis is of an illness, the person moves to the next stage. If the medical diagnosis does not support illness, the client may return to normal functioning or may seek validation from a different health care provider.

4. *Assuming a dependent role.* The stage of assuming a dependent role begins when a person accepts the diagnosis and planned treatment of the illness. As the severity of the illness increases, so does the dependent role. It is during this stage that the person may enter the hospital for treatment and care. The responses of the person to care depend on many different variables: the severity of the illness, the

degree of anxiety or fear about the outcome, the loss of roles, the support systems available, individualized reactions to stress, and previous experiences with illness care.

5. *Achieving recovery and rehabilitation.* The final stage of an acute illness is recovery and rehabilitation. Institutional health care focuses on the acute care needs of the ill client, with recovery beginning in the hospital and completed at home. This focus makes client education and continuity of care a major goal for nursing. It has also contributed to the shift in settings for nursing care, with increasing numbers of nurses providing care in community settings and the home. The person now gives up the dependent role and resumes normal roles and responsibilities. As a result of education during treatment and care, the person may be at a higher level of wellness after recovery is complete. There is no set timetable for recovery from an illness. The degree of severity of the illness and the method of treatment both affect the length of time required, as does the person's compliance with treatment plans and motivation to return to normal health.

CHRONIC ILLNESS.   **Chronic illness** is a term that encompasses many different lifelong pathologic and psychologic alterations in health. It is the leading health problem in the world today, and the number of people with chronic illnesses is estimated to triple by the year 2040. Current trends affecting an increased incidence of chronic illnesses include diseases of aging, diseases of lifestyle and behavior, and environmental factors.

Most descriptions of chronic illness are based on the definition by the National Commission on Chronic Illness, which states that a chronic illness is any impairment or deviation from normal functioning that has one or more of the following characteristics:

- It is permanent.
- It leaves permanent disability.
- It is caused by nonreversible pathologic alterations.
- It requires special training of the client for rehabilitation.
- It may require a long period of care.

Chronic illness is also characterized by impaired function in more than one body system; responses to this impaired function may occur in sensory perception, self-care abilities, mobility, cognition, and social skills. The demands on the individual and family as a result of these responses are often lifelong (Miller, 2000).

The intensity of a chronic illness and its related manifestations range from mild to severe, and the illness is usually characterized by periods of remission and exacerbation. During periods of **remission,** the person does not experience symptoms, even though the disease is still clinically present. During periods of **exacerbation,** the symptoms reappear. These periods of change in symptoms do not appear in all chronic diseases.

Needs of the Chronically Ill Person.   Each person with a chronic illness has a unique set of responses and needs. The response of the person to the illness is influenced by the following factors:

- The point in the life cycle at which the onset of the illness occurs
- The type and degree of limitations imposed by the illness
- The visibility of impairment or disfigurement
- The pathophysiology causing the illness
- The relationship between the impairment and functioning in social roles
- Pain and fear

These factors are highly complex. They are interrelated within each person, resulting in individualized illness behaviors and needs. Because there are so many different chronic diseases and because the experience of each person with the illness is a composite of individualized responses, it is difficult to generalize about needs. However, almost all people with a chronic illness will need to:

- Live as normally as possible, despite the symptoms and treatment that make the person with a chronic illness feel alienated, lonely, and different from others without the illness.
- Learn to adapt activities of daily living and self-care activities.
- Grieve the loss of physical function and structure, income, status, roles, and dignity.
- Learn to live with chronic pain.
- Comply with a medical treatment plan.
- Maintain a positive self-concept and a sense of hope.
- Maintain a feeling of being in control.
- Confront the inevitability of death. (Miller, 2000; Pollock, 1986)

Some people with chronic illness successfully meet health-related needs, whereas others do not. Research indicates that adaptation is influenced by variables such as anger, depression, denial, self-concept, locus of control, hardiness, and disability. Nursing interventions for the person with a chronic illness focus on education to promote independent functioning, reduce health care costs, and improve well-being and quality of life.

The Family of the Client with a Chronic Illness.   The client with a chronic illness may be hospitalized for diagnosis and treatment of acute exacerbations, but the care of the client is primarily provided at home. Chronic illness in a family member is a major stressor that may cause changes in family structure and function, as well as changes in performing family developmental tasks.

Many different factors affect family responses to chronic illness; family responses in turn affect the client's response to and perception of the illness. Factors influencing response to chronic illness include personal, social, and economic resources; the nature and course of the disease; and demands of the illness as perceived by family members.

Support for the family is essential. The following information should be considered when performing any family assessment and developing a client's plan of care:

- Cohesiveness and communication patterns within the family
- Family interactions that support self-care

- Number of friends and relatives available
- Family values and beliefs about health and illness
- Cultural and spiritual beliefs
- Developmental level of the client and family

It is important to remember that standardized teaching plans may not be effective. Rather, chronically ill clients and families should be given the freedom to choose appropriate literature, self-help or support groups, and interactions with others who have the same illness.

REHABILITATION

Rehabilitation is the process of learning to live to one's maximum potential with a chronic impairment and its resultant functional disability. Rehabilitation nursing is based on a philosophy that each person has a unique set of strengths and abilities that can enable that person to live with dignity, self-worth, and independence. Nursing care to promote rehabilitation primarily focuses on clients with chronic illnesses or impairments.

The terms *impairment, disability,* and *handicap* are often used as synonyms, but they have different meanings. An **impairment** is a disturbance in structure or function resulting from physiologic or psychologic abnormalities. A **disability** is the degree of observable and measurable impairment. A **handicap** is the total adjustment to disability that limits functioning at a normal level (Stanhope & Lancaster, 1999). For example, following a motorcycle accident, Kim Rushin had damage to her left leg that resulted in an impairment in the ability to flex her knee. This resulted in a 50% disability of that leg and caused a handicap, because Kim was a school bus driver and could no longer operate the bus safely.

A Team Approach to Care

Rehabilitation promotes reintegration into the client's family and community through a team approach. Many different aspects of the client's life are included in the plan of care, including physical function, mental health, interpersonal relationships, social interactions, and vocational status. This comprehensive consideration of the client requires the expertise of a team of health care providers.

The rehabilitation team usually meets weekly to discuss the achievement of client goals (Figure 2–4 ■). As a part of this comprehensive plan of care, the team assesses the client's level of function, develops an individualized plan of care, maintains ongoing evaluation of outcomes, and includes the family in the plan of care.

Nursing in Rehabilitation

The nurse provides care for the chronically ill client of all ages and with many types of disability. The 20-year-old

Figure 2–4 ■ The rehabilitation team discusses the individualized plan of care and achievement of goals.

man with quadriplegia from a spinal cord injury has different needs than the 75-year-old woman who has had a stroke and is unable to move her left arm or speak. However, the plan of care developed for each of these clients considers common factors in assessing and planning individualized interventions.

Assessment of the client and family includes functional level and self-care abilities, educational needs, psychosocial needs, and the home environment. It is critical to determine the priorities of needs from the client and family perspective before establishing any plan of care. The nurse assesses the client's level of physical function, goals, concerns, stage of loss, home environment, and available resources.

Interventions to facilitate rehabilitation are revised to meet client and family needs as the client progresses toward reintegration. General areas of interventions include the following:

- Preventing complications
- Providing care as necessary and appropriate, with the goal of achieving a level of independence that is realistic for the client
- Implementing individualized teaching plans, with emphasis on care at home
- Making referrals to community agencies (for nursing care, special equipment or supplies, support groups, counseling, physical therapy, occupational therapy, respiratory therapy, vocational guidance, house cleaning, meals)

To ensure continuity of care during rehabilitation, the community health nurse is involved in the plan of care during the acute care stage. Continued education and support of the client and family are essential; the achievement of self-care and mobility does not guarantee independence in all areas of human functioning.

EXPLORE MediaLink

NCLEX review questions, case studies, care plan activities, MediaLink applications, and other interactive resources for this chapter can be found on the Companion Website at www.prenhall.com/lemone.

Click on Chapter 2 to select the activities for this chapter. For animations, video clips, more NCLEX review questions, and an audio glossary, access the Student CD-ROM accompanying this textbook.

TEST YOURSELF

1. Which of the following physical stressors increases the risk for illness in the young adult?

   a. Sexually transmitted diseases
   b. Motor vehicle accidents
   c. Financial difficulties
   d. Exposure to environmental pollutants

2. Mr. Jones, age 50, is 20 pounds overweight, smokes, and rarely exercises. As a middle adult, these factors increase his risk for disorders of which body system?

   a. Cardiovascular
   b. Renal
   c. Gastrointestinal
   d. Nervous

3. You have been asked to present a health-related program at the local senior center. What would be an appropriate topic?

   a. The Hazards of Substance Abuse
   b. Accident Prevention in the Home
   c. Family Roles and Tasks
   d. Treating Acute Illness

4. Which of the following illustrates the primary level of prevention of illness?

   a. Health screenings for hypertension
   b. Stopping smoking
   c. Annual physical examination
   d. Rehabilitation programs

5. You call your instructor to say you have the "flu" and will not be in class. What level of illness behavior are you demonstrating?

   a. Experiencing symptoms
   b. Assuming the sick role
   c. Seeking medical care
   d. Assuming a dependent role

See Test Yourself answers in Appendix C.

BIBLIOGRAPHY

Administration on Aging. (2002). *Profile of older Americans: 2002.* Bethesda, MD: National Aging Information Center, US Department of Health and Human Services.

American Association of Retired Persons. (2001). *Profile of older Americans: 2001.* Washington, DC: Resource Services Group.

American Cancer Society. (2002). *Summary of American Cancer Society recommendations for the early detection of cancer in asymptomatic people.* Atlanta, GA: American Cancer Society.

Artinian, N. (1994). Selecting a model to guide family assessment. *Dimensions in Critical Care Nursing, 14*(1), 4–12.

Burckhardt, C. (1987). Coping strategies of the chronically ill. *Nursing Clinics of North America, 22,* 543–550.

Centers for Disease Control and Prevention. (1999a). Births and deaths. *Monthly Vital Statistics Report, 47*(28). Washington, DC: US Department of Health and Human Services.

———. (1999b). *Deaths/mortality.* Washington, DC: National Center for Health Statistics.

Clemen-Stone, S., McGuire, S., & Eigsti, D. (1998). *Comprehensive community health nursing* (5th ed.). St. Louis: Mosby.

Crooks, E., & Clochesy, J. (2001, May). Special needs: Nurses can provide hope and quality care for the chronically, critically ill adult. *American Journal of Nursing* (Suppl.), 21–24, 48–50.

Dewar, A. L., & Lee, E. A. (2000). Bearing illness and injury. *Western Journal of Nursing Research, 22*(8), 912–926.

Duffy, B. (1997). Using a creative teaching process with adult patients. *Home Healthcare Nurse, 15*(2), 102–108.

Dunn, H. (1959). High-level wellness for man and society. *American Journal of Public Health, 49,* 786–972.

Duvall, E. (1977). *Marriage and family development.* Philadelphia: Lippincott.

Edelman, C., & Mandle, C. (2002). *Health promotion throughout the lifespan* (5th ed.). St. Louis: Mosby.

Eliopolous, C. (2000). *Gerontological nursing* (5th ed.). Philadelphia: Lippincott.

Erikson, E. (1963). *Childhood and society* (2nd ed.). New York: Norton.

Fowler, J. (1981). *Stages of faith: The psychology of human development and the quest for meaning.* New York: Harper & Row.

Fowler, S. (1997). Health promotion in chronically ill older adults. *Journal of Neuroscience Nursing, 29*(1), 39–43.

Freidman, M. (1981). *Family nursing: Theory and assessment.* New York: Appleton-Century-Crofts.

Grbich, C., Parker, D., & Maddocks, I. (2001). The emotions and coping strategies of caregivers of family members with a terminal cancer. *Journal of Palliative Care, 17*(1), 30–36.

Havighurst, R. (1972). *Human development and education* (3rd ed.). New York: Longman.

Kohlberg, L. (1979). *The meaning and measurement of moral development.* New York: Clark University.

Kozier, B., Erb, G., Berman, A., & Burke, K. (2000). *Fundamentals of nursing: Concepts, process and practice* (6th ed.). Upper Saddle River, NJ: Prentice Hall.

Leavell, H., & Clark, A. (1965). *Preventive medicine for doctors in the community.* New York: McGraw-Hill.

Lipson, J., Dibble, S., & Minarik, P. (1996). *Culture & nursing care: A pocket guide.* San Francisco: UCSF Nursing Press.

Lubkin, I. (1999). *Chronic illness: Impact and interventions* (4th ed.). Boston: Jones and Bartlett.

Lueckenotte, A. G. (2000). *Gerontologic nursing* (2nd ed.). St. Louis: Mosby.

Miller, C. (1998). *Nursing care of the older adult: Theory and practice* (3rd ed.). Philadelphia: Lippincott.

Miller, J. (2000). *Coping with chronic illness: Overcoming powerlessness* (3rd ed.). Philadelphia: F. A. Davis.

O'Neill, E. S., & Morrow, L. L. (2001). The symptom experience of women with chronic illness. *Journal of Advanced Nursing, 33*(2), 257–268.

Paterson, B. L. (2001). The shifting perspectives model of chronic illness. *Journal of Nursing Scholarship, 33*(1), 21–26.

Pender, N., Parsons, M., & Murdaugh, C. (2002). *Health promotion in nursing practice* (4th ed.). Upper Saddle River, NJ: Prentice Hall.

Pollock, S. (1986). Human responses to chronic illness: Physiologic and psychosocial adaptation. *Nursing Research, 35*(5), 90–95.

Stanhope, M., & Lancaster, J. (1999). *Community health nursing: Process and practice for promoting health* (5th ed.). St. Louis: Mosby.

Strauss, A., et al. (1984). *Chronic illness and the quality of life.* St. Louis: Mosby.

Suchman, E. (1972). Stages of illness and medical care. In E. Jaco (Ed.), *Patients, physicians and illness.* New York: Free Press.

Swanson, E., & Tripp-Reimer, T. (1997). *Chronic illness and the older adult.* New York: Springer.

US Census Department. (1999). *Statistical abstract of the United States.* Washington, DC: US Government Printing Office.

US Department of Health and Human Services. (2000). *Healthy people 2010.* Washington, DC: US Department of Health and Human Services.

_____. (1997). *Administration on aging: Aging into the 21st century.* Washington, DC: Department of Health and Human Services.

Weitzel, E. A. (2001). Risk for poisoning: Drug toxicity. In M. Maas, K. Buckwalter, M. Hardy, T. Tripp-Reimer, M. Titler, & J. Specht (Eds.), *Nursing care of older adults: Diagnoses, outcomes, & interventions* (pp. 34–46). St. Louis: Mosby.

Westerhoff, J. (1976). *Will our children have faith?* New York: Seabury Press.

Woods, N., Yates, B., & Primomo, J. (1989). Supporting families during chronic illness. *Image: Journal of Nursing Scholarship, 21*(1), 46–50.

World Health Organization. (1974). *Constitution of the World Health Organization: Chronicle of the World Health Organization.* Geneva: World Health Organization.

Wu, R. (1973). *Behavior and illness.* Englewood Cliffs, NJ: Prentice Hall.

Community-Based and Home Care of the Adult Client

LEARNING OUTCOMES

After completing this chapter, you will be able to:

- Define community-based nursing care.
- Discuss factors affecting health status in the community.
- Describe community-based health care services.
- Describe home health nursing and the roles of the home health nurse.
- Describe the components of the home health care system, including agencies, clients, referrals, physicians, reimbursement, and legal considerations.
- Discuss the effect of the home setting on nursing practice.
- Apply the nursing process to care of the client in the home.

MediaLink

www.prenhall.com/lemone
Additional resources for this chapter can be found on the Student CD-ROM accompanying this textbook, and on the Companion Website at www.prenhall.com/lemone. Click on Chapter 3 to select the activities for this chapter.

CD-ROM
- Audio Glossary
- NCLEX Review

Companion Website
- More NCLEX Review
- Case Study
    Home Health Nursing
- Care Plan Activity
    Home Health Assessment
- MediaLink Application
    Hospice: Purpose and Benefits

BOX 3-1	■ Community-Based Nursing Care Settings

- Hospitals
  - Inpatient care
  - Outpatient (ambulatory) surgery
  - Outpatient diagnostics and treatments
  - Cardiac rehabilitation
  - Support groups
  - Education groups
- County health departments
- Senior centers
- Long-term care
- Parish nursing
- Adult day care centers
- Homeless shelters
- Mobile vans

- Mental health centers
- Schools
- Crisis intervention centers
- Ambulatory surgery centers
- Alcohol/drug rehabilitation
- Health care provider offices
- Health care clinics
- Free clinics
- Urgent care centers
- Rural health centers
- Home care
- Hospice care
- Industry
- Jails and prisons

Hospitals have become primarily acute care providers with services focused on high-technology care for severely ill or injured people or for people having major surgery. Even those clients rarely remain in the hospital for long. They are moved as rapidly as possible to less acute care settings within the hospital and then to community-based care. Health care has become a managed care, community-based system. Although many nurses are still employed in hospitals, they are increasingly providing nursing care outside of the acute care, in-hospital setting.

COMMUNITY-BASED NURSING CARE

A **community** may be a small neighborhood in a major urban city or a large area of rural residents. Communities are formed by the characteristics of people, area, social interaction, and common ties. Each community, however, is unique. People who live in a community may share a culture, history, or heritage. Although a community is where people live, have homes, raise families, and carry on daily activities, its members often cross community boundaries to work or to seek health care. Nurses who provide care within a community must know the composition and characteristics of the clients with whom they will work.

In contrast to *community health nursing,* which focuses on the health of the community, **community-based nursing** centers on individual and family health care needs. The nurse practicing community-based care provides direct services to individuals to manage acute or chronic health problems and to promote self-care. The care is provided in the local community, is culturally competent, and is family centered. The philosophy of community-based nursing directs nursing care for clients wherever they are, including where they live, work, play, worship, and go to school (Zotti, Brown, & Stotts, 1996).

Nurses provide community-based care in many different ways and locations, ranging from leading support groups in a hospital (for individuals and family members diagnosed with such illnesses as cancer or diabetes) to managing a freestanding clinic to

providing care at the client's home. Box 3–1 illustrates the varied settings within the community in which a nurse may provide care.

FACTORS AFFECTING HEALTH IN THE COMMUNITY

Many factors affect health in a community. These factors include social support systems, the community health care structure, environmental factors, and economic resources.

Social Support Systems

A person's social support system consists of the people who lend assistance to meet financial, personal, physical, or emotional needs. In most instances, family, friends, and neighbors provide the best social support within the community. To understand the community social structure, the nurse needs to know:

- The degree to which men and women are seen as equals and partners in health care.
- Available support for health care for the client and family, including neighbors, friends, their church, organizations, self-help groups, and professional providers.
- Cultural and ethnic background of the community.
- Level of neighborhood cooperation and communication.

Community Health Care Structure

The health care structure of a community has a direct effect on the health of the people living and working within it. The size of the community often determines the type of services provided as well as the access to the services. For example, urban residents have various means of transportation to a variety of community health care providers, whereas rural residents must often travel long distances for any type of care. The financial base of the community is also important, often determining state and county funding of services.

Nurses who provide community-based care must know about public health services, the number and kind of health screenings offered, the location and specialty of health care professionals within the community, and the availability and accessibility of services and supplies. Other factors to consider include facilities (e.g., day care and long-term care), housing, and the number and kind of support agencies providing assistance (e.g., housing, shelter, and food).

Environmental Factors

The environment within which a person lives and works may have both helpful and harmful effects on health. Air and water quality differs across communities. Air pollution may occur across a large area, or may be limited to the home. Within the home, pollution may occur from such sources as molds, pesticides, and fumes from new carpet. The water source also varies, with water supplies coming from rivers, lakes, reservoirs, or wells. No matter the source, chemical runoff or bacteria may contaminate water. It is critical to determine whether clients have a safe supply of running water.

Household and community safety and health resource accessibility are also important. Nurses must consider lighting, street and sidewalk or road upkeep and conditions, effects of ice and snow, condition of stairs and floors, and usefulness and availability of bathroom facilities. Physical barriers to accessing community resources include lack of transportation, distance to services, and location of services.

Economic Resources

Economic resources encompass the financial and insurance coverages that provide the means to have health care within the community. As private medical insurance becomes more and more expensive, fewer citizens have it; and many U.S. citizens have no insurance at all. Most unskilled jobs do not provide health care benefits, resulting in a substantial percentage of what might be labeled "the working poor," those who have no financial assistance for illness care or health care screenings from an employer. Older adults on limited incomes often find their monthly income consumed by medicines and medical supplies.

Medicare and Medicaid are health assistance programs created by 1965 Social Security amendments. Medicare is a federal health insurance plan for acute care needs of the disabled and those over 65 years. This plan covers some services provided in hospitals, long-term facilities, and the home; however, many necessary health care components are not covered fully or at all, including prescribed and over-the-counter medications and adaptive equipment for safety, such as shower seats or raised toilet seats. Coverage for care at home continues only as long as skilled providers are needed, and the person is not considered homebound even if he or she needs a wheelchair and assistance from others to leave the home. Medicaid is a state-run health insurance program for people with limited incomes. Each state has different benefits and criteria for coverage.

COMMUNITY-BASED HEALTH CARE SERVICES

Community-based health care services can take many forms. Some are discussed here, but a more detailed discussion of home health care is provided later in the chapter.

Home Health Care

Home health care encompasses both health and social services provided to the chronically ill, disabled, or recovering person in his or her own home. Home care is usually provided when a person needs help that cannot be provided by a family member or friend. Among clients who benefit from home health care services are those who:

- Cannot live independently at home because of age, illness, or disability.
- Have chronic, debilitating illnesses such as congestive heart failure, heart disease, kidney disease, respiratory diseases, diabetes mellitus, or muscle-nerve disorders.
- Are terminally ill and want to die with comfort and dignity at home.
- Do not need in-patient hospital or nursing home care but require additional assistance.
- Need short-term help at home for postoperative care.

The services provided in the home may include professional nursing care, care provided by home health care aides, physical therapy, speech therapy, occupational therapy, medical social worker services, and nutritional services. Clients receiving home health care services are usually under the care of a physician, with the focus of care being treatment or rehabilitation. Registered nurses or licensed practical nurses provide nursing care based on physician orders. These nurses give direct care, supervise other health care providers, coordinate client care with the physician, advocate for the client and family, and teach family members and friends how to care for the client to assist the nurse as well as when professional services are no longer necessary.

Hospice care is a special component of home care, designed to provide medical, nursing, social, psychological, and spiritual care for terminally ill clients and their families. Hospice care relies on a philosophy of relieving pain and suffering and allowing the client to die with dignity in a comfortable environment. Licensed nurses, medical social workers, physicians, occupational and physical therapists, and volunteers provide care. Hospice care is discussed in Chapter 11. ⊝⊙

Respite Care

Respite care provides short-term or intermittent home care, often using volunteers. These services exist primarily to give the family member or friend who is the primary caregiver some time away from care. Respite care does much to relieve the burden of full-time caregiving.

Community Centers and Clinics

Community centers and clinics may be directed by physicians, advanced practice nurses in collaboration with physicians, or advanced practice nurses working independently (depending on state regulations). These health care settings may be located within a hospital, be part of a hospital but located in another area, or be independent of a hospital base. Health care centers and clinics provide a wide range of services and often meet the health needs of clients who are unable to access care elsewhere. This group includes the homeless, the poor, those with substance abuse problems, those with sexually transmitted diseases, and the victims of violent or abusive behavior.

Day Care Programs

Day care programs, such as senior centers, are usually located where people gather for social, nutritional, and recreational purposes. These programs vary among communities. Meals may be provided at low cost.

Parish Nursing and Block Nursing

Parish nursing and block nursing are nontraditional, community-based ways of providing health promotion and health restoration nursing interventions to specific groups of people. Both types of care meet the needs of people who are often underserved by the traditional health care system.

A nurse who practices **parish nursing** works with the pastor and staff of a faith community to promote health and healing through counseling, referrals, teaching, and assessment of health care needs. A parish nurse may be employed by a hospital and contracted by a church, be employed directly by a church, or work as a volunteer with the congregation of a church. The parish nurse helps bridge gaps between members of the church and the health care system.

Block nursing is nursing care provided to people who live on the same block as the nurse. Services are administered based on need rather than on eligibility for reimbursement. Other residents of the block often provide volunteer services to assist the nurse, with funding for care often coming from grants and demonstration projects.

Meals-on-Wheels

Many communities have a food service, usually called Meals-on-Wheels, for older people who do not have assistance in the home for food preparation. A hot, nutritionally balanced meal is delivered once a day, usually at noon. Volunteers often deliver the meals, providing not only nutrition but also a friendly, caring visit each day.

HOME HEALTH CARE

Home care is not easily defined. It is not simply illness care at home, nor is it the act of setting up a hospital room in someone's house. The National Association for Home Care (NAHC) 2000 defines **home care** as services for recovering, disabled, or chronically ill people who are in need of treatment or support to function effectively in the home environment. Home care is appropriate for adults and children in danger of abuse or neglect or for any person who needs either short-term or long-term assistance that cannot be provided by family members or friends.

The U.S. Department of Health and Human Services places home care along a continuum of health care. Home care is provided in the client's place of residence for the purpose of promoting, maintaining, or restoring health or of maximizing the level of independence while minimizing the effects of disability and illness, including terminal illness.

Home care is both professional and technical. Professional home care is provided by people who are practice driven, licensed, certified, and/or have special qualifications. Nurses, therapists, social workers, and home health aides are considered professional providers. Technical home care providers are business and product driven. Customer satisfaction, field service, reimbursement, and profits are their primary concerns. Durable medical equipment companies (businesses that deliver medical equipment to homes) are technical providers.

Many milestones marked the growth and development of home health care in the United States. The passage of Medicare in 1965, Medicaid in 1970, the addition of hospice benefits in 1973, and the introduction of diagnosis-related groups (DRGs) in 1983 dramatically affected home care. Medicare legislation entitled the nation's elderly to home care services, primarily skilled nursing and other curative or restorative therapies. This same benefit was extended to certain disabled younger Americans in 1973.

The introduction of DRGs to help control health care costs greatly increased home health care. DRGs are categories for reimbursement of inpatient services. The DRG system pays the same predetermined amount of money for the care of different persons with the same medical diagnosis. Many changes in the health care system have been attributed to the introduction of DRGs, including earlier discharge from hospitals and the increased need for home care services.

Roles of the Home Health Nurse

The role expectations of the home health nurse are similar to those of the professional nurse in any setting. On behalf of clients in the home, the nurse serves as an advocate, a provider of direct care, an educator, and a coordinator of services (see Chapter 1).

Advocate

As client advocate, the nurse explores, informs, supports, and affirms the choices of clients. Advocacy begins on the first visit, when the nurse discusses advanced directives, living wills, and durable power of attorney for health care. The home health agency's bill of rights also needs to be discussed. During the course of care, clients may need help negotiating the complex medical system (especially in regard to medical insurance), accessing community resources, recognizing and coping with required changes in lifestyle, and making informed decisions. When the family's desires differ from the client's, advocacy can be a challenge. If a conflict arises, the nurse must remain the client's primary advocate.

Provider of Direct Care

Home health nurses usually are not involved in providing personal care for clients (bathing, changing linens, and so on). The family usually provides routine personal care, or the nurse may arrange for a home health aide. If a personal care need arises during the course of the skilled visit (e.g., if a client has an in-

Figure 3–1 ■ The home health nurse often provides client education. This nurse is teaching the client and a family member how to apply dressings.

continent episode), the nurse typically either bathes and changes the client or assists the caregiver to do so before moving on to the skilled activities planned for the visit.

As a provider of direct care, the nurse uses the nursing process to assess, diagnose, plan care, intervene, and evaluate client needs. During the course of this process, home health nurses frequently are involved in performing specific procedures and treatments such as physical assessments, care of intravenous lines, ostomy care, wound care, and pain management.

Educator

Most of the home health nurse's time is spent teaching. Many nurses believe that their role as teacher is the crux of their nursing practice and that nurses in the home are always teaching (Figure 3–1 ■). For this reason, it is important that home health nurses develop expertise in the theory and principles of client education.

The greatest educational challenge may be motivating the client. Discovering what it takes to make the client want to learn and focusing the client on what is most important can tax the ingenuity of even the most dedicated nurse. Despite the work involved, nurses are rewarded by the knowledge that through their efforts, clients have learned to manage independently. Because the nurse's role as educator is becoming increasingly important, guidelines for home care are included in the discussion of each major disorder addressed in this textbook.

Coordinator of Services

As coordinator of services, the home health nurse is the main contact with the client's physician and all other providers involved in the treatment plan. It is the responsibility of the registered nurse case coordinator (or clinical case manager) to report client changes, discuss responses, and develop and secure treatment plan revisions on an ongoing basis. This is accomplished both formally, through scheduled case and team con-

ferences, and informally (often over the phone) with concerned providers. Documentation of all coordination activities is legally required.

Standards for Nursing Practice in the Home

Home health nurses are responsible for adhering to the same codes and standards that guide all other nurses. These codes and standards, provided in Chapter 1, guide nursing practice and protect the public. In addition to these guidelines, other codes and statements give specific guidance on issues that affect care in the home. ∞

ANA Standards for Home Health Nursing Practice

The ANA Standards for Home Health Nursing Practice are used in conjunction with the ANA Standards of Community Health Nursing as a basis for the practice of nursing in the home. The standards address the nursing process, interdisciplinary collaboration, quality assurance, professional development, and research (see Box 3–2). The standards speak to two levels of practitioners (generalist, who is prepared on the baccalaureate level, and specialist, who is prepared on the graduate level) and outline what achievements are expected of the professional nurse in the home.

NAHC Bill of Rights

Another source of guidance regarding home care is the NAHC Bill of Rights. Its use is a federal requirement for all home health agencies. Although they are permitted to make additions to the NAHC's original bill of rights, home health agencies are required by law to address the concepts in the NAHC Bill of Rights with all home health clients on the initial visit. Box 3–3 provides an example of a home health agency's bill of rights.

ANA Position Statements

The ANA has published position statements addressing moral, ethical, and legal issues faced by home and community health nurses. Examples are as follows:

- *A Statement on the Scope of Home Health Nursing Practice*
- *Risk Versus Responsibility in Providing Nursing Care*
- *Cultural Diversity in Nursing Practice*
- *Foregoing Artificial Nutrition and Hydration*

The Home Health Care System

Nurses who practice home care do so within a system that includes home health agencies, clients, referral sources, physicians, reimbursement sources, and legal considerations. The system is interactive and, like any other, functions best when its members communicate, cooperate, and collaborate with one another.

Home Health Agencies

Home health agencies are either public or private organizations engaged in providing skilled nursing and other therapeutic services in the client's home. The several different types of

BOX 3–2	■ ANA Standards for Home Health Nursing Practice

STANDARD I. ORGANIZATION OF HOME HEALTH SERVICES

All home health services are planned, organized, and directed by a master's-prepared professional nurse with experience in community health and administration.

STANDARD II. THEORY

The nurse applies theoretical concepts as a basis for decisions in practice.

STANDARD III. DATA COLLECTION

The nurse continuously collects and records data that are comprehensive, accurate, and systematic.

STANDARD IV. DIAGNOSIS

The nurse uses health assessment data to determine nursing diagnoses.

STANDARD V. PLANNING

The nurse develops care plans that establish goals. The care plan is based on nursing diagnoses and incorporates therapeutic, preventive, and rehabilitative nursing actions.

STANDARD VI. INTERVENTION

The nurse, guided by the care plan, intervenes to provide comfort, to restore, improve, and promote health, to prevent complications and sequelae of illness, and to effect rehabilitation.

STANDARD VII. EVALUATION

The nurse continually evaluates the client's and family's responses to interventions in order to determine progress toward goal at-tainment and to revise the database, nursing diagnoses, and plan of care.

STANDARD VIII. CONTINUITY OF CARE

The nurse is responsible for the client's appropriate and uninterrupted care along the health care continuum, and therefore uses discharge planning, case management, and coordination of community resources.

STANDARD IX. INTERDISCIPLINARY COLLABORATION

The nurse initiates and maintains a liaison relationship with all appropriate health care providers to assure that all efforts effectively complement one another.

STANDARD X. PROFESSIONAL DEVELOPMENT

The nurse assumes responsibility for professional development and contributes to the professional growth of others.

STANDARD XI. RESEARCH

The nurse participates in research activities that contribute to the profession's continuing development of knowledge of home care.

STANDARD XII. ETHICS

The nurse uses the code for nurses established by the American Nurses Association as a guide for ethical decision making in practice.

Note. From Standards for Home Health Nursing Practice by American Nurses Association, 1986, Kansas City, MO: ANA.

home health agencies differ only in the way their programs are organized and administered. All home health agencies are similar in that they must meet uniform standards for licensing, certification, and accreditation. Home health agencies include the following:

- *Official or public agencies.* State or local governments operate these agencies, which are financed primarily by tax funds. Most official agencies offer home care, health education, and disease-prevention programs in the community.
- *Voluntary or private not-for-profit agencies.* Donations, endowments, charities such as the United Way, and third-party (insurance company) reimbursement support these agencies. They are governed by a volunteer board of directors, which usually represents the community they serve.
- *Private, proprietary agencies.* Most of these agencies are for-profit organizations governed by either individual owners or national corporations. Although some participate in third-party reimbursement, others rely on clients paying their own bills (often called out-of-pocket expenses).
- *Institution-based agencies.* These agencies operate under a parent organization, such as a hospital. The home health

agency is governed by the sponsoring organization and the mission of both is similar. Often, the majority of home health referrals come from the parent organization.

Home health agency personnel typically include administrators, managers, professional providers, paraprofessionals, and business office staff. Depending on the agency and geographic location, professional providers may include registered nurses, practical nurses, nurse practitioners, enterostomal therapists, physical therapists, occupational therapists, speech therapists, respiratory therapists, social workers, a chaplain or pastoral minister, dietitians, and home health aides. It is not unusual for clients to require the services of several professionals simultaneously. No matter how many providers are in the home, the responsibility for case coordination (also called case management) remains with the registered nurse.

Clients

The client in home health is the person receiving care and the person's family. The recognition that the family is also a client acknowledges the powerful influence that families exert on

BOX 3–3 ■ A Home Health Agency's Bill of Rights

The agency acknowledges the client's rights and encourages the client and family to participate in their plan of care through informed decision making. In accordance with this belief, each client/family member will receive, prior to admission, the following bill of rights and responsibilities.

1. The client and the client's property will be treated with respect by the program's staff.
2. The client will receive care without regard to race, color, creed, age, sex, religion, national origin, or mental or physical handicap.
3. The client has the right to be free from mental and physical abuse.
4. The client's medical record and related information is maintained in a confidential manner by the program.
5. The client will receive a written statement of the program's objectives, scope of services, and grievance process prior to admission.
6. The client, family, or guardian has the right to file a complaint regarding the services provided by the program without fear of disruption of service, coercion, or discrimination.
7. The client will be advised of the following in advance of service:
   a. Description of services and proposed visit frequency
   b. Overview of the anticipated plan of care and its likely outcome
   c. Options that may be available
8. The client/family is encouraged to participate in the plan of care. The client will receive the necessary information concerning the client's condition and will be encouraged to participate in changes that may arise in care.
9. The program shall provide for the right of the client to refuse any portion of planned treatment to the extent permitted by law without relinquishing other portions of the treatment plan, except where medical contraindications exist. The client will be informed of the expected consequences of such action.
10. The client has a right to continuity of care:
    a. Services provided within a reasonable time frame

   b. A program that is capable of providing the level of care required by the client
   c. Timely referral to alternative services, as needed
   d. Information regarding impending discharge, continuing care requirements, and other services, as needed
11. The client will be informed of the extent to which payment will be expected for items or services to be furnished to clients by Medicare, Medicaid, and any other program that is funded partially or fully with federal funds. Upon admission, the client will be informed orally and in writing of any charges for items and services that the program expects will not be covered upon admission. The client will be informed of any change in this amount as soon as possible, but no later than within 25 days after the program is made aware of the change.
12. Upon request, the client may obtain:
    a. An itemized bill.
    b. The program's policy for uncompensated care.
    c. The program's policy for disclosure of the medical record.
    d. Identity of health care providers with which the program has contractual agreements, insofar as the client's care is concerned.
    e. The name of the responsible person supervising the client's care and how to contact this person during regular business hours.
13. The client has the right to obtain medical equipment and other health-related items from the company of the client's choice and assumes financial responsibility for such. The program's staff will assist in obtaining supplies and physician approvals as needed.
14. The client/family is responsible for:
    a. Giving the program accurate, necessary information.
    b. Being available and cooperative during scheduled visits.
    c. Assisting, as much as possible, in the plan of care.
    d. Alerting the staff to any problems as soon as possible.

Note. Adapted from the Patient Bill of Rights and Responsibilities, Bon Secours Home Health Hospice Program, Baltimore, MD.

health. A client's family is not limited to persons related by birth, adoption, or marriage. In the home, family members may include lovers, friends, colleagues, other significant people, and even animals that hold the potential of greatly affecting the health care environment.

Age and functional disability are the primary predictors of need for home care services. Information from a national survey conducted by the Agency for Health Care Policy and Research found that about half of all home care clients are over the age of 65 and that the number of home care services that clients need seems to increase with age (NAHC, 2000).

PREPARING CLIENTS FOR CARE AT HOME. The old adage that discharge plans begin at admission makes more

sense today than ever before. With shortened lengths of hospital stay, it is imperative for nurses to evaluate all clients for their ability to manage at home. Nurses preparing to send clients home must consider many of the questions outlined in the Meeting Individualized Needs Box on page 44.

MEETING PRIORITY NEEDS. When preparing clients for discharge to home, the nurse focuses on safety and survival first. Even if health education is to continue with home care, a day or two may elapse before the nurse arrives, and clients must be able to manage by themselves until then. The nurse must not discharge clients without giving them the correct information and supplies to get them through the first few days at home. Additionally, clients should not be discharged without complete

Meeting Individualized Needs

THE CLIENT BEING DISCHARGED FROM ACUTE CARE TO HOME CARE

QUESTIONS FOR CONSIDERATION:

- Does the client need follow-up therapy, treatments, or additional education?
- What equipment, supplies, or information about community resources is necessary?
- What teaching materials can be sent home? Are they written at an acceptable reading level? Do they come in other languages?
- What cognitive abilities do the client and the caregiver seem to have? Are there any sensory deprivations that impede learning?

- Who will be the principal caregiver in the home? Is there one? Are all caregivers comfortable in doing what needs to be done? If not, what support do they need to become comfortable?
- Was the caregiver present during and included in instruction? How have the client and caregiver responded to health teaching thus far? Have they comprehended what has been taught? Was their stress level such that they could not listen?
- Has a devastating diagnosis and/or prognosis just been determined?
- Is high-technology intervention necessary?

---

information about their medications and the manifestations of complications they should report to their doctor. Finally, all clients should be able to at least minimally manage any necessary treatments. Management includes not only performing procedures safely but also knowing how to obtain necessary supplies in the community.

Clients need help understanding their situations, making health care decisions, and changing health behaviors. It is unrealistic, however, to believe that clients can be taught everything they need to know during today's shortened hospital stays. The nurse should therefore recommend a home health referral for anyone in need of follow-up teaching. Prioritized teaching is essential: Even under the best of circumstances, clients generally forget about one-third of what is said to them, and their recall of specific instructions and advice is less than 50%. Comprehensive information related to client and family teaching is included in most of the following chapters in this textbook. This can be used as a guide in planning teaching.

Referrals

A referral source is a person recommending home health services and supplying the agency with details about the client's needs. The source may be a physician, nurse, social worker, therapist, or discharge planner. Families sometimes generate their own referrals, either by approaching one of the sources already mentioned or by calling a home health agency directly to make an inquiry. When the family seeks a referral and the agency believes that the client qualifies for services, usually the agency contacts the client's physician and requests a referral on the client's behalf.

The nurse may make a referral to either a home health agency, a hospice, or a community resource if the client seems to need formal follow-up beyond the present clinical setting. Hospital discharge planners, social workers, organizations for older adults, and local nonprofit agencies usually have a good command of the services and support groups available in their communities.

The nurse must talk to clients and their caregivers about concerns related to home management. It is not unusual for one family member to think that no additional help is necessary and for another to feel differently.

The nurse can facilitate an informal family meeting in which everyone shares concerns and can make inquiries about the family's insurance coverage for home health care. Suggesting services that families cannot afford only adds to the problem. For clients with limited means, the nurse can consult with staff in the institution who are most knowledgeable about funding. In every instance, it is important that the nurse avoid making assumptions: Well-educated and financially secure clients can be just as overwhelmed by illness as clients who are poor and less learned. Everyone is a referral candidate.

If the family believes that no help is necessary and the nurse believes otherwise, then the nurse may ask the family to consider an evaluation visit, explaining how the situation may look different once the client is home. If family members continue to refuse, the nurse can let them know that the door is never closed and give them contacts in the community that they can access independently should their needs change.

Physicians

Home care cannot begin without a physician's order, nor can it proceed without a physician-approved treatment plan. This is a legal and reimbursement requirement. Only after a referral is made and an initial set of physician orders is obtained can a nursing assessment visit be scheduled to identify the client's needs. If the input of another provider, such as a physical therapist, is necessary to complete the initial assessment, then the nurse arranges for this visit.

At the nursing assessment visit, the nurse begins to formulate the plan of care. Box 3–4 lists Medicare's required data for the nursing plan of care. Once formulated, the nurse sends the plan of care back to the physician for review and approval. The physician's signature on the plan of care authorizes the home health agency's providers to continue with services and also

BOX 3–4 ■ Medicare's Required Data for the Plan of Care

1. All pertinent diagnoses
2. A notation of the beneficiary's mental status
3. Types of services, supplies, and equipment ordered
4. Frequency of visits to be made
5. Client's prognosis
6. Client's rehabilitation potential
7. Client's functional limitations
8. Activities permitted
9. Client's nutritional requirements
10. Client's medications and treatments
11. Safety measures to protect against injuries
12. Discharge plans
13. Any other items the home health agency or physician wishes to include

Note. From Medicare Health Insurance Manual-11, Section 204.2.

Figure 3–2 ■ Demystifying high-technology home care equipment is a nursing challenge. This nurse demonstrates the use of a patient-controlled analgesia (PCA) pump used in management of chronic pain.

serves as a contract indicating agreement to participate in the care of the client on an ongoing basis. The plan is reviewed as necessary, but at least once every 60 days.

Reimbursement for Services

A reimbursement source pays for home health services. Medicare is home care's largest single reimbursement source, although other sources exist (Medicaid, other public funding, private insurance, and public donation). The reimbursement source evaluates each treatment plan to determine if the goals and plans set forth by the professional providers match the needs assessed. Only interventions identified on the treatment plan are covered. Periodically the reimbursement source may ask for the home health provider's notes to substantiate what is being done in the home. This is one reason why accurate documentation is critical.

Medicare does not reimburse visits made to support general health maintenance, health promotion, or clients' emotional or socioeconomic needs. Both client and nurse must meet specific criteria to secure Medicare reimbursement. The client must meet all of the following criteria:

- The physician must decide that the client needs care at home and make a plan for home care.
- The client must need at least one of the following: intermittent (not full time) skilled nursing care, physical therapy, speech language pathology services, or occupational therapy.
- The client must be homebound. This means leaving the home is a major effort. When leaving the home, it must be infrequent, for a short time, to get medical care, or to attend religious services.
- The home health agency must be Medicare approved.

Medicare will reimburse only when the skilled provider performs at least one of the following tasks:

- Teaching about a new or acute situation.
- Assessing an acute process or a change in the client's condition.

- Performing a skilled procedure or a hands-on service requiring the professional skill, knowledge, ability, and judgment of a licensed nurse (Figure 3–2 ■).

The reimbursement guidelines present problems because they are not sensitive to the full scope of nursing practice. Many of the client and family needs that nurses encounter during home visits are complex and time consuming, reflecting both intense psychosocial and economic concerns. This situation presents a profound dilemma. How are nurses to reconcile spending time on issues for which their agency will receive no payment? How are they to meet agency home visit productivity standards when each home they enter requires more and more from them? How are they to document activities and interventions that are not considered "skilled"? There are no easy answers to these questions.

Legal Considerations

The legal considerations in home health center around issues of privacy and confidentiality, the client's access to health information, the client's freedom from unreasonable restraint, witnessing of documents, informed consent, and matters of negligence and/or malpractice. Numerous sources suggest that nurses can best avoid lawsuits by familiarizing themselves with the standards of practice, providing care that is consistent with both the standards and their agency's policies, and documenting all care fully and accurately according to agency guidelines.

Differences in Inpatient Care and Home Care

Nursing practice in the home is a unique experience that differs in many ways from nursing practice in a hospital setting. These differences include the following:

- *Nurses are invited into homes.* Nurses are guests and cannot assume entry, as they do in formal clinical settings. The environment belongs to the client, who retains control. Every nursing action must communicate respect for these boundaries. To negotiate both repeated entry and a share of power in the client's domain, the nurse must establish trust and rapport quickly. This is often difficult, because most home health nurses are with each client for only 1 hour a few times a week.

- *Home health nursing is solitary.* In the home, there are no colleagues present to consult, to assist, or to rely on for support. The home is a practice setting where nurses learn to trust their theoretical and intuitive knowledge and to be totally accountable.

- *The home is one of the richest symbols in Western culture.* The word *home* generates strong feelings of ownership, control, security, family history, independence, comfort, protection, and conflict. The family perceives a sharing of self when they consistently allow entry to a stranger. Because clients and nurses most often meet during periods of vulnerability and crisis, and because socializing is such an integral part of the home visit process, nurse providers are often perceived as friends or extended family members, blurring the boundaries of practice.

- *Intimacy and shared humanity are nurtured in the home.* During the course of establishing rapport and getting to know each other as people, the nurse-client relationship often becomes something more. Nurses and clients end up giving to each other and learning from each other. By connecting as human beings, they touch each other's spirits in profound ways (Carson, 1989). In home health, it is not unusual for nurses to realize suddenly not only that they do things to create a healing environment but also that their very presence has become the healing environment.

- *Family issues and relationships are more visible in the home.* Over time, as the nurse becomes a familiar presence and the family's behavior relaxes, the nurse can gain a clearer and more complete picture of family relationships, dynamics, lifestyle choices, and coping patterns. Multigenerational behavior patterns are more obvious, and working around them can become quite a feat.

- *Nurses play a variety of roles.* Although they focus on providing health care, home health nurses also understand that promoting the client's optimal wellness often necessitates interventions that are not treatment oriented. Nurses report that they find themselves functioning as social workers, friends, spiritual comforters, psychologists, financial counselors, and interpreters of medical information.

- *"Families of one" are a worrisome reality.* Today more older adults are living alone. Some may have current or potential caregivers nearby, whereas others, for any of various reasons, have no one. These people often require considerable nursing support to remain strong, independent, and resourceful. Caring for "families of one" can take a toll on even the strongest home health nurse. Some nurses have reported calling between visits, keeping in touch after discharge, and driving by on days off because they have such difficulty "letting go" their concerns about these clients.

- *Caregiver burden is not easily hidden in the home.* In more than 22 million American households, people are taking care of disabled relatives and friends (Health Care Financing Administration [HCFA], 1997). Many of these caregivers are themselves older adults. Health care planners visualize the home as a place where all kinds of medical services can occur but may give little thought to how people manage. Few ever ask whether families can cope with the level of care they are expected to assume. Caregiving has only recently been acknowledged as a complex activity, requiring adjustment in family living patterns, relationships, and finances. For some families, the crisis of caregiving is short lived, but for others it lasts for years. As a result, caregivers are at great risk for both physical and emotional illness. Because the success of home care heavily depends on the supports in place, addressing the needs of the support network is imperative.

- *Care in the home sometimes is inadequate.* Personal health habits, living conditions, resources, and support systems may leave much to be desired. It is not unusual for home health nurses to face unchanged dressings, undertreated infections, off-and-on self-medication, poor nutrition, filthy conditions, and unreliable caregivers. No matter how vigilant nurses may be, practice settings like these work against their best efforts. If the conditions cannot be changed, the nurse usually has two choices: to withdraw from the situation or to continue to practice within the environment.

Practical Information from Home Health Nurses

A study (Stulginsky, 1993a, 1993b) of practicing home health nurses solicited knowledge about the art and science of home health nursing from their lived experience. The results have added a practical dimension to many of the interventions home health nurses typically implement during client care. The practical information gleaned from this research and from other home health experts follows.

Establish Trust and Rapport

To establish trust and rapport in the client's home, nurses must try to find common ground and to let go of ethnocentric ("My culture's way is the best way") views. Nurses must be sure everything they say and do communicates an understanding that they are guests—offering suggestions in a way that acknowledges the client's right to say no, sensing and honoring "where people are in their situation," maintaining a respectful distance, and noticing and honoring family customs ("Gee, no one wears shoes in your house; I'll take mine off, too."). Nurses should try to negotiate their schedules around the family's needs; nursing should enhance family coping, not complicate it. Above all, nurses should validate clients' illness experiences, remembering that everyone needs someone who is willing to listen and say, "I hear what you are saying, and I think I have a sense of how you feel."

Proceed Slowly

The nurse must enter the home with an awareness that the first contact is important. On the first nursing visit, the nurse can suggest to clients that they have someone else present "to help them listen." To avoid overwhelming clients with too much information, the nurse stresses the essential information and repeats it on subsequent visits. When making suggestions, the nurse offers clients the pluses and minuses of each alternative. Informed decisions are difficult to make if people are too overwhelmed to think of their options. The nurse speaks slowly, directly, and within the client's range of vision (the client may have to lip-read) and refrains from shouting at clients who are hearing-impaired. The nurse must allow time for families to process new information.

Set Goals and Boundaries

The nurse explores clients' expectations of home care. In particular, the nurse explains the primary goal (to achieve self-care), defines nurse and client roles within this framework, and discusses limitations. The nurse may make statements such as, "No, a home health nurse is not the same as a private duty nurse" and "Home health nurses do not routinely do that, but today I will make an exception." It is important that the nurse stresses mutual accountability, choice, and negotiation as part of the process.

Assess the Home Environment

The nurse surveys the overall home environment, using common sense, intuition, and imagination. Among the variables to note are sights, sounds, smells, dress, tone of voice, body language, and the use of touch; visiting patterns among family members; significant relationships; what is sacred and what is not; the appearance of the house, yard, sidewalk, and neighborhood; and the effect of illness on the family. The nurse asks questions and listens carefully to stories and offhand remarks.

Set Priorities

It is important that nurses be flexible and realize they cannot tackle everything. Although it is necessary to enter the home with a plan in mind, nurses must be prepared to modify the plan according to conditions they encounter once inside. Safety, issues that are of concern to clients, and those problems that can most easily be solved should be addressed first. Alternatively, the nurse can focus on safety first, then short-term and long-term goals. If the priorities that are set are primarily the nurse's and not the client's, then they may not be met.

Promote Learning

Instead of just teaching the client, the nurse tries actively to promote the client's ability to learn by, for example, identifying what is most important to the client and teaching that. Survival takes first priority; the nurse teaches the information people need to ensure their safety until the next visit. The nurse prioritizes material on a needs-to-know, wants-to-know, ought-to-know basis, assessing and responding to learner readiness.

Timing is important; people who are not ready to listen cannot be taught. In addition, the nurse must allow a sufficient amount of time to teach, ask clients how and when they learn best, use appropriate methods and materials when possible, and capitalize on clients' frustrations and desires to regain control of self-care. When possible, the nurse teaches while providing care.

The nurse can empower clients to learn by talking them through learning tasks, encouraging them to listen to their own bodies and to ask questions, and urging them to write thoughts and questions about their care and bring them to the next visit or doctor's appointment.

Limit Distractions

Homes are full of events or circumstances that may divert attention from the job at hand. Such distractions as children, animals, noise, clutter, and mannerisms that are controlling, manipulative, or aggressive can try even the most experienced nurse. However, environmental and behavioral distractions can yield useful information about people, their relationships, and their values. For example, a dirty house could indicate a lack of interest in housekeeping, outright neglect and abuse, depression, or increased disability.

Distractions should be limited as much as possible. For example, the nurse might ask a client, "May I please turn off your television while we visit?" or "I would like to schedule my next visit for a time when the children are in school. Is that all right with you?" The nurse must be truthful about allergies, fear of a client's pet, or difficulty hearing in a particular room, but should not debate the priority of the visit over the distraction (such as a favorite television show). The nurse may not change the client's views and may also risk losing the client's trust and rapport. If all efforts at limiting distractions fail, the nurse should leave the home and return on another day: "I can see this is not going to work for us today. I will need to leave."

If any distraction originates with the nurse, such as fear of harm, reaction to the client's lifestyle, preoccupation with role or a feeling of being overwhelmed by the situation in the home, the nurse should seek out a colleague to discuss the problem. Often, another perspective helps when dealing with the issue.

Put Safety First

Nurses must focus on safety and survival first, for themselves as well as their clients, in all that they do. When traveling in the community, the nurse takes such precautions as keeping car doors locked, having a cellular phone, keeping supplies out of sight, and staying inside the car in potentially dangerous situations. Colleagues, families, and community members can offer useful guidelines for maintaining safety and self-protection.

It is important to avoid overwhelming families with numerous health care providers in the home. Most people dislike having strangers in their home, no matter how helpful they may seem to be. The nurse can help families manage moments of crisis by staying as close as possible. If abuse is suspected, the nurse must notify authorities and/or remove clients from potentially dangerous situations.

BOX 3–5 ■ Home Safety Assessment Checklist

GENERAL HOUSEHOLD SAFETY
1. Do stairwells and halls have good lighting?
2. Do staircases have handrails on both sides?
3. Are rugs securely tacked down?
4. Is the telephone readily accessible? Is the dial easy to read?
5. Are electrical cords in good condition and out of the way?
6. Is furniture sturdy?
7. Is the temperature of the home comfortable?
8. Are protective screens in front of fireplaces or heating devices?
9. Are smoke detectors present and working?

BATHROOM
1. Are grab bars present in the tub and/or shower? Around the toilet?
2. Are toilet seats high enough?
3. Are nonskid materials (rugs, mats) on the floor, tub/shower?
4. Are medications stored safely? Out of the reach of children?
5. Is the water temperature safe?
6. Are electrical outlets and appliances a safe distance from the tub?

KITCHEN
1. Are floors slippery? Are nonskid rugs used?
2. Is the stove in good working order?
3. Is the refrigerator in good working order? Clean?
4. Are electrical outlets overloaded with appliances?
5. Are sharp objects kept in a special container or safe area?
6. Is food storage adequate? Clean?
7. Are cleaning materials stored safely?

Make Do

Nurses must learn to be resourceful and cost conscious with equipment, supplies, and services in the home. When needing to make do or improvise, they should do so in a low-key manner to avoid causing the family additional anxiety. The nurse must make every effort to convey the message that the situation is under control; after leaving the home, the nurse can react as necessary.

Special Considerations in Home Care

Ensuring Home Safety

Safety assessment in the home is a nursing responsibility and a legal requirement. Nurses cannot close their eyes to an unsafe environment. Upon entering the home and on a continuing basis, it is imperative that the nurse alert the family to unsafe and hazardous conditions, suggest remedies, and document in the clinical record the family's response to the nurse's suggestions. See Box 3–5 for a sample home safety assessment list. In particular, nurses must remain alert to:

- How clients handle stairs.
- How clients manage their own care if they are alone.
- The presence of a smoke detector in the home.
- The presence of bathroom safety equipment.
- Electrical hazards.
- Slippery throw rugs, clutter, or a furniture arrangement that may cause a fall.
- A supply of expired medications.
- Inappropriate clothing or shoes.
- Cooking habits that may precipitate a fire.
- An inadequate food supply.
- Poorly functioning utilities.
- Chipping paint.
- Signs of abusive behavior.

Nurses cannot go into homes and change the family's living space and lifestyle, but they can register their concern and re-act appropriately if the situation suggests that an injury is about to occur or if they suspect abuse or neglect. In the home and community setting, ignoring an unsafe environment is considered nursing negligence.

The disposal of toxic medications and sharp objects (such as needles used for injections) is also a safety issue in the home, especially if young children are present. Once again, it is imperative that the nurse address this with the client, demonstrate safe disposal, and provide the necessary equipment to accomplish that end. Documentation should address what information the nurse has covered, the family's response to the teaching, and assessment of the family's ongoing practice of safety precautions.

Infection Control

Infection control in the home centers around protecting clients, caregivers, and the community from the spread of disease. Within the home, nurses may encounter clients with infectious or communicable diseases, clients who are immunocompromised, and/or clients having multiple access devices, drainage tubes, or draining wounds. The home presents a challenging environment in which to practice infection control for several reasons: Families typically are set in their own ways of doing things; caregivers often lack any formal education on the subject; the setting itself may not be conducive; and the facilities for even the most basic of aseptic practices (handwashing) may be lacking. Without a doubt, the single most important nursing intervention in controlling infection is health teaching. Clients and caregivers need to know the importance of effective handwashing, the use of gloves, the disposal of wastes and soiled dressings, the handling of linens, and the practice of standard precautions. Unfortunately, the imparting of important information does not always bring about a change in behavior. Trying to change a family's values frequently demands a great deal of ingenuity from the nurse.

THE NURSING PROCESS IN HOME CARE

The nursing process used in home care is no different from that practiced in any other setting. The unique challenges of home care present themselves chiefly in the implementation step. Generally, the differences lie in assessing how the home's unique environment affects the need or problem and using outcome criteria and mutual participation to plan goals and interventions.

Assessment

In home health care, nursing assessment and data collection center chiefly around the first home visit. This is not to say that nurses do not collect information on an ongoing basis, but because most agencies require the submission of a plan of care within 48 hours of the initial evaluation, the first visit carries tremendous weight. Under ideal circumstances, a preliminary review of background information initiates the assessment process; the reality in home health, however, is that few clients are referred with copies of either their medical records or their discharge summaries. If the client has received home health services in the past, records may be available, but often all the nurse has prior to initiating care is the referral form describing the present problem, some notations about past medical history, and a projection of the skilled interventions needed. Therefore, it falls to the nurse to try to obtain as complete a clinical picture as possible when meeting the client.

Assessment begins when the nurse calls the client to arrange a visit. This initial telephone call can yield much information to the nurse who pays close attention. For example:

- How alert, oriented, and stressed does the client (and/or family) seem to be?
- Does the client know the reason for the home health referral?
- How open to intervention do the client and family seem to be?
- Have they encountered any difficulties since discharge from the prior setting?
- Do they need any supplies on the first visit?

During the visit, much of the assessment process centers around collecting the information requested on the tools and forms contained in the agency's admission packet. These packets usually include a physical and psychosocial database; a medication sheet; forms for pain assessment, spiritual assessment, and financial assessment; and a family roster. It is extremely important that the data collected be as complete and accurate as possible and reflect subjective, objective, current, and historical information. Through interviewing, direct observation, and physical assessment, the nurse can achieve the goal of the initial visit, namely, to gain as clear and accurate a clinical picture of the client as possible.

Diagnosis

After completing the initial assessment, the nurse identifies the real and/or potential client problems that emerge from the data. Nursing diagnoses describing the client's health problems and needs, based on data collection, must be part of the home health record both to organize care and to justify reimbursement.

In almost all home care situations, *deficient knowledge* is an appropriate nursing diagnosis. Nursing interventions for this diagnosis specific to a client with Alzheimer's disease and the client's family can be found in the Nursing Care of the Older Adult box on page 50.

Planning

Planning in home health includes setting priorities, establishing goals, and deciding on intervention strategies designed to meet the needs of the client. The greatest level of success is achieved when clients feel an ownership of the suggested plan. For this reason, planned interventions and outcome criteria should be client centered, realistic, achievable, and mutually accepted. The nurse works with the client to:

- Identify significant issues and needs.
- Set mutually agreed-upon goals (outcome criteria).
- Make and initiate acceptable plans to meet the goals.

Outcome criteria should be verbally stated to clients and documented clearly and concisely, in timed, measurable, and observable terms. These measures help clients and care providers to better focus their work together and evaluate the effectiveness of care. In addition, outcome criteria provide the reimbursement source a measurable standard from which to judge the appropriateness of the plan of care.

Implementation

The home health nurse implements most of the planned interventions, although some may be carried out by another agency provider, a paraprofessional introduced into the setting by the nurse case manager, or the client.

Nurses and clients reach an agreement about the implementation of care through a process called **contracting,** the negotiation of a cooperative working agreement between the nurse and client that is continuously renegotiated. Contracting is a concept used often in, but not exclusive to, many home and community health settings. Contracting can occur both formally and informally. It involves exploring a need, establishing goals, evaluating resources, developing a plan, assigning responsibilities, agreeing on a time frame, and, evaluating or terminating. Contracting requires the nurse to relinquish control as the expert and consider the client as an equal partner in the process.

Contracting is not appropriate with all clients. It is certainly inadvisable if the nurse-client relationship is to be no more than two visits or if the client has limited cognitive abilities. However, contracting is useful for clients who demonstrate a willingness to be active participants in their health care. It is empowering, can save time, and keeps the nursing goals directed and focused. Box 3–6 provides an example of verbal contracting.

Nursing Care of the Older Adult

HOME CARE BY FAMILY CAREGIVERS FOR THE OLDER ADULT WITH A DEMENTING DISORDER

NURSING DIAGNOSIS

Deficient knowledge related to lack of information about Alzheimer's disease process and care

OUTCOME CRITERIA

Short term: Adequate knowledge, as evidenced by family's stating of disease progression and treatment (expected within 1 week)

Long term: Adequate knowledge, as evidenced by family's following of the recommended interventions throughout illness course (within 1 month) or by discharge from home health

INTERVENTIONS

- Alert the family to both environmental hazards and client habits that could threaten safety. (first visit)
- Provide the family with specific recommendations for keeping the client safe, for example, serving foods warm, not hot; allowing the client to eat with fingers; cutting food in small pieces; wearing an ID bracelet; discouraging daytime sleep. (first visit)
- Discuss the disease course (degenerative), the prognosis (incurable), typical issues of concern (promoting adequate nutrition, activity, rest, safety, and independence); supporting cognitive function; communication, socialization, and family caregiving; the supportive care available; and the ultimate need for long-term placement with disease progression. (first visit)
- Discuss local resources, including adult day care, support groups, and Alzheimer's Disease Association. Give family a list of these resources. (first visit)

- Include all family members or significant persons in teaching and planning care. (each visit)
- Prepare the family for typical types of Alzheimer's disease behaviors: forgetfulness, disorientation, agitation, screaming, crying, physical or verbal abuse, accusations of infidelity. (subsequent visits)
- Teach the family specific interventions for dealing with these behaviors: calm, unhurried manner, music, stroking, rocking, structuring the environment, distracting the client. (subsequent visits)
- Stress the importance of both exercise and recreation in terms of quality of life and decreasing nighttime restlessness. (subsequent visits)
- Reinforce the client's continued needs for socialization and intimacy. (subsequent visits)
- Suggest specific interventions for meeting socialization needs: limiting visitors to one or two at a time, pet therapy, use of the phone. (subsequent visits)
- Suggest useful interventions that are described in the literature and/or that are utilized in more formal Alzheimer's disease settings and may also be helpful in the home. (subsequent visits)
- Keep the environment safe for the client.
- Use reality orientation with client several times a day, and post clocks, calendars, and telephone numbers within easy sight of the client.
- Give client simple directions, using simple sentences and a quiet, monotone voice so as not to excite the client.
- Allow the use of the telephone, because calls will help orient the client.

BOX 3–6 ■ Contracting

Nurse: Mr. Ford, your mother is no longer safe alone in her home and requires help performing many of her activities of daily living. I can initiate home health aide services three times a week for 2 hours a day under Medicare, but she will need more assistance than that. Services beyond what Medicare provides must be contracted for by you on a private-pay basis.

Mr. Ford: Can you arrange that for us?

Nurse: I can give you a list of agencies here in the community that provide home health aide services, and I can recommend the ones that our clients have used successfully in the past, but the responsibility for choosing a service and negotiating hours and fees belongs to the family.

Mr. Ford: I really don't know much about this. I'd really feel better if you did this for us.

Nurse: Why don't the two of us discuss your mother's needs so that you'll have a clearer understanding of what type of help you

want to try to arrange. I can tell you about the local agencies we frequently refer our clients to, and I can give you suggestions about what questions to ask. We can also discuss the typical costs involved. This way, when you call to make inquiries, you'll be equipped with the right information.

Mr. Ford: I still would rather you do this.

Nurse: Mr. Ford, this is something the family must do. What I will do is teach whomever you hire what they will need to know about caring for your mother. Can we agree that by my next visit, you will have made some inquiries and will be ready to discuss what agency will best meet your family's situation?

Mr. Ford: All right. I'll start making some calls. Give me 2 or 3 days.

Nurse: Fine, then I'll plan for a longer visit Thursday so we can discuss what you find out.

Evaluation

Evaluation in home health is both formative and summative. Formative evaluation is the systematic ongoing comparison of the plan of care with the goals actually being achieved from visit to visit. In summative evaluation, the nurse reviews the total plan of care and the client's progress toward goals to determine the client's eligibility for discharge.

Reimbursement guidelines may be helpful in driving the evaluation process. Because reimbursement sources require that all skilled services be justified, many home health agencies have designed their clinical notes to include areas for evaluation of the client's response to the visit's interventions and documentation of a plan of care for the next scheduled visit.

 EXPLORE MediaLink

NCLEX review questions, case studies, care plan activities, MediaLink applications, and other interactive resources for this chapter can be found on the Companion Website at www.prenhall.com/lemone.

Click on Chapter 3 to select the activities for this chapter. For animations, video clips, more NCLEX review questions, and an audio glossary, access the Student CD-ROM accompanying this textbook.

TEST YOURSELF

1. What is the name given to nursing care provided by a faith community to promote health and healing?

   a. Respite care
   b. Parish nursing
   c. Block nursing
   d. Day care

2. While making the first home health visit, the nurse discusses advanced directives, living wills, and durable power of attorney for health care. These topics are part of which nursing role?

   a. Provider of direct care
   b. Coordinator of services
   c. Educator
   d. Advocate

3. Which of the following home health agency personnel is responsible for care coordination?

   a. Physician
   b. Social worker
   c. Registered nurse
   d. Home health aide

4. What agency is the largest single reimbursement source for home care?

   a. Medicare
   b. Medicaid
   c. Private insurance
   d. Self-pay

5. Nurses practicing in the home provide teaching for a variety of topics. Which of the following areas is essential to maintaining infection control?

   a. Fire and smoke detectors
   b. Handwashing
   c. Uncluttered floors and stairs
   d. Medications

See Test Yourself answers in Appendix C.

BIBLIOGRAPHY

American Association of Retired People. (2000). Caregiving and long-term care. Available www.research.aarp.org

American Nurses Association. (1986). *Standards of home health nursing practice.* Kansas City, MO: Author.

_____ . (2000). Reading room: Position statements. Available www.nursingworld.org

Boland, D., & Sims, S. (1996). Family care giving at home. *Image: Journal of Nursing Scholarship, 28*(1), 55–58.

Capone, L. (1997). Client challenge: Home care—a family affair. *Home Healthcare Nurse, 15*(1), 49–51.

Carson, V. (1989). *Spiritual dimensions of nursing practice.* Philadelphia: Saunders.

Chafey, K. (1996). "Caring" is not enough: Ethical paradigms for community-based care. *N & HC: Perspectives on Community, 17*(1), 10–15.

Clemen-Stone, S., McGuire, S., & Eigsti, D. (1998). *Comprehensive community health nursing* (5th ed.). St. Louis: Mosby.

Costello, M., & Todd-Magel, C. (1997). Bridging the gap: Hospital to home nutrition support. *MEDSURG Nursing, 6*(6), 328–337.

DeSavorgnani, A., & Haring, R. (1999). The impact of cultural issues on home care personnel and patients. *Caring, 18*(4), 22–27.

Grossman, D. (1996). Cultural dimensions in home health nursing. *American Journal of Nursing, 96*(7), 33–36.

Health Care Financing Administration. (1997). *Managed care in Medicare and Medicaid. Fact sheet*. Washington, DC: USDHHS.

_____ . (2001). *Medicare and home health care*. Washington, DC: USDHHS.

_____ . (2001). *Medicare & You 2001*. Washington, DC: USDHHS.

Jones, A., & Foster, N. (1997). Transitional care: Bridging the gap. *MEDSURG Nursing, 6*(1), 32–38.

National Association for Home Care. (2000). How to choose a home care provider. What are my rights as a patient? Available www.nahc.org

Paladichuk, A., & McNeal, G. (1997). Breaking down the walls: Critical care at home and on the road. *Critical Care Nurse, 17*(2), 94–99.

Rice, R. (2000). Home health care. Resources for home care nurses. *Geriatric Nursing, 21*(5), 276–279.

Roush, C., & Cox, J. (2000). The meaning of home. How it shapes the practice of home and hospice care. *Home Healthcare Nurse, 18*(6), 388–394.

Schoen, M., & Koenig, R. (1997). Home health care nursing: Past and present—part 1. *MEDSURG Nursing, 6*(4), 230–232.

Schumacher, K., Stewart, B., & Archbold, P. (1998). Conceptualization and measurement of doing family caregiving well. *Image: Journal of Nursing Scholarship, 30*(1), 63–69.

Shoultz, J., & Hatcher, P. (1997). Looking beyond primary care to primary health care: An approach to community-based action. *Nursing Outlook, 45*(1), 23–26.

Stulginsky, M. (1993a). Nurses' home health experience: Part I—The practice setting. *Nursing & Health Care, 14*(8), 402–407.

_____ . (1993b). Nurses' home health experience: Part II—The unique demands of home visits. *Nursing & Health Care, 14*(9), 476–485.

Swavely, D., Peter, D., & Stephens, D. (1999). Improving smooth sailing between hospital and home. *MEDSURG Nursing, 8*(5), 304–308.

Watson, J. (2000). Home health care. Reconsidering caring in the home. *Geriatric Nursing, 21*(6), 330–331.

Zotti, M., Brown, P., & Stotts, R. (1996). Community-based nursing versus community health nursing: What does it all mean? *Nursing Outlook, 44*(5), 211–217.

ALTERATIONS IN PATTERNS OF HEALTH

Nursing Care
of Clients in Pain

MediaLink

www.prenhall.com/lemone
Additional resources for this chapter
can be found on the Student CD-ROM
accompanying this textbook, and on
the Companion Website at www.
prenhall.com/lemone. Click on Chapter 4
to select the activities for this chapter.

CD-ROM
• Audio Glossary
• NCLEX Review

Animations
• Components of a Reflex Arc
• Morphine

Companion Website
• More NCLEX Review
• Case Study
   Assessing the Client in Pain
• Care Plan Activity
   Nursing Care for the Client in Pain
• MediaLink Application
   Complementary Therapies

LEARNING OUTCOMES

After completing this chapter, you will be able to:

■ Describe the neurophysiology of pain.

■ Compare and contrast definitions and characteristics of acute, chronic, central, phantom, and psychogenic pain.

■ Discuss factors affecting individualized responses to pain.

■ Clarify myths and misconceptions about pain.

■ Discuss collaborative care for the client in pain, including medications, surgery, and transcutaneous electrical nerve stimulation, and complementary therapies.

■ Use the nursing process as a framework for providing individualized nursing care for clients experiencing pain.

Pain is a subjective response to both physical and psychologic stressors. All people experience pain at some point during their lives. Although pain usually is experienced as uncomfortable and unwelcome, it also serves a protective role, warning of potentially health-threatening conditions. For this reason, pain is increasingly referred to as the *fifth* vital sign, with recommendations to assess pain with each vital sign assessment. The JCAHO (2000) has established pain standards that identify the relief of pain as a client right and requires health care facilities to implement specific procedures for, and provider education on, pain assessment and management.

Each individual pain event is a distinct and personal experience influenced by physiologic, psychologic, cognitive, sociocultural, and spiritual factors. Pain is the symptom most associated with describing oneself as ill, and it is the most common reason for seeking health care. Among the many definitions and descriptors of pain is the one most relevant: Pain is "whatever the person experiencing it says it is, and existing whenever the person says it does" (McCaffery, 1979, p. 11). This definition acknowledges the client as the only person who can accurately define and describe his or her own pain and serves as the basis for nursing assessment and care of clients in pain. It also supports the values and beliefs about pain necessary for holistic nursing care, including the following:

- Only the person affected can experience pain; that is, pain has a personal meaning.
- If the client says he or she has pain, the client is in pain. All pain is real.
- Pain has physical, emotional, cognitive, sociocultural, and spiritual dimensions.
- Pain affects the whole body, usually negatively.
- Pain may serve as both a response to and a warning of actual or potential trauma.

THEORIES AND NEUROPHYSIOLOGY OF PAIN

One well-known theory, gate control, suggests that the interaction of two systems determines pain and its perception (Melzack & Wall, 1965, 1968). The first of these interrelated systems is the substantia gelatinosa in the dorsal horns of the spinal cord (Figure 4–1 ■). The substantia gelatinosa regulates impulses entering or leaving the spinal cord. The second system is an inhibitory system within the brainstem.

Small-diameter A-delta and C fibers in the spinal cord carry fast and slow pain impulses. In addition, large-diameter A-beta fibers carry impulses for tactile stimulation from the skin. In the substantia gelatinosa, these impulses encounter a "gate" that is thought to be opened and closed by the domination of either the large-diameter touch fibers or the small-diameter pain fibers. If impulses along the small-diameter pain fibers outnumber impulses along the large-diameter touch fibers, then the gate is open and pain impulses travel unimpeded to the brain. If impulses from the touch fibers predominate, then they will close the gate and the pain impulses will be turned away there. This explains why massaging a stubbed toe can reduce the intensity and duration of the pain.

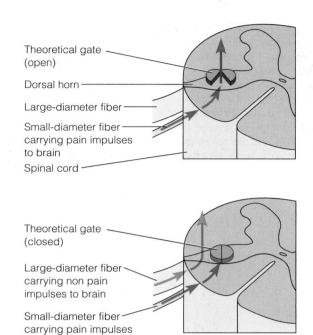

Figure 4–1 ■ The spinal cord component of the gate control theory. Pain transmission by small-diameter fibers is blocked when large-diameter fibers carrying touch impulses dominate, closing the gate in the substantia gelatinosa.

The second system described by the gate control theory, the inhibitory system, is thought to be located in the brainstem. It is believed that cells in the midbrain, activated by a variety of stimuli such as opiates, psychologic factors, or even simply the presence of pain itself, signal receptors in the medulla. These receptors in turn stimulate nerve fibers in the spinal cord to block the transmission of impulses from pain fibers.

Ongoing research has demonstrated that the control and modulation of pain is much more complex than the description in the gate control theory, which served as a base for further research about pain-modulating systems. Tactile information is now known to be transmitted by both large-diameter and small-diameter fibers, and interactions between sensory neurons is known to occur at multiple levels of the central nervous system (Porth, 2002).

Stimuli

Nerve receptors for pain are called *nociceptors* (Figure 4–2 ■). They are located at the ends of small afferent neurons and are woven throughout all the tissues of the body except the brain. Nociceptors are especially numerous in the skin and muscles. Pain occurs when biologic, mechanical, thermal, electrical, or chemical factors stimulate nociceptors (Table 4–1). The intensity and duration of the stimuli determine the sensation. Long-lasting, intense stimulation produces greater pain than brief, mild stimulation.

Nociceptors are stimulated either by direct damage to the cell or by the local release of biochemicals secondary to cell injury. *Bradykinin,* an amino acid, appears to be the most

Figure 4–2 ■ *A,* Cutaneous nociceptors generate pain impulses that travel via A-delta and C fibers to the spinal cord's dorsal horn. *B,* Secondary neurons in dorsal horn pass impulses across spinal cord to anterior spinothalamic tract. *C,* Slow pain impulses ascend to the thalamus, while fast pain impulses ascend to the cerebral cortex. The reticular formation in the brainstem integrates the emotional, cognitive, and autonomic responses to pain.

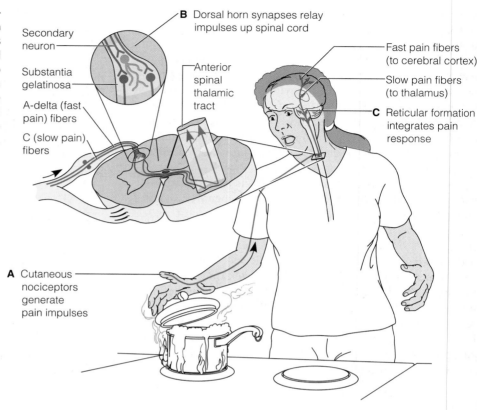

abundant and potent pain-producing chemical; other biochemical sources of pain include prostaglandins, histamine, hydrogen ions, and potassium ions. These biochemicals are thought to bind to nociceptors in response to noxious stimuli, causing the nociceptors to initiate pain impulses.

Pain Pathway

The neural pathway of pain illustrated in Figure 4–2 is summarized as follows:

1. Pain is perceived by the nociceptors in the periphery of the body (e.g., in the skin or viscera). Cutaneous pain is transmitted through small afferent A-delta and even smaller C nerve fibers to the spinal cord. A-delta fibers are myelinated and transmit impulses rapidly. They produce sharp, well-defined pain sensations, such as those that result from cuts, electric shocks, or the impact of a blow. A-delta fibers are associated with acute pain. C fibers are not myelinated and thus transmit pain impulses more slowly. The pain from deep body structures (such as muscles and viscera) is primarily transmitted by C fibers, producing diffuse burning or aching sensations. C fibers are associated with chronic pain. Both A-delta and C fibers are involved in most injuries. For example, if a person bangs the elbow, A-delta fibers transmit this pain stimulus within 0.1 second. The person feels this pain as a sharp, localized, smarting sensation. One or more seconds after the blow, the person experiences a duller, aching, diffuse sensation of pain impulses carried by the C fibers.

TABLE 4–1 Pain Stimuli	
Causative Factor	**Example**
Microorganisms (e.g., bacteria, viruses)	Meningitis
Inflammation	Sore throat
Impaired blood flow	Angina
Invasive tumor	Colon cancer
Radiation	Radiation for cancer
Heat	Sunburn
Obstruction	Kidney stone
Spasm	Colon cramping
Compression	Carpal tunnel syndrome
Decreased movement	Pain after cast removal
Stretching or straining	Sprained ankle
Fractures	Fractured hip
Swelling	Arthritis
Deposits of foreign tissue	Endometriosis
Chemicals	Skin rash
Electricity	Electrical burn
Conflict, difficulty in life	Psychogenic pain

2. Secondary neurons transmit the impulses from the afferent neurons through the dorsal horn of the spinal cord, where they synapse in the substantia gelatinosa. The impulses then cross over to the anterior and lateral spinothalamic tracts.

3. The impulses ascend the anterior and lateral spinothalamic tracts and pass through the medulla and midbrain to the thalamus.

4. In the thalamus and cerebral cortex, the pain impulses are perceived, described, localized, and interpreted, and a response is formulated. A noxious impulse becomes pain when the sensation reaches conscious levels and is perceived and evaluated by the person experiencing the sensation.

Some pain impulses ascend along the paleospinothalamic tract in the medial section of the spinal cord. These impulses enter the reticular formation and the limbic systems, which integrate emotional and cognitive responses to pain. Interconnections in the autonomic nervous system may also cause an autonomic response to the pain. In addition, deep nociceptors often converge on the same spinal neuron, resulting in pain that is experienced in a part of the body other than its origin.

Inhibitory Mechanisms

Efferent fibers run from the reticular formation and midbrain to the substantia gelatinosa in the dorsal horns of the spinal cord. Along these fibers, pain may be inhibited or modulated. The analgesia system is a group of midbrain neurons that transmits impulses to the pons and medulla, which in turn stimulate a pain inhibitory center in the dorsal horns of the spinal cord. The exact nature of this inhibitory mechanism is unknown.

The most clearly defined chemical inhibitory mechanism is fueled by *endorphins* (endogenous morphines), which are naturally occurring opioid peptides present in neurons in the brain, spinal cord, and gastrointestinal tract. Endorphins in the brain are released in response to afferent noxious stimuli, whereas endorphins in the spinal cord are released in response to efferent impulses. Endorphins work by binding with opiate receptors on the neurons to inhibit pain impulse transmission (Figure 4–3 ■).

TYPES AND CHARACTERISTICS OF PAIN
Acute Pain

Acute pain has a sudden onset, is usually temporary, and is localized. Pain that lasts for less than 6 months and has an identified cause is classified as acute pain. The sudden onset usually results from tissue injury from trauma, surgery, or inflammation. The pain is usually sharp and localized, although it may radiate. The three major types of acute pain are:

- **Somatic pain,** which arises from nerve receptors originating in the skin or close to the surface of the body. Somatic pain may be either sharp and well localized or dull and diffuse. It is often accompanied by nausea and vomiting.
- **Visceral pain,** which arises from body organs. Visceral pain is dull and poorly localized because of the low number of nociceptors. The viscera are sensitive to stretching, inflammation, and ischemia but relatively insensitive to cutting and

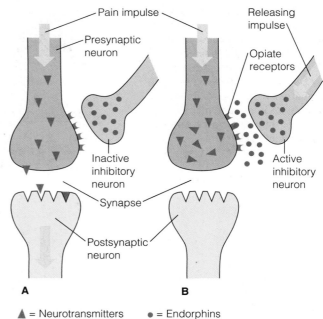

▲ = Neurotransmitters   ● = Endorphins

Figure 4–3 ■ *A,* Pain impulse causes presynaptic neuron to release burst of neurotransmitters across synapse. These bind to postsynaptic neuron and propagate impulse. *B,* Inhibitory neuron releases endorphins, which bind to presynaptic opiate receptors. Neurotransmitter release is inhibited; pain impulse is interrupted.

temperature extremes. Visceral pain is associated with nausea and vomiting, hypotension, and restlessness. It often radiates or is referred.

- **Referred pain,** which is perceived in an area distant from the site of the stimuli. It commonly occurs with visceral pain, as visceral fibers synapse at the level of the spinal cord, close to fibers innervating other subcutaneous tissue areas of the body (Figure 4–4 ■). Pain in a spinal nerve may be felt over the skin in any body area innervated by sensory neurons that share that same spinal nerve route. Body areas defined by spinal nerve routes are called dermatomes (see Chapter 40). ⊙

Acute pain warns of actual or potential injury to tissues. As a stressor, it initiates the fight-or-flight autonomic stress response. Characteristic physical responses include tachycardia, rapid and shallow respirations, increased blood pressure, dilated pupils, sweating, and pallor. The person experiencing the pain responds to this threat with anxiety and fear. This psychologic response may further increase the physical responses to acute pain.

Chronic Pain

Chronic pain is prolonged pain, usually lasting longer than 6 months. It is not always associated with an identifiable cause and is often unresponsive to conventional medical treatment. Chronic pain is often described as dull, aching, and diffuse. Unlike acute pain, chronic pain has a much more complex and poorly understood purpose.

MediaLink | REFLEX ARC ANIMATION

Figure 4-4 ■ Referred pain is the result of the convergence of sensory nerves from certain areas of the body before they enter the brain for interpretation. For example, a toothache may be felt in the ear, pain from inflammation of the diaphragm may be felt in the shoulder, and pain from ischemia of the heart muscle (angina) may be felt in the left arm.

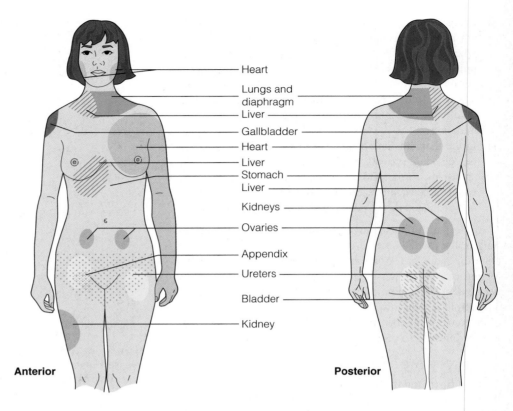

Heart
Lungs and diaphragm
Liver
Gallbladder
Heart
Liver
Stomach
Liver
Kidneys
Ovaries
Appendix
Ureters
Bladder
Kidney

Anterior

Posterior

Chronic pain can be subdivided into four categories:

- *Recurrent acute pain* is characterized by relatively well-defined episodes of pain interspersed with pain-free episodes. Examples of recurrent acute pain include migraine headaches and sickle cell crises.
- *Ongoing time-limited pain* is identified by a defined time period. Some examples are cancer pain, which ends with control of the disease or death, and burn pain, which ends with rehabilitation or death.
- *Chronic nonmalignant pain* is non-life-threatening pain that nevertheless persists beyond the expected time for healing. Chronic lower back pain falls into this category.
- *Chronic intractable nonmalignant pain syndrome* is similar to simple chronic nonmalignant pain, but is characterized by the person's inability to cope well with the pain and sometimes by physical, social, and/or psychologic disability resulting from the pain.

The client with chronic pain often is depressed, withdrawn, immobile, irritable, and/or controlling. Although chronic pain may range from mild to severe and may be continuous or intermittent, the unrelenting presence of the pain often results in the pain itself becoming the pathologic process requiring intervention. The most common chronic pain condition is lower back pain. Other common chronic pain conditions include the following (McCance & Huether, 2002):

- *Neuralgias* are painful conditions that result from damage to a peripheral nerve caused by infection or disease. Postherpetic neuralgia (following shingles) is an example.
- Reflex sympathetic *dystrophies* are characterized by continuous severe, burning pain. These conditions follow peripheral nerve damage and present the symptoms of pain, vasospasm, muscle wasting, and vasomotor changes (vasodilation followed by vasoconstriction).
- *Hyperesthesias* are conditions of oversensitivity to tactile and painful stimuli. Hyperesthesias result in diffuse pain that is usually increased by fatigue and emotional lability.
- Myofascial pain syndrome is a common condition marked by injury to or disease of muscle and fascial tissue. Pain results from muscle spasm, stiffness, and collection of lactic acid in the muscle. Fibromyalgia is an example.
- Cancer often produces chronic pain, usually due to factors associated with the advancing disease. These factors include a growing tumor that presses on nerves or other structures, stretching of viscera, obstruction of ducts, or metastasis to bones. The malignant tumor also may mechanically stimulate pain or the production of biochemicals that cause pain. Pain also may be associated with chemotherapy and radiation therapy.
- Chronic postoperative pain is rare but may occur following incisions in the chest wall, radical mastectomy, radical neck dissection, and surgical amputation.

Central Pain

Central pain is related to a lesion in the brain that may spontaneously produce high-frequency bursts of impulses that are perceived as pain. A vascular lesion, tumor, trauma, or inflammation may cause central pain. Thalamic pain, one of the most common types, is severe, spontaneous, and often continuous. Hyperesthesia (an abnormal sensitivity to touch, pain, or other sensory stimuli) may occur on the side of the body opposite to the lesion in the thalamus. The perception of body position and movement may also be lost.

Phantom Pain

Phantom pain is a syndrome that occurs following amputation of a body part. The client experiences pain in the missing body part even though he or she is completely mentally aware that it is gone. This pain may include itching, tingling, or pressure sensations, or it may be more severe, including burning or stabbing sensations. In some cases, the client may describe a sensation that an amputated limb is twisted or cramped. It is thought that this type of pain may be due to stimulation of the severed nerves at the site of the amputation. Treatment is complex and often unsuccessful.

Psychogenic Pain

Psychogenic pain is experienced in the absence of any diagnosed physiologic cause or event. Typically psychogenic pain involves a long history of severe pain. It is thought that the client's emotional needs prompt the pain sensations. Psychogenic pain is real, and may in turn lead to physiologic changes, such as muscle tension, which may produce further pain. This condition may result from interpersonal conflicts, a need for support from others, or a desire to avoid a stressful or traumatic situation. Depression is often present.

FACTORS AFFECTING RESPONSES TO PAIN

Physical response to pain involves specific and often predictable neurologic changes. In fact, everyone has the same pain threshold and perceives pain stimuli at the same stimulus intensity. For example, heat is perceived as painful at 44° to 46° C, the range at which it begins to damage tissue. What varies is the person's perception of and reaction to pain. The individualized response to pain is shaped by multiple and interacting factors including age, sociocultural influences, emotional state, past experiences with pain, source and meaning of the pain, and knowledge base.

When describing a person as being highly sensitive to pain, one is referring to the person's **pain tolerance,** which is the amount of pain a person can endure before outwardly responding to it. The ability to tolerate pain may be decreased by repeated episodes of pain, fatigue, anger, anxiety, and sleep deprivation. Medications, alcohol, hypnosis, warmth, distraction, and spiritual practices may increase pain tolerance.

Age

Age influences a person's perception and expression of pain. The older adult with normal age-related changes in neurophysiology may have decreased perception of sensory stimuli and a higher pain tolerance. In addition, chronic disease processes more common in the older adult, such as peripheral vascular disease or diabetes, may interfere with normal nerve impulse transmission. Individuals in this age group may have atypical responses to pain: decreased perception of acute pain, heightened perceptions of chronic pain, and/or increased incidence of referred pain.

Often believing that pain is a part of growing older, the client may ignore pain or self-medicate with over-the-counter medications. As a result of these behaviors, the older adult is at increased risk of injury or serious illness. Table 4–2 lists age-related changes and their effects on pain.

Sociocultural Influences

Each person's response to pain is strongly influenced by the family, community, and culture. Sociocultural influences affect the way in which a person tolerates pain, interprets the meaning of pain, and reacts verbally and nonverbally to the pain. For example, if the client's family believes that males should not cry and must tolerate pain stoically, then the male client often will appear withdrawn and refuse pain medication. If a family encourages open and intense emotional expression, then the client may cry freely and appear comfortable requesting pain medication.

Cultural standards also teach an individual how much pain to tolerate, what types of pain to report, to whom to report the pain, and what kind of treatment to seek. For example, clients of northern European ancestry may value "being a good patient," which may cause them to avoid "complaining" about their pain, whereas clients of Jewish ancestry may value seeking information about their pain, which may cause them to discuss their pain often and in detail. Note, however, that behaviors vary greatly within a culture and from generation to generation. The nurse should approach each client as an individual, observing the client carefully, taking the time to ask questions, and avoiding assumptions.

TABLE 4–2   Nursing Care of the Older Adult: Age-Related Changes and Their Effects on Pain

Factors Related to Aging	Effects	Outcomes
Decreased blood flow	Ischemia, decreases in brain function	Client forgets to take medication
Changes in neurotransmitters related to sleep and mood	Decreased sleep resulting in vulnerability to pain	Greater risk of chronic pain, fatigue, increased withdrawal
Reduced levels of norepinephrine	Lowered transmission of pain	Less likely to notice an injury
Changes in sensory interpretation	Lowered pain sensation	Client may not take appropriate protective action
Decreased peripheral nerve conduction	Lowered response to pain	Not seeking appropriate care
Slowed reaction time	Slower avoidance response	Client receives more serious injury
Reduced movement	Increased risk for muscle wasting	May cause immobility

The nurse also has a set of sociocultural values and beliefs about pain. If these values and beliefs differ from those of the client, the assessment and management of pain may be based on the values of the nurse rather than on the needs of the client. The nurse must be familiar with ethnic and cultural diversity in pain expression and management and respect cultural differences. It is particularly important to remember that pain behaviors are not an objective indicator of the amount of pain present for any individual client. Finally, most experts agree that cultural differences in the expression of, response to, and interpretation of the meaning of pain need further research.

Emotional Status

Emotional status influences the pain perception. The sensation of pain may be blocked by intense concentration (e.g., during sports activities) or may be increased by anxiety or fear. Pain often is increased when it occurs in conjunction with other illnesses or physical discomforts such as nausea or vomiting. The presence or absence of support people or caregivers that genuinely care about pain management also may alter emotional status and the perception of pain.

Anxiety may increase the perception of pain, and pain in turn may cause anxiety. In addition, the muscle tension common with anxiety can create its own source of pain. This association explains why nonpharmacologic interventions such as relaxation or guided imagery are helpful in relieving or decreasing pain.

Fatigue, lack of sleep, and depression also are related to pain experiences. Pain interferes with a person's ability to fall asleep and stay asleep and thus induces fatigue. In turn, fatigue can lower pain tolerance. Depression is clearly linked to pain: Serotonin, a neurotransmitter, is involved in the modulation of pain in the central nervous system (CNS). In clinically depressed people, serotonin is decreased, leading to an increase in pain sensations. The reverse is also true: In the presence of pain, depression is common.

Past Experiences with Pain

Previous experiences with pain are likely to influence the person's response to a current pain episode. If supportive adults responded to childhood experiences with pain appropriately, the adult usually will have a healthy attitude to pain. If, however, the person's pain was responded to with exaggerated emotions or neglectful indifference, that person's future responses to pain may be exaggerated or denied.

The responses of health care providers to the person in pain can influence the person's response during the next pain episode. If providers respond to pain with effective strategies and a caring attitude, the client will remain more comfortable during any subsequent pain episode, and anxiety will be avoided. If, however, the pain is not adequately relieved, or if the client feels that empathetic care was not given, anxiety about the next pain episode sets up the client for a more complex and therefore more painful event.

Source and Meaning

The meaning associated with the pain influences the experience of pain. For example, the pain of labor to deliver a baby is experienced differently from the pain following removal of a major organ for cancer. Because pain is the major signal for health problems, it is strongly linked to all associated meanings of health problems, such as disability, loss of role, and death. For this reason, it is important to explain to clients the etiology and prognosis for the pain assessed.

If the client perceives the pain as deserved (e.g., "just punishment for sins"), then the client may actually feel relief that the "punishment" has commenced. If the client believes that the pain will relieve him or her from an unrewarding job, dangerous military service, or even stressful social obligations, there may similarly be a feeling of relief. In contrast, pain that is perceived as meaningless (e.g., chronic low back pain or the unrelieved pain of arthritis) can cause anxiety and depression.

Knowledge

A lack of understanding of the source, outcome, and meaning of the pain can contribute negatively to the pain experience. It is important to assess the client's readiness to learn, use methods of teaching that are effective for the client and family, and evaluate learning carefully. Teaching must include the process of the pain, its predictable course (if possible), and the proposed plan of care. In addition, encourage clients to communicate preferences for pain relief. Learning how to let significant others know of the presence of pain and how to use their help can also promote effective pain management.

MYTHS AND MISCONCEPTIONS ABOUT PAIN

Myths and misconceptions about pain and its management are common in both health care providers and clients. Following are some of the most common of these myths.

Myth 1: Pain is a result, not a cause. According to the traditional view, pain is only a symptom of a condition. However, it is now recognized that unrelieved or poorly relieved pain itself sets up further responses, such as immobility, anger, and anxiety; pain may also delay healing and rehabilitation.

Myth 2: Chronic pain is really a masked form of depression. Serotonin plays a chemical role in pain transmission and is also the major modulator of depression. Therefore, pain and depression are chemically related, not mutually exclusive. It is common to find them coexisting.

Myth 3: Narcotic medication is too risky to be used in chronic pain. This common misconception often deprives clients of the most effective source of pain relief. It is true that other methods should be tried first; if, however, they prove ineffective, narcotics should be considered as an appropriate alternative.

Myth 4: It is best to wait until a client has pain before giving medication. It is now widely accepted that anticipating pain has a noticeable effect on the amount of pain a client experiences. Offering pain relief before a pain event is well on its way can lessen the pain.

Myth 5: Many clients lie about the existence or severity of their pain. Very few clients lie about their pain.

Myth 6: Postoperative pain is best treated with intramuscular injections. The most commonly used postoperative pain relief for many years was meperidine (Demerol) given intramuscularly. However, meperidine has many adverse effects, such as irritating tissues and producing the CNS stimulant normeperidine. In addition, meperidine is short acting. Most contemporary experts do not recommend its use to manage postoperative pain.

COLLABORATIVE CARE

Effective pain relief results from collaboration among health care providers. Pain clinics are centers staffed by a team of health care professionals who use a multidisciplinary approach to managing chronic pain. Therapies may include traditional pharmacologic agents as well as herbs, vitamins, and other dietary supplements; nutritional counseling; psychotherapy; biofeedback; hypnosis; acupuncture; massage; and other treatments. Hospices for dying clients also provide a multifaceted approach to pain management. Chapter 11 provides information about pain management during end-of-life care.

Medications

Medication is the most common approach to pain management. Various drugs with many kinds of delivery systems are available. These drugs include nonnarcotic analgesics, nonsteroidal anti-inflammatory drugs (NSAIDs), narcotics, synthetic narcotics, antidepressants, and local anesthetic agents. In addition to administering prescribed medications, the nurse may act independently in choosing the dosage and timing. The nurse is also responsible for assessing the side effects of medications, evaluating a medication's effectiveness, and providing client teaching. The nurse's role in pain relief is client advocate and direct caregiver.

The World Health Organization "ladder of analgesia" effectively guides the use of medications (WHO, 1986/1990) (Figure 4–5 ■). NSAIDs and narcotic pain medications are used progressively until pain is relieved, reflecting the interactive nature of these two types of analgesics. Box 4–1 describes terms associated with pain medication.

Nonnarcotic Analgesics

Nonnarcotic analgesics such as acetaminophen (Tylenol) produce analgesia and reduce fever. The exact mechanism of action is unknown. They are used to treat mild to moderate pain.

NSAIDs

NSAIDs act on peripheral nerve endings and minimize pain by interfering with prostaglandin synthesis. Examples are aspirin, ibuprofen, and celecoxib (Celebrex). The NSAIDs have anti-inflammatory, analgesic, and antipyretic actions. NSAIDs are the treatment of choice for mild to moderate pain and continue to be effective when combined with narcotics for moderate to severe pain. Examples of NSAIDs and factors to consider when selecting an NSAID are provided in Table 4–3. Nursing implications for NSAIDs are found in the Medication Administration box on page 63.

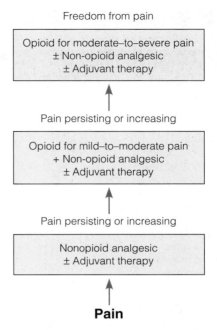

Freedom from pain

Opioid for moderate–to–severe pain
± Non-opioid analgesic
± Adjuvant therapy

Pain persisting or increasing

Opioid for mild–to–moderate pain
+ Non-opioid analgesic
± Adjuvant therapy

Pain persisting or increasing

Nonopioid analgesic
± Adjuvant therapy

Pain

Figure 4–5 ■ The WHO analgesic ladder illustrates the process for selection of analgesic medications for pain management.

From Cancer Pain Relief and Palliative Care *by World Health Organization, 1990, (Technical Report Series, no. 804) Geneva: WHO. Reprinted by permission.*

BOX 4–1	■ Terms Associated with Pain Medication

■ *Addiction:* The compulsive use of a substance despite negative consequences, such as health threats or legal problems.

■ *Drug abuse:* The use of any chemical substance for other than a medical purpose.

■ *Physical drug dependence:* A biologic need for a substance. If the substance is not supplied, physical withdrawal symptoms occur.

■ *Psychologic drug dependence:* A psychologic need for a substance. If the substance is not supplied, psychologic withdrawal symptoms occur.

■ *Drug tolerance:* The process by which the body requires a progressively greater amount of a drug to achieve the same results.

■ *Equianalgesic:* Having the same pain-killing effect when administered to the same individual. Drug dosages are equianalgesic if they have the same effect as morphine sulfate 10 mg administered intramuscularly.

■ *Pseudoaddiction:* Behavior involving drug seeking; a result of receiving inadequate pain relief.

Narcotics (Opioids)

Narcotics, or opioids, are derivatives of the opium plant. These drugs (and their synthetic forms) are the pharmacologic treatment of choice for moderate to severe pain. Examples are morphine, codeine, and fentanyl (Durgesic, Actiq). Narcotic analgesics produce analgesia by binding to opioid receptors both within and outside the CNS. A summary of narcotic drugs, their

MediaLink | PAIN CONTROL GUIDELINES

TABLE 4-3   Factors to Consider When Selecting an NSAID

Chemical Class	Half Life (Hours)	Onset of Action (Hours)	Usual Dosing Interval (Times per Day)	Usual Daily Dose (Mg)
Salicylates				
Acetylated				
Aspirin	0.25	0.25–0.50	4–6	325–1000
Aspirin, buffered				
Aspirin, enteric coated				
Aspirin, sustained release				
Nonacetylated				
Choline salicylate (Arthropan)		1–2	2–4	1200
Choline magnesium trisalicylate				
(Trilisate)	2–19	2	2–4	1200
Diflunisal (Dolobid)	8–12	2–3	2–3	250–500
Salsalate (Disalcid)	2–19	—	2–3	325–3000
Magnesium salicylate			3–4	various
Sodium salicylate			4–6	various
Propionic Acids				
Fenoprofen (Nalfon)	2–3	—	3–4	300–600
Flurbiprofen (Ansaid)	5.7	—	2–3	100
Ibuprofen (Motrin, others)	2	0.5	3–4	300–800
Ketoprofen (Orudis)	1.6–4	—	3–4	25–75
Ketoprofen SR (Oruvail)		—	1	200
Naproxen (Naprosyn)	13	1	2	250–500
Naproxen sodium (Anaprox)	13–15	1–2	2	250–500
Oxaprozin (Daypro)	21–25	1–2	1–2	600
Acetic Acids				
Diclofenac sodium (Voltaren)	1.2–2	0.5	3	50
Etodolac (Lodine)	6–7	0.5	3	200–400
Indomethacin (Indocin)	4–6	0.5	2–4	25–50
Indomethacin SR (Indocin SR)	—	2–4		150
Ketoralac (Toradol)	4–6	0.5–1	4–6	10–30
Sulindac (Clinoril, others)	8	—	2	150–200
Tolmetin (Tolectin)	5	—	3	400
Fenamates (Anthranilic Acids)				
Meclofenamate (Meclomen)	2–3	—	3–4	50
Mefenamic acid (Ponstel)	2	—	4	250
Oxicams				
Piroxican (Feldene)	24	2–4	1–2	10–20
Nonacidic (Naphthylkanone)				
Nabumetone (Relafon)	22	—	1–2	500–1000
Pyrazolones				
Phenylbutazone (Butazolidin)	40–60	0.5–1	3–4	100–600

usual dosages, peak effect, and nursing implications is provided in Table 4–4.

A common myth among health care professionals is that using narcotics for pain treatment poses a real threat of addiction. Actually, when the medications are used as recommended, there is little to no risk of addiction. Rather, if pain is not adequately treated, the client may seek more and more narcotic relief, thus increasing the risk of tolerance. Nursing implications for narcotics are found in the Medication Administration box on page 65.

Antidepressants

Antidepressants within the tricyclic and related chemical groups act on the production and retention of serotonin in the CNS, thus inhibiting pain sensation. They also promote normal sleeping patterns, further alleviating the suffering of the client in pain.

Local Anesthetics

Drugs such as benzocaine and zylocaine are part of a large group of substances that block the initiation and transmission of nerve impulses in a local area, thus blocking pain as well. Local anesthetics can be delivered by a variety of methods. They are sometimes used to enable a client to begin moving and using a painful area to diminish long-term pain.

Duration of Action

Each of the pharmacologic agents has a unique absorption and duration of action. The nurse caring for the client in pain must

Medication Administration
Nonsteroidal Anti-Inflammatory Drugs

Examples of NSAIDs are:

    aspirin (acetylsalicylic acid)
    fenoprofen calcium (Nalfon)
    ibuprofen (Motrin)
    rofecoxib (Vioxx)
    diflunisal (Dolobid)
    ketorolac tromethamine (Toradol)
    naproxen (Naprosyn)
    indomethacin (Indocin)
    celecoxib (Celebrex)

The NSAIDs have anti-inflammatory, analgesic, and antipyretic effects. It is believed that they inhibit the enzyme cyclooxygenase, thereby decreasing synthesis of prostaglandins. These drugs provide analgesic effects by reducing inflammation and by perhaps blocking the generation of noxious impulses.

Nursing Responsibilities
- Do not administer aspirin with other NSAIDs.
- Assess and document if the client is taking a hypoglycemic agent or insulin; the NSAIDs may increase the hypoglycemic effect.
- Administer with meals, milk, or a full glass of water to decrease gastric irritation.
- Assess clients who are also taking anticoagulants for bleeding; the NSAIDs increase this risk.

Client and Family Teaching
- Drugs may cause gastrointestinal bleeding (report nausea, vomiting of blood, dark stools), visual disturbances (report blurred or diminished vision), hearing problems, dizziness, skin rash, and renal problems (report weight gain or edema).
- Take medications with meals to decrease gastric irritation.
- Avoid drinking alcohol or taking any over-the-counter drug unless approved by the health care provider.
- The desired effects may not appear for 3–5 days, and the full effects may not appear for 2–4 weeks.
- Maintain regular health care appointments.

---

understand that no drug will have a totally predictable course of action, because each person absorbs, metabolizes, and excretes medications at different dosage levels. The only way to obtain reliable data about the effectiveness of the medication for the individual client is to assess how that client responds. Therefore, the best choice is to individualize the dosing schedule.

The two major descriptors of dosing schedules are *around the clock* (ATC) or *as necessary* (PRN). (The abbreviation PRN stands for *pro re nata,* Latin for "as circumstances may require.") An ATC administration is appropriate if the client experiences pain constantly and predictably during a 24-hour period. A PRN administration is appropriate for pain that is not predictable or constant. The PRN medication should be administered as soon as the pain begins.

Giving analgesics before the pain occurs or increases gives the client confidence in the certainty of pain relief and thereby avoids some of the untoward effects of pain. The benefits of a preventive approach can be summarized as follows:

- The client may spend less time in pain.
- Frequent analgesic administration may allow for smaller doses and less analgesic administration.
- Smaller doses will in turn mean fewer side effects.
- The client's fear and anxiety about the return of pain will decrease.
- The client will probably be more physically active and avoid the difficulties caused by immobility.

The side effects of a drug can become difficult to manage if the dosage is too high. The best formula for adequate dosage is a balance between effective pain relief and minimal side effects. Within prescribed limits, the nurse can choose the correct dose according to the client's response. It is also the role of the nurse to inform the physician if the prescribed dosage does not meet the client's needs.

Routes of Administration

The route of administration significantly affects how much of the medication is needed to relieve pain. For example, oral doses of some narcotics must be up to 5 times greater than parenteral doses to achieve the same degree of pain relief. Different narcotics have different recommended dosages. Consulting an equianalgesic dosage chart helps ensure that dosages of different narcotics administered by different routes will have the same analgesic effect when administered to the same client. These charts are based on a comparison of an analgesic to 10 mg (IM) of morphine. Table 4–4 is an example of an equianalgesic chart.

ORAL. The simplest route for both client and nurse is the oral (PO) route. Special nursing care is still required, because some medications must be given with food, some are irritating to the gastrointestinal system, and some clients have trouble swallowing pills. Liquid and timed-release forms are available for special applications.

RECTAL. The rectal route is helpful for clients who are unable to swallow. Several of the opioid narcotics are available in this form. The rectal route is effective and simple, but the client and family may not accept it. To be effective, any rectal medication must be placed above the rectal sphincter.

TRANSDERMAL. The transdermal, or patch, form of medication is increasingly being used because it is simple, painless, and delivers a continuous level of medication (Figure 4–6 ■). Although expensive, transdermal medications are easy to store and apply. Additional short-acting medication is often needed for breakthrough pain.

To apply a medication transdermally, the nurse or client must clip any hair from the area, clean the site (which should be on the upper torso) with clear water, dry the cleansed area,

TABLE 4-4   Equianalgesic Drug Chart

Analgesic	Dosage (mg)	Peak (min)	Duration (h)	Nursing Considerations
Morphine sulfate	10 IM 30–60 PO	30–60 IM 60–120 PO	4–5 IM 4–5 PO	PO dose is 3–6 times the IM dose. A lower dose may be appropriate for older clients with chronic pain. Contraindicated in clients with acute bronchial asthma or upper-airway obstruction.
Butorphanol tartrate (Stadol)	2 IM N/A PO	30–60 IM	3–4 IM	May cause withdrawal in clients physically dependent on narcotics. May cause hallucinations. Increases cardiac workload. Contraindicated in clients with myocardial infarction.
Codeine	130 IM 200 PO	30–60 IM 60–120 PO	4 IM 4 PO	PO dose is about 1.5 times the IM dose. Often given synergistically with aspirin or acetaminophen for best effect. More toxic in high doses than morphine. Causes more nausea and vomiting than morphine and is constipating.
Hydromorphone HCl (Dilaudid)	1.5 IM 7.5 PO	15–30 IM 30 PO	4 IM 4 PO	PO dose is 5 times IM dose. Shorter acting than morphine. May cause loss of appetite. Contraindicated in clients with increased intracranial pressure or status asthmaticus.
Levorphanol tartrate (Levo-Dromoran)	2 IM 4 PO	60 IM 90–120 PO	4–5 IM 4–5 PO	Longer acting than morphine when given in repeated, regular doses. Accumulates, so analgesic effect may increase. SC recommended over IM route. Warn client drug has bitter taste. Contraindicated in clients with respiratory depression, asthma, alcoholism, or increased intracranial pressure.
Meperidine HCl (Demerol)	75 IM 300 PO	30–50 IM 60–90 PO	2–4 IM 2–4 PO	Metabolized to normeperidine, a toxic CNS stimulant which may cause CNS hyperexcitability. Normeperidine's effects increased, not reversed, by naloxone. Use with caution in clients with renal disease. PO dose of 300 not recommended.
Methadone HCl (Dolophine)	10 IM 20 PO	60–120 IM 90–120 PO	4–6 IM 4–6 PO	Initial PO dose is twice IM dose. Accumulates, so analgesic effect may increase. Warn client drug has bitter taste. Also used for heroin detoxification and temporary maintenance. Oral liquid form is legally required in maintenance programs.
Nalbuphine HCl (Nubain)	10 IM N/A PO	30–60 IM	3–6 IM	Longer acting and less likely to cause hypotension than morphine. Respiratory depression does not increase with increased dosages as compared to morphine. Similar to butorphanol, but does not increase cardiac workload.
Oxycodone HCl	N/A IM 30 PO	60 PO	3–6 PO	Now available as a single-entity product in tablet or liquid form. Also available in 5-mg dose in drugs such as Percodan and Percocet. Has faster onset and higher peak effect than most PO narcotics.
Oxymorphone HCl (Numorphan)	1–1.5 IM N/A PO	30–60 IM	3–6 IM	Also available as rectal suppository (10 mg equianalgesic), but more effective if given IM.
Pentazocine HCl	60 IM 180 PO	30–60 IM 30–90 PO	3–4 IM 3–4 PO	PO dose is 3 times IM dose. May produce withdrawal in clients physically dependent on narcotics. May cause confusion, hallucinations, anxiety. Contraindicated in clients with head injury or increased intracranial pressure. Use with caution in clients with cardiac problems.
Propoxyphene HCl (Darvon)	N/A IM 500 PO	120 PO	4–6 PO	Available only in oral form in United States. Never give as much as 500 mg PO. PO dose of 65–130 mg recommended. Used for mild to moderate pain. May cause false decreases in urinary steroid excretion tests. Report suspected propoxyphene abuse; propoxyphene in excessive doses ranks second to barbiturates as a cause of drug-related deaths.

Note: Morphine sulfate 10 mg IM is the analgesic dose to which all other IM and PO doses in this table are considered equianalgesic.

Medication Administration
Narcotic Analgesics

Examples of narcotic analgesics are:

buprenorphine HCl (Buprenex)
codeine
hydromorphone HCl (Dilaudid)
meperidine HCl (Demerol)
morphine sulfate
nalbuphine HCl (Nubain)
oxymorphone HCl (Numorphan)
pentazocine (Talwin)
propoxyphene napsylate (Darvocet-N)

Narcotic analgesics are used to treat severe pain. The drugs in this category include opium, morphine, codeine, opium derivatives, and synthetic substances. Morphine and codeine are pure chemical substances isolated from opium. These drugs decrease the awareness of the sensation of pain by binding to opiate receptors in the brain and spinal cord. It is also believed that they diminish the transmission of pain impulses by altering cell membrane permeability to sodium and by affecting the release of neurotransmitters for efferent nerves sensitive to noxious stimuli. Narcotic analgesics affect the central nervous system; causing analgesia, euphoria, drowsiness, mental clouding, and lethargy. They also have various other effects: Depending on the drug used, the narcotics depress respirations, stimulate the vomiting center, depress the cough reflex, induce peripheral vasodilatation (resulting in hypotension), constrict the pupil, and decrease intestinal peristalsis. The narcotics are addictive, causing psychologic and physical dependence.

Nursing Responsibilities
- Narcotics are regulated by federal law; the nurse must record the date, time, client name, type and amount of the drug used, and sign the entry in a narcotic inventory sheet. If the drug must be wasted after it is signed out, the act must be witnessed and the narcotic sheet signed by the nurse and the witness. Computerized narcotic documentation methods are also available.
- Keep a narcotic antagonist, such as naloxone, immediately available to treat respiratory depression.

- Assess allergies or adverse effects from narcotics previously experienced by the client.
- Meperidine (Demerol) is associated with CNS toxicity and thus involves significant patient risk. For any client who is receiving more than one dose, monitor for nervousness, restlessness, tremors, twitching, shakiness, myoclonic jerks, diaphoresis, changes in level of awareness, agitation, disorientation, confusion, delirium, hallucinations, violent shivering, and/or seizures. This toxicity can occur with any route of administration or any dosing regimen. This risk is increased with oral administration and in clients with decreased renal function (including normal changes with aging). Report these manifestations to the physician.
- Assess for any respiratory disease, such as asthma, that might increase the risk of respiratory depression.
- Assess the characteristics of the pain and the effectiveness of drugs that have been previously used to treat the pain.
- Take and record baseline vital signs before administering the drug.
- Administer the drugs, following established guidelines.
- Monitor vital signs, level of consciousness, pupillary response, nausea, bowel function, urinary function, and effectiveness of pain management.
- Teach noninvasive methods of pain management for use in conjunction with narcotic analgesics.
- Provide for client safety.

Client and Family Teaching
- The use of narcotics to treat severe pain is unlikely to cause addiction.
- Do not drink alcohol.
- Do not take over-the-counter medications unless approved by the health care provider.
- Increase intake of fluids and fiber in the diet to prevent constipation.
- The drugs often cause dizziness, drowsiness, and impaired thinking; use caution when driving or making decisions.
- Report decreasing effectiveness or the appearance of side effects to the physician.

Figure 4–6 ■ The transdermal patch administers medication in predictable doses.

apply the patch immediately upon opening the package, and ensure that the contact is complete, especially around the edges. The effectiveness of a patch lasts for a variable amount of time, and the next patch should be applied on a different site.

INTRAMUSCULAR. Once the most popular route for pain medication administration, the intramuscular (IM) route is being reconsidered. Its disadvantages include uneven absorption from the muscle, discomfort on administration, and time consumed to prepare and administer the medication.

INTRAVENOUS. The intravenous (IV) route provides the most rapid onset, usually ranging from 1 to 15 minutes. Medication can be given by drip, bolus, or **patient-controlled analgesia (PCA),** a pump with a control mechanism that affords the client self-management of pain (Figure 4–7 ■). Studies of PCA use for postoperative pain have shown that clients require less

Figure 4–7 ■ PCA units allow the client to self-manage severe pain. The units may be portable or mounted on intravenous poles.

Courtesy of Baxter Healthcare Corporation.

overall medication because of the even blood level of medication maintained, the feeling of control maintained by the client, and the absence of anxiety. Several drugs are available for this route. The disadvantages are the nursing care needed for any intravenous line, the potential for infection, and the cost of disposable supplies. The PCA method of administration requires careful client teaching.

SUBCUTANEOUS. The subcutaneous (SC) route is accepted, but it is less commonly used than other methods. Its advantages and disadvantages are similar to those of the intravenous route.

INTRASPINAL. The intraspinal route is invasive and requires more extensive nursing care. Nursing implications for clients receiving intraspinal analgesia can be found in box below.

NERVE BLOCKS. In a nerve block, anesthetics, sometimes in combination with steroidal anti-inflammatory drugs, are injected by a physician or nurse anesthetist into or near a nerve,

NURSING CARE OF THE CLIENT RECEIVING INTRASPINAL ANALGESIA

Intraspinal analgesia is used to manage chronic and intractable cancer and severe postoperative pain. The intraspinal route may be either intrathecal (into the subarachnoid space) or epidural (into the epidural space). With the infusion of a narcotic into these spaces, there is a direct effect on the opiate receptors in the dorsal horn of the spinal cord; the narcotics are also absorbed systemically and affect the brain. This method provides complete pain relief but has some potentially dangerous side effects.

PROCEDURE

The physician places a catheter into the epidural space. Tubing is attached to an infusion pump, and the prescribed medication is administered. A portable or implantable pump may be used for narcotic administration that lasts more than a few days.

NURSING CARE

- Monitor vital signs every 15 minutes for the first 2–3 hours and every hour for the first 24 hours; the client is at risk for respiratory depression, which may not manifest itself for several hours.
- Ensure that naloxone, a narcotic antagonist, is immediately available to reverse respiratory depression.
- Monitor the effectiveness of the pain management.
- Monitor intake and output. Intraspinal narcotics may block the micturition reflex, causing urinary retention and necessitating the insertion of a Foley catheter.
- Use sterile technique to care for the catheter.

Spinal cord
Pia mater
Subarachnoid space
Dura mater and arachnoid mater
Epidural space
Catheter in epidural space

Epidural analgesia

Vertebra
Spinal cord
L_2-L_3 intervertebral space

Placement of the catheter in the epidural space.

usually in an area between the nociceptor and the dorsal root. The procedure may be performed to determine the precise location of the pain source: Pain relief indicates that the injection site is the site of the source of the pain.

Temporary (local) nerve blocks may give the client enough relief to (1) develop a more hopeful attitude that pain relief is possible, (2) allow local procedures to be performed without causing discomfort, or (3) exercise and move the affected part. Nerve blocks may also be performed to predict the results of neurosurgery. For long-term pain relief, a permanent neurolytic agent is used. Neurolytic blocks usually are reserved for terminally ill clients because of the risks of weakness, paralysis, and bowel and bladder dysfunction.

Surgery

As a pain relief measure, surgery usually is performed only after all other methods have failed. Clients need thorough knowledge of the implications of the use of surgery for pain relief. For example, motor function loss is an unwelcome side effect of some surgeries. Surgical procedures used to relieve pain are shown in Figure 4–8 ■ and include cordotomy, neurectomy, sympathectomy, and rhizotomy.

Cordotomy

A cordotomy is an incision into the anterolateral tracts of the spinal cord to interrupt the transmission of pain. Because it is difficult to isolate the nerves responsible for upper body pain, this surgery is most often performed for pain in the abdominal region and legs, including severe pain from terminal cancer. A percutaneous cordotomy produces lesions of the anterolateral surface of the spinal cord by means of a radio frequency current.

Neurectomy

A neurectomy is the removal of a nerve. It is sometimes used for pain relief. A peripheral neurectomy is the severing of a nerve at any point distal to the spinal cord.

Sympathectomy

The sympathetic nerves play an important role in producing and transmitting the sensation of pain. A sympathectomy involves destruction by injection or incision of the ganglia of sympathetic nerves, usually in the lumbar region or the cervicodorsal region at the base of the neck.

Rhizotomy

Rhizotomy is surgical severing of the dorsal spinal roots. It is most often performed to relieve the pain of cancer of the head, neck, or lungs. A rhizotomy may be performed not only by surgically cutting the nerve fibers but also by injecting a chemical such as alcohol or phenol into the subarachnoid space or by using a radio frequency current to selectively destroy pain fibers.

Transcutaneous Electrical Nerve Stimulation

A **transcutaneous electrical nerve stimulation (TENS)** unit consists of a low-voltage transmitter connected by wires to electrodes placed by the client as directed by the physical therapist (Figure 4–9 ■). The client experiences a gentle tapping or vibrating sensation over the electrodes. The client can adjust the voltage to achieve maximum pain relief.

The gate control theory clarifies how TENS works. It is believed that TENS electrodes stimulate the large-diameter A-beta touch fibers to close the gate in the substantia gelatinosa. It is also theorized that TENS stimulates endorphin release by inhibitory neurons.

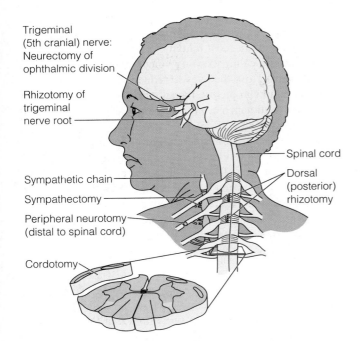

Trigeminal (5th cranial) nerve: Neurectomy of ophthalmic division

Rhizotomy of trigeminal nerve root

Sympathetic chain

Sympathectomy

Peripheral neurotomy (distal to spinal cord)

Cordotomy

Spinal cord

Dorsal (posterior) rhizotomy

Figure 4–8 ■ Surgical procedures are used to treat severe pain that does not respond to other types of management.

Figure 4–9 ■ The TENS unit is believed to assist in pain management through the gate control theory. Electrodes that deliver low-voltage electrical stimuli are placed directly on the client over painful areas.

Source: Rehabilicare, Inc./Complex Technologies.

A TENS unit is most commonly used to relieve chronic benign pain and acute postoperative pain. In either case, thorough client teaching is essential, including an explanation of manufacturer's directions, instructions on where to place the electrodes, and the importance of placing the electrodes on clean, unbroken skin. The client should assess the skin daily for signs of irritation.

TENS offers several advantages: avoidance of drug side effects, client control, and good interaction with other therapies. Disadvantages are its cost and the need for expert training for initiation.

Complementary Therapies

Acupuncture

Acupuncture is an ancient Chinese system involving the stimulation of certain specific points on the body to enhance the flow of vital energy (chi) along pathways called meridians. Acupuncture points can be stimulated by the insertion and withdrawing of needles; the application of heat, massage, laser, or electrical stimulation; or a combination of these methods. Only care providers with special training can use this method. Acupuncture is becoming a more widely accepted therapy, especially for the treatment of pain.

Biofeedback

Biofeedback is an electronic method of measuring physiologic responses such as brain waves, muscle contraction, and skin temperature, and then "feeding" this information back to the client. Most biofeedback units consist of electrodes placed on the client's skin and an amplification unit that transforms data into visual cues, such as colored lights. The client thus learns to recognize stress-related responses and to replace them with relaxation responses. Eventually, the client learns to repeat independently those actions that produce the desired brain wave effect.

Relaxation helps the client avoid the anxiety that often accompanies and complicates pain. Additionally, biofeedback gives the client a measure of control over the response to pain.

Hypnotism

Hypnosis is a trance state in which the mind becomes extremely suggestible. To achieve hypnosis, the client sits or lies down in a dimly lighted, quiet room. The therapist suggests that the client relax and fix attention on an object. The therapist then repeats in a calm, soothing voice simple phrases, such as instructions to relax and listen to the therapist's voice. The client gradually becomes more and more relaxed and falls into a trance in which the client is no longer aware of the physical environment and hears only the therapist's voice. During this state, the therapist may make suggestions to encourage pain relief. It is possible to achieve complete anesthesia or to modify pain in a variety of ways through hypnotism. For the technique to work, however, the client must be fully relaxed and must want to be hypnotized.

Advantages include client control and lack of side effects. Disadvantages include the need for a skilled practitioner; however, some clients can learn to hypnotize themselves to achieve pain relief.

Relaxation

Relaxation involves learning activities that deeply relax the body and mind. Relaxation distracts the client, lessens the effects of stress from pain, increases pain tolerance, increases the effectiveness of other pain relief measures, and increases perception of pain control. In addition, by teaching the client relaxation techniques, the nurse acknowledges the client's pain and provides reassurance that the client will receive help in managing the pain (McCaffery & Beebe, 1999). Examples of relaxation activities are as follows:

- Diaphragmatic breathing can relax muscles, improve oxygen levels, and provide a feeling of release from tension. The use of diaphragmatic breathing is more effective when the client either lies down or sits comfortably, remains in a quiet environment, and keeps the eyelids closed. Inhaling and exhaling slowly and regularly is also helpful. The technique for diaphragmatic breathing is described and illustrated in Chapter 7.
- Progressive muscle relaxation may be used alone or in conjunction with deep breathing to help manage pain. The client should be taught to tighten one group of muscles (such as those of the face), hold the tension for a few seconds, and then relax the muscle group completely. The client should repeat these actions for all parts of the body. This method is also more effective when the client lies or sits comfortably, is in a quiet environment, and keeps the eyelids closed. Audiotapes are available to help the client with this relaxation process.
- Guided imagery, also called creative visualization, is the use of the imaginative power of the mind to create a scene or sensory experience that relaxes the muscles and moves the attention of the mind away from the pain experience. To use guided imagery, the client must be able to concentrate, use the imagination, and follow directions. The nurse can facilitate this technique by asking the client to describe places or situations that are most relaxing. The nurse then speaks to the client in a calm, soothing voice about them. The client usually must close the eyes to reduce visual stimulation so that the mind can picture the situation in as much detail as possible. Audiotapes are available to assist the client with guided imagery.
- Meditation is a process whereby the client empties the mind of all sensory data and, typically, concentrates on a single object, word, or idea. This activity produces a deeply relaxed state in which oxygen consumption decreases, muscles relax, and endorphins are produced. At its deepest level, the meditative state may resemble a trance. A variety of exercises can induce the meditative state, and all are relatively easy to learn. Many books and audiotapes are available commercially.

Distraction

Distraction involves the redirection of the client's attention away from the pain and onto something that the client finds more pleasant. Examples of distracting activities are practicing focused breathing, listening to music, or doing some form of rhythmic activity to music. For example, the client using recorded music for distraction may sing along with the song, tap out the rhythm with the fingers or foot, clap to the music, conduct the music, or add harmony. Full participation in the music is key to pain relief.

Participating in an activity that promotes laughter, such as reading a joke book or viewing a comedy, has been found to be highly effective in pain relief. Laughing for 20 minutes or more is known to produce an increase in endorphins that may continue pain relief even after the client stops laughing.

Cutaneous Stimulation

It is believed that stimulation of the skin is effective in relieving pain because it prompts closure of the gate in the substantia gelatinosa. Cutaneous stimulation may be accomplished by massage, vibration, application of heat and cold, and therapeutic touch (see Table 4–5).

NURSING CARE

Nursing care of the client with pain presents perhaps more of a challenge than almost any other type of illness or injury. Regardless of the type of pain, the goal of nursing care is to assist the client to achieve optimal control of the pain.

Assessment

A comprehensive approach to pain assessment is essential to ensure adequate and appropriate interventions. The assessment areas are client perceptions, physiologic responses, behavioral responses, and self-management of pain and the effectiveness of pain management strategies.

Client Perceptions

The most reliable indicator of the presence and degree of pain is the client's own statement about the pain. The McGill Pain Questionnaire is a useful tool in assessing the client's subjective experience of the pain. It asks the client to locate the pain, to describe the quality of the pain, to indicate how the pain changes with time, and to rate the intensity of the pain (Figure 4–10 ■).

The client's perception of the pain can also be assessed by using the following PQRST technique.

- P = What precipitated (triggered, stimulated) the pain? Has anything relieved the pain? What is the pattern of the pain?
- Q = What are the quality and quantity of the pain? Is the pain sharp, stabbing, aching, burning, stinging, deep, crushing, viselike, gnawing?
- R = What is the region (location) of the pain? Does the pain radiate to other areas of the body?
- S = What is the severity of the pain?
- T = What is the timing of the pain? When does it begin, how long does it last, and how is it related to other events in the client's life?

The most common method to assess the severity of pain is a pain rating scale. Several scales are illustrated in Figure 4–11 ■.

TABLE 4–5   Methods of Cutaneous Stimulation

Method	Technique	Advantages	Disadvantages
Touch	Nurse places hands on client's body or less than 1 inch (about 2.5 cm) above client's body to realign energy.	May initiate gate closure. Communicates caring.	None.
Pressure	Nurse places hand firmly on or around the area where the client feels the pain.	May relieve pain, decrease bleeding, and prevent swelling.	Benefits are temporary—when pressure is lifted, pain returns.
Massage	Nurse gently or briskly stimulates client's subcutaneous tissues by kneading, pulling, or pressing with fingers, palms, or knuckles.	May initiate gate closure. Promotes relaxation and sedation. Minimal side effects.	Time consuming.
Vibration	Nurse uses an electrical or battery-operated vibrator to stimulate the client's subcutaneous tissues.	May initiate gate closure. Low risk of tissue damage. Less costly than TENS.	Expense of equipment.
Heat	Nurse applies a hot-water bottle, heating pad, or hot towels to client's body. A hot shower or hot bath may also be effective. A heat lamp or other heat-generating device may also be used.	May reduce muscle spasm and pain. Works best for localized pain.	Contraindicated if bleeding or swelling is present.
Cold	Nurse applies dry or moist cold packs, gel packs, towels, or bags of ice chips to the client's body.	May reduce muscle spasm and pain. Cold may slow the transmission of pain impulses, and is more effective than heat for pain relief.	Cannot be used on ischemic tissues.

Figure 4–10 ■ The McGill Pain Questionnaire.

From Pain Measurement and Assessment *by R. Melzack, 1983, New York: Raven. Reprinted by permission.*

Figure 4–11 ■ Examples of commonly used pain scales.

For clients who do not understand English or numerals, a scale using colors (e.g., light blue for no pain through bright red for worst possible pain) or pictures may be helpful. The following nursing interventions will help the nurse use a pain rating scale to achieve optimal results.

- To ensure consistent communication, explain the specific pain rating scale being used. If a word descriptor scale is used, verify that the client can read the language being used. If a numerical scale is used, be sure the client can count to 10. If the client is not able to report pain because of communication difficulties, intubation, emotional disturbances, or cognitive impairments, follow these guidelines (Pasero & McCaffrey, 2000):
  - Be sure the client is unable to report pain. Researchers have found that even residents in a nursing home who are cognitively impaired can validly self-report pain.
  - Consider pathologic conditions and procedures that might cause pain and treat the client for pain.
  - Look for indicators of pain, such as grimacing, restlessness, stillness, verbal or nonverbal vocalizations, and grasping an object.

- Ask a family member or caretaker about the client's pain to serve as a proxy pain rating.
- Discuss the definition of the word *pain* to ensure that the client and the provider are communicating on the same level. It is often helpful to use the client's own words when describing the pain.
- Explain that the report of pain is important for promoting recovery, not just for achieving temporary comfort.

Physiologic Responses

Predictable physiologic changes occur in the presence of acute pain. These may include muscle tension; tachycardia; rapid, shallow respirations; increased blood pressure; dilated pupils; sweating; and pallor. Over time, however, the body adapts to the pain stimulus, and these physiologic changes may be extinguished in clients with chronic pain.

Behavioral Responses

Some behaviors are so typical of people in pain that the behaviors are referred to as *pain behaviors.* They include bracing or guarding the painful part, taking medication, crying, moaning, grimacing, withdrawing from activity and socialization, becoming immobile, talking about pain, holding the painful area, breathing with increased effort, exhibiting a sad facial expression, and being restless.

Behavioral responses to pain may or may not coincide with the client's report of pain and are not reliable cues to the pain experience. For example, one client may rate pain at an 8 on a 1 to 10 scale while laughing or walking down the hall; another may deny pain completely while tachycardic, hypertensive, and grimacing. Discrepancies between the client's report of pain and behavioral responses may be the result of cultural factors, coping skills, fear, denial, or the utilization of relaxation or distraction techniques.

Clients may deny pain for a variety of reasons, including fear of injections, fear of drug/narcotic addiction, misinterpretation of terms (the client may not think that aching, soreness, or discomfort qualify as pain), or the misconception that health care providers know when clients experience pain. Some clients may deny pain as part of an attempt to deny that there is something wrong with them. Other clients, by contrast, may think that "as needed" medications will be given only if their pain rating is high. Clients may also use pain as a mechanism to gain attention from family and health care providers.

Self-Management of Pain

The client's attempts to manage pain are useful additions to the assessment database. This information is individualized and client specific, including many factors such as culture, age, and client knowledge. Collect detailed descriptions of actions the client or significant others took, when and how these measures were applied, and how well they worked.

Nursing Diagnoses and Interventions

The primary nursing diagnoses for clients in pain are acute pain and chronic pain. The interventions for these diagnoses are combined in this discussion.

Acute Pain or Chronic Pain

- Assess the characteristics of the pain by asking the client to:
  - Point to the pain location or to mark the pain location on a figure drawing. *Pain location provides information about the etiology of the pain and the type of pain being experienced.*
  - Rate the intensity of the pain by using a pain scale (1 to 10, with 10 being the worst pain ever experienced), a visual analog scale (a scale on which pain is marked on a continuum from no pain to severe pain), or with word descriptors (such as the McGill Pain Questionnaire). Use the same scale with each assessment. *The intensity of pain is a subjective experience. The perception of the intensity of pain is affected by the client's degree of concentration or distraction, state of consciousness, and expectations. Some body tissues are more sensitive than others.*

> **PRACTICE ALERT** *Do not assume that the older client or the cognitively impaired client is not having pain or is unable to identify the intensity of pain.* ■

- Describe the quality of the pain, saying, for example, "Describe what your pain feels like." If necessary, provide word descriptors for the client to select. *Descriptive terms provide insight into the nature and perception of the pain. In addition, the location and type of pain (e.g., acute versus chronic) affect the quality.*
- Describe the pattern of the pain, including time of onset, duration, persistence, and times without pain. It is also important to ask if the pain is worse at regular times of the day and if it has any relationship to activity. *The pattern of pain provides clues about cause and location.*
- Describe any precipitating or relieving factors such as *sleep deficits, anxiety, temperature extremes, excessive noise, anxiety, fear, depression, and activity.*
- Describe the meaning of the pain, including its effects on lifestyle, self-concept, roles, and relationships. *Clients with acute pain may believe the pain is a normal response to injury or that it signals serious illness and death. Pain is a stressor that may affect the ability of the client to cope effectively. The client with chronic pain often has concerns about addiction to pain medication, costs, social interactions, sexual activities, and relationships with significant others.*
- Monitor manifestations of pain by taking vital signs; assessing skin temperature and moisture; observing pupils; observing facial expressions, position in bed, guarding of body parts; and noting restlessness. *Autonomic responses to pain may result in an increased blood pressure, tachycardia, rapid respirations, perspiration, and dilated pupils. Other responses to pain include grimacing, clenching the hands, muscle rigidity, guarding, restlessness, and nausea. The client with chronic pain may have an unexpressive, tired facial appearance.*

> **PRACTICE ALERT** *Consider pain the fifth vital sign and assess clients for pain every time you check temperature, pulse, respirations, and blood pressure.* ■

MediaLink | PAIN CARE PLAN

- Communicate belief in the client's pain by verbally acknowledging the presence of the pain, listening carefully to the description of pain, and acting to help the client manage the pain. *Because pain is a personal, subjective experience, the nurse must convey belief in the client's pain. By doing so, the nurse reduces anxiety and thereby lessens pain (see the Nursing Research box on this page for related research).*
- Provide optimal pain relief with prescribed analgesics, determining the preferred route of administration. Provide pain-relieving measures for severe pain on a regular around-the-clock basis or by self-administration (such as with a PCA pump). *The client is a part of the decision-making process and can exert some control over the situation by choosing the administration route. Analgesics are usually most effective when they are administered before pain occurs or becomes severe. Around-the-clock administration has been proven to provide better pain management for both acute and chronic pain.*
- Teach the client and family nonpharmacologic methods of pain management, such as relaxation, distraction, and cutaneous stimulation. *These techniques are especially useful when used in conjunction with pain medications and may also be useful in managing chronic pain.*
- Provide comfort measures, such as changing positions, back massage, oral care, skin care, and changing bed linens. *Basic comfort measures for personal cleanliness, skin care, and mobility promote physical and psychosocial well-being, lessening the perception of pain.*
- Provide client and family teaching and make referrals if necessary to assist with coping, financial resources, and home care. *The client (and family) with pain requires information about medications, noninvasive techniques for pain management, and sources of assistance with home-based care. The client with acute pain requires information about the expected course of pain resolution.*

Using NANDA, NIC, and NOC

Chart 4–1 shows links between NANDA nursing diagnosis, NIC, and NOC when caring for the client in pain.

Home Care

Teaching the client and family includes:

- Specific drugs to be taken, including the frequency, potential side effects, possible drug interactions, and any special precautions to be taken (such as taking with food or avoiding alcohol).
- How to take or administer the drugs (see Box 4–2).
- The importance of taking pain medications before the pain becomes severe.
- An explanation that the risk of addiction to pain medications is small when they are used for pain relief and management.
- The importance of scheduling periods of rest and sleep.

Suggest the following resources:

- Pain clinics
- Community support groups
- American Cancer Society
- American Pain Society

Nursing Research

Evidence-Based Practice for the Client Experiencing Pain

Pain is individualized to each person and to each painful experience. Nurses play a major role in assessing and managing pain, and must attend to the subjective quality of pain in order to successfully provide effective pain relief. The responses of the nurse to the client's expressions of pain may influence pain management, but limited research has explored this relationship. This study (Watt-Watson, Garkinel, Gallop, Stevens, & Streiner, 2000) was conducted to examine the relationship between nurses' empathic responses and their clients' pain intensity and analgesic administration after uncomplicated coronary artery bypass graft surgery. At the same time, the nurses' empathy and pain knowledge and beliefs were assessed.

The nurses were moderately empathic, and their responses did not significantly affect the clients' pain intensity or analgesia administered. The nurses showed a deficit of knowledge and misbeliefs about pain. It was postulated that the nurses may not have recognized the levels of pain intensity that occur with internal thoracic artery grafts. The researchers recommended having a better understanding of strategies to encourage clients to describe their pain experiences and to seek help. They also recommended that strategies are needed to encourage nurses to address the clients' pain experiences.

IMPLICATIONS FOR NURSING

Findings from this study support other research that nurses (and other health care providers) are prone to undertreat pain. It is necessary for nurses to make greater efforts to understand the experiences of others. It is also necessary to make additional or more specific pain assessments; for example, although the clients' pain greatly increased with movement, this specific assessment was rarely conducted. Educational programs for nurses, related to pain, should include specific postoperative pain assessments, explore myths and misconceptions about pain medications, and clarify the individualized experiences of and responses to pain.

Critical Thinking in Client Care

1. Reflect on your own experiences with pain. Will those experiences facilitate or hinder your assessments and interventions for clients in pain?
2. You are caring for a young man who has multiple injuries from a motorcycle accident. He tells you his pain is so bad that he "just wants to die." How would you respond?
3. You are caring for an 80-year-old man with diabetes who has had his left foot amputated for gangrene. He is restless and moaning. Another nurse tells you to give only one-half of the ordered dose of narcotics because "he is old and there is a danger of respiratory depression." What would you do?
4. Why do you think nurses tend to underestimate and undermedicate pain?

Note. Adapted from The Impact of Nurses' Empathic Responses on Patients' Pain Management in Acute Care *by J. Watt-Watson et al., 2000,* Nursing Research, *49(4), pp. 191–200.*

CHART 4-1 NANDA, NIC, AND NOC LINKAGES

The Client Experiencing Pain

NURSING DIAGNOSES	NURSING INTERVENTIONS	NURSING OUTCOMES
• Acute Pain • Chronic Pain	• Pain Management • Analgesic Administration • Conscious Sedation • PCA Assistance • Cutaneous Stimulation • Anxiety Reduction • TENS • Heat/Cold Application • Accupressure • Progressive Muscle Relaxation • Environmental Management: Comfort	• Pain Control Behavior • Pain: Disruptive Effects • Pain Level

Note. Data from Nursing Outcomes Classification (NOC) by M. Johnson & M. Maas (Eds.), 1997, St. Louis: Mosby; Nursing Diagnoses: Definitions & Classification 2001–2002 by North American Nursing Diagnosis Association, 2001, Philadelphia: NANDA; Nursing Interventions Classification (NIC) by J.C. McCloskey & G. M. Bulechek (Eds.), 2000, St. Louis: Mosby. Reprinted by permission.

BOX 4-2 ■ Providing Long-Term Analgesia at Home

Route	Drug	Nursing Implications
Oral	Oxycodone (OxyContin)	■ Available in a timed-release formulation for 12-hour dosing and as fast-acting formulations (OxyIR, Oxyfast) for breakthrough pain.
Oral	Morphine (Kadian)	■ Formulated of timed-release particles in a capsule. If client cannot swallow the capsule, it may be sprinkled over food or given by nasogastric or gastric tube.
Transdermal	Fentanyl (Duragesic)	■ Absorbed slowly through the skin, allows 72-hour dose schedule.
Transdermal	Liocaine (Lidoderm)	■ Effective for 12 hours for various neuropathic pains. Monitor clients also taking Class 1 antiarrhythmic drugs for increased effects.
Transmucosal	Fentanyl citrate (Actiq)	■ A lozenge formulation used to treat breakthrough cancer pain in opioid-tolerant clients.

Nursing Care Plan
A Client with Chronic Pain

Susan Akers, age 37, is currently being seen at an outpatient clinic for chronic nonmalignant pain. She works at a local paper factory. She has a 3-year history of neck and shoulder pain that usually is accompanied by headaches. She believes the pain is related to lifting objects at work, but it is now precipitated by activities of daily living. Susan is absent from work approximately three times a month and states that the absences are due to her pain and headaches. She has been seeking care in the local emergency department on the average of twice monthly for injections for pain. She does not regularly use medications but does take Darvocet-N 100 and Valium as needed (usually two to three times a day). Ms. Akers is divorced and has two children. She states that she has several friends in the area, but her parents and siblings live in another part of the United States.

ASSESSMENT

During the nursing history, Susan rates her pain during an acute episode as a 7 on a 1 to 10 scale. She states that lifting objects and moving her hands and arms above shoulder level precipitates sharp pain. The pain never really goes away, but it does decrease with upper extremity rest. She says that when she lifts a lot at work, she has difficulty sleeping that night. She takes two Darvocet-N 100 tablets every 4 hours when the pain is severe, but does not get complete relief.

DIAGNOSIS

• *Chronic pain* related to muscle inflammation

EXPECTED OUTCOMES

• Return for follow-up visits with a journal of activities and pain experiences.
• After 3 to 5 days on regularly scheduled doses of pain medication, report a decrease in the level of pain from 7 to 3 or 4 on a 1 to 10 scale.
• Decrease number of absences from work.
• Modify activities at work and at home, especially when pain is intense.

(continued on page 74)

Nursing Care Plan
A Client with Chronic Pain *(continued)*

PLANNING AND IMPLEMENTATION

- Encourage discussion of pain, and acknowledge belief in Susan's report of pain.
- Consult with a physician for a nonnarcotic analgesic with a minimum of side effects, and instruct in maintaining regular dosing schedules.
- For episodes of acute pain, take narcotic analgesics as soon as the pain begins and every 4 hours, while continuing the dosage of nonnarcotic analgesic.
- Teach one relaxation technique that is personally useful.
- Explore distraction techniques such as listening to music, watching comedies, or reading.
- Provide clinic phone number and instruct to call if pain is unrelieved with narcotic and nonnarcotic analgesics.

EVALUATION

Susan returns for scheduled follow-up visits with a completed journal of her activities and associated pain. She reports that taking oral narcotic analgesics has relieved her pain and that within 3 weeks nonnarcotic analgesics brought her pain under control. She also reports that her supervisor has reassigned her to a position that requires no lifting. She now rates her pain at 2 or 3 on a 1 to 10 scale. She has missed only 1 day of work in the last 3 months and reports that her children and friends have helped with her household tasks when she has requested they do so.

Critical Thinking in the Nursing Process

1. Describe three factors that support the statement, "Pain is a personal experience."
2. Susan asks you how often she should take her pain medications. You tell her to (a) take them on a regular basis or (b) wait until she experiences pain. Which action would you choose, and why?
3. Develop a care plan for Susan for the nursing diagnosis of *risk for constipation.* Why is this necessary?

See Evaluating Your Response in Appendix C.

EXPLORE MediaLink

NCLEX review questions, case studies, care plan activities, MediaLink applications, and other interactive resources for this chapter can be found on the Companion Website at www.prenhall.com/lemone.

Click on Chapter 4 to select the activities for this chapter. For animations, video clips, more NCLEX review questions, and an audio glossary, access the Student CD-ROM accompanying this textbook.

TEST YOURSELF

1. Your neighbor has had lower back pain for 9 months. How would this pain be categorized?
   a. Acute pain
   b. Chronic pain
   c. Referred pain
   d. Somatic pain

2. Which of the following statements is a pain myth?
   a. "It is best to wait until a client has pain before giving medication."
   b. "Anxiety can cause pain; pain can cause anxiety."
   c. "Meperidine (Demerol) is no longer recommended for postoperative pain."
   d. "The rationale for use of a TENS unit is supported by the gate control theory."

3. You are taking a health history for a client who has taken an NSAID for several years. What would be an appropriate question to ask?
   a. "Do you understand what this drug could do to you?"

   b. "Have you ever vomited blood or had very dark stools?"
   c. "Do you know that you may become addicted to this drug?"
   d. "Have you noticed any problems with your breathing?"

4. You are replacing a transdermal pain medication. Where on the body would you place it?
   a. On one side of the buttocks
   b. Below the navel, midline on the abdomen
   c. On the anterior thigh
   d. On the upper torso

5. Which of the following statements would be most useful in determining the *quality* of a client's pain?
   a. "Tell me where you hurt."
   b. "Rate your pain on a scale of 0 to 10."
   c. "Describe what your pain feels like."
   d. "Tell me how this pain affects your sleep."

See Test Yourself answers in Appendix C.

BIBLIOGRAPHY

Acello, B. (2000). Controlling pain. Facing fears about opioid addiction. *Nursing, 30*(5), 72.

Ackerman, C., & Turkoski, B. (2000). Using guided imagery to reduce pain and anxiety. *Home Healthcare Nurse, 18*(8), 524–530.

American Pain Society. 2001. *Pain: The fifth vital sign.* Available www.ampainsoc.org

American Pain Society Quality of Care Committee. (1995). Quality improvement guidelines for the treatment of acute pain and cancer pain. *Journal of the American Medical Association, 274*(23), 1874–1880.

Anonymous. (1997). The use of opioids for the treatment of chronic pain: A consensus statement from the American Academy of Pain Medicine and the American Pain Society. *Clinical Journal of Pain, 13*(1), 6–8.

Berkowitz, C. (1997). Epidural pain control—your job, too. *RN, 60*(8), 22–27.

Carpenito, L. (2000). *Nursing diagnosis: Application to clinical practice* (8th ed.). Philadelphia: Lippincott.

Coyne, M., Smith, J., Stein, D., Hieser, M., & Hoover, L. (1998). Describing pain management documentation. *MEDSURG Nursing, 7*(1), 45–51.

Dellasega, C., & Keiser, C. (1997). Pharmacologic approaches to chronic pain in the older adult. *American Journal of Primary Health Care, 22*(5), 20, 22–24, 26.

Joint Commission on Accreditation of Healthcare Organizations. (2000). *Joint Commission on Accreditation of Healthcare Organizations pain standards for 2001.* Available www.jcaho.org

Kodiath, M. (1997). Chronic pain: Contrasting two cultures. *Clinical Excellence for Nurse Practitioners, 1*(1), 59–61.

Lipson, J., Dibble, S., & Minarik, P. (1996). *Culture & nursing care: A pocket guide.* San Francisco: UCSF Nursing Press.

McCaffery, M. (1979). *Nursing management of the patient with pain.* Philadelphia: Lippincott.

McCaffery, M., & Beebe, A. (1999). *Pain: Clinical manual.* St. Louis: Mosby.

McCance, K., & Huether, S. (2002). *Pathophysiology: The biologic basic for disease in adults and children* (4th ed.). St. Louis: Mosby.

McKenry, L., & Salerno, E. (1998). *Pharmacology in nursing* (20th ed.). St. Louis: Mosby.

Melzack, R. (1975). The McGill Pain Questionnaire: Major properties and scoring methods. *Pain, 1,* 277.

Melzack, R., & Wall, P. (1965). Pain mechanisms: A new theory. *Science, 150,* 971–979.

_____ . (1968). Gate control theory of pain. In A. Soulairac, J. Cahn, & J. Carpentier (Eds.), *Pain: Proceedings of the International Association on Pain.* Baltimore: Williams & Wilkins.

Merboth, M. K., & Barnason, S. (2000). Managing pain: The fifth vital sign. *Nursing Clinics of North America, 35*(2), 375–383.

Pasero, C. (1999). Using agonist-antagonist opioids and antagonist drugs. *American Journal of Nursing, 99*(1), 20–21.

_____ . (2000). Oral patient-controlled analgesia. *American Journal of Nursing, 100*(3), 24.

Pasero, C., & McCaffrey, M. (1999). Opioids by the rectal route. *American Journal of Nursing, 99*(11), 20.

_____ . (2000). When patients can't report pain. *American Journal of Nursing, 100*(9), 22–23.

Porth, C. (2002). *Pathophysiology: Concepts of altered health states* (6th ed.). Philadelphia: Lippincott.

Seal, R. (1997). Choosing the right step on the analgesic ladder. *Community Nurse, 3*(2), 58–59.

U.S. Department of Health and Human Services. (1992). *Acute pain management: Operative or medical procedures and trauma* (AHCPR Publication No. 92-0032). Rockville, MD: Agency for Health Care Policy and Research, Public Health Service, USDHHS.

Victor, K. (2001). Properly assessing pain in the elderly. *RN, 64*(5), 45–49.

Waitman, J., & McCaffery, M. (2001). Meperidine—A liability. *American Journal of Nursing, 101*(1), 57–58.

Watt-Watson, J., Garfinkel, P., Gallop, R., Stevens, B., & Streiner, D. (2000). The impact of nurses' empathic responses on patients' pain management in acute care. *Nursing Research, 49*(4), 191–200.

Wilson, B. A., Shannon, M. T., & Stang, C. L. (2001). *Nursing drug guide 2001.* Upper Saddle River, NJ: Prentice Hall.

World Health Organization. (1986/1990). *Cancer pain relief.* Geneva: WHO.

CHAPTER | 5

Nursing Care of Clients with Altered Fluid, Electrolyte, or Acid-Base Balance

MediaLink

www.prenhall.com/lemone

Additional resources for this chapter can be found on the Student CD-ROM accompanying this textbook, and on the Companion Website at www.prenhall.com/lemone. Click on Chapter 5 to select the activities for this chapter.

CD-ROM
- Audio Glossary
- NCLEX Review

Animations
- Membrane Transport
- Acid-Base Balance
- Fluid Balance

Companion Website
- More NCLEX Review
- Case Study
    Hypernatremia
- Care Plan Activity
    Fluid Volume Deficit
    Hypocalcemia
- MediaLink Application
    Metabolic Acidosis and Type 1 Diabetes

LEARNING OUTCOMES

After completing this chapter, you will be able to:

- Discuss the functions and regulatory mechanisms that maintain water and electrolyte balance in the body.

- Compare and contrast the causes, effects, and care of the client with fluid volume or electrolyte imbalance.

- Describe the pathophysiology and manifestations of imbalances of sodium, potassium, calcium, magnesium, and phosphorus.

- Discuss the causes and effects of acid-base imbalances.

- Identify laboratory and diagnostic tests used to diagnose and monitor treatment of fluid, electrolyte, and acid-base disorders.

- Recognize normal and abnormal values of electrolytes in the blood.

- Use arterial blood gas findings to identify the type of acid-base imbalance present in a client.

- Provide teaching about diet and medications used to treat or prevent electrolyte disorders.

- Use the nursing process as a framework to provide individualized nursing care to clients with fluid, electrolyte, and acid-base disorders.

Changes in the normal distribution and composition of body fluids often occur in response to illness and trauma. These changes affect fluid balance of the intracellular and extracellular compartments of the body, the concentration of electrolytes within fluid compartments, and the body's hydrogen ion concentration (pH). Normal physiologic processes depend on a relatively stable state in the internal environment of the body. The fluid volume, electrolyte composition, and pH of both intracellular and extracellular spaces must remain constant within a relatively narrow range to maintain health and life.

Homeostasis is the body's tendency to maintain a state of physiologic balance in the presence of constantly changing conditions. Homeostasis is necessary if the body is to function optimally at a cellular level and as a total organism. Homeostasis depends on multiple factors in both the external and internal environments, such as available oxygen in the air and nutrients in food, as well as normal body temperature, respiration, and digestive processes. The normal volume, composition, distribution, and pH of body fluids reflect a state of homeostasis.

The goal in managing fluid, electrolyte, and acid-base imbalances is to reestablish and maintain a normal balance. Nursing care includes assessing clients who are likely to develop imbalances, monitoring clients for early manifestations, and implementing collaborative and nursing interventions to prevent or correct imbalances. Effective nursing interventions require an understanding of the multiple processes that maintain fluid, electrolyte, and acid-base balance and an understanding of the causes and treatment of imbalances that occur.

Mechanisms that maintain normal fluid and electrolyte balance are discussed first, followed by sections on fluid imbalances and electrolyte imbalances. Discussion of normal acid-base balance precedes discussion of acid-base imbalances. Case studies related to selected fluid, electrolyte, and acid-base disorders are found throughout the chapter.

OVERVIEW OF NORMAL FLUID AND ELECTROLYTE BALANCE

Fluid and electrolyte balance in the body involves regulatory mechanisms that maintain the composition, distribution, and movement of fluids and electrolytes. This section provides an overview of fluid and electrolyte balance in the body. It is followed by discussion of fluid volume and electrolyte balance disorders.

Body Fluid Composition

Body fluid is composed of water and various dissolved substances (solutes).

Water

Water is the primary component of body fluids. It functions in several ways to maintain normal cellular function. Water:

- Provides a medium for the transport and exchange of nutrients and other substances such as oxygen, carbon dioxide, and metabolic wastes to and from cells.
- Provides a medium for metabolic reactions within cells.
- Assists in regulating body temperature through the evaporation of perspiration.

- Provides form for body structure and acts as a shock absorber.
- Provides insulation.
- Acts as a lubricant.

Total body water constitutes about 60% of the total body weight, but this amount varies with age, gender, and the amount of body fat. Total body water decreases with aging; in people over age 65, body water may decrease to 45% to 50% of total body weight. Fat cells contain comparatively little water: In the person who is obese, the proportion of water to total body weight is less than in the person of average weight; in a person who is very thin, the proportion of water to total body weight is greater than in the person of average weight. Adult females have a greater ratio of fat to lean tissue mass than adult males; therefore, they have a lower percentage of body water content.

To maintain normal fluid balance, body water intake and output should be approximately equal. The average fluid intake and output usually is about 2500 mL over a 24-hour period. Table 5–1 shows the sources of fluid gain and loss.

Electrolytes

Body fluids contain both water molecules and chemical compounds. These chemical compounds can either remain intact in solution or separate (dissociate) into discrete particles. **Electrolytes** are substances that dissociate in solution to form charged particles called ions. *Cations* are positively charged electrolytes; *anions* are negatively charged electrolytes. For example, sodium chloride (NaCl) in solution dissociates into a sodium ion, a cation carrying a positive charge (Na^+); and a chloride ion, an anion carrying a negative charge (Cl^-). Electrolytes may be *univalent*, with only one unit of electrical charge, such as sodium (Na^+) and chloride (Cl^-); or they may be *divalent*, carrying two units of electrical charge, such as magnesium (Mg^{2+}) and phosphate (HPO_4^{2-}).

Electrolytes have many functions. They:

- Assist in regulating water balance.
- Help regulate and maintain acid-base balance.
- Contribute to enzyme reactions.
- Are essential for neuromuscular activity.

The concentration of electrolytes in body fluids generally is measured in milliequivalents per liter of water (mEq/L).

TABLE 5–1 Balanced Fluid Gain and Loss for an Adult

	Source	Amount (mL)
Gain	Fluids taken orally	1200
	Water in food	1000
	Water as by-product of food metabolism	300 ↓
	Total	2500
Loss		↑
	Urine	1500
	Feces	200
	Perspiration	300
	Respiration	500

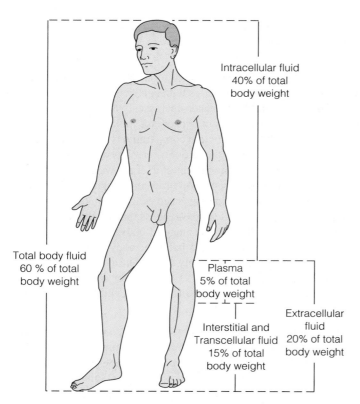

Figure 5–1 ■ The major fluid compartments of the body.

A milliequivalent is a measure of the chemical combining power of the ion. For example, 100 mEq of sodium (Na^+) can combine with 100 mEq of chloride (Cl^-) to form sodium chloride (NaCl). Sodium, potassium, and chloride usually are measured in milliequivalents. In some cases, the amount of an electrolyte in body fluid may be measured by weight in milligrams per 100 mL (1 deciliter [dL]) of water (mg/dL). Calcium, magnesium, and phosphorus often are measured by weight in milligrams per deciliter.

Body Fluid Distribution

Body fluid is classified by its location inside or outside of cells. *Intracellular fluid (ICF)* is found within cells. It accounts for approximately 40% of total body weight (Figure 5–1 ■). ICF is essential for normal cell function, providing a medium for metabolic processes. *Extracellular fluid (ECF)* is located outside of cells. It accounts for approximately 20% of the total body weight. ECF is classified by location.

- Interstitial fluid is located in the spaces between most of the cells of the body. It accounts for approximately 15% of total body weight.
- Intravascular fluid, called plasma, is contained within the arteries, veins, and capillaries. It accounts for approximately 5% of total body weight.
- Transcellular fluid includes urine; digestive secretions; perspiration; and cerebrospinal, pleural, synovial, intraocular, gonadal, and pericardial fluids.

A trace amount of water is found in bone, cartilage, and other dense connective tissues; this water is not exchangeable with other body fluids.

ECF is the transport medium that carries oxygen and nutrients to and waste products from the cells. For example, plasma transports oxygen from the lungs and glucose from the digestive system to the tissues. These solutes diffuse through the capillary wall into the interstitial space, and from there across the cell membrane into the cells. Waste products of metabolism (e.g., carbon dioxide and hydrogen ion) diffuse from the intracellular space into the interstitial space, and from there into plasma via the capillary walls. Plasma then transports these waste products to the lungs and kidneys for elimination.

The concentration of various electrolytes in ICF and ECF differs significantly, as shown in Figure 5–2 ■. ICF contains high concentrations of potassium (K^+), magnesium (Mg^{2+}), and phosphate (PO_4^{2-}), as well as other solutes such as glucose and oxygen. Sodium (Na^+), chloride (Cl^-), and bicarbonate (HCO_3^-) are the principal extracellular electrolytes. The high sodium concentration in ECF is essential to regulating body fluid volume. The concentration of potassium in ECF is low. There is a minimal difference in electrolyte concentration between plasma and interstitial fluid. Normal values for electrolytes in plasma are shown in Table 5–2.

The body fluid compartments are separated by several types of membranes.

- Cell membranes separate interstitial fluid from intracellular fluid.
- Capillary membranes separate plasma from interstitial fluid.
- Epithelial membranes separate transcellular fluid from interstitial fluid and plasma. These membranes include the mucosa of the stomach, intestines, and gallbladder; the pleural, peritoneal, and synovial membranes; and the tubules of the kidney.

A cell membrane consists of layers of lipid and protein molecules. The layering of these molecules controls the passage of fluid and solutes between the cell and interstitial fluid. The cell membrane is selectively permeable; that is, it allows the passage of water, oxygen, carbon dioxide, and small water-soluble molecules, but bars proteins and other intracellular colloids.

The capillary membrane separating the plasma from the interstitial space is made of squamous epithelial cells. Pores in the membrane allow solute molecules (such as glucose and sodium), dissolved gases, and water to cross the membrane. Minute amounts of albumin and other proteins can also pass through the pores of a capillary membrane, but normally plasma proteins stay in the intravascular compartment.

Body Fluid Movement

Four chemical and physiologic processes control the movement of fluid, electrolytes, and other molecules across membranes between the intracellular and interstitial space and the interstitial space and plasma. These processes are osmosis, diffusion, filtration, and active transport.

OSMOSIS. The process by which water moves across a selectively permeable membrane from an area of lower solute concentration to an area of higher solute concentration is **osmosis** (Figure 5–3 ■). A *selectively permeable membrane* allows water molecules to cross but is relatively impermeable to dissolved substances (*solutes*). Osmosis continues until the solute

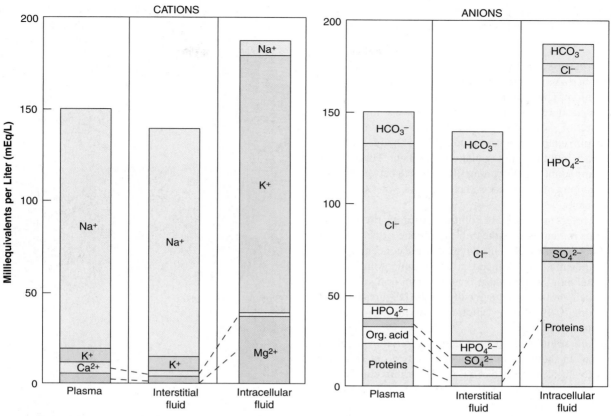

Figure 5–2 ■ Electrolyte composition (cations and anions) of body fluid compartments.

From Fundamentals of Anatomy and Physiology 4e, *by Martini, Frederic. © Reprinted by permission of Pearson Education, Inc., Upper Saddle River, NJ.*

TABLE 5-2	Normal Values for Electrolytes and Serum Osmolality	
Serum Component	**Values**
Electrolytes	
Sodium (Na⁺)	135–145 mEq/L
Chloride (Cl⁻)	98–106 mEq/L
Bicarbonate (HCO₃)	22–26 mEq/L
Calcium (Ca²⁺) (total)	8.5–10 mg/dL
Potassium (K⁺)	3.5–5.0 mEq/L
Phosphate/inorganic phosphorus (PO₄⁻²)	1.7–2.6 mEq/L (2.5–4.5 mg/dL)
Magnesium (Mg²⁺)	1.6–2.6 mg/dL (1.3–2.1 mEq/L)
Serum osmolality	275–295 mOsm/kg

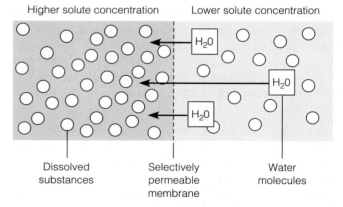

Figure 5–3 ■ Osmosis. Water molecules move through a selectively permeable membrane from an area of low solute concentration to an area of high solute concentration.

concentration on both sides of the membrane is equal. For example, if pure water and a sodium chloride solution are separated by a selectively permeable membrane, then water molecules will move across the membrane to the sodium chloride solution. Osmosis is the primary process that controls body fluid movement between the ICF and ECF compartments.

Osmolarity and Osmolality. The concentration of a solution may be expressed as the osmolarity or osmolality of the solution. *Osmolarity* refers to the amount of solutes per liter of solution (by volume); it is reported in milliosmoles per liter (mOsm/L) in a solution. *Osmolality* refers to the number of solutes per kilogram of water (by weight); it is reported in milliosmoles per kilogram (mOsm/kg). Because osmotic activity in the body is regulated by the number of active particles (solutes) per kilogram of water, osmolality is used to describe the concentration of body fluids. The normal osmolality of both ICF and ECF ranges between 275 and 295 mOsm/kg. The osmolality of the extracellular fluid depends chiefly on sodium concentration. Serum osmolality may be estimated by doubling the serum sodium concentration (approximately 142 mEq/L).

Osmotic Pressure and Tonicity.   The power of a solution to draw water across a membrane is known as the *osmotic pressure* of the solution. The composition of interstitial fluid and intravascular plasma is essentially the same except for a higher concentration of proteins in the plasma. These proteins (especially albumin) exert osmotic pressure, pulling fluid from the interstitial space into the intravascular compartment. This osmotic activity is important in maintaining fluid balance between the interstitial and intravascular spaces, helping hold water within the vascular system.

Tonicity refers to the effect a solution's osmotic pressure has on water movement across the cell membrane of cells within that solution. *Isotonic* solutions have the same concentration of solutes as plasma. Cells placed in an isotonic solution will neither shrink nor swell as there is no net gain or loss of water within the cell, and no change in cell volume (Figure 5–4 A ■). Normal saline (0.9% sodium chloride solution) is an example of an isotonic solution.

Hypertonic solutions have a greater concentration of solutes than plasma. In their presence, water is drawn out of a cell, causing it to shrink (Figure 5–4B). A 3% sodium chloride solution is hypertonic. *Hypotonic* solutions (such as 0.45% sodium chloride) have a lower solute concentration than plasma (Figure 5–4C). When red blood cells are placed in a hypotonic solution, water moves into the cells, causing them to swell and rupture (*hemolyze*).

The concepts of osmotic draw and tonicity are important in understanding the pathophysiologic changes that occur with fluid and electrolyte imbalances, as well as treatment measures. For example, an increased sodium concentration of extracellular fluid causes water to shift from the ICF compartment to the ECF compartment. In this case, administering a hypotonic intravenous solution will facilitate water movement back into the intracellular space.

DIFFUSION.   The process by which solute molecules move from an area of high solute concentration to an area of low solute concentration to become evenly distributed is **diffusion** (Figure 5–5 ■). The two types of diffusion are simple and facilitated diffusion. *Simple diffusion* occurs by the random movement of particles through a solution. Water, carbon dioxide, oxygen, and solutes move between plasma and the interstitial space by simple diffusion through the capillary membrane. Water and solutes move into the cell by passing through protein channels or by dissolving in the lipid cell membrane. *Facilitated diffusion*, also called carrier-mediated diffusion, allows large water-soluble molecules, such as glucose and amino acids, to diffuse across cell membranes. Proteins embedded in the cell membrane function as *carriers*, helping large molecules cross the membrane.

The rate of diffusion is influenced by a number of factors, such as the concentration of solute and the availability of carrier proteins in the cell membrane. The effect of both simple and facilitated diffusion is to establish equal concentrations of the molecules on both sides of a membrane.

A Isotonic solution

B Hypertonic solution

C Hypotonic solution

Figure 5–4 ■ The effect of tonicity on red blood cells. *A,* In an isotonic solution, RBCs neither gain nor lose water. *B,* In a hypertonic solution, cells lose water and shrink in size. *C,* In a hypotonic solution, cells absorb water and may burst (hemolysis).

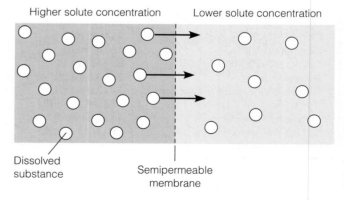

Figure 5–5 ■ Diffusion. Solute molecules move through a semipermeable membrane from an area of high solute concentration to an area of low solute concentration.

FILTRATION.   The process by which water and dissolved substances (solutes) move from an area of high hydrostatic pressure to an area of low hydrostatic pressure is **filtration.** This usually occurs across capillary membranes. *Hydrostatic pres-*

Figure 5–6 ■ Fluid balance between the intravascular and interstitial spaces is maintained in the capillary beds by a balance of filtration at the arterial end and osmotic draw at the venous end.

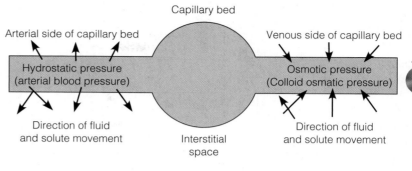

Medialink | MEMBRANE TRANSPORT ANIMATION

sure is created by the pumping action of the heart and gravity against the capillary wall. Filtration occurs in the glomerulus of the kidneys, as well as at the arterial end of capillaries.

A balance of hydrostatic (filtration) pressure and osmotic pressure regulates the movement of water between the intravascular and interstitial spaces in the capillary beds of the body. Hydrostatic pressure within the arterial end of the capillary pushes water into the interstitial space. Hydrostatic pressure within the interstitial space opposes this movement to some degree. At the venous end of the capillary, the osmotic force of plasma proteins draws fluid back into the capillary (Figure 5–6 ■).

ACTIVE TRANSPORT. **Active transport** allows molecules to move across cell membranes and epithelial membranes against a concentration gradient. This movement requires energy (adenosine triphosphate, or ATP) and a carrier mechanism to maintain a higher concentration of a substance on one side of the membrane than on the other. The sodium-potassium pump is an important example of active transport (Figure 5–7 ■). High concentrations of potassium in intracellular fluids and of sodium in extracellular fluids are maintained because cells actively transport potassium from interstitial fluid (where the concentration of potassium is about 5 mEq/L) into intracellular fluid (where the potassium concentration is about 150 mEq/L).

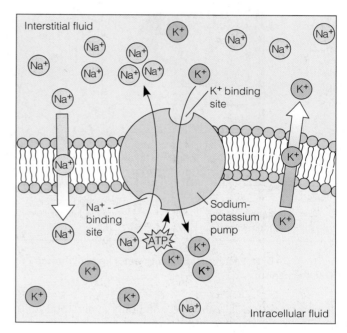

Figure 5–7 ■ The sodium-potassium pump. Sodium and potassium ions are moved across the cell membranes against their concentration gradients. This active transport process is fueled by energy from adenosine triphosphate (ATP).

Body Fluid Regulation

Homeostasis requires several regulatory mechanisms and processes to maintain the balance between fluid intake and excretion. These include thirst, the kidneys, renin-angiotensin-aldosterone mechanism, antidiuretic hormone, and atrial natriuretic factor. These mechanisms affect the volume, distribution, and composition of body fluids.

Thirst

Thirst is the primary regulator of water intake. Thirst plays an important role in maintaining fluid balance and preventing dehydration. The thirst center, located in the brain, is stimulated when the blood volume drops because of water losses or when serum osmolality (solute concentration) increases (Figure 5–8 ■).

The thirst mechanism is highly effective in regulating extracellular sodium levels. Increased sodium in ECF causes the serum osmolality to increase, stimulating the thirst center. Fluid intake in turn reduces the sodium concentration of ECF

and lowers serum osmolality. Conversely, a drop in serum sodium and low serum osmolality inhibit the thirst center.

> **PRACTICE ALERT** *The thirst mechanism declines with aging, making older adults more vulnerable to dehydration and hyperosmolality (high serum osmolality). Clients with an altered level of consciousness or who are unable to respond to thirst also are at risk.* ■

Kidneys

The kidneys are primarily responsible for regulating fluid volume and electrolyte balance in the body. They regulate the volume and osmolality of body fluids by controlling the excretion of water and electrolytes. In adults, about 170 L of plasma are filtered through the glomeruli every day. By selectively reabsorbing water and electrolytes, the kidneys maintain the volume and osmolality of body fluids. About 99% of the

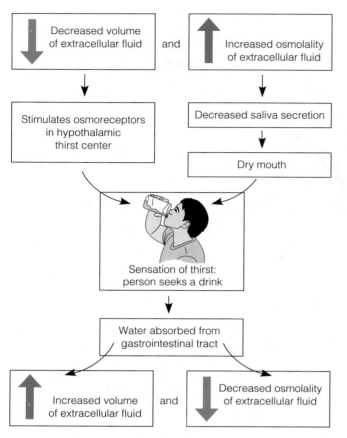

Figure 5–8 ■ Factors stimulating water intake through the thirst mechanism.

Figure 5–9 ■ The renin-angiotensin-aldosterone system. Decreased blood volume and renal perfusion set off a chain of reactions leading to release of aldosterone from the adrenal cortex. Increased levels of aldosterone regulate serum K^+ and Na^+, blood pressure, and water balance through effects on the kidney tubules.

glomerular filtrate is reabsorbed, and only about 1500 mL of urine is produced over a 24-hour period.

Renin-Angiotensin-Aldosterone System

The renin-angiotensin-aldosterone system works to maintain intravascular fluid balance and blood pressure. A fall in blood flow or blood pressure to the kidneys stimulates specialized receptors in the juxtaglomerular cells of the nephrons to produce *renin*, an enzyme. Renin converts angiotensinogen (a plasma protein) in the circulating blood into angiotensin I. Angiotensin I travels through the bloodstream to the lungs, where it is converted to angiotensin II by angiotensin-converting enzyme (ACE). Angiotensin II is a potent vasoconstrictor; it raises the blood pressure. It also stimulates the thirst mechanism to promote fluid intake and acts directly on the kidneys, causing them to retain sodium and water. Angiotensin II stimulates the adrenal cortex to release aldosterone. Aldosterone promotes sodium and water retention in the distal nephron of the kidney, restoring blood volume (Figure 5–9 ■).

Antidiuretic Hormone

Antidiuretic hormone (ADH) regulates water excretion from the kidneys. Osmoreceptors in the hypothalamus respond to increases in serum osmolality and decreases in blood volume, stimulating ADH production and release. ADH acts on the distal tubules of the kidney, making them more permeable to water and thus increasing water reabsorption. With increased water reabsorption, urine output falls, blood volume is restored, and serum osmolality drops as the water dilutes body fluids (Figure 5–10 ■).

Two disorders of ADH production illustrate this effect. First, diabetes insipidus is a condition characterized by a deficiency in ADH production. The lack of ADH causes the distal tubules and collecting ducts of the kidney to be impermeable to water, resulting in copious, very dilute urine output. ADH is not released in response to resulting serum hyperosmolality, but the thirst mechanism is stimulated and the client drinks additional fluids, maintaining high urine output. Second, in the syndrome of inappropriate ADH secretion (SIADH), excess ADH is released. Increased water reabsorption causes increased fluid volume and scant, concentrated urine output. These diseases of the pituitary gland are discussed in Chapter 17. ∞

Atrial Natriuretic Factor

Atrial natriuretic factor (ANF) is a hormone released by atrial muscle cells in response to distension from fluid overload. ANF affects several body systems, including the cardiovascular, renal, neural, gastrointestinal, and endocrine systems, but it primarily affects the renin-angiotensin-aldosterone system. ANF opposes this system by inhibiting renin secretion and blocking the secretion and sodium-retaining effects of aldosterone. As a result, ANF promotes sodium wasting and diuresis (increased urine output) and causes vasodilation.

↓ Blood pressure
↓ Blood volume
↑ Blood osmolality

Osmoreceptors in hypothalamus stimulate posterior pituitary to secrete ADH

ADH increases distal tubule permeability to ↑ reabsorption of H_2O

Urine output
↑ Blood pressure
↑ Blood volume
↓ Blood osmolality

Figure 5–10 ■ Antidiuretic hormone (ADH) release and effect. Increased serum osmolality or a fall in blood volume stimulates the release of ADH from the posterior pituitary. ADH increases the permeability of distal tubules, promoting water reabsorption.

FLUID AND ELECTROLYTE IMBALANCES

THE CLIENT WITH FLUID VOLUME DEFICIT

Fluid volume deficit (FVD) is a decrease in intravascular, interstitial, and/or intracellular fluid in the body. Fluid volume deficits may be due to excessive fluid losses, insufficient fluid intake, or failure of regulatory mechanisms and fluid shifts within the body. Fluid volume deficit is a relatively common problem that may exist alone or in combination with other electrolyte or acid-base imbalances. The term **dehydration** refers to loss of water alone, even though it often is used interchangeably with fluid volume deficit.

PATHOPHYSIOLOGY

The most common cause of fluid volume deficit is excessive loss of gastrointestinal fluids from vomiting, diarrhea, gastrointestinal suctioning, intestinal fistulas, and intestinal drainage. Other causes of fluid losses include:

- Excessive renal losses of water and sodium from diuretic therapy, renal disorders, or endocrine disorders.
- Water and sodium losses during sweating from excessive exercise or increased environmental temperature.
- Hemorrhage.
- Chronic abuse of laxatives and/or enemas.

Inadequate fluid intake may result from lack of access to fluids, inability to request or to swallow fluids, oral trauma, or altered thirst mechanisms. Older adults are at particular risk for fluid volume deficit (see Nursing Care of the Older Adult box on page 84).

Fluid volume deficit can develop slowly or rapidly, depending on the type of fluid loss. Loss of extracellular fluid volume can lead to **hypovolemia,** decreased circulating blood volume. Electrolytes often are lost along with fluid, resulting in an **isotonic fluid volume deficit.** When both water and electrolytes are lost, the serum sodium level remains normal, although levels of other electrolytes such as potassium may fall. Fluid is drawn into the vascular compartment from the interstitial spaces as the body attempts to maintain tissue perfusion. This eventually depletes fluid in the intracellular compartment as well.

Hypovolemia stimulates regulatory mechanisms to maintain circulation. The sympathetic nervous system is stimulated, as is the thirst mechanism. ADH and aldosterone are released, prompting sodium and water retention by the kidneys.

Third Spacing

Third spacing is a shift of fluid from the vascular space into an area where it is not available to support normal physiologic processes. The trapped fluid represents a volume loss and is

Nursing Care of the Older Adult

FLUID VOLUME DEFICIT

The older adult is at risk for fluid volume deficit from a variety of factors. Physical changes include the following:

- The perception of thirst decreases with aging.
- As muscle tissue declines with aging, the amount of total body water decreases.
- Renal blood flow and glomerular filtration decline with aging, and the ability to concentrate urine decreases.
- Body temperature regulation is less effective with aging.

Functional changes of aging also affect fluid balance:

- Fear of incontinence can lead to self-limiting of fluid intake.

- Physical disabilities associated with age-related illnesses, such as arthritis or stroke, may limit access to fluids.
- Cognitive impairments can interfere with recognition of thirst and the ability to respond to it.

Older adults who have self-care deficits, or who are confused, depressed, tube fed, on bed rest, or taking medications (such as sedatives, tranquilizers, diuretics, and laxatives) are at greatest risk for fluid volume deficits. Older adults without air conditioning are at risk during extremely hot weather.

---

unavailable for normal physiologic processes. Fluid may be sequestered in the abdomen or bowel, or in such other actual or potential body spaces as the pleural or peritoneal space. Fluid may also become trapped within soft tissues following trauma or burns. Assessing the extent of fluid volume deficit resulting from third spacing is difficult. It may not be reflected by changes in weight or intake-and-output records, and it may not become apparent until after organ malfunction occurs (Metheny, 2000).

MANIFESTATIONS

With a rapid fluid loss (such as hemorrhage or uncontrolled vomiting), manifestations of hypovolemia develop rapidly. When the loss of fluid occurs more gradually, the client's fluid volume may be very low before symptoms develop. The *Multisystem Effects of Fluid Volume Deficit* are illustrated on page 85.

Rapid weight loss is a good indicator of fluid volume deficit. Each liter of body fluid weighs about 1 kg (2.2 lb). Loss of interstitial fluid causes skin turgor to diminish. When pinched, the skin of a client with FVD remains elevated. Loss of skin elasticity with aging makes this assessment finding less accurate in older adults. Tongue turgor is not generally affected by age; therefore, assessing the size, dryness, and longitudinal furrows of the tongue may be a more accurate indicator of fluid volume deficit.

Postural or orthostatic hypotension is a sign of hypovolemia. A drop of more than 15 mmHg in systolic blood pressure when changing from a lying to standing position often indicates loss of intravascular volume. Venous pressure falls as well, causing flat neck veins, even when the client is recumbent. Loss of intravascular fluid causes the hematocrit to increase.

Compensatory mechanisms to conserve water and sodium and maintain circulation account for many of the manifestations of fluid volume deficit, such as tachycardia; pale, cool skin (vasoconstriction); and decreased urine output. The specific gravity of urine increases as water is reabsorbed in the tubules. Table 5–3 compares assessment findings for fluid deficit and fluid excess.

COLLABORATIVE CARE

The primary goals of care related to fluid volume deficit are to prevent deficits in clients at risk and to correct deficits and their underlying causes. Depending on the acuity of the imbalance, treatment may include replacement of fluids and electrolytes by the intravenous, oral, or enteral route. When possible, the oral or enteral route is preferred for administering fluids. In acute situations, however, intravenous fluid administration is necessary.

Diagnostic Tests

Laboratory and diagnostic tests may be ordered when fluid volume deficit is suspected. Such tests measure:

- *Serum electrolytes.* In an isotonic fluid deficit, sodium levels are within normal limits; when the loss is water only, sodium levels are high. Decreases in potassium are common.
- *Serum osmolality.* To help differentiate isotonic fluid loss from water loss. With water loss, osmolality is high; it may be within normal limits with an isotonic fluid loss.
- *Serum hemoglobin and hematocrit.* The hematocrit often is elevated due to loss of intravascular volume and hemoconcentration.
- *Urine specific gravity and osmolality.* As the kidneys conserve water, both the specific gravity and osmolality of urine increase.
- *Central venous pressure (CVP).* The CVP measures the mean pressure in the superior vena cava or right atrium, providing an accurate assessment of fluid volume status. The technique for measuring CVP is outlined in Box 5–1.

Fluid Management

A fluid challenge may be done to evaluate fluid volume when urine output is low and cardiac or renal function is questionable. A fluid challenge helps prevent fluid volume overload resulting from intravenous fluid therapy when cardiac or renal function is compromised. Nursing responsibilities for a fluid challenge are as follows:

1. Obtain and document baseline vital signs, breath sounds, urine output, and mental status.

Multisystem Effects of Fluid Volume Deficit (FVD)

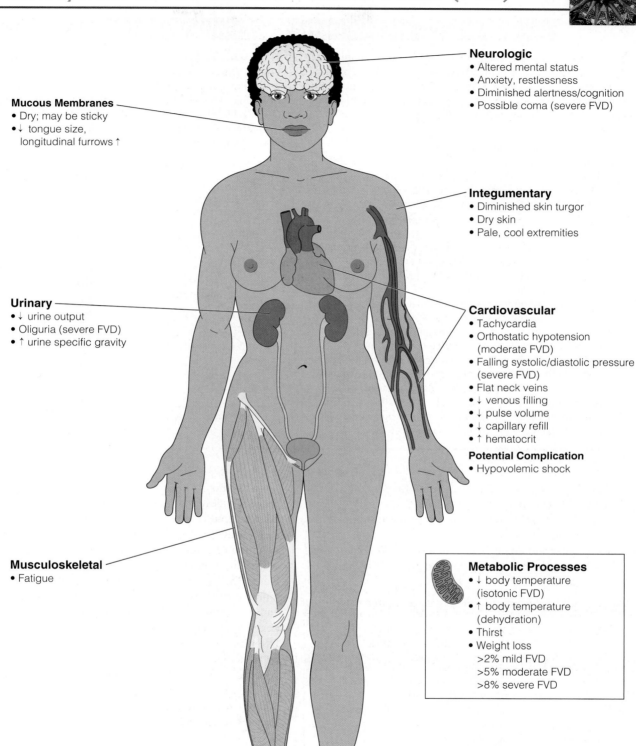

Neurologic
- Altered mental status
- Anxiety, restlessness
- Diminished alertness/cognition
- Possible coma (severe FVD)

Mucous Membranes
- Dry; may be sticky
- ↓ tongue size, longitudinal furrows ↑

Integumentary
- Diminished skin turgor
- Dry skin
- Pale, cool extremities

Urinary
- ↓ urine output
- Oliguria (severe FVD)
- ↑ urine specific gravity

Cardiovascular
- Tachycardia
- Orthostatic hypotension (moderate FVD)
- Falling systolic/diastolic pressure (severe FVD)
- Flat neck veins
- ↓ venous filling
- ↓ pulse volume
- ↓ capillary refill
- ↑ hematocrit

Potential Complication
- Hypovolemic shock

Musculoskeletal
- Fatigue

Metabolic Processes
- ↓ body temperature (isotonic FVD)
- ↑ body temperature (dehydration)
- Thirst
- Weight loss
  >2% mild FVD
  >5% moderate FVD
  >8% severe FVD

BOX 5–1 ■ Measuring Central Venous Pressure (CVP) with a Manometer

CVP is a hemodynamic monitoring method for evaluating fluid volume status. It measures mean right atrial pressure by means of a catheter. The CVP catheter is inserted by a physician, most often at the client's bedside, into the antecubital, internal jugular, or subclavian vein. Nursing responsibilities in measuring CVP are as follows:

1. Explain to the client and family what is being done.
2. Prior to the first measurement, take baseline vital signs, and measure the level of the right atrium on the client's thorax. This is usually at the fourth intercostal space on the lateral chest wall, midway between the anterior and posterior chest. This site is marked and used as the reference point for all measurements.
3. Place the bed in the same position for each reading, usually with the client supine and the head of the bed flat.
4. Use a carpenter's level to check the level of the measuring device to make sure the 0 on the manometer is level with the reference point on the client's chest (see figure).
5. Remove any air bubbles in the line.
6. Turn the stopcock on the manometer so that fluid flows into the manometer, filling it a few centimeters above the expected reading. Then turn the stopcock to open the line between the manometer and the client. The fluid level will fall and then reach a point at which it fluctuates with the client's respirations. This point is recorded as the CVP.
7. After the measurement is taken, turn the stopcock so that the fluid can again flow from the fluid source to the client.

NORMAL VALUES

When CVP is measured by a manometer, normal values range from 2 to 8 cm water. A low CVP indicates inadequate venous return from fluid deficit and hypovolemia or due to peripheral vasodilation. A high CVP indicates fluid overload, cardiac problems that decrease cardiac contractility, or pulmonary disorders that increase pulmonary vascular resistance.

2. Administer (by IV infusion) an initial fluid volume of 200 to 300 mL over 5 to 10 minutes.
3. Reevaluate baseline data at the end of the 10-minute infusion period.
4. Administer additional fluid until a specified volume is infused or the desired hemodynamic parameters are achieved.

TABLE 5–3 Comparison of Assessment Findings in Clients with Fluid Imbalance

Assessment	Fluid Deficit	Fluid Excess
Blood pressure	Decreased systolic Postural hypotension	Increased
Heart rate	Increased	Increased
Pulse amplitude	Decreased	Increased
Respirations	Normal	Moist crackles Wheezes
Jugular vein	Flat	Distended
Edema	Rare	Dependent
Skin turgor	Loose, poor turgor	Taut
Output	Low, concentrated	May be low or normal
Urine specific gravity	High	Low
Weight	Loss	Gain

Intravenous fluids are often prescribed to correct FVD. Table 5–4 describes the types, tonicity, and uses of commonly administered intravenous fluids. Isotonic electrolyte solutions (0.9% NaCl or Ringer's solution) are used to expand plasma volume in hypotensive clients or to replace abnormal losses, which are usually isotonic in nature. Five percent dextrose in water (D5W) is given to provide water to treat total body water deficits. D5W is isotonic (similar in tonicity to the plasma) and thus does not provoke hemolysis of red blood cells. The dextrose is metabolized to carbon dioxide and water, leaving free water available for tissue needs.

Hypotonic saline solution (0.45% NaCl with or without added electrolytes) or hypotonic mixed electrolyte solutions are used as maintenance solutions. These solutions provide additional electrolytes such as potassium, a buffer (lactate or acetate) as needed, and water.

NURSING CARE

Nurses are responsible for identifying clients at risk for fluid volume deficit, initiating and carrying out measures to prevent and treat fluid volume deficit, and monitoring the effects of therapy.

Health Promotion

Health promotion activities focus on teaching clients to prevent fluid volume deficit. Discuss the importance of maintaining ad-

TABLE 5–4 Commonly Administered Intravenous Fluids

	Fluid and Tonicity	Uses
Dextrose in Water Solutions	5% dextrose in water (D5W) Isotonic	Replaces water losses Provides free water necessary for cellular rehydration Lowers serum sodium in hypernatremia
	10% dextrose in water (D10W) Hypertonic	Provides free water Provides nutrition (supplies 340 kcal/L)
	20% dextrose in water (D20W) Hypertonic	Supplies 680 kcal/L May cause diuresis
	50% dextrose in water (D50W) Hypertonic	Supplies 1700 kcal/L Used to correct hypoglycemia
Saline Solutions	0.45% sodium chloride Hypotonic	Provides free water to replace hypotonic fluid losses Maintains levels of plasma sodium and chloride
	0.9% sodium chloride Isotonic	Expands intravascular volume Replaces water lost from extracellular fluid Used with blood transfusions Replaces large sodium losses (as from burns)
	3% sodium chloride Hypertonic	Corrects serious sodium depletion
Combined Dextrose and Saline Solution	5% dextrose & 0.45% sodium chloride Isotonic	Provides free water Provides sodium chloride Maintenance fluid of choice if there are no electrolyte imbalances
Multiple Electrolyte Solutions	Ringer's solution Isotonic (electrolyte concentrations of sodium, potassium, chloride, and calcium are similar to plasma levels)	Expands the intracellular fluid Replaces extracellular fluid losses
	Lactated Ringer's solution Isotonic (similar in composition of electrolytes to plasma but does not contain magnesium)	Replaces fluid losses from burns and the lower gastrointestinal tract Fluid of choice for acute blood loss

equate fluid intake, particularly when exercising and during hot weather. Advise clients to use commercial sports drinks to replace both water and electrolytes when exercising during warm weather. Instruct clients to maintain fluid intake when ill, particularly during periods of fever or when diarrhea is a problem.

Discuss the increased risk for fluid volume deficit with older adults (see p. 84) and provide information about prevention. Teach older adults (and their caretakers) that thirst decreases with aging and urge them to maintain a regular fluid intake of about 1500 mL per day, regardless of perception of thirst.

Carefully monitor clients at risk for abnormal fluid losses through routes such as vomiting, diarrhea, nasogastric suction, increased urine output, fever, or wounds. Monitor fluid intake in clients with decreased level of consciousness, disorientation, nausea and anorexia, and physical limitations.

Assessment

Collect assessment data through the health history interview and physical examination.

• Health history: Risk factors such as medications, acute or chronic renal or endocrine disease; precipitating factors such

as hot weather, extensive exercise, lack of access to fluids, recent illness (especially if accompanied by fever, vomiting, and/or diarrhea); onset and duration of symptoms.
• Physical assessment: Weight; vital signs including orthostatic blood pressure and pulse; peripheral pulses and capillary refill; jugular neck vein distention; skin color, temperature, turgor; level of consciousness and mentation; urine output. See Box 5–2 for physical assessment changes in the older adult.

BOX 5–2 ■ Assessing Older Adults

FLUID VOLUME DEFICIT
With aging, the elasticity of skin decreases. As a result, turgor diminishes, even in the well-hydrated older adult. This makes skin turgor less reliable when assessing for fluid volume deficit. In addition, some older adults experience postural hypotension, even when well hydrated. Allow the older adult to stand quietly for a full minute before rechecking blood pressure and pulse when measuring orthostatic vital signs.

Nursing Diagnoses and Interventions

The focus for nursing diagnoses and interventions for the client with fluid volume deficit is on managing the effects of the deficit and preventing complications.

Deficient Fluid Volume

Clients with fluid volume deficit due to abnormal losses, inadequate intake, or impaired fluid regulation require close monitoring as well as immediate and ongoing fluid replacement.

- Assess intake and output accurately, monitoring fluid balance. In acute situations, hourly intake and output may be indicated. *Urine output should be 30 to 60 mL per hour (unless renal failure is present). Urine output of less than 30 mL per hour indicates inadequate renal perfusion and an increased risk for acute renal failure and inadequate tissue perfusion.*

PRACTICE ALERT *Report a urine output of less than 30 mL per hour to the primary health care provider.* ■

- Assess vital signs, CVP, and peripheral pulse volume at least every 4 hours. *Hypotension, tachycardia, low CVP, and weak, easily obliterated peripheral pulses indicate hypovolemia.*
- Weigh daily under standard conditions (time of day, clothing, and scale). *In most instances (except third spacing), changes in weight accurately reflect fluid balance.* See the Nursing Research box on this page.
- Administer and monitor the intake of oral fluids as prescribed. Identify beverage preferences and provide these on a schedule. *Oral fluid replacement is preferred when the client is able to drink and retain fluids.*
- Administer intravenous fluids as prescribed using an electronic infusion pump. Monitor for indicators of fluid overload if rapid fluid replacement is ordered: dyspnea, tachypnea, tachycardia, increased CVP, jugular vein distension, and edema. *Rapid fluid replacement may lead to hypervolemia, resulting in pulmonary edema and cardiac failure, particularly in clients with compromised cardiac and renal function.*
- Monitor laboratory values: electrolytes, serum osmolality, BUN, and hematocrit. *Rehydration may lead to changes in serum electrolytes, osmolality, BUN, and hematocrit. In some cases, electrolyte replacement may be necessary during rehydration.*

Ineffective Tissue Perfusion

A fluid volume deficit can lead to decreased perfusion of renal, cerebral, and peripheral tissues. Inadequate renal perfusion can lead to acute renal failure. Decreased cerebral perfusion leads to changes in mental status and cognitive function, causing restlessness, anxiety, agitation, excitability, confusion, vertigo, fainting, and weakness.

- Monitor for changes in level of consciousness and mental status. *Restlessness, anxiety, confusion, and agitation may indicate inadequate cerebral blood flow and circulatory collapse.*
- Monitor serum creatinine, BUN, and cardiac enzymes, reporting elevated levels to the physician. *Elevated levels may indicate impaired renal function or cardiac perfusion related to circulatory failure.*

Nursing Research

Evidence-Based Practice for Clients with Imbalanced Fluid Volume

Nurses caring for clients with a fluid volume imbalance frequently monitor both 24-hour intake and output records and daily weights. These measurements require caregiver time, and may be providing redundant data. Nurse managers on three nursing units compared the results of continuous 48-hour intake and output records with daily weights for a total of 73 selected clients on their units. Their findings suggest that even when compliance with recording accurate intake and output is optimal, it is an unreliable measure of actual fluid balance (Wise, Mersch, Racioppi, Crosier, & Thompson, 2000).

IMPLICATIONS FOR NURSING

A significant shortage of licensed nurses is predicted for the early part of the 21st century. Tight nursing resources will require efficient nursing practice to maintain quality care. This study suggests that for the majority of clients (the exceptions being clients with kidney disease or who are on a fluid restriction), measuring accurate daily weights is a better indicator of fluid balance than intake and output records.

Critical Thinking

1. What factors can you identify that would affect the accuracy of intake and output records?
2. What measures can you and your institution take to ensure accurate daily weight measurements?
3. Compare intake and output records and daily weights for your assigned clients. Is the balance between intake and output accurately reflected by day-to-day weight changes? If not, what factors can you identify that might account for this discrepancy?

Note. Adapted from "Evaluating the Reliability and Utility of Cumulative Intake and Output" by L.C. Wise et al., 2000, Journal of Nursing Care Quality, 14(3), pp. 37–42.

- Turn at least every 2 hours. Provide good skin care and monitor for evidence of skin or tissue breakdown. *Impaired circulation to peripheral tissues increases the risk of skin breakdown. Turn frequently to relieve pressure over bony prominences. Keep skin clean, dry, and moisturized to help maintain integrity.*

Risk for Injury

The client with fluid volume deficit is at risk for injury because of dizziness and loss of balance resulting from decreased cerebral perfusion secondary to hypovolemia.

- Institute safety precautions, including keeping the bed in a low position, using side rails as needed, and slowly raising the client from supine to sitting or sitting to standing position. *Using safety precautions and allowing time for the blood pressure to adjust to position changes reduce the risk of injury.*
- Teach client and family members how to reduce orthostatic hypotension:
  a. Move from one position to another in stages; for example, raise the head of the bed before sitting up, and sit for a few minutes before standing.

CHART 5–1 NANDA, NIC, AND NOC LINKAGES

The Client with Fluid Volume Deficit

NURSING DIAGNOSES	NURSING INTERVENTIONS	NURSING OUTCOMES
• Deficient Fluid Volume • Decreased Cardiac Output	• Fluid Management • Hypovolemia Management • Circulatory Care	• Fluid Balance • Hydration • Circulatory Status • Vital Signs Status

Note. Data from Nursing Outcomes Classification (NOC) *by M. Johnson & M. Maas (Eds.), 1997, St. Louis: Mosby;* Nursing Diagnoses: Definitions & Classification 2001–2002 *by North American Nursing Diagnosis Association, 2001, Philadelphia: NANDA;* Nursing Interventions Classification (NIC) *by J.C. McCloskey & G. M. Bulechek (Eds.), 2000, St. Louis: Mosby. Reprinted by permission.*

b. Avoid prolonged standing.

c. Rest in a recliner rather than in bed during the day.

d. Use assistive devices to pick up objects from the floor rather than stooping.

Teaching measures to reduce orthostatic hypotension reduces the client's risk for injury. Prolonged bed rest increases skeletal muscle weakness and decreases venous tone, contributing to postural hypotension. Prolonged standing allows blood to pool in the legs, reducing venous return and cardiac output.

Using NANDA, NIC, and NOC

Chart 5–1 shows the links between NANDA nursing diagnoses, nursing interventions classification (NIC), and nursing outcomes classification (NOC) when caring for the client with fluid volume deficit.

Home Care

Depending on the severity of the fluid volume deficit, the client may be managed in the home or residential facility, or may be admitted to an acute care facility. Assess the client's understanding of the cause of the deficit and the fluids necessary for providing replacement. Address the following topics when preparing the client and family for home care.

- The importance of maintaining adequate fluid intake (at least 1500 mL per day; more if extra fluid is being lost through perspiration, fever, or diarrhea)
- Manifestations of fluid imbalance, and how to monitor fluid balance
- How to prevent fluid deficit:
   Avoid exercising during extreme heat.
   Increase fluid intake during hot weather.
   If vomiting, take small frequent amounts of ice chips or clear liquids, such as weak tea, flat cola, or ginger ale.
   Reduce intake of coffee, tea, and alcohol, which increase urine output and can cause fluid loss.
- Replacement of fluids lost through diarrhea with fruit juices or bouillon, rather than large amounts of tap water
- Alternate sources of fluid (such as gelatin, frozen juices, or ice cream) for effective replacement of lost fluids

THE CLIENT WITH FLUID VOLUME EXCESS

Fluid volume excess results when both water and sodium are retained in the body. Fluid volume excess may be caused by fluid overload (excess water and sodium intake) or by impairment of the mechanisms that maintain homeostasis. The excess fluid can lead to excess intravascular fluid (**hypervolemia**) and excess interstitial fluid (**edema**).

PATHOPHYSIOLOGY

Fluid volume excess usually results from conditions that cause retention of both sodium and water. These conditions include heart failure, cirrhosis of the liver, renal failure, adrenal gland disorders, corticosteroid administration, and stress conditions causing the release of ADH and aldosterone. Other causes include an excessive intake of sodium-containing foods, drugs that cause sodium retention, and the administration of excess amounts of sodium-containing intravenous fluids (such as 0.9% NaCl or Ringer's solution). This iatrogenic cause of fluid volume excess primarily affects clients with impaired regulatory mechanisms.

In fluid volume excess, both water and sodium are gained together in about the same proportions as normally exists in extracellular fluid. The total body sodium content is increased, which in turn causes an increase in total body water. Because the increase in sodium and water is isotonic, the serum sodium and osmolality remain normal, and the excess fluid remains in the extracellular space.

MANIFESTATIONS AND COMPLICATIONS

Excess extracellular fluid leads to hypervolemia and circulatory overload. Excess fluid in the interstitial space causes peripheral or generalized edema. The following manifestations of fluid volume excess relate to both the excess fluid and its effects on circulation.

- The increase in total body water causes weight gain (more than 5% of body weight) over a short period.
- Circulatory overload causes manifestations such as:
  - A full, bounding pulse.
  - Distended neck and peripheral veins.

- Increased central venous pressure (> 11–12 cm of water).
- Cough, **dyspnea** (labored or difficult breathing), **ortho-pnea** (difficulty breathing when supine).
- Moist crackles (rales) in the lungs; pulmonary edema (excess fluid in pulmonary interstitial spaces and alveoli) if severe.
- Increased urine output (**polyuria**).
- **Ascites** (excess fluid in the peritoneal cavity).
- Peripheral edema, or if severe, **anasarca** (severe, generalized edema).
- Dilution of plasma by excess fluid causes a decreased hematocrit and BUN.
- Possible cerebral edema (excess water in brain tissues) can lead to altered mental status and anxiety.

Heart failure is not only a potential cause of fluid volume excess, but it is also a potential complication of the condition if the heart is unable to increase its workload to handle the excess blood volume. Severe fluid overload and heart failure can lead to pulmonary edema, a medical emergency. See Chapter 30 for more information about heart failure and pulmonary edema.

COLLABORATIVE CARE

Managing fluid volume excess focuses on prevention in clients at risk, treating its manifestations, and correcting the underlying cause. Management includes limiting sodium and water intake and administering diuretics.

Diagnostic Tests

The following laboratory tests may be ordered.

- *Serum electrolytes* and *serum osmolality* are measured. Serum sodium and osmolality usually remain within normal limits.
- *Serum hematocrit* and *hemoglobin* often are decreased due to plasma dilution from excess extracellular fluid.

Additional tests of *renal* and *liver function* (such as serum creatinine, BUN, and liver enzymes) may be ordered to help determine the cause of fluid volume excess if it is unclear.

Medications

Diuretics are commonly used to treat fluid volume excess. They inhibit sodium and water reabsorption, increasing urine output. The three major classes of diuretics, each of which acts on a different part of the kidney tubule, are as follows:

- Loop diuretics act in the ascending loop of Henle.
- Thiazide-type diuretics act on the distal convoluted tubule.
- Potassium-sparing diuretics affect the distal nephron.

The nursing implications for diuretics are outlined in the box below.

Treatments

Fluid Management

Fluid intake may be restricted in clients who have fluid volume excess. The amount of fluid allowed per day is prescribed by the primary care provider. All fluid intake must be calculated,

Medication Administration

Diuretics for Fluid Volume Excess

Diuretics increase urinary excretion of water and sodium. They are categorized into three major groups: loop diuretics, thiazide and thiazide-like diuretics, and potassium-sparing diuretics. Diuretics are used to enhance renal function and to treat vascular fluid overload and edema. Common side effects include orthostatic hypotension, dehydration, electrolyte imbalance, and possible hyperglycemia. Diuretics should be used with caution in the older adult. Examples of each major type follow.

LOOP DIURETICS

Furosemide (Lasix)	Ethacrynic Acid (Edecrin)
Bumetanide (Bumex)	Torsemide (Demadex)

Loop diuretics inhibit sodium and chloride reabsorption in the ascending loop of Henle (see Chapter 25 for the anatomy of the kidneys). As a result, loop diuretics promote the excretion of sodium, chloride, potassium, and water.

THIAZIDE AND THIAZIDELIKE DIURETICS

Bendroflumethiazide (Naturetin)	Polythiazide (Renese)
Chlorothiazide (Diuril)	Chlorthalidone (Hygroton)
Hydrochlorothiazide (HydroDIURIL, Oretic)	Trichlormethiazide (Naqua)
Metolazone (Zaroxolyn)	Indapamide (Lozol)

Thiazide and thiazidelike diuretics promote the excretion of sodium, chloride, potassium, and water by decreasing absorption in the distal tubule.

POTASSIUM-SPARING DIURETICS

Spironolactone (Aldactone)
Amiloride HCl (Midamor)
Triamterene (Dyrenium)

Potassium-sparing diuretics promote excretion of sodium and water by inhibiting sodium-potassium exchange in the distal tubule.

Client and Family Teaching

- The drug will increase the amount and frequency of urination.
- The drugs must be taken even when you feel well.
- Take the drugs in the morning and afternoon to avoid having to get up at night to urinate.
- Change position slowly to avoid dizziness.
- Report the following to your primary health care provider: dizziness; trouble breathing; or swelling of face, hands, or feet.
- Weigh yourself every day, and report sudden gains or losses.
- Avoid using the salt shaker when eating.
- If the drug increases potassium loss, eat foods high in potassium, such as orange juice and bananas.
- Do not use salt substitute if you are taking a potassium-sparing diuretic.

BOX 5–3 ■ Fluid Restriction Guidelines

- Subtract requisite fluids (e.g., ordered IV fluids, fluid used to dilute IV medications) from total daily allowance.
- Divide remaining fluid allowance:
  - Day shift: 50% of total
  - Evening shift: 25% to 33% of total
  - Night shift: Remainder
- Explain the fluid restriction to the client and family members.
- Identify preferred fluids and intake pattern of client.
- Place allowed amounts of fluid in small glasses (gives perception of a full glass).
- Offer ice chips (when melted, ice chips are approximately half the frozen volume).
- Provide frequent mouth care.
- Provide sugarless chewing gum (if allowed) to reduce thirst sensation.

BOX 5–4 ■ Foods High in Sodium

HIGH IN ADDED SODIUM

Processed Meat and Fish
- Bacon
- Luncheon meat and other cold cuts
- Sausage
- Smoked fish

Selected Dairy Products
- Buttermilk
- Cheeses
- Cottage cheese
- Ice cream

Processed Grains
- Graham crackers
- Most dry cereals

Most Canned Goods
- Meats
- Soups
- Vegetables

Snack Foods
- Salted popcorn
- Potato chips/pretzels
- Nuts
- Gelatin desserts

Condiments and Food Additives
- Barbecue sauce
- Catsup
- Chili sauce
- Meat tenderizers
- Worcestershire sauce
- Saccharin
- Pickles
- Soy sauce
- Salted margarine
- Salad dressings

NATURALLY HIGH IN SODIUM
- Brains
- Kidney
- Clams
- Crab
- Lobster
- Oysters
- Shrimp
- Dried fruit
- Spinach
- Carrots

including meals and that used to administer medications orally or intravenously. Box 5–3 provides guidelines for clients with a fluid restriction.

Dietary Management

Because sodium retention is a primary cause of fluid volume excess, a sodium-restricted diet often is prescribed. Americans typically consume about 4 to 5 grams (g) of sodium every day; recommended sodium intake is 500 to 2400 mg per day. The primary dietary sources of sodium are the salt shaker, processed foods, and foods themselves (see Box 5–4).

A mild sodium restriction can be achieved by instructing the client and primary food preparer in the household to reduce the amount of salt in recipes by half, avoid using the salt shaker during meals, and avoid foods that contain high levels of sodium (either naturally or because of processing). In moderate and severely sodium-restricted diets, salt is avoided altogether, as are all foods containing significant amounts of sodium.

NURSING CARE

Nursing care focuses on preventing fluid volume excess in clients at risk and on managing problems resulting from its effects.

Health Promotion

Health promotion related to fluid volume excess focuses on teaching preventive measures to clients who are at risk (e.g., clients who have heart or kidney failure). Discuss the relationship between sodium intake and water retention. Provide guidelines for a low-sodium diet, and teach clients to carefully read food labels to identify "hidden" sodium, particularly in processed foods. Instruct clients at risk to weigh themselves on a regular basis, using the same scale, and to notify their primary care provider if they gain more than 5 lb in a week or less.

Carefully monitor clients receiving intravenous fluids for signs of hypervolemia. Reduce the flow rate and promptly report manifestations of fluid overload to the physician.

Assessment

Collect assessment data through the health history interview and physical examination.

- Health history: Risk factors such as medications, heart failure, acute or chronic renal or endocrine disease; precipitating factors such as a recent illness, change in diet, or change in medications. Recent weight gain; complaints of persistent cough, shortness of breath, swelling of feet and ankles, or difficulty sleeping when lying down.
- Physical assessment: Weight; vital signs; peripheral pulses and capillary refill; jugular neck vein distention; edema; lung sounds (crackles or wheezes), dyspnea, cough, and sputum; urine output; mental status.

Nursing Diagnoses and Interventions

Nursing diagnoses and interventions for the client with fluid volume excess focus on the multisystem effects of the fluid overload.

Excess Fluid Volume

Nursing care for the client with fluid volume excess includes collaborative interventions such as administering diuretics and maintaining a fluid restriction, as well as monitoring the status and effects of the fluid volume excess. This is particularly critical in older clients because of the age-related decline in cardiac and renal compensatory responses.

- Assess vital signs, heart sounds, CVP, and volume of peripheral arteries. *Hypervolemia can cause hypertension, bounding peripheral pulses, a third heart sound (S_3) due to the volume of blood flow through the heart, and high CVP readings.*
- Assess for the presence and extent of edema, particularly in the lower extremities, the back, sacral, and periorbital areas. *Initially, edema affects the dependent portions of the body— the lower extremities of ambulatory clients and the sacrum in bedridden clients. Periorbital edema indicates more generalized edema.*

PRACTICE ALERT *Assess urine output hourly. Maintain accurate intake and output records. Note urine output less than 30 ml per hour or a positive fluid balance on 24-hour total intake and output calculations. Heart failure and inadequate renal perfusion may result in decreased urine output and fluid retention.* ■

- Obtain daily weights at the same time of day, using approximately the same clothing and a balanced scale. *Daily weights are one of the most important gauges of fluid balance. Acute weight gain or loss represents fluid gain or loss. Weight gain of 2 kg is equivalent to 2 L of fluid gain.*
- Administer oral fluids cautiously, adhering to any prescribed fluid restriction. Discuss the restriction with the client and significant others, including the total volume allowed, the rationale, and the importance of reporting all fluid taken. *All sources of fluid intake, including ice chips, are recorded to avoid excess fluid intake.*
- Provide oral hygiene at least every 2 hours. *Oral hygiene contributes to client comfort and keeps mucous membranes intact; it also helps relieve thirst if fluids are restricted.*
- Teach client and significant others about the sodium-restricted diet, and emphasize the importance of checking before bringing foods to the client. *Excess sodium promotes water retention; a sodium-restricted diet is ordered to reduce water gain.*
- Administer prescribed diuretics as ordered, monitoring the client's response to therapy. *Loop or high-ceiling diuretics such as furosemide can lead to rapid fluid loss and signs of hypovolemia and electrolyte imbalance.*

Risk for Impaired Skin Integrity

Tissue edema decreases oxygen and nutrient delivery to the skin and subcutaneous tissues, increasing the risk of injury.

- Frequently assess skin, particularly in pressure areas and over bony prominences. *Skin breakdown can progress rapidly when circulation is impaired.*
- Reposition the client at least every 2 hours. Provide skin care with each position change. *Frequent position changes minimize tissue pressure and promote blood flow to tissues.*
- Provide an eggcrate mattress or alternating pressure mattress, foot cradle, heel protectors, and other devices to reduce pressure on tissues. *These devices, which distribute pressure away from bony prominences, reduce the risk of skin breakdown.*

Risk for Impaired Gas Exchange

With fluid volume excess, gas exchange may be impaired by edema of pulmonary interstitial tissues. Acute pulmonary edema is a serious and potentially life-threatening complication of pulmonary congestion.

- Auscultate lungs for presence or worsening of crackles and wheezes; auscultate heart for extra heart sounds. *Crackles and wheezes indicate pulmonary congestion and edema. A gallop rhythm (S_3) may indicate diastolic overloading of the ventricles secondary to fluid volume excess.*
- Place in Fowler's position if dyspnea or orthopnea is present. *Fowler's position improves lung expansion by decreasing the pressure of abdominal contents on the diaphragm.*
- Monitor oxygen saturation levels and **arterial blood gases (ABGs)** for evidence of impaired gas exchange (SaO_2 < 92%–95%; PaO_2 < 80 mmHg). Administer oxygen as indicated. *Edema of interstitial lung tissues can interfere with gas exchange and delivery to body tissues. Supplemental oxygen promotes gas exchange across the alveolar-capillary membrane, improving tissue oxygenation.*

Using NANDA, NIC, and NOC

Chart 5–2 shows links between NANDA nursing diagnoses, NIC, and NOC when caring for a client with fluid volume excess.

CHART 5–2 NANDA, NIC, AND NOC LINKAGES

The Client with Fluid Volume Excess

NURSING DIAGNOSES	NURSING INTERVENTIONS	NURSING OUTCOMES
• Excess Fluid Volume	• Fluid Management • Fluid Monitoring	• Fluid Balance
• Impaired Gas Exchange	• Oxygen Therapy • Respiratory Monitoring	
• Activity Intolerance	• Energy Management	• Respiratory Status: Gas Exchange • Activity Tolerance

Note. Data from Nursing Outcomes Classification (NOC) by M. Johnson & M. Maas (Eds.), 1997, St. Louis: Mosby; Nursing Diagnoses: Definitions & Classification 2001–2002 by North American Nursing Diagnosis Association, 2001, Philadelphia: NANDA; Nursing Interventions Classification (NIC) by J.C. McCloskey & G. M. Bulechek (Eds.), 2000, St. Louis: Mosby. Reprinted by permission.

Home Care

Teaching for home care focuses on managing the underlying cause of fluid volume excess and preventing future episodes of excess fluid volume. Address the following topics when preparing the client and family for home care.

- Signs and symptoms of excess fluid and when to contact the care provider
- Prescribed medications: when and how to take, intended and adverse effects, what to report to care provider
- Recommended or prescribed diet; ways to reduce sodium intake; how to read food labels for salt and sodium content; use of salt substitutes, if allowed. (See Box 5–5)
- If restricted, the amount and type of fluids to take each day; how to balance intake over 24 hours
- Monitoring weight; changes reported to care provider
- Ways to decrease dependent edema:
  a. Change position frequently.
  b. Avoid restrictive clothing.
  c. Avoid crossing the legs when sitting.
  d. Wear support stockings or hose.
  e. Elevate feet and legs when sitting.
- How to protect edematous skin from injury:
  a. Do not walk barefoot.
  b. Buy well-fitting shoes; shop in the afternoon when feet are more likely to be swollen.
- Using additional pillows or a recliner to sleep, to relieve orthopnea

---

BOX 5–5   ■ Client Teaching

LOW-SODIUM DIET

- Reducing sodium intake will help the body excrete excess sodium and water.
- The body needs less than one-tenth of a teaspoon of salt per day.
- Approximately one-third of sodium intake comes from salt added to foods during cooking and at the table; one-fourth to one-third comes from processed foods; and the rest comes from food and water naturally high in sodium.
- Sodium compounds are used in foods as preservatives, leavening agents, and flavor enhancers.
- Many nonprescription drugs (such as analgesics, cough medicine, laxatives, and antacids) as well as toothpastes and mouthwashes contain high amounts of sodium.
- Low-sodium salt substitutes are not really sodium free and may contain half as much sodium as regular salt.
- Use salt substitutes sparingly; larger amounts often taste bitter instead of salty.
- The preference for salt will eventually diminish.
- Salt, monosodium glutamate, baking soda, and baking powder contain substantial amounts of sodium.
- Read labels.
- In place of salt or salt substitutes, use herbs, spices, lemon juice, vinegar, and wine as flavoring when cooking.

Nursing Care Plan
A Client with Fluid Volume Excess

Dorothy Rainwater is a 45-year-old Native American woman hospitalized with acute renal failure that developed as a result of acute glomerulonephritis. She is expected to recover, but she has very little urine output. Ms. Rainwater is a single mother of two teenage sons. Until her illness, she was active in caring for her family, her career as a high school principal, and community activities.

ASSESSMENT

Mike Penning, Ms. Rainwater's nurse, notes that she is in the oliguric phase of acute renal failure, and that her urine output for the previous 24 hours is 250 mL; this low output has been constant for the past 8 days. She gained 1 lb (0.45 kg) in the past 24 hours. Laboratory test results from that morning are: sodium, 155 mEq/L (normal 135 to 145 mEq/L); potassium, 5.3 mEq/L (normal 3.5 to 5.0 mEq/L); calcium, 7.6 mg/dL (normal 8.0 to 10.5 mg/dL), and urine specific gravity 1.008 (normal 1.010 to 1.030). Ms. Rainwater's serum creatinine and blood urea nitrogen (BUN) are high; however, her ABGs are within normal limits.

In his assessment of Ms. Rainwater, Mike notes the following:

- BP 160/92; P 102, with obvious neck vein distention; R 28, with crackles and wheezes; head of bed elevated 30 degrees; T 98.6° F.
- Periorbital and sacral edema present; 3+ pitting bilateral pedal edema; skin cool, pale, and shiny.
- Alert, oriented; responds appropriately to questions.
- Client states she is thirsty, slightly nauseated, and extremely tired.

Ms. Rainwater is receiving intravenous furosemide and is on a 24-hour fluid restriction of 500 mL plus the previous day's urine output to manage her fluid volume excess.

DIAGNOSES

- *Excess fluid volume* related to acute renal failure
- *Risk for impaired skin integrity* related to fluid retention and edema
- *Risk for impaired gas exchange* related to pulmonary congestion
- *Activity intolerance* related to fluid volume excess, fatigue, and weakness

EXPECTED OUTCOMES

- Regain fluid balance, as evidenced by weight loss, decreasing edema, and normal vital signs.
- Experience decreased dyspnea.
- Maintain intact skin and mucous membranes.
- Increase activity levels as prescribed.

PLANNING AND IMPLEMENTATION

- Weigh at 0600 and 1800 daily.

(continued on page 94)

Nursing Care Plan
A Client with Fluid Volume Excess *(continued)*

- Assess vital signs and breath sounds every 4 hours.
- Measure intake and output every 4 hours.
- Obtain urine specific gravity every 8 hours.
- Restrict fluids as follows: 350 mL from 0700 to 1500; 300 mL from 1500 to 2300; 100 mL from 2300 to 0700. Prefers water or apple juice.
- Turn every 2 hours, following schedule posted at the head of bed. Inspect and provide skin care as needed; avoid vigorous massage of pressure areas.
- Provide oral care every 2 to 4 hours (can brush her own teeth, caution not to swallow water); use moistened applicators as desired.
- Elevate head of bed to 30 to 40 degrees; prefers to use own pillows.
- Assist to recliner chair at bedside for 20 minutes two or three times a day. Monitor ability to tolerate activity without increasing dyspnea or fatigue.

EVALUATION

At the end of the shift, Mike evaluates the effectiveness of the plan of care and continues all diagnoses and interventions. Ms. Rainwater gained no weight, and her urinary output during his shift is 170 mL. Her urine specific gravity remains 1.008. Her vital signs are unchanged, but her crackles and wheezes have decreased slightly. Her skin and mucous membranes are intact. Ms. Rainwater tolerated the bedside chair without dyspnea or fatigue.

Critical Thinking in the Nursing Process

1. What is the pathophysiologic basis for Ms. Rainwater's increased respiratory rate, blood pressure, and pulse?
2. Explain how elevating the head of the bed 30 degrees facilitates respirations.
3. Suppose Ms. Rainwater says, "I would really like to have all my fluids at once instead of spreading them out." How would you reply, and why?
4. Outline a plan for teaching Ms. Rainwater about diuretics.

See Evaluating Your Response in Appendix C.

SODIUM IMBALANCE

Sodium is the most plentiful electrolyte in ECF, with normal serum sodium levels ranging from 135 to 145 mEq/L. Sodium is the primary regulator of the volume, osmolality, and distribution of ECF. It also is important to maintain neuromuscular activity. Because of the close interrelationship between sodium and water balance, disorders of fluid volume and sodium balance often occur together. Sodium imbalances affect the osmolality of ECF and water distribution between the fluid compartments. When sodium levels are low (**hyponatremia**), water is drawn into the cells of the body, causing them to swell. In contrast, high levels of sodium in ECF (**hypernatremia**) draw water out of body cells, causing them to shrink.

OVERVIEW OF NORMAL SODIUM BALANCE

Most of the body's sodium comes from dietary intake. Although a sodium intake of 500 mg per day is usually sufficient to meet the body's needs, the average intake of sodium by adults in the United States is about 6 to 15 g per day (Porth, 2002). Other sources of sodium include prescription drugs and certain self-prescribed remedies. Sodium is primarily excreted by the kidneys. A small amount is excreted through the skin and the gastrointestinal tract.

The kidney is the primary regulator of sodium balance in the body. The kidney excretes or conserves sodium in response to changes in vascular volume. A fall in blood volume prompts several mechanisms that lead to sodium and water retention.

- The renin-angiotensin-aldosterone system (see Figure 5–9) is stimulated. Angiotensin II prompts the renal tubules to reabsorb sodium. It also causes vasoconstriction, slowing blood flow through the kidney and reducing glomerular filtration. This further reduces the amount of sodium excreted. Angiotensin II promotes the release of aldosterone from the adrenal cortex. In the presence of aldosterone, more sodium is reabsorbed in the cortical collecting tubules of the kidney, and more potassium is eliminated in the urine.
- Antidiuretic hormone (ADH) is released from the posterior pituitary (see Figure 5–10). ADH promotes sodium and water reabsorption in the distal tubules of the kidney, reducing urine output and expanding blood volume.

In contrast, when blood volume expands, sodium and water elimination by the kidneys increases.

- The **glomerular filtration rate** (the rate at which plasma is filtered through the glomeruli of the kidney) increases, allowing more water and sodium to be filtered and excreted.
- Atrial natriuretic peptide (ANP) is released by cells in the atria of the heart. ANP increases sodium excretion by the kidneys.
- ADH release from the pituitary gland is inhibited. In the absence of ADH, the distal tubule is relatively impermeable to water and sodium, allowing more to be excreted in the urine. Table 5–5 summarizes the causes and effects of sodium imbalances.

THE CLIENT WITH HYPONATREMIA

Hyponatremia is a serum sodium level of less than 135 mEq/L. Hyponatremia usually results from a loss of sodium from the body, but it may also be caused by water gains that dilute ECF.

TABLE 5–5 Causes and Manifestations of Sodium Imbalances

Imbalance	Possible Causes	Manifestations
Hyponatremia Serum sodium <135 mEq/L *Other Lab Values* Serum osmolality <280 mOsm/kg	• Excess sodium loss through kidneys, GI tract, or skin • Water gains related to renal disease, heart failure, or cirrhosis of the liver • Syndrome of inappropriate secretion of antidiuretic hormone (SIADH) • Excessive hypotonic IV fluids	• Anorexia, nausea, vomiting, abdominal cramping, and diarrhea • Headache • Altered mental status • Muscle cramps, weakness, and tremors • Seizures and coma
Hypernatremia Serum sodium >145 mEq/L *Other Lab Values* Serum osmolality >295 mOsm/kg	• Altered thirst • Inability to respond to thirst sensation or obtain water • Profuse sweating • Diarrhea • Diabetes insipidus • Oral electrolyte solutions or hyperosmolar tube-feeding formulas • Excess IV fluids such as normal saline, 3% or 5% sodium chloride, or sodium bicarbonate	• Thirst • Increased temperature • Dry, sticky mucous membranes • Restlessness • Weakness • Altered mental status • Decreasing level of consciousness • Muscle twitching • Seizures

PATHOPHYSIOLOGY AND MANIFESTATIONS

Excess sodium loss can occur through the kidneys, gastrointestinal tract, or skin. Diuretic medications, kidney diseases, or adrenal insufficiency with impaired aldosterone and cortisol production can lead to excessive sodium excretion in urine. Vomiting, diarrhea, and gastrointestinal suction are common causes of excess sodium loss through the GI tract. Sodium may also be lost when gastrointestinal tubes are irrigated with water instead of saline, or when repeated tap water enemas are administered (Porth, 2002). Excessive sweating or loss of skin surface (as with an extensive burn) can also cause excessive sodium loss.

Water gains that can lead to hyponatremia may occur with:

• Systemic diseases such as heart failure, renal failure, or cirrhosis of the liver.
• Syndrome of inappropriate secretion of antidiuretic hormone (SIADH), in which water excretion is impaired.
• Excessive administration of hypotonic intravenous fluids.

Hyponatremia causes a drop in serum osmolality. Water shifts from ECF into the intracellular space, causing cells to swell and reducing the osmolality of intracellular fluid. Many of the manifestations of hyponatremia can be attributed to cellular edema and hypo-osmolality.

The manifestations of hyponatremia depend on the rapidity of onset, the severity, and the cause of the imbalance. If the condition develops slowly, manifestations are usually not experienced until the serum sodium levels reach 125 mEq/L. In addition, the manifestations of hyponatremia vary, depending on extracellular fluid volume. Early manifestations of hyponatremia include muscle cramps, weakness, and fatigue from its effects on muscle cells. Gastrointestinal function is affected, causing anorexia, nausea and vomiting, abdominal cramping, and diarrhea.

As sodium levels continue to decrease, the brain and nervous system are affected by cellular edema. Neurologic manifestations progress rapidly when the serum sodium level falls below 120 mEq/L, and include headache, depression, dulled sensorium, personality changes, irritability, lethargy, hyperreflexia, muscle twitching, and tremors. If serum sodium falls to very low levels, convulsions and coma are likely to occur.

When hyponatremia is associated with decreased ECF volume, the manifestations are those of hypovolemia. In hyponatremia associated with fluid volume excess, manifestations include those of hypervolemia.

COLLABORATIVE CARE

Collaborative management of hyponatremia focuses on restoring normal blood volume and serum sodium levels.

Diagnostic Tests

The following laboratory tests may be ordered.

• *Serum sodium* and *osmolality* are decreased in hyponatremia (serum sodium <135 mEq/L; serum osmolality <275 mOsm/kg).
• A *24-hour urine specimen* is obtained to evaluate sodium excretion. In conditions associated with normal or increased extracellular volume (such as SIADH), urinary sodium is increased; in conditions resulting from losses of isotonic fluids (e.g., sweating, diarrhea, vomiting, and third-space fluid accumulation), by contrast, urinary sodium is decreased.

Medications

When both sodium and water have been lost (hyponatremia with hypovolemia), sodium-containing fluids are given to replace both water and sodium. These fluids may be given by mouth, nasogastric tube, or intravenously. Isotonic Ringer's solution or isotonic saline (0.9% NaCl) solution may be administered. Cautious administration of intravenous 3% or 5% NaCl solution may be necessary in clients who have very low plasma sodium levels (110 to 115 mEq/L).

Loop diuretics are administered to clients who have hyponatremia with normal or excess ECF volume. Loop diuretics promote an isotonic diuresis and fluid volume loss without hyponatremia (see p. 90). Thiazide diuretics are avoided because they cause a relatively greater sodium loss in relation to water loss.

In addition, drugs to treat the underlying cause of hyponatremia may be administered.

Fluid and Dietary Management

If hyponatremia is mild, increasing the intake of foods high in sodium may restore normal sodium balance (see Box 5–4). Fluids often are restricted to help reduce ECF volume and correct hyponatremia (see Box 5–3).

NURSING CARE

Nursing care of the client with hyponatremia focuses on identifying clients at risk and managing problems resulting from the systemic effects of the disorder.

Health Promotion

People at risk for mild hyponatremia include those who participate in activities that increase fluid loss through excessive perspiration (diaphoresis) and then replace those losses by drinking large amounts of water. This includes athletes, people who do heavy labor in high environmental temperatures, and older adults living in non-air-conditioned settings during hot weather. Teach the following to clients who are at risk.

- Manifestations of mild hyponatremia, including nausea, abdominal cramps, and muscle weakness
- The importance of drinking liquids containing sodium and other electrolytes at frequent intervals when perspiring heavily, when environmental temperatures are high, and/or if watery diarrhea persists for several days

Assessment

Assessment data related to hyponatremia include the following:

- Health history: Current manifestations, including nausea and vomiting, abdominal discomfort, muscle weakness, headache, other symptoms; duration of symptoms and any precipitating factors such as heavy perspiration, vomiting, or diarrhea; chronic diseases such as heart or renal failure, cirrhosis of the liver, or endocrine disorders; current medications.
- Physical assessment: Mental status and level of consciousness; vital signs including orthostatic vitals and peripheral pulses; presence of edema or weight gain.

Nursing Diagnoses and Interventions
Risk for Imbalanced Fluid Volume
Because of its role in maintaining fluid balance, sodium imbalances often are accompanied by water imbalances. In addition, treatment of hyponatremia can affect the client's fluid balance.

- Monitor intake and output, weigh daily, and calculate 24-hour fluid balance. *Fluid excess or deficit may occur with hyponatremia.*

PRACTICE ALERT   *Carefully monitor clients receiving sodium-containing intravenous solutions for signs of hypervolemia (increased blood pressure and CVP, tachypnea, tachycardia, gallop rhythm, shortness of breath, crackles). Hypertonic saline solutions can lead to hypervolemia, particularly in clients with cardiovascular or renal disease.* ■

- Use an intravenous flow control device to administer hypertonic saline (3% and 5% NaCl) solutions; carefully monitor flow rate and response. *Hypertonic solutions can increase the risk of pulmonary and cerebral edema due to water retention. Careful monitoring is vital to prevent these complications and possible permanent damage.*
- If fluids are restricted, explain the reason for the restriction, the amount of fluid allowed, and how to calculate fluid intake. *Teaching increases the client's sense of control and compliance.*

For additional nursing interventions that may apply to the client with hyponatremia, review the discussions of fluid volume deficit and fluid volume excess.

Risk for Decreased Intracranial Adaptive Capacity
The client with severe hyponatremia experiences fluid shifts that cause an increase in intracellular fluid volume. This can cause brain cells to swell, increasing pressure within the cranial vault.

- Monitor serum electrolytes and serum osmolality. Report abnormal results to the care provider. *As serum sodium levels fall, the manifestations and neurologic effects of hyponatremia become increasingly severe.*
- Assess for neurologic changes, such as lethargy, altered level of consciousness, confusion, and convulsions. Monitor mental status and orientation. Compare baseline data with continuing assessments. *Serum sodium levels of 115 to 120 mEq/L can cause headache, lethargy, and decreased responsiveness; sodium levels less than 110 to 115 mEq/L may cause seizures and coma.*
- Assess muscle strength and tone, and deep tendon reflexes. *Increasing muscle weakness and decreased deep tendon reflexes are manifestations of increasing hyponatremia.*

PRACTICE ALERT   *Maintain a quiet environment, and institute seizure precautions in clients with severe hyponatremia. Severe hyponatremia can lead to seizures. A quiet environment reduces neurologic stimulation. Safety precautions, such as ensuring that side rails are up and having an airway readily available, reduce risk of injury from seizure.* ■

Using NANDA, NIC, and NOC

Chart 5–3 shows links between NANDA nursing diagnoses, NIC, and NOC when caring for a client with a sodium imbalance.

Home Care

Teaching for home care focuses on the underlying cause of the sodium deficit and often on prevention. Teach clients who have experienced hyponatremia and those who are at risk for developing hyponatremia about the following:

CHART 5–3 NANDA, NIC, AND NOC LINKAGES

The Client with a Sodium Imbalance

NURSING DIAGNOSES	NURSING INTERVENTIONS	NURSING OUTCOMES
• Risk for Imbalanced Fluid Volume	• Electrolyte Management • Fluid Monitoring	• Fluid Balance • Electrolyte Balance
• Fatigue	• Energy Management	• Energy Conservation
• Risk for Injury	• Environmental Management: Safety • Fall Prevention	• Risk Control • Safety Status: Physical Injury
• Risk for Impaired Oral Mucous Membrane	• Oral Health Maintenance	• Tissue Integrity: Skin and Mucous Membranes

Note. Data from Nursing Outcomes Classification (NOC) by M. Johnson & M. Maas (Eds.), 1997, St. Louis: Mosby; Nursing Diagnoses: Definitions & Classification 2001–2002 by North American Nursing Diagnosis Association, 2001, Philadelphia: NANDA; Nursing Interventions Classification (NIC) by J.C. McCloskey & G. M. Bulechek (Eds.), 2000, St. Louis: Mosby. Reprinted by permission.

- Manifestations of mild and more severe hyponatremia to report to the primary care provider
- The importance of regular serum electrolyte monitoring if taking a potent diuretic or on a low-sodium diet
- Types of foods and fluids to replace sodium orally if dietary sodium is not restricted

THE CLIENT WITH HYPERNATREMIA

Hypernatremia is a serum sodium level greater than 145 mEq/L. It may develop when sodium is gained in excess of water, or when water is lost in excess of sodium. Either fluid volume deficit or fluid volume excess often accompany hypernatremia.

PATHOPHYSIOLOGY AND MANIFESTATIONS

Two regulatory mechanisms protect the body from hypernatremia: (1) Excess sodium in ECF stimulates the release of ADH so more water is retained by the kidneys; and (2) the thirst mechanism is stimulated to increase the intake of water (Metheny, 2000). These two factors increase extracellular water, diluting the excess sodium and restoring normal levels. Because of the effectiveness of these mechanisms, hypernatremia almost never occurs in clients who have an intact thirst mechanism and access to water.

Water deprivation is a cause of hypernatremia in clients who are unable to respond to thirst due to altered mental status or physical disability. Excess water loss may occur with watery diarrhea or increased insensible losses (due to fever, hyperventilation, excessive perspiration, or massive burns). Unless water is adequately replaced, clients with diabetes insipidus also may develop hypernatremia. Excess sodium intake can result from ingestion of excess salt or hypertonic intravenous solutions. Clients who experience near-drowning in seawater are at risk for hypernatremia, as are clients with heatstroke.

Hypernatremia causes hyperosmolality of ECF. As a result, water is drawn out of cells, leading to cellular dehydration. The most serious effects of cellular dehydration are seen in the brain. As brain cells contract, neurologic manifestations develop. The brain itself shrinks, causing mechanical traction on cerebral vessels. These vessels may tear and bleed. Although the brain rapidly adapts to hyperosmolality to minimize the water loss, acute hypernatremia can cause widespread cerebral vascular bleeding (Metheny, 2000).

Thirst is the first manifestation of hypernatremia. If thirst is not relieved, the primary manifestations relate to altered neurologic function (see Table 5–5). Initial lethargy, weakness, and irritability can progress to seizures, coma, and death in severe hypernatremia. Both the severity of the sodium excess and the rapidity of its onset affect the manifestations of hypernatremia.

COLLABORATIVE CARE

Treatment of hypernatremia depends on its cause. Hypernatremia is corrected slowly (over a 48-hour period) to avoid development of cerebral edema secondary to a shift of water into the brain cells.

Diagnostic Tests

The following laboratory and diagnostic tests may be ordered.

- *Serum sodium levels* are greater than 145 mEq/L in hypernatremia.
- *Serum osmolality* is greater than 295 mOsm/kg in hypernatremia.
- The *water deprivation test* may be conducted to identify diabetes insipidus. Water and all other fluids are withheld for a specified period of time. During this time, urine specimens are obtained for osmolality and specific gravity. No change in these values supports the diagnosis of diabetes insipidus.

Medications

The principal treatment for hypernatremia is oral or intravenous water replacement. Hypotonic intravenous fluids such as 5% dextrose in water or 0.45% NaCl solution may be administered to correct the water deficit. Diuretics may also be given to increase sodium excretion.

NURSING CARE

Health Promotion

Clients at risk for hypernatremia, as well as their care providers, need teaching to prevent this electrolyte disorder. Instruct caregivers of debilitated clients who are unable to perceive thirst or unable to respond to it to offer fluids at regular intervals. If the client is unable to maintain adequate fluid intake, contact the primary care provider about an alternate route for fluid intake (e.g., a feeding tube). Teach care providers the importance of providing adequate water for clients receiving tube feedings (many of which are hypertonic).

Assessment

Assessment data related to hypernatremia include the following:

- Health history: Duration of symptoms and any precipitating factors such as water deprivation, increased water loss due to heavy perspiration, temperature or rapid breathing, diarrhea, excess salt intake, or diabetes insipidus; current medications; perception of thirst.
- Physical assessment: Vital signs including temperature; mucous membranes; altered mental status or level of consciousness; manifestations of fluid volume excess or fluid volume deficit.

Nursing Diagnoses and Interventions

Risk for Injury

Mental status and brain function may be affected by hypernatremia itself or by rapid correction of the condition that leads to cerebral edema. In either case, closely monitor the client and take precautions to reduce risk of injury.

- Monitor and maintain fluid replacement to within the prescribed limits. Monitor serum sodium levels and osmolality; report rapid changes to the care provider. *Rapid water replacement or rapid changes in serum sodium or osmolality*

can cause fluid shifts within the brain, increasing the risk of bleeding or cerebral edema.

- Monitor neurologic function, including mental status, level of consciousness, and other manifestations such as headache, nausea, vomiting, elevated blood pressure, and decreased pulse rate. *Both hypernatremia and rapid correction of hypernatremia affect the brain and brain function. Careful monitoring is vital to detect changes in mental status that may indicate cerebral bleeding or edema.*
- Institute safety precautions as necessary: Keep the bed in its lowest position, side rails up and padded, and an airway at bedside. *Clients with sodium disorders are at risk for injury due to seizure activity and changes in mental status.*
- Keep clocks, calendars, and familiar objects at bedside. Orient to time, place, and circumstances as needed. Allow significant others to remain with the client as much as possible. *An unfamiliar environment and altered thought processes can further increase the client's risk for injury. Significant others provide a sense of security and reduce the client's anxiety.*

Using NANDA, NIC, and NOC

Chart 5–3 shows links between NANDA nursing diagnoses, NIC, and NOC when caring for a client with a sodium imbalance.

Home Care

When preparing the client who has experienced hypernatremia for home care, discuss the following topics.

- The importance of responding to thirst and consuming adequate fluids (If the client is dependent on a caregiver, stress the importance of regularly offering fluids to the caregiver.)
- If prescribed, guidelines for following a low-sodium diet (see Box 5–5)
- Use and effects (intended and unintended) of any prescribed diuretic or other medication
- The importance of following a schedule for regular monitoring of serum electrolyte levels and reporting manifestations of imbalance to care provider

POTASSIUM IMBALANCE

Potassium, the primary intercellular cation, plays a vital role in cell metabolism, cardiac, and neuromuscular function. The normal serum (ECF) potassium level is 3.5 to 5.0 mEq/L.

OVERVIEW OF NORMAL POTASSIUM BALANCE

Most potassium in the body is found within the cells (ICF), which have a concentration of 140 to 150 mEq/L. This significant difference in the potassium concentrations of ICF and ECF helps maintain the resting membrane potential of nerve and muscle cells; either a deficit or an excess of potassium can adversely affect neuromuscular and cardiac function. The higher intracellular potassium concentration is maintained by the sodium-potassium pump.

To maintain its balance, potassium must be replaced daily. Normally, potassium is supplied in food. Virtually all foods contain potassium, although some foods and fluids are richer sources of this element than others (see Box 5–6).

The kidneys eliminate potassium very efficiently; even when potassium intake is stopped, the kidneys continue to excrete it. Because the kidneys do not conserve potassium well, significant amounts may be lost through this route. However, because the kidneys are the principal organs involved in the elimination of potassium, renal failure can lead to potentially serious elevations of serum potassium.

Aldosterone helps regulate potassium elimination by the kidneys. An increased potassium concentration in ECF stimulates aldosterone production by the adrenal gland. The kidneys respond to aldosterone by increasing potassium excretion.

BOX 5–6	■ Foods High in Potassium	

FRUITS

■ Apricots	■ Cantaloupe	■ Oranges
■ Avocados	■ Dates	■ Raisins
■ Bananas		

VEGETABLES AND VEGETABLE JUICES

■ Carrots	■ Peas	■ Tomatoes
■ Cauliflower	■ Potatoes	■ V-8 Juice
■ Mushrooms	■ Spinach	

MEATS AND FISH

■ Beef	■ Liver	■ Tuna
■ Chicken	■ Lobster	■ Turkey
■ Kidney	■ Pork loin	■ Salmon

MILK PRODUCTS

■ Buttermilk	■ Low-fat yogurt
■ Chocolate milk	■ Milk
■ Evaporated milk	

Changes in aldosterone secretion can profoundly affect the serum potassium level.

Normally only small amounts of potassium are lost in the feces, but substantial amounts may be lost from the gastrointestinal tract with diarrhea or through drainage from an ileostomy (a permanent opening into the small bowel).

Potassium constantly shifts into and out of the cells. This movement between ICF and ECF can significantly affect the serum potassium level. For example, potassium shifts into or out of the cells in response to changes in hydrogen ion concentration (pH, discussed later in this chapter) as the body strives to maintain a stable acid-base balance. Table 5–6 summarizes potassium imbalances, their causes, and manifestations.

THE CLIENT WITH HYPOKALEMIA

Hypokalemia is an abnormally low serum potassium (less than 3.5 mEq/L). It usually results from excess potassium loss, although hospitalized clients may be at risk for hypokalemia because of inadequate potassium intake.

PATHOPHYSIOLOGY AND MANIFESTATIONS

Excess potassium may be lost through the kidneys or the gastrointestinal tract. These losses cause depletion of total potassium stores in the body.

• Excess potassium loss through the kidneys often is secondary to drugs such as potassium-wasting diuretics, corticosteroids, amphotericin B, and large doses of some antibiotics. Hyperaldosteronism, a condition in which the adrenal glands secrete excess aldosterone, also causes excess elimination of potassium through the kidneys. Glucosuria and osmotic diuresis (e.g., associated with diabetes mellitus) also cause potassium wasting through the kidneys (Metheny, 2000).

• Gastrointestinal losses of potassium result from severe vomiting, gastric suction, or loss of intestinal fluids through diarrhea or ileostomy drainage.

TABLE 5–6 Causes and Manifestations of Potassium Imbalances

Imbalance	Causes	Manifestations
Hypokalemia Serum potassium <3.5 mEq/L	• Excess GI losses: vomiting, diarrhea, ileostomy drainage • Renal losses: diuretics, hyperaldosteronism • Inadequate intake • Shift into cells: Alkalosis, rapid tissue repair	Cardiovascular • Dysrhythmias • ECG changes Gastrointestinal • Nausea and vomiting • Anorexia • Decreased bowel sounds • Ileus Musculoskeletal • Muscle weakness • Leg cramps
Hyperkalemia Serum potassium >5.0 mEq/L	• Renal failure • Potassium-sparing diuretics • Adrenal insufficiency • Excess potassium intake (e.g., excess potassium replacement) • Aged blood • Shift out of cells: Cell and tissue damage, acidosis	Cardiovascular • Tall, peaked T waves, widened QRS • Dysrhythmias • Cardiac arrest Gastrointestinal • Nausea and vomiting • Abdominal cramping • Diarrhea Neuromuscular • Muscle weakness • Paresthesias • Flaccid paralysis

Potassium intake may be inadequate in clients who are unable or unwilling to eat for prolonged periods. Hospitalized clients are at risk, especially those on extended parenteral fluid therapy with solutions that do not contain potassium. Clients with anorexia nervosa or alcoholism may develop hypokalemia due to both inadequate intake and loss of potassium through vomiting, diarrhea, or laxative or diuretic use.

A *relative* loss of potassium occurs when potassium shifts from ECF into the cells. This usually is due to loss of hydrogen ion and alkalosis, although it also may occur during periods of rapid tissue repair (e.g., following a burn or trauma), in the presence of excess insulin (insulin promotes potassium entry into skeletal muscle and liver cells), during acute stress, or because of hypothermia. In these instances, the total body stores of potassium remain adequate.

Hypokalemia affects the transmission of nerve impulses, interfering with the contractility of smooth, skeletal, and cardiac muscle, as well as the regulation and transmission of cardiac impulses.

- Characteristic electrocardiogram (ECG) changes of hypokalemia include flattened or inverted T waves, the development of U waves, and a depressed ST segment (Figure 5–11 ■). The most serious cardiac effect is an increased risk of atrial and ventricular **dysrhythmias** (abnormal rhythms). Hypokalemia increases the risk for digitalis toxicity in clients receiving this drug used to treat heart failure (see Chapter 30). ⊘
- Hypokalemia affects both the resting membrane potential and intracellular enzymes in skeletal and smooth muscle cells. This causes skeletal muscle weakness and slowed peristalsis of the gastrointestinal tract. Muscles of the lower extremities are affected first, then the trunk and upper extremities.

Hypokalemia also can affect kidney function, particularly the ability to concentrate urine. Severe hypokalemia can lead to **rhabdomyolysis,** a condition in which muscle fibers disintegrate, releasing myoglobin to be excreted in the urine. The *Multisystem Effects of Hypokalemia* are summarized on page 101.

COLLABORATIVE CARE

The management of hypokalemia focuses on prevention and treatment of a deficiency.

Diagnostic Tests

The following laboratory and diagnostic tests may be ordered.

- *Serum potassium (K⁺)* is used to monitor potassium levels in clients who are at risk for or who are being treated for hypokalemia. A serum K⁺ of 3.0 to 3.5 mEq/L is considered mild hypokalemia. Moderate hypokalemia is defined as a serum K⁺ of 2.5 to 3.0 mEq/L, and severe hypokalemia as a serum K⁺ of less than 2.5 mEq/L (Metheny, 2000).
- *Arterial blood gases (ABGs)* are measured to determine acid-base status. An increased pH (alkalosis) often is associated with hypokalemia.

A Normal ECG

B ECG in hypokalemia

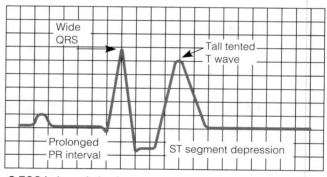

C ECG in hyperkalemia

Figure 5–11 ■ The effects of changes in potassium levels on the electrocardiogram (ECG). *A,* Normal ECG; *B,* ECG in hypokalemia; *C,* ECG in hyperkalemia.

- *ECG recordings* are obtained to evaluate the effects of hypokalemia on the cardiac conduction system.

Medications

Oral and/or parenteral potassium supplements are given to prevent and, as needed, treat hypokalemia. To prevent hypokalemia in the client taking nothing by mouth, 40 mEq of potassium chloride per day is added to intravenous fluids. The dose used to treat hypokalemia includes the daily maintenance requirement, replacement of ongoing losses (e.g., gastric suction), and additional potassium to correct the existing deficit.

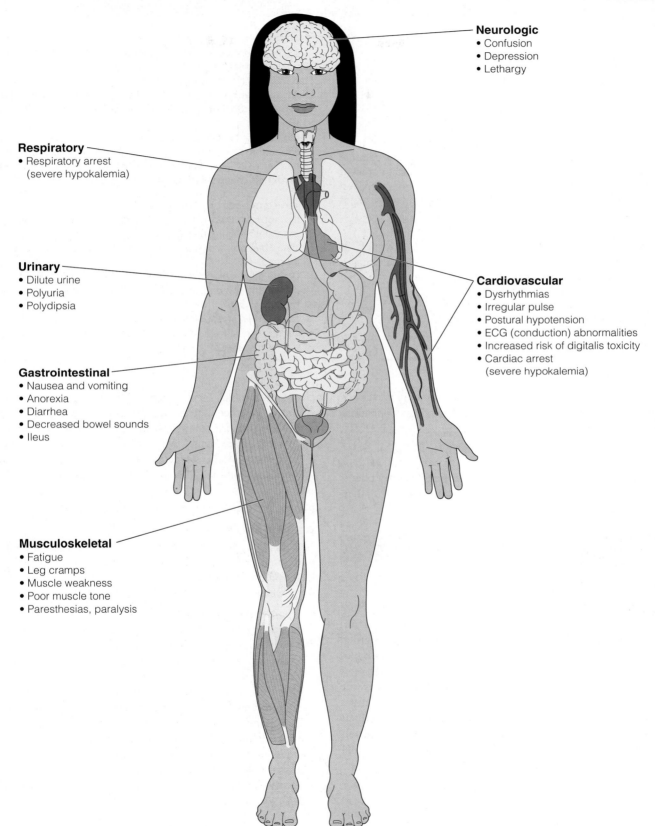

Neurologic
- Confusion
- Depression
- Lethargy

Respiratory
- Respiratory arrest
  (severe hypokalemia)

Urinary
- Dilute urine
- Polyuria
- Polydipsia

Cardiovascular
- Dysrhythmias
- Irregular pulse
- Postural hypotension
- ECG (conduction) abnormalities
- Increased risk of digitalis toxicity
- Cardiac arrest
  (severe hypokalemia)

Gastrointestinal
- Nausea and vomiting
- Anorexia
- Diarrhea
- Decreased bowel sounds
- Ileus

Musculoskeletal
- Fatigue
- Leg cramps
- Muscle weakness
- Poor muscle tone
- Paresthesias, paralysis

Medication Administration
Hypokalemia

POTASSIUM SOURCES
Potassium acetate (Tri-K)
Potassium bicarbonate (K + Care ET)
Potassium citrate (K-Lyte)
Potassium chloride (K-Lease, Micro-K 10, Apo-K)
Potassium gluconate (Kaon Elixir, Royonate)

Potassium is rapidly absorbed from the gastrointestinal tract; potassium chloride is the agent of choice, because low chloride often accompanies low potassium. Potassium is used to prevent and/or treat hypokalemia (e.g., with parenteral nutrition and potassium-wasting diuretics, and prophylactically after major surgery).

Nursing Responsibilities
- When giving oral forms of potassium:
  a. Dilute or dissolve effervescent, soluable, or liquid potassium in fruit or vegetable juice or cold water.
  b. Chill to increase palatability.
  c. Give with food to minimize GI effects.
- When giving parenteral forms of potassium:
  a. Administer slowly
  b. *Do not* administer undiluted.

  c. Assess injection site frequently for signs of pain and inflammation.
  d. Use an infusion control device.
- Assess for abdominal pain, distention, gastrointestinal bleeding; if present, do not administer medication. Notify health care provider.
- Monitor fluid intake and output.
- Assess for manifestations of hyperkalemia: weakness, feeling of heaviness in legs, mental confusion, hypotension, cardiac arrhythmias, changes in ECG, increased serum potassium levels.

Client and Family Teaching
- Do not take potassium supplements if you are also taking a potassium-sparing diuretic.
- When parenteral potassium is discontinued, eat potassium-rich foods.
- Do not chew enteric-coated tablets or allow them to dissolve in the mouth; this may affect the potency and action of the medications.
- Take potassium supplements with meals.
- Do not use salt substitutes when taking potassium (most salt substitutes are potassium based).

Several days of therapy may be required. Commonly prescribed potassium supplements, their actions, and nursing implications are described in the box above.

Dietary Management

A diet high in potassium-rich foods is recommended for clients at risk for developing hypokalemia or to supplement drug therapy (see Box 5–6).

NURSING CARE

Health Promotion

When providing general health education, discuss using balanced electrolyte solutions (e.g., Pedialyte or sports drinks) to replace abnormal fluid losses (excess perspiration, vomiting, or severe diarrhea). Discuss the necessity of preventing hypokalemia with clients at risk. Provide diet teaching and refer clients with anorexia nervosa for counseling. Stress the potassium-losing effects of taking diuretics and using laxatives to enhance weight loss. Discuss the potassium-wasting effects of most diuretics with clients taking these drugs, and encourage a diet rich in high-potassium foods, as well as regular monitoring of serum potassium levels.

Assessment

Assessment data related to hypokalemia include the following:

- Health history: Current manifestations, including anorexia, nausea and vomiting, abdominal discomfort, muscle weakness or cramping, other symptoms; duration of symptoms and any precipitating factors such as diuretic use, prolonged vomiting or diarrhea; chronic diseases such as diabetes, hyperaldosteronism, or Cushing's syndrome; current medications.
- Physical assessment: Mental status; vital signs including orthostatic vitals, apical and peripheral pulses; bowel sounds, abdominal distension; muscle strength and tone.

Nursing Diagnoses and Interventions
Activity Intolerance

Muscle cramping and weakness are common early manifestations of hypokalemia. The lower extremities are usually affected initially. This muscle weakness can cause the client to fatigue easily, particularly with activity.

- Monitor skeletal muscle strength and tone, which are affected by moderate hypokalemia. *Increasing weakness, paresthesias, or paralysis of muscles or progression of affected muscles to include the upper extremities or trunk can indicate a further drop in serum potassium levels.*
- Monitor respiratory rate, depth, and effort; heart rate and rhythm; and blood pressure at rest and following activity. *Tachypnea, dyspnea, tachycardia, and/or a change in blood pressure may indicate decreasing ability to tolerate activities. Report changes to the care provider.*
- Assist with self-care activities as needed. *Increasing muscle weakness can lead to fatigue and affect the ability to meet self-care needs.*

Decreased Cardiac Output

Hypokalemia affects the strength of cardiac contractions and can lead to dysrhythmias that further impair cardiac output.

Hypokalemia also alters the response to cardiac drugs, such as digitalis and the antidysrhythmics.

- Monitor serum potassium levels, particularly in clients at risk for hypokalemia (those with excess losses due to drug therapy, gastrointestinal losses, or who are unable to consume a normal diet). Report abnormal levels to the care provider. *Potassium must be replaced daily, as the body is unable to conserve it. Either lack of intake or abnormal losses of potassium in the urine or gastric fluids can lead to hypokalemia.*
- Monitor vital signs, including orthostatic vitals and peripheral pulses. *As cardiac output falls, the pulse becomes weak and thready. Orthostatic hypotension may be noted with decreased cardiac output.*

PRACTICE ALERT *Pace clients with severe hypokalemia on a cardiac monitor. Closely monitor cardiac rhythm and observe for characteristic ECG changes of hypokalemia (ST segment depression, flattened T waves, and U waves). Report rhythm changes and treat as indicated. Severe hypokalemia can cause life-threatening dysrhythmias.* ■

- Monitor clients taking digitalis for toxicity. Monitor response to antidysrhythmic drugs. *Hypokalemia potentiates digitalis effects and increases resistance to certain antidysrhythmics.*
- Dilute intravenous potassium and administer using an electronic infusion device. In general, potassium is given no faster than 10 to 20 mEq/hour. Closely monitor intravenous flow rate and response to potassium replacement. *Rapid potassium administration is dangerous and can lead to hyperkalemia and cardiac arrest.*

PRACTICE ALERT *Never administer undiluted potassium directly into the vein.* ■

Risk for Imbalanced Fluid Volume

- Maintain accurate intake and output records. *Gastrointestinal fluid losses can lead to significant potassium losses.*

- Monitor bowel sounds and abdominal distention. *Hypokalemia affects smooth muscle function and can lead to slowed peristalsis and paralytic ileus.*

Acute Pain

Discomfort is common when intravenous potassium chloride at a concentration of more than 40 mEq/L is given into a peripheral vein.

- When possible, administer intravenous KCl through a central line. *The rapid blood flow through central veins dilutes the KCl solution, decreasing discomfort.*
- Spread the total daily dose of KCl over 24 hours to minimize the concentration of intravenous solutions. *High concentrations of KCl are irritating to vein walls, particularly if inflammation is present.*
- Discuss with the physician using a small amount of lidocaine prior to or with the infusion. *Both a lidocaine bolus given at the infusion site and a small amount of lidocaine in the intravenous infusion have been shown to at least partially relieve discomfort associated with concentrated potassium solutions* (Metheny, 2000).

Using NANDA, NIC, and NOC

Chart 5–4 shows links between NANDA nursing diagnoses, NIC, and NOC for clients with a potassium imbalance.

Home Care

The focus in preparing the client with or at risk for hypokalemia is prevention. Discharge planning focuses on teaching self-care practices. Include the following topics when preparing the client and family for home care.

- Recommended diet, including a list of potassium-rich foods
- Prescribed medications and potassium supplements, their use, and desired and unintended effects
- Using salt substitutes (if recommended) to increase potassium intake; avoiding substitutes if taking a potassium supplement or potassium-sparing diuretic

CHART 5–4 NANDA, NIC, AND NOC LINKAGES

The Client with Potassium Imbalance

NURSING DIAGNOSES	NURSING INTERVENTIONS	NURSING OUTCOMES
• Decreased Cardiac Output	• Cardiac Care • Electrolyte Management: Hyperkalemia • Electrolyte Management: Hypokalemia	• Cardiac Pump Effectiveness • Vital Signs Status
• Activity Intolerance	• Energy Management	• Energy Conservation • Activity Tolerance
• Risk for Ineffective Health Maintenance	• Health Education • Risk Identification	• Health-Seeking Behavior

Note. Data from Nursing Outcomes Classification (NOC) by M. Johnson & M. Maas (Eds.), 1997, St. Louis: Mosby; Nursing Diagnoses: Definitions & Classification 2001–2002 by North American Nursing Diagnosis Association, 2001, Philadelphia: NANDA; Nursing Interventions Classification (NIC) by J.C. McCloskey & G. M. Bulechek (Eds.), 2000, St. Louis: Mosby. Reprinted by permission.

- Manifestations of potassium imbalance (hypokalemia or hyperkalemia) to report to health care provider
- Recommendations for monitoring serum potassium levels
- If taking digitalis, manifestations of digitalis toxicity to report to health care provider
- Managing gastrointestinal disorders that cause potassium loss (vomiting, diarrhea, ileostomy drainage) to prevent hypokalemia

THE CLIENT WITH HYPERKALEMIA

Hyperkalemia is an abnormally high serum potassium (greater than 5 mEq/L). Hyperkalemia can result from inadequate excretion of potassium, excessively high intake of potassium, or a shift of potassium from the intracellular to the extracellular space. *Pseudohyperkalemia* (an erroneously high serum potassium reading) can occur if the blood sample hemolyzes, releasing potassium from blood cells, before it is analyzed. Hyperkalemia affects neuromuscular and cardiac function.

PATHOPHYSIOLOGY AND MANIFESTATIONS

Impaired renal excretion of potassium is a primary cause of hyperkalemia. Untreated renal failure, adrenal insufficiency (e.g., Addison's disease or inadequate aldosterone production), and medications (such as potassium-sparing diuretics, the antimicrobial drug trimethoprim, and some NSAIDs) impair potassium excretion by the kidneys.

In clients with normal renal excretion of potassium, excess oral potassium (e.g., by supplement or use of salt substitutes) rarely leads to hyperkalemia. Rapid intravenous administra-

Nursing Care Plan
A Client with Hypokalemia

Rose Ortiz is a 72-year-old widow who lives alone, although close to her daughter's home. Ms. Ortiz has mild heart failure and is being treated with digoxin (Lanoxin) 0.125 mg, furosemide (Lasix) 40 mg PO daily, and a mildly restricted sodium diet (2 g daily). For the last several weeks, Ms. Ortiz has complained that she feels weak and sometimes faint, light headed, and dizzy. Serum electrolyte tests ordered by her physician reveal a potassium level of 2.4 mEq/L. Potassium chloride solution (Kaochlor 10%, 20 mEq/15 mL) PO twice daily is prescribed, and Ms. Ortiz is referred to Nancy Walters, RN, for follow-up care.

ASSESSMENT
Ms. Ortiz's health history reveals that she has rigidly adhered to her sodium-restricted diet and has been compliant in taking her prescribed medications, with the exception of occasionally taking an additional "water pill" when her ankles swell. She takes a laxative every evening to ensure a daily bowel movement. She states that she is reluctant to take the potassium chloride the doctor has ordered because her neighbor complains that his potassium supplement upsets his stomach. Physical assessment findings included T 98.4, P 70, R 20, and BP 138/84. Muscle strength in her upper extremities is normal and equal; lower extremity strength is weak but equal. Sensation is normal.

DIAGNOSES
- *Risk for injury* related to muscle weakness
- *Risk for ineffective health maintenance* related to lack of knowledge about how diuretic therapy and laxative affect potassium levels

EXPECTED OUTCOMES
- Maintain potassium level within normal limits (3.5 to 5.0 mEq/L).
- Regain normal muscle strength.
- Remain free of injury.
- Verbalize understanding of the effects of diuretic therapy and laxatives on potassium levels.

- Identify measures to avoid gastrointestinal irritation when taking oral potassium.
- Identify potassium-rich foods.

PLANNING AND IMPLEMENTATION
- Explain need to use caution when ambulating, particularly when climbing or descending stairs.
- Discuss side effects of furosemide, and explain how taking additional tablets may have contributed to hypokalemia.
- Discuss alternative measures to prevent constipation without using laxatives on a regular basis (e.g., high-fiber diet, adequate fluid intake).
- Explain purpose of the prescribed potassium and its role in reversing muscle weakness.
- Teach to take potassium supplement after breakfast and supper, diluted in 4 oz of juice or water, and to sip it slowly over a 5- to 10-minute period. Advise to call if gastric irritation occurs.
- Discuss dietary sources of potassium; provide a list of potassium-rich foods.

EVALUATION
On a follow-up visit 1 week later, Ms. Ortiz states that her muscle weakness, dizziness, and other symptoms have resolved. She is taking the prescribed drugs as directed and is using laxatives only two or three times a week. Ms. Ortiz reports that she has increased her intake of potassium-rich foods and fluids and of high-fiber foods. Her potassium level is within normal limits.

Critical Thinking in the Nursing Process
1. What is the pathophysiologic basis for Rose's muscle weakness and dizziness?
2. How may the chronic overuse of laxatives contribute to hypokalemia?
3. Describe the interaction of digitalis, diuretics, and potassium.
4. Develop a plan of care for Ms. Ortiz for the nursing diagnosis *Constipation*.

See Evaluating Your Response in Appendix C.

tion of potassium or transfusion of aged blood can lead to hyperkalemia.

A shift of potassium ions from the intracellular space can occur in acidosis, with severe tissue trauma, during chemotherapy, and due to starvation. In acidosis, excess hydrogen ions enter the cells, causing potassium to shift into the extracellular space. The extent of this shift is greater with metabolic acidosis than with respiratory acidosis (see "Acid-Base Disorders" later in this chapter).

Hyperkalemia alters the cell membrane potential, affecting the heart, skeletal muscle function, and the gastrointestinal tract. The most harmful consequence of hyperkalemia is its effect on cardiac function. The cardiac conduction system is affected first, with slowing of the heart rate, possible heart blocks, and prolonged depolarization. ECG changes include peaked T waves, a prolonged PR interval, and widening of the QRS complex (see Figure 5–11). Ventricular dysrhythmias develop, and cardiac arrest may occur. Severe hyperkalemia decreases the strength of myocardial contractions.

Skeletal muscles become weak and paralysis may occur with very high serum potassium levels. Hyperkalemia causes smooth muscle hyperactivity, leading to gastrointestinal disturbances.

The seriousness of hyperkalemia is based on the serum potassium (K^+) level and ECG changes.

- Mild hyperkalemia: serum K^+ between 5 and 6.5 mEq/L; ECG changes limited to peaked T wave.
- Moderate hyperkalemia: serum K^+ between 6.5 and 8 mEq/L; ECG changes limited to peaked T wave.
- Severe hyperkalemia: serum K^+ greater than 8 mEq/L; ECG shows absent P waves and widened QRS pattern.

The manifestations of hyperkalemia result from its effects on the heart, skeletal, and smooth muscles. Early manifestations include diarrhea, colic (abdominal cramping), anxiety, paresthesias, irritability, and muscle tremors and twitching. As serum potassium levels increase, muscle weakness develops, progressing to flaccid paralysis. The lower extremities are affected first, progressing to the trunk and upper extremities.

COLLABORATIVE CARE

The management of hyperkalemia focuses on returning the serum potassium level to normal by treating the underlying cause and avoiding additional potassium intake. The choice of therapy for existing hyperkalemia is based on the severity of the hyperkalemia.

Diagnostic Tests

The following laboratory and diagnostic tests may be ordered.

- *Serum electrolytes* show a serum potassium level greater than 5.0 mEq/L. Low calcium and sodium levels may increase the effects of hyperkalemia; therefore, these electrolytes are usually measured as well.
- *ABGs* are measured to determine if acidosis is present.
- An *ECG* is obtained and *continuous ECG monitoring* is instituted to evaluate the effects of hyperkalemia on cardiac conduction and rhythm.

Medications

Medications are administered to lower the serum potassium and to stabilize the conduction system of the heart. For moderate to severe hyperkalemia, calcium gluconate is given intravenously to counter the effects of hyperkalemia on the cardiac conduction system. While the effect of calcium gluconate lasts only for 1 hour, it allows time to initiate measures to lower serum potassium levels. To rapidly lower these levels, regular insulin and 50 g of glucose are administered. Insulin and glucose promote potassium uptake by the cells, shifting potassium out of ECF. In some cases, a β_2-agonist such as albuterol may be given by nebulizer to temporarily push potassium into the cells. Sodium bicarbonate may be given to treat acidosis. As the pH returns toward normal, hydrogen ions are released from the cells and potassium returns into the cells.

To remove potassium from the body, sodium polystyrene sulfonate (Kayexalate), a resin that binds potassium in the gastrointestinal tract, may be administered orally or rectally. If renal function is normal, diuretics such as furosemide are given to promote potassium excretion. Commonly prescribed drugs, their actions, and nursing implications are summarized on page 106.

Dialysis

When renal function is severely limited, either peritoneal dialysis or hemodialysis may be implemented to remove excess potassium. These measures are invasive and typically used only when other measures are ineffective. See Chapter 27 for more information about dialysis. ⊘

NURSING CARE

Nursing care focuses related to hyperkalemia include identifying clients at risk, preventing hyperkalemia, and addressing problems resulting from the systemic effects of hyperkalemia.

Health Promotion

Clients at the greatest risk for developing hyperkalemia include those taking potassium supplements (prescribed or over-the-counter), using potassium-sparing diuretics or salt substitutes, and experiencing renal failure. Athletes participating in competition sports such as body building and using anabolic steroids, muscle-building compounds, or "energy drinks" also may be at risk for hyperkalemia.

Teach all clients to carefully read food and dietary supplement labels. Discuss the importance of taking prescribed potassium supplements as ordered, and not increasing the dose unless prescribed by the care provider. Advise clients taking a potassium supplement or potassium-sparing diuretic to avoid salt substitutes, which usually contain potassium. Discuss the importance of maintaining an adequate fluid intake (unless a fluid restriction has been prescribed) to maintain renal function to eliminate potassium from the body.

Assessment

Assessment data related to hyperkalemia include the following:

- Health history: Current manifestations, including numbness and tingling, nausea and vomiting, abdominal cramping,

muscle weakness, palpitations; duration of symptoms and any precipitating factors such as use of salt substitutes, potassium supplements, or reduced urine output; chronic diseases such as renal failure or endocrine disorders; current medications.
- Physical assessment: Apical and peripheral pulses; bowel sounds; muscle strength in upper and lower extremities; ECG pattern.

Nursing Diagnoses and Interventions

Risk for Activity Intolerance

Both hypokalemia (low serum potassium levels) and hyperkalemia (high serum potassium levels) affect neuromuscular activity and the function of cardiac, smooth, and skeletal muscles. Hyperkalemia can cause muscle weakness and even paralysis.

- Monitor skeletal muscle strength and tone. *Increasing weakness, muscle paralysis, or progression of affected muscles to affect the upper extremities or trunk can indicate increasing serum potassium levels.*
- Monitor respiratory rate and depth. Regularly assess lung sounds. *Muscle weakness due to hyperkalemia can impair ventilation. In addition, medications such as sodium bicarbonate or sodium polystyrene sulfonate can cause fluid re-*

tention and pulmonary edema in clients with preexisting cardiovascular disease.
- Assist with self-care activities as needed. *Increasing muscle weakness can lead to fatigue and affect the ability to meet self-care needs.*

Risk for Decreased Cardiac Output

Hyperkalemia affects depolarization of the atria and ventricles of the heart. Severe hyperkalemia can cause dysrhythmias with ventricular fibrillation and cardiac arrest. The cardiac effects of hyperkalemia are more pronounced when the serum potassium level rises rapidly. Low serum sodium and calcium levels, high serum magnesium levels, and acidosis contribute to the adverse effects of hyperkalemia on the heart muscle.

PRACTICE ALERT *Monitor the ECG pattern for development of peaked, narrow T waves, prolongation of the PR interval, depression of the ST segment, widened QRS interval, and loss of the P wave. Notify the physician of changes. Progressive ECG changes from a peaked T wave to loss of the P wave and widening of the QRS complex indicate an increasing risk of dysrhythmias and cardiac arrest.* ∎

Medication Administration

Hyperkalemia

DIURETICS
Potassium-wasting diuretics, such as furosemide (Lasix), may be used to enhance renal excretion of potassium.

Nursing Responsibilities
- Monitor serum electrolytes.
- Monitor and record weight at regular intervals under standard conditions (same time of day, balanced scale, same clothing).
- Monitor intake and output.

INSULIN, HYPERTONIC DEXTROSE, AND SODIUM BICARBONATE
Insulin, hypertonic dextrose (10% to 50%), and sodium bicarbonate are used in the emergency treatment of moderate to severe hyperkalemia. Insulin promotes the movement of potassium into the cell, and glucose prevents hypoglycemia. The onset of action of insulin and hypertonic dextrose occurs within 30 minutes and is effective for approximately 4 to 6 hours.

Sodium bicarbonate elevates the serum pH; potassium is moved into the cell in exchange for hydrogen ion. Sodium bicarbonate is particularly useful in the client with metabolic acidosis. Onset of effects occurs within 15 to 30 minutes and is effective for approximately 2 hours.

Nursing Responsibilities
- Administer intravenous insulin and dextrose over prescribed interval of time using an infusion pump.
- Administer sodium bicarbonate as prescribed. It may be administered as an intravenous bolus or added to a dextrose-in-water solution and given by infusion.
- In clients receiving sodium bicarbonate, monitor for sodium overload, particularly in clients with hypernatremia, heart failure, and renal failure.

- Monitor the ECG pattern closely.
- Monitor serum electrolytes (K^+, Na^+, Ca^{2+}, Mg^{2+}) frequently during treatment.

CALCIUM GLUCONATE AND CALCIUM CHLORIDE
Intravenous calcium gluconate or calcium chloride is used as a temporary emergency measure to counteract the toxic effects of potassium on myocardial conduction and function.

Nursing Responsibilities
- Closely monitor the ECG of the client receiving intravenous calcium, particularly for bradycardia.
- Calcium should be used cautiously in clients receiving digitalis, because calcium increases the cardiotonic effects of digitalis and may precipitate digitalis toxicity, leading to dysrhythmias.

SODIUM POLYSTYRENE SULFONATE (KAYEXALATE) AND SORBITOL
Sodium polystyrene sulfonate (Kayexalate) is used to treat moderate or severe hyperkalemia. Categorized as a cation exchange resin, Kayexalate exchanges sodium or calcium for potassium in the large intestine. Sorbitol is given with Kayexalate to promote bowel elimination. Kayexalate and sorbitol may be administered orally, through a nasogastric tube, or rectally as a retention enema. The usual dosage is 20 g three or four times a day with 20 mL of 70% sorbitol solution.

Nursing Responsibilities
- Because Kayexalate contains sodium, monitor clients with heart failure and edema closely for water retention.
- Monitor serum electrolytes (K^+, Na^+, Ca^{2+}, Mg^{2+}) frequently during therapy.
- Restrict sodium intake in clients who are unable to tolerate increased sodium load (e.g., those with CHF or hypertension).

- Closely monitor the response to intravenous calcium gluconate, particularly in clients taking digitalis. *Calcium increases the risk of digitalis toxicity.*

Risk for Imbalanced Fluid Volume

Renal failure is a major cause of hyperkalemia. Clients with renal failure also are at risk for fluid retention and other electrolyte imbalances.

- Closely monitor serum potassium, BUN, and serum creatinine. Notify the physician if serum potassium level is greater than 5 mEq/L, or if serum creatinine and BUN levels are increasing. *Serum creatinine and BUN are the primary indicators of renal function. Levels of these substances rise rapidly in acute renal failure, more slowly in chronic renal failure* (see Chapter 27). ⟲
- Maintain accurate intake and output records. Report an imbalance of 24-hour totals and/or urine output less than 30 mL/hour. *Oliguria (scant urine) or anuria (no urine output) may indicate renal failure and an increased risk for hyperkalemia and fluid volume excess.*
- Monitor clients receiving sodium bicarbonate for fluid volume excess. *Increased sodium from injection of a hypertonic sodium bicarbonate solution can cause a shift of water into the extracellular space.*
- Monitor clients receiving cation exchange resins and sorbitol for fluid volume excess. *The resin exchanges potassium for sodium or calcium in the bowel. Excessive sodium and water retention may occur.*

Using NANDA, NIC, and NOC

Chart 5–4 shows links between NANDA nursing diagnoses, NIC, and NOC when caring for a client with a potassium imbalance.

Home Care

Preventing future episodes of hyperkalemia is the focus when preparing the client for home care. Include the family, a significant other, or a caregiver when teaching the following topics.

- Recommended diet and any restrictions including salt substitutes and foods high in potassium
- Medications to be avoided, including over-the-counter and fitness supplements
- Follow-up appointments for lab work and evaluation

Nursing Care Plan
A Client with Hyperkalemia

Montigue Longacre, a 51-year-old African American male, has end-stage renal failure. He arrives at the emergency clinic complaining of shortness of breath on exertion and extreme weakness.

ASSESSMENT

Mr. Longacre tells the nurse, Janet Allen, RN, that he normally receives dialysis three times a week. He missed his last treatment, however, to attend his father's funeral. During the last several days, he has eaten a number of fresh oranges he received as a gift. Physical assessment findings include T 99.2, P 100, R 28, BP 168/96, 2+ pretibial edema, and a 6 lb (3.6 kg) weight gain since his last hemodialysis treatment 4 days ago. Laboratory and diagnostic tests show the following abnormal results.

- K^+ 6.5 mEq/L (normal 3.5 to 5 mEq/L)
- BUN 118 mg/dL (normal 7 to 18 mg/dL)
- Creatinine 14 mg/dL (normal 0.7 to 1.3 mg/dL)
- HCO_3^- 17 mEq/L (normal 22 to 26 mEq/L)
- Peaked T wave noted on ECG

Mr. Longacre is placed on continuous ECG monitoring, and the physician prescribes hemodialysis. As an interim measure to lower the serum potassium, the physician prescribes D50W (25 g of dextrose), one ampule, to be administered intravenously with 10 units of regular insulin over 30 minutes.

DIAGNOSIS

- *Activity intolerance* related to skeletal muscle weakness
- *Risk for decreased cardiac output* related to hyperkalemia
- *Risk for ineffective health maintenance* related to inadequate knowledge of recommended diet
- *Excess fluid volume* related to renal failure

EXPECTED OUTCOMES

- Gradually resume usual physical activities.
- Maintain serum potassium level within normal range.

- Verbalize causes of hyperkalemia, the importance of hemodialysis treatments as scheduled, and the role of diet in preventing hyperkalemia.

PLANNING AND IMPLEMENTATION

- Monitor intake and output.
- Monitor serum potassium and ECG closely during treatment.
- Teach causes of hyperkalemia and the relationship between hemodialysis and hyperkalemia.
- Discuss the importance of avoiding foods high in potassium to prevent or control hyperkalemia.

EVALUATION

Following emergency treatment and hemodialysis, Mr. Longacre's ECG and serum potassium level have returned to normal. His muscle strength has returned to near normal, and he verbalizes an understanding of his prescribed hemodialysis regimen. Janet Allen provides verbal and written information about hyperkalemia, the importance of complying with the hemodialysis regimen, and the importance of limiting intake of dietary sources of potassium in renal failure. She also furnishes a list of foods high in potassium and cautions against using potassium-containing salt substitutes and nonprescription drugs.

Critical Thinking in the Nursing Process

1. What information given by Mr. Longacre indicated that he might be experiencing hyperkalemia?
2. Why was continuous ECG monitoring instituted as an emergency measure?
3. What additional emergency measures might have been instituted if Mr. Longacre's serum potassium level was 8.5 mEq/L and his ECG showed changes in impulse conduction?
4. Develop a care plan for Mr. Longacre for the nursing diagnosis *anxiety.*

See Evaluating Your Response in Appendix C.

CALCIUM IMBALANCE

Calcium is one of the most abundant ions in the body. The normal adult total serum calcium concentration is 8.5 to 10.0 mg/dL.

OVERVIEW OF NORMAL CALCIUM BALANCE

Calcium is obtained from dietary sources, although only about 20% of the calcium ingested is absorbed into the blood. The remainder is excreted in feces. Extracellular calcium is excreted by the kidneys. Approximately 99% of the total calcium in the body is bound to phosphorus to form the minerals in bones and teeth. The remaining 1% is in extracellular fluid. About half of this extracellular calcium is ionized (free); it is this ionized calcium that is physiologically active. The remaining extracellular calcium is bound to protein or other ions.

Ionized calcium is essential to a number of processes:

- Stabilizing cell membranes
- Regulating muscle contraction and relaxation
- Maintaining cardiac function
- Blood clotting

Serum calcium levels are regulated by the interaction of three hormones: parathyroid hormone (PTH), calcitonin, and calcitriol (a metabolite of vitamin D). When serum calcium levels fall, the parathyroid glands secrete PTH, which mobilizes skeletal calcium stores, increases calcium absorption in the intestines, and promotes calcium reabsorption by the kidneys (Figure 5–12 ■). Calcitriol facilitates this process by stimulating calcium release from the bones, absorption in the intestines, and reabsorption by the kidneys. Calcitonin is secreted by the thyroid gland in response to high serum calcium levels. Its effect on serum calcium levels is the opposite of PTH: It inhibits the movement of calcium out of bone, reduces intestinal absorption of calcium, and promotes calcium excretion by the kidneys.

Serum calcium levels are also affected by acid-base balance. When hydrogen ion concentration falls and the pH rises (**alkalosis**), more calcium is bound to protein. While the total serum calcium remains unchanged, less calcium is available in the ionized, active form. Conversely, when hydrogen ion concentration increases and the pH falls (**acidosis**), calcium is released from protein, making more ionized calcium available. Table 5–7 summarizes the causes and manifestations of calcium imbalances.

THE CLIENT WITH HYPOCALCEMIA

Hypocalcemia is a total serum calcium level of less than 8.5 mg/dL. Hypocalcemia can result from decreased total body calcium stores or low levels of extracellular calcium with normal amounts of calcium stored in bone. The systemic effects of hypocalcemia are caused by decreased levels of ionized calcium in extracellular fluid.

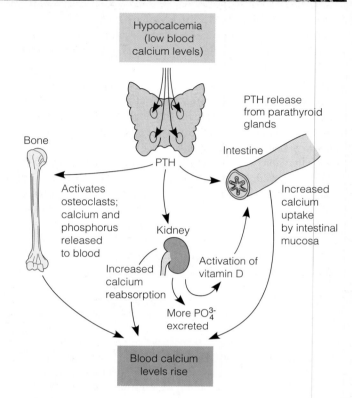

Figure 5–12 ■ Low calcium levels (hypocalcemia) trigger the release of parathyroid hormone (PTH), increasing calcium ion levels through stimulation of bones, kidneys, and intestines.

RISK FACTORS

Certain populations of people are at greater risk for hypocalcemia: people who have had a parathyroidectomy (removal of the parathyroid glands), older adults (especially women), people with lactose intolerance, and those with alcoholism. Older adults often consume less milk and milk products (good sources of calcium) and may have less exposure to the sun (a source of vitamin D). Older adults also may be less active, promoting calcium loss from bones. They are more likely to be taking drugs that interfere with calcium absorption or promote calcium excretion (e.g., furosemide). Older women are at particular risk after menopause because of reduced estrogen levels. Intolerance to lactose (found in milk and milk products) causes diarrhea and often limits the intake of milk and milk products, leading to possible calcium deficiency. Ethanol, or drinking alcohol, has a direct effect on calcium balance, reduces its intestinal absorption, and interferes with other processes involved in regulating serum calcium levels.

PATHOPHYSIOLOGY

Common causes of hypocalcemia are hypoparathyroidism (see Chapter 17 ⊙⊙) resulting from surgery (parathyroidectomy, thyroidectomy, radical neck dissection) and acute pancreatitis.

TABLE 5-7 Causes and Manifestations of Calcium Imbalances

Imbalance	Causes	Manifestations

Hypocalcemia
Serum calcium <4.3 mEq/L
or 8.5 mg/dL
	• Parathyroidectomy or neck surgery
	• Acute pancreatitis
	• Inadequate dietary intake
	• Lack of sun exposure
	• Lack of weight-bearing exercise
	• Drugs: loop diuretics, calcitonin
	• Hypomagnesemia, alcohol abuse
		Neuromuscular
		  • Tetany
		    • Paresthesias
		    • Muscle spasms
		    • Positive Chvostek's sign
		    • Positive Trousseau's sign
		    • Laryngospasm
		    • Seizures
		  • Anxiety, confusion, psychoses
		Cardiovascular
		  • Decreased cardiac output
		  • Hypotension
		  • Dysrhythmias
		Gastrointestinal
		  • Abdominal cramping
		  • Diarrhea

Hypercalcemia
Serum calcium >5.3 mEq/L
or 10 mg/dL
	• Hyperparathyroidism
	• Some cancers
	• Prolonged immobilization
	• Paget's disease
	• Excess milk or antacid intake
	• Renal failure
		Neuromuscular
		  • Muscle weakness, fatigue
		  • Decreased deep tendon reflexes
		Behavioral
		  • Personality changes
		  • Altered mental status
		  • Decreasing level of consciousness
		Gastrointestinal
		  • Abdominal pain
		  • Constipation
		  • Anorexia, nausea, vomiting
		Cardiovascular
		  • Dysrhythmias
		  • Hypertension
		Renal
		  • Polyuria, thirst

In the client who has undergone surgery, symptoms of hypocalcemia usually occur within the first 24 to 48 hours, but may be delayed.

PRACTICE ALERT *Carefully monitor clients who have undergone neck surgery for manifestations of hypocalcemia. Check serum calcium levels, and report changes to the care provider.* ■

Additional causes of hypocalcemia include other electrolyte imbalances (such as hypomagnesemia or hyperphosphatemia), alkalosis, malabsorption disorders that interfere with calcium absorption in the bowel, and inadequate vitamin D (due to lack of sun exposure or malabsorption). Massive transfusion of banked blood also can lead to hypocalcemia. Citrate is added to blood to prevent clotting and as a preservative. When blood is administered faster than the liver can metabolize the citrate, it can bind with calcium, temporarily removing ionized calcium from circulation. Many drugs increase the risk for hypocalcemia, including loop diuretics (such as furosemide), anticonvulsants (such as phenytoin and phenobarbital), phosphates (including phosphate enemas), and drugs that lower serum magnesium levels (such as cisplatin and gentamycin) (Metheny, 2000).

Hypocalcemia affects neuromuscular cell membranes, increasing neuromuscular irritability. The threshold of excitation of sensory nerve fibers is lowered as well, leading to paresthesias (altered sensation). The nervous system becomes more excitable, and muscle spasms develop. In the heart, this change in cell membranes can lead to dysrhythmias such as ventricular tachycardia and cardiac arrest. Hypocalcemia decreases the contractility of cardiac muscle fibers, leading to decreased cardiac output.

MANIFESTATIONS AND COMPLICATIONS

The most serious manifestations of hypocalcemia are **tetany** (tonic muscular spasms) and convulsions. Numbness and tingling around the mouth (circumoral) and in the hands and feet develop. Muscle spasms of the face and extremities occur, and deep tendon reflexes become hyperactive. Chvostek's sign, contraction of the facial muscles produced by tapping the facial nerve in front of the ear (Figure 5–13A ■), and Trousseau's sign, carpal spasm induced by inflating a blood pressure cuff on the upper arm to above systolic blood pressure for 2 to 5 minutes (Figure 5–13B), indicate increased neuromuscular excitability in clients without obvious symptoms.

A

B

Figure 5–13 ■ *A,* Positive Chvostek's sign. *B,* Positive Trousseau's sign.

Tetany can cause bronchial muscle spasms, simulating an asthma attack, and visceral muscle spasms, producing acute abdominal pain. Cardiovascular manifestations include hypotension, possible bradycardia (slow heart rate), and ventricular dysrhythmias.

Serious complications of hypocalcemia include airway obstruction and possible respiratory arrest from laryngospasm, ventricular dysrhythmias and cardiac arrest, heart failure, and convulsions.

COLLABORATIVE CARE

Management of hypocalcemia is directed toward restoring normal calcium balance and correcting the underlying cause.

Diagnostic Tests

The following laboratory and diagnostic tests may be ordered when hypocalcemia is known or suspected. Measurements include:

- *Total serum calcium* is the amount of ionized (active) calcium available usually is estimated. In critically ill clients, however, *ionized calcium* may be directly measured using ion-selective electrodes. Direct measurement of ionized calcium requires special handling of the blood specimen, including placing the specimen on ice and analyzing it immediately.
- *Serum albumin,* because the albumin level affects serum calcium results. When the albumin level is low (hypoalbuminemia), the amount of ionized calcium may remain normal even though the total calcium level is low.
- *Serum magnesium,* because hypocalcemia is often associated with hypomagnesemia (serum magnesium <1.6 mg/dL). In this case, normal magnesium levels must be restored to correct the hypocalcemia.
- *Serum phosphate* hyperphosphatemia (serum phosphate > 4.5 mg/dL) can lead to hypocalcemia because of the inverse relationship between phosphorus and calcium (as phosphate levels rise, calcium levels fall).
- *Parathyroid hormone (PTH),* to identify the possible diagnoses of hyperparathyroidism.
- An *ECG,* to evaluate the effects of hypocalcemia on the heart, such as a prolonged ST segment.

Medications

Hypocalcemia is treated with oral or intravenous calcium. The client with severe hypocalcemia is treated with intravenous calcium to prevent life-threatening problems such as airway obstruction. The most common intravenous calcium preparations include calcium chloride and calcium gluconate. Although calcium chloride contains more elemental calcium than calcium gluconate, it also is more irritating to the veins and may cause venous sclerosis (hardening of the vein walls) if given into a peripheral vein. Intravenous calcium preparations can cause necrosis and sloughing of tissue if they extravasate into subcutaneous tissue. Rapid drug administration can lead to bradycardia and possible cardiac arrest due to overcorrection of hypocalcemia with resulting hypercalcemia. See page 111 for further information about calcium administration.

Oral calcium preparations (calcium carbonate, calcium gluconate, or calcium lactate) are used to treat chronic, asymptomatic hypocalcemia. Calcium supplements may be combined with vitamin D, or vitamin D may be given alone to increase gastrointestinal absorption of calcium.

Dietary Management

A diet high in calcium-rich foods may be recommended for clients with chronic hypocalcemia or with low total body stores of calcium. Box 5–7 lists foods that are high in calcium.

NURSING CARE

Health Promotion

Because of the large stores of calcium in bones, most healthy adults have a very low risk of developing hypocalcemia. A deficit of total body calcium is often associated with aging,

Medication Administration
Calcium Salts

CALCIUM SALTS

Calcium carbonate (BioCal, Calsam, Caltrate, OsCal, Tums, others)
Calcium chloride
Calcium citrate (Citrical)
Calcium glubionate
Calcium gluceptate
Calcium gluconate (Calcinate)
Calcium lactate

Calcium salts are given to increase calcium levels when there is a deficit (a total body deficit or inadequate levels of extracellular calcium). Calcium is necessary to maintain bone structure and for multiple physiologic processes including neuromuscular and cardiac function as well as blood coagulation. In the presence of vitamin D, calcium is well absorbed from the gastrointestinal tract. Severe hypocalcemia is treated with intravenous calcium preparations.

Nursing Responsibilities

Oral calcium salts
- Administer 1 to 1.5 hours after meals and at bedtime.
- Give calcium tablets with a full glass of water.

Intravenous calcium salts
- Assess IV site for patency. Do not administer calcium if there is a risk of leakage into the tissues.
- May be given by slow IV push (dilute with sterile normal saline for injection prior to administering) or added to compatible parenteral fluids such as NS, lactated Ringer's solution, or D_5W.
- Administer into the largest available vein; use a central line if available.
- Do not administer with bicarbonate of phosphate.
- Continuously monitor ECG when administering IV calcium to clients taking digitalis due to increased risk of digitalis toxicity.
- Frequently monitor serum calcium levels and response to therapy.

Client and Family Teaching
- Take calcium tablets with a full glass of water 1 to 2 hours after meals. Do not take with food or milk. If possible, do not take within 1 to 2 hours of other medications.
- Maintain adequate vitamin D intake through diet or exposure to the sun to promote calcium absorption.
- Calcium carbonate can cause constipation. Eat a high-fiber diet and maintain a generous fluid intake to prevent constipation.

---

however, increasing the risk of osteoporosis, fractures, and disability. Women have a higher risk for developing osteoporosis than men due to lower bone density and hormonal influences. Teach women of all ages the importance of maintaining adequate calcium intake through diet and, as needed, calcium supplements. Stress the relationship between weight-bearing exercise and bone density, and encourage women to engage in a regular aerobic and weight-training exercise regime. Discuss hormone replacement therapy and its potential benefits during and after menopause. See Chapter 39 ⊙ for more information about osteoporosis.

Assessment

Assessment data related to hypocalcemia include the following:

- Health history: Current manifestations, including numbness and tingling around mouth and of hands and feet, abdominal pain, shortness of breath; acute or chronic diseases such as pancreatitis, liver or kidney disease; current medications.
- Physical assessment: Muscle spasms; deep tendon reflexes; Chvostek's sign and Trousseau's sign; respiratory rate and

depth; vital signs and apical pulse; heart rate and rhythm; presence of convulsions.

Nursing Diagnoses and Interventions
Risk for Injury

The client with hypocalcemia is at risk for injury from possible laryngospasm, cardiac dysrhythmias, or convulsions. In addition, too rapid administration of intravenous calcium or extravasation of the medication into subcutaneous tissues can lead to injury.

- Frequently monitor airway and respiratory status. Report changes such as respiratory **stridor** (a high-pitched, harsh inspiratory sound indicative of upper airway obstruction) or increased respiratory rate or effort to the physician. *These changes may indicate laryngeal spasm due to tetany.*

PRACTICE ALERT *Laryngeal spasm is a respiratory emergency, requiring immediate intervention to maintain ventilation and gas exchange.* ■

- Monitor cardiovascular status including heart rate and rhythm, blood pressure, and peripheral pulses. *Hypocalcemia decreases myocardial contractility, causing reduced cardiac output and hypotension. It also can cause bradycardia or ventricular dysrhythmias. Cardiac arrest may occur in severe hypocalcemia.*
- Continuously monitor ECG in clients receiving intravenous calcium preparations, especially if the client also is taking digitalis. *Rapid administration of calcium salts can lead to hypercalcemia and cardiac dysrhythmias. Calcium administration increases the risk of digitalis toxicity and resultant dysrhythmias.*

BOX 5–7	■ Foods High in Calcium
■ Cottage cheese	■ Canned sardines and salmon
■ Cheese	■ Rhubarb
■ Milk	■ Broccoli
■ Cream	■ Collard greens
■ Yogurt	■ Soy flour
■ Ice cream	■ Spinach
■ Molasses	■ Tofu

MediaLink | HYPOCALCEMIA CARE PLAN

- Provide a quiet environment. Institute seizure precautions such as raising the side rails and keeping an airway at bedside. *A quiet environment reduces central nervous system stimuli and the risk of convulsions in the client with tetany.*

Using NANDA, NIC, and NOC

Chart 5–5 shows links between NANDA nursing diagnoses, NIC, and NOC for the client with a calcium imbalance.

Home Care

In preparing the client with hypocalcemia for discharge and home care, consider the circumstances leading to low serum calcium levels. Discuss risk factors for hypocalcemia specific to the client, and provide information about managing these risk factors to avoid future episodes of hypocalcemia. Teach about prescribed medications, including calcium supplements. Provide a list of foods high in calcium, as well as sources of vitamin D if recommended. Discuss symptoms to report to the care provider, and stress the importance of follow-up care as scheduled.

THE CLIENT WITH HYPERCALCEMIA

Hypercalcemia is a serum calcium value greater than 10.0 mg/dL. Excess ionized calcium in ECF can have serious widespread effects.

PATHOPHYSIOLOGY

Hypercalcemia usually results from increased resorption of calcium from the bones. The two most common causes of bone resorption are hyperparathyroidism and malignancies. In hyperparathyroidism, excess PTH is produced. This causes calcium to be released from bones, as well as increased calcium absorption in the intestines and retention of calcium by the kidneys. Hypercalcemia is a common complication of malignancies. It may develop as a result of bone destruction by the tu-

mor or due to hormonelike substances produced by the tumor itself. Prolonged immobility and lack of weight bearing also cause increased resorption of bone with calcium release into extracellular fluids. Self-limiting hypercalcemia also may follow successful kidney transplant.

Increased intestinal absorption of calcium also can lead to hypercalcemia. This may result from excess vitamin D, overuse of calcium-containing antacids, or excessive milk ingestion. Renal failure and some drugs such as thiazide diuretics and lithium can interfere with elimination of calcium by the kidneys, causing high serum calcium levels.

The effects of hypercalcemia largely depend on the degree of serum calcium elevation and the length of time over which it develops. In general, higher serum calcium levels are associated with more serious effects. Calcium has a stabilizing effect on the neuromuscular junction; hypercalcemia decreases neuromuscular excitability, leading to muscle weakness and depressed deep tendon reflexes. Gastrointestinal motility is reduced as well. In the heart, calcium exerts an effect similar to digitalis (see Chapter 30), strengthening contractions and reducing the heart rate. Hypercalcemia affects the conduction system of the heart, leading to bradycardia and heart blocks. The ability of the kidneys to concentrate urine is impaired by hypercalcemia, causing excess sodium and water loss and increased thirst.

Extremely high serum calcium levels affect mental status. This is thought to be due to increased calcium in cerebrospinal fluid (CSF). Behavior differences range from personality changes to confusion, impaired memory, and acute psychoses.

MANIFESTATIONS AND COMPLICATIONS

Manifestations of hypercalcemia relate to its effects on neuromuscular activity, the central nervous system, the cardiovascular system, and the kidneys. Decreased neuromuscular excitability causes muscle weakness and fatigue, as well as gastrointestinal manifestations such as anorexia, nausea, vom-

CHART 5–5 NANDA, NIC, AND NOC LINKAGES

The Client with Calcium Imbalance

NURSING DIAGNOSES	NURSING INTERVENTIONS	NURSING OUTCOMES
• Risk for Injury	• Seizure Precautions • Environmental Management: Safety	• Risk Control • Safety Status: Physical Injury
• Decreased Cardiac Output	• Cardiac Precautions • Electrolyte Management: Hypocalcemia	• Cardiac Pump Effectiveness • Vital Signs Status
• Disturbed Thought Processes	• Anxiety Reduction • Delusion Management	• Cognitive Orientation • Information Processing
• Risk for Ineffective Breathing Pattern	• Airway Management • Respiratory Monitoring	• Respiratory Status: Ventilation • Airway Patency

Note. Data from Nursing Outcomes Classification (NOC) by M. Johnson & M. Maas (Eds.), 1997, St. Louis: Mosby; Nursing Diagnoses: Definitions & Classification 2001–2002 by North American Nursing Diagnosis Association, 2001, Philadelphia: NANDA; Nursing Interventions Classification (NIC) by J.C. McCloskey & G. M. Bulechek (Eds.), 2000, St. Louis: Mosby. Reprinted by permission.

iting, and constipation. CNS effects may include confusion, lethargy, behavior or personality changes, and coma. Cardiovascular effects include dysrhythmias, ECG changes, and possible hypertension. Hypercalcemia causes polyuria, and, as a result, increased thirst.

Complications of hypercalcemia can affect several different organ systems. Peptic ulcer disease may develop due to increased gastric acid secretion. Pancreatitis can occur as a result of calcium deposits in pancreatic ducts. Excess calcium can precipitate to form kidney stones. Hypercalcemic crisis, an acute increase in the serum calcium level, can lead to cardiac arrest.

COLLABORATIVE CARE

The management of hypercalcemia focuses on correcting the underlying cause and reducing the serum calcium level. Treatment is particularly important in clients who have one or more of the following: serum calcium levels greater than 12 mg/dL, overt symptoms of hypercalcemia, compromised renal function, and an inability to maintain an adequate fluid intake.

Diagnostic Tests

The laboratory and diagnostic tests that may be ordered and the resultant findings are as follows:

- *Serum electrolytes* show a total serum calcium greater than 10.0 mg/dL.
- *Serum PTH levels* are measured to identify or rule out hyperparathyroidism as the cause of hypercalcemia.
- *ECG* changes in hypercalcemia include a shortened QT interval, shortened and depressed ST segment, and widened T wave. Bradycardia or heart block may be identified on the ECG.

Medications

Measures to promote calcium elimination by the kidneys and reduce calcium resorption from bone are used to treat hypercalcemia. In acute hypercalcemia, intravenous fluids are given (see "Fluid Management" that follows) with a loop diuretic such as furosemide to promote elimination of excess calcium. Calcitonin, which promotes the uptake of calcium into bones, also may be used to rapidly lower serum calcium levels.

A number of drugs that inhibit bone resorption are available. The bisphosphonates (pamidronate and etidronate) are commonly used to treat hypercalcemia associated with malignancies. These drugs also are used to prevent and treat osteoporosis. Their nursing implications for calcitonin and bisphosphonate drugs are presented in the boxes on pages 1226 and 1232. When a bisphosphonate drug is ineffective to correct hypercalcemia, mithramycin, a chemotherapeutic agent, may be used. Glucocorticoid drugs (see Chapter 17 ⟳) may be used in combination with other therapies to lower serum calcium levels by inhibiting intestinal calcium absorption and bone resorption.

Rapid reversal of hypercalcemia in emergency situations may be accomplished by intravenous administration of sodium phosphate or potassium phosphate. Calcium binds to phosphate, and serum calcium levels thereby decrease. Paradoxically, complications of this therapy can include fatal hypocalcemia resulting from binding of the ionized calcium and soft tissue calcifications.

Other drug therapies include the use of intravenous plicamycin (Mithracin) to inhibit bone resorption. Glucocorticoids (cortisone), which compete with vitamin D, and a low-calcium diet may be prescribed to decrease gastrointestinal absorption of calcium and to increase urinary calcium excretion. Also, calcitonin may be prescribed to decrease skeletal mobilization of calcium and phosphorus and to increase renal output of calcium and phosphorus.

Fluid Management

Intravenous fluids, usually isotonic saline, are administered to clients with severe hypercalcemia to restore vascular volume and promote renal excretion of calcium. Isotonic saline is used because sodium excretion is accompanied by calcium excretion. Careful assessment of cardiovascular and renal function is done prior to fluid therapy; the client is carefully monitored for evidence of fluid overload during treatment.

NURSING CARE

Health Promotion

Identify and monitor clients at risk for hypercalcemia. Promote mobility in clients when possible. Ambulate hospitalized clients as soon as possible. In the home setting, discuss the benefits of weight-bearing activity with clients, families, and caregivers. Encourage a generous fluid intake of up to 3 to 4 quarts per day. Encourage clients at risk to limit their intake of milk and milk products, as well as calcium-containing antacids and supplements.

Assessment

Assessment data related to hypercalcemia include the following:

- **Health history:** Current manifestations, including weakness or fatigue, abdominal discomfort, nausea or vomiting, increased urination and thirst; changes in memory or thinking; duration of symptoms and any risk factors such as excess intake of milk or calcium products, prolonged immobility, malignancy, renal failure, or endocrine disorders; current medications.
- **Physical assessment:** Mental status and level of consciousness; vital signs including apical pulse; bowel sounds; muscle strength of upper and lower extremities; deep tendon reflexes.

PRACTICE ALERT *Remember, calcium has a stabilizing or sedative effect on neuromuscular transmission. Therefore:*

Hypo*calcemia* → Increased *neuromuscular excitability, muscle twitching, spasms, and possible tetany*

Hyper*calcemia* → Decreased *neuromuscular excitability, muscle weakness, and fatigue* ∎

Nursing Diagnoses and Interventions

Risk for Injury

Clients with hypercalcemia are at risk for injury due to changes in mental status, the effects of hypercalcemia on muscle strength, and loss of calcium from bones.

- Institute safety precautions if confusion or other changes in mental status are noted. *Changes in mental status may impair judgment and the client's ability to maintain own safety.*

> **PRACTICE ALERT** *Monitor cardiac rate and rhythm, treating and/or reporting dysrhythmias as indicated. Prepare for possible cardiac arrest; keep emergency resuscitation equipment readily available. Hypercalcemia can cause bradycardia, various heart blocks, and cardiac arrest. Immediate treatment may be necessary to preserve life.* ■

- Observe for manifestations of digitalis toxicity, including vision changes, anorexia, and changes in heart rate and rhythm. Monitor serum digitalis levels. *Hypercalcemia increases the risk of digitalis toxicity.*
- Promote fluid intake (oral and/or intravenous) to keep the client well hydrated and maintain dilute urine. Encourage fluids such as prune or cranberry juice to help maintain acid urine. *Acidic, dilute urine reduces the risk of calcium salts precipitating out to form kidney stones.*
- If excess bone resorption has occurred, use caution when turning, positioning, transferring, or ambulating. *Bones that have lost excess calcium may fracture with minimal stress or trauma* (pathologic fractures).

Risk for Excess Fluid Volume

Large amounts of isotonic intravenous fluid often are administered to help correct acute hypercalcemia, leading to a risk for hypervolemia. Clients with preexisting cardiac or renal disease are at particular risk.

- Closely monitor intake and output. *A loop diuretic such as furosemide may be necessary if urinary output does not keep up with fluid administration.*
- Frequently assess vital signs, respiratory status, and heart sounds. *Increasing pulse rate, dyspnea, adventitious lung sounds, and an S_3 on auscultation of the heart may indicate excess fluid volume and potential heart failure.*
- Place in semi-Fowler's to Fowler's position. *Elevating the head of the bed improves lung expansion and reduces the work of breathing.*
- Administer diuretics as ordered, monitoring response. *Loop diuretics may be ordered to help eliminate excess fluid and calcium.*

Using NANDA, NIC, and NOC

Chart 5–5 shows links between NANDA nursing diagnoses, NIC, and NOC when caring for a client with a calcium imbalance.

Home Care

Discuss the following topics when preparing the client for discharge.

- Avoid excess intake of calcium-rich foods and antacids.
- Use of prescribed drugs to prevent excess calcium resorption, their dose, use, and desired and possible adverse effects.
- Increase fluid intake to 3 to 4 quarts per day; increase the intake of acid ash foods (meats, fish, poultry, eggs, cranberries, plums, prunes); increase dietary fiber and fluid intake to prevent constipation.
- Maintain weight-bearing physical activity to prevent hypercalcemia.
- Early manifestations of hypercalcemia to report to care provider.
- Follow recommended schedule for monitoring serum electrolyte levels.

MAGNESIUM IMBALANCE

Only about 1% of the magnesium in the body is in extracellular fluid; the rest is found within the cells and in bone. The normal serum concentration of magnesium ranges from 1.6 to 2.6 mg/dL (1.3 to 2.1 mEq/L).

OVERVIEW OF NORMAL MAGNESIUM BALANCE

Magnesium is obtained through the diet (it is plentiful in green vegetables, grains, nuts, meats, and seafood) and excreted by the kidneys. Magnesium is vital to many intracellular processes, including enzyme reactions and synthesis of proteins and nucleic acids. Magnesium exerts a sedative effect on the neuromuscular junction, decreasing acetylcholine release. It is an essential ion for neuromuscular transmission and cardiovascular function. The physiologic effects of magnesium are affected by both potassium and calcium levels. Approximately 65% of extracellular magnesium is ionized; the re-

mainder is bound to protein. Table 5–8 summarizes common causes and manifestations of magnesium imbalances.

THE CLIENT WITH HYPOMAGNESEMIA

Hypomagnesemia is a magnesium level of less than 1.6 mg/dL. It is a common problem, particularly in critically ill clients. Hypomagnesemia may be caused by deficient magnesium intake, excessive losses, or a shift between the intracellular and extracellular compartments.

RISK FACTORS

Loss of gastrointestinal fluids, particularly from diarrhea, an ileostomy, or intestinal fistula is a major risk factor for hypomagnesemia. Disruption of nutrient absorption in the small intestine also increases the risk. Chronic alcoholism is the most

TABLE 5-8 Causes and Manifestations of Magnesium Imbalances

Imbalance	Causes	Manifestations
Hypomagnesemia Serum magnesium <1.6 mg/dL	• Chronic alcoholism • GI losses: intestinal suction, diarrhea, ileostomy • Impaired absorption • Inadequate replacement • Increased excretion: drugs, renal disease, osmotic diuresis	Neuromuscular • Muscle weakness, tremors • Tetany, seizures Gastrointestinal • Dysphagia • Anorexia, nausea, vomiting, diarrhea Cardiovascular • Tachycardia • Dysrhythmias • Hypertension CNS • Mood and personality changes • Paresthesias
Hypermagnesemia Serum magnesium >2.1 mEq/L or 2.6 mg/dL	• Renal insufficiency or failure • Excess intake of antacids, laxatives • Excess magnesium administration	Neuromuscular • Muscle weakness • Depressed deep tendon reflexes Gastrointestinal • Nausea and vomiting Cardiovascular • Hypotension • Bradycardia • Cardiac arrest CNS • Respiratory depression • Coma

common cause of deficient magnesium levels in the United States (Metheny, 2000). Multiple factors associated with alcoholism contribute to hypomagnesemia: deficient nutrient intake, increased gastrointestinal losses, impaired absorption, and increased renal excretion. Other risk factors for hypomagnesemia include:

- Protein-calorie malnutrition or starvation.
- Endocrine disorders including diabetic ketoacidosis.
- Drugs such as loop or thiazide diuretics, aminoglycoside antibiotics, amphotericin B, and cyclosporine.
- Rapid administration of citrated blood (banked blood).
- Kidney disease.

PATHOPHYSIOLOGY

Magnesium deficiency usually occurs along with low serum potassium and calcium levels. The effects of hypomagnesemia relate not only to the magnesium deficiency but also to hypokalemia and hypocalcemia.

Hypomagnesemia causes increased neuromuscular excitability, with muscle weakness and tremors. The accompanying hypocalcemia contributes to this effect. In the central nervous system, this increased neural excitability can lead to seizures and changes in mental status.

Deficient intracellular magnesium in the myocardium increases the risk of cardiac dysrhythmias and sudden death. Hypokalemia increases this risk. Hypomagnesemia also increases the risk of digitalis toxicity. Chronic hypomagnesemia

may contribute to hypertension, probably due to increased vasoconstriction.

MANIFESTATIONS AND COMPLICATIONS

Neuromuscular manifestations of hypomagnesemia include tremors, hyperreactive reflexes, positive Chvostek's and Trousseau's signs, tetany, paresthesias, and seizures. CNS effects include confusion, mood changes (apathy, depression, agitation), hallucinations, and possible psychoses.

An increased heart rate and ventricular dysrhythmias are common, especially when hypokalemia is present or the client is taking digitalis. Cardiac arrest and sudden death may occur. Gastrointestinal manifestations include nausea, vomiting, anorexia, diarrhea, and abdominal distention.

COLLABORATIVE CARE

Hypomagnesemia is diagnosed by measuring serum electrolyte levels. The ECG shows a prolonged PR interval, widened QRS complex, and depression of the ST segment with T wave inversion.

Treatment is directed toward prevention and identification of an existing deficiency. Magnesium is added to intravenous total parenteral nutrition solutions to prevent hypomagnesemia.

In clients able to eat, a mild deficiency may be corrected by increasing the intake of foods rich in magnesium (see Box 5–8), or with oral magnesium supplements. Oral magnesium supplements may cause diarrhea, however, limiting their use.

BOX 5–8	■ Foods High in Magnesium
■ Green, leafy vegetables ■ Seafood ■ Meat ■ Wheat bran ■ Milk ■ Legumes ■ Bananas	■ Oranges ■ Grapefruit ■ Chocolate ■ Molasses ■ Coconut ■ Refined sugar

Clients with manifestations of hypomagnesemia are treated with parenteral magnesium sulfate. Treatment is continued for several days to restore intracellular magnesium levels. Magnesium may be given intravenously or by deep intramuscular injection. Renal function is evaluated prior to administration, and serum magnesium levels are monitored during treatment. The intravenous route is used for severe magnesium deficiency or if neurologic changes or cardiac dysrhythmias are present. See the box below for the nursing implications of parenteral magnesium sulfate.

NURSING CARE

Health Promotion

Discuss the importance of maintaining adequate magnesium intake through a well-balanced diet, particularly with clients at risk (people with alcoholism, malabsorption, or bowel surgery). Many hospitalized clients are at risk for hypomagnesemia due to protein-calorie malnutrition and other disorders. Monitor serum magnesium levels, reporting changes to the health care provider.

Medication Administration

Magnesium Sulfate

Magnesium sulfate is used to prevent or treat hypomagnesemia. It also is used as an anticonvulsant in severe eclampsia or preeclampsia. It may be given intravenously or by intramuscular injection.

Nursing Responsibilities
- Assess serum magnesium levels and renal function tests (BUN and serum creatinine) prior to administering. Notify the care provider if magnesium levels are above normal limits or renal function is impaired.
- Frequently monitor neurologic status and deep tendon reflexes during therapy. Withhold magnesium and notify the care provider if deep tendon reflexes are hypoactive or absent.
- Monitor intake and output.
- Administer IM doses deep into the ventral or dorsal gluteal sites.
- Intravenous magnesium sulfate may be given by direct IV push or by continuous infusion.

Client and Family Teaching
Explain purpose and duration of treatment. Discuss reason for frequent neurologic and reflex assessments.

Assessment

In addition to asking questions related to risk factors for hypomagnesemia, use the guidelines for assessing clients with hypokalemia and hypocalcemia for subjective and objective assessment data.

Nursing Diagnoses and Interventions

Nursing care for clients with hypomagnesemia focuses on careful monitoring of manifestations and responses to treatment, promoting safety, client and family teaching, and administering prescribed medications.

Risk for Injury
- Monitor serum electrolytes, including magnesium, potassium, and calcium. *Magnesium deficiency often is accompanied by deficiencies of potassium and calcium.*
- Monitor gastrointestinal function, including bowel sounds and abdominal distention. *Hypomagnesemia reduces gastrointestinal motility.*
- Initiate cardiac monitoring, reporting and treating (as indicated) ECG changes and dysrhythmias. In clients receiving digitalis, monitor for digitalis toxicity. *Low magnesium levels can precipitate ventricular dysrhythmias, including lethal dysrhythmias such as ventricular fibrillation.*
- Assess deep tendon reflexes frequently during intravenous magnesium infusions and prior to each intramuscular dose. *Depressed tendon reflexes indicate a high serum magnesium level.*
- Maintain a quiet, darkened environment. Institute seizure precautions. *Increased neuromuscular and CNS irritability can lead to seizures. A quiet, dark environment reduces stimuli.*

Home Care

Prior to discharge, instruct the client to increase dietary intake of foods high in magnesium and provide information about magnesium supplements. In addition, if alcohol abuse has precipitated a magnesium deficit, discuss alcohol treatment options, including inpatient treatment and support groups such as Alcoholics Anonymous, Al-Anon, and/or Al-a-Teen.

THE CLIENT WITH HYPERMAGNESEMIA

Hypermagnesemia is a serum magnesium level greater than 2.6 mg/dL. It is much less common than hypomagnesemia. Hypermagnesemia can develop in renal failure, particularly if magnesium is administered parenterally or orally (e.g., magnesium-containing antacids or laxatives). Older adults are at risk for hypermagnesemia as renal function declines with aging and they are more likely to use over-the-counter laxatives and other preparations that contain magnesium.

PATHOPHYSIOLOGY AND MANIFESTATIONS

Elevated serum magnesium levels interfere with neuromuscular transmission and depress the central nervous system. Hypermagnesemia also affects the cardiovascular system, potentially causing hypotension, flushing, sweating, and bradydysrhythmias.

Predictable manifestations occur with increasing serum magnesium levels. With lower levels, nausea and vomiting, hypotension, facial flushing, sweating, and a feeling of warmth occur. As levels increase, signs of central nervous system depression appear (weakness, lethargy, drowsiness, weak or absent deep tendon reflexes). Marked elevations cause respiratory depression, coma, and compromised cardiac function (ECG changes, bradycardia, heart block, and cardiac arrest).

COLLABORATIVE CARE

The management of hypermagnesemia focuses on identifying and treating the underlying cause. All medications or compounds containing magnesium (such as antacids, intravenous solutions, or enemas) are withheld. In the client with renal failure, hemodialysis or peritoneal dialysis is instituted to remove the excess magnesium.

Calcium gluconate is administered intravenously to reverse the neuromuscular and cardiac effects of hypermagnesemia. The client may require mechanical ventilation to support respiratory function, and a pacemaker to maintain adequate cardiac output.

NURSING CARE

Nursing care includes instituting measures to prevent and identify hypermagnesemia in clients at risk, monitoring for critical effects of hypermagnesemia, and providing measures to ensure the client's safety. Consider the following nursing diagnoses for the client with hypermagnesemia.

- *Decreased cardiac output* related to altered myocardial conduction
- *Risk for ineffective breathing pattern* related to respiratory depression
- *Risk for injury* related to muscle weakness and altered level of consciousness
- *Risk for ineffective health maintenance* related to lack of knowledge about use of magnesium-containing supplements, antacids, laxatives, and enemas

Home Care

Discharge teaching and planning focuses on instructions to avoid magnesium-containing medications, including antacids, mineral supplements, cathartics, and enemas (see Box 5–9).

| **BOX 5–9** | ■ **Medications Containing Magnesium** |

Antacids	**Laxatives**
■ Gelusil	■ Milk of Magnesia
■ Maalox No. 1	■ Magnesium oxide
■ Maalox Plus	■ Haley's M-O
■ Riopan	■ Magnesium citrate
■ Milk of Magnesia	■ Epsom salts
■ Mylanta	
■ Di-Gel	
■ Gaviscon	

PHOSPHATE IMBALANCE

Although most phosphate (85%) is found in bones, it is the primary intracellular anion. About 14% is in intracellular fluid, and the remainder (1%) is in extracellular fluid. The normal serum phosphate (or phosphorus) level in adults is 2.5 to 4.5 mg/dL. Phosphorus levels vary with age, gender, and diet.

OVERVIEW OF NORMAL PHOSPHATE BALANCE

Phosphate is essential to intracellular processes such as the production of adenosine triphosphate (ATP), the fuel that supports muscle contraction, nerve cell transmission, and electrolyte transport. Phosphate is vital for red blood cell function and oxygen delivery to tissues; nervous system and muscle function; and the metabolism of fats, carbohydrates, and protein. It also assists in maintaining acid-base balance.

Phosphorus is ingested in the diet, absorbed in the jejunum, and primarily excreted by the kidneys. When phosphate intake is low, the kidneys conserve phosphorus, excreting less. An inverse relationship exists between phosphate and calcium levels: When one increases, the other decreases. Regulatory mechanisms for calcium levels (parathyroid hormone, calci-tonin, and vitamin D) also influence phosphate levels. The causes and manifestations of phosphate imbalances are summarized in Table 5–9.

THE CLIENT WITH HYPOPHOSPHATEMIA

Hypophosphatemia is a serum phosphorus of less than 2.5 mg/dL. Low serum phosphate levels may indicate a total body deficit of phosphate or a shift of phosphate into the intracellular space, the most common cause of hypophosphatemia. Decreased gastrointestinal absorption of phosphate or increased renal excretion of phosphate also can cause low phosphate levels. Hypophosphatemia often is *iatrogenic,* that is, related to treatment. Selected causes of hypophosphatemia include the following:

- *Refeeding* syndrome can develop when malnourished clients are started on enteral or total parenteral nutrition. Glucose in the formula or solution stimulates insulin release, which promotes the entry of glucose and phosphate into the cells, depleting extracellular phosphate levels.

TABLE 5-9 Causes and Manifestations of Phosphate Imbalances

Imbalance	Causes	Manifestations
Hypophosphatemia Serum phosphorus <2.5 mg/dL	• Shift of phosphorus into cells • IV glucose administration • Total parenteral nutrition without phosphorus • Aluminum- or magnesium-based antacids • Diuretic therapy • Alcoholism	• Paresthesias • Muscle weakness • Muscle pain and tenderness • Confusion, decreasing LOC • Seizures • Bone pain, osteomalacia • Anorexia, dysphagia • Decreased bowel sounds • Possible acute respiratory failure
Hyperphosphatemia Serum phosphate >4.5 mg/dL	• Renal failure • Chemotherapy • Muscle tissue trauma • Sepsis • Severe hypothermia • Heat stroke	• Circumoral and peripheral paresthesias • Muscle spasms • Tetany • Soft tissue calcification

• Medications frequently contribute to hypophosphatemia, including intravenous glucose solutions, antacids (aluminum- or magnesium-based antacids bind with phosphate), anabolic steroids, and diuretics.
• Alcoholism affects both the intake and absorption of phosphate.
• Hyperventilation and respiratory alkalosis cause phosphate to shift out of extracellular fluids into the intracellular space.
• Other causes include diabetic ketoacidosis with excess phosphate loss in the urine, stress responses, and extensive burns.

PATHOPHYSIOLOGY AND MANIFESTATIONS

Most effects of hypophosphatemia result from depletion of ATP and impaired oxygen delivery to the cells due to a deficiency of the red blood cell enzyme 2,3-DPG. Severe hypophosphatemia affects virtually every major organ system.

• Central nervous system: Reduced oxygen and ATP synthesis in the brain causes neurologic manifestations such as irritability, apprehension, weakness, paresthesias, lack of coordination, confusion, seizures, and coma.
• Hematologic: Oxygen delivery to the cells is reduced. Hemolytic anemia may develop due to lack of ATP in red blood cells.
• Musculoskeletal: Decreased ATP causes muscle weakness and release of creatinine phosphokinase (CPK, a muscle enzyme); acute rhabdomyolysis (muscle cell breakdown) can develop.
• Respiratory: Chest muscle weakness can interfere with effective ventilation, leading to respiratory failure.
• Cardiovascular: Hypophosphatemia decreases myocardial contractility; decreased oxygenation of the heart muscle can cause chest pain and dysrhythmias.
• Gastrointestinal: Anorexia can occur, as well as dysphagia (difficulty swallowing), nausea and vomiting, decreased bowel sounds, and possible ileus due to reduced gastrointestinal motility.

COLLABORATIVE CARE

Treatment for hypophosphatemia is directed at prevention, treating the underlying cause of the disorder, and replacing phosphate. An improved diet and oral phosphate supplement (such as Neutra-Phos or Neutra-Phos K capsules) may restore normal phosphate levels in clients with a mild to moderate deficiency. Intravenous phosphate (sodium phosphate or potassium phosphate) is given when serum phosphate levels are less than 1 mg/dL. Oral phosphate supplements are then continued for up to 1 week to restore intracellular phosphate levels (Metheny, 2000).

NURSING CARE

Nurses can be instrumental in identifying clients at risk for phosphate deficiency and preventing it from developing. Nurses should closely monitor serum electrolyte values in clients at risk, including those who are malnourished, receiving intravenous glucose solutions or total parenteral nutrition, or being treated with diuretic therapy or antacids that bind with phosphate. Nursing diagnoses that may be appropriate for the client with hypophosphatemia include:

• *Impaired physical mobility* related to muscle weakness and poor coordination
• *Ineffective breathing pattern* related to weakened muscles of respiration
• *Decreased cardiac output* related to reduced myocardial contractility
• *Risk for injury* related to muscle weakness and altered mental status

Home Care

In preparing for discharge, teach the client and family about the causes and manifestations of hypophosphatemia. Discuss the importance of avoiding phosphorus-binding antacids, unless prescribed. Stress a well-balanced diet to maintain an adequate intake of phosphate.

THE CLIENT WITH HYPERPHOSPHATEMIA

Hyperphosphatemia is a serum phosphate level greater than 4.5 mg/dL. As with other electrolyte imbalances, it may be the result of impaired phosphate excretion, excess intake, or a shift of phosphate from the intracellular space into extracellular fluids.

- Acute or chronic renal failure is the primary cause of impaired phosphate excretion.
- Rapid administration of phosphate-containing solutions can increase serum phosphate levels. This can include phosphate enemas. In addition, excess vitamin D increases phosphate absorption and can lead to hyperphosphatemia in clients with impaired renal function.
- A shift of phosphate from the intracellular to extracellular space can occur during chemotherapy, due to sepsis or hypothermia, or because of extensive trauma or heat stroke.
- Because phosphate levels are affected by serum calcium concentrations, disruption of the mechanisms that regulate calcium levels (e.g., hypoparathyroidism, hyperthyroidism, or vitamin D intoxication) can lead to hyperphosphatemia.

PATHOPHYSIOLOGY AND MANIFESTATIONS

Excessive serum phosphate levels cause few specific symptoms. The effects of high serum phosphate levels on nerves and muscles (muscle cramps and pain, paresthesias, tingling around the mouth, muscle spasms, tetany) are more the result of hypocalcemia that develops secondary to an elevated serum phosphorus level. The phosphate in the serum combines with ionized calcium, and the ionized serum calcium level falls.

Calcification of soft tissues can occur with high phosphate levels. Phosphates bind with calcium to precipitate in soft tissues such as the kidneys and other organs. Soft tissue calcification can impair the function of affected organs.

COLLABORATIVE CARE

Treatment of the underlying disorder often corrects hyperphosphatemia. When this is not feasible, phosphate-containing drugs are eliminated and intake of phosphate-rich foods such as organ meats and milk and milk products is restricted. Agents that bind with phosphate in the gastrointestinal tract (such as calcium-containing antacids) may be prescribed. If renal function is adequate, intravenous normal saline may be given to promote renal excretion of phosphate. Dialysis may be necessary to reduce phosphate levels in clients with renal failure.

NURSING CARE

When providing nursing care for the client with hyperphosphatemia, monitor the client for laboratory data revealing an excess of phosphorus and a deficit of calcium, as well as the signs of hypocalcemia.

Home Care

Discuss the risk of hyperphosphatemia related to using phosphate preparations as laxatives or enemas, particularly with clients who have other risk factors for the disorder. When preparing the client for discharge, teach about the use of phosphate-binding preparations as ordered and dietary phosphate restrictions.

ACID-BASE DISORDERS

Homeostasis and optimal cellular function require maintenance of the hydrogen ion (H^+) concentration of body fluids within a relatively narrow range. Hydrogen ions determine the relative acidity of body fluids. **Acids** release hydrogen ions in solution; **bases** (or **alkalis**) accept hydrogen ions in solution. The hydrogen ion concentration of a solution is measured as its pH. The relationship between hydrogen ion concentration and pH is inverse; that is, as hydrogen ion concentration increases, the pH falls, and the solution becomes more acidic. As hydrogen ion concentration falls, the pH rises, and the solution becomes more alkaline or basic. The pH of body fluids is slightly basic, with the normal pH ranging from 7.35 to 7.45 (a pH of 7 is neutral).

REGULATION OF ACID-BASE BALANCE

A number of mechanisms work together to maintain the pH of the body within this normal range. Metabolic processes in the body continuously produce acids, which fall into two categories: volatile acids and nonvolatile acids. **Volatile acids** can be eliminated from the body as a gas. Carbonic acid (H_2CO_3) is the only volatile acid produced in the body. It dissociates (separates) into carbon dioxide (CO_2) and water (H_2O); the carbon dioxide is then eliminated from the body through the lungs. All other acids produced in the body are *nonvolatile acids* that must be metabolized or excreted from the body in fluid. Lactic acid, hydrochloric acid, phosphoric acid, and sulfuric acid are examples of nonvolatile acids. Most acids and bases in the body are weak; that is, they neither release nor accept a significant amount of hydrogen ion.

Three systems work together in the body to maintain the pH despite continuous acid production: buffers, the respiratory system, and the renal system.

Buffer Systems

Buffers are substances that prevent major changes in pH by removing or releasing hydrogen ions. When excess acid is present

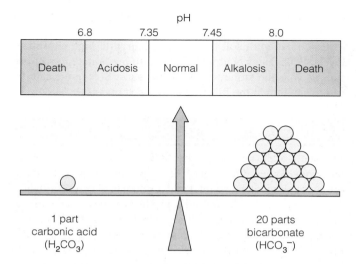

Figure 5–14 ■ The normal ratio of bicarbonate to carbonic acid is 20:1. As long as this ratio is maintained, the pH remains within the normal range of 7.35 to 7.45.

in body fluid, buffers bind with hydrogen ions to minimize the change in pH. If body fluids become too basic or alkaline, buffers release hydrogen ions, restoring the pH. Although buffers act within a fraction of a second, their capacity to maintain pH is limited. The major buffer systems of the body are the bicarbonate-carbonic acid buffer system, phosphate buffer system, and protein buffers.

The bicarbonate-carbonic acid buffer system can be illustrated by the following equation:

$$CO_2 + H_2O \leftrightarrow H_2CO_3 \leftrightarrow H^+ + HCO_3^-$$

Bicarbonate (HCO_3^-) is a weak base; when an acid is added to the system, it combines with bicarbonate, and the pH changes only slightly. Carbonic acid (H_2CO_3) is a weak acid produced when carbon dioxide dissolves in water. If a base is added to the system, it combines with carbonic acid, and the pH remains within the normal range. Although the amounts of bicarbonate and carbonic acid in the body vary to a certain extent, as long as a ratio of 20 parts bicarbonate (HCO_3^-) to 1 part carbonic acid (H_2CO_3) is maintained, the pH remains within the 7.35 to 7.45 range (Figure 5–14 ■). The normal serum bicarbonate level is 24 mEq/L, and that of carbonic acid is 1.2 mEq/L. Thus, the ratio of bicarbonate to carbonic acid is 20:1. It is this ratio that maintains the pH within the normal range. Adding a strong acid to extracellular fluid depletes bicarbonate, changing the 20:1 ratio and causing the pH to drop below 7.35. This is known as acidosis. Addition of a strong base depletes carbonic acid as it combines with the base. The 20:1 ratio again is disrupted and the pH rises above 7.45, a condition known as alkalosis.

Intracellular and plasma proteins also serve as buffers. Plasma proteins contribute to buffering of extracellular fluids. Proteins in intracellular fluid provide extensive buffering for organic acids produced by cellular metabolism. In red blood cells, hemoglobin acts as a buffer for hydrogen ion when carbonic acid dissociates. Inorganic phosphates also serve as extracellular buffers, al-

though their roles are not as important as the bicarbonate-carbonic acid buffer system. Phosphates are, however, important intracellular buffers, helping to maintain a stable pH.

Respiratory System

The respiratory system (and the respiratory center of the brain) regulates carbonic acid in the body by eliminating or retaining carbon dioxide. Carbon dioxide is a potential acid; when combined with water, it forms carbonic acid (see previous equation). Acute increases in either carbon dioxide or hydrogen ions in the blood stimulate the respiratory center in the brain. As a result, both the rate and depth of respiration increase. The increased rate and depth of lung ventilation eliminates carbon dioxide from the body, and carbonic acid levels fall, bringing the pH to a more normal range. Although this compensation for increased hydrogen ion concentration occurs within minutes, it becomes less effective over time. Clients with chronic lung disease may have consistently high carbon dioxide levels in their blood.

Alkalosis, by contrast, depresses the respiratory center. Both the rate and depth of respiration decrease, and carbon dioxide is retained. The retained carbon dioxide then combines with water to restore carbonic acid levels and bring the pH back within the normal range.

Renal System

The renal system is responsible for the long-term regulation of acid-base balance in the body. Excess nonvolatile acids produced during metabolism normally are eliminated by the kidneys. The kidneys also regulate bicarbonate levels in extracellular fluid by regenerating bicarbonate ions as well as reabsorbing them in the renal tubules. Although the kidneys respond more slowly to changes in pH (over hours to days), they can generate bicarbonate and selectively excrete or retain hydrogen ions as needed. In acidosis, when excess hydrogen ion is present and the pH falls, the kidneys excrete hydrogen ions and retain bicarbonate. In alkalosis, the kidneys retain hydrogen ions and excrete bicarbonate to restore acid-base balance.

Assessment of Acid-Base Balance

Acid-base balance is evaluated primarily by measuring arterial blood gases.

PRACTICE ALERT *Arteries are high-pressure vessels in contrast to veins. Obtaining an arterial blood sample requires specialized training. It may be done by a registered nurse, respiratory therapist, or laboratory technician who has been trained in drawing ABGs. Apply firm pressure to the puncture site for 5 minutes after the needle is withdrawn to prevent bleeding into the surrounding tissues.* ■

Arterial blood is used because it reflects acid-base balance throughout the entire body better than venous blood. Arterial blood also provides information about the effectiveness of the lungs in oxygenating blood. The elements measured are pH, the $Paco_2$, the Pao_2, and bicarbonate level.

TABLE 5–10 Normal Arterial Blood Gas Values

Value	Normal Range	Significance
pH	7.35 to 7.45	Reflects hydrogen ion (H$^+$) concentration • <7.35 = acidosis • >7.45 = alkalosis
PaCO_2	35 to 45 mmHg	Partial pressure of carbon dioxide (CO_2) in arterial blood • <35 mmHg = hypocapnia • >45 mmHg = hypercapnia
PaO_2	80 to 100 mmHg	Partial pressure of oxygen (O_2) in arterial blood • <80 mmHg = hypoxemia
HCO_3^-	22 to 26 mEq/L	Bicarbonate concentration in plasma
BE	−3 to +3	Base excess; a measure of buffering capacity

PRACTICE ALERT *You will see the abbreviations PaCO_2 and PaO_2 used interchangeably with PCO_2 and PO_2. The P stands for partial pressure: the pressure exerted by the gas dissolved in the blood. The a indicates that the sample is arterial blood. Because these measurements rarely are done on venous blood, the a often is deleted from the abbreviation.* ■

The PaCO_2 measures the pressure exerted by dissolved carbon dioxide in the blood. The PaCO_2 reflects the respiratory component of acid-base regulation and balance. The PaCO_2 is regulated by the lungs. The normal value is 35 to 45 mmHg. A PaCO_2 of less than 35 mmHg is known as *hypocapnia;* a PaCO_2 greater than 45 mmHg is *hypercapnia.*

The PaO_2 is a measure of the pressure exerted by oxygen that is dissolved in the plasma. Only about 3% of oxygen in the blood is transported in solution; most is combined with hemoglobin. However, it is the dissolved oxygen that is available to the cells for metabolism. As dissolved oxygen diffuses out of plasma into the tissues, more is released from hemoglobin. The normal value for PaO_2 is 80 to 100 mmHg. A PaO_2 less than 80 mmHg is indicative of *hypoxemia.* The PaO_2 is valuable for evaluating respiratory function, but is not used as a primary measurement in determining acid-base status.

The **serum bicarbonate** (HCO_3^-) reflects the renal regulation of acid-base balance. It is often called the metabolic component of arterial blood gases. The normal HCO_3^- value is 22 to 26 mEq/L.

The **base excess (BE)** is a calculated value also known as buffer base capacity. The measurement of base excess reflects the degree of acid-base imbalance by indicating the status of the body's total buffering capacity. It represents the amount of acid or base that must be added to a blood sample to achieve a pH of 7.4. This is essentially a measure of increased or decreased bicarbonate. The normal value for base excess for arterial blood is − 3.0 to + 3.0. Normal ABG values are summarized in Table 5–10.

ABGs are analyzed to identify acid-base disorders and their probable cause, to determine the extent of the imbalance, and to monitor treatment. When analyzing ABG results, it is important to use a systematic approach. First evaluate each individual measurement, then look at the interrelationships to determine the client's acid-base status (see Box 5–10).

ACID-BASE IMBALANCE

Acid-base disorders fall into two major categories: acidosis and alkalosis. Acidosis occurs when the hydrogen ion concentration increases above normal (pH below 7.35). Alkalosis occurs when the hydrogen ion concentration falls below normal (pH above 7.45).

Acid-base imbalances are further classified as *metabolic* or *respiratory* disorders. In metabolic disorders, the primary change is in the concentration of bicarbonate. In **metabolic acidosis,** the amount of bicarbonate is decreased in relation to the amount of acid in the body (Figure 5–15A ■). It can develop as a result of abnormal bicarbonate losses or because of excess nonvolatile acids in the body. The pH falls below 7.35 and the bicarbonate concentration is less than 22 mEq/L. **Metabolic alkalosis,** by contrast, occurs when there is an excess of bicarbonate in relation to the amount of hydrogen ion (Figure 5–15B). The pH is above 7.45 and the bicarbonate concentration is greater than 26 mEq/L.

In respiratory disorders, the primary change is in the concentration of carbonic acid. **Respiratory acidosis** occurs when carbon dioxide is retained, increasing the amount of carbonic acid in the body (Figure 5–16A ■). As a result, the pH falls to less than 7.35, and the PaCO_2 is greater than 45 mmHg. When too much carbon dioxide is "blown off," carbonic acid levels fall and **respiratory alkalosis** develops (Figure 5–16B). The pH rises to above 7.45 and the PaCO_2 is less than 35 mmHg.

Acid-base disorders are further defined as *primary* (simple) and *mixed.* Primary disorders usually are due to one cause. For example, respiratory failure often causes respiratory acidosis due to retained carbon dioxide; renal failure usually causes metabolic acidosis due to retained hydrogen ion and impaired bicarbonate production. Table 5–11 summarizes primary acid-base imbalances with common causes

BOX 5–10 ■ Interpreting Arterial Blood Gases

1. Look at the pH.
   - pH < 7.35 = acidosis
   - pH > 7.45 = alkalosis
2. Look at the Pa_{CO_2}.
   - Pa_{CO_2} < 35 mmHg = hypocapnia; more carbon dioxide is being exhaled than normal
   - Pa_{CO_2} > 45 mmHg = hypercapnia; carbon dioxide is being retained
3. Evaluate the pH–Pa_{CO_2} relationship for a possible respiratory problem.
   - If the pH is < 7.35 (acidosis) and the Pa_{CO_2} is > 45 mmHg (hypercapnia), retained carbon dioxide is causing increased H^+ concentration and *respiratory acidosis.*
   - If the pH is > 7.45 (alkalosis) and the Pa_{CO_2} is < 35 mmHg (hypocapnia), low carbon dioxide levels and decreased H^+ concentration are causing *respiratory alkalosis.*
4. Look at the bicarbonate.
   - If the HCO_3^- is < 22 mEq/L, bicarbonate levels are lower than normal.
   - If the HCO_3^- is > 26 mEq/L, bicarbonate levels are higher than normal.
5. Evaluate the pH, HCO_3^-, and BE for a possible metabolic problem.
   - If the pH is < 7.35 (acidosis), the HCO_3^- is < 22 mEq/L, and the BE is < −3 mEq/L, then low bicarbonate levels

and high H^+ concentrations are causing *metabolic acidosis.*
   - If the pH is > 7.45 (alkalosis), the HCO_3^- is > 26 mEq/L, and the BE is > + 3 mEq/L, then high bicarbonate levels are causing *metabolic alkalosis.*
6. Look for compensation.
   - *Renal compensation:*
     - In respiratory acidosis (pH < 7.35, Pa_{CO_2} > 45 mmHg), the kidneys retain HCO_3^- to buffer the excess acid, so the HCO_3^- is > 26 mEq/L.
     - In respiratory alkalosis (pH > 7.45, Pa_{CO_2} < 35 mmHg), the kidneys excrete HO_3^- to minimize the alkalosis, so the HCO_3^- is < 22 mEq/L.
   - *Respiratory compensation*
     - In metabolic acidosis (pH < 7.35, HCO_3^- < 22 mEq/L), the rate and depth of respirations increase, increasing carbon dioxide elimination, so the Pa_{CO_2} is < 35 mmHg.
     - In metabolic alkalosis (pH > 7.45, HCO_3^- > 26 mEq/L), respirations slow, carbon dioxide is retained, so the Pa_{CO_2} is > 45 mmHg.
7. Evaluate oxygenation.
   - Pa_{O_2} < 80 mmHg = hypoxemia; possible hypoventilation
   - Pa_{O_2} > mmHg = hyperventilation

of each. Mixed disorders occur from combinations of respiratory and metabolic disturbances. For example, a client in cardiac arrest develops a mixed respiratory and metabolic acidosis due to lack of ventilation (and retained CO_2) and hypoxia of body tissues that leads to anaerobic metabolism and acid by-products (excess nonvolatile acids).

Compensation

With primary acid-base disorders, compensatory changes in the other part of the regulatory system occur to restore a normal pH and homeostasis. In metabolic acid-base disorders, the change in pH affects the rate and depth of respirations. This, in turn, affects carbon dioxide elimination and the Pa_{CO_2}, helping restore the carbonic acid to bicarbonate ratio. The kidneys

Figure 5–15 ■ Metabolic acid-base imbalances. *A,* Metabolic acidosis. *B,* Metabolic alkalosis.

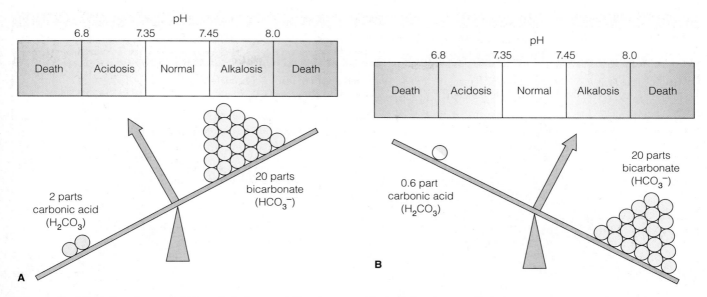

Figure 5–16 ■ Respiratory acid-base imbalances. *A*, Respiratory acidosis. *B*, Respiratory alkalosis.

TABLE 5-11 Common Causes of Primary Acid-Base Imbalances

Imbalance	Common Causes
Metabolic acidosis pH < 7.35 HCO_3^- <22 mEq/L	↑ Acid production • Lactic acidosis • Ketoacidosis related to diabetes, starvation, or alcoholism • Salicylate toxicity ↓ Acid excretion • Renal failure ↑ Bicarbonate loss • Diarrhea, ileostomy drainage, intestinal fistula • Biliary or pancreatic fistulas ↑ Chloride • Sodium chloride IV solutions • Renal tubular acidosis • Carbonic anhydrase inhibitors
Metabolic alkalosis pH >7.45 HCO_3^- >26 mEq/L	↑ Acid loss or excretion • Vomiting, gastric suction • Hypokalemia ↑ Bicarbonate • Alkali ingestion (bicarbonate of soda) • Excess bicarbonate administration
Respiratory acidosis pH <7.35 Pa_{CO_2} >45 mmHg	Acute respiratory acidosis • Acute respiratory conditions (pulmonary edema, pneumonia, acute asthma) • Opiate overdose • Foreign body aspiration • Chest trauma Chronic respiratory acidosis • Chronic respiratory conditions (COPD, cystic fibrosis) • Multiple sclerosis, other neuromuscular diseases • Stroke
Respiratory alkalosis pH >7.45 Pa_{CO_2} <35 mmHg	• Anxiety-induced hyperventilation (e.g., anxiety) • Fever • Early salicylate intoxication • Hyperventilation with mechanical ventilator

TABLE 5-12 Compensation for Simple Acid-Base Imbalances

Primary Disorder	Cause	Compensation	Effect on ABGs
Metabolic acidosis	Excess nonvolatile acids; bicarbonate deficiency	Rate and depth of respirations increase, eliminating additional CO_2	↓ pH ↓ HCO_3^- ↓ $Paco_2$
Metabolic alkalosis	Bicarbonate excess	Rate and depth of respirations decrease, retaining CO_2	↑ pH ↑ HCO_3^- ↑ $Paco_2$
Respiratory acidosis	Retained CO_2 and excess carbonic acid	Kidneys conserve bicarbonate to restore carbonic acid:bicarbonate ratio of 1:20	↓ pH ↑ $Paco_2$ ↑ HCO_3^-
Respiratory alkalosis	Loss of CO_2 and deficient carbonic acid	Kidneys excrete bicarbonate and conserve H^+ to restore carbonic acid:bicarbonate ratio	↑ pH ↓ $Paco_2$ ↓ HCO_3^-

compensate for simple respiratory imbalances. The change in pH affects both bicarbonate conservation and hydrogen ion elimination (see Table 5–12).

Compensatory changes in respirations occur within minutes of a change in pH. These changes, however, become less effective over time. The renal response takes longer to restore the pH, but is a more effective long-term mechanism. If the pH is restored to within normal limits, the disorder is said to be *fully compensated*. When these changes are reflected in ABG values but the pH remains outside normal limits, the disorder is said to be *partially compensated*.

THE CLIENT WITH METABOLIC ACIDOSIS

Metabolic acidosis (bicarbonate deficit) is characterized by a low pH (< 7.35) and a low bicarbonate (< 22 mEq/L). It may be caused by excess acid or loss of bicarbonate from the body. When metabolic acidosis develops, the respiratory system attempts to return the pH to normal by increasing the rate and depth of respirations. Carbon dioxide elimination increases, and the $Paco_2$ falls (< 35 mmHg).

RISK FACTORS

Metabolic acidosis rarely is a primary disorder; it usually develops during the course of another disease.

- *Acute lactic acidosis* usually results from tissue hypoxia due to shock or cardiac arrest.
- Clients with type 1 diabetes mellitus are at risk for developing *diabetic ketoacidosis* (see Chapter 18 ⊙ for more information about diabetes and its complications).
- *Acute or chronic renal failure* impairs the excretion of metabolic acids.
- Diarrhea, intestinal suction, or abdominal fistulas increase the risk for excess *bicarbonate loss*.

Other common causes of metabolic acidosis are listed in Table 5–11.

PATHOPHYSIOLOGY

Three basic mechanisms that can cause metabolic acidosis are:

- Accumulation of metabolic acids.
- Excess loss of bicarbonate.
- An increase in chloride levels.

An accumulation of metabolic acids can result from excess acid production or impaired elimination of metabolic acids by the kidney. Lactic acidosis develops due to tissue hypoxia and a shift to anaerobic metabolism by the cells. Lactate and hydrogen ions are produced, which form lactic acid. Both oxygen and glucose are necessary for normal cell metabolism. When intracellular glucose is inadequate due to starvation or a lack of insulin to move it into cells, the body breaks down fatty tissue to meet its metabolic needs. In this process, fatty acids are released, which are converted to ketones; ketoacidosis develops. Aspirin (acetylsalicylic acid) breaks down into salicylic acid in the body. Substances such as aspirin, methanol (wood alcohol), and ethylene (contained in antifreeze and solvents) cause a toxic increase in body acids by either breaking down into acid products (salicylic acid) or stimulating metabolic acid production (Porth, 2002). Renal failure impairs the body's ability to excrete excess hydrogen ions and form bicarbonate.

Excess metabolic acids increase the hydrogen ion concentration of body fluids. The excess acid is buffered by bicarbonate, leading to what is known as a high **anion gap** acidosis (see Box 5–11).

The pancreas secretes bicarbonate-rich fluid into the small intestine. Intestinal suction, severe diarrhea, ileostomy drainage, or fistulas can lead to excess losses of bicarbonate. Hyperchloremic acidosis can develop when excess chloride solutions (such as NaCl or ammonium chloride) are infused, causing a rise in chloride concentrations. It also may be related to renal disease or administration of carbonic anhydrate inhibitor diuretics. The anion gap remains normal in metabolic acidosis due to bicarbonate loss or excess chloride.

BOX 5–11 ■ Unraveling the Anion Gap

Calculation of the anion gap can help identify the underlying mechanism in metabolic acidosis if it is unclear.

The number of cations (positively charged ions) and anions (negatively charged ions) in ECF normally is equal (refer to Figure 5–2). Not all of these ions, however, are measured in laboratory testing (e.g., organic acids and proteins). The anion gap is calculated by subtracting the sum of two measured anions, chloride and bicarbonate, from the concentration of the major cation, sodium (see accompanying Figure 5–17 ■). The normal anion gap is 8 to 12 mEq/L.

Excess acids in ECF are buffered by bicarbonate, reducing serum bicarbonate levels and the total measured concentration of anions. This increases the anion gap (B in figure). When bicarbonate is lost from the body or chloride levels increase, however, the anion gap remains within normal limits (C in figure). This occurs because an increase or decrease in one of these negatively charged ions causes a corresponding change in the other to maintain balance (e.g., $\downarrow HCO_3^- \leftrightarrow \uparrow Cl^-$), and there is no change in the amount of unmeasured anions.

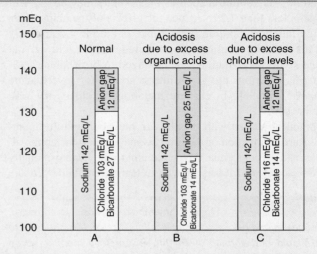

Figure 5–17 ■ Illustration of the anion gap in metabolic acidosis. A, Normal anion gap. B, High anion gap caused by excess acids. C, Normal anion gap with hyperchloremia.

Acidosis depresses cell membrane excitability, affecting neuromuscular function. It also increases the amount of free calcium in ECF by interfering with protein binding. Severe acidosis (pH of 7.0 or less) depresses myocardial contractility, leading to a fall in cardiac output. If kidney function is normal, acid excretion and ammonia production increase to eliminate excess hydrogen ions.

Acid-base imbalances also affect electrolyte balance. In acidosis, potassium is retained as the kidney excretes excess hydrogen ion. Excess hydrogen ions also enter the cells, displacing potassium from the intracellular space to maintain the balance of cations and anions within the cells. The effect of both processes is to increase serum potassium levels. Also in acidosis, calcium is released from its bonds with plasma proteins, increasing the amount of ionized (free) calcium in the blood. Magnesium levels may fall in acidosis (Bullock & Henze, 2000).

MANIFESTATIONS

Metabolic acidosis affects the function of many body systems. Its general manifestations include weakness and fatigue, headache, and general malaise. Gastrointestinal function is affected, causing anorexia, nausea, vomiting, and abdominal pain. The level of consciousness declines, leading to stupor and coma. Cardiac dysrhythmias develop, and cardiac arrest may occur. The skin is often warm and flushed. Skeletal problems may develop in chronic acidosis, as calcium and phosphate are released from the bones. Manifestations of compensatory mechanisms are seen. The respirations are deep and rapid, known as **Kussmaul's respirations.** The client may complain of shortness of breath or dyspnea. See the box on this page.

COLLABORATIVE CARE

Management of metabolic acidosis focuses on treating the underlying cause of the disorder and correcting the acid-base imbalance.

Diagnostic Tests

The following laboratory and diagnostic tests may be ordered.

- *ABGs* generally show a pH of less than 7.35 and a bicarbonate level of less than 22 mEq/L. A compensatory decrease in $PaCO_2$ to less than 35 mmHg is usually present.
- *Serum electrolytes* demonstrate elevated serum potassium levels and possible low magnesium levels. The total calcium may remain unchanged, although more physiologically active ionized calcium is available. Sodium, chloride, and bicarbonate levels are used to calculate the anion gap.
- The *ECG* may show changes which reflect both the acidosis (particularly when severe) and the accompanying hyperkalemia.

Manifestations of Metabolic Acidosis

- Anorexia
- Nausea and vomiting
- Abdominal pain
- Weakness
- Fatigue
- General malaise

- Decreasing levels of consciousness
- Dysrhythmias
- Bradycardia
- Warm, flushed skin
- Hyperventilation (Kussmaul's respirations)

Medications

An alkalinizing solution such as bicarbonate may be given if the pH is less than 7.2 to reduce the effects of the acidosis on cardiac function. Sodium bicarbonate is the most commonly used alkalinizing solution; others include lactate, citrate, and acetate solutions (which are metabolized to bicarbonate). Alkalinizing solutions are given intravenously for severe acute metabolic acidosis. In chronic metabolic acidosis, the oral route is used.

The client treated with bicarbonate must be carefully monitored. Rapid correction of the acidosis may lead to metabolic alkalosis and hypokalemia. Hypernatremia and hyperosmolality may develop as well, leading to water retention and fluid overload.

PRACTICE ALERT *As metabolic acidosis is corrected, potassium shifts back into the intracellular space. This can lead to hypokalemia and cardiac dysrhythmias. Carefully monitor serum potassium levels during treatment.* ■

Treatment for diabetic ketoacidosis includes intravenous insulin and fluid replacement. Alcoholic ketoacidosis is treated with saline solutions and glucose. Treatment for lactic acidosis from decreased tissue perfusion (e.g., shock or cardiac arrest) focuses on correcting the underlying problem and improving tissue perfusion. Clients with chronic renal failure and mild or moderate metabolic acidosis may or may not require treatment, depending on the pH and bicarbonate levels. When metabolic acidosis is due to diarrhea, treatment includes correcting the underlying cause and providing fluid and electrolyte replacement.

NURSING CARE

Health Promotion

To promote health in clients at risk for metabolic acidosis, discuss management of their underlying disease process (e.g., type 1 diabetes or renal failure) to prevent complications such as diabetic ketoacidosis and metabolic acidosis. Because early manifestations of metabolic acidosis (e.g., fatigue, general malaise, anorexia, nausea, abdominal pain) resemble those of common viral disorders such as "the flu," stress the importance of promptly seeking treatment if these symptoms develop.

Assessment

Assessment data related to metabolic acidosis include the following:

- Health history: Current manifestations, including anorexia, nausea, vomiting, abdominal discomfort, fatigue, lethargy, other symptoms; duration of symptoms and any precipitating factors such as diarrhea, ingestion of a toxin such as aspirin, methanol, or ethylene; chronic diseases such as diabetes or renal failure, cirrhosis of the liver, or endocrine disorders; current medications.

- Physical assessment: Mental status and level of consciousness; vital signs including respiratory rate and depth; apical and peripheral pulses; skin color and temperature; abdominal contour and distention; bowel sounds; urine output.

Nursing Diagnoses and Interventions
Decreased Cardiac Output

Metabolic acidosis affects cardiac output by decreasing myocardial contractility, slowing the heart rate, and increasing the risk for dysrhythmias. The accompanying hyperkalemia increases the risk for decreased cardiac output as well (see earlier discussion about hyperkalemia).

- Monitor vital signs, including peripheral pulses and capillary refill. *Hypotension, diminished pulse strength, and slowed capillary refill may indicate decreased cardiac output and impaired tissue perfusion. Poor tissue perfusion can increase the risk for lactic acidosis.*
- Monitor the ECG pattern for dysrhythmias and changes characteristic of hyperkalemia. Notify the physician of changes. *Progressive ECG changes such as widening of the QRS complex indicate an increasing risk of dysrhythmias and cardiac arrest. Dysrhythmias further decrease cardiac output, possibly intensifying the degree of acidosis.*
- Monitor laboratory values, including arterial blood gases, serum electrolytes, and renal function studies (serum creatinine and BUN). *Frequent monitoring of laboratory values allows evaluation of the effectiveness of treatment as well as early identification of potential problems.*

Risk for Excess Fluid Volume

Administering bicarbonate to correct acidosis increases the risk for hypernatremia, hyperosmolality, and fluid volume excess.

- Monitor and maintain fluid replacement as ordered. Monitor serum sodium levels and osmolality. *Bicarbonate administration can cause hypernatremia and hyperosmolality, leading to water retention.*
- Monitor heart and lung sounds, CVP, and respiratory status. *Increasing dyspnea, adventitious lung sounds, a third heart sound (S_3) due to the volume of blood flow through the heart, and high CVP readings are indicative of hypervolemia and should be reported to the care provider.*
- Assess for edema, particularly in the back, sacral, and periorbital areas. *Initially, edema affects dependent tissues—the back and sacrum in clients who are bedridden. Periorbital edema indicates more generalized edema.*
- Assess urine output hourly. Maintain accurate intake and output records. Note urine output less than 30 mL/hour or a positive fluid balance on 24-hour total intake and output calculations. *Heart failure and inadequate renal perfusion may lead to decreased urine output.*
- Obtain daily weights using consistent conditions. *Daily weights are an accurate indicator of fluid balance.*
- Administer prescribed diuretics as ordered, monitoring the client's response to therapy. *Loop or high-ceiling diuretics such as furosemide can lead to further electrolyte imbal-*

CHART 5–6 NANDA, NIC, AND NOC LINKAGES

The Client with Metabolic Acidosis

NURSING DIAGNOSES	NURSING INTERVENTIONS	NURSING OUTCOMES
• Decreased Cardiac Output	• Acid-Base Management • Vital Signs Monitoring	• Cardiac Pump Effectiveness
• Risk for Excess Fluid Volume	• Electrolyte Management • Fluid Management	• Electrolyte & Acid-Base Balance • Vital Signs Status
• Risk for Injury	• Environmental Management: Safety	• Safety Status: Physical Injury

Note. Data from Nursing Outcomes Classification (NOC) by M. Johnson & M. Maas (Eds.), 1997, St. Louis: Mosby; Nursing Diagnoses: Definitions & Classification 2001–2002 by North American Nursing Diagnosis Association, 2001, Philadelphia: NANDA; Nursing Interventions Classification (NIC) by J.C. McCloskey & G. M. Bulechek (Eds.), 2000, St. Louis: Mosby. Reprinted by permission.

---

ances, especially hypokalemia. This is a significant risk as during correction of metabolic acidosis.

Risk for Injury

Mental status and brain function are affected by acidosis, increasing the risk for injury.

- Monitor neurologic function, including mental status, level of consciousness, and muscle strength. *As the pH falls, mental functioning declines, leading to confusion, stupor, and a decreasing level of consciousness.*
- Institute safety precautions as necessary; keep the bed in its lowest position, side rails raised. *These measures help protect the client from injury resulting from confusion or disorientation.*
- Keep clocks, calendars, and familiar objects at bedside. Orient to time, place, and circumstances as needed. Allow significant others to remain with the client as much as possible. *An unfamiliar environment and altered thought processes can further increase the risk for injury. Significant others provide a sense of security and reduce anxiety.*

Nursing care also includes measures to treat the underlying disorder, such as diabetic ketoacidosis. Refer to the chapters on diabetes (Chapter 18) and renal failure (Chapter 27) for specific interventions. ⌘

Using NANDA, NIC, and NOC

Chart 5–6 shows links between potential NANDA nursing diagnoses, NIC, and NOC when caring for a client with metabolic acidosis.

Home Care

Discharge planning and teaching focuses on the underlying cause of the imbalance. The client who has developed ketoacidosis as a result of diabetes mellitus, starvation, or alcoholism needs interventions and teaching to prevent future episodes of acidosis. Diet, medication management, and alcohol dependency treatment are vital teaching areas. When metabolic acidosis is related to renal failure, the client should be referred for management of the renal failure itself. Clients who have experienced diarrhea or excess ileostomy drainage leading to bicarbonate loss need information about appropriate diarrhea treatment strategies and when to call their primary care provider.

THE CLIENT WITH METABOLIC ALKALOSIS

Metabolic alkalosis (bicarbonate excess) is characterized by a high pH (>7.45) and a high bicarbonate (>26 mEq/L). It may be caused by loss of acid or excess bicarbonate in the body. When metabolic alkalosis develops, the respiratory system attempts to return the pH to normal by slowing the respiratory rate. Carbon dioxide is retained, and the $PaCO_2$ increases (>45 mmHg).

RISK FACTORS

As is the case with other acid-base imbalances, metabolic alkalosis rarely occurs as a primary disorder. Risk factors include hospitalization, hypokalemia, and treatment with alkalinizing solutions (e.g., bicarbonate).

PATHOPHYSIOLOGY

Hydrogen ions may be lost via gastric secretions, through the kidneys, or because of a shift of H^+ into the cells. Metabolic alkalosis due to loss of hydrogen ions usually occurs because of vomiting or gastric suction. Gastric secretions are highly acidic (pH 1 to 3). When these are lost through vomiting or gastric suction, the alkalinity of body fluids increases. This increased alkalinity results both from the loss of acid and selective retention of bicarbonate by the kidneys as chloride is depleted (chloride is the major anion in ECF; when it is lost, bicarbonate is retained as a replacement anion).

Increased renal excretion of hydrogen ions can be prompted by hypokalemia as the kidneys try to conserve potassium, excreting hydrogen ion instead. Hypokalemia contributes to metabolic alkalosis in another way as well. When potassium shifts out of cells to maintain extracellular potassium levels, hydrogen ions shift into the cells to maintain the balance between cations and anions within the cell.

Manifestations of Metabolic Alkalosis

- Confusion
- Decreasing levels of consciousness
- Hyperreflexia
- Tetany
- Dysrhythmias
- Hypotension
- Seizures
- Respiratory failure

Excess bicarbonate usually occurs as a result of ingesting antacids that contain bicarbonate (such as soda bicarbonate or Alka-Seltzer) or overzealous administration of bicarbonate to treat metabolic acidosis. Common causes of metabolic alkalosis are summarized in Table 5–11.

In alkalosis, more calcium combines with serum proteins, reducing the amount of ionized (physiologically active) calcium in the blood. This accounts for many of the common manifestations of metabolic alkalosis. Alkalosis also affects potassium balance: Hypokalemia not only can cause metabolic alkalosis (see above), but it also can result from metabolic alkalosis. Hydrogen ions shift out of the intracellular space to help restore the pH, prompting more potassium to enter the cells and depleting ECF potassium. The high pH depresses the respiratory system as the body retains carbon dioxide to restore the carbonic acid to bicarbonate ratio.

MANIFESTATIONS AND COMPLICATIONS

Manifestations of metabolic alkalosis occur as a result of decreased calcium ionization and are similar to those of hypocalcemia, including numbness and tingling around the mouth and of fingers and toes, dizziness, Trousseau's sign, and muscle spasm (see box above). As the respiratory system compensates for metabolic alkalosis, respirations are depressed and respiratory failure with hypoxemia and respiratory acidosis may develop.

COLLABORATIVE CARE

The management of metabolic alkalosis focuses on diagnosing and correcting the underlying cause.

Diagnostic Tests

The following laboratory and diagnostic tests may be ordered.

- *ABGs* show a pH greater than 7.45 and bicarbonate level greater than 26 mEq/L. With compensatory hypoventilation, carbon dioxide is retained, and the $PaCO_2$ is greater than 45 mmHg.
- *Serum electrolytes* often demonstrate decreased serum potassium (< 3.5 mEq/L) and decreased chloride (< 95 mEq/L) levels. The serum bicarbonate level is high. Although the total serum calcium may be normal, the ionized fraction of calcium is low.
- *Urine pH* may be low (pH 1 to 3) if metabolic acidosis is caused by hypokalemia. The kidneys selectively retain potassium and excrete hydrogen ion to restore ECF potassium levels. Urinary chloride levels may be normal or greater than 250 mEq/24 hours.

- The *ECG pattern* shows changes similar to those seen with hypokalemia. These changes may be due to hypokalemia or to the alkalosis.

Medications

Treatment of metabolic alkalosis includes restoring normal fluid volume and administering potassium chloride and sodium chloride solution. The potassium restores serum and intracellular potassium levels, allowing the kidneys to more effectively conserve hydrogen ions. Chloride promotes renal excretion of bicarbonate. Sodium chloride solutions restore fluid volume deficits that can contribute to metabolic alkalosis. In severe alkalosis, an acidifying solution such as dilute hydrochloric acid or ammonium chloride may be administered. In addition, drugs may be used to treat the underlying cause of the alkalosis.

NURSING CARE

Health Promotion

Health promotion activities focus on teaching clients the risks of using sodium bicarbonate as an antacid to relieve heartburn or gastric distress. Stress the availability of other effective antacid preparations and the need to seek medical evaluation for persistent gastric symptoms.

In the hospital setting, carefully monitor laboratory values for clients at risk for developing metabolic alkalosis, particularly clients undergoing continuous gastric suction.

Assessment

Focused assessment data related to metabolic alkalosis include the following:

- Health history: Current manifestations, such as numbness and tingling, muscle spasms, dizziness, other symptoms; duration of symptoms and any precipitating factors such as bicarbonate ingestion, vomiting, diuretic therapy, or endocrine disorders; current medications.
- Physical assessment: Vital signs including apical pulse and rate and depth of respirations; muscle strength; deep tendon reflexes.

Nursing Diagnoses and Interventions
Risk for Impaired Gas Exchange

Respiratory compensation for metabolic alkalosis depresses the respiratory rate and reduces the depth of breathing to promote carbon dioxide retention. As a result, the client is at risk for impaired gas exchange, especially in the presence of underlying lung disease.

- Monitor respiratory rate, depth, and effort. Monitor oxygen saturation continuously, reporting an oxygen saturation level of less than 95% (or as ordered). *The depressed respiratory drive associated with metabolic alkalosis can lead to hypoxemia and impaired oxygenation of tissues. Oxygen saturation levels of less than 90% indicate significant oxygenation problems.*

- Assess skin color; note and report cyanosis around the mouth. *Central cyanosis, seen around the mouth and oral mucous membranes, indicates significant hypoxia.*
- Monitor mental status and level of consciousness. Report decreasing LOC or behavior changes such as restlessness, agitation, or confusion. *Changes in mental status or behavior may be early signs of hypoxia.*
- Place in semi-Fowler's or Fowler's position as tolerated. *Elevating the head of the bed facilitates alveolar ventilation and gas exchange.*
- Schedule nursing care activities to allow rest periods. *The client who is hypoxemic has limited energy reserves, necessitating frequent rest and limited activities.*
- Administer oxygen as ordered or necessary to maintain oxygen saturation levels. *Supplemental oxygen can help maintain blood and tissue oxygenation despite depressed respirations.*

Deficient Fluid Volume

Clients with metabolic alkalosis often have an accompanying fluid volume deficit.

PRACTICE ALERT *Assess intake and output accurately, monitoring fluid balance. In acute situations, hourly intake and output may be indicated. Urine output less than 30 mL/hour indicates inadequate tissue perfusion, inadequate renal perfusion and an increased risk for acute renal failure.* ■

- Assess vital signs, CVP, and peripheral pulse volume at least every 4 hours. *Hypotension, tachycardia, low CVP, and weak, easily obliterated peripheral pulses indicate hypovolemia.*
- Weigh daily under standard conditions (time of day, clothing, and scale). *Rapid weight changes accurately reflect fluid balance.*
- Administer intravenous fluids as prescribed using an electronic infusion pump. Monitor for indicators of fluid overload if rapid fluid replacement is ordered: dyspnea, tachypnea, tachycardia, increased CVP, jugular vein distension, and edema. *Rapid fluid replacement may lead to hypervolemia, resulting in pulmonary edema and cardiac failure, particularly in clients with compromised cardiac and renal function.*

- Monitor serum electrolytes, osmolality, and ABG values. *Rehydration and administration of potassium chloride will affect both acid-base and fluid and electrolyte balance. Careful monitoring is important to identify changes.*

Nursing care also includes interdependent care measures to treat the underlying disorder, such as excessive vomiting or hypokalemia.

Using NANDA, NIC, and NOC

Chart 5–7 shows links between potential NANDA nursing diagnoses, NIC, and NOC when caring for a client with metabolic alkalosis.

Home Care

When preparing the client with metabolic alkalosis for discharge and home care, consider the cause of the alkalosis and any underlying factors. For example, provide teaching about the following:

- Using appropriate antacids for heartburn and gastric distress
- Using potassium supplements as ordered or eating high-potassium foods to avoid hypokalemia if taking a potassium-wasting diuretic or if aldosterone production is impaired
- Contacting the primary care provider if uncontrolled or extended vomiting develops

THE CLIENT WITH RESPIRATORY ACIDOSIS

Respiratory acidosis is caused by an excess of dissolved carbon dioxide, or carbonic acid. It is characterized by a pH of less than 7.35 and a $Paco_2$ greater than 45 mmHg. Respiratory acidosis may be either acute or chronic. In chronic respiratory acidosis, the bicarbonate is higher than 26 mEq/L as the kidneys compensate by retaining bicarbonate.

RISK FACTORS

Acute or chronic lung disease (e.g., pneumonia or chronic obstructive pulmonary disease) is the primary risk factor for respiratory acidosis. Other conditions that depress or interfere with ventilation, such as excess narcotic analgesics, airway

CHART 5–7 NANDA, NIC, AND NOC LINKAGES

The Client with Metabolic Alkalosis

NURSING DIAGNOSES	NURSING INTERVENTIONS	NURSING OUTCOMES
• Risk for Impaired Gas Exchange	• Acid-Base Management • Fluid Management	• Respiratory Status: Gas Exchange
• Deficient Fluid Volume	• Intravenous Therapy	• Electrolyte & Acid-Base Balance • Fluid Balance

Note. Data from Nursing Outcomes Classification (NOC) by M. Johnson & M. Maas (Eds.), 1997, St. Louis: Mosby; Nursing Diagnoses: Definitions & Classification 2001–2002 by North American Nursing Diagnosis Association, 2001, Philadelphia: NANDA; Nursing Interventions Classification (NIC) by J.C. McCloskey & G. M. Bulechek (Eds.), 2000, St. Louis: Mosby. Reprinted by permission.

obstruction, or neuromuscular disease, also are risk factors for respiratory acidosis. Selected causes of respiratory acidosis are listed in Table 5–11.

PATHOPHYSIOLOGY

Both acute and chronic respiratory acidosis result from carbon dioxide retention caused by alveolar hypoventilation. Hypoxemia (low oxygen in the arterial blood) frequently accompanies respiratory acidosis.

Acute Respiratory Acidosis

Acute respiratory acidosis occurs due to a sudden failure of ventilation. Chest trauma, aspiration of a foreign body, acute pneumonia, and overdoses of narcotic or sedative medications can lead to this condition. Because acute respiratory acidosis occurs with the sudden onset of hypoventilation—as, for example, with cardiac arrest—the $PaCO_2$ rises rapidly and the pH falls markedly. A pH of 7 or lower can occur within minutes (Metheny, 2000). The serum bicarbonate level initially is unchanged because the compensatory response of the kidneys occurs over hours to days.

Hypercapnia (increased carbon dioxide levels) affects neurologic function and the cardiovascular system. Carbon dioxide rapidly crosses the blood-brain barrier. Cerebral blood vessels dilate, and if the condition continues, intracranial pressure increases and papilledema (swelling and inflammation of the optic nerve where it enters the retina) develops (Porth, 2002). Peripheral vasodilation also occurs, and the pulse rate increases to maintain cardiac output.

Chronic Respiratory Acidosis

Chronic respiratory acidosis is associated with chronic respiratory or neuromuscular conditions such as chronic obstructive pulmonary disease (COPD), asthma, cystic fibrosis, or multiple sclerosis. These conditions affect alveolar ventilation because of airway obstruction, structural changes in the lung, or limited chest wall expansion. Most clients with chronic respiratory acidosis have COPD with chronic bronchitis and emphysema. In chronic respiratory acidosis, the $PaCO_2$ increases over time and remains elevated. The kidneys retain bicarbonate, increasing bicarbonate levels, and the pH often remains close to the normal range.

The acute effects of hypercapnia may not develop because carbon dioxide levels rise gradually, allowing compensatory changes to occur. When carbon dioxide levels are chronically elevated, the respiratory center becomes less sensitive to the gas as a stimulant of the respiratory drive. The PaO_2 provides the primary stimulus for respirations. Clients with chronic respiratory acidosis are at risk for developing *carbon dioxide narcosis* with manifestations of acute respiratory acidosis, if the respiratory center is suppressed by administering excess supplemental oxygen.

PRACTICE ALERT *Carefully monitor neurologic and respiratory status in clients with chronic respiratory acidosis who are receiving oxygen therapy. Immediately report decreasing level of consciousness or depressed respirations.* ■

Manifestations of Respiratory Acidosis

ACUTE RESPIRATORY ACIDOSIS
- Headache
- Warm, flushed skin
- Blurred vision
- Irritability, altered mental status
- Decreasing level of consciousness
- Cardiac arrest

CHRONIC RESPIRATORY ACIDOSIS
- Weakness
- Dull headache
- Sleep disturbances with daytime sleepiness
- Impaired memory
- Personality changes

MANIFESTATIONS

The manifestations of acute and chronic respiratory acidosis differ. In acute respiratory acidosis, the rapid rise in $PaCO_2$ levels causes manifestations of hypercapnia. Cerebral vasodilation causes manifestations such as headache, blurred vision, irritability, and mental cloudiness. If the condition continues, the level of consciousness progressively decreases. Rapid and dramatic changes in ABGs can lead to unconsciousness and ventricular fibrillation, a potentially lethal cardiac dysrhythmia. The skin of the client with acute respiratory acidosis may be warm and flushed, and the pulse rate is elevated.

The manifestations of chronic respiratory acidosis include weakness and a dull headache. Sleep disturbances, daytime sleepiness, impaired memory, and personality changes also may be manifestations of chronic respiratory acidosis (see the box above).

COLLABORATIVE CARE

Clients with acute respiratory failure usually require treatment in the emergency department or intensive care unit. The focus is on restoring adequate ventilation and gas exchange. Hypoxemia often accompanies acute respiratory acidosis, so oxygen is administered as well. Supplemental oxygen is administered with caution to clients with chronic respiratory acidosis.

Diagnostic Tests

The following laboratory and diagnostic tests may be ordered.

- *ABGs* show a pH of less than 7.35 and a $PaCO_2$ of more than 45 mmHg. In acute respiratory acidosis, the bicarbonate level is initially within normal range but increases to greater than 26 mEq/L if the condition persists. In chronic respiratory acidosis, both the $PaCO_2$ and the HCO_3^- may be significantly elevated.
- *Serum electrolytes* may show hypochloremia (chloride level < 98 mEq/L) in chronic respiratory acidosis.
- *Pulmonary function tests* may be done to determine if chronic lung disease is the cause of the respiratory acidosis. These studies would not be done during the acute period, however.

Medications

Bronchodilator drugs may be administered to open the airways and antibiotics prescribed to treat respiratory infections. If excess narcotics or anesthetic has caused acute respiratory acidosis, drugs to reverse their effects (such as naloxone) may be given.

Respiratory Support

Treatment of respiratory acidosis, either acute or chronic, focuses on improving alveolar ventilation and gas exchange. Clients with severe respiratory acidosis and hypoxemia may require intubation and mechanical ventilation (see Chapter 36 for more information about these procedures). ∞ The $PaCO_2$ level is lowered slowly to avoid complications such as cardiac dysrhythmias and decreased cerebral perfusion. In clients with chronic respiratory acidosis, oxygen is administered cautiously to avoid carbon dioxide narcosis.

Pulmonary hygiene measures, such as breathing treatments or percussion and drainage, may be instituted. Adequate hydration is important to promote removal of respiratory secretions.

NURSING CARE

Health Promotion

Health promotion activities related to respiratory acidosis focus on identifying, monitoring, and teaching clients at risk. Carefully monitor clients receiving anesthesia, narcotic analgesics, or sedatives for signs of respiratory depression. Monitor the response of clients with a history of chronic lung disease to oxygen therapy. Teach clients who have an identified risk for respiratory acidosis (such as people using narcotic analgesia for cancer pain and people with chronic lung disease) and their families about early manifestations of respiratory depression and acidosis, and instruct them to immediately contact their care provider if manifestations develop.

Assessment

Assessment data related to respiratory acidosis include the following:

- Health history: Current manifestations, including headache, irritability or lethargy, difficulty thinking, blurred vision, and other symptoms; duration of symptoms and any precipitating factors such as drug use or respiratory infection; chronic diseases such as cystic fibrosis or COPD; current medications.
- Physical assessment: Mental status and level of consciousness; vital signs; skin color and temperature; rate and depth of respirations, pulmonary excursion, lung sounds; examination of optic fundus for possible papilledema.

Nursing Diagnoses and Interventions

Impaired Gas Exchange

- Frequently assess respiratory status, including rate, depth, effort, and oxygen saturation levels. *Decreasing respiratory rate and effort along with decreasing oxygen saturation levels may signal worsening respiratory failure and respiratory acidosis.*

PRACTICE ALERT *Frequently assess level of consciousness. A decline in level of consciousness may indicate increasing hypercapnia and the need for increasing ventilatory support (such as intubation and mechanical ventilation).* ■

- Promptly evaluate and report ABG results to the physician and respiratory therapist. *Rapid changes in carbon dioxide or oxygen levels may necessitate modification of the treatment plan to prevent complications of overcorrection of respiratory acidosis.*
- Place in semi-Fowler's to Fowler's position as tolerated. *Elevating the head of the bed promotes lung expansion and gas exchange.*
- Administer oxygen as ordered. Carefully monitor response. Reduce the oxygen flow rate or percentage and immediately report increasing somnolence. *Supplemental oxygen can suppress the respiratory drive in clients with chronic respiratory acidosis.*

Ineffective Airway Clearance

- Frequently auscultate breath sounds (whether on or off a mechanical ventilator). *Increasing adventitious sounds or decreasing breath sounds (faint or absent) may indicate worsening airway clearance due to obstruction or fatigue.*
- Encourage the client with chronic respiratory acidosis to use pursed-lip breathing. *Pursed-lip breathing helps maintain open airways throughout exhalation, promoting carbon dioxide elimination.*
- Frequently reposition and encourage out of bed as tolerated. *Repositioning, sitting at the bedside, and ambulation promote airway clearance and lung expansion.*
- Encourage fluid intake of up to 3000 mL per day as tolerated or allowed. *Fluids help liquify secretions and hydrate respiratory mucous membranes, promoting airway clearance.*
- Administer medications such as inhaled bronchodilators as ordered. *Inhaled bronchodilators help relieve bronchial spasm, dilating airways.*
- Provide percussion, vibration, and postural drainage as ordered. *Pulmonary hygiene measures such as these help loosen respiratory secretions so they can be coughed out of airways.*

Using NANDA, NIC, and NOC

Chart 5–8 shows links between NANDA nursing diagnoses, NIC, and NOC when caring for a client with respiratory acidosis.

Home Care

Planning and teaching for home care focuses on the problem that caused the client to develop respiratory acidosis. The client who developed acute respiratory acidosis as a result of acute pneumonia or chest trauma may only require teaching to prevent future problems. If acute respiratory acidosis occurred secondarily to a narcotic overdose, determine if the drug was prescribed for pain or if it was an illicit street drug. Provide teaching to the client who requires narcotic medication on a continuing basis. Refer the client using illicit drugs to a substance abuse counselor, treatment center, or Narcotics Anonymous as appropriate.

CHART 5–8 NANDA, NIC, AND NOC LINKAGES

The Client with Respiratory Acidosis

NURSING DIAGNOSES	NURSING INTERVENTIONS	NURSING OUTCOMES
• Impaired Gas Exchange • Ineffective Airway Clearance	• Acid-Base Management: Respiratory Acidosis • Respiratory Monitoring • Ventilation Assistance	• Electrolyte & Acid-Base Balance • Respiratory Status: Gas Exchange • Respiratory Status: Ventilation

Note. Data from Nursing Outcomes Classification (NOC) *by M. Johnson & M. Maas (Eds.), 1997, St. Louis: Mosby;* Nursing Diagnoses: Definitions & Classification 2001–2002 *by North American Nursing Diagnosis Association, 2001, Philadelphia: NANDA;* Nursing Interventions Classification (NIC) *by J.C. McCloskey & G. M. Bulechek (Eds.), 2000, St. Louis: Mosby. Reprinted by permission.*

For clients with chronic lung disease, discuss ways to avoid future episodes of acute respiratory failure. Encourage the client to be immunized against pneumococcal pneumonia and influenza. Discuss ways to avoid acute respiratory infections and measures to take when respiratory status is further compromised.

THE CLIENT WITH RESPIRATORY ALKALOSIS

Respiratory alkalosis is characterized by a pH greater than 7.45 and a $PaCO_2$ of less than 35 mmHg. It is always caused by hyperventilation leading to a carbon dioxide deficit.

Nursing Care Plan
A Client with Acute Respiratory Acidosis

Marlene Hitz, age 76, is eating lunch with her friends when she suddenly begins to choke and is unable to breathe. After several minutes of trying, an attendant at the senior center successfully dislodges some meat caught in Ms. Hitz's throat using the Heimlich maneuver. Ms. Hitz is taken by ambulance to the emergency department for follow-up because she was apneic for 3 to 4 minutes, her respirations are shallow, and she is disoriented.

ASSESSMENT

Ms. Hitz is placed in an observation room. Oxygen is started at 4 L/min per nasal cannula. David Love, the nurse admitting Ms. Hitz, makes the following assessments: T 98.2, P 102, R 36 and shallow, BP 146/92. Skin is warm and dry. Alert but restless and not oriented to time or place; she responds slowly to questions. Stat ABGs are drawn, a chest X-ray is done, and D5 ½ NS is started intravenously at 50 mL/hr.

The chest X-ray shows no abnormality. ABG results are pH 7.38 (normal: 7.35 to 7.45), $PaCO_2$ 48 mmHg (normal: 35 to 45 mmHg), PaO_2 92 mmHg (normal: 80 to 100 mmHg), and HCO_3^- 24 mEq/L (normal: 22 to 26 mEq/L).

DIAGNOSES

- *Impaired gas exchange* related to temporary airway obstruction
- *Anxiety* related to emergency hospital admission
- *Risk for injury* related to confusion

EXPECTED OUTCOMES

- Regain normal gas exchange and ABG values.
- Be oriented to time, place, and person.

- Regain baseline mental status.
- Remain free of injury.

PLANNING AND IMPLEMENTATION

- Monitor ABGs, to be redrawn in 2 hours.
- Monitor vital signs and respiratory status (including oxygen saturation) every 15 minutes for the first hour then every hour.
- Assess color of skin, nail beds, and oral mucous membranes every hour.
- Assess mental status and orientation every hour.
- Monitor anxiety level as evidenced by restlessness and agitation.
- Maintain a calm, quiet environment.
- Provide reorientation and explain all activities.
- Keep side rails in place, and place call bell within reach.

EVALUATION

Ms. Hitz remains in the emergency department for 6 hours. Her ABGs are still abnormal, and David Love now notes the presence of respiratory crackles and wheezes. She is less anxious and responds appropriately when asked who and where she is. Because she has not regained normal gas exchange, Ms. Hitz is admitted to the hospital for continued observation and treatment.

Critical Thinking in the Nursing Process

1. Describe the pathophysiologic process that leads to acute respiratory acidosis in Marlene Hitz.
2. Describe the effect of acidosis on mental function.
3. What teaching would you provide to Marlene Hitz to prevent future episodes of choking?

See Evaluating Your Response in Appendix C.

RISK FACTORS

Anxiety with hyperventilation is the most common cause of respiratory alkalosis; therefore, anxiety disorders increase the risk for this acid-base imbalance. In the client who is critically ill, mechanical ventilation is a risk factor for respiratory alkalosis.

PATHOPHYSIOLOGY

In acute respiratory alkalosis, the pH rises rapidly as the $Paco_2$ falls. Because the kidneys are unable to rapidly adapt to the change in pH, the bicarbonate level remains within normal limits. Anxiety-based hyperventilation is the most common cause of acute respiratory alkalosis. Other physiologic causes of hyperventilation include high fever, hypoxia, gram-negative bacteremia, and thyrotoxicosis. Early salicylate intoxication (aspirin overdose), encephalitis, and high progesterone levels in pregnancy directly stimulate the respiratory center, potentially leading to hyperventilation and respiratory alkalosis. Hyperventilation also can occur during anesthesia or mechanical ventilation if the rate and tidal volume (depth) of ventilations is excessive.

If hyperventilation continues, the kidneys compensate by eliminating bicarbonate to restore the bicarbonate to carbonic acid ratio. The bicarbonate level is lower than normal in chronic respiratory alkalosis, and the pH may be close to the normal range.

Alkalosis increases binding of extracellular calcium to albumin, reducing ionized calcium levels. As a result, neuromuscular excitability increases and manifestations similar to hypocalcemia develop. Low carbon dioxide levels in the blood cause vasoconstriction of cerebral vessels, increasing the neurologic manifestations of the disorder.

MANIFESTATIONS

The manifestations of respiratory alkalosis include lightheadedness, a feeling of panic and difficulty concentrating, circumoral and distal extremity paresthesias, tremors, and positive Chvostek's and Trousseau's signs. The client also may experience tinnitus, a sensation of chest tightness, and palpitations (cardiac dysrhythmias). Seizures and loss of consciousness may occur. See the box below.

COLLABORATIVE CARE

Management of respiratory alkalosis focuses on correcting the imbalance and treating the underlying cause.

Manifestations of Respiratory Alkalosis

- Dizziness
- Numbness and tingling around mouth, of hands and feet
- Palpitations
- Dyspnea
- Chest tightness
- Anxiety/panic
- Tremors
- Tetany
- Seizures, loss of consciousness

Diagnostic Tests

ABGs generally show a pH greater than 7.45 and a $Paco_2$ less than 35 mmHg. In chronic hyperventilation, there is a compensatory decrease in serum bicarbonate to less than 22 mEq/L and the pH may be near normal.

Medications

A sedative or antianxiety agent may be necessary to relieve anxiety and restore a normal breathing pattern. Additional drugs to correct underlying problems other than anxiety-induced hyperventilation may be ordered.

Respiratory Therapy

The usual treatment for anxiety-related respiratory alkalosis involves instructing the client to breathe more slowly and having the client breathe into a paper bag or rebreather mask. This allows rebreathing of exhaled carbon dioxide, increasing $Paco_2$ levels and reducing the pH. If excessive ventilation by a mechanical ventilator is the cause of respiratory alkalosis, ventilator settings are adjusted to reduce the respiratory rate and tidal volume as indicated. When hypoxia is the underlying cause of hyperventilation, oxygen is administered.

NURSING CARE

Health Promotion

Identify clients at risk in the hospital (e.g., clients on mechanical ventilation or who have a fever or infection), and monitor assessment data and ABGs to identify early manifestations of hyperventilation and respiratory alkalosis.

Assessment, Diagnoses, and Interventions
Ineffective Breathing Pattern

The usual cause of hyperventilation and respiratory alkalosis is psychologic, although physiologic disorders also can lead to hyperventilation. It is important to not only address the hyperventilation, but also to identify the underlying cause.

- Assess respiratory rate, depth, and ease. Monitor vital signs (including temperature) and skin color. *Assessment data can help identify the underlying cause, such as a fever or hypoxia.*
- Obtain subjective assessment data such as circumstances leading up to the current situation, current health and recent illnesses or medication use, and current manifestations. *Subjective data provide cues to the cause and circumstances of the hyperventilation response.*
- Reassure the client that he or she is not experiencing a heart attack and that symptoms will resolve when breathing returns to normal. *Manifestations of hyperventilation and respiratory alkalosis such as dyspnea, chest tightness or pain, and palpitations can mimic those of a heart attack.*
- Instruct the client to maintain eye contact and breathe with you to slow the respiratory rate. *These measures help to make*

CHART 5–9   NANDA, NIC, AND NOC LINKAGES

The Client with Respiratory Alkalosis

NURSING DIAGNOSES	NURSING INTERVENTIONS	NURSING OUTCOMES
• Ineffective Breathing Pattern • Risk for Injury	• Acid-Base Management: Respiratory Alkalosis • Anxiety Reduction	• Anxiety Control • Respiratory Status: Gas Exchange

Note. Data from Nursing Outcomes Classification (NOC) by M. Johnson & M. Maas (Eds.), 1997, St. Louis: Mosby; Nursing Diagnoses: Definitions & Classification 2001–2002 by North American Nursing Diagnosis Association, 2001, Philadelphia: NANDA; Nursing Interventions Classification (NIC) by J.C. McCloskey & G. M. Bulechek (Eds.), 2000, St. Louis: Mosby. Reprinted by permission.

the client aware of respirations and provide a sense of support and control (Ackley & Ladwig, 2002).

- Have the client breathe into a paper bag. *This allows the client to rebreathe exhaled carbon dioxide, increasing the $Paco_2$ and decreasing the pH.*
- Protect the client from injury. *If hyperventilation continues to the point at which the client loses consciousness, respirations will return to normal, as will acid-base balance.*
- If the client has experienced repeated episodes of hyperventilation or has a chronic anxiety disorder, refer for counseling. *Counseling can help the client develop alternative strategies for dealing with anxiety.*

Using NANDA, NIC, and NOC

Chart 5–9 shows links between NANDA nursing diagnoses, NIC, and NOC when caring for a client with respiratory alkalosis.

Home Care

Planning and teaching for home care is directed toward the underlying cause of hyperventilation. If anxiety precipitated the episode, discuss anxiety-management strategies with the client. Refer the client and family to a counselor if appropriate. Teach the client to identify a hyperventilation reaction, and how to breathe into a paper bag to manage it at home.

 EXPLORE MediaLink

NCLEX review questions, case studies, care plan activities, MediaLink applications, and other interactive resources for this chapter can be found on the Companion Website at www.prenhall.com/lemone.

Click on Chapter 5 to select the activities for this chapter. For animations, video clips, more NCLEX review questions, and an audio glossary, access the Student CD-ROM accompanying this textbook.

TEST YOURSELF

1. Isotonic intravenous fluids are recommended to restore intravascular fluid volume. Which solution would the nurse identify as an isotonic intravenous solution?

   a. Ringer's solution
   b. 10% dextrose in water
   c. 3% sodium chloride
   d. 0.45% sodium chloride

2. When assessing a client with fluid volume deficit, the nurse would expect to find:

   a. Increased pulse rate and blood pressure
   b. Dyspnea and respiratory crackles
   c. Headache and muscle cramps
   d. Orthostatic hypotension and flat neck veins

3. Laboratory results for a client show a serum potassium level of 2.2 mEq/L. Which of the following nursing actions is of highest priority for this client?

   a. Keep the client on bed rest
   b. Initiate cardiac monitoring
   c. Start oxygen at 2 L/min
   d. Initiate seizure precautions

4. The nurse evaluates teaching about calcium supplement therapy as effective when the client states that she will take her calcium tablets:

   a. All at one time in the morning
   b. With meals
   c. As needed for tremulousness
   d. With a full glass of water

5. Arterial blood gas results for a client show pH 7.21, PaO_2 98 mmHg, $PaCO_2$ 32 mmHg, and HCO_3^- 17 mEq/L. The nurse correctly interprets these values as indicative of which of the following acid-base imbalances?

   a. Metabolic acidosis
   b. Metabolic alkalosis
   c. Respiratory acidosis
   d. Respiratory alkalosis

See Test Yourself answers in Appendix C.

BIBLIOGRAPHY

Ackley, B. J., & Ladwig, G. B. (2002). *Nursing diagnosis handbook: A guide to planning care* (5th ed.). St. Louis: Mosby.

Braunwald, E., Fauci, A. S., Kasper, D. L., Hauser, S. L., Longo, D. L., & Jameson, J. L. (2001). *Harrison's principles of internal medicine* (15th ed.). New York: McGraw-Hill.

Bullock, B. A., & Henze, R. L. (2000). *Focus on pathophysiology.* Philadelphia: Lippincott.

Call-Schmidt, T. (2001). Interpreting lab results: A primer. *MEDSURG Nursing, 10*(4), 179–184.

Castiglione, V. (2000). Emergency. Hyperkalemia. *American Journal of Nursing, 100*(1), 55–56.

Cook, L. (1999). The value of lab values. *American Journal of Nursing, 99*(5), 66–69, 71, 73, 75.

Danner, K. (2000). Acid/base balance: Making sense of pH. *CIN PLUS* (On-line serial), *3*(1), 3.

Deglin, J. H., & Vallerand, A. H. (2001). *Davis's drug guide for nurses* (7th ed.). Philadelphia: F. A. Davis.

Edwards, S. (2001). Regulation of water, sodium and potassium: Implications for practice. *Nursing Standard, 15*(22), 36–44.

Gallo, J. J., Busby-Whitehead, J., Rabins, P. V., Silliman, R. A., & Murphy, J. B. (Eds.). (1999). *Reichel's care of the elderly: Clinical aspects of aging* (5th ed.). Philadelphia: Lippincott Williams & Wilkins.

Heater, D. W. (1999). If ADH goes out of balance: Diabetes insipidus. *RN, 62*(7), 42–46.

_____. (1999). If ADH goes out of balance: SIADH. *RN, 62*(7), 47–49.

Horne, C., & Derrico, D. (1999). Mastering ABGs. *American Journal of Nursing, 99*(8), 26–32.

Iggulden, H. (1999). Dehydration and electrolyte balance. *Nursing Standard, 13*(19), 48–56.

Incredibly easy! Understanding imbalances caused by GI fluid loss. (1999). *Nursing, 29*(8), 72.

Johnson, M., Bulechek, G., Dochterman, J. M., Maas, M., & Moorhead, S. (2001). *Nursing diagnoses, outcomes, & interventions: NANDA, NOC, and NIC linkages.* St. Louis: Mosby.

Kuhn, M. A. (1999). *Complementary therapies for health care providers.* Philadelphia: Lippincott.

Lehne, R. A. (2001). *Pharmacology for nursing care* (4th ed.). Philadelphia: Saunders.

Malarkey, L. M., & McMorrow, M. E. (2000). *Nurse's manual of laboratory tests and diagnostic procedures* (2nd ed.). Philadelphia: Saunders.

Meeker, M. H., & Rothrock, J. C. (1999). *Alexander's care of the patient in surgery* (11th ed.). St. Louis: Mosby.

Metheny, N. M. (2000). *Fluid and electrolyte balance: Nursing considerations* (4th ed.). Philadelphia: Lippincott.

Morrison, C. (2000). Helping patients maintain a healthy fluid balance. *Nursing Times,* (NTplus), *96*(31), 3–4.

Naxarko, L. (2000). How age affects fluid intake. *Nursing Times* (NTplus), *96*(31), 11–12.

North American Nursing Diagnosis Association. (2001). *NANDA nursing diagnoses: Definitions & classification 2001–2002.* Philadelphia: NANDA.

Porth, C. M. (2002). *Pathophysiology: Concepts of altered health states* (6th ed.). Philadelphia: Lippincott.

Powers, F. (1999). The role of chloride in acid-base balance. *Journal of Intravenous Nursing, 22*(5), 286–291.

Roper, M. (1996). Assessing orthostatic vital signs. *American Journal of Nursing, 96*(8), 43–46.

Rosenberger, K. (1998). Pharmacology update. Management of electrolyte abnormalities: Hypocalcemia, hypomagnesemia, and hypokalemia. *Journal of the American Academy of Nurse Practitioners, 10*(5), 209–217.

Sheehy, C. M., Perry, P. A., & Cromwell, S. L. (1999). Dehydration: Biological considerations, age-related changes, and risk factors in older adults. *Biological Research for Nuring, 1*(1), 30–37.

Shepherd, E. (2000). Fluids: A balancing act. *Nursing Times* (NTplus), *96*(31), 1.

Sheppard, M. (2001). Assessing fluid balance. *Nursing Times* (NTplus), *97*(6), XI–XII.

Shoulders-Odom, B. (2000). Using an algorithm to interpret arterial blood gases. *Dimensions of Critical Care Nursing, 19*(1), 36–41.

Springhouse. (1999). *Nurse's handbook of alternative & complementary therapies.* Springhouse, PA: Author.

Tasota, F. J., & Wesmiller, S. W. (1998). Balancing act: Keeping blood pH in equilibrium. *Nursing, 28*(12), 34–41.

Terpstra, T. L., & Terpstra, T. L. (2000). Syndrome of inappropriate antidiuretic hormone secretion: Recognition and management. *MEDSURG Nursing, 9*(2), 61–68.

Tierney, L. M., McPhee, S. J., & Papadakis, M. A. (2001). *Current medical diagnosis & treatment* (40th ed.). New York: Lange Medical Books/McGraw-Hill.

Wallace, L. S. (2000). Using color to simplify ABG interpretation. *MEDSURG Nursing, 9*(4), 205–208.

Whitney, E. N., & Rolfes, S. R. (2002). *Understanding nutrition* (9th ed.). Belmont, CA: Wadsworth.

Wilkinson, J. M. (2000). *Nursing diagnosis handbook with NIC interventions and NOC outcomes* (7th ed.). Upper Saddle River, NJ: Prentice Hall Health.

Wise, L. C., Mersch, J., Racioppi, J., Crosier, J., & Thompson, C. (2000). Evaluating the reliability and utility of cumulative intake and output. *Journal of Nursing Care Quality, 14*(3), 37–42.

Wong, F. W. (1999). A new approach to ABG interpretation. *American Journal of Nursing, 99*(8), 34–36.

CHAPTER | 6

Nursing Care of Clients Experiencing Trauma and Shock

www.prenhall.com/lemone

Additional resources for this chapter can be found on the Student CD-ROM accompanying this textbook, and on the Companion Website at www.prenhall.com/lemone. Click on Chapter 6 to select the activities for this chapter.

CD-ROM
- Audio Glossary
- NCLEX Review

Animation
- Hypovolemic Shock

Companion Website
- More NCLEX Review
- Case Study
    A Client Experiencing Trauma
- MediaLink Applications
    Organ Donation
    Injury Prevention

LEARNING OUTCOMES

After completing this chapter, you will be able to:

- Describe the components and types of trauma.

- Discuss causes, effects, and initial management of trauma.

- Discuss diagnostic tests used in assessing clients experiencing trauma and shock.

- Describe collaborative interventions for clients experiencing trauma and shock, including medications, blood transfusion, and intravenous fluids.

- Discuss organ donation and forensic implications of traumatic injury or death.

- Discuss cellular homeostasis and basic hemodynamics.

- Discuss the risk factors, etiologies, and pathophysiologies of hypovolemic shock, cardiogenic shock, obstructive shock, and distributive shock.

- Use the nursing process as a framework for providing individualized care to clients experiencing trauma and shock.

THE CLIENT EXPERIENCING TRAUMA

Many different accidental or purposeful acts may cause trauma, including motor vehicle and farm machinery accidents, gunshot wounds, falls, violence toward others, or self-inflicted violence. The injuries, disabilities, and deaths resulting from these acts constitute a major health care challenge.

Trauma usually occurs suddenly, leaving the client and family with little time to prepare for its consequences. Nurses provide a vital link in both the physical and psychosocial care for the injured client and family. In caring for the client who has experienced trauma, nurses must consider not only the initial physical injury, but also its long-term consequences, including rehabilitation and the client's return to a previous way of life.

COMPONENTS OF TRAUMA

Trauma results from an abnormal exchange of energy between a host and a mechanism in a predisposing environment. The *host* is the person or group at risk of injury. Multiple factors influence the host's potential for injury: age, sex, race, economic status, preexisting illnesses, and use of substances such as alcohol. Most trauma victims are young and unemployed, involved in substance abuse, likely to be reinjured within 5 years of their first injury, and at greater risk of dying young. Statistics show that trauma primarily afflicts males.

The *mechanism* is the source of the energy transmitted to the host. The energy exchanged can be mechanical, gravitational, thermal, electrical, physical, or chemical. Table 6–1 lists the most common mechanisms for each type of energy. Mechanical energy is the most common type of energy transferred to a host in trauma. The most common mechanical source of injury in all adult age groups is the motor vehicle.

Guns are another common mechanical source of injury. Trauma from gunshot wounds has steadily increased over the past 20 years and has become a major reason for emergency department and trauma center admissions, especially in large cities.

When describing a traumatic injury, *intention* is included as a component. Most gunshot and stab wounds are examples of intentional injuries. It is important to remember, however, that some gunshot wounds are unintentional, such as those that occur when children play with their parents' guns. Other common unintentional injuries result from motor vehicle crashes, falls, drowning, and fires.

The final component of trauma is the *environment.* For example, a road that has become slippery after a snowstorm is a physical environment that may contribute to an injury. Occupation is an important environmental factor to consider. Those in certain occupations face a high risk of trauma; examples include police officers, professional athletes, and racecar drivers. One's social environment also influences risk for injury. (See the box below for one example, domestic violence.)

TABLE 6–1	Common Mechanisms of Injury by Energy Source
Energy Source	**Common Mechanisms of Injury**
Mechanical	Motor vehicles Firearms Machines
Gravitational	Falls
Thermal	Heating appliances Fire Freezing temperatures
Electrical	Wires, sockets, and other electrical objects Lightning
Physical	Fists, feet, and other body parts (as in physical assault) Sharp objects, such as knives Ultraviolet radiation Ionizing radiation Water (drowning) Other submersion agents (e.g., grain) Explosions
Chemical	Drugs Poisons Industrial chemicals

Meeting Individualized Needs

ASSESSING DOMESTIC VIOLENCE

Although domestic violence may involve either men or women, most victims are women. Domestic violence is the leading cause of injury to women, causing more injuries than muggings, stranger rapes, and car accidents combined. More than 4 million women are beaten by male partners every year. Health care is affected by this phenomenon, with women who were abused requiring 100,000 hospital days, 30,000 emergency room visits, and 40,000 trips to health care providers every year. These numbers mean that incorporating domestic violence awareness into nursing assessment is essential. The following guidelines (Speck & Whalley, 1996) are useful:

1. Include questions about domestic violence in a non-threatening way, such as with the question, "When you are arguing or fighting, does anyone ever get pushed or shoved?"
2. Use more specific open-ended questions once violence is disclosed, such as, "Tell me more" or "and then what happened?"
3. Evaluate the danger for the client by asking about the number and severity of past incidents, the use of alcohol and drugs, the presence of weapons in the home, and the desire of the couple to solve disputes in nonviolent ways.
4. Include in the physical assessment evidence of bruises, scars, or deformities, signs of neglect or malnutrition; presence of choke marks, wire marks, or cigarette burns.

MediaLink | INJURY PREVENTION APPLICATION

TYPES OF TRAUMA

Whether intentional or accidental, trauma causes injury to one or more parts of the body. **Minor trauma** causes injury to a single part or system of the body and is usually treated in the hospital or emergency department. A fracture of the clavicle, a small second-degree burn, and a cut requiring stitches are considered minor trauma. Major or multiple trauma involves serious single-system injury (such as the traumatic amputation of a leg) or multiple-system injuries. **Multiple trauma** (which is most often the result of a motor vehicle accident) requires immediate intervention specifically focused on ensuring survival. Clients who suffer multiple trauma receive immediate emergency care and often require long periods of intensive collaborative and nursing care.

Trauma also may be classified as either blunt or penetrating. **Blunt trauma** occurs when there is no communication from the damaged tissues to the outside environment. It is caused by a combination of forces including *deceleration* (a decrease in the speed of a moving object), *acceleration* (an increase in the speed of a moving object), *shearing* (forces occurring across a plane, with structures slipping across each other), *compression,* and *crushing*. Blunt forces often cause multiple injuries. Common blunt forces are motor vehicle accidents, falls, assaults, and sports activities. Blunt trauma often causes alterations in the anatomy and physiology of the head, spinal cord, bones, thorax, and abdomen.

Penetrating trauma occurs as the result of foreign objects set in motion. Penetration of tissues causes damage to body structures, most commonly the intestines, liver, spleen, and vascular system. Examples of penetrating trauma are gunshot or stab wounds and impalement.

Other types of trauma occur from inhalation, thermal changes, and blast forces. Inhalation of gases, smoke, and steam may injure the respiratory system. Thermal injuries are manifested as burns or freezing. Injuries from blasts (explosions) result from the velocity of air movement and the force of projectiles from the explosion. Blast injuries are more severe in water than in air (the blast wave travels farther and faster in water) and enclosed spaces. The trauma from blast injuries includes pulmonary edema and hemorrhage, damage to abdominal organs, burns, penetrating injuries, and ruptured tympanic membranes.

EFFECTS OF TRAUMATIC INJURY

Death is a common result of serious traumatic injury, and may be immediate, early, or late. Immediate death happens at the scene from such injuries as a torn thoracic aorta or decapitation. Early death occurs within several hours of the injury from, for example, shock or delay in recognizing injuries. Late death generally occurs 1 or more days after the injury and results from complications or multiple organ failure.

Because of the serious consequences of trauma, it is important to rapidly identify the client's injuries and institute appropriate interventions quickly. Following are common effects of trauma and health care interventions at the scene of the accident or in the emergency department.

Figure 6–1 ■ Placement of an oral endotracheal tube (ETT) for intubation. When the ETT is in place, air or oxygen can be blown into the external opening of the tube and enter the trachea.

Airway Obstruction

The trauma client's airway may become obstructed by the presence of blood, teeth, the tongue, direct injury, or vomitus. After the client's cervical spine is immobilized (a procedure discussed later in this chapter), oxygen must be supplied. Airway interventions may include clearing the airway by suctioning, using airway adjuncts such as an oropharyngeal airway, or intubating with an oral endotracheal airway (Figure 6–1 ■). Intubation is the preferred method of airway management.

Tension Pneumothorax

A **pneumothorax** results when air enters the pleural space due to blunt and penetrating injuries to the chest. When a one-way valve is created, most often by blunt trauma, air can enter the pleural space but not exit; thus, a **tension pneumothorax** may develop. Immediate needle thoracostomy (insertion of a large-bore needle into the appropriate thoracic space) and chest tube insertion are performed. Most often, the needle is inserted into the second intercostal space at the midclavicular line or a chest tube is placed into the fifth intercostal space at the midaxillary line (Figure 6–2 ■).

Hemorrhage

When the client has suffered an injury that causes external hemorrhage, such as severing of an artery, the bleeding must be controlled immediately. This may be done by applying direct pressure over the wound and applying pressure over arterial pressure points (Figure 6–3 ■).

Internal hemorrhage may result from either blunt or penetrating traumatic injury. Discovering the cause and location of the injury, as well as the extent of related blood loss, are the most important concerns. Several potential spaces in the body

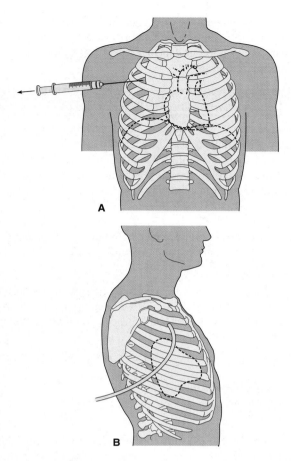

A

B

Figure 6–2 ■ A needle thoracostomy may be used in the emergency treatment of a tension pneumothorax. *A,* A large-gauge needle is introduced, and air and fluid are aspirated. *B,* Alternatively, a chest tube may be inserted and connected to a chest drainage system.

can accommodate large amounts of blood that may accumulate (called *third spacing*) following injury. For example, bleeding into the pleural space may occur with chest trauma, and bleeding into the abdominal cavity may occur with abdominal trauma. A pelvic fracture may cause massive hemorrhage in the retroperitoneal region. Once the source of internal hemorrhage has been recognized, interventions are initiated, including operative control of bleeding and continual assessment of the client. Hemorrhage may result in hypovolemic shock (discussed later in the chapter).

Integumentary Effects

Injuries to the integument generally are not as serious as other injuries, with the exception of burns (see Chapter 15). The primary organ involved in integumentary trauma is the skin; however, underlying structures may also be injured. Injuries may result from either blunt or penetrating sources. It is important to evaluate all injuries to the integument, because they may indicate a more serious injury such as an open fracture. Additionally, large wounds may contribute to significant blood loss.

Four specific injuries to the integument are contusions, abrasions, puncture wounds, and lacerations (Figure 6–4 ■).

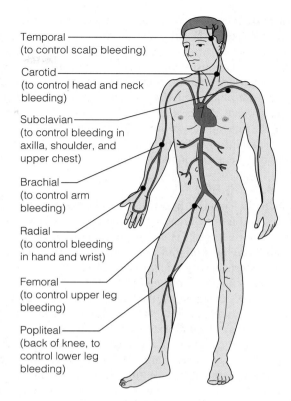

Temporal
(to control scalp bleeding)

Carotid
(to control head and neck bleeding)

Subclavian
(to control bleeding in axilla, shoulder, and upper chest)

Brachial
(to control arm bleeding)

Radial
(to control bleeding in hand and wrist)

Femoral
(to control upper leg bleeding)

Popliteal
(back of knee, to control lower leg bleeding)

Figure 6–3 ■ The major pressure points used for the control of bleeding.

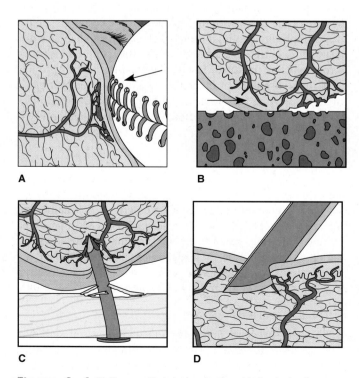

A

B

C

D

Figure 6–4 ■ Traumatic injuries to the skin include: *A,* contusion; *B,* abrasion; *C,* puncture wound; and *D,* laceration.

Contusions, or superficial tissue injuries, result from blunt trauma that causes the breakage of small blood vessels and bleeding into the surrounding tissue. **Abrasions,** or partial-thickness denudations of an area of integument, generally result from falls or scrapes. **Puncture** wounds occur when a sharp or blunt object penetrates the integument. **Lacerations** are open wounds that result from sharp cutting or tearing. Injuries to the integument are at risk for contamination from dirt, debris, or foreign objects. Infection may cause further physical stress to the client with multiple injuries.

Abdominal Effects

The abdomen contains both solid organs (liver, spleen, and pancreas) and hollow organs (stomach and intestines). Direct trauma to the abdomen can lacerate and compress the solid organs and cause burst injuries to the hollow organs. Blood vessels may be torn and organs may be displaced from their blood supply, producing life-threatening hemorrhage. Damage to the mesenteric vessels supplying the bowel can result in bowel ischemia and infarction. Injury to the stomach, pancreas, and small bowel may allow digestive enzymes to leak out into the abdominal cavity. Rupture of the large bowel results in escape of feces which causes peritonitis. Blunt or penetrating trauma to the abdomen may also cause rupture of the diaphragm with herniation of the abdominal organs into the thoracic cavity. The immediate threat following abdominal trauma is hemorrhage; the later threat is peritonitis.

Musculoskeletal Effects

Musculoskeletal injuries may occur alone or with multiple injuries as the result of blunt or penetrating trauma. Musculoskeletal injuries usually are not considered a high priority in the care of the client with multiple injuries. Exceptions are the life- or limb-threatening musculoskeletal injury, such as a dislocated hip, pulseless extremity, or significant blood loss such as from a pelvic fracture. Musculoskeletal injuries may provide clues to the presence of other serious injuries; for example, a fractured clavicle may indicate an associated thoracic injury. Care of the client who has suffered a musculoskeletal injury is discussed in Chapter 38. ∞

Neurologic Effects

Head injuries are a common type of injury sustained as the result of trauma. Injuries to the spinal cord resulting in loss of neurologic function are devastating outcomes of trauma, but they are much less common than head injuries. Most head and spinal cord injuries result from blunt trauma and are sustained in motor vehicle crashes. Falls, sports injuries, and assault are other sources of neurologic injury. Care of the client with a neurologic injury is discussed in Chapters 41 and 42. ∞

Effects on the Family

Trauma usually occurs suddenly and with little warning. It may result in death or cause injury serious enough to alter both the client's and the family's lives. The suddenness and seriousness of the event are precipitating factors in the development of a psychologic crisis. Over the past decade, some emergency departments have instituted care plans that allow families to participate as active members of the resuscitation team. This type of care is not without controversy, but it should be considered when appropriate.

COLLABORATIVE CARE

Collaborative care of the trauma client depends on a team approach. Providing trauma care with a team focus helps each team member know his or her role. Prompt delegation of tasks and responsibilities improves the client's chances for survival and decreases the morbidity that may result from traumatic injuries.

Prehospital Care

The major functions of prehospital care include injury identification, critical interventions, and rapid transport.

Injury Identification

Emergency care of the client experiencing trauma is based on rapid assessment to identify injuries and begin appropriate interventions. Injuries that indicate the need for trauma center care include:

- Penetrating injuries to the abdomen, pelvis, chest, neck, or head.
- Spinal cord injuries with deficit.
- Crushing injuries to the abdomen, chest, or head.
- Major burns.

Many methods help health care providers determine the seriousness of the client's injuries and the potential for survival. Scoring systems such as the Champion Revised Trauma Scoring System can be helpful (Table 6–2). A rapid

TABLE 6–2 Champion Revised Trauma Scoring System		
Test	**Score**	**Coded Value**
Glasgow Coma Scale*	13 to 15	4
	9 to 12	3
	6 to 8	2
	4 to 5	1
	3	0
Systolic blood pressure	> 89	4
	76 to 89	3
	50 to 75	2
	1 to 49	1
	0	0
Respiratory rate	10 to 29	4
	> 29	3
	6 to 9	2
	1 to 5	1
	0	0
	Total score:	_____

The highest possible total score is 12. The lowest possible score is 0. The higher the total score, the greater the chance of survival.

* See Chapter 40 for instructions for using the Glasgow Coma Scale.

Note. From "A Revision of the Trauma Score" by H. Champion et al., 1989, Journal of Trauma, 29(5): 624. Used with permission.

Figure 6–5 ■ Immobilization of the cervical spine at the scene of the accident is essential to preventing further injury to the spinal cord. The combined use of a hard cervical collar, sandbags, and tape best restricts flexion, extension, rotation, and lateral bending of the neck.

Source: Spencer Grant/Photo Researchers, Inc.

but comprehensive trauma assessment, completed on the scene, includes:

- Airway and breathing assessments to determine if the airway is patent, maintainable, or nonmaintainable, and if ventilations are impeded, such as by rib fractures or a collapsed lung.
- Circulation assessment to palpate peripheral and central pulses; to assess capillary refill, skin color, and temperature; and to identify any external sources of bleeding.
- Level of consciousness and pupillary function.
- Any obvious injuries.

Critical Interventions

As life-threatening problems are identified during the primary assessment, appropriate on-the-scene interventions must be performed immediately. These include providing life support, immobilizing the cervical spine, managing the airway, and treating hemorrhage and shock.

Immobilization of the client's cervical spine is a primary intervention. The client is placed on a spine board, and a cervical collar and a head immobilizer are applied (Figure 6–5 ■). The cervical spine may also be immobilized by logrolling the client onto a board, placing towel rolls or a head immobilizer along the sides of the client's head, and securing the client to the board. If the client was wearing a helmet at the time of injury, the helmet should remain on until the client arrives at the hospital, unless the client's airway is at risk. If necessary, health care personnel at the scene will remove the helmet by manipulating it over the client's nose and ears while holding the client's head and neck immobile; safe removal requires at least two people. Improper removal risks injury or additional injury to the spinal cord.

If the client's airway is patent, oxygen is administered. Ventilations may be assisted with a bag-valve-mask resuscitator until airway management is achieved. Active external bleeding is controlled by direct pressure. Measures to reverse shock (discussed later in the chapter) are initiated.

Rapid Transport

Clients who have multiple injuries must be transported as soon as possible to a regional trauma center. The most common modes of rapid transport are ground ambulance and air ambulance, which includes helicopters specially staffed and equipped to care

for trauma victims. Figure 6–6 ■ shows a flight nurse assessing a client. Stable clients within access of a ground ambulance are best transported by ground. Unstable clients and those injured in the wilderness or other areas in which ground access is difficult may best be transported by air. When these transport systems are unavailable, the client is transported by any possible means.

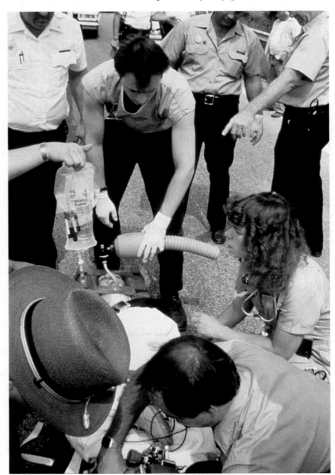

Figure 6–6 ■ Flight nurses provide initial assessment, stabilization, and support for clients with trauma.

Courtesy of University Air Care/University of Cincinnati Hospital.

Emergency Department Care

Diagnostic Tests

The diagnostic tests ordered once the client reaches the hospital depend on the type of injury the client has sustained. Tests that may be ordered for victims of trauma include the following:

- *Blood type and crossmatch* involves typing the client's blood for ABO antigens and Rh factor, screening the blood for antibodies, and crossmatching the client's serum and donor red blood cells.
- *Blood alcohol level* measures the amount of alcohol in a client's blood. It has been found that between 20% and 50% of people who are injured may be intoxicated. Alcohol alters the client's level of consciousness and response to pain.
- *Urine drug screen* may also be ordered. Like alcohol, such drugs as cocaine alter the client's level of consciousness and overall response to the primary survey.
- *Pregnancy test* for any woman of childbearing age rules out the potential for pregnancy and fetal injury.
- *Diagnostic peritoneal lavage* determines the presence of blood in the peritoneal cavity, which may indicate abdominal injury. The test is generally done in the emergency department. A local anesthetic (such as lidocaine) is injected subcutaneously, and a small incision is made in the lower abdomen. A catheter is placed into the peritoneal cavity, and any free blood is aspirated. If 10 mL of blood is found, the client is taken to the operating room for exploratory surgery. If no free blood is aspirated, 1 L of a warm isotonic solution (Ringer's solution or normal saline) is rapidly infused into the peritoneal cavity and then allowed to drain by gravity. If the solution returns pink and is found to have a red blood cell count of 100,000 mm^3, a white blood cell count of > 500, or bile, food, or feces, the test is considered positive and the client is taken to the operating room for exploratory surgery.
- *Computerized tomography (CT) scans* can discover injuries to the brain, skull, spine, spinal cord, chest, and abdomen.
- *Magnetic resonance imaging (MRI) scans* can discover injuries to the brain and spinal cord.

Medications

Medications used to treat the client who has experienced trauma depend on the type and severity of the injuries, as well as the degree of traumatic shock that is present. The following general categories of medications may be used. (Fluid administration and the drugs listed are covered later in the chapter in discussion of the collaborative care of the client in shock.)

- Blood components and crystalloids are administered intravenously in the initial treatment of traumatic shock to replace intravascular volume.
- Inotropic drugs (drugs that increase myocardial contractility) are given to increase cardiac output and improve tissue perfusion. These drugs, administered only after fluid volume restoration, include dopamine (Dopastat, Intropin), dobutamine (Dobutrex), and isoproterenol (Isuprel).
- Vasopressors may be administered in conjunction with fluid replacement to treat neurogenic, septic, or anaphylactic shock. Examples of vasopressors include dopamine, epinephrine, norepinephrine, and phenylephrine.
- Opioids, administered by bolus or continuous infusion, are used to treat pain as soon as possible. However, the effects of the pain medications may alter client responses to injury and mask potential injuries. If pain medications are administered, they must be carefully regulated, and the client must be closely monitored. If the client has penetrating and open wounds, tetanus immunization status must be determined. If the client is unable to remember when the last tetanus immunization was given or is unable to answer, tetanus prophylaxis is given.

Blood Transfusions

Blood and blood components are initially produced in the body and then donated for use by another person through a **transfusion** (an infusion of blood or blood components). A client may be given whole blood, packed red blood cells (RBCs), platelets, plasma, albumin, clotting factors, prothrombin, or cryoprecipitate (Table 6–3). Blood and blood components increase the amount of hemoglobin available to carry oxygen to the cells, improve hemoglobin and hematocrit levels during active bleeding, increase intravascular volume, and replace deficient substances such as platelets and clotting factors.

Each person has one of four blood types: A, B, AB, or O. The blood group antigens A and B, present on RBC membranes, form the basis for the ABO blood categorization. The presence or absence of these inherited antigens determines one's blood type. People with blood type A have A antigens, those with type B have B antigens, those with type AB have both antigens, and those with neither antigen have blood type O (called a universal donor).

ABO antibodies develop in the serum of people whose RBCs lack the corresponding antigen; these antibodies are called anti-A and anti-B. The person with blood type B has A antibodies, the person with type A has B antibodies, the person with type O has both types of antibodies, and the person with blood type AB has no antibodies (called a universal recipient).

A third antigen on the RBC membrane is D. People who are Rh positive have the D antigen, whereas people who are Rh negative do not. These antigens and antibodies may cause ABO and Rh incompatibilities.

A transfusion of incompatible blood causes hemolysis (breakdown) of the RBCs and agglutination of erythrocytes. (Agglutination is the clumping of cells that results from their interaction with specific antibodies.) The ABO blood group names and compatibilities are listed in Table 6–4.

Before RBCs or whole blood can be administered, a series of procedures determine donor and recipient ABO types and Rh groups. These procedures, called a type and crossmatch, are performed by mixing the donor cells with the recipient's serum and watching for agglutination. If none occurs, the blood is considered compatible.

Despite meticulous procedures for matching blood types and antigens, blood transfusion reactions may still occur. The most common is a *febrile reaction*. Antibodies within the client

TABLE 6–3	Types of Blood Components Used in Transfusion Therapy	
Type	**Use**	**Limitations**
Whole blood	Replaces blood volume and oxygen-carrying capacity in hemorrhage and shock. Contains RBCs, plasma proteins, clotting factors, and plasma.	Contains few platelets or granulocytes; deficient in clotting factors V and VII. Greatest risks are for incompatibility or circulatory overload.
Red cells	Increase oxygen-carrying capacity in slow bleeding or in clients with anemia, with leukemia, or having surgery.	Has no viable platelets or granulocytes. Incompatibility may cause hemolytic reactions.
Platelets	Used to control or prevent bleeding in clients with platelet deficiencies.	If given for an extended period of time, antibodies may develop. Hypersensitivity reactions may occur.
Plasma	Expands blood volume; can be administered to any blood group or type. Contains all clotting factors and is used to restore those deficient in bleeding disorders.	May cause vascular overload, hypersensitivity reactions, or hemolytic reactions.
Albumin	Expands blood volume in shock and trauma. Used to treat clients in shock from trauma or infection and in surgery to replace blood volume and proteins.	Is not a substitute for whole blood. May cause hypersensitivity reactions.
Clotting factors	Factor VIII concentrate is used to treat clients with hemophilia A and von Willebrand's disease. Factor IX concentrate is used to treat clients with hemophilia B and other clotting factor deficiencies.	
Prothrombin complex	Contains prothrombin, clotting factors VII, IX, X, and part of XI. Used to treat clients with deficiencies of these factors.	
Cryoprecipitate	Contains factor VIII, factor XIII, von Willebrand's factor, and fibrinogen. Used to treat clients with clotting factor deficiencies.	May cause ABO incompatibilities.

receiving the blood are directed against the donor's white blood cells, causing fever and chills. Febrile reactions typically begin during the first 15 minutes of the transfusion. Using leukocyte-poor blood avoids future febrile reactions.

Hypersensitivity reactions result when antibodies in the client's blood react against proteins, such as immunoglobulin A, in the donor blood. Hypersensitivity reactions may appear during or after the transfusion. The manifestations of hypersensitivity reaction include *urticaria* (the appearance of reddened wheals of various sizes on the skin) and itching.

Hemolytic reactions, the most dangerous transfusion reactions, usually result from an ABO incompatibility. Clumping RBCs block capillaries, decreasing blood flow to vital organs. In addition, macrophages engulf the clumped RBCs, releasing free hemoglobin into the circulating blood; the hemoglobin is

then filtered by the kidneys and may block the renal tubules, causing renal failure. Hemolytic reactions usually begin after infusion of 100 to 200 mL of the incompatible blood. Manifestations of a hemolytic reaction include flushing of the face, a burning sensation along the vein, headache, urticaria, chills, fever, lumbar pain, abdominal pain, chest pain, nausea and vomiting, tachycardia, hypotension, and dyspnea. If any of these manifestations appear, the blood transfusion must be immediately discontinued.

Other risks to clients receiving blood include circulatory overload, electrolyte imbalances, and infectious diseases such as hepatitis or cytomegalovirus.

Clients who have experienced trauma of any severity have had substantial blood loss and are usually in hypovolemic shock. Blood replacement is the treatment of choice to restore

TABLE 6–4	Blood Group Types and Compatibilities			
Blood Group	**RBC Agglutinogens**	**Serum Agglutinogens**	**Compatible Donor Blood Groups**	**Incompatible Donor Blood Groups**
A	A	Anti-B	A, O	B, AB
B	B	Anti-A	B, O	A, AB
AB	A, B	None	A, B, AB, O	None
O	None	Anti-A, Anti-B	O	A, B, AB

Note: Group O is often called the universal donor, and group AB is called the universal recipient.

Medication Administration

Blood Transfusion

The risk for and seriousness of blood transfusion reactions require that extreme caution be taken when blood is administered. Most fatal transfusion reactions are the result of human error. Although general guidelines are provided here, each institution has specific policies and procedures that must be followed. Prior to beginning the transfusion, the nurse must determine that typed and cross-matched blood is available and collect the needed equipment a Y-tubing blood administration set with a filter, a large-bore intravenous catheter, Usually 18 or 19 gauge, and normal saline solution. Only normal saline is used with a blood transfusion. Dextrose causes clumping of RBCs, and distilled water causes hemolysis.

Nursing Responsibilities

- Assess for any previous reactions to blood.
- Explain the procedure to the client, and answer any questions.
- Prepare the intravenous equipment. Shut off one side of the Y tubing, and attach the other side to the saline solution. Flush the tubing and filter with the saline.
- If venous access is not already in place, insert the intravenous needle (following body substance precautions), and begin administering the saline.
- Using institutional procedure, obtain the blood from the blood bank or laboratory. Administer the blood immediately; if this is not possible, return it to the blood bank or laboratory.
- Check and document that the donor and recipient blood have been tested and are compatible. This usually involves two nurses, each verifying that:
  a. An order for blood has been written.
  b. Type and crossmatch have been done.
  c. The name of the client and the name on the blood bag are identical.
  d. The number assigned to the unit of blood is identical to the one on the requisition for the blood.
  e. Blood type and Rh factor are compatible.
  f. The blood has not exceeded its expiration date.
  g. The unit of blood is intact and has no bubbles or discoloration.
- Identify the client by reading the arm band and asking the client to tell you his or her name. Check the arm band against the unit of blood.
- Gently invert the blood bag several times to mix the plasma and RBCs.
- Take and record vital signs as a baseline.
- Attach the open side of the Y tubing to the blood unit, and begin the transfusion at a slow rate of about 2 mL per minute. (Some trauma clients may have blood infused at a rapid rate. If blood is infused rapidly, it may need to be warmed prior to administration to prevent hypothermia.) Stay with the client for at least the first 15 minutes of the transfusion, monitoring for manifestations of a reaction and taking the client's vital signs.
- Continue to monitor the client during the transfusion, assessing for manifestations of hypersensitivity or hemolytic reactions and taking and recording vital signs as directed by institutional policy.
- After the first 15 minutes, the rate of infusion is increased. If there is no danger of fluid volume overload, most clients can tolerate an infusion of a unit of blood (ranging from 250 to 500 mL, depending on the blood component administered) in 2 hours. The unit of blood should be administered in 3 to 4 hours; after this time, it has warmed and begins to deteriorate.

oxygen-carrying capacity. Clients in severe shock with active bleeding are given universal, type O red blood cells immediately. Clients with less severe injuries or bleeding may be stabilized with other types of fluids until type-specific or cross-matched blood is available.

Some emergency departments and trauma centers use autotransfusion to provide blood for transfusions for the client with multiple injuries and/or severe shock. Autotransfusion is a method of blood administration in which special equipment collects and returns the client's own blood. The chest cavity is the typical source of blood to be autotransfused.

Nursing considerations for blood transfusion therapy are described in the Medication Administration box above.

Emergency Surgery

Immediate surgical intervention is indicated when the client remains in shock despite resuscitation and there is no obvious external sign of blood loss. Abdominal and chest X-ray studies and a diagnostic peritoneal lavage or CT scan may be performed to help identify the potential source of the blood loss. It is important that the emergency or trauma nurse speak with the family as soon as possible and keep them informed about what is happening to their family member. Unfortunately, the need for emergency surgery may not allow time for family members or significant others to see their loved one before transfer to the operating room.

Organ Donation

The **Uniform Anatomical Gift Act** (1968, 1987) requires that people be informed about their options for organ donation. Under this act, consent for organ donation may be given not only by the donor but also by a spouse, adult children, parents, adult siblings, guardian, or any adult authorized to do so. The act also encourages people to carry donor cards.

The increased success of organ transplant has made it a more common and valuable method of prolonging and improving life; however, many people are still waiting for organs, and many people who may be suitable organ donors die each year from trauma. Organs and tissues that may be transplanted include bones, eyes, liver, lungs, skin, muscles and tendons, pancreas, kidneys, heart, and heart valves.

The organ donation process begins with identification of the potential organ donor. Most people are potential organ donors. Exceptions include those who:

- Currently abuse intravenous drugs.
- Have preexisting untreated infections, such as septicemia.

MediaLink | ORGAN DONATION APPLICATION

Medication Administration

Blood Transfusion (continued)

- Take the following actions if manifestations of a reaction occur:
  a. Stop the infusion of blood immediately, and notify the physician. Continue to infuse the saline.
  b. Take vital signs and assess manifestations.
  c. Compare the blood slip with the unit of blood to ensure that an identification error was not made.
  d. Save the blood bag and any remaining blood for return to the laboratory for further tests to determine the cause of the reaction.
  e. Follow institutional policy for collecting urine and venous blood samples.
  f. Continue to monitor the client and provide prescribed interventions to treat hypersensitivity or hemolytic manifestations.
- Do not add medications to blood infusions or tubing.
- When the blood is totally infused, use the saline to flush the tubing to ensure complete administration of the blood.
- Return the empty blood bag to the blood bank or laboratory.

Client and Family Teaching
- The possible risks of blood transfusions include infectious diseases and acquired immune deficiency syndrome (AIDS). However, because of careful handling and storage of blood, bacterial contamination is rare. Although hepatitis may be transmitted by contaminated blood, new tests for hepatitis antibodies in the donor blood are reducing this risk. Many people are afraid of contracting AIDS from blood; however, donor screening and HIV-antibody testing of donor blood has virtually eliminated the transmission of HIV by blood transfusion.
- During the transfusion, immediately report any warm feelings, chills, itching, feelings of weakness or fainting, or difficulty breathing.
- Report any signs of a delayed transfusion reaction: chills, fever, cough, difficulty breathing, hives, itching, or changes in circulation. Report difficulty with breathing, and seek medical care immediately.

Y-tubing blood administration set with filter. Spikes, Upper clamps, Drip chamber, Blood filter chamber, Main flow rate clamp, Slide clamp, Y-Injection site, Adapter

- Are HIV positive.
- Have any malignancy other than a primary brain tumor.
- Have active tuberculosis.

The family needs to be made aware of the client's prognosis and presented with the option of donating the client's organs. Both the family's and the client's feelings about organ donation must be explored. Even if the client carries an organ donation card, many institutions will not remove any organs without a signature from a family member or other authorized person. The nurse must always respect the family's concerns and feelings in this process. Some members of certain cultural groups may have religious constraints or issues of mistrust that may interfere with the donation process.

Before any organs can be removed, the client must be declared brain dead. Box 6–1 lists **brain death criteria**. Once

BOX 6–1 ■ Brain Death Criteria

CLINICAL SIGNS
- Irreversible condition
- Apnea with a $PaCO_2$ greater than 60 mmHg
- No response to deep stimuli
- No spontaneous movement (some spinal cord reflexes may be present)
- No gag or corneal reflex
- No oculocephalic or oculovestibular reflex
- Absence of toxic or metabolic disorders

CONFIRMATORY TESTS
- Cerebral blood flow study
- Electroencephalogram

brain death has been confirmed, the family must also understand the diagnosis and be allowed time to accept the client's death.

When caring for an adult client who is brain dead and an organ donor, the nurse carries out the following:

- Maintain systolic blood pressure of 90 mmHg to keep the client's organs perfused until removal.
- Maintain urine output at more than 30 mL per hour. This is usually accomplished by administering fluids and/or in-otropic agents such as dopamine.
- Maintain oxygen saturation at 90% or greater.

Forensic Considerations

Injuries often happen under circumstances that require legal investigation. Many injuries, particularly penetrating trauma, may involve criminal activity. Therefore, the nurse must recognize the need to identify, store, and properly transfer potential evidence for medical-legal investigations.

Each item of clothing removed from the client must be placed in a breathable container, such as a paper bag, and documented appropriately. Bullets or knives should be labeled, with their source specified, and given to the proper authorities.

The client's hands may yield important evidence, such as powder burns on the skin or tissue or hair samples beneath the fingernails. In the case of death, it is recommended that paper bags be placed over the client's hands if the presence of evidence is suspected; otherwise, the evidence should be collected by nail clippings.

Look for entrance and exit wounds and document these findings with pictures, diagrams, or written descriptions. Once the evidence has been collected, identified, and properly stored, ensure that it is given to the appropriate authorities. A chain of custody needs to be maintained throughout the entire process. All evidence must be identified and labeled, and documentation procedures must chronicle where and in whose possession the evidence has been. For the chain of custody to remain intact, the evidence must remain in the continuous possession of identified people and be marked and sealed in tamper-proof containers.

NURSING CARE

Nursing care of the client who has been injured begins with a primary assessment and the initiation of collaborative interventions for any life-threatening injuries. Nursing care is directed toward the client's specific responses to trauma.

Health Promotion

Prevention efforts can reduce the incidence and severity of trauma. Areas of health promotion and trauma prevention interventions for individuals and communities include the following (Bucher & Melander, 1999):

- Motor vehicle safety: seatbelts, airbags, helmets, driving under the influence of alcohol or drugs, reckless driving, visual or cognitive deficits in the older adult
- Home safety: snow and ice removal, electrical wiring, falls, burns, drowning
- Farm safety: operating heavy equipment
- Work safety: operating work equipment, wearing safety equipment
- Relationships: domestic violence, child abuse, elder abuse, or neglect
- Communities: gun control, gangs, condition of streets, neighborhood safety

(In providing information about trauma prevention to members of the community, the nurse serves as a health care educator, political activist, and safety advocate.)

Assessment

Assessment of the client experiencing trauma was discussed with collaborative care.

Nursing Diagnoses and Interventions

The trauma client has many complex and interrelated actual or potential alterations in health. The nursing care in this section focuses on client and family problems with respirations, infection, immobility, and spirituality. Nursing interventions for decreased cardiac output and altered perfusion are discussed in the section of the chapter on nursing care of the client in shock.

Ineffective Airway Clearance

The client with multiple injuries is at great risk for developing airway obstruction and apnea. Facial injuries, loose teeth, blood, and vomitus increase the risk for aspiration and obstruction. Neurologic injuries and cerebral edema alter the client's respiratory drive and ability to keep the airway clear.

- Assess if airway is patent, maintainable, or nonmaintainable. Assess for manifestations of airway obstruction: stridor, tachypnea, bradypnea, cough, cyanosis, dyspnea, decreased or absent breath sounds, changes in oxygen levels, and changes in level of consciousness. *Assessing the airway and initiating interventions are the first steps in managing the client with multiple injuries.*
- Monitor oxygen saturation by applying a pulse oximeter. Adjust oxygen flow to maintain oxygen saturation from 94% to 100%. *Changes in oxygen saturation as measured by the pulse oximeter indicate the effectiveness of the client's airway.*
- Monitor level of consciousness. *An early sign of an ineffective airway is change in the client's behavior. If the client becomes restless, anxious, combative, or unresponsive, the effectiveness of the airway needs to be immediately evaluated and appropriate interventions initiated.*

Risk for Infection

Traumatic injuries are considered dirty wounds. Projectiles enter the body through dirty surfaces and clothing, carrying dirt and debris into the wound. Open fractures provide a portal for the entry of bacteria and dirt. Even with surgical intervention, the wounds often remain contaminated.

- Use careful handwashing practices. *Handwashing remains the single most important factor in preventing the spread of infection.*
- Use strict standard precautions and aseptic technique when caring for wounds. *Standard precautions are essential to protect the client and the nurse from infection.* In addition:

- Monitor wounds for odor, redness, heat, swelling, and copious or purulent drainage.
- Monitor hidden wounds, such as those under casts, by asking the client whether the pain has increased and observing for increased drainage and heat over the area of the wound.
- Ensure that cross-contamination between wounds does not occur. Collect drainage in ostomy bags if it is copious. *The skin is the first line of defense against infection. Wounds provide a portal of entry for organisms. Risk factors for wound infection include contamination, inadequate wound care, and the condition of the wound at the time of closure. Aseptic techniques used in applying and changing dressings reduce the entry of organisms.*
- Take and record vital signs, including temperature, every 2 to 4 hours. *Vital signs, particularly an elevated body temperature, indicate the presence of an infection.*
- Provide adequate fluids and nutrition. *Adequate fluids, calories, and protein are essential to wound healing.*
- Assess for manifestations of gas gangrene: fever, pain, and swelling in traumatized tissues; drainage with a foul odor. *Gas gangrene is usually caused by the organism* Clostridium perfringens. *This bacterium is found in the soil and can be introduced into the body during a traumatic injury. The organism grows in the tissues, causing necrosis; hydrogen and carbon dioxide are released, with resultant swelling of tissues. If the infection continues, tissues are progressively destroyed, and sepsis and death may result.*
- Assess status of tetanus immunization and administer tetanus toxoid or human toxin-antitoxin (TAT) as prescribed. *Tetanus is caused by an exotoxin produced by* Clostridium tetani, *usually introduced through an open wound. The organism is commonly found in the soil.*
- Use strict aseptic technique when inserting catheters, suctioning, administering parenteral medications, or performing any other invasive procedure. *Using aseptic technique during invasive procedures reduces the risk of entry of organisms.*

Impaired Physical Mobility

The client with trauma injuries is often unable to change positions independently and is at risk for complications of the integumentary, cardiovascular, gastrointestinal, respiratory, musculoskeletal, and renal systems. Clients at greatest risk are those who have had multiple injuries, spinal cord injuries, peripheral nerve injuries, and traumatic amputations. Collaborate with the physical therapist and occupational therapist (if available) to determine the most effective types and schedule of exercises and assistive devices.

- If active bleeding or edema is not present, provide active or passive exercises to affected and unaffected extremities at least once every 8 hours. *Exercise improves muscle tone, maintains joint mobility, improves circulation, and prevents contractures.*
- Help the client turn, cough, and deep breathe and use the incentive spirometer at least every 2 hours. *Changing positions, coughing, deep breathing and incentive spirometry reduce the risk of integumentary and respiratory complications.*

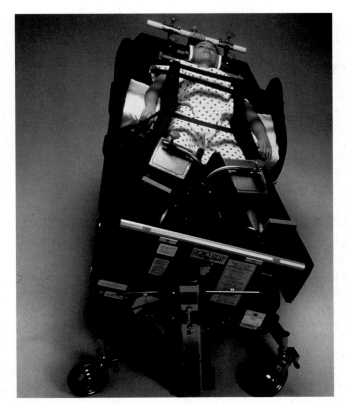

Figure 6–7 ■ A kinetic continuous rotation bed provides a means of turning the client with multiple injuries to decrease the hazards of immobility.

Courtesy of Kinetic Concepts, Inc.

- If the client is unable to be moved and positioned, consider a specialty bed, such as the kinetic continuous rotation bed (Figure 6–7 ■). *The kinetic continuous rotation bed allows continuous turning of the client; the motion decreases pulmonary complications, venous stasis, postural hypotension, urinary stasis, muscle wasting, and bone demineralization.*
- Monitor the lower extremities each day for manifestations of deep vein thrombosis: heat, swelling, and pain. Measure and record the circumference of the thigh and calf each day. If antiemboli stockings are used, remove them for 1 hour during each shift and assess the skin. *Venous stasis results when surrounding muscles are unable to contract and help move the blood through the veins. Thrombus (clot) formation in deep veins is a major risk for pulmonary embolism.*

Spiritual Distress

Trauma generally strikes without warning and carries potentially devastating consequences, including severe alterations in the lives of the victim and family, and death. The traumatic death of a loved one may be the most difficult event a family may ever experience. The decision to cease life support systems or to donate organs challenges the family's belief systems and psychologic stability. Nursing care of the family (or client) experiencing spiritual distress includes the following:

- Give the family information about the option to donate the client's organs. *The decision to donate organs needs to be based on information about the client's condition, prognosis, and criteria by which brain death is determined. It is important to convey to family members that organ donation is only an option and that they should not feel they are obligated to consent or are doing something wrong if they do not consent.*

- Encourage the family to ask questions and express their feelings about the traumatic event and/or organ donation. *Allowing families to express their feelings may help prevent long-term consequences such as guilt.*
- Refer the family for follow-up care. Long-term follow-up is important for the family facing the sudden death of a loved one. *Grieving is not an overnight process, and providing the family with resources that may be used in the future may help prevent future crises and dysfunction.* (For more information, see Chapter 11.) ⬭

Risk for Posttrauma Syndrome

Posttrauma syndrome is an intense, sustained emotional response to a disastrous event. It is characterized by emotions that range from anger to fear and by flashbacks or psychic numbing. In the initial stage, the client may be calm or may express feelings of anger, disbelief, terror, and shock. In the long-term phase, which begins anywhere from a few days to several months after the event, the client often experiences flashbacks and nightmares of the traumatic event. The client may call on ineffective coping mechanisms, such as alcohol or drugs, and withdraw from relationships.

- Assess emotional responses while providing physical care. Observe for crying, sleep problems, suspiciousness, and fear during the initial phase of treatment. If the client is unconscious, encourage family members and friends to express their feelings. *These assessments provide valuable information about the client's ability to cope with the trauma.*

- Be available if the client wishes to talk about the trauma, and encourage expression of feelings. *The client may initially deny negative feelings; this denial is a coping mechanism in the initial phase of recovery.*
- Teach relaxation techniques, such as deep breathing, progressive muscle relaxation, or imagery (see Chapter 4). ⬭ *These techniques are often useful in coping when thoughts of the trauma recur.*
- Refer the client and family members for counseling, psychotherapy, or support groups as appropriate. *Continued therapy may be necessary in assisting the client and family to resolve the acute and long-term effects of trauma.*

Using NANDA, NIC, and NOC

Chart 6–1 shows links between NANDA nursing diagnoses, NIC, and NOC when caring for the patient with multiple injuries.

Home Care

Address the following topics to prepare the client and family for home care.

- The type of home environment to which the client will be returning, including any changes that will be required to let the client function in that environment
- Medications, dressings, wound care, equipment, and supplies
- Special diet, if needed
- Rehabilitation plan and its effect on the client's family
- Follow-up appointments with the physician or at the trauma clinic
- Emotional changes that the client may undergo as a result of the trauma
- Helpful resources:
  - Home health care
  - Community support groups
  - National Institute of Neurological Disorders and Stroke

CHART 6–1 NANDA, NIC, AND NOC LINKAGES

The Client Experiencing Trauma

NURSING DIAGNOSES	NURSING INTERVENTIONS	NURSING OUTCOMES
• Risk for Falls • Risk for Injury	• Fall Prevention • Surveillance: Safety	• Safety Behavior: Fall Prevention • Safety Behavior: Personal • Risk Control
• Posttrauma Syndrome	• Counseling	• Coping • Grief Resolution
• Risk for Trauma	• Environmental Management: Safety • Vehicle Safety Promotion	• Safety Status: Physical Injury
• Impaired Tissue Integrity	• Bleeding Reduction • Blood Products Administration • Fluid Management • Hemorrhage Control • Infection Protection	• Tissue Integrity: Skin and Mucous Membranes • Wound Healing • Fluid Balance • Circulation Status • Infection Control

Note. Data from Nursing Outcomes Classification (NOC) by M. Johnson & M. Maas (Eds.), 1997, St. Louis: Mosby; Nursing Diagnoses: Definitions & Classification 2001–2002 by North American Nursing Diagnosis Association, 2001, Philadelphia: NANDA; Nursing Interventions Classification (NIC) by J.C. McCloskey & G. M. Bulechek (Eds.), 2000, St. Louis: Mosby. Reprinted by permission.

Nursing Care Plan
A Client with Multiple Injuries

Jane Souza is a 25-year-old married woman with two children who provides day care for preschool children in her home. As she is driving the interstate at 65 miles per hour, a car crosses the median and strikes her vehicle head-on. Jane, who is not wearing a seat belt, is thrown forward against the steering wheel. The front of her car is pushed up against her by the car that struck her, entrapping her lower extremities.

After extensive efforts to extricate her from the car, Jane is transported to the local trauma center. She is still conscious, is receiving high-flow oxygen by mask, and has one intravenous line in place. Her vital signs are a palpable systolic blood pressure of 80, a pulse rate of 120, and a respiratory rate of 36. On arrival, she states that she is having difficulty breathing.

ASSESSMENT
- Airway: Maintainable with high-flow oxygen in place.
- Breathing: Respiratory rate of 36, multiple bruising and abrasions on right side of her chest, decreased breath sounds on the right side.
- Circulation: No palpable radial pulses; palpable brachial pulses. Monitor shows sinus tachycardia. No active external bleeding noted. Skin color pale, cool to the touch, and diaphoretic.
- Neurologic: Moved her fingers when asked; complains of difficulty breathing; denies that she is hurt. Pupils 4 mm, equal, and react to light. Has a broken right arm and an open fracture of the left ankle; because of these injuries, extremity movement is limited.

Because of Jane's respiratory distress, she is intubated and ventilated with 100% oxygen. Another intravenous line is inserted and O-negative blood administered.

DIAGNOSES
- *Ineffective breathing pattern* related to multiple bruises and abrasions on the right side of the chest, and respiratory difficulty
- *Deficient fluid volume* related to acute internal blood loss (presumed because no active bleeding can be found)

- *Risk for injury* related to trauma resuscitation

EXPECTED OUTCOMES
- Maintain adequate oxygenation.
- Maintain adequate circulating blood volume.

PLANNING AND IMPLEMENTATION
- Monitor airway and assist in any needed airway management.
- Explain all procedures.
- Monitor the effects of fluid and blood administration, including any changes in blood pressure and pulse.
- Prepare for transfer to the operating room for emergency surgery.
- Keep family informed about her condition.

EVALUATION
Jane is transferred to the operating room, where it is determined that she has a ruptured spleen and a serious pelvic fracture. Jane's treatment continues in the operating room.

Critical Thinking in the Nursing Process
1. Is the nursing diagnosis deficient fluid volume appropriate for Jane Souza? Why or why not?
2. The assessment of a client who has experienced trauma is, in order: A = airway, B = breathing, and C = circulation. What is the rationale for this sequence?
3. Following surgery, Jane is moved to the surgical intensive care unit. She is very anxious and restless. What assessments would you make to identify the cause of her restlessness?
4. Infection is a common complication for the trauma client. Describe five risks for infection that are present from the time of injury to the time of hospital discharge.

See Evaluating Your Response in Appendix C.

THE CLIENT EXPERIENCING SHOCK

Shock is a clinical syndrome characterized by a systemic imbalance between oxygen supply and demand. This imbalance results in a state of inadequate blood flow to body organs and tissues, causing life-threatening cellular dysfunction.

OVERVIEW OF CELLULAR HOMEOSTASIS AND HEMODYNAMICS

To maintain cellular metabolism, cells of all body organs and tissues require a regular and consistent supply of oxygen and the removal of metabolic wastes. This homeostatic regulation is maintained primarily by the cardiovascular system and depends on four physiologic components.

1. A cardiac output sufficient to meet bodily requirements

2. An uncompromised vascular system, in which the vessels have a diameter sufficient to allow unimpeded blood flow and have good tone (the ability to constrict or dilate to maintain normal pressure)
3. A volume of blood sufficient to fill the circulatory system, and a blood pressure adequate to maintain blood flow
4. Tissues that are able to extract and use the oxygen delivered through the capillaries

In a healthy person, these components function as a system to maintain tissue perfusion. During shock, however, one or more of these components are disrupted. An understanding of basic hemodynamics is necessary to understand the pathophysiology of shock.

- **Stroke volume (SV)** is the amount of blood pumped into the aorta with each contraction of the left ventricle.
- **Cardiac output (CO)** is the amount of blood pumped per minute into the aorta by the left ventricle. CO is determined

by multiplying the stroke volume (SV) by the heart rate (HR): CO = SV × HR.

- **Mean arterial pressure (MAP)** is the product of cardiac output and systemic vascular resistance (SVR): MAP = CO × SVR. When CO, SVR, or total blood volume rises, MAP and tissue perfusion increase. Conversely, when CO, SVR, or total blood volume falls, MAP and tissue perfusion decrease.
- The sympathetic nervous system maintains the smooth muscle surrounding the arteries and arterioles in a state of partial contraction called sympathetic tone. Increased sympathetic stimulation increases vasoconstriction and SVR; decreased sympathetic stimulation allows vasodilatation, which decreases SVR.

PATHOPHYSIOLOGY

When one or more cardiovascular components do not function properly, the body's hemodynamic properties are altered. Consequently, tissue perfusion may be inadequate to sustain normal cellular metabolism. The result is the clinical syndrome known as shock. The manifestations of shock result from the body's attempts to maintain vital organs (heart and brain) and to preserve life following a drop in cellular perfusion. However, if the injury or condition triggering shock is severe enough or of long enough duration, then cellular hypoxia and cellular death occur.

Shock is triggered by a sustained drop in mean arterial pressure. This drop can occur after a decrease in cardiac output, a decrease in the circulating blood volume, or an increase in the size of the vascular bed due to peripheral vasodilatation. If intervention is timely and effective, the physiologic events that characterize shock may be stopped; if not, shock may lead to death.

Stage I: Early, Reversible, and Compensatory Shock

The initial stage of shock begins when baroreceptors in the aortic arch and the carotid sinus detect a sustained drop in MAP of less than 10 mmHg from normal levels. The circulating blood volume may decrease (usually to less then 500 mL), but not enough to cause serious effects.

The body reacts to the decrease in arterial pressure as it would to any physical stressor. The cerebral integration center initiates the body's response systems, causing the sympathetic nervous system to increase the heart rate and the force of cardiac contraction, thus increasing cardiac output. Sympathetic stimulation also causes peripheral vasoconstriction, resulting in increased systemic vascular resistance and a rise in arterial pressure. The net result is that the perfusion of cells, tissues, and organs is maintained.

Symptoms are almost imperceptible during the early stage of shock. The pulse rate may be slightly elevated. If the injury is minor or of short duration, arterial pressure is usually maintained, and no further symptoms occur.

Compensatory shock begins after the MAP falls 10 to 15 mmHg below normal levels. The circulating blood volume is reduced by 25% to 35% (1000 mL or more), but compensatory mechanisms are able to maintain blood pressure and tissue perfusion to vital organs, thereby preventing cell damage.

- Stimulation of the sympathetic nervous system results in the release of epinephrine from the adrenal medulla and the release of norepinephrine from the adrenal medulla and the sympathetic fibers. Both hormones rapidly stimulate the alpha- and beta-adrenergic fibers. Stimulated alpha-adrenergic fibers cause vasoconstriction in the blood vessels supplying the skin and most of the abdominal viscera. Perfusion of these areas decreases. Stimulated beta-adrenergic fibers cause vasodilatation in vessels supplying the heart and skeletal muscles (beta one response), and increase the heart rate and force of cardiac contraction (beta two response). Further, blood vessels in the respiratory system dilate, and the respiratory rate increases (beta two response). Thus, stimulation of the sympathetic nervous system results in increased cardiac output and oxygenation of these tissues.
- The renin-angiotensin response occurs as the blood flow to the kidneys decreases. Renin released from the kidneys converts a plasma protein to angiotensin II, which causes vasoconstriction and stimulates the adrenal cortex to release aldosterone. Aldosterone causes the kidneys to reabsorb water and sodium and to lose potassium. The absorption of water maintains circulating blood volume while increased vasoconstriction increases SVR, maintaining central vascular volume and raising blood pressure.
- The hypothalamus releases adrenocorticotropic hormone (ACTH), causing the adrenal glands to secrete aldosterone. Aldosterone promotes the reabsorption of water and sodium by the kidneys, preserving blood volume and pressure.
- The posterior pituitary gland releases antidiuretic hormone (ADH), which increases renal reabsorption of water to increase intravascular volume. The combined effects of hormones released by the hypothalamus and posterior pituitary glands work to conserve central vascular volume.
- As MAP falls in the compensatory stage of shock, decreased capillary hydrostatic pressure causes a fluid shift from the interstitial space into the capillaries. The net gain of fluid raises the blood volume.

Working together, these compensatory mechanisms can maintain MAP for only a short period of time. During this period, the perfusion and oxygenation of the heart and brain are adequate. If effective treatment is provided, the process is arrested, and no permanent damage occurs. However, unless the underlying cause of shock is reversed, these compensatory mechanisms soon become harmful, and shock perpetuates shock.

Stage II: Intermediate or Progressive Shock

The progressive stage of shock occurs after a sustained decrease in MAP of 20 mmHg or more below normal levels and a fluid loss of 35% to 50% (1800 to 2500 mL of fluid). Although the compensatory mechanisms in the previous state remain activated, they are no longer able to maintain MAP at a level sufficient to ensure perfusion of vital organs.

The vasoconstriction response that first helped sustain MAP eventually limits blood flow to the point that cells become oxygen deficient. To remain alive, the affected cells switch from aerobic to anaerobic metabolism. The lactic acid formed as a by-product of anaerobic metabolism contributes to an acidotic state at the cellular level. As a result, adenosine triphosphate (ATP), the source of cellular energy, is produced inefficiently. Lacking energy, the sodium-potassium pump fails. Potassium moves out of the cell, while sodium and water move inward. As this process continues, the cell swells, cell membrane integrity is lost, and cell organelles are damaged. Lysosomes within the cell spill out their digestive enzymes, which disintegrate any remaining organelles. Some enzymes spread to adjacent cells, where they erode and rupture cell membranes.

The acid by-products of anaerobic metabolism dilate the precapillary arterioles and constrict the postcapillary venules. This causes increased hydrostatic pressure within the capillary, and fluid shifts back into the interstitial space. The capillaries also become increasingly permeable, allowing serum proteins to shift from the vascular space into the interstitium. The buildup of plasma proteins increases the osmotic pressure in the interstitium, further accelerating the fluid shift out of the capillaries.

Throughout this period, the heart rate and vasoconstriction increase; however, perfusion of the skin, skeletal muscles, kidneys, and gastrointestinal organs is greatly diminished. Cells in the heart and brain become hypoxic while other body cells and tissues become ischemic and anoxic. A generalized state of acidosis and hyperkalemia ensues (see Chapter 5 ⊕). Unless this stage of shock is treated rapidly, the client's chances of survival are poor.

Stage III: Refractory or Irreversible Shock

If shock progresses to the irreversible stage, tissue anoxia becomes so generalized and cellular death so widespread that no treatment can reverse the damage. Even if MAP is temporarily restored, too much cellular damage has occurred to maintain life. Death of cells is followed by death of tissues, which results in death of organs. Death of vital organs contributes to subsequent death of the body.

Effects of Shock on Body Systems

Whatever its causes, shock produces predictable effects on the body's organ systems. (See *Multisystem Effects of Shock* on page 152.)

Cardiovascular System

The perfusion and oxygenation of the heart are adequate in the early stages of shock. As shock progresses, myocardial cells become hypoxic, and myocardial muscle function diminishes. Initially, the blood pressure may be normal or even slightly elevated (as a result of compensatory mechanisms) and the heart rate only slightly increased. Sympathetic stimulation increases the heart rate (a sinus tachycardia of 120 beats per minute is common) in an effort to increase cardiac output. As a result of vasoconstriction and decreased blood volume, the palpated pulse is rapid, weak, and thready; as shock progresses, peripheral pulses are usually nonpalpable.

Tachycardia reduces the time available for left ventricular filling and coronary artery perfusion, further reducing cardiac output. With progressive shock, altered acid-base balance, hypoxia, and hyperkalemia damage the heart's electrical systems and contractility. Consequently, cardiac dysrhythmias may develop. Decreased blood volume with decreased venous return also decreases cardiac output, and blood pressure falls.

The blood pressure changes produced by shock are characterized by a progressive decrease in both systolic and diastolic pressures and a narrowing pulse pressure. Auscultation of blood pressure is often difficult or impossible and is an inaccurate reflection of blood pressure status. For this reason, hemodynamic monitoring is usually instituted to follow the client's cardiovascular status accurately.

Respiratory System

During shock, oxygen delivery to cells may be impaired by a drop in circulating blood volume or, in the case of blood loss, by an insufficient number of red blood cells that carry oxygen. Although the respiratory rate increases because of compensatory mechanisms that promote oxygenation, the number of alveoli that are perfused decreases, and gas exchange is impaired. As a result, oxygen levels in the blood decrease, and carbon dioxide levels increase. As perfusion of the lungs diminishes, carbon dioxide is retained, and respiratory acidosis occurs.

A complication of decreased perfusion of the lungs is acute respiratory distress syndrome (ARDS), or "shock lung." The exact mechanism that produces ARDS is unknown, but some contributing factors have been identified. The pulmonary capillaries become increasingly permeable to proteins and water, resulting in noncardiogenic pulmonary edema. Production of surfactant (which controls surface tension within alveoli) is impaired, and the alveoli collapse or fill with fluid. This potentially lethal form of respiratory failure may result from any condition that causes hypoperfusion of the lungs, but it is more common in shock caused by hemorrhage, severe allergic responses, trauma, and infection. (ARDS is discussed further in Chapter 36.) ⊕

Gastrointestinal and Hepatic Systems

The gastrointestinal organs normally receive 25% of the cardiac output through the splanchnic circulation. Shock constricts the splanchnic arterioles and redirects arterial blood flow to the heart and brain. Consequently, gastrointestinal organs become ischemic and may be irreversibly damaged.

Gastric mucosa tends to ulcerate when it becomes ischemic. Lesions of the gastric and duodenal mucosa (called *stress ulcers*) can develop within hours of severe trauma, sepsis, or burns (Porth, 2002). Gastrointestinal ulcers may hemorrhage within 2 to 10 days following the original cause of shock. In addition, the permeability of damaged mucosa increases, allowing enteric bacteria or their toxins to enter the abdominal cavity and then progress to the circulation, resulting in sepsis.

Gastric and intestinal motility is impaired during shock, and paralytic ileus may result. If the episode of shock is prolonged, necrosis of the bowel may occur. In many cases, alterations in the structure and function of the gastrointestinal tract impair absorption of nutrients, such as protein and glucose.

Shock also alters the metabolic functions of the liver. Initially, *gluconeogenesis* (the process of forming glucose from noncarbohydrate sources) and *glycogenolysis* (the breakdown of glycogen into glucose) increase. This process allows blood glucose

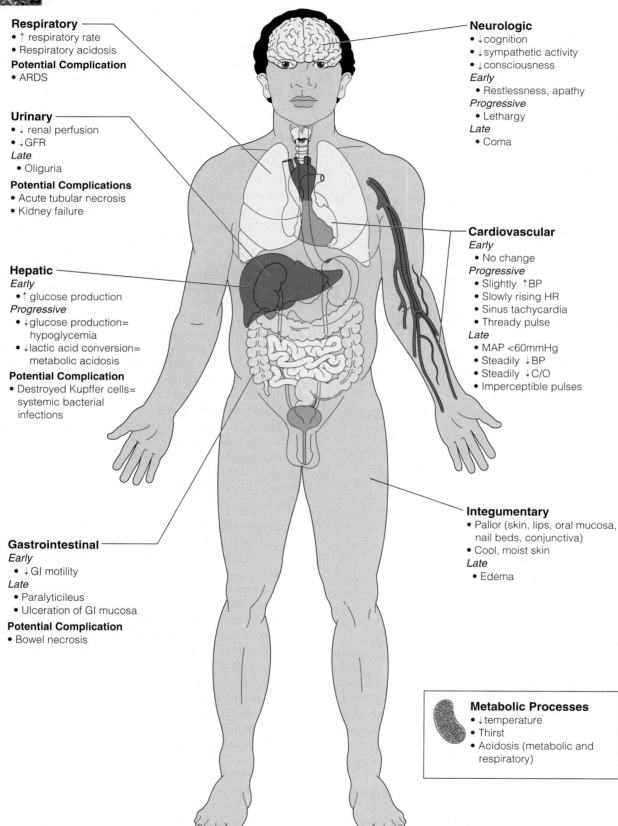

Respiratory
- ↑ respiratory rate
- Respiratory acidosis

Potential Complication
- ARDS

Urinary
- ↓ renal perfusion
- ↓GFR

Late
- Oliguria

Potential Complications
- Acute tubular necrosis
- Kidney failure

Hepatic
Early
- ↑ glucose production

Progressive
- ↓glucose production=
  hypoglycemia
- ↓lactic acid conversion=
  metabolic acidosis

Potential Complication
- Destroyed Kupffer cells=
  systemic bacterial
  infections

Gastrointestinal
Early
- ↓GI motility

Late
- Paralyticileus
- Ulceration of GI mucosa

Potential Complication
- Bowel necrosis

Neurologic
- ↓cognition
- ↓sympathetic activity
- ↓consciousness

Early
- Restlessness, apathy

Progressive
- Lethargy

Late
- Coma

Cardiovascular
Early
- No change

Progressive
- Slightly ↑BP
- Slowly rising HR
- Sinus tachycardia
- Thready pulse

Late
- MAP <60mmHg
- Steadily ↓BP
- Steadily ↓C/O
- Imperceptible pulses

Integumentary
- Pallor (skin, lips, oral mucosa,
  nail beds, conjunctiva)
- Cool, moist skin

Late
- Edema

Metabolic Processes
- ↓temperature
- Thirst
- Acidosis (metabolic and
  respiratory)

levels to increase as the body attempts to respond to the stressor; however, as shock progresses, liver functions are impaired, and hypoglycemia develops. Metabolism of fats and protein is impaired, and the liver can no longer effectively remove lactic acid, contributing to the development of metabolic acidosis.

The destruction of the liver's reticuloendothelial Kupffer cells (phagocytes that destroy bacteria) causes a further problem. Bacteria may proliferate within the circulatory system, causing overwhelming bacterial infection and toxicity.

Neurologic System

The primary effects of shock on the neurologic system involve changes in mental status and orientation. Cerebral hypoxia produces altered levels of consciousness, beginning with apathy and lethargy and progressing to coma. A common early symptom of cerebral hypoxia is restlessness. Continued ischemia of brain cells eventually causes swelling, resulting in cerebral edema, neurotransmitter failure, and irreversible brain cell damage.

As cerebral ischemia worsens, the sympathetic activity and vasomotor centers are depressed. This leads to a loss of sympathetic tone, causing systemic vasodilatation and pooling of blood in the periphery. As a result, venous return and cardiac output further decrease.

Renal System

Blood that normally perfuses the kidneys is shunted to the heart and brain during the progressive stage of shock, resulting in renal hypoperfusion. The drop in renal perfusion is reflected in a corresponding decrease in the glomerular filtration rate. Urine output is reduced, and the urine that is produced is highly concentrated. Oliguria of less than 20 mL per hour indicates progressive shock.

Healthy kidneys can tolerate a drop in perfusion for only about 20 minutes; thereafter, acute tubular necrosis develops (Porth, 2002). As tubular necrosis occurs, epithelial cells slough off and block the tubules, disrupting nephron function. The accumulating loss of functional nephrons eventually causes renal failure. Without normal renal function, metabolic waste products are retained in the plasma.

If treatment restores renal perfusion, the kidneys can regenerate the lost epithelial cells in the tubules, and renal function usually returns to normal. However, in the older or chronically ill client or in the client with sustained shock, loss of renal function may become permanent.

Effects on Skin, Temperature, and Thirst

In most types of shock, blood vessels supplying the skin are vasoconstricted, and the sweat glands are activated. As a result, changes in skin color occur. The skin of Caucasian clients becomes pale. In people with darker skin (such as those of African, Hispanic, or Mediterranean descent), shock-related skin color changes may be assessed as paleness of the lips, oral mucous membranes, nail beds, and conjunctiva. The skin is usually cool and moist and, in the later stages of shock, often edematous.

The body temperature decreases as shock progresses, the result of a decrease in overall body metabolism. Some people in shock become thirsty, probably a response to decreased blood volume and increased serum osmolality (Porth, 2002).

TYPES OF SHOCK

Shock is identified according to its underlying cause. All types of shock progress through the same stages and exert similar effects on body systems. Any differences are noted in the following discussion.

Hypovolemic Shock

Hypovolemic shock is caused by a decrease in intravascular volume of 15% or more (Porth, 2002). In hypovolemic shock, the venous blood returning to the heart decreases, and ventricular filling drops. As a result, stroke volume, cardiac output, and blood pressure decrease. Hypovolemic shock is the most common type of shock, and it often occurs simultaneously with other types.

The decrease in circulating blood volume that triggers hypovolemic shock may result from:

- Loss of blood volume from hemorrhage (from surgery, trauma, gastrointestinal bleeding, blood coagulation disorders, ruptured esophageal varices).
- Loss of intravascular fluid from the skin due to injuries such as burns (see Chapter 15). 🔗
- Loss of blood volume from severe dehydration.
- Loss of body fluid from the gastrointestinal system due to persistent and severe vomiting or diarrhea, or continuous nasogastric suctioning.
- Renal losses of fluid due to the use of diuretics or to endocrine disorders such as diabetes insipidus.
- Conditions causing fluid shifts from the intravascular compartment to the interstitial space.
- Third spacing due to such disorders as liver diseases with ascites, pleural effusion, or intestinal obstruction.

Hypovolemic shock affects all body systems. Its effects vary depending on the client's age, general state of health, extent of injury or severity of illness, length of time before treatment is provided, and the rate of volume loss.

The manifestations of hypovolemic shock result directly from the decrease in circulating blood volume and the initiation of compensatory mechanisms (Figure 6–8 ■). The loss of circulating blood volume reduces cardiac output by decreasing venous return to the heart. As a result, blood pressure drops. The carotid and cardiac baroreceptors sense the decrease in blood pressure and communicate it to the vasomotor centers in the brainstem. The vasomotor centers then induce the sympathetic compensatory responses. If the fluid loss is less than 500 mL, activation of the sympathetic response is generally adequate to restore cardiac output and blood pressure to near normal, although the heart rate may remain elevated.

With a sustained loss of blood volume (1000 mL or more), the shock stage progresses. Heart rate and vasoconstriction increase, and blood flow to the skin, skeletal muscles, kidneys, and abdominal organs decreases. Several renal mechanisms and a decline in capillary pressure help conserve blood volume. Eventually, the amount of blood flowing to cells is too low to oxygenate them and sustain production of cellular energy. Anaerobic metabolism begins, producing an acidotic environment for cells. As a result, cells lose their physical integrity.

MediaLink | HYPOVOLEMIC SHOCK ANIMATION

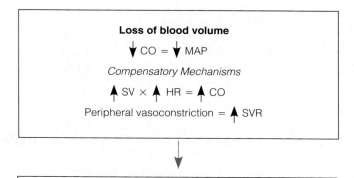

Loss of blood volume

$\downarrow$ CO = $\downarrow$ MAP

Compensatory Mechanisms

$\uparrow$ SV $\times$ $\uparrow$ HR = $\uparrow$ CO

Peripheral vasoconstriction = $\uparrow$ SVR

Continued loss of blood volume

Compensatory Mechanisms

Vasoconstriction: periphery, skin, abdominal organs

Vasodilation: heart, skeletal muscles, respiratory

retention of H_2O and Na^+

$\uparrow$ SV $\times$ $\uparrow$ HR = $\uparrow$ CO + $\uparrow$ SVR = $\uparrow$ MAP

Continued loss of blood volume

$\downarrow$ CO = $\downarrow$ MAP

$\downarrow$ Tissue perfusion and oxygenation

Cellular anaerobic metabolism

Cellular hypoxia and death

Irreversible shock

Multisystem organ failure

Death

Key CO: Cardiac output
HR: Heart rate
MAP: Mean arterial pressure
SV: Stroke volume
SVR: Systemic vascular resistance

Figure 6–8 ■ The stages of hypovolemic shock.

If untreated, shock causes multiple organ failure, and death results. Manifestations of various stages of hypovolemic shock are listed in Box 6–2.

Cardiogenic Shock

Cardiogenic shock occurs when the heart's pumping ability is compromised to the point that it cannot maintain cardiac output and adequate tissue perfusion. Cardiac disorders are discussed in Chapters 29 and 30; this section focuses only on the effects of shock caused by these disorders.

BOX 6–2 ■ **Assessment Findings in Clients in Hypovolemic Shock**

INITIAL STAGE
- Blood pressure: normal to slightly decreased
- Pulse: slightly increased from baseline
- Respirations: normal (baseline)
- Skin: cool, pale (in periphery), moist
- Mental status: alert and oriented
- Urine output: slight decrease
- Other: thirst, decreased capillary refill time

COMPENSATORY AND PROGRESSIVE STAGES
- Blood pressure: hypotension
- Pulse: rapid, thready
- Respirations: increased
- Skin: cool, pale (includes trunk); poor turgor with fluid loss, edematous with fluid shift
- Mental status: restless, anxious, confused, or agitated
- Urine output: oliguria (less than 30 mL/hour)
- Other: marked thirst, acidosis, hyperkalemia, decreased capillary refill time, decreased or absent peripheral pulses

IRREVERSIBLE STAGE
- Blood pressure: severe hypotension (often, systolic pressure is below 80 mmHg)
- Pulse: very rapid, weak
- Respirations: rapid, shallow; crackles and wheezes
- Skin: cool, pale, mottled with cyanosis
- Mental status: disoriented, lethargic, comatose
- Urine output: anuria
- Other: loss of reflexes, decreased or absent peripheral pulses

---

The loss of the pumping action of the heart may be caused by the following conditions.

- Myocardial infarction
- Cardiac tamponade
- Restrictive pericarditis
- Cardiac arrest
- Dysrhythmias, such as fibrillation or ventricular tachycardia
- Pathologic changes in the valves
- Cardiomyopathies from hypertension, alcohol, bacterial or viral infections, or ischemia
- Complications of cardiac surgery
- Electrolyte imbalances (especially changes in normal potassium and calcium levels)
- Drugs affecting cardiac muscle contractility
- Head injuries causing damage to the cardioregulatory center

Myocardial infarction is the most common cause of cardiogenic shock. Clients admitted to the hospital for treatment of myocardial infarction or cardiac surgery are at risk for cardiogenic shock. The severity and progression of shock are related to the amount of myocardial damage.

Whatever the cardiogenic cause, the decrease in cardiac output causes a decrease in MAP. Heart rate may increase in response to compensatory mechanisms. However, tachycardia increases myocardial oxygen consumption and decreases coronary perfusion. The myocardium becomes progressively de-

---

BOX 6–3 ■ **Assessment Findings in Clients in Cardiogenic Shock**

■ Blood pressure: hypotension
■ Pulse: rapid, thready; distention of veins of hands and neck
■ Respirations: increased, labored; crackles and wheezes; pulmonary edema
■ Skin: pale, cyanotic, cold, moist
■ Mental status: restless, anxious, lethargic progressing to comatose
■ Urine output: oliguria to anuria
■ Other: dependent edema; elevated CVP; elevated pulmonary capillary wedge pressure; arrhythmias

---

pleted of oxygen, causing further myocardial ischemia and necrosis. The typical sequence of shock is essentially unchanged in cardiogenic shock.

Cyanosis, however, is more common in cardiogenic shock, because stagnating blood increases extraction of oxygen from the hemoglobin at the capillary beds. As a result, the skin, lips, and nail beds may appear cyanotic. As cardiac failure (and cardiogenic shock) progresses, left ventricular end-diastolic pressure increases. The increase is transmitted to the pulmonary capillary bed, and pulmonary edema may occur. Retention of blood in the right side of the heart increases right atrial pressure, which leads to jugular venous distention as a result of backflow through the vena cava. Manifestations of cardiogenic shock are listed in Box 6–3.

Obstructive Shock

Obstructive shock is caused by an obstruction in the heart or great vessels that either impedes venous return or prevents effective cardiac pumping action. The causes of obstructive shock are impaired diastolic filling (e.g., pericardial tamponade or pneumothorax), increased right ventricular afterload (e.g., pulmonary emboli), and increased left ventricular afterload (e.g., aortic stenosis, abdominal distention). The manifestations are the result of decreased cardiac output and blood pressure, with reduced tissue perfusion and cellular metabolism.

Distributive Shock

Distributive shock (also called **vasogenic shock**) includes several types of shock that result from widespread vasodilatation and decreased peripheral resistance. As the blood volume does not change, relative hypovolemia results.

Septic Shock

Septic shock, the leading cause of death for clients in intensive care units, is one part of a progressive syndrome called systemic inflammatory response syndrome (SIRS). This condition is most often the result of gram-negative bacterial infections (i.e., *Pseudomonas, E. coli, Klebsiella*), but may also follow gram-positive infections from *Staphyloccus* and *Streptococcus* bacteria. Gram-negative sepsis has greatly increased in the past 10 years, with a 60% mortality rate despite treatment. The pathophysiology of septic shock is complex and not completely understood.

Clients at risk for developing infections leading to septic shock include those who are hospitalized, have debilitating chronic illnesses, or have poor nutritional status. The risk is heightened after invasive procedures or surgery. Other clients at risk of septic shock include older adults and those who are immunocompromised. Portals of entry for infection that may lead to septic shock are as follows:

• Urinary system: catheterizations, suprapubic tubes, cystoscopy
• Respiratory system: suctioning, aspiration, tracheostomy, endotracheal tubes, respiratory therapy, mechanical ventilators
• Gastrointestinal system: peptic ulcers, ruptured appendix, peritonitis
• Integumentary system: surgical wounds, intravenous catheters, intra-arterial catheters, invasive monitoring, decubitus ulcers, burns, trauma
• Female reproductive system: elective surgical abortion, ascending infections from transmission of bacteria during the intrapartal and postpartal periods, tampon use, sexually transmitted diseases

Septic shock begins with *septicemia* (the presence of pathogens and their toxins in the blood). As pathogens are destroyed, their ruptured cell membranes allow endotoxins to leak into the plasma. The endotoxins disrupt the vascular system, coagulation mechanism, and immune system and trigger an immune and inflammatory response (see Chapter 8 🔗 for more information). For this reason, the initial effects of septic shock differ from those of hypovolemic and cardiogenic shock; cardiac output is high and systemic vascular resistance is low.

Endotoxins directly damage the endothelial lining of small blood vessels first; the small blood vessels of the kidneys and lungs are most susceptible. Cellular damage stimulates the release of vasoactive proteins and activates coagulation factor XII. The vasoactive proteins stimulate peripheral vasodilatation and increase capillary permeability; the activation of coagulation factors results in the production of multiple intravascular blood clots.

As a result of the increased capillary permeability and vasodilatation, fluid shifts from the intravascular space to the interstitial space. Hypovolemia results as fluid volume is lost from the circulating blood. Hypovolemia and intravascular coagulation alter oxygenation and cellular metabolism, leading to anaerobic metabolism, lactic acidosis, and cellular death.

Septic shock has an early phase and a late phase. In early septic shock (sometimes called the *warm* phase), vasodilatation results in weakness and warm, flushed skin, and the septicemia often causes high fever and chills. In late septic shock (sometimes called the *cold* phase), hypovolemia and activity of the compensatory mechanisms result in typical shock manifestations, including cold, moist skin; oliguria; and changes in mental status. Death may result from respiratory failure, cardiac failure, or renal failure. Manifestations of septic shock are listed in Box 6–4.

Toxic shock syndrome is an especially virulent form of septic shock, occurring most frequently in menstruating women who use tampons. It is thought that bacterial toxins diffuse

BOX 6–4	■ Assessment Findings in Clients in Septic Shock

EARLY (WARM) SEPTIC SHOCK
- Blood pressure: normal to hypotension
- Pulse: increased, thready
- Respirations: rapid and deep
- Skin: warm, flushed
- Mental status: alert, oriented, anxious
- Urine output: normal
- Other: increased body temperature; chills; weakness; nausea, vomiting, diarrhea; decreased CVP

LATE (COLD) SEPTIC SHOCK
- Blood pressure: hypotension
- Pulse: tachycardia, arrhythmias
- Respirations: rapid, shallow, dyspneic
- Skin: cool, pale, edematous
- Mental status: lethargic to comatose
- Urine output: oliguria to anuria
- Other: normal to decreased body temperature; decreased CVP

BOX 6–5	■ Assessment Findings in Clients in Neurogenic Shock

- Blood pressure: hypotension
- Pulse: slow and bounding
- Respirations: vary
- Skin: warm, dry
- Mental status: anxious, restless, lethargic progressing to comatose
- Urine output: oliguria to anuria
- Other: lowered body temperature

from the site of infection in the vagina into the circulation. The toxins then trigger a widespread inflammatory response and septic shock. The manifestations of toxic shock syndrome include extreme hypotension, hyperpyrexia, headache, myalgia, confusion, skin rash, vomiting, and diarrhea (Porth, 2002).

Disseminated intravascular coagulation (DIC), a generalized response to injury, is a potential risk in septic shock. This condition is characterized by simultaneous bleeding and clotting throughout the vasculature. Sepsis injures blood cells, causing platelet aggregation and decreased blood flow. As a result, blood clots form throughout the microcirculation. The clotting slows circulation further while stimulating excess fibrinolysis. As the body's stores of clotting factors are depleted, generalized bleeding begins. DIC is further discussed in Chapter 32.

Neurogenic Shock

Neurogenic shock is the result of an imbalance between parasympathetic and sympathetic stimulation of vascular smooth muscle. If parasympathetic overstimulation or sympathetic understimulation persists, sustained vasodilatation occurs, and blood pools in the venous and capillary beds.

Neurogenic shock causes dramatic reduction in systemic vascular resistance as the size of the vascular compartment increases. As systemic vascular resistance decreases, pressure in the blood vessels becomes too low to drive nutrients across capillary membranes, and cellular metabolism is impaired.

The following conditions can cause neurogenic shock by increasing parasympathetic stimulation or inhibiting sympathetic stimulation of the smooth muscle of blood vessels.

- Head injury
- Trauma to the spinal cord (spinal shock, a form of neurogenic shock, is described in Chapter 41)
- Insulin reactions (which cause hypoglycemia, decreasing glucose to the medulla)
- Central nervous system depressant drugs (such as sedatives, barbiturates, or narcotics)

- Anesthesia (spinal and general)
- Severe pain
- Prolonged exposure to heat

Bradycardia occurs early, but tachycardia begins as compensatory mechanisms are initiated. Central venous pressure drops as veins dilate, venous return to the heart decreases, stroke volume decreases, and MAP falls. In early stages, the extremities are warm and pink (from the pooling of blood), but as shock progresses, the skin becomes pale and cool. Manifestations of neurogenic shock are listed in Box 6–5.

Anaphylactic Shock

Anaphylactic shock is the result of a widespread hypersensitivity reaction (called *anaphylaxis*). The pathophysiology in this type of shock includes vasodilatation, pooling of blood in the periphery, and hypovolemia with altered cellular metabolism. These physiologic alterations occur when a sensitized person has contact with an *allergen* (a foreign substance to which an individual is hypersensitive). Many different allergens can cause anaphylactic shock, including medications, blood administration, latex, foods, snake venom, and insect stings.

Anaphylactic shock does not occur with the first exposure to an allergen. With the first exposure to a foreign substance (the *antigen*), the body produces specific immunoglobulin E (IgE) antibodies against this antigen. The person is thus sensitized to that specific antigen. With subsequent exposure, the antigen reacts with the already formed IgE antibodies, disrupting cellular integrity. In addition, large amounts of histamine and other vasoactive amines are released and distributed through the circulatory system. These substances cause increased capillary permeability and massive vasodilatation, resulting in profound hypotension and eventual vascular collapse.

Histamine also causes constriction of smooth muscles in the bladder, uterus, intestines, and bronchioles. Respiratory distress, bronchospasm, laryngospasm, and severe abdominal cramping result. Serotonin (a neurotransmitter with vasoconstrictive properties) is released, further affecting respiratory status by increasing capillary permeability in the lungs. As a result, plasma leaks into the alveoli, gas exchange is impaired, and pulmonary edema may occur.

Anaphylactic shock begins and progresses rapidly. Manifestations may begin within 20 minutes of contact with an antigen. Unless appropriate intervention is provided, death can occur within a matter of minutes. Because anaphylaxis is rapid and potentially lethal, people with known allergies should carry some form of

> **BOX 6–6** ■ **Assessment Findings in Clients in Anaphylactic Shock**
>
> ■ Blood pressure: hypotension
> ■ Pulse: increased, dysrhythmias
> ■ Respirations: dyspnea, stridor, wheezes, laryngospasm, bronchospasm, pulmonary edema
> ■ Skin: warm, edematous (lips, eyelids, tongue, hands, feet, genitals)
> ■ Mental status: restless, anxious, lethargic to comatose
> ■ Urine output: oliguria to anuria
> ■ Other: paresthesias; pruritus; abdominal cramps, vomiting, diarrhea

warning (such as a MedicAlert bracelet) informing others of their susceptibility. Health care providers should be extremely careful to assess and document allergies or previous drug reactions. Manifestations of anaphylactic shock are listed in Box 6–6.

COLLABORATIVE CARE

Medical care for the client in shock focuses on treating the underlying cause, increasing arterial oxygenation, and improving tissue perfusion. Depending on the cause and type of shock, interventions include emergency care measures, oxygen therapy, fluid replacement, and medications. Emergency care is often the first course of collaborative action taken to arrest shock, as discussed earlier in this chapter.

Diagnostic Tests

The following diagnostic tests can help identify the type of shock and assess the client's physical status. Measurements include:

- *Blood hemoglobin* and *hematocrit.* Changes in hemoglobin and hematocrit concentrations usually occur in hypovolemic shock. These changes reflect the underlying etiology. In hypovolemic shock resulting from hemorrhage, the hemoglobin and hematocrit concentrations are lower than normal; in hypovolemic shock resulting from intravascular fluid loss, by contrast, the hemoglobin and hematocrit concentrations are higher than normal.
- *Arterial blood gases (ABGs),* to determine oxygen and carbon dioxide levels and pH. The effects of shock and of the body's compensatory mechanisms cause a decrease in pH (indicating acidosis), a decrease in the partial pressure of oxygen (Pao_2) and in total oxygen saturation, and an increase in the partial pressure of carbon dioxide ($Paco_2$).
- *Serum electrolytes,* to monitor the severity and progression of shock. As shock progresses, glucose levels decrease, sodium levels decrease, and potassium levels increase.
- *Blood urea nitrogen (BUN), serum creatinine levels, urine specific gravity,* and *osmolality,* to check renal function. As perfusion of the kidneys is decreased and renal function is reduced, the BUN and creatinine levels increase as does urine specific gravity and osmolality.
- *Blood cultures,* to identify the causative organism in septic shock.

- *White blood cell count* and *differential,* in the client with septic or anaphylactic shock. The total WBC count is increased in septic shock. Elevated neutrophils indicate acute infection, increased monocytes indicate a bacterial infection, and increased eosinophils indicate an allergic response.
- *Serum cardiac enzymes,* which are elevated in cardiogenic shock: lactate dehydrogenase (LDH), creatine phosphokinase (CPK), and serum glutamic-oxaloacetic transaminase (SGOT).
- *Central venous catheter,* to aid in the differential diagnosis of shock and to provide information about the preload of the heart. A pulmonary artery catheter may be inserted to monitor cardiac dynamics, fluid balance, and the effects of vasoactive medications.

Other diagnostic tests may be ordered to determine the extent of injury or damage or to locate the site of internal hemorrhage. These tests might include X-ray studies, computerized tomography (CT) scans, magnetic resonance imaging (MRI), endoscopic examinations, and echocardiograms. Newer diagnostic methods for hypoperfusion include gastric tonometry and sublingual Pco_2. Gastric tonometry measures the partial pressure of carbon dioxide in the gastric lumen. The measurement of sublingual carbon dioxide correlates well with decreased MAP (Sole, Lamborn, & Hartshorn, 2001).

Medications

When fluid replacement alone is not sufficient to reverse shock, vasoactive drugs (drugs causing vasoconstriction or vasodilatation) and inotropic drugs (drugs improving cardiac contractility) may be administered. When used to treat shock, these drugs increase venous return through vasoconstriction of peripheral vessels; they also improve the pumping ability of the heart by facilitating myocardial contractility and by dilating coronary arteries to increase perfusion of the myocardium.

Drugs used to treat shock are discussed in the Medication Administration box on page 158. Other drugs that may be administered to the client in shock include:

- Diuretics to increase urine output after fluid replacement has been initiated.
- Sodium bicarbonate to treat acidosis.
- Calcium to replace calcium lost as a result of blood transfusions.
- Antiarrhythmic agents to stabilize heart rhythm.
- Antibiotics to suppress organisms responsible for septic shock.
- A cardiotonic glycoside (such as digitalis) to treat cardiac failure.
- Steroids to treat anaphylactic shock.

Oxygen Therapy

Establishing and maintaining a patent airway and ensuring adequate oxygenation are critical interventions in reversing shock. All clients in shock (even those with adequate respirations) should receive oxygen therapy (usually by mask or nasal cannula) to maintain the Pao_2 at greater than 80 mmHg during the first 4 to 6 hours of care. If the client's unassisted respiration cannot maintain Pao_2 at this level, ventilatory assistance may be necessary. Care of the client requiring ventilatory assistance is discussed in Chapter 36.

Medication Administration

The Client in Shock

ADRENERGICS (SYMPATHOMIMETICS)

Adrenergic drugs (also called sympathomimetics) mimic the fight-or-flight response of the sympathetic nervous system, selectively stimulating alpha-adrenergic and beta-adrenergic receptors. Many of these drugs have both vasopressor (vasoconstricting) effects and positive inotropic effects (Table 6–5). Stimulation of alpha-adrenergic receptors results in vasoconstriction and increased systemic blood pressure. Stimulation of beta-adrenergic receptors increases the force and rate of myocardial contraction.

The physiologic effect of these drugs includes improved perfusion and oxygenation of the heart, with increased stroke volume and heart rate, and increased cardiac output. Increased cardiac output in turn increases tissue perfusion and oxygenation. The major disadvantage is that increases in stroke volume and heart rate also increase the oxygen requirements of the myocardium. These drugs may be used in the early stages of shock, especially in types of shock characterized by vasodilation.

Nursing Responsibilities

- Carefully monitor responses in the older adult, who may be especially sensitive to sympathomimetics and require lower doses.
- When administering these drugs by the subcutaneous route, carefully aspirate the injection site to avoid injecting the drug directly into a blood vessel.
- Use the intravenous route only with continuous infusion pumps. Carefully adjust the dose to accommodate the client's cardiovascular status (as ordered by the physician or by written protocol).
- Document lung sounds, vital signs, and hemodynamic parameters before starting the medication, and then according to institutional policy (usually every 5 to 15 minutes).
- Record and monitor urine output, report output of less than 30 mL per hour.
- Be aware that the sympathomimetics are incompatible with sodium bicarbonate or alkaline solutions.

Table 6–5   Adrenergic Drugs Used to Treat Shock

Action	Drug	Receptor
Vasoconstrictors	Norepinephrine (Levophed)	A
	Metaraminol (Aramine)	A
Inotropes	Dopamine (Inotropin)*	A, B[1]
	Dobutamine (Dobutrex)	B[1]
	Isoprotenernol (Isuprel)	B[1], B[2]

*Receptors are dose dependent.

- When administering drugs that cause vasoconstriction, such as norepinephrine (Levophed) and metaraminol (Aramine), monitor the intravenous insertion site for infiltration. If infiltration does occur, stop the infusion and notify the physician immediately. (Infiltration may cause ischemia and necrosis of tissue.)

Client Teaching

- Because these drugs mimic a physiologic reaction to stress, they may cause feelings of anxiety.
- Close monitoring to adjust the dose will be carried out by qualified nurses using written protocols.
- Report heart palpitations or chest pain immediately.

VASODILATORS

  Nitroglycerin (Tridil)
  Nitroprusside (Nipride)

Drugs that cause vasodilation act directly on smooth muscle, affecting both arterioles and veins. Peripheral resistance, cardiac output, and pulmonary wedge pressure are all reduced as a result of the vasodilation. These effects decrease the oxygen need of the heart and decrease pulmonary congestion. Vasodilators are used primarily in the treatment of cardiogenic shock and may be combined with a sympathomimetic (e.g., dopamine).

Nursing Responsibilities

- Protect these drugs from light by wrapping the intravenous bag in the package that is provided.
- Mix with D5W only.
- Infuse with an infusion pump, and use within 4 hours of reconstitution.
- Do not add other medications to the solution.
- Assess mental status, blood pressure, and pulse prior to initiating medication. Thereafter, assess blood pressure and pulse according to institutional policy (usually every 5 minutes initially, then every 15 minutes until stable, and then every hour).
- Monitor for confusion, dizziness, tachycardia, arrhythmias, hypotension, and adventitious breath sounds. Report these immediately if they occur, and slow infusion to a keep-open rate.
- Monitor for signs of thiocyanate poisoning (nausea, disorientation, muscle spasms, decreased or absent reflexes) if infusion lasts longer than 72 hours.
- Keep client in bed with side rails up.

Client and Family Teaching

- It is important to stay in bed and change positions slowly to avoid dizziness.
- The blood pressure and pulse are taken frequently to adjust the dose of medication.
- Headache is a common side effect.

Fluid Replacement

The most effective treatment for the client in hypovolemic shock is the administration of intravenous fluids or blood. Fluids also treat septic and neurogenic shock. However, the client with cardiogenic shock may require either fluid replacement or restriction, depending on pulmonary artery pressure.

Various fluids may be administered alone or in combination as part of fluid replacement therapy in treating shock. Whole blood or blood products increase the oxygen-carrying capacity of the blood and thus increase oxygenation of cells. Fluid replacements, such as crystalloid and colloid solutions, increase circulating blood volume and tissue perfusion. Fluid replacements are administered in massive amounts through two large-bore peripheral lines or through a central line.

Crystalloid Solutions

Crystalloid solutions contain dextrose or electrolytes dissolved in water; they are either isotonic or hypotonic. Isotonic solutions include normal saline (0.9%), lactated Ringer's solution, and Ringer's solution. Hypotonic solutions include one-half normal saline (0.45%) and 5% dextrose in water (D5W).

All crystalloid solutions increase fluid volume in both the intravascular and the interstitial space. Of the total amount infused, only about 25% remains in the intravascular system; the remaining 75% moves into the interstitial space. Consequently, fluid volume is only minimally expanded and the potential for peripheral edema is increased when crystalloid solutions are used. However, Ringer's lactate (an electrolyte solution) and 0.9% saline are the fluids of choice in treating hypovolemic shock, especially in the emergency phase of care while blood is being typed and crossmatched. Large amounts of these solutions may be infused rapidly, increasing blood volume and tissue perfusion.

Colloid Solutions

Colloid solutions contain substances (colloids) that should not diffuse through capillary walls. Hence, colloids tend to remain in the vascular system and increase the osmotic pressure of the serum, causing fluid to move into the vascular compartment from the interstitial space. As a result, plasma volume expands.

Colloid solutions used to treat shock include 5% albumin, 25% albumin, hetastarch, plasma protein fraction, and dextran.

Colloid products reduce platelet adhesiveness and have been associated with reductions in blood coagulation. Consequently, the client's prothrombin time (PT), INR, platelet count, and activated partial thromboplastin time (PTT) should be monitored when these solutions are administered. Normal values are as follows:

PT	10–15 seconds
INR	1–1.2 seconds
Platelets	150,000–400,000
APTT	< 35 seconds

See the box below for further information about colloid solutions and associated nursing responsibilities and client teaching.

Blood and Blood Products

If hypovolemic shock is due to hemorrhage, the infusion of blood and blood products may be indicated. The goal of blood administration is to keep the hematocrit at 30% to 35% and the hemoglobin level between 12.5 and 14.5 g/100 mL. Available blood and blood products include fresh whole blood, stored whole blood, packed red blood cells, platelet concentrate, fresh-frozen plasma, and cryoprecipitate. Often, packed red blood cells are given to provide hemoglobin concentration and are supplemented with crystalloids to maintain an adequate circulatory volume (see discussion of blood administration earlier in the chapter).

Medication Administration

Colloid Solutions

COLLOID SOLUTIONS (PLASMA EXPANDERS)

Albumin 5% (Albuminar-5, Buminate 5%)
Albumin 25% (Albuminar-25, Buminate 25%)
Dextran 40 (Gentran 40)
Dextran 70 (Gentran 70, Macrodex)
Dextran 75 (Gentran 75)
Hetastarch (Hespan [HES])
Plasma protein fraction (Plasmanate, Plasma-Plex, Plasmatein, Protenate)

These solutions are blood volume expanders and are used to treat hypovolemic shock due to surgery, hemorrhage, burns, or other trauma. Albumin and plasma protein fraction are prepared from healthy blood donors. Dextran and hetastarch are synthetically prepared large molecules. The solutions promote circulatory volume and tissue perfusion by rapidly expanding plasma volume. Dextran solutions are infrequently used.

Nursing Responsibilities
- Before infusion begins, establish baseline of vital signs, lung sounds, heart sounds, and (if possible) CVP and pulmonary artery wedge pressure.
- Start administration of ordered intravenous fluids, using a large-gauge (18 or 19 gauge) infusion needle.
- Take and record vital signs as required by institutional policy (usually every 15 to 60 minutes) and client status.
- Take and record intake and output every 1 to 2 hours.

- Monitor for manifestations of congestive heart failure or pulmonary edema (dyspnea, cyanosis, cough, crackles, wheezes). If these manifestations appear, stop the fluids and notify the physician immediately.
- Monitor for bleeding from new sites; an increase in blood pressure may cause bleeding in severed vessels that did not bleed with decreased blood pressure.
- Monitor for manifestations of dehydration (dry lips; scant, dark-colored urine; loss of skin turgor). Increased intravenous fluids are usually ordered if the client becomes dehydrated.
- Monitor for manifestations of circulatory overload (jugular vein distention, increase in CVP, increase in pulmonary artery wedge pressure). If these manifestations occur, slow rate of infusion and notify physician.
- Monitor prothrombin time, partial thromboplastin time, and platelet counts.
- If administering dextran or plasma protein fraction, have epinephrine and antihistamines readily available for any manifestations of a hypersensitivity reaction (fever, chills, rash, headache, wheezing, flushing).
- Maintain client on bed rest with side rails elevated.

Client and Family Teaching
- The solutions are given to replace lost serum protein, which helps maintain the volume of blood.
- The vital signs are taken frequently to ensure the safety of the client.

NURSING CARE

Nursing assessments and interventions to prevent shock are an essential part of the nursing care of every client. The primary nursing interventions to prevent shock are assessment and monitoring.

Health Promotion and Assessment

Nursing assessments are critical in preventing shock. Identifying clients at risk and making focused assessments are essential. Although shock may occur at any age, physiologic changes with aging make the older adult a high-risk population (see the box below).

- *Hypovolemic shock:* Clients who have undergone surgery, have sustained multiple traumatic injuries, or have been seriously burned are most likely to develop hypovolemic shock. Monitoring fluid status is essential in preventing shock and includes daily assessments of weight, fluid intake by all routes, measurable fluid loss (e.g., urine, vomitus, wound drainage, gastric drainage, and chest tube drainage), and fluid loss that must be estimated, such as profuse perspiration and wound drainage. Assessments for the critically ill client are ongoing and include fluid balance, hemodynamic values, and vital signs.
- *Cardiogenic shock:* Clients with left anterior wall myocardial infarctions are at risk for developing cardiogenic shock. Nursing care to prevent the development of cardiogenic shock focuses on maintaining or improving myocardial oxygen supply by providing immediate pain relief, maintaining rest, and administering supplemental oxygen.
- *Neurogenic shock:* The risk of neurogenic shock is increased in clients who have spinal cord injuries and those who have received spinal anesthesia. Preventive nursing care includes maintaining immobility of clients with spinal cord trauma and elevating the head of the bed 15 to 20 degrees following spinal anesthesia. Elevations of more than 20 degrees, however, can potentiate headaches following spinal anesthesia and should be avoided.
- *Anaphylactic shock:* Prevent anaphylactic shock by collecting information about allergies and drug reactions during the health history. Note these allergies clearly on all documents and place a special armband on the client. Careful and frequent assessments during blood administration may prevent serious reactions to blood or blood products.

- *Septic shock:* Clients who are hospitalized, are debilitated, are chronically ill, or have undergone invasive procedures or tube insertions are at high risk for septic shock. Nursing care to prevent septic shock includes careful and consistent handwashing, the use of aseptic techniques for procedures (e.g., catheterizations, suctioning, changing dressings, starting and maintaining intravenous fluids or medications), and monitoring for local and systemic manifestations (e.g., white blood cell and differential counts) of infection.

Nursing Diagnoses and Interventions

Nursing care for the client in shock focuses on assessing and monitoring overall tissue perfusion and on meeting psychosocial needs of the client and the family. This section discusses nursing diagnoses that are appropriate for the client with hypovolemic shock.

Decreased Cardiac Output

Decreased cardiac output is the primary problem for the client in shock. Although much of the care related to this diagnosis is collaborative, many independent nursing interventions are critical to the care of the client in shock.

- *Assess and monitor cardiovascular function via the following:*
  - Blood pressure
  - Heart rate and rhythm
  - Pulse oximetry
  - Peripheral pulses
  - Hemodynamic monitoring of arterial pressures, pulmonary artery pressures, and central venous pressures (CVPs)

    A baseline assessment is necessary to establish the stage of shock. If palpable peripheral pulses and audible (to auscultation) blood pressure are lost, inserting central arterial, venous, and pulmonary artery catheters is essential to establish progression of shock accurately and to evaluate the client's response to therapy.
- Measure and record intake and output (total output and urinary output) hourly. *A decrease in circulating blood volume with hypotension and the effect of the compensatory mechanisms associated with shock can cause renal failure. Urinary output of less than 30 mL per hour in an acutely ill adult indicates reduced renal blood flow.*
- Monitor bowel sounds, abdominal distention, and abdominal pain. *Decreased splanchnic blood flow reduces bowel motility and peristalsis; paralytic ileus may result.*

Nursing Care of the Older Adult

VARIATIONS IN ASSESSMENT FINDINGS—SHOCK

- Cardiac changes may include a thickened left ventricular wall, decreased elasticity of the myocardium, and more rigid valves. These changes result in a decreased stroke volume and cardiac output, thus decreasing responses to shock in general and increasing the risk of cardiogenic shock.
- Decreased arterial wall elasticity and vasomotor tone reduce the older adult's ability to respond to a decrease in oxygenation.

- Decreased elasticity and turgor of the skin make assessments of skin turgor more difficult.
- Previous medication and blood administration increase the risk of anaphylactic shock.
- Decreased immune system response increases the risk of septic shock.

Figure 6–9 ■ The client in shock should be positioned with the lower extremities elevated approximately 20 degrees (knees straight), trunk horizontal, and the head elevated about 10 degrees.

- Monitor for sudden sharp chest pain, dyspnea, cyanosis, anxiety, and restlessness. *Hemoconcentration and increased platelet aggregation may result in pulmonary emboli.*
- Maintain bed rest and provide (to the extent possible) a calm, quiet environment. Place in a supine position with the legs elevated to about 20 degrees, trunk flat, and head and shoulders elevated higher than the chest (Figure 6–9 ■). *Limiting activity and ensuring rest decreases the workload of the heart. The supine position with legs elevated increases venous return; however, this position should not be used for clients in cardiogenic shock. The Trendelenburg position is no longer recommended, because it causes the abdominal organs to press against the diaphragm (limiting respirations), decreases filling of the coronary arteries, and initiates aortic and carotid sinus reflexes.*

Altered Tissue Perfusion

As shock progresses, diminished tissue perfusion causes ischemia and hypoxia of major organ systems. As shock worsens, blood flow and oxygenation of the lungs, heart, and brain are also impaired. Hypoxia and ischemia result from decreased tissue perfusion in the kidneys, brain, heart, lungs, gastrointestinal tract, and the periphery.

- Monitor skin color, temperature, turgor, and moisture. *Decreased tissue perfusion is evidenced by the skin's becoming pale, cool, and moist; as hemoglobin concentrations decrease, cyanosis occurs.*
- Monitor cardiopulmonary function by assessing/monitoring the following:
  - Blood pressure (by auscultation or by hemodynamic monitoring)
  - Rate and depth of respirations
  - Lung sounds
  - Pulse oximetry
  - Peripheral pulses (brachial, radial, dorsalis pedis, and posterior tibial); include presence, equality, rate, rhythm, and quality (If unable to palpate pulses, use a device such as a Doppler ultrasound flowmeter to assess peripheral arterial blood flow.)
  - Jugular vein distention
  - CVP measurements

Baseline vital signs are necessary to determine trends in subsequent findings. As shock progresses, the blood pressure decreases, and the pulse becomes rapid, weak, and thready. As perfusion of the lungs decreases, crackles, wheezes, and dyspnea are commonly assessed. Capillary refill is prolonged, and peripheral pulses are weak or nonpalpable. Neck veins that cannot be seen when the client is in the supine position indicate decreased intravascular volume. CVP is an accurate means of determining fluid status in the client in shock; the findings will be low (5 to 15 cm of water is normal) in hypovolemic shock because of the decreased blood volume. (See Chapter 5 ⊙ for a discussion of CVP.)

- Monitor body temperature. *An elevated body temperature increases metabolic demands, depleting reserves of bodily energy. It also increases myocardial oxygen demand and may place the client with previous cardiac problems at even greater risk for hypoperfusion.*
- Monitor urinary output per Foley catheter hourly, using a urimeter. *Urine output is a reliable indicator of renal perfusion.*
- Assess mental status and level of consciousness. *The appropriateness of the client's behavior and responses reflects the adequacy of cerebral circulation. Restlessness and anxiety are common early in shock; in later stages, the client may become lethargic and progress to a comatose state. Altered levels of consciousness are the result of both cerebral hypoxia and the effects of acidosis on brain cells.*

Anxiety

Many clients in hypovolemic shock have experienced some form of major trauma and may have life-threatening, multiple injuries. Following on-the-scene treatment, the client is usually admitted to the health care setting through the emergency department. Surgery may be required to treat injuries, followed by care in a critical care unit. Throughout this sequence of crisis events, treatment is invasive, and contact with family is minimal. Client and family responses to these situations of uncertainty, instability, and change include anxiety, fear, and powerlessness (see page 162). These responses are affected by age, developmental level, cultural and ethnic group, experience with illness and the health care system, and support systems.

- Assess the cause(s) of the anxiety, and manipulate the environment to provide periods of rest. *Reducing stimuli that cause anxiety is calming and facilitates rest, which is necessary in the client at risk for bleeding.*
- Administer prescribed pain medications on a regular basis. *Pain precipitates and/or aggravates anxiety.*
- Provide interventions to increase comfort and reduce restlessness:
  - Maintain a clean environment.
  - Provide skin and oral care.
  - Monitor the effectiveness of ventilation or oxygen therapy.
  - Eliminate all nonessential activities.
  - Remain with the client during procedures.
  - Speak slowly and calmly, using short sentences.
  - Use touch to provide support.

Unfamiliar sounds, sights, and odors can increase anxiety. Damp skin or a dry mouth increases discomfort. Inadequate gas exchange with a decrease in oxygen or an increase in carbon dioxide in the blood may cause the client to experience a "feeling of doom." Activity increases the body's need

Nursing Research

Evidence-Based Practice for Care of ICU Clients

The purpose of this study (Hupcey, 2000) was to describe the psychosocial needs of critically ill clients and behaviors of family members, friends, and ICU staff who helped or hindered meeting those needs. Data were collected by interviewing 45 adult clients who were in a medical or surgical ICU for a minimum of 3 days, and grounded theory methodology was used to analyze and conceptualize the experiences of the patients. A model of the psychosocial needs of this population was developed around the overarching need of all subjects in this study to feel safe. This core variable encompassed the four categories of identified needs: knowing, regaining control, hoping, and trusting.

- Knowing what was happening provided reassurance and helped the subjects "get through a terrible experience." Those who did not know or understand refused treatments, felt frightened, and even fought with staff.
- Regaining control emerged from an initial sense of total loss of control. Loss of control was frustrating and led to feelings of insecurity.
- Maintaining hope was essential to not giving up and survival. Sources of hope included family members, friends, staff, and religious beliefs.
- Trusting the ICU staff was essential to feel safe.

IMPLICATIONS FOR NURSING

Nurses in the ICU can provide interventions to make clients feel safe. Nurses can incorporate family members as part of the team to provide support and can encourage the use of hospital or individual resources of spiritual strength. Hope can be assessed, and interventions designed to meet individualized needs. Control and independence can be fostered by having clients make decisions about such areas as control of lights and television. Based on the findings of this study, feeling safe is also fostered in ICU clients when nurses are technically competent and genuinely caring. In addition, nurses need to be aware that clients require frequent and repeated explanations and reorientations.

Critical Thinking in Client Care

1. Make a list of the barriers to feeling safe for clients who are in the ICU. Consider the physical environment, the client's physical condition, and factors such as medications. Do you believe any of these barriers could be changed? If not, why not?
2. Consider the verbal and nonverbal methods of demonstrating genuine caring. Conversely, think about the verbal and nonverbal ways that health care providers may not demonstrate caring. If you were a nurse manager in an ICU unit, how could you encourage caring?
3. Considering the information from this study, what level of health care provider would you delegate to provide care for a 75-year-old woman who has had a stroke and is unable to verbally communicate? How would your decision differ if it were a 55-year-old woman who had suffered serious head trauma in an automobile crash (driving while intoxicated)?

---

for oxygen. Listening and touch provide support in an environment in which the client often feels alone and abandoned. Severe anxiety interferes with the ability to understand others and to respond appropriately.

- Provide support for the client and family:
  - Provide time, space, and privacy for family members.

- Allow family members access to the client when feasible.
- Encourage the expression of feelings and concerns. Provide anticipatory guidance to prepare for recovery or death and to support realistic hope.
- Acknowledge the beliefs, values, and expectations of the client and family.

CHART 6–2   NANDA, NIC, AND NOC LINKAGES

The Client Experiencing Shock

NURSING DIAGNOSES	NURSING INTERVENTIONS	NURSING OUTCOMES
• Ineffective Tissue Perfusion	• Cardiac Care: Acute • Shock Management • Acid-Base Monitoring • Fluid Management • Hypovolemia Management • Hemodynamic Regulation • Vital Signs Monitoring	• Tissue Perfusion: Cardiac • Electrolyte and Acid-Base Balance • Fluid Balance • Tissue Perfusion: Peripheral • Vital Sign Status
• Decreased Cardiac Output	• Cardiac Care • Hemodynamic Regulation	• Circulatory Pump Effectiveness • Circulatory Status • Tissue Perfusion: Abdominal Organs • Tissue Perfusion: Peripheral • Vital Signs Status

Note. Data from Nursing Outcomes Classification (NOC) *by M. Johnson & M. Maas (Eds.), 1997, St. Louis: Mosby;* Nursing Diagnoses: Definitions & Classification 2001–2002 *by North American Nursing Diagnosis Association, 2001, Philadelphia: NANDA;* Nursing Interventions Classification (NIC) *by J.C. McCloskey & G. M. Bulechek (Eds.), 2000, St. Louis: Mosby. Reprinted by permission.*

Allowing the family access to the client reduces anxiety and gives both the client and the family some feeling of control. If prognosis is poor, access and involvement allow the family to begin the grieving process. If recovery is expected, contact provides the client and family with a feeling of hope. Supporting the client and family facilitates concrete problem solving, promotes acceptance of the illness and its implications, and helps them begin to establish ways of managing the illness experience.

- Provide information about the current setting to both the client and family; give the family information about available resources (such as pastoral care, social services, temporary housing, meals). *Knowing what to expect and how to control the environment to meet basic needs reduces anxiety.*

Using NANDA, NIC, and NOC

Chart 6–2 shows links between NANDA nursing diagnoses, NIC, and NOC when caring for the client who is experiencing shock.

Home Care

Home care for the client who has experienced shock is highly individualized, depending on the cause and the illness or injury that caused shock. Therefore, topics for consideration are not included in this section.

Nursing Care Plan
A Client with Septic Shock

Huang Mei Lan is a 43-year-old unmarried female who lives alone in a major West Coast city. Ms. Huang came to America 15 years ago from China and now speaks English well. Her family still lives in China. She worked in a neighborhood sewing shop until 3 years ago, when she was diagnosed with breast cancer. Her treatment included mastectomy of the affected breast and follow-up chemotherapy.

Last month, Ms. Huang experienced a recurrence of cancer in the lymph glands of the affected side. Surgery to remove the glands was performed and chemotherapy started. Ms. Huang has a central line, a urinary catheter, and a surgical incision. She is underweight, weak, and depressed. Although she has multiple physical problems, she never complains or asks for any kind of medication.

ASSESSMENT

Ms. Huang's primary nurse, Robert O'Brien, enters her room early in the morning to make an initial assessment. He finds Ms. Huang huddled in the middle of the bed, shivering violently. Her vital signs are T 104° F, P 110, R 30, and BP 106/66. Her skin is hot, dry, and flushed with poor turgor. She is alert and oriented, but is restless and appears anxious. Ms. Huang states she is nauseated and suddenly begins vomiting and is incontinent of liquid stool. Laboratory data indicate leukocytosis, respiratory alkalosis, and reduced platelet count. Blood cultures, as well as cultures of Ms. Huang's sputum, urine, and wound drainage, are conducted. She is diagnosed as having septic shock.

Hetastarch is ordered per intravenous line, and intravenous broad-spectrum antibiotics are begun until the organism and its portal of entry can be determined. Despite treatment, Ms. Huang's condition worsens. Her blood pressure continues to drop, her skin becomes cool and cyanotic, and she begins to have periods of disorientation. She is transferred to the critical care unit. As she is being prepared for the transfer, she begins to cry and asks, "Am I going to die?"

DIAGNOSES

- *Deficient fluid volume* related to vomiting, diarrhea, high fever, and shift of intravascular volume to interstitial spaces
- *Ineffective breathing pattern* related to rapid respirations and progression of septic shock
- *Ineffective tissue perfusion* related to progression of septic shock with decreased cardiac output, hypotension, and massive vasodilatation
- *Anxiety* related to feelings that illness is worsening and is potentially life threatening, and the transfer to the critical care unit

EXPECTED OUTCOMES

- Maintain adequate circulating blood volume.
- Regain and maintain blood gas parameters within normal limits.
- Regain and maintain stable hemodynamic levels.
- Verbalize increased ability to cope with stressors.

PLANNING AND IMPLEMENTATION

- Monitor neurologic status, including mental status and level of consciousness.
- Monitor cardiovascular status, including arterial blood pressure; rate, rhythm, and quality of pulses; central venous pressure; pulmonary artery pressure; and cardiac output.
- Monitor color and character of skin.
- Monitor results of arterial blood gases, blood counts, clotting times, and platelet counts.
- Monitor respiratory status, including respiratory rate, rhythm, and breath sounds.
- Monitor body temperature every 2 hours.
- Monitor urinary output hourly, reporting any output of less than 30 mL per hour.
- Explain procedures and provide comfort measures (oral care, skin care, turning, positioning).

EVALUATION

Despite intensive nursing and medical care, Ms. Huang's condition remains critical. The interventions are continued.

Critical Thinking in the Nursing Process

1. Vasopressors may be used in the treatment of septic shock. Explain the rationale for their use.
2. While monitoring Ms. Huang's arterial blood gases, the nurse notes that her PaO_2 is < 60 mmHg and her $PaCO_2$ is > 50. What do these findings indicate, and why have they occurred?
3. Ms. Huang has been given large amounts of colloids intravenously. Hemodynamic monitoring indicates a higher than normal CVP and pulmonary artery pressure. What do these findings indicate? What physical assessments would you make to confirm the changes?

See Evaluating Your Response in Appendix C.

EXPLORE MediaLink

NCLEX review questions, case studies, care plan activities, MediaLink applications, and other interactive resources for this chapter can be found on the Companion Website at www.prenhall.com/lemone.

Click on Chapter 6 to select the activities for this chapter. For animations, video clips, more NCLEX review questions, and an audio glossary, access the Student CD-ROM accompanying this textbook.

TEST YOURSELF

1. What is the most common mechanical source of injury in adults of all ages?

   a. Gunshot wounds
   b. Fire
   c. Drowning
   d. Motor vehicles

2. Severe facial injuries, such as those resulting from going through a windshield, increase the risk for all of the following. What would you assess first?

   a. Airway obstruction
   b. Hemorrhage
   c. Contusions
   d. Fractures

3. Which on-the-scene intervention would be a priority?

   a. Determine cause of injury
   b. Assess airway patency

   c. Assess peripheral capillary refill
   d. Palpate for internal hemorrhage

4. You are monitoring blood administration to a trauma victim in shock. Which of the following assessments indicate a dangerous transfusion reaction?

   a. Red raised areas (wheals) on the skin that itch
   b. An increase in body temperature by 3°
   c. Decreasing blood pressure and dyspnea
   d. Increasing blood pressure and pulse

5. What type of shock causes widespread vasodilatation and decreased peripheral resistance?

   a. Cardiogenic shock
   b. Septic shock
   c. Hypovolemic shock
   d. Obstructive shock

See Test Yourself answers in Appendix C.

BIBLIOGRAPHY

A crash course in skin trauma. (1998). *Homecare Education Management, 3*(2), 24–25.

American College of Surgeons. Committee on Trauma. (1997). *Advanced trauma life support manual.* Chicago: ACS.

Asuncion, M., & Koushik, V. (2000). Shock states in the elderly40. *Clinical Geriatriacs, 8*(8), 40–42, 45–48.

Bucher, L., & Melander, S. (1999). *Critical care nursing.* Philadelphia: Saunders.

Carpenito, L. (2000). *Nursing diagnoses: Application to clinical practice* (8th ed.). Philadelphia: Lippincott.

Champion, H., Copes, W., Gann, D., Gennarelli, T., & Flanagan, M. (1989). A revision of the trauma score. *Journal of Trauma, 29*(5), 624.

Craven, A. (1998). Trauma. In C. Hudak, B. Gall, & P. Morton (Eds.), *Critical care nursing: A holistic approach* (7th ed.) (pp. 973–990). Philadelphia: Lippincott-Raven.

DeJong, M. (1997). Emergency! Cardiogenic shock. *American Journal of Nursing, 97*(6), 40–41.

Emergency Nurses Association. (1992). *Trauma resource document.* Park Ridge, IL: ENA.

Fitzpatrick, L., & Fitzpatrick, T. (1997). Blood transfusions: Keeping your patient safe. *Nursing 97, 27*(8), 34–42.

Hupcey, J. (2000). Feeling safe: The psychosocial needs of ICU patients. *Journal of Nursing Scholarship, 32*(4), 361–367.

Huston, C. (1996). Emergency! Hemolytic transfusion reaction. *American Journal of Nursing, 96*(3), 47.

Johnson, M., & Maas, M. (Eds.). (1997). *Nursing outcomes classification (NOC).* St. Louis: Mosby.

Jordan, K. S. (2000). Fluid resuscitation in acutely injured patients. *Journal of Intravenous Nursing, 23*(2), 81–87.

Labovich, T. (1997). Transfusion therapy: Nursing implications. *Clinical Journal of Oncology Nursing, 1*(3), 61–72.

Liepert, D., & Rosenthal, M. (2000). Management of cardiogenic, hypovolemic, and hyperdynamic shock. *Current Reviews for Perianesthesia Nurses, 22*(9), 1–3, 113, back cover.

Lisanti, P. (1996). Emergency! Anaphylaxis. *American Journal of Nursing, 96*(11), 51.

McCloskey, J. C., & Bulechek, G. M. (Eds.). (2000). *Nursing interventions classification (NIC).* St. Louis: Mosby.

McConnell, E. (1997). Safely administering a blood transfusion. *Nursing 97, 27*(6), 30.

McCracken, L. (2001). The forensic ABC's of trauma care. *Canadian Nurse, 97*(3), 30–33.

McKenny, L., & Salerno, E. (1998). *Pharmacology in nursing* (20th ed.). St. Louis: Mosby.

Mower-Wade, D., Bartley, M., & Chiari-Allwein, J. (2001). How to respond to shock. *Dimensions of Critical Care Nursing, 20*(2), 22–27.

North American Nursing Diagnosis Association. (2001). *Nursing diagnoses: Definitions & classification 2001–2002.* Philadelphia: NANDA.

Porth, C. (2002). *Pathophysiology: Concepts of altered health states* (6th ed.). Philadelphia: Lippincott.

Sole, M., Lamborn, M., & Hartshorn, J. (2001). *Introduction to critical care nursing* (3rd ed.). Philadelphia: Saunders.

Speck, P., & Whalley, A. (1996). Domestic violence: Role of the RN. *Tennessee Nurse, 59*(3), 27, 31.

Stamatos, C., Sorensen, P., & Tefler, K. (1996). Meeting the challenge of the older trauma patient. *American Journal of Nursing, 96*(5), 40–47.

Stoll, E. (2001). Sepsis and septic shock. *Clinical Journal of Oncology Nursing, 5*(2), 71–72.

Tierney, L., McPhee, S., & Papadakis, M. (Eds.). (2001). *Current diagnosis & treatment* (40th ed.). Stamford, CT: Appleton & Lange.

Waldsburger, W. J. (1999). Massive transfusion in trauma. *AACN Clinical Issues: Advanced Practice in Acute & Critical Care, 10*(1), 69–84.

Watts, D., Abrahams, E., MacMillan, C., Sanat, J., Silver, R., VanGorder, S., Waller, M., & York, D. (1998). Insult after injury: Pressure ulcers in trauma patients. *Orthopaedic Nursing, 17*(4), 84–91.

Wilson, B., Shannon, M., & Stang, C. (2001). *Nursing drug guide 2001.* Upper Saddle River, NJ: Prentice Hall.

Nursing Care of Clients Having Surgery

www.prenhall.com/lemone
Additional resources for this chapter
can be found on the Student
CD-ROM accompanying this
textbook, and on the Companion
Website at www.prenhall.com/lemone.
Click on Chapter 7 to select the activities
for this chapter.

CD-ROM
• Audio Glossary
• NCLEX Review

Companion Website
• More NCLEX Review
• Case Study
   The Circulating Nurse
• Care Plan Activity
   Providing Postoperative Care
• MediaLink Application
   Anesthesia and Outpatient Surgery

LEARNING OUTCOMES

After completing this chapter, you will be able to:

- Describe the various classifications of surgical procedures.

- Identify diagnostic tests used in the perioperative period.

- Describe nursing implications for medications prescribed for the surgical client.

- Provide appropriate nursing care for the client in the perioperative, intraoperative, and postoperative phases of surgery.

- Identify variations in perioperative care for the older adult.

- Describe principles of pain management specific to acute postoperative pain control.

- Discuss the differences and similarities between outpatient and inpatient surgery.

- Use the nursing process as a framework for providing individualized care for the client undergoing surgery.

TABLE 7–1 Classification of Surgical Procedures

	Classification	Function	Examples
Purpose	Diagnostic	Determine or confirm a diagnosis	Breast biopsy, bronchoscopy
	Ablative	Remove diseased tissue, organ, or extremity	Appendectomy, amputation
	Constructive	Build tissue/organs that are absent (congenital anomalies)	Repair of cleft palate
	Reconstructive	Rebuild tissue/organ that has been damaged	Skin graft after a burn, total joint replacement
	Palliative	Alleviate symptoms of a disease (not curative)	Bowel resection in client with terminal cancer
	Transplant	Replace organs/tissue to restore function	Heart, lung, liver, kidney transplant
Risk Factor	Minor	Minimal physical assault with minimal risk	Removal of skin lesions, dilation and curettage (D&C), cataract extraction
	Major	Extensive physical assault and/or serious risk	Transplant, total joint replacement, cholecystectomy, colostomy, nephrectomy
Urgency	Elective	Suggested, though no foreseen ill effects if postponed	Cosmetic surgery, cataract surgery, bunionectomy
	Urgent	Necessary to be performed within 1 to 2 days	Heart bypass surgery, amputation resulting from gangrene, fractured hip
	Emergency	Performed immediately	Obstetric emergencies, bowel obstruction, ruptured aneurysm, life-threatening trauma

Surgery is an invasive medical procedure performed to diagnose or treat illness, injury, or deformity. Although surgery is a medical treatment, the nurse assumes an active role in caring for the client before, during, and after surgery. **Collaborative care** and **independent nursing care** together prevent complications and promote the surgical client's optimal recovery.

Perioperative nursing is a specialized area of practice. It incorporates the three phases of the surgical experience: preoperative, intraoperative, and postoperative. The **preoperative phase** begins when the decision for surgery is made and ends when the client is transferred to the operating room. The **intraoperative phase** begins with the client's entry into the operating room and ends with admittance to the postanesthesia care unit (PACU), or recovery room. The **postoperative phase** begins with the client's admittance to the PACU and ends with the client's complete recovery from the surgical intervention.

Surgical procedures can be classified according to purpose, risk factor, and urgency (Table 7–1). Based on this information, nursing care can be individualized to best meet client needs.

Although the perioperative nurse works in collaboration with other health care professionals to identify and meet the client's needs, the perioperative nurse has the primary responsibility and accountability for nursing care of the client undergoing surgery.

SETTINGS FOR SURGERY

Surgical patients may be inpatients or outpatients. The complexity of the surgery and recovery and the expected disposition of the client following the surgery are the major differences. Sometimes outpatients, clients intending to be discharged home immediately, are admitted to the hospital. Cataract removal with or without lens implants, hernia repairs, tubal ligations, vasectomies, dilation and curettage (D&C), hemorrhoidectomies, and biopsies are commonly performed outpatient surgeries.

Inpatient and outpatient surgeries are performed in the same operating suites in most hospitals. There are also **freestanding outpatient surgical facilities**, which are not physically or financially connected to a hospital. Surgeons may practice in both hospital and freestanding surgical facilities. The number of outpatient surgeries has rapidly grown in the past decade as part of the effort to contain the high costs of surgery. Moreover, increasingly complex surgeries on clients with complicated medical problems are now commonly performed on an outpatient basis. This increase in number of procedures and acuity level of the clients has presented a challenge to the perioperative nurse, the patient, and the family.

Outpatient surgery offers several advantages:

- Decreased cost to the client, hospital, and insuring agency
- Reduced risk of hospital-acquired infection
- Less interruption in the client's and family's routine
- Possible reduction in time lost from work and/or other responsibilities
- Less physiologic stress to the client and family

Outpatient surgery also presents some disadvantages:

- Less time for the nurse to establish rapport with client and family
- Less time for the nurse to assess, evaluate, and teach the client and family
- Lack of opportunity for the nurse to assess for the risk of postoperative complications that may occur after discharge

Many similarities exist between nursing care of the inpatient and outpatient surgical clients. Physical care is provided in much the same manner in the preoperative, intraoperative, and postoperative phases of surgery. The major differences lie in the degree of teaching and emotional support that must be provided for outpatient surgical clients and their families. In addition to the physiologic insult of surgery, the outpatient surgical client must cope with the additional stress of needing to learn a great deal of information in a short span of time. The nurse teaches the client and family in both the preoperative and postoperative periods to enable the client to perform self-care following discharge. More extensive teaching and emotional support is mandated as clients requiring more complex surgical procedures and experiencing more complicated health problems undergo outpatient surgery.

PRACTICE ALERT *Clients having outpatient surgery should wear or bring clothing that will be easy to put on after surgery and accommodate any dressings or appliances. Furthermore, despite being NPO, clients must bring any medications they regularly use (especially those prescribed by other providers), such as steroids, antibiotics, anticoagulants, antivirals, diuretics, oral contraceptives, hypotensives, cardiotonics, hypoglycemics, asthma medications, seizure medications, and analgesics. Clients should consult with the surgeon and anesthesiologist before taking these medications.* ■

Following outpatient surgery, the client is discharged after meeting the institution's criteria:

- Vital signs are stable.
- Client is able to stand and begin to walk without dizziness or nausea.
- Pain is controlled or alleviated.
- Client is able to urinate.
- Client is oriented.
- Client demonstrates understanding of postoperative instructions.

LEGAL REQUIREMENTS

It is the responsibility of the surgeon who performs the procedure to obtain the client's consent for care. The surgeon should discuss the above information with the client and family in language they can understand. **Informed consent** (or an **operative permit**) is a legal document required for certain diagnostic procedures or therapeutic measures, including surgery. This legal document protects the client, nurse, physician, and health care facility. Informed consent includes the following information:

- Need for the procedure in relation to the diagnoses
- Description and purpose of the proposed procedure
- Possible benefits and potential risks
- Likelihood of a successful outcome
- Alternative treatments or procedures available
- Anticipated risks should the procedure not be performed
- Physician's advice as to what is needed
- Right to refuse treatment or withdraw consent

Ideally, the nurse should be present when the information is provided. Later, the nurse can discuss the information with the client and family, if necessary. If the client has questions or concerns that were not discussed or made clear, or if the nurse questions the client's understanding, the surgeon is responsible for supplying further information. If these situations arise, the nurse should contact the surgeon before having the client give informed consent. Following a thorough discussion of the informed consent, the nurse witnesses the client's signature on the informed consent form (Figure 7–1 ■). The nurse also signs the form, indicating that the correct person is signing the form and that the client was alert and aware of what was being signed.

SURGICAL RISK FACTORS

Prior to planning and implementing care for the surgical client, the nurse must first assess the client's needs and the factors that may increase the risks associated with surgery. The type of surgical procedure directs the assessment and interventions planned by the nurse. However, a complete assessment is also necessary to identify *risk factors* and to determine the client's overall health status. Table 7–2 lists common risk factors for the client undergoing surgery, and the related nursing interventions and implications. For example, when a client is admitted for surgery on the right knee, it should be of concern to the nurse if this client has diabetes, smokes 1.5 packs of cigarettes per day, has numbness in the right foot, and takes insulin. This information should be incorporated into a care plan, using appropriate nursing diagnoses and interventions to meet all of the client's needs and assist the client toward full postoperative recovery.

Interpreting and responding to identified risk factors requires nursing judgment. It is important to bring information to the attention of the surgeons and anesthesiologists prior to surgery, so necessary modifications can be made for the patient.

PRACTICE ALERT *Remind diabetic clients that the stress of surgery increases rather than decreases blood sugar. Coordinate insulin injection and/or hypoglycemic medication with the client, surgeon, and anesthesiologist.* ■

COLLABORATIVE CARE

The client undergoing surgery receives care from a number of health care providers. This collaborative approach focuses on placing the client in the best possible health status before, during, and after surgery.

Diagnostic Tests

Diagnostic tests performed prior to surgery provide baseline data or detect problems that may place the client at additional risk during and after surgery. Because of the trend toward shortened hospital stays, many diagnostic studies and procedures are performed in a preadmission clinic within a week prior to elective surgery.

M.R. # _____

**Informed Consent to Operation, Administraton of Anesthetics,
and to the Rendering of Other Medical Services**

Saint
Francis
Medical
Center

1.   I do hereby authorize and direct _____ M.D./D.O./D.D.S., my physician, and/or such associates or assistants of his choice, to perform the following operation or procedure:

_____

_____

upon _____ (patient's name). I understand that the above named physician and his associates or assistants are employed by me and will be occupied solely with performing such operation or procedure.

2.   The nature of the operation or procedure has been explained to me and no warranty or guarantee has been made as to result or cure. I have been advised that additional surgical and/or medical procedures or treatment may be deemed necessary during the course of the operation or procedure consented hereto, and I fully consent to such additional procedures and treatment which, in the opinion of my physician, are deemed necessary or desirable for the well being of the patient. The possible risks and complications of the operation or procedure have been explained to me. The physician has explained to me the above medical terminology and I satisfactorily understand the type of operation/procedure.

3.   I hereby authorize and direct the above named physician and/or his associates or assistants or those working under his direction to provide for _____ (patient's name) such additional services as he or they may deem reasonable and necessary, including, but not limited to, the administration and maintenance of anesthesia, blood or blood derivatives, and the performance of services involving pathology and radiology and I hereby consent thereto. The possible risks and complications of blood transfusions and the administration of anesthetics have also been explained to me.

4.   I understand also that the persons in attendance at such operation or procedure for the purpose of administering anesthesia, and the radiologists in attendance at such operation or procedure for the purpose of performing radiological (x-ray) service are not the agents, servants or employees of St. Francis Medical Center nor of any physician, but are independent health care providers who are employed by me in the same way that my surgeon and physician are employed by me.

5.   I hereby authorize the Medical Center pathologist or personnel to use their discretion in the disposal of any severed tissue or member.

6.   I hereby grant permission for St. Francis Medical Center to obtain clinical photographs for educational purposes or for my patient record as deemed necessary by my physician.

7.   **The exception to this consent:** (If none, write "none".) _____
_____ and I assume full responsibility for these exceptions.

_____   _____

PATIENT'S SIGNATURE   **DATE**

If the patient is a minor or incompetent or is unable to sign, the following must be completed:

I hereby certify that I am the (relationship) _____ of the above named patient
who is unable to sign because _____ ,
and I am fully authorized to give the consent herein granted.

_____   _____

SIGNATURE   **DATE**

_____   _____

WITNESSED BY/date   **WITNESSED BY/date**

If signed in the physician's office, the following MUST be completed by the Medical Center.

_____   _____

REVIEWED BY (patient name) **/date**   **WITNESSED BY /date**

Figure 7–1 ■ Informed consent form.

TABLE 7–2   Nursing Implications for Surgical Risk Factors

Factor	Associated Risk	Nursing Implications
Advanced age	Older adults have age-related changes that affect physiologic, cognitive, and psychosocial responses to the stress of surgery; decrease tolerance of general anesthesia and postoperative medications; and delay wound healing.	Selected nursing interventions are summarized in Table 7–6.
Obesity	The obese client is at increased risk for delayed wound healing, wound dehiscence, infection, pneumonia, atelectasis, thrombophlebitis, arrhythmias, and heart failure.	Promote weight reduction if time permits. Monitor closely for wound, pulmonary, and cardiovascular complications postoperatively. Encourage coughing, turning, and diaphragmatic breathing exercises and early ambulation.
Malnutrition	Reserves may not be sufficient to allow the body to respond satisfactorily to the physical assault of surgery; organ failure and shock may result. Increased metabolic demands may result in poor wound healing and infection.	With the physician and dietitian, promote weight gain by providing a well-balanced diet high in calories, protein, and vitamin C. Administer total parenteral nutrition intravenously, nutritional supplements, and tube feedings as prescribed. Daily weights and calorie counts also may be ordered.
Dehydration/electrolyte imbalance	Depending on the degree of dehydration and/or type of electrolyte imbalance, cardiac dysrhythmia or heart failure may occur. Liver and renal failure may also result.	Administer intravenous fluids as ordered. Monitor I&O. Monitor client for evidence of electrolyte imbalance (see Chapter 5). ⌘
Cardiovascular disorders	Presence of cardiovascular disease increases the risk of hemorrhage and shock, hypotension, thrombophlebitis, pulmonary embolism, stroke (especially in the older client), and fluid volume overload.	Diligently monitor vital signs, especially pulse rate, regularity, and rhythm, and general condition of the client. Closely monitor fluid intake (oral and parenteral) to prevent circulatory overload. Assess skin color. Assess for chest pain, lung congestion, and peripheral edema. Observe for signs of hypoxia, and administer oxygen as ordered. Early postoperative ambulation and leg exercises reduce the risk of vascular problems, such as thrombophlebitis and pulmonary embolism.
Respiratory disorders	Respiratory complications such as bronchitis, atelectasis, and pneumonia are some of the most common and serious postoperative complications. Respiratory depression from general anesthesia and acid-base imbalance may also occur. Clients with pulmonary disease are more at risk for developing these complications.	Closely monitor respirations, pulse, and breath sounds. Also assess for hypoxia, dyspnea, lung congestion, and chest pain. Encourage coughing, turning, and diaphragmatic breathing exercises and early postoperative ambulation. Encourage the client to quit smoking or at least to reduce the number of cigarettes smoked.
Diabetes mellitus	Diabetes causes an increased risk for fluctuating blood glucose levels, which can lead to life-threatening hypoglycemia or ketoacidosis. Diabetes also increases the risk for cardiovascular disease, delayed wound healing, and wound infection.	Monitor the client closely for signs and symptoms of hypoglycemia and hyperglycemia. Monitor blood glucose levels every 4 hours or as ordered. Administer insulin as prescribed. Encourage intake of food at the designated meal and snack times.
Renal and liver dysfunction	The client with renal or liver dysfunction may poorly tolerate general anesthesia, have fluid/electrolyte and acid-base imbalances, decreased metabolism and excretion of drugs, increased risk for hemorrhage, and delayed wound healing.	Monitor for fluid volume overload, I&O, and response to medication. Evaluate closely for drug side effects and evidence of acidosis or alkalosis.
Alcoholism	The client may be malnourished and experience delirium tremens (acute withdrawal symptoms). More general anesthesia may be required. Hemorrhage and delayed wound healing can result from liver damage and poor nutritional status.	Monitor closely for signs of delirium tremens. Encourage well-balanced diet. Monitor for wound complications. Administer supplemental nutrients parenterally as ordered.

(continued on page 170)

TABLE 7–2 Nursing Implications for Surgical Risk Factors (continued)

Factor	Associated Risk	Nursing Implications
Nicotine use	Cigarette smokers are at increased risk for respiratory complications such as pneumonia, atelectasis, and bronchitis because of increased mucous secretions and a decreased ability to expel them.	Ideally, the client should quit smoking. Be supportive of the client, and monitor closely for respiratory difficulties. Coughing, turning, and diaphragmatic breathing exercises with early ambulation are very important. Increase daily fluid intake to 2500–3000 mL (unless contraindicated) to help liquefy respiratory secretions to aid expectoration.
Adolescence	Diversity in age, and physical, cognitive, and psychological maturation makes preparation for surgery vary in content and inclusion of significant others. Increased need for control, privacy, and peer interaction poses special challenges in the acute care setting.	Adapt assessment and interventions to the development level of individual clients, involving them in preparation and care to the extent possible. Allow for regressive and independent behavior including rejection of adult support.
Medications	Anesthesia interaction with some medications can cause respiratory difficulties, hypotension, and circulatory collapse. Other medications can produce side effects that may increase surgical risk.	Inform the anesthesiologist of all prescribed or over-the-counter medications.
Anticoagulants (including aspirin)	May cause intraoperative and postoperative hemorrhage.	Monitor for bleeding. Assess PT/PTT values.
Diuretics (particularly thiazides)	May lead to fluid and electrolyte imbalances, producing altered cardiovascular response and respiratory depression.	Monitor I&O and electrolytes. Assess cardiovascular and respiratory status.
Antihypertensives (particularly phenothiazines)	Increase the hypotensive effects of anesthesia.	Closely monitor blood pressure.
Antidepressants (particularly monoamine oxidase inhibitors)	Increase the hypotensive effects of anesthesia.	Closely monitor blood pressure.
Antibiotics (particularly the "mycin" group)	May cause apnea and respiratory paralysis.	Monitor respirations.
Herbal supplements	Some may prolong the effects of anesthesia. Others may increase the risks of bleeding or raise blood pressure.	Inquire about the use of herbs or other dietary supplements. These should be discontinued at least 1 week before surgery.

Complete blood counts, electrolyte studies, coagulation studies, and urinalysis are the most commonly performed preoperative laboratory tests. Table 7–3 discusses the significance and nursing implications of abnormal findings for these common tests. Additional diagnostic tests may be performed as the history and physical findings indicate. For example, if the client has a low hemoglobin and hematocrit, and significant blood loss during surgery is anticipated, then the surgeon may order a type and crossmatch of the client's blood for a possible transfusion.

In addition to laboratory tests, elderly clients or those with risk factors related to heart and lung function typically have a chest X-ray. This radiologic procedure provides baseline information about the size, shape, and condition of the heart and lungs. Pulmonary complications such as lung disease, tuberculosis, calcification, infiltration, or pneumonia may require that surgery be postponed to allow the client to

undergo further evaluation or treatment. If findings are abnormal and the surgery cannot be postponed, information from the chest X-ray study can be used to determine the safest form of anesthesia.

Another commonly performed preoperative diagnostic procedure is the electrocardiogram (ECG). This test is ordered routinely on clients undergoing general anesthesia when they are over 40 years of age or have cardiovascular disease. The ECG provides data for evaluation about either new or preexisting cardiac conditions. The client's surgery may be cancelled or postponed if a life-threatening cardiac condition is discovered.

In addition to the chest X-ray study and ECG, other diagnostic tests may be performed preoperatively to gather further assessment data. For example, for clients who have chronic obstructive pulmonary disease, pulmonary function studies often are performed to determine the extent of respiratory dysfunction. This information guides the anesthesiologist before

TABLE 7–3 Laboratory Tests for Perioperative Assessment

Test	Significance of Increased Values	Significance of Decreased Values	Nursing Implications
Hemoglobin (Hgb) and hematocrit (Hct)	Dehydration, excessive fluid plasma loss, polycythemia vera	Fluid overload, excessive blood loss, anemia	Monitor oxygenation, intake and output (I&O), and vital signs; assess for bleeding.
White blood cell (WBC) count	Infectious/inflammatory processes, leukemia	Immune deficiencies	Monitor for signs of inflammation; monitor drainage, temperature, and pulse. Use strict universal precautions.
Platelet count	Malignancies, polycythemia vera	Clotting deficiency disorders, chemotherapy	If decreased, assess for bleeding at incision sites and drainage tubes, and assess for hematomas.
Carbon dioxide (CO₂)	Emphysema, chronic bronchitis, asthma, pneumonia, respiratory acidosis, vomiting, nasogastric suctioning	Metabolic acidosis, hyperventilation	Monitor respiratory status and arterial blood gases (ABGs).
Electrolytes Potassium (K⁺)	Kidney dysfunction, dehydration, suctioning	Side effects of diuretics, vomiting, NG suctioning	Monitor K⁺ level, cardiac and neurologic function, and preoperative diuretic therapy.
Sodium (Na⁺)	Kidney dysfunction, normal saline-containing intravenous fluids	Side effects of diuretics, vomiting, NG suctioning	Monitor Na⁺ level and I&O; assess for peripheral edema and effects of perioperative diuretic therapy.
Chloride (Cl⁻)	Kidney dysfunction, dehydration, alkalosis	Side effects of diuretics, vomiting, NG suctioning	Monitor Cl⁻ level and I&O; assess for peripheral edema and perioperative diuretic therapy.
Prothrombin time (protime, or PT) and partial thromboplastin time (PTT)	Defect in mechanism for blood clotting, anticoagulant therapy (aspirin, heparin, warfarin), side effect of other drugs affecting clotting time	Hypercoagulability of the blood may lead to thrombus formation in the veins	If clotting time is elevated, monitor PT/PTT values. Assess for bleeding at incision site and drainage tubes and for hematomas. If clotting time is decreased, monitor for thrombus formation (pulmonary emboli, thrombophlebitis), and evaluate PT and PTT values.
Urinalysis	Varied	Varied	Used to detect abnormal substances (e.g., protein, glucose, red blood cells, or bacteria) in the urine. Notify surgeon if abnormalities are detected.

and during surgery in choosing the type of anesthetic to be used, and it guides the surgeon and nursing staff in the recovery phase.

Medications

The client having surgery receives medications before, during, and after surgery to achieve specific therapeutic outcomes. Traditionally, all medication orders are cancelled when the client goes to surgery and must be rewritten by the physician when the client returns to the postsurgical care unit.

Preoperative Medications

The surgical client usually is given preoperative medications 45 to 70 minutes before the scheduled surgery. Any delay in administration should be reported promptly to the surgical department. Preoperative medications may also be given in the surgical holding room to produce the desired effects.

A combination of preoperative drugs may be ordered to achieve the desired outcomes with minimal side effects. Such outcomes include sedation, reducing anxiety, inducing amnesia to minimize unpleasant surgical memories, increasing comfort during preoperative procedures, reducing gastric acidity and volume, increasing gastric emptying, decreasing nausea and

vomiting, and reducing the incidence of aspiration by drying oral and respiratory secretions. Table 7–4 outlines commonly prescribed preoperative medications.

Intraoperative Medications

Anesthesia is used to produce unconsciousness, analgesia, reflex loss, and muscle relaxation during a surgical procedure. General anesthesia produces these effects, whereas regional anesthesia results in analgesia, reflex loss, and muscle relaxation but does not cause the client to lose consciousness. An anesthesiologist (physician) or certified registered nurse anesthetist (CRNA) administers the anesthetics during the intraoperative phase of surgery.

GENERAL ANESTHESIA. **General anesthesia** is most commonly administered by inhalation and, to a lesser extent, by the intravenous route. It produces central nervous system depression. As a result, the client loses consciousness and does not perceive pain, skeletal muscles relax, and reflexes diminish.

Advantages to general anesthesia include rapid excretion of the anesthetic agent and prompt reversal of its effects when desired. Additionally, general anesthesia can be used with all age groups and any type of surgical procedure. It produces amnesia.

TABLE 7–4   Preoperative Medications

Generic	Trade	Dose and Route	Action by Category	Nursing Implications
Benzodiazepines Midazolam Diazepam Lorazepam	Versed Valium Ativan	3–5 mg IM 5–2 mg PO 1–4 mg IM or IV	Decreases anxiety and produces sedation to some extent Induces amnesia May induce substantial amnesia	Monitor for respiratory depression, hypotension, drowsiness, and lack of coordination.
Opioid Analgesics Morphine Meperidine	Morphine Demerol	5–15 mg IM 50–150 mg IM	Decreases anxiety, provides analgesia, allows decreased anesthetics	Monitor for respiratory depression, nausea, vomiting, orthostatic hypotension, and pruritus. Smaller doses may be given to frail or older clients.
Antacids Sodium citrate	Bicitra	15–30 mL PO	Increases the pH and reduces volume of gastric fluid; used in clients with GERD and/or trauma	No significant factors in this setting
H$_2$-Receptor Antagonists Cimetidine Famotidine Ranitidine	Tagamet Pepcid Zantac	300 mg IV, IM, or PO 20 mg IV 50 mg IV, IM, or PO	Reduces gastric acid volume and concentration	Monitor for confusion and dizziness in older adults.
Gastric Acid Pump Inhibitors Lansoprazole Omeprazole	Prevacid Prilosec	15–60 mg PO 20–40 mg PO	Suppresses gastric acid secretion	Monitor for dizziness and headache, rash, or thirst.
Antiemetics Metoclopramide Droperidol	Reglan Inapsine	10 mg IV 10–15 mg PO 0.625–2.5 mg IM	Enhances gastric emptying Tranquilizer	Monitor for sedation and extrapyramidal reaction (involuntary movement, muscle tone changes, and abnormal posture).
Anticholinergics Atropine sulfate Glycopyrrolate Scopolamine	Atropine Sulfate Robinul Scopolamine	0.4–0.6 mg IM or IV 0.1–0.3 IM mg or IV 0.4–0.6 mg IM or IV	Reduces oral and respiratory secretions to decrease risk of aspiration; decreases vomiting and laryngospasm	Monitor for confusion, restlessness, and tachycardia. Prepare client to expect a dry mouth.

Disadvantages of general anesthesia include risks associated with circulatory and respiratory depression. Clients with serious respiratory or circulatory diseases, such as emphysema or congestive heart failure, are at greater risk for complications.

The phases of general anesthesia are divided into three distinct categories: induction, maintenance, and emergence. During the induction phase, the client receives the anesthetic agent intravenously or by inhalation. During this phase, airway patency is achieved with endotracheal intubation. The next phase of general anesthesia is maintenance. During this period, the client is positioned, the skin is prepared, and surgery is performed. The anesthesiologist maintains the proper depth of anesthesia while constantly monitoring physiologic parameters such as heart rate, blood pressure, respiratory rate, temperature, and oxygen and carbon dioxide levels. The final phase of anesthesia is the client's emergence from this altered physiologic state. As the anesthetic agents are withdrawn or the effects reversed pharmacologically, the client begins to awaken. The endotracheal tube is removed (extubated) once the client is able to reestablish voluntary breathing. It is critical to ensure airway patency in this period, because extubation may cause bronchospasm or laryngospasm.

REGIONAL ANESTHESIA.   **Regional anesthesia** is a type of local anesthesia in which medication instilled around the nerves blocks transmission of nerve impulses in a particular area. Regional anesthesia produces analgesia, relaxation, and reduced reflexes. The client is awake and conscious during the surgical procedure but does not perceive pain. Regional anesthesia may be classified in several ways:

• Surface or topical anesthesia is applied to the skin or mucous membranes to block nerve impulses at that site. Skin wounds or burns are anesthetized using a cocaine solution, lidocaine (Xylocaine), or benzocaine.

- Local nerve infiltration is achieved by injecting lidocaine or tetracaine around a local nerve to depress nerve sensation over a limited area of the body. This technique may be used when a skin or muscle biopsy is obtained or when a small wound is sutured.
- Nerve blocks are accomplished by injecting an anesthetic agent at the nerve trunk to produce a lack of sensation over a specific area, such as an extremity.
- Epidural blocks are local anesthetic agents injected into the epidural space, outside the dura mater of the spinal cord. This type of intraspinal anesthesia can be used for surgeries of the abdomen and lower extremities.
- Spinal anesthesia is accomplished by injecting a local anesthetic agent into the subarachnoid space. Surgeries of the lower abdomen, perineum, and lower extremities are likely to use this type of regional anesthesia. Leakage of cerebrospinal fluid (CSF) from the needle insertion site may cause reduced CSF pressure and postoperative headaches. Bed rest, hydration, and pressure to the infusion site combat this common side effect.

CONSCIOUS SEDATION. Conscious sedation is described in Box 7–1.

Postoperative Medications

Management of acute postoperative pain by medication follows the principles outlined later in the chapter. For more information on pain management, see the nursing care section on managing acute postoperative pain, and see Chapter 4. ∞

BOX 7–1   ■ Conscious Sedation

An increased number of surgical and diagnostic procedures are being performed using **conscious sedation.** This type of anesthesia provides analgesia and amnesia, but the client remains conscious. The pharmacologic effects are produced by administering a combination of intravenous medications with opioids (such as morphine sulfate, meperidine hydrochloride [Demerol], and fentanyl [Sublimaze]) and sedatives (such as diazepam [Valium] and midazolam [Versed]). During conscious sedation the client is able to independently maintain an open airway. This allows the client to respond to verbal and physical stimulation.

Common adverse side effects include venous thrombosis, phlebitis, local irritation, confusion, drowsiness, hypotension, and apnea. Reversal agents (naloxone hydrochloride [Narcan] and flumazenil [Romazicon]) are used as needed to enhance the safety of conscious sedation.

The American Society of Perianesthesia Nurses (1995) and the Association of Operating Room Nurses (1993) include management and monitoring before, during, and after the procedure using conscious sedation. Included in the standards are knowledge of anatomy, physiology, and complications; physiologic monitoring; use of oxygen delivery devices and airway management; and understanding of legal ramifications of administering or monitoring clients receiving intravenous conscious sedation.

Established, severe pain is more difficult to treat than pain that is at its onset. Therefore, postoperative analgesics should be administered initially at regular intervals to maintain a therapeutic blood level. Administering analgesics as needed (prn) lowers this therapeutic level; delays in the medication administration further increase pain intensity. Therefore, prn administration of analgesics is not recommended in the first 36 to 48 hours postoperatively.

> **PRACTICE ALERT** *Nurses are responsible for assessing clients' pain level and administering pain medication. Work collaboratively with surgeons to schedule postoperative analgesics rather than rely on prn administration orders.* ■

Nonsteroidal anti-inflammatory drugs (NSAIDs) treat mild to moderate postoperative pain. This category of drugs should be given soon after surgery (orally, parenterally, or rectally) along with opioids unless contraindicated. Although NSAIDs may not be sufficient to control pain completely, they allow lower doses of opioid analgesics and, therefore, fewer side effects. NSAIDs can be given safely to older clients, but observe closely for side effects, particularly gastric and renal toxicity.

Opioid analgesics, such as morphine and meperidine (Demerol), are considered the foundation for managing moderate to severe postoperative pain. Opioid dosage requirements vary greatly from one client to another, so the dosage must be individually tailored. Later in the postoperative recovery period, opioid analgesics (oral or intramuscular) may be given prn. In this way, pain relief can be maintained, while the potential for drug side effects is decreased.

Contrary to the belief of many health care providers (including nurses), physical dependence and tolerance to opioid analgesics is uncommon in short-term postoperative use. Additionally, opioid analgesics, when used to treat acute pain, rarely lead to psychologic dependence and addiction.

Older clients tend to be more sensitive to the analgesic effects of opioids, experiencing a higher peak effect with a longer duration of pain control. The Nursing Research box on page 174 provides additional information.

> **PRACTICE ALERT** *Oral analgesia requires a significantly greater dose than parenteral for most analgesics. Teach clients who are being discharged, and their caregivers, the relative strength of oral analgesics. (Caution them to not rely on trade names to gauge effectiveness. Two Tylenol with codeine (30 mg) is equianalgesia to 10 mg parenteral morphine; however, oral Demerol 100 mg does not provide equianalgesia with 10 mg parenteral morphine.)* ■

Surgery

Members of the Surgical Team

Because of the complexity of the intraoperative environment, members of the surgical team must function as a coordinated unit. The surgeon, surgical assistant(s), anesthesiologist or *certified registered nurse anesthetist* (CRNA), *circulating* nurse, and *scrub*

Nursing Research

Evidence-Based Practice for Managing Postoperative Pain in Frail Older Women

As the population continues to age, increasing numbers of older adults are hospitalized for surgical procedures. Older adults, and especially those over age 75, are more likely to have a longer postoperative period of pain, find analgesics less helpful, and have more confusion. It is not known if pain perception in this population is decreased, if pain tolerance is different, or if pain relief is adequate. Zalon (1997) conducted a study to understand postoperative pain from the perspective of frail, older women after surgery. Analysis of data from 16 women revealed three themes: (1) the immediate reality of pain, (2) security, and (3) dealing with pain.

The women in the study found it difficult to put the pain experience into words, suggesting it was a unique and solitary experience. Feeling secure was manifested by seeking comfort and was influenced by trust. The comfort of nursing care was valued, and was facilitated by the nurses' demeanor, words, and actions. The women dealt with pain through endurance, asking for medication for intolerable pain. Other strategies for handling pain included using medication for sleep and lying still.

Implications for Nursing

Findings from this study highlight the importance of assessing pain in postoperative older adults, and asking probing questions if nonverbal cues are different than verbal reports of pain. Establishing trust within the nurse-client relationship is critical to relieving pain. Teaching is necessary to dispel myths about addiction, and to allow clients control and independence so they ask for pain medications. Exploring with older clients their perception of pain, as well as the significance it has for recovery from illness, are necessary elements in providing adequate pain relief and restoring health.

Critical Thinking in Client Care

1. What physiologic changes make pain management more difficult for an 80-year-old client following surgery than for a 30 year old?
2. Your older client says: "I deserved this pain, so I don't want to take anything to make it better." What would be your response and why?
3. A man of Native American descent, age 76, replies that "something doesn't feel right" when asked to rate his pain on a scale of 0 to 10. His pulse is increased and he is protective of his abdominal incision. What could you ask or do to accurately assess his pain?
4. If your grandfather was having surgery tomorrow, what would you like him to be taught about pain management?
5. An independent, 85-year-old woman has a PCA pump for analgesia following major surgery. She continuously presses the pump button, but continues to complain of severe pain. What do you do now?

---

nurse or operating room technician (Figure 7–2 ■) constitute the surgical team. Each member provides specialized skills and is essential to the successful outcome of the surgery. Risks to members of the surgical team from bloodborne pathogens or injury are minimized when the surgical team is well organized and prepared.

The surgeon is the physician performing the procedure. As head of the surgical team, the surgeon is responsible for all medical actions and judgments.

The surgical assistant works closely with the surgeon in performing the operation. The number of assistants varies according to the complexity of the procedure. The assistant may be another physician, a nurse, a physician assistant, or other trained personnel. The assistant performs such duties as exposing the operative site, retracting nearby tissue, sponging and/or suctioning the wound, ligating bleeding vessels, and suturing or helping suture the surgical wound.

The anesthesiologist or CRNA relieves the surgeon of the responsibility for the client's general well-being, thus allowing the surgeon to focus on the technical aspects of the procedure. The anesthesiologist or CRNA evaluates the client preoperatively, administers the anesthesia and other required medications, transfuses blood or other blood products, infuses intravenous fluids, continuously monitors the client's physiologic status, alerts the surgeon to developing problems and treats them as they arise, and supervises the client's recovery in the PACU.

The circulating nurse is a highly experienced registered nurse who coordinates and manages a wide range of activities before, during, and after the surgical procedure. For example,

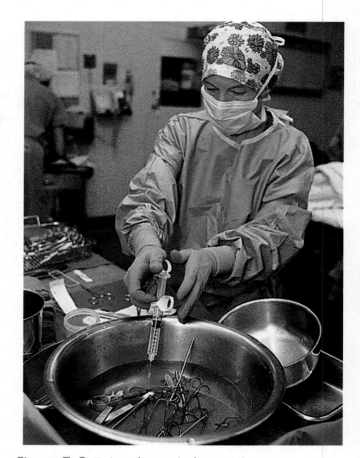

Figure 7–2 ■ A scrub nurse in the operating room.

the circulating nurse oversees the physical aspects of the operating room itself, including the equipment. The circulating nurse also assists with transferring and positioning the client, prepares the client's skin, ensures that no break in aseptic technique occurs, and counts all sponges and instruments. The circulating nurse assists all other team members, including the anesthesiologist or CRNA. Thorough documentation in the surgical area is essential, and the circulating nurse is responsible for documenting intraoperative nursing activities, medications, blood administration, placement of drains and catheters, and length of the procedure. The circulating nurse also formulates a care plan based on physiologic and psychosocial assessments of the client. Finally, the circulating nurse is at all times an advocate for the safety and well-being of the client.

The role of the scrub nurse primarily involves technical skills, manual dexterity, and in-depth knowledge of the anatomic and mechanical aspects of a particular surgery. The scrub nurse handles sutures, instruments, and other equipment immediately adjacent to the sterile field. Although the title implies that the person who performs these duties is a nurse, the role of the scrub nurse may also be assumed by an operating room technician (ORT), depending on hospital policy and the complexity of the surgery.

The role of nurses in surgery continues to evolve to improve client care. In recent years, nurses have begun to specialize within the already specialized field of perioperative nursing. Specialty surgical teams have developed in response to the demands of increasingly complex technical surgeries. For example, a designated open heart surgical team may be responsible for all open heart cases and ordinarily not be involved with other procedures. The use of specialty surgical teams allows nurses to become highly skilled in a particular range of procedures.

Surgical Attire

Strict dress codes are necessary in the surgical department to provide infection control within the operating room suites, reduce cross-contamination between the surgery department and other hospital units or departments, and promote both personnel and client health and safety. Based on research and recommendations by hospital infection control authorities, guidelines for attire differ among surgical facilities. Following institutional guidelines, all personnel in the surgical department must be in proper surgical attire. The design and composition of the surgical attire minimize bacterial shedding, thus reducing wound contamination. The area in the surgical department is divided into *unrestricted, semirestricted,* and *restricted* zones. The unrestricted zones permit access by those in hospital uniforms or street clothes. These areas may also allow limited access for communicating with operating room personnel.

The semirestricted zones require scrub attire, including a scrub suit, shoe covers, and a cap or hood (Figure 7–3 ■). Hallways, work areas, and storage areas are considered semirestricted.

Restricted zones are within operating rooms. Personnel wear masks, sterile gowns, and gloves in addition to appropriate scrub attire (Figure 7–3). The entire surgical attire is changed between procedures or when it becomes soiled or wet.

Figure 7–3 ■ Surgical attire. *A,* Scrub attire includes scrub suit, shoe covers, and cap or hood to cover hair. *B,* Sterile attire includes scrub suit, shoe covers, and cap or hood, plus gown, gloves, and mask.

The Surgical Scrub

The surgical scrub is performed to render hands and arms as clean as possible in preparation for a procedure. All personnel who participate directly in the procedure must perform a surgical scrub with a brush and antimicrobial soap. Skin cannot be rendered sterile, but it can be considered "surgically clean" following the scrub. The purposes of the surgical scrub are to:

- Remove dirt, skin oils, and transient microorganisms from hands and forearms.
- Increase client safety by reducing microorganisms on surgical personnel.
- Leave an antimicrobial residue on the skin to inhibit growth of microbes for several hours.

Following the 5- to 10-minute surgical scrub, hands and arms are dried with sterile towels.

Preparing the Client

Although much preparation has taken place prior to the client's transfer to the surgical department, additional activities such as shaving and positioning may be performed. The skin preparation, which usually includes cleansing the area with a prescribed antimicrobial agent, already may have been performed either by the client or by nursing personnel before the transfer to the surgical department. Additional skin cleansing is performed in the surgical department to further decrease microorganisms on the skin and thereby reduce the possibility of wound infection.

Figure 7–4 ■ Areas to be shaved. *A*, Head surgery. *B*, Abdominal surgery. *C*, Thoracoabdominal surgery. *D*, Gynecologic surgery. *E*, Genitourinary surgery. *F*, Forearm, elbow, or hand surgery. *G*, Hip surgery. *H*, Lower leg or foot surgery.

The surgeon also may order the skin shaved in and around the proposed incision area (Figure 7–4 ■). Shaving may be completed preoperatively, but more often it is performed in the surgical department. The extent of shaving varies. Generally, the area shaved is wider than the planned incision because of the possibility of unexpected extension of the incision. Disposable, sterile supplies are used, in accordance with aseptic techniques. However, the benefit of shaving the incisional site has become controversial. Physical trauma to the shaved area can weaken the client's defense against organisms, thus increasing the chance of wound infection. An altered body image

also may result from the physiologic trauma of a surgical shave, particularly if the shave involves the head or groin area. Hospital policy and surgeon preference should be followed.

Preparing the client for surgery also includes **positioning** the client on the operating table. Table 7–5 shows frequently used positions and describes corresponding surgical procedures and possible adverse effects. Positioning exposes the operative site and gives access for anesthesia administration. Proper positioning is imperative to prevent injury to the client. Pressure, rubbing, and/or shearing forces can cause injury to the tissue over bony prominences. If positioning

TABLE 7-5 Common Surgical Positions

Position and Use	Possible Adverse Effects and Nursing Interventions
(a) The *dorsal recumbent* (or *supine*) *position* is used for many abdominal surgeries (e.g., colostomy and herniorrhaphy) as well as for some thoracic surgeries (e.g., open heart surgery) and some surgeries on the extremities.	This position may cause excessive pressure on posterior bony prominences, such as the back of the head, scapulae, sacrum, and heels. Pad these areas with soft materials. To avoid compression of blood vessels and sluggish circulation, ensure that the knees are not flexed. Use trochanter rolls or other padding to avoid internal or external rotation of the hips and shoulders.
(b) The *semisitting position* is used for surgeries on the thyroid and neck areas.	This position can lead to postural hypotension and venous pooling in the legs. It may promote skin breakdown on the buttocks. Sciatic nerve injury is possible. Assess for hypotension. Ensure that knees are not sharply flexed. Use soft padding to prevent nerve compression.
(c) The *prone position* is used for spinal fusions and removal of hemorrhoids.	This position causes pressure on the face, knees, thighs, anterior ankles, and toes. Pad bony prominences, and support the feet under the ankles. To promote optimum respiratory function, raise the client's chest and abdomen, and support with padding. Corneal abrasion could occur if the eyes are not closed or are insufficiently padded.
(d) The *lateral chest position* is used for some thoracic surgeries, as well as hip replacements.	This may cause excessive pressure on the bony prominences on the side on which the client is positioned. Ensure adequate padding and support, especially of the downside arm. The weight of the upper leg may cause peroneal nerve injury on the downside leg. Both legs must therefore be padded.
(e) The *lithotomy position* is used for gynecologic, perineal, or rectal surgeries.	This position causes an 18% decrease (from a standing position) in vital capacity of the lungs. Monitor respirations, and assess for hypoxia and dyspnea. The lithotomy position can lead to joint damage, peroneal nerve damage, and damage to peripheral blood vessels. To avoid injury, ensure adequate padding, and manipulate both legs into the stirrups simultaneously.
(f) The *jackknife position* is used for proctologic surgeries, such as removal of hemorrhoids, and for some spinal surgeries.	This position causes a 12% decrease (from a standing position) in vital capacity of the lungs. Monitor respirations, and assess for hypoxia and dyspnea. In this position, the greatest pressure is felt at the bends in the table. Therefore, the client is supported with pads at the groin and knees, as well as at the ankles. Padding of the chest and knees helps prevent skin breakdown. Padding and proper positioning help prevent pressure on the ear, the neck, and the nerves of the upper arm.

causes normal joint range of motion to be exceeded, injury to muscles and joints can occur. Improper positioning also can lead to sensory and motor dysfunction, resulting in nerve damage. Pressure on peripheral blood vessels can decrease venous return to the heart and negatively affect the client's blood pressure. Additionally, oxygenation of the blood can be decreased if the client is not properly positioned to promote lung expansion.

Because the anesthetized client cannot respond to discomfort, it is the surgical team's responsibility to position the client not only for the best surgical advantage but also for client safety and comfort. The circulating nurse refers to hospital policy, the surgeon's preference, and the client's history to ensure optimal positioning, and continuously assesses the client.

Intraoperative Awareness

Prior to induction of anesthesia, the circulating nurse establishes rapport with the client to assess the client's psychologic status. This assessment is continued throughout the surgical procedure. After anesthetic medications have been given, the client may appear oblivious to the surroundings; however, studies have shown that the client's awareness during the intraoperative period may be greater than once believed. Intraoperative awareness is the client's subconscious awareness of what is being said and done during surgery. Although most clients do not consciously remember what happened or what was said, psychologic trauma can result. Because there is no reliable method of preventing this phenomenon, conversations during surgery should be professional.

PRACTICE ALERT *Do not say anything while the client is unconscious that would be inappropriate if the client were awake. Maintain a respectful, professional demeanor throughout the operative period.* ■

Special Considerations for the Older Adult

Because of cardiovascular and tissue changes that result from aging, surgeries longer than 2 hours place the older adult at increased risk for complications. The older adult is more prone to hypotension, hypothermia, and hypoxemia resulting from anesthesia and the cool temperature in the operating room.

Positioning may also cause complications in the older adult. Intraoperative positioning of arthritic joints can cause postoperative joint pain unrelated to the operative site. Also, the longer the surgery, the greater the chance of decubitus ulcer (pressure sore) formation. The older client is at increased risk for developing pressure sores because of decreased subcutaneous fat tissue and reduced peripheral circulation.

Finally, the older adult often has some degree of hearing and/or visual impairment. These impairments coupled with a strange environment can make the operating room a frightening, disorienting place. By effectively communicating with the client, the nurse can provide support and reassurance to minimize these factors. To decrease confusion and assist in communication, hearing aids and glasses should be used when appropriate and possible.

Dietary Management

Wound healing after surgery depends on adequate nutritional intake. During the immediate postoperative phase, dietary intake is withheld until evidence of peristalsis is found and the client can tolerate liquids without nausea and vomiting. While intravenous fluids maintain hydration and electrolyte balance, they do not provide nutrition. Some clients believe that intravenous fluids are the same as intravenous "feeding," but this is a myth. Unless balanced nutrition through the gastrointestinal intake can be reestablished within 3 to 4 days, parenteral hyperalimentation is critical for homeostasis and wound healing.

- Protein and calories are needed for wound healing and recovery from surgery.
- Low-fat, high-fiber diets are important for chronic cardiovascular fitness, but are contraindicated in the wound healing phase following surgery.
- Failure to use the gastrointestinal tract for more than 4 or 5 days allows the intestinal mucosa to atrophy, putting the client at risk for infection.

Fluid administered through peripheral veins must be isotonic or only moderately hypertonic to prevent sclerosing the small peripheral veins. Solutions of 10% dextrose are tolerable peripherally for a short time but do not provide adequate calories for healing and maintenance. To provide adequate nutrition, central vein access must be established and solutions must be prepared with protein, carbohydrates, lipids, vitamins, and minerals. This is important for clients who have extended recovery periods without eating after surgery.

Parenteral nutrition has serious risks. Central vein access may cause infection and sepsis. Normal stimulation to the intestinal tract is lost when the parenteral approach is used alone. Using the gut is better than using the vein because it (1) prevents intestinal atrophy, which results in a very thin bowel wall poorly suited to absorb nutrients; (2) prevents bacteria and inert particles from translocating across the bowel lining into the bloodstream; (3) introduces fats and other large particles into the lymphatic circulation and stimulates the immune system; and (4) is safer and far less expensive than parenteral nutritional support (Hiemburger & Weinsier, 1997). Education and counseling to support adequate nutritional intake should be ongoing throughout the preoperative and postoperative period.

NURSING CARE

The following section will discuss nursing care in each of the three phases of surgery. A case study at the end of the section follows one client through the postoperative experience, bringing this information together. Perioperative nursing diagnoses are provided in Box 7–2 to assist in identifying the needs of the surgical client. This is not an exhaustive list, but it can serve as a guide in identifying possible nursing diagnoses.

Preoperative Nursing Care

The client's response to planned surgery varies greatly. When planning and implementing nursing care, consider individual

BOX 7–2 ■ Examples of Perioperative Nursing Diagnoses

Preoperative
- Knowledge, Deficient
- Anxiety
- Fear
- Anticipatory Grieving
- Decisional Conflict
- Coping, Ineffective
- Sexuality Patterns, Ineffective
- Sleep Pattern, Disturbed
- Thought Processes, Disturbed
- Family Processes, Interrupted

Intraoperative
- Knowledge, Deficient
- Anxiety
- Fear
- Airway Clearance, Ineffective
- Aspiration, Risk for
- Decreased Cardiac Output
- Hypothermia
- Infection, Risk for
- Thought Processes, Disturbed
- Gas Exchange, Impaired
- Urinary Elimination, Impaired
- Fluid Volume, Deficient
- Fluid Volume, Excessive
- Verbal Communication, Impaired

Postoperative
- Knowledge, Deficient
- Pain
- Breathing Pattern, Ineffective
- Airway Clearance, Ineffective
- Skin Integrity, Impaired
- Nutrition Imbalanced: Less Than Body Requirements
- Sexuality Patterns, Ineffective
- Sleep Pattern, Disturbed
- Fatigue
- Urinary Retention
- Urinary Elimination, Impaired
- Adjustment, Impaired
- Body Image, Disturbed
- Physical Mobility, Impaired
- Activity Intolerance, Risk for
- Injury, Risk for
- Self-Care, Deficient
- Health Maintenance, Ineffective
- Diversional Activity, Deficient
- Social Isolation

psychologic and physical differences, the type of surgery, and the circumstances surrounding the need for surgery. A thorough nursing assessment is needed to determine the most appropriate care for each client undergoing surgery.

Before planning and implementing care for the surgical client, gather assessment information by taking a nursing history and performing a physical examination. Use this information to establish baseline data, identify physical needs, determine teaching needs and psychologic support for the client and family, and prioritize nursing care. The type of surgical procedure directs the assessment and intervention planned by the nurse.

PRACTICE ALERT *Be sure to assess information about use of over-the-counter medications including herbal supplements. These drugs can interact with medications administered in the perioperative period. ■*

Surgery is a significant and stressful event. Regardless of the nature of the surgery (whether major or minor), the client and family will be anxious. The degree of anxiety they will feel is not necessarily proportional to the magnitude of the surgical procedure. For example, a client scheduled to have a biopsy to rule out cancer, which is considered minor surgery, may be more anxious than a client undergoing gallbladder removal, which is considered major surgery.

The nurse's ability to listen actively to both verbal and nonverbal messages is imperative to establishing a trusting relationship with the client and family. Therapeutic communication can help the client and family identify fears and concerns. The nurse can then plan nursing interventions and supportive care to reduce the client's anxiety level and assist the client to cope successfully with the stressors encountered during the perioperative period.

Preoperative Client and Family Teaching

Client teaching is an essential nursing responsibility in the preoperative period. Client education and emotional support have a positive effect on the client's physical and psychologic well-being, both before and after surgery. In an analysis of 102 studies, surgical clients receiving client education and/or supportive interventions had less pain and anxiety, experienced fewer complications, were discharged sooner, were more satisfied with their care, and returned to normal activities sooner than clients who did not receive this type of care. These positive outcomes may be attributed in part to the sense of control the client gains through the nurse's teaching.

Client teaching should begin as soon as the client learns of the upcoming surgery. Teaching may begin as early as in the physician's office or at the time of preadmission testing. Although education continues during postoperative care, most teaching is done before surgery, because pain and the effects of anesthesia can greatly diminish the client's ability to learn.

The amount of information desired varies from client to client. Therefore, assess the client's need for and readiness to accept information. The teaching will be directed in part by the particular surgical procedure that is being performed. The information in Box 7–3 is relevant to most clients undergoing major surgery.

In addition to teaching the client and family about measures that will decrease the risk of complications, provide other preoperative information to prepare the client and family for surgery. This information should include the following:

- Diagnostic tests—reasons and preparations
- Arrival time if surgery is scheduled in early morning
- Preparations for the day of surgery after midnight prior to a morning surgery, skin preparation, indwelling catheter or bladder elimination, start of intravenous infusion, preoperative medication, handling of valuables (rings, watch, money)

BOX 7–3 ■ **Preoperative Client Teaching**

DIAPHRAGMATIC BREATHING EXERCISE

Diaphragmatic (abdominal) breathing exercises are taught to the client who is at risk for developing pulmonary complications, such as atelectasis or pneumonia. Risk factors for pulmonary complications include general anesthesia, abdominal or thoracic surgery, history of smoking, chronic lung disease, obesity, and advanced age.

In diaphragmatic breathing, the client inspires deeply while allowing the abdomen to expand outward. On expiration, the abdomen contracts inward as air from the lungs is expelled.

1. Explain to the client that the diaphragm is a muscle that makes up the floor of the abdominal cavity and assists in breathing. The purpose of diaphragmatic breathing is to promote lung expansion and ventilation and enhance blood oxygenation.
2. Position the client in a high or semi-Fowler's position (see figure below).
3. Ask the client to place the hands lightly on the abdomen.
4. Instruct the client to breathe in deeply through the nose, allowing the chest and abdomen to expand.
5. Have the client hold the breath for a count of 5.
6. Tell the client to exhale completely through pursed (puckered) lips, allowing the chest and abdomen to deflate.

7. Have the client repeat the exercise five times consecutively.

Encourage the client to perform diaphragmatic breathing exercises every 1 to 2 waking hours, depending on the client's needs and institutional protocol.

COUGHING EXERCISE

Coughing exercises are also taught to the client who is at risk for developing pulmonary complications. The purpose of coughing is to loosen, mobilize, and remove pulmonary secretions. Splinting the incision decreases the physical and psychologic discomfort associated with coughing.

1. Assist the client in following steps 1 through 4 for diaphragmatic breathing.
2. Ask the client to splint the incision with interlocked hand or pillow (see figure below).
3. Tell the client to take three deep breaths and then cough forcefully.
4. Have the client repeat the exercise five times consecutively every 2 hours while awake, taking short rest periods between coughs, if necessary.

Diaphragmatic breathing exercise.

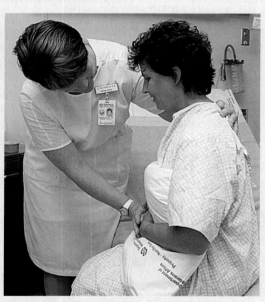

Splinting abdomen while coughing.

- Sedative/hypnotic medication to be taken the night before surgery to promote rest and sleep
- Counseling on whether to take significant medications the morning of surgery
- Informed consent
- Expected timetable for surgery and the recovery room
- Transfer to the surgery department
- Location of the surgical waiting room
- Transfer to recovery room
- Anticipated postoperative routine and devices or equipment (drains, tubes, equipment for IV infusions, oxygen or humidifying mask, dressings, splints, casts)
- Plans for postoperative pain control

PRACTICE ALERT *Researchers report that many patients experience unnecessarily long preoperative fasts.* ■

The American Society of Anesthesiologists guidelines for preoperative fasting in healthy patients undergoing elective procedures are available online at www.asahq.org/practice/npo/npoguide.html. Withdrawal from caffeine in beverages such as coffee or colas may cause headaches and irritability. Dehydration, hypovolemia, and hypoglycemia are other recognized side effects. Thirst, worry, and hunger are reported by patients to be related to fasting. Fasting does not ensure that the stomach will be empty or that the gastric contents will be less acidic.

BOX 7–3   ■ Preoperative Client Teaching (continued)

LEG, ANKLE, AND FOOT EXERCISES

Leg exercises are taught to the client who is at risk for developing thrombophlebitis (inflammation of a vein, which is associated with the formation of blood clots). Risk factors for developing thrombophlebitis include decreased mobility preoperatively and/or postoperatively; a history of difficulties with peripheral circulation; and cardiovascular, pelvic, or lower extremity surgeries.

The purpose of leg exercises is to promote venous blood return from the extremities. As the leg muscles contract and relax, blood is pumped back to the heart, promoting cardiac output and reducing venous stasis. These exercises also maintain muscle tone and range of motion, which facilitate early ambulation.

Teach the client to perform the following exercises while lying in bed:

1. Muscle pumping exercise: Contract and relax calf and thigh muscles at least 10 times consecutively.
2. Leg exercises:
   a. Bend the knee and raise it toward the chest (see figure below).
   b. Straighten out leg and hold for a few seconds before lowering the leg back to the bed.
   c. Repeat exercise five times consecutively prior to alternating to the other foot.
3. Ankle and foot exercises:
   a. Rotate both ankles by making complete circles, first to the right and then to the left (see figure below).
   b. Repeat five times and then relax.
   c. With feet together, point toes toward the head and then to the foot of the bed (see figure below).
   d. Repeat this pumping action 10 times, and then relax.

Leg exercises.

Encourage the client to perform leg, ankle, and foot exercises every 1 to 2 hours while awake, depending on the client's needs and ambulatory status, the physician's preference, and institutional protocol.

TURNING IN BED

The client who is at risk for circulatory, respiratory, or gastrointestinal dysfunction following surgery is taught to turn in bed. Although this may be a simple task prior to surgery, after surgery (particularly after abdominal surgery) the client may find it a difficult procedure. To make the procedure more comfortable, the client may need to splint the incision by using the hand placed on a small pillow or blanket. Additionally, the client should be taught that analgesics can be given to ease postoperative discomfort involved with turning. Encourage the client to turn every 2 hours while awake.

1. Tell the client to grasp the side rail toward the direction to be turned, to rest the opposite foot on the mattress, and to bend the knee.
2. Instruct the client to roll over in one smooth motion by pulling on the side rail while pushing off with the bent knee.
3. Pillows may need to be positioned behind the client's back to help the client maintain a side-lying position. The older client may also need padding over pressure points between the knees and ankles to decrease the chance of decubitus ulcer formation from pressure.

Ankle and foot exercises.

Preoperative Client Preparation

A preoperative surgical checklist serves as an outline for finalizing preparation of the client for surgery in most institutions. Complete the checklist before the client is transported to surgery. Nursing responsibilities the day of surgery are as follows:

- Assist with bathing, grooming, and changing into operating room gown.
- Ensure that the client takes nothing by mouth (NPO). Provide additional teaching, and reinforce prior teaching.
- Remove nail polish, lipstick, and makeup to facilitate circulatory assessment during and after surgery.

- Ensure that identification, blood, and allergy bands are correct, legible, and secure.
- Remove hair pins and jewelry; a wedding ring may be worn if it is removed from the finger, covered with gauze, and then taped to the finger.
- Complete skin or bowel preparation as ordered.
- Insert an indwelling catheter, intravenous line, or nasogastric tube as ordered.
- Remove dentures, artificial eye, and contact lenses, and store them in a safe place.
- Leave a hearing aid in place if the client cannot hear without it, and notify the operating room nurse.

- Verify that the informed consent has been signed prior to administering preoperative medications.
- Verify that the client's height and weight are recorded in the chart (for dosage of anesthesia).
- Verify that all ordered diagnostic test reports are in the chart.
- Have the client empty the bladder immediately before the preoperative medication is administered (unless an indwelling catheter is in place).
- Administer preoperative medication as scheduled (refer to "Preoperative Medications" earlier in the chapter).
- Ensure the safety of the client once the medication has been given by placing the client on bed rest with raised side rails and by placing the call light within reach.
- Obtain and record vital signs.
- Provide ongoing supportive care to the client and the client's family.
- Document all preoperative care in the appropriate location, such as the preoperative surgical checklist, the medication record, or the narrative preoperative nursing notes.
- Verify with the surgical personnel the client's identity, and verify that all client information is documented appropriately.
- Help the surgical personnel transfer the client from the bed to the gurney.
- Prepare the client's room for postoperative care, including making the surgical bed and ensuring that the anticipated supplies and equipment are in the room.

Intraoperative Nursing Care

The intraoperative phase of surgery begins when the client enters the operating room and ends when the client is transferred to the postanesthesia care unit (PACU). Nursing care in this phase focuses on keeping the client and the environment safe and providing physiologic monitoring and psychologic support. Circulating nurses and scrub nurses, according to specific role definitions, support and care for the patient and assist the surgeons.

PRACTICE ALERT *Objects on the sterile drape are considered sterile. Remain a minimum of 12 inches away from draped tables and sterile fields to avoid contamination if you are not attired in sterile gown and gloves.* ■

Postoperative Nursing Care
Immediate Postoperative Care

Immediate postoperative care begins when the client has been transferred from the operating room to the PACU. The nurse monitors the client's vital signs and surgical site to determine the response to the surgical procedure and to detect significant changes. Assessing mental status and level of consciousness is another ongoing nursing responsibility, and the client may require repeated orientation to time, place, and person. Emotional support also is essential, because the client is in a vulnerable and dependent position. Assessing and evaluating hydration status by monitoring intake and output is crucial to detecting cardiovascular or renal complications. In addition, the PACU nurse assesses the client's pain

level. Careful administration of analgesics provides comfort without compounding the potential side effects from the anesthesia.

Care When the Client Is Stable

After being stabilized and awake, the client is transferred to his or her room. The PACU nurse communicates information about the client's condition and postoperative orders to the floor nurse prior to the client's arrival. This prepares the floor nurse for additional problems or needed equipment.

Immediate and continuing assessment is essential to detect and/or prevent complications. In documenting assessment findings, the nurse completes a flow record of the individual client's situation. Baseline data are obtained and compared with preoperative data. A postoperative head-to-toe assessment includes but may not be limited to the following:

- General appearance
- Vital signs
- Level of consciousness
- Emotional status
- Quantity of respirations
- Skin color and temperature
- Discomfort/pain
- Nausea/vomiting
- Type of intravenous fluids and flow rate
- Dressing site
- Drainage on the dressing and/or bed linen
- Urinary output (catheter or ability to urinate)
- Ability to move all extremities

The hospital policy or physician's orders dictate the frequency of follow-up assessments. After major surgery, the nurse generally assesses the client every 15 minutes during the first hour and, if the client is stable, every 30 minutes for the next 2 hours, and then every hour during the subsequent 4 hours. Assessments are then carried out every 4 hours, subject to change according to the client's condition and protocol for the particular surgical procedure. It is critically important to inform the surgeon immediately if the assessment reveals any signs of impending shock or other life-threatening changes.

After carrying out the initial assessment and ensuring the client's safety by lowering the bed, raising the side rails, and placing the call light within reach, the nurse notes the physician's postoperative orders. These orders guide the nurse in the care of the postoperative client. For example, the orders specify activity level, diet, medications for pain and nausea, antibiotics, continuation of preoperative medications, frequency of vital sign assessments, administration of intravenous fluids, and laboratory tests such as hemoglobin and potassium level. In most institutions, orders written prior to surgery must be reordered following surgery because the client's condition is presumed to have changed.

Common Postoperative Complications

Several factors place the client at risk for postoperative complications. Nursing care before, during, and after surgery is aimed at preventing and/or minimizing the effects of these complications.

Preoperative care and teaching to decrease postoperative complications have been discussed. Let us now address postoperative cardiovascular, respiratory, and wound complications, and problems associated with elimination.

Cardiovascular Complications

Common postoperative cardiovascular complications include shock, hemorrhage, deep venous thrombosis, and pulmonary embolism.

SHOCK.   Shock is a life-threatening postoperative complication. It results from an insufficient blood flow to vital organs, an inability to use oxygen and nutrients, or the inability to rid tissues of waste material. Hypovolemic shock, the most common type in the postoperative client, results from a decrease in circulating fluid volume. Decreased fluid volume develops with blood or plasma loss or, less commonly, from severe prolonged vomiting or diarrhea. Symptoms vary according to the severity of the shock; the greater the loss of fluid volume, the more severe the symptoms. Chapter 6 ⊖⊙ provides a detailed discussion of nursing care of the client with various types of shock.

HEMORRHAGE.   Hemorrhage is an excessive loss of blood. A concealed hemorrhage occurs internally from a blood vessel that is no longer sutured or cauterized or from a drainage tube that has eroded a blood vessel. An obvious hemorrhage occurs externally from a dislodged or ill-formed clot at the wound. Hemorrhage also may result from abnormalities in the blood's ability to clot; these abnormalities may result from a pathologic condition, or they may be a side effect of medications.

Hemorrhage from a venous source oozes out quickly and is dark red, whereas an arterial hemorrhage is characterized by bright red spurts of blood pulsating with each heartbeat. Whether the hemorrhage is from a venous or an arterial source, hypovolemic shock will occur if sufficient blood is lost from the circulation.

Common assessment with hemorrhage depends on the amount and rate of blood loss. Restlessness and anxiety are observed in the early stage of hemorrhage. Frank bleeding will be present if the hemorrhage is external. The client will have symptoms characteristic of shock.

Care of the client who is hemorrhaging centers around stopping the bleeding and replenishing the circulating blood volume. Nursing care includes providing care for shock and one or more of the following:

- Applying one or more sterile gauze pads and a snug pressure dressing to the area
- Applying pressure with gloved hands (may be necessary for severe external bleeding)
- Preparing client and family for emergency surgery (in severe situations when bleeding cannot be stopped)

DEEP VEIN THROMBOSIS.   Deep venous thrombosis (DVT) is the formation of a thrombus (blood clot) in association with inflammation in deep veins. This complication most often occurs in the lower extremities of the postoperative client. It may

result from the combination of several factors, including trauma during surgery, pressure applied under the knees, and sluggish blood flow during and after surgery. Clients particularly at risk for developing DVT include those who are over age 40 and who:

- Have undergone orthopedic surgery to lower extremities; urologic, gynecologic, or obstetric surgeries; or neurosurgery.
- Have varicose veins.
- Have a history of thrombophlebitis or pulmonary emboli.
- Are obese.
- Have an infection.
- Have a malignancy.

Common assessment findings reveal pain or cramping in the involved calf or thigh. Redness and edema of the entire extremity may occur along with a slightly elevated temperature. The client may have a positive Homans' sign (pain in the calf on dorsiflexion of the affected foot).

Nursing care of the client with DVT focuses on preventing a portion of the clot from dislodging and becoming an embolus (traveling blood clot) circulating to the heart, brain, or lungs; preventing other clots from forming; and supporting the client's own physiologic mechanism for dissolving clots. Nursing care includes the following measures:

- Administer anticoagulants and analgesics as prescribed. (NSAIDs are not usually given along with anticoagulants, because doing so increases the anticoagulant effects.)
- Monitor laboratory values for clotting times.
- Maintain bed rest and keep affected extremity at or above heart level.
- Apply thigh-high antiemboli stockings or devices to stimulate venous return.
- Ensure that the affected area is not rubbed or massaged.
- Apply heat as prescribed.
- Record bilateral calf or thigh circumferences every shift.
- Teach and support the client and family.
- Assess color and temperature of involved extremity every shift.

PULMONARY EMBOLISM.   A pulmonary embolism is a dislodged blood clot or other substance that lodges in a pulmonary artery. For the postoperative client with DVT, the threat that a portion of the thrombus may dislodge from the vein wall and travel to the lung, heart, or brain is a constant concern. Early detection of this potentially life-threatening complication depends on the nurse's astute, continuing assessment of the postoperative client.

Common assessment findings of the client experiencing a pulmonary embolism include mild to moderate dyspnea, chest pain, diaphoresis, anxiety, restlessness, rapid respirations and pulse, dysrhythmias, cough, and cyanosis. The severity of the symptoms is determined by the degree of pulmonary vascular blockage. Sudden death can occur if a major pulmonary artery becomes completely blocked.

Stabilizing respiratory and cardiovascular functioning while preventing the formation of additional emboli is of utmost importance in the care of the client with a pulmonary embolism. Nursing care includes the following measures:

- Immediately notify the physician and nursing supervisor.
- Frequently assess and record general condition and vital signs.
- Maintain the client on bed rest, and keep the head of the bed elevated.
- Provide oxygen as ordered and monitor pulse oximetry.
- Administer prescribed intravenous fluids to maintain fluid balance while preventing fluid overload.
- Administer prescribed anticoagulants.
- Maintain comfort by administering analgesics and sedatives (use caution to prevent respiratory depression).
- Provide supportive measures for the client and family.

Refer to Chapter 36 for a detailed discussion of pulmonary embolism.

Respiratory Complications

Common postoperative respiratory complications include pneumonia and atelectasis.

PNEUMONIA. Pneumonia is an inflammation of lung tissue. Inflammation is caused either by a microbial infection or by a foreign substance in the lung, which leads to an infection. Numerous factors may be involved in the development of pneumonia, including aspiration infection, retained pulmonary secretions, failure to cough deeply, and impaired cough reflex and decreased mobility.

Common assessment findings of the client with pneumonia are as follows:

- High fever
- Rapid pulse and respirations
- Chills (may be present initially)
- Productive cough (may be present depending on the type of pneumonia)
- Dyspnea
- Chest pain
- Crackles and wheezes

Treating the pulmonary infection, supporting the client's respiratory efforts, promoting lung expansion, and preventing the organisms' spread are the goals in the care of the client with pneumonia. Nursing care includes the following measures:

- Obtain sputum specimens for culture and sensitivity testing.
- Position client with the head of the bed elevated.
- Encourage the client to turn, cough, and perform deep-breathing exercises at least every 2 hours.
- Assist with incentive spirometry, intermittent positive pressure breathing (IPPB), and/or nebulizer treatments as ordered.
- Ambulate client as condition permits and as prescribed.
- Administer oxygen as ordered.
- Assess vital signs, breath sounds, and general condition.
- Maintain hydration to help liquefy pulmonary secretions.
- Administer antibiotics, expectorants, antipyretics, and analgesics as ordered.
- Provide or assist with frequent oral hygiene.

- Prevent the spread of microorganisms by teaching proper disposal of tissues, covering mouth when coughing, and good handwashing technique.
- Provide supportive measures for the client and family.

Chapter 36 provides a detailed discussion of pneumonia.

ATELECTASIS. Atelectasis is an incomplete expansion or collapse of lung tissue resulting in inadequate ventilation and retention of pulmonary secretions. Common assessment findings include dyspnea, diminished breath sounds over the affected area, anxiety, restlessness, crackles, and cyanosis.

Promoting lung expansion and systemic oxygenation of tissues is a goal in the care of the client with atelectasis. Nursing care includes:

- Positioning the client with the head of bed elevated.
- Administering oxygen as prescribed.
- Encouraging coughing, turning, and deep breathing every 2 hours.
- Ambulating the client as condition permits and as prescribed.
- Assisting with incentive spirometry or other pulmonary exercises, such as inflating a balloon, as ordered.
- Administering analgesics as prescribed.
- Promoting hydration.
- Providing supportive measures to the client and family.

Wound Complications

Discussion of the complications associated with surgical wounds follows an overview of wound healing, wound drainage, and nursing care of wounds.

Wounds heal by either *primary, secondary,* or *tertiary intention* (Figure 7–5 ■). Healing by primary intention takes place when the wound is uncomplicated and clean and has sustained little tissue loss. The edges of the incision are well approximated (have come together well) with sutures or staples. This type of surgical incision heals quickly, and very little scarring is expected.

Secondary intention refers to the healing that occurs when the wound is large, gaping, and irregular. Tissue loss prevents wound edges from approximating; therefore, granulation fills in the wound. This type of wound takes longer to heal, is more prone to infection, and develops more scar tissue.

If enough time passes before a wound is sutured, healing by tertiary intention occurs. Infection is more likely to take place. Because the wound edges are not approximated, tissue is regenerated by the granulation process. Closure of the wound results in a wide scar.

From the time the surgical incision is made until the wound is completely healed, all wounds progress through four stages of healing. However, healing time varies according to many factors, such as age, nutritional status, general health, and the type and location of the wound. Figure 7–5 also provides a summary of the stages of wound healing.

Wound drainage (exudate) results from the inflammatory process in the first two stages of wound healing. The drainage is from the rich blood supply that surrounds the wound tissue and is composed of escaped fluid and cells. The drainage is described as serous, sanguineous, or purulent.

Stages of Wound Healing

- *Stage I: from surgery through day 2.* Inflammatory process occurs to prepare the surrounding tissue for healing. Blood vessels constrict, and clotting occurs. Vasodilation follows, bringing more blood, white blood cells, and fibroplastin to the wound site. Epithelial cells begin to form and reestablish blood flow in the wound tissue. A mild temperature elevation is normal.
- *Stage II: day 3 through day 14 following surgery.* Fewer white blood cells are present. Collagen tissue forms in the wound tissue. Granulation tissue, red with a rich blood supply, is established.
- *Stage III: day 15 to week 6 following surgery.* Collagen fibers continue to strengthen the wound. As the blood supply decreases, the scar tissue appears pink and somewhat raised.
- *Stage IV: several months to a year following surgery.* As the wound tissue constricts, the scar becomes flat, smaller, and white.

Primary intention

Clean incision   Early suture   "Hairline" scar

Secondary intention

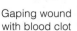

Gaping wound   Granulation tissue   Large scar
with blood clot   fills in wound

Tertiary intention

Contaminated wound   Granulation tissue   Closure with
                                                    wide scar

Figure 7–5 ■ Wound healing by primary, secondary, and tertiary intention.

- Serous drainage contains mostly the clear serous portion of the blood. The drainage appears clear or slightly yellow and is thin in consistency.
- Sanguineous drainage contains a combination of serum and red blood cells and has a thick, reddish appearance. This is the most common type of drainage from a noncomplicated surgical wound.
- Purulent drainage is composed of white blood cells, tissue debris, and bacteria. Purulent drainage is the result of infection and tends to be of a thicker consistency, with various colors specific to the type of organism. It also may have an unpleasant odor.

Box 7–4 describes and illustrates various types of wound drainage devices. These devices decrease pressure in the wound area by removing excess fluid, which promotes healing and decreases complications.

Nursing care of the postoperative client with a surgical wound focuses on preventing and monitoring for wound complications. The nurse assumes a leading role in supporting the wound healing process, providing emotional support to the client and teaching wound care to the client.

Common assessment findings of an infected wound include purulent, odorous discharge and redness, warmth, and edema around the edges of the incision. Additionally, the client may have a fever, chills, and increased respiratory and pulse rates. Nursing care includes the following measures:

- Maintain medical asepsis (e.g., by using a good handwashing technique).
- Follow Centers for Disease Control and Prevention (CDC) guidelines for wound care.
- Observe aseptic technique during dressing changes and handling of tubes and drains.
- Assess vital signs, especially temperature.
- Evaluate the characteristics of wound discharge (color, odor, and amount).
- Assess the condition of the incision (approximation of the edges, sutures, staples, or drains).
- Clean, irrigate, and pack the wound in the prescribed manner. Sterile normal saline is often prescribed; povidone-iodine (Betadine) is no longer recommended for wound care.
- Maintain the client's hydration and nutritional status.
- Culture the wound prior to beginning antibiotic therapy.
- Administer antibiotics and antipyretics as prescribed.
- Provide supportive measures to client and family.

Dehiscence is a separation in the layers of the incisional wound (Figure 7–6A ■). Treatment depends on the extent of wound disruption. If the dehiscence is extensive, the incision must be resutured in surgery. **Evisceration** is the protrusion of body organs from a wound dehiscence (Figure 7–6B). These serious complications may result from delayed wound healing or may occur immediately following surgery. They also may occur after forceful straining (coughing, sneezing, or vomiting). When dehiscence occurs, immediately cover the wound with a sterile dressing moistened with normal saline. Emergency surgery is performed to repair these conditions.

BOX 7-4 ■ Wound Drainage Devices ■

A Penrose drain, used for passive wound drainage, promotes healing from the inside to the outside (see figure *A* below). The use of the drain decreases the chance of abscess formation. The safety pin in the Penrose drain prevents the exposed end from slipping down into the wound. Wound care focuses on cleaning around the drain with a prescribed solution, such as sterile normal saline, and replacing the precut gauze dressing as necessary to keep the surrounding skin dry and encourage further drainage. An absorbent dressing is placed over the drain and gauze (not shown).

Wound suction devices promote drainage of fluid from the incision site, decreasing pressure on healing tissues and reducing abscess formation. Shown are the Jackson-Pratt and Hemovac wound suction devices (see figures *B* and *C* below).

The frequency with which the nurse empties the device depends on the time elapsed since surgery, type of surgery, amount of drainage, and hospital policy. For example, immediately after surgery the nurse may empty the device every 15 to 60 minutes. With time, as drainage decreases, the device is emptied every 2 to 4 hours (per hospital policy). Amount, color, consistency, and odor of drainage are documented.

Usually, the nurse removes the drain on the second to fourth day after surgery (depending on hospital policy). Removal causes minor client discomfort. The drain site is cleaned, and a sterile dressing is applied.

Wound drainage devices. *A,* Penrose passive wound drainage device. *B,* Jackson-Pratt wound suction device. *C,* Hemovac wound suction device.

Either the nurse or physician removes sutures or staples after the wound has healed sufficiently (usually 5 to 10 days after surgery). Removal is performed using medical aseptic technique. Additional support may be provided to the incision by applying strips of tape (or Steri-Strips) as directed by institutional policy or by the physician.

Complications Associated with Elimination

Common postoperative complications associated with elimination include urinary retention and altered bowel elimination. The inability to urinate with urinary retention may occur postoperatively as a result of the recumbent position, effects of anesthesia and narcotics, inactivity, altered fluid balance, nervous tension, or surgical manipulation in the pelvic area. Nursing care centers around promoting normal urinary elimination and includes the following measures.

- Assess for bladder distention if the client has not voided within 7 to 8 hours after surgery or if the client is urinating small amounts frequently.
- Assess the amount of urine in the bladder with a portable ultrasound scanner. This noninvasive procedure decreases the potential for urinary tract infections and urethral trauma from repeated catheterizations.
- Monitor intake and output.

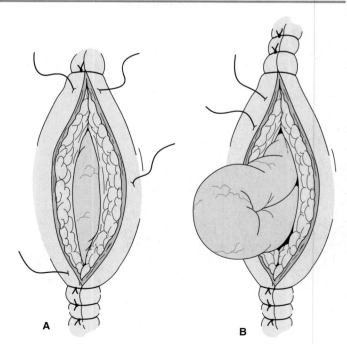

Figure 7-6 ■ Wound complications. *A,* Dehiscence is a disruption in the incision resulting in a separation of the layers of the wound. *B,* Evisceration is a protrusion of a body organ through a surgical incision.

- Maintain intravenous infusion if fluids are prescribed.
- Increase daily oral fluid intake to 2500 to 3000 mL if the client's condition permits.
- Insert a straight or indwelling catheter if ordered.
- Promote normal urinary elimination by:
  a. Assisting and providing privacy when the client uses a bedpan.
  b. Helping the client use the bedside commode or walk to the bathroom.
  c. Assisting male clients to stand to void.
  d. Pouring a measured amount of warm water over the peritoneal area. (If urination occurs, subtract the amount of water from the total amount for an accurate output measurement.)

  Bowel elimination frequently is altered after abdominal or pelvic surgery and sometimes after other surgeries. Return to normal gastrointestinal function may be delayed by general anesthesia, narcotic analgesia, decreased mobility, or altered fluid and food intake during the perioperative period.

  Nursing care centers around the return of normal bowel function and includes the following measures.
- Assess for the return of normal peristalsis:
  a. Auscultate bowel sounds every 4 hours while the client is awake.

b. Assess the abdomen for distention. (A distended abdomen with absent or high-pitched bowel sounds may indicate paralytic ileus.)
  c. Determine whether the client is passing flatus.
  d. Monitor for passage of stool, including amount and consistency.
- Encourage early ambulation within prescribed limits.
- Facilitate a daily fluid intake of 2500 to 3000 mL (unless contraindicated).
- Provide privacy when the client is using the bedpan, bedside commode, or bathroom.

If no bowel movement has occurred within 3 to 4 days after surgery, a suppository or an enema may be ordered.

Special Considerations for Older Adults

Physiologic, cognitive, and psychosocial changes associated with the aging process place the older adult at increased risk for postoperative complications. These age-related changes with selected nursing interventions are summarized in Table 7–6. With an ever-increasing population of older adults, particularly the very old, the nurse must be aware of these normal changes and modify nursing care accordingly in an effort to provide safe, supportive care.

TABLE 7–6   Nursing Interventions for Older Surgical Clients

System	Age-Related Changes	Nursing Interventions
General appearance	Change in height, weight, and fat distribution	Assess physical parameters. Provide for warmth. Turn frequently.
Integument	Diminished integrity secondary to loss of subcutaneous fat and decreased oil production, elasticity, and hydration	Provide careful preoperative preparation to avoid trauma. Use other means to assess oxygenation and hydration, such as evaluation of mucous membranes, laboratory studies, and urine output.
Sensory-perceptual	Decline in vision and hearing ability; dryness of mouth	Compensate for sensory deficits: speak low, not loud; minimize noise in environment; provide adequate room light; stay within client's field of vision when speaking; encourage client to wear hearing aid to the operating room. Provide comfort measures when NPO.
Respiratory	Decreased efficiency of cough reflex and decreased aeration of lung fields	Teach and encourage coughing and diaphragmatic breathing exercises. Assess baseline parameters. Constantly monitor lung sounds and respiratory status.
Cardiovascular	Less efficient, decreased adaptation to stress	Monitor for hypotension and shock. Assess for thrombus formation, cardiac dysrhythmias, peripheral pulses, and edema.
Gastrointestinal	Decline in gastric motility	Encourage intake of adequate fluids, nutritious meals, soft diet. Assist with feeding; monitor bowel function.
Genitourinary	Decreased efficiency of kidney; loss of bladder control	Monitor I&O and electrolyte levels. Assess for drug side effects. Assist with voiding as needed.
Musculoskeletal	Stiffness of joints; decrease in strength; brittleness of bones	Carefully position on OR table. Move carefully and gently. Prevent pressure sores.
Cognitive-psychosocial	Decreased reaction time; stable intellectual ability stable; proneness to delirium and altered mental status while in hospital	Provide ample time for making decisions. Implement safety measures. Talk to client as adult, not as child. Orient frequently.

Note. Adapted from "Perioperative Nursing Care for the Elderly Surgical Patient" by C. Dellasea and C. Burgunder, 1991, Today's O.R. Nurse, 13(6): 12–17.

Managing Acute Postoperative Pain

Pain is expected after surgery. It is neither realistic nor practical to eliminate postoperative pain completely. Nevertheless, the client should receive substantial relief from and control of this discomfort. Controlling postoperative pain not only promotes comfort but also facilitates coughing, turning, deep-breathing exercises, earlier ambulation, and decreased length of hospitalization, resulting in fewer postoperative complications, and therefore reducing health care costs. Despite the apparent benefits of effective pain control, recent studies indicate that about 50% of postoperative clients do not receive adequate pain relief or control (Acute Pain Management Guideline Panel, 1992).

Managing acute postoperative pain is an important nursing role before, during, and after surgery. Successful pain manage-

ment involves the cooperative efforts of the client, physician, and nurse. Preoperatively, the client should learn how much pain to anticipate and what methods are available to control pain. After discussing options with the client, health care providers must respect the client's personal preferences. The information that follows is based on *Acute Pain Management in Adults: Operative Procedures* (Acute Pain Management Guideline Panel, 1992).

Postoperative medications were discussed earlier in the chapter. Various nonpharmacologic approaches to pain management are used alone or in combination to control acute postoperative pain. Relaxation, distraction, and imagery techniques can decrease mild pain and anxiety. Massage and the application of heat or cold can also relieve postoperative pain. Transcutaneous electrical nerve stimulation (TENS) has been used

CHART 7–1 NANDA, NIC, AND NOC LINKAGES

The Postoperative Client

NURSING DIAGNOSES	NURSING INTERVENTIONS	NURSING OUTCOMES
• Acute Pain	• Analgesic Administration • Pain Management • Patient-Controlled Analgesia (PCA) Assistance • Postanesthesia Care	• Pain Level • Comfort Level • Pain Control Behavior
• Risk for Infection	• Infection Protection • Infection Control • Cough Enhancement • Nutrition Management • Wound Care • Incision Site Care • Vital Signs Monitoring	• Risk Control • Tissue Integrity: Skin • Immobility Consequences: Physiological • Nutritional Status
• Risk for Imbalanced Fluid Volume	• Electrolyte Management • Fluid Management • Fluid Monitoring • Intravenous (IV) Therapy • Vital Signs Monitoring	• Fluid Balance • Hydration
• Nausea	• Nausea Management • Vomiting Management • Medication Administration • Pain Management	• Nausea Level
• Ineffective Protection	• Surgical Precautions • Postanesthesia Care • Infection Control • Wound Care • Surveillance: Safety	• Infection Status • Neurological Status: Consciousness • Wound Healing • Cognitive Orientation
• Delayed Surgical Recovery	• Exercise Management: Ambulation • Incision Site Care • Infection Control • Nutrition Management • Pain Management • Urinary Elimination Management • Sleep Enhancement • Discharge Planning	• Immobility Consequences: Physiological • Wound Healing • Nutritional Status • Comfort Level • Urinary Elimination • Sleep • Knowledge: Diet, Health Resources, Infection Control, Medication, Prescribed Activity, Treatment Regimen

Note. Data from Nursing Outcomes Classification (NOC) by M. Johnson & M. Maas (Eds.), 1997, St. Louis: Mosby; Nursing Diagnoses: Definitions & Classification 2001–2002 by North American Nursing Diagnosis Association, 2001, Philadelphia: NANDA; Nursing Interventions Classification (NIC) by J.C. McCloskey & G. M. Bulechek (Eds.), 2000, St. Louis: Mosby. Reprinted by permission.

successfully to decrease postoperative incisional pain. Other approaches include acupuncture, acupressure, and therapeutic touch. Additional information on pain management techniques is found in Chapter 4. ⬭

Opioid dosage requirements vary greatly from one client to another and by the route they are taken. Remember that oral doses of analgesics are not equal to parenteral doses. Oral doses need to be higher to provide equianalgesia. See Table 4–4 regarding equianalgesics.

The client's input and participation in assessing pain and pain relief is essential to a successful pain control regime. For example, the client can rate the pain on a scale of 0 to 10 (where 0 signifies no pain and 10 signifies unbearable pain). Assess and document pain at scheduled intervals to determine the degree of pain control, to observe for drug side effects, and to assess the need for changes in the dosage and/or frequency of medication administration.

Using NANDA, NIC, and NOC

Chart 7–1 shows links between NANDA nursing diagnoses, NIC, and NOC when caring for the postoperative client.

Home Care

Because the postoperative phase does not end until the client has recovered completely from the surgical intervention, the nurse plays a vital role as the client nears discharge. As the client prepares to recuperate at home, provide information and support to help the client successfully meet self-care demands. All aspects of teaching should be accompanied by written guidelines, directions, and information. This is particularly helpful when a large amount of unfamiliar, detailed information is presented. Because the hospital stay is often brief, make an organized, coordinated effort to educate the client and family. Teaching needs vary, but the most common needs include:

- How to perform wound care. Teaching is more effective if the nurse first demonstrates and explains the procedure for the client and family or other caregiver. The client and family should then participate in the care. To evaluate the effectiveness of the teaching, ask the client or caregiver to demonstrate the procedure in return. Ideally, teaching is carried out over several days, evaluated, and periodically reinforced.
- Signs and symptoms of a wound infection. The client should be able to determine what is normal and what should be reported to the physician.
- Method and the frequency of taking one's temperature.
- Limitations or restrictions that may be imposed on such activities as lifting, driving, bathing, sexual activity, and other physical activities.
- Control of pain. If analgesics are prescribed, instruct the client in the dosage, frequency, purpose, common side effects, and other side effects to report to the physician. Reinforce the use of relaxation, distraction, imagery, or other pain control techniques that the client has found useful in controlling postoperative pain.

Nursing Care Plan
A Client Having Surgery

Martha Overbeck is a 74-year-old widow of German descent who lives alone in a senior citizens' housing complex. She is active there, as well as in the Lutheran Church. She has been in good health and is independent, but she has become progressively less active as a result of arthritic pain and stiffness. Mrs. Overbeck has degenerative joint changes that have particularly affected her right hip. On the recommendation of her physician and following a discussion with her friends, Mrs. Overbeck has been admitted to the hospital for an elective right total hip replacement. Her surgery has been scheduled for 8:00 A.M. the following day.

Mrs. Eva Jackson, a close friend and neighbor, accompanies Mrs. Overbeck to the hospital. Mrs. Overbeck explains that her friend will help in her home and assist her with the wound care and prescribed exercises.

ASSESSMENT
Gloria Nobis, RN, is assigned to Mrs. Overbeck's care on return to her room. Ms. Nobis performs a complete head-to-toe assessment and determines that Mrs. Overbeck is drowsy but oriented. Her skin is pale and slightly cool. Mrs. Overbeck states she is cold and requests additional covers. Ms. Nobis places a warmed cotton blanket next to Mrs. Overbeck's body, adds another blanket to her covers, and adjusts the room's thermostat to increase the room temperature. Mrs. Overbeck states that she is in no pain and would like to sleep. She has even, unlabored respirations and stable vital signs as compared to preoperative readings.

Mrs. Overbeck is NPO. An intravenous solution of dextrose and water is infusing at 100 mL/h per infusion pump. No redness or edema is noted at the infusion site. Ms. Nobis notes that the antibiotic ciprofloxacin hydrochloride (Cipro) is to be administered by mouth when the client is able to tolerate fluids. Mrs. Overbeck has a large gauze dressing over her right upper lateral thigh and hip with no indications of drainage from the wound. Tubing protrudes from the distal end of the dressing and is attached to a passive suctioning device (Hemovac). Ms. Nobis empties 50 mL of dark red drainage from the suctioning device and records the amount and characteristics on a flow record. Mrs. Overbeck has a Foley catheter in place with 250 mL of clear, light amber urine in the dependent gravity drainage bag.

When assessing Mrs. Overbeck's lower extremities, Ms. Nobis finds her feet slightly cool and pale with rapid capillary refill time bilaterally. Dorsalis pedis and posterior tibial pulses are strong and equal bilaterally. Ms. Nobis notes slight pitting edema in the right foot and ankle as compared with the left extremity. She also notes sensation and ability to move both feet and toes, without numbness or tingling (paresthesia).

Ms. Nobis records the above findings on a postoperative flow sheet. After ensuring that Mrs. Overbeck is safely positio reach her call light, Ms. Nobis gives Mrs. Overbeck's Jackson, a progress report. They then go into Mrs. Over

(continued

Nursing Care Plan
A Client Having Surgery (continued)

DIAGNOSES

Ms. Nobis makes the following postoperative nursing diagnoses for Mrs. Overbeck.

- *Risk for infection* of right hip wound related to disruption of normal skin integrity by the surgical incision
- *Risk for injury* related to potential dislocation of right hip prosthesis secondary to total hip replacement
- *Pain* related to right hip incision and positioning of arthritic joints during surgery

EXPECTED OUTCOMES

The expected outcomes established in the plan of care specify that Mrs. Overbeck will:

- Regain skin integrity of the right hip incision without experiencing signs or symptoms of infection.
- Demonstrate (along with Mrs. Jackson) proper aseptic technique while performing the dressing change.
- Verbalize signs and symptoms of infection to be reported to her physician.
- Describe measures to be taken to prevent dislocation of right hip prosthesis.
- Report control of pain at incision and in arthritic joints.
- Remain afebrile.

PLANNING AND IMPLEMENTATION

Ms. Nobis develops a care plan that includes the following interventions to assist Mrs. Overbeck during her postoperative recovery.

- Use aseptic technique while changing dressing.
- Monitor temperature and pulse every 4 hours to assess for elevation.
- Assess wound every 8 hours for purulent drainage and odor. Assess edges of wound for approximation, edema, redness, or inflammation in excess of expected inflammatory response.
- Teach Mrs. Overbeck and Mrs. Jackson how to use aseptic technique while assessing the wound and performing the dressing change.
- Teach Mrs. Overbeck and Mrs. Jackson the signs and symptoms of infection and when to report findings to the physician.

- Review and discuss with Mrs. Overbeck the written materials on total hip replacement.
- Convey empathetic understanding of Mrs. Overbeck's incisional and arthritic joint pain.
- Medicate Mrs. Overbeck every 4 hours (or as ordered) to maintain a therapeutic analgesic blood level.

EVALUATION

Throughout Mrs. Overbeck's hospitalization, Ms. Nobis works with Mrs. Overbeck and Mrs. Jackson to ensure that Mrs. Overbeck can care for herself after discharge from the hospital. Five days after her surgery, Mrs. Overbeck is discharged with a well-approximated incision with no indications of an infection. Prior to discharge, Ms. Nobis is confident that with Mrs. Jackson's help, Mrs. Overbeck can properly assess the incision. With minimal help, Mrs. Overbeck is able to replace the dressing using aseptic technique. She can cite the signs and symptoms of an infection, take her own oral temperature, and describe preventive measures to decrease the chances of dislocating her prosthetic hip. Because of her reduced mobility the past 5 days, Mrs. Overbeck says she can tell the arthritis in her "old bones" is "acting up." She reports less pain in her right hip than before the surgery. Mrs. Overbeck tells Ms. Nobis she will be back the following winter to have her left hip replaced.

Critical Thinking in the Nursing Process

1. Describe risk factors for Mrs. Overbeck's safety; what changes in her home environment would you suggest to promote safety until she recovers more fully?
2. Why is Mrs. Overbeck placed on the antibiotic Cipro although she has no indications of an infection? What teaching would you do?
3. Mrs. Overbeck's clotting time is slightly elevated as a result of an ordered anticoagulant. Why would this medication be ordered? Consider the client's age and the area of surgery.
4. Mrs. Overbeck is 30 pounds above her ideal weight and has osteoarthritis. Develop a care plan for the nursing diagnosis *altered health maintenance* related to intake in excess of metabolic requirements.

See Evaluating Your Response in Appendix C.

EXPLORE MediaLink

NCLEX review questions, case studies, care plan activities, MediaLink applications, and other interactive resources for this chapter can be ınd on the Companion Website at www.prenhall.com/lemone.

Click on Chapter 7 to select the activities for this chapter. For animations, video clips, more NCLEX review questions, and an audio glossary, access the Student CD-ROM accompanying this textbook.

TEST YOURSELF

1. The nurse's primary responsibility related to informed consent is:
   a. Defining the risks and benefits of the surgery
   b. Witnessing the client's signature on the consent form
   c. Explaining the right to refuse treatment or withdraw consent
   d. Advising the client and family about what is needed for the diagnosis

2. Obtaining a preoperative blood pressure measurement serves the following purpose:
   a. Fulfills a legal requirement
   b. Informs anesthesiologist so proper level of anesthesia can be given
   c. Prevents atelectasis
   d. Provides a baseline to compare postoperative blood pressure levels

3. Nonsteroidal anti-inflammatory drugs are given in the postoperative period to:
   a. Stimulate appetite
   b. Increase amnesia
   c. Potentiate analgesia
   d. Improve renal function

4. Discharge planning for a client with a total knee replacement will include dietary management guidelines. Specifically, the client will eat a diet:
   a. Low in cholesterol, high in fat
   b. High in protein, moderate in calories
   c. Low in fat, high in fiber
   d. Regular diet without dairy products

5. In the immediate postoperative period for knee surgery, assessment distal to the site includes:
   a. Urinary pH
   b. Rebound tenderness
   c. Chvostek's sign
   d. Neurovascular assessment

See Test Yourself answers in Appendix C.

BIBLIOGRAPHY

Acute Pain Management Guideline Panel. (1992). *Acute pain management in adults: Operative procedures* (AHCPR Publication No. 92-0019). Rockville, MD: Agency for Health Care Policy and Research, Public Health Service, USDHHS.

American Society of Perianesthesia Nurses. (1995). *Standards of perianesthesia nursing practice.* Thorofare, NJ: ASPAN.

Arndt, K. (1999). Inadvertent hypothermia in the OR. *AORN Journal, 70,* 204–214.

Association of Operating Room Nurses. (1993). *AORN standards and recommended practices for perioperative nursing.* Denver, CO: AORN.

Bailes, B.K. (2000). Perioperative care of the elderly surgical patient. *AORN Journal, 72,* 186–207.

Brown, B., Riippa, M., & Shaneberger, K. (2001). Promoting patient safety through preoperative patient verification. *AORN Journal, 74*(5), 690–698.

Busen, N.H. (2001). Perioperative preparation of the adolescent surgical patient. *AORN Journal, 73,* 337–363.

Carpenito, L. (1997). *Nursing diagnosis: Application to clinical practice* (7th ed.). Philadelphia: Lippincott.

Crensha, J.T., & Winslow, E.H. (2002). Preoperative fasting: Old habits die hard. *American Journal of Nursing, 102*(5), 36–45.

Cuzzell, J. (1994). Back to basics: Test your wound assessment. *American Journal of Nursing, 94*(6), 34–35.

DeFazio-Quinn, D. (1997). Ambulatory surgery . . . an evolution. *Nursing Clinics of North America, 32*(2), 377–386.

Fairchild, S. (1996). *Perioperative nursing: Principles and practice* (2nd ed.). Boston: Little, Brown and Company.

Flanagan, M. (1997). *Wound management.* New York: Churchill Livingstone.

Heimberger, D.C., & Weinsier, R.L. (1997). *Handbook of clinical nutrition* (3rd ed.). St. Louis: Mosby.

Hollingsworth, H. (1995). Nurses' assessment and management of pain at wound dressing changes. *Journal of Wound Care, 4*(2), 77–83.

Ireland, D. (1997). Legal issues in ambulatory surgery. *Nursing Clinics of North America, 32*(2), 469–476.

Kee, J. (1995). Laboratory & diagnostic tests with nursing implications. Upper Saddle River, NJ: Prentice Hall.

Kreger, C. (2001). Getting to the root of pain: Spinal anesthesia and analgesia. *Nursing 2001, 31*(6), 37–42.

Lancaster, K. (1997). Patient teaching in ambulatory surgery. *Nursing Clinics of North America, 32*(2), 417–427.

McKenry, L., & Salerno, E. (1998). *Pharmacology in nursing* (20th ed.). St. Louis: Mosby.

Nash, P., & O'Malley, M. (1997). Streamlining the perioperative process. *Nursing Clinics of North America, 32*(1), 141–151.

New, S., & Gutierrez, L. (1997). Quality improvement in the ambulatory surgical setting. *Nursing Clinics of North America, 32*(2), 477–488.

Ozawa, S., Shander, A., & Ochani, T.D. (2001). A practical approach to achieving bloodless surgery. *AORN Journal, 74*(1), 34–47.

Pasero, C., & McCaffery, M. (1996). Managing postoperative pain in the elderly. *American Journal of Nursing, 96*(10), 38–45.

Pontieri-Lewis, V. (1997). The role of nutrition in wound healing. *MEDSURG Nursing, 6*(4), 187–190, 221.

Porth, C. (1998). *Pathophysiology: Concepts of altered health states* (5th ed.). Philadelphia: Lippincott.

Ruzicka, S. (1997). The impact of normal aging processes and chronic illness on perioperative care of the elderly. *Seminars in Perioperative Nursing, 6*(1), 3–13.

Schick, L. (1998). The postanesthesia patient. In C. Hudak, B. Gallo, & P. Morton (Eds.), *Critical care nursing: A holistic approach* (7th ed.) (pp. 137–150). Philadelphia: Lippincott.

Scott, E.M., Leaper, D.J., Clark, N., & Kelly, P.J. (2001). Effects of warming therapy on pressure ulcers—A randomized trial. *AORN Journal, 73*(5), 921–928.

Steelman, V., Bulechek, G., & McCloskey, J. (1994). Toward a standardized language to describe perioperative nursing. *AORN Journal, 60*(5), 786–795.

Stringer, B., Infante-Revard, C., & Hanley, J. (2001). Quantifying and reducing the risk of bloodborne pathogen exposure. *AORN Journal, 73,* 1135–1146.

Tappen, R.M., Muzic, J., & Kennedy, P. (2001). Preoperative assessment and discharge planning for older adults undergoing ambulatory surgery. *AORN Journal, 73,* 464–474.

Walton, J. (2001). Helping high-risk surgical patients beat the odds. *Nursing 2001, 31*(3), 54–59.

Whitman, M. (2000). The starving patient. *Clinical Journal of Oncology Nursing, 4*(3), 121–125.

Williams, G. (1997). Preoperative assessment and health history review. *Nursing Clinics of North America, 32*(2), 395–416.

Zalon, M. (1997). Pain in frail, elderly women after surgery. *Image: Journal of Nursing Scholarship, 29*(1), 21–26.

Nursing Care of Clients with Infection

MediaLink

www.prenhall.com/lemone
Additional resources for this chapter can be found on the Student CD-ROM accompanying this textbook, and on the Companion Website at www.prenhall.com/lemone. Click on Chapter 8 to select the activities for this chapter.

CD-ROM
• Audio Glossary
• NCLEX Review

Animations
• Inflammatory Response
• White Blood Cells
• Penicillin

Companion Website
• More NCLEX Review
• Case Study
   Bioterrorism Preparedness
• Care Plan Activity
   Postoperative Infection
• MediaLink Application
   Antibiotic-Resistant Organisms

LEARNING OUTCOMES

After completing this chapter, you will be able to:

■ Discuss the components and functions of the immune system and the immune response.

■ Compare antibody-mediated and cell-mediated immune response.

■ Describe the pathophysiology of wound healing, inflammation, and infection.

■ Compare natural and acquired immunity and active and passive immunity.

■ Identify factors responsible for nosocomial infections.

■ Provide teaching for clients with inflammation or an infection and their families.

■ Use the nursing process as a framework to provide individualized care to clients with inflammation and infection.

The human body is continually threatened by foreign substances, infectious agents, and abnormal cells. The immune system is the body's major defense mechanism against infectious organisms and abnormal or damaged cells. Recent years have seen the emergence of resistant microorganisms such as methicillin-resistant *Staphylococcus aureus* and altered strains of familiar diseases, such as multiple-drug-resistant tuberculosis. New diseases have also emerged, such as Lyme disease and human immunodeficiency virus (HIV).

A thorough knowledge of the immune system increases understanding of the local and systemic inflammatory response, resistance to infectious disease, and the importance of immunization. This foundation can help the nurse teach clients and families to follow recommended treatment regimens, to promote and maintain health, and to prevent disease. In addition, the nurse can prescribe appropriate rehabilitative measures, such as increased rest and attention to optimal nutrition.

OVERVIEW OF THE IMMUNE SYSTEM

The immune system is a complex and intricate network of specialized cells, tissues, and organs. Cells of the immune system seek out and destroy damaged cells and foreign tissue, yet recognize and preserve host cells (Porth, 2002). The immune system performs the following functions:

- Defending and protecting the body from infection by bacteria, viruses, fungi, and parasites

- Removing and destroying damaged or dead cells
- Identifying and destroying malignant cells, thereby preventing their further development into tumors

The immune system is activated by minor injuries, such as small lacerations or bruises, or by major injuries, such as burns, surgeries, and systemic diseases (e.g., pneumonia). The response of the immune system may be nonspecific or specific. Nonspecific responses prevent or limit the entry of invaders into the body, thereby limiting the extent of tissue damage and reducing the workload of the immune system. **Inflammation** is a nonspecific response activated by both minor and major injuries. When the inflammatory process is unable to destroy invading organisms or toxins, a more specific response, called the immune response, is activated.

Immune System Components

The immune system consists of molecules, cells, and organs that produce the immune response (Table 8–1). These components may be involved in the nonspecific inflammatory response, the specific immunologic response, or both.

Leukocytes

Leukocytes, or white blood cells (WBCs), are the primary cells involved in both nonspecific and specific immune system responses. Like all blood cells, leukocytes derive from stem cells, the hemocytoblasts, in the bone marrow (Figure 8–1 ■). Unlike red blood cells (RBCs), which are confined to the circulation,

TABLE 8–1   Cells and Tissues of the Immune System

Component	Location	Function
Leukocytes		
Granulocytes		
Neutrophils	Circulation	Phagocytosis and chemotaxis
Eosinophils	Circulation, respiratory tract, and gastrointestinal tract	Phagocytosis Protection against parasites Involved in allergic response
Basophils	Circulation	Release of chemotactic substances
Monocytes and macrophages	Circulation (monocytes) and body tissue, such as skin (histocytes), liver (Kupffer's cells), alveoli, spleen, tonsils, lymph nodes, bone marrow, brain	Trapping and phagocytizing of foreign substances and cellular debris Secretion of interleukin-1 to stimulate lymphocyte growth
Lymphocytes		
T cells (mature in thymus gland)	Circulation, lymph system, tissues	Activation of T and B cells Control of viral infections and destruction of cancer cells Involved in hypersensitivity reactions and graft tissue rejection
B cells (mature in bone marrow)	Circulation, spleen	Production of antibodies (immunoglobulins) to specific antigens
NK (natural killer) cells	Circulation	Cytotoxic; killing of tumor cells, fungi, viral-infected cells, and foreign tissue
Lymphoid Tissues		
Primary or central lymphoid structures	Bone marrow and thymus gland	Production of immune cells; sites for cell maturation
Secondary or peripheral lymphoid structures	Lymph nodes, spleen, tonsils, intestinal lymphoid tissue, lymphoid tissue in other organs	Sites for activation of immune cells by antigens

Figure 8–1 ■ The development and differentiation of leukocytes from hemocytoblasts.

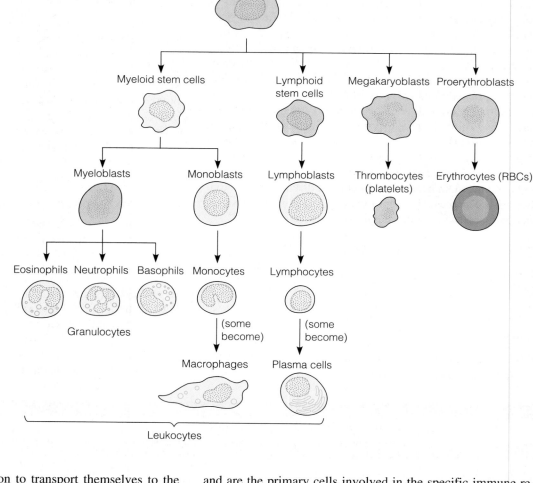

leukocytes use the circulation to transport themselves to the site of an inflammatory or immune response. As the mobile units of the immune system, leukocytes detect, attack, and destroy anything that is recognized as "foreign." They are able to move through tissue spaces, locating damaged tissue and infection by responding to chemicals released by other leukocytes and damaged tissue.

The normal number of circulating leukocytes is 4,500 to 10,000 cells per cubic millimeter (mm^3) of blood (Kee, 2001). Many more leukocytes are marginated; that is, they adhere to vascular epithelial cells along the vessel walls, in other tissue spaces, or in the lymph system. In the presence of an attack such as an infection, additional WBCs are released from the bone marrow, leading to **leukocytosis,** a WBC count of greater than 10,000/mm^3. As WBCs move out of the bone marrow into the blood, the bone marrow increases its production of additional leukocytes. A decrease in the number of circulating leukocytes, known as **leukopenia,** occurs when bone marrow activity is suppressed or when leukocyte destruction increases.

Leukocytes are divided into three major groups: granulocytes, monocytes, and lymphocytes. The granulocytes and monocytes derive from the myeloid stem cells of the bone marrow and are instrumental in the inflammatory response. Lymphocytes derive from the lymphoid stem cells of the bone marrow

and are the primary cells involved in the specific immune response. In laboratory tests, the WBC count indicates the total number of circulating leukocytes. The WBC differential identifies the portion of the total represented by each type of leukocyte.

GRANULOCYTES. Granulocytes constitute 60% to 80% of the total number of normal blood leukocytes. Their cytoplasm has a granular appearance, and their nuclei are distinctively multilobular (see Figure 8–1). Granulocytes have a short life span, measured in hours to days, compared to the life span of monocytes, which is measured in months to years. Granulocytes play a key role in protecting the body from harmful microorganisms during acute inflammation and infection. There are three types of granulocytes: neutrophils, eosinophils, and basophils.

Neutrophils, also called polymorphonuclear leukocytes (PMNs or polys), are the most plentiful of the granulocytes, constituting 55% to 70% of the total number of circulating leukocytes. Neutrophils are *phagocytic* cells, responsible for engulfing and destroying foreign agents, particularly bacteria and small particles. Neutrophils are the first phagocytic cells to arrive at the site of invasion, drawn by chemicals released by damaged tissue and invading organisms.

Neutrophils are produced in the bone marrow and released into the circulation when they mature. Segmented neutrophils (or segs) are mature forms, and usually account for about 55% of total leukocytes. *Bands* are immature neutrophils and usually comprise 5% of leukocytes. It takes about 10 days for a neutrophil to mature and be released into the circulation. Once released, neutrophils have a circulating half-life of 6 to 10 hours. They cannot replicate and must be replaced constantly to maintain adequate numbers in the circulation. They do not return to the bone marrow.

Eosinophils account for 1% to 4% of the total number of circulating leukocytes. They mature in the bone marrow in 3 to 6 days before being released into the circulation. Eosinophils have a circulating half-life of 30 minutes and a tissue half-life of 12 days. They too are phagocytic cells, but are less efficient at this process than neutrophils. Eosinophils are found in large numbers in the respiratory and gastrointestinal tracts, where they are thought to be responsible for protecting the body from parasitic worms, including tapeworms, flukes, pinworms, and hookworms. Eosinophils surround the parasite and release toxic enzymes from their cytoplasmic granules. The parasite, although too large to be phagocytized, is destroyed. Eosinophils are also involved in a hypersensitivity response, inactivating some of the inflammatory chemicals released during the inflammatory response.

Basophils constitute about 0.5% to 1% of the circulating leukocytes. These cells are not phagocytic. Granules within basophils contain proteins and chemicals such as heparin, histamine, bradykinin, serotonin, and a slow-reacting substance of anaphylaxis (leukotrienes). These substances are released into the bloodstream during an acute hypersensitivity reaction or stress response.

MONOCYTES AND MACROPHAGES.
Monocytes are the largest of the leukocytes and constitute 2% to 3% of circulating leukocytes. After their release from the bone marrow, monocytes are mobile for 1 to 2 days. They then migrate to various tissues throughout the body, attaching themselves to the tissues, where they remain for months or even years until they are activated. Monocytes mature into **macrophages** after settling into the tissues. Once they have migrated and matured, macrophages are differentiated by the tissues in which they reside. *Histiocytes* are tissue macrophages in loose connective tissue, *Kupffer cells* are found in the liver, *alveolar macrophages* in the lungs, and *microglia* in the brain. Tissue macrophages are also found in the spleen, tonsils, lymph nodes, and bone marrow.

Monocytes and macrophages are actively phagocytic, with the capacity to phagocytize large foreign particles and cell debris. Once they are in the tissue, macrophages can multiply to encapsulate and trap foreign matter that cannot be phagocytized. Like neutrophils, macrophages are drawn to an inflamed area by chemicals released from damaged tissue, a process known as chemotaxis. Monocytes and macrophages are particularly important in the body's defense against chronic infections such as tuberculosis, viral infections, and certain intracellular parasitic infections.

LYMPHOCYTES.
Small and nondescript cells, the **lymphocytes** account for 20% to 40% of circulating leukocytes. Lymphocytes are the principal effector and regulator cells of specific immune responses. Along with monocytes and macrophages, lymphocytes protect the body from microorganisms, foreign tissue, and cell mutations or alterations. Through a process known as immune surveillance, lymphocytes monitor the body for cancerous cells and eliminate or destroy them.

Like other leukocytes, lymphocytes derive from the stem cells in the bone marrow (Figure 8–2 ■). Lymphocytes have "homing" patterns: They constantly circulate, then return to concentrate in lymphoid tissues (the lymph nodes, spleen, thymus, tonsils, Peyer's patches in the submucosa of the distal ileum, and the appendix). On contact with an **antigen,** lymphocytes are activated and mature into either effector cells (e.g., plasma cells or cytotoxic cells), which are instrumental in destruction of the antigen, or memory cells. Memory cells stay inactive, sometimes for years, but activate immediately with subsequent exposure to the same antigen. They then proliferate rapidly, producing an intense immune response. Memory cells are responsible for providing acquired immunity.

Lymphocyte types are difficult to distinguish by appearance. They have distinct differences in how and where they mature, and in life cycle, surface characteristics, and function.

The three types of lymphocytes are **T lymphocytes (T cells), B lymphocytes (B cells),** and **natural killer cells (NK cells or null cells).** None of these cells acts independently. Their functions are closely interrelated.

T cells mature in the thymus gland, whereas B cells complete their maturation in the bone marrow. T cells and B cells are integral to the specific immune response and are discussed further in that section of this chapter.

NK cells are large, granular cells found in the spleen, lymph nodes, bone marrow, and blood. They constitute 15% of circulating lymphocytes. NK cells provide immune surveillance and resistance to infection, and they play an important role in the destruction of early malignant cells. Like B cells and T cells, NK cells are cytotoxic, but whereas T cells and B cells can attack only specific infected cells or malignant cells, NK cells can attack any target.

ANTIGENS.
Substances that are recognized as foreign or "nonself" are called antigens; they provoke a specific immune response when introduced into the body. Typically, antigens are large protein molecules, although polysaccharides, polypeptides, and nucleic acids may also be antigenic. Many antigens are proteins found on the cell membrane or cell wall of microorganisms or tissues such as transplanted tissue or organs, incompatible blood cells, vaccines, pollen, egg white, and insect or snake venom.

Complete antigens, known as immunogens, have two characteristics:

- *Immunogenicity* is the ability to stimulate a specific immune response.
- *Specific reactivity* is the stimulation of specific immune system components.

The portion of an antigen that incites a specific immune response is called its antigenic determinant site (epitope). Complete antigens typically are large molecules with multiple antigenic sites; examples include proteins and certain polysaccharides. Small molecules (e.g., chemical toxins, drugs, and

Figure 8–2 ■ The development and differentiation of lymphocytes from the lymphoid stem cell (lymphoblasts).

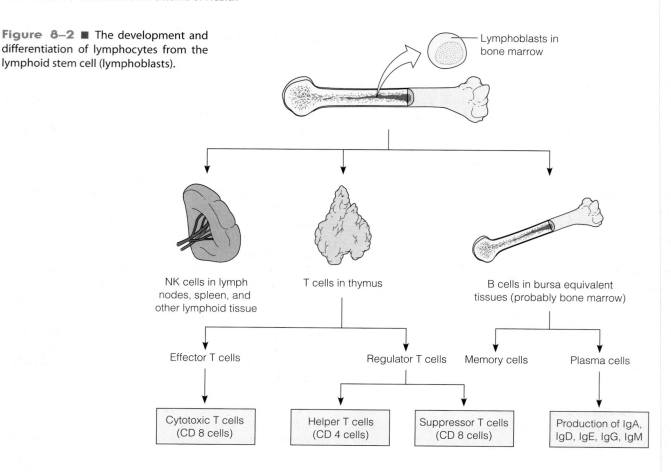

dust) that cannot evoke an antigenic response alone may link to proteins to function as complete antigens. These substances are known as haptans.

When an antigen is encountered in the body, a specific receptor on a lymphocyte "recognizes" it, and an immune response is generated. Two separate but overlapping immune responses may occur, depending on the antigen itself and the type of immune cell activated by contact with the antigen. Antigens such as bacteria, bacterial toxins, and free viruses usually activate B cells to produce **antibodies,** molecules that bind with the antigen and inactivate it. This is the **antibody-mediated (humoral) immune response.** Other antigens, such as viral-infected cells, cancer cells, and foreign tissue, activate T cells, which are the primary agents of the **cell-mediated (cellular) immune response.** In this immune response, the lymphocytes themselves inactivate the antigen, either directly or indirectly.

Lymphoid System

The *lymphoid system* consists of the lymph nodes, spleen, thymus, tonsils, lymphoid tissue scattered in connective tissues and mucosa, and the bone marrow. The thymus and bone marrow, in which T cells and B cells mature, are considered central lymphoid organs. The spleen, lymph nodes, tonsils, and other peripheral lymphoid tissue are peripheral lymphoid organs (Figure 8–3 ■).

Lymph nodes, the most numerous elements of the lymphoid system, are small, round or bean-shaped encapsulated bodies that vary in size from 1 mm to 2 cm. Distributed throughout the

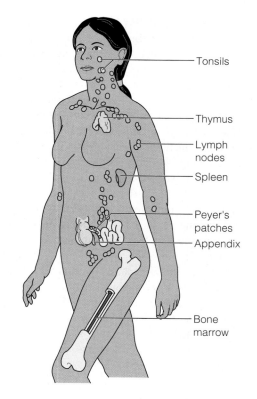

Figure 8–3 ■ The lymphoid system: the central organs of the thymus and bone marrow, and the peripheral organs, including the spleen, tonsils, lymph nodes, and Peyer's patches.

body, lymph nodes generally occur in groups at the junction of the lymphatic vessels. They can be found in the neck, axillae, abdomen, and groin.

Lymph nodes have two functions: (1) to filter foreign products or antigens from the lymph, and (2) to house and support proliferation of lymphocytes and macrophages. Lymph, a clear, protein-containing fluid transported by lymph vessels, enters the node through afferent lymphatic vessels. Inside the node, the lymph flows through sinuses in the cortex of the lymph node where T and B lymphocytes and macrophages are abundant, then through sinuses of the medulla of the lymph node, which contains macrophages and plasma cells. The presence of a foreign antigen stimulates lymphocytes and macrophages to proliferate in the lymph nodes. Macrophages destroy the antigen by phagocytosis. Immune cells and lymph then leave the lymph node through efferent vessels. An abundant blood supply to the node also facilitates lymphocyte movement.

The *spleen* is the largest lymphoid organ in the body and the only lymphoid organ that can filter blood. The spleen is located in the upper left quadrant of the abdomen. The spleen has two kinds of tissue, white pulp and red pulp. White pulp is lymphoid tissue that serves as a site for lymphocyte proliferation and immune surveillance. B cells predominate in the white pulp. Blood filtration occurs in the red pulp. In blood-filled venous sinuses, phagocytic cells dispose of damaged or aged RBCs and platelets. Other debris and foreign matter, such as bacteria, viruses, and toxins, are also removed from the blood. The spleen also stores blood and the breakdown products of RBCs for future use. The spleen is not essential for life. If it is removed because of disease or trauma, the liver and the bone marrow assume its functions.

The *thymus gland* is located in the superior anterior mediastinal cavity beneath the sternum. It reaches its maximum size at puberty, then begins to atrophy slowly. By adulthood, it is difficult to differentiate from surrounding adipose tissue even though it remains active. In the elderly, the vast majority of thymus tissue has been replaced by adipose and fibrous connective tissue. During fetal life and childhood, the thymus serves as a site for the maturation and differentiation of thymic lymphoid cells, the T cells. Thymosin, an immunoregulatory hormone of the thymus, stimulates lymphopoiesis, the formation of lymphocytes or lymphoid tissue.

Bone marrow is soft organic tissue found in the hollow cavity of the long bones, particularly the femur and humerus, as well as the flat bones of the skull, sternum, ribs, and vertebrae. Bone marrow produces and stores hematopoietic stem cells, from which all cellular components of the blood are derived (see Figure 8–1).

Lymphoid tissues are also located at key sites of potential invasion by microorganisms: the submucosa of the genitourinary, respiratory, and gastrointestinal tracts and the skin. Plasma cells in these lymphoid tissues defend the body against bacterial invasion at areas exposed to the external environment. In general, these tissues are known as *mucosa-associated lymphoid tissue* (MALT). Diffuse collections of lymphocytes, plasma cells, and phagocytes are scattered throughout the respiratory tract, concentrating at bifurcations of the bronchi and bronchioles. Gas-

trointestinal lymphoid tissue occurs as both diffusely scattered MALT and in more clearly defined tissues, such as the appendix and Peyer's patches, which are lymph nodules located on the distal ileum near its junction with the colon. Tonsils and adenoids protect the body from inhaled or ingested foreign agents. Skin-associated lymphoid tissue contains lymphocytes and Langerhans cells in the epidermis, which transport antigens to regional lymph nodes for phagocytosis.

Nonspecific Inflammatory Response

Barrier protection is the body's first line of defense against infection. The skin is the primary barrier. When intact, it prevents invasion by external organisms. When the skin is damaged or lost (e.g., as a result of injury, surgery, or burns), infection is much more likely. The membranes lining inner surfaces of the body are protected by a barrier of mucus, which traps microorganisms and other foreign substances. These can then be removed by other protective mechanisms, such as ciliary movement or the washing action of tears or urine. In addition, many body fluids contain bactericidal substances that provide barrier protection. These include acid in gastric fluid, zinc in prostatic fluid, and lysozyme in tears, nasal secretions, saliva, and sweat (Copstead & Banasik, 2000).

When these first-line defenses are breached, resulting tissue damage or foreign material entering the body induces a nonspecific immune response known as inflammation. Inflammation is an adaptive response to injury that brings fluid, dissolved substances, and blood cells into the interstitial tissues where the invasion or damage has occurred. The response is called nonspecific because the same events occur regardless of cause of the inflammatory process. Through the inflammatory reaction, the invader is neutralized and eliminated, destroyed tissue removed, and the process of healing and repair initiated.

There are three stages in the inflammatory response: (1) a vascular response characterized by vasodilation and increased permeability of blood vessels, (2) a cellular response and phagocytosis, and (3) tissue repair.

Vascular Response

After tissue cells are damaged, local blood vessels briefly constrict. Vasodilation follows almost immediately as inflammatory mediators such as histamine and kinins are released from damaged tissue (see Box 8–1). Increased blood flow causes vasocongestion at the injury site with resultant redness and heat. The congestion also increases local hydrostatic pressure. This, along with increased vessel permeability that results from chemical mediators, moves fluid out of the capillaries and into the interstitial spaces of the tissue. The escaping fluid, called fluid exudate, contains large amounts of protein and causes local edema. Fluid exudate has three functions: (1) It provides protection to the injured tissue by bringing certain nutrients needed for tissue healing; (2) it dilutes bacterial toxins; and (3) it transports cells needed for phagocytosis. Mild tissue damage such as a blister produces a *serous* exudate of primarily plasma fluid and a few proteins. With moderate to severe tissue damage, fluid exudate is *sanguineous* or *hemorrhagic,* containing large amounts of RBCs. A mixture of RBCs and

Medialink | INFLAMMATORY RESPONSE ANIMATION

BOX 8–1 ■ Inflammatory Mediators

Many of the manifestations of inflammation are produced by *inflammatory mediators,* which are chemicals released as a result of immunologic processes or tissue injury or damage. These inflammatory mediators are broadly classified as follows:

■ Vasoactive substances produce smooth muscle constriction, postcapillary vasodilation, and increased capillary permeability.
■ Chemotactic factors attract leukocytes to the damaged tissue.
■ Plasma enzymes activate the clotting cascade, plasminogen system, and complement system.
■ Miscellaneous cell products (e.g., oxygen metabolites and lysosomal enzymes) damage surrounding tissue.

Many of the outward manifestations of inflammation result from vasoactive substances such as *histamine, serotonin,* and *leukotrienes* (formerly known as slow-reacting substance of anaphylaxis, or SRS-A). Stored in mast cells, basophils, and platelets, histamine is released when an injury occurs or with stimulation by the immune system. An important component of the early inflammatory response, histamine causes vasodilation and vascular permeability in the affected area. Histamine is also a key factor in

many hypersensitivity reactions. Serotonin is released from platelets and produces effects similar to those of histamine. The leukotrienes play a significant vasoactive role in the later stages of the inflammatory response.

Prostaglandins are chemotactic substances drawing leukocytes to the inflamed tissue. In addition, they play a vasoactive role and are pain and fever inducers. Aspirin and other nonsteroidal anti-inflammatory drugs (NSAIDs) as well as the glucocorticoids inhibit prostaglandin synthesis, thereby reducing fever, pain, and inflammation.

Plasma factors such as Hageman factor activate the clotting cascade, plasminogen system (involved in the lysis of clots), and complement system. With activation of the clotting cascade, bacteria and other foreign substances are trapped in the area of tissue damage. Fibrin, which has vasoactive by-products, is also released. (See Chapter 32 for a full description of the clotting process.) The complement system serves a chemotactic role and facilitates the phagocytic process.

Major chemical mediators of inflammation are summarized in Table 8–4.

serum is referred to as *serosanguineous* exudate. *Fibrinous* exudate forms a thick, sticky meshwork of fibrinogen, in effect "walling off" inflamed tissues and preventing the spread of infection (Porth, 2002). In more severe or acute inflammation, the fluid contains fibrin, RBCs, and dead and live bacteria. This type of exudate, called *purulent* exudate, has an odor and color characteristic of the bacteria present.

The vascular response localizes invading bacteria and keeps them from spreading. Increased capillary permeability enhances the release of clotting factors such as fibrinogen, which converts to fibrin threads, entrapping the bacteria and walling them off from contact with the rest of the body.

Cellular Response

The cellular stage of the inflammatory process begins within less than an hour after the injury. This stage is marked by the margination and emigration of leukocytes into the damaged tissue, chemotaxis, and phagocytosis (Porth, 2002).

As serous fluid escapes the capillaries, the viscosity of blood in the area increases and its flow becomes more sluggish. Leukocytes marginate, moving to the edges of the blood vessels, and begin to adhere to the capillary endothelium. This process is known as pavementing. After margination and pavementing, leukocytes emigrate from the blood vessel into the tissue spaces (Figure 8–4 ■). Within hours, millions of leukocytes emigrate into the area of inflammation (Price & Wilson, 1997).

Once leukocytes have emigrated, they are drawn to the damaged or inflamed tissues by chemotactic signals. Infectious agents, damaged tissues, and activated plasma substances such as complement fractions provide chemotaxic signals that attract an army of neutrophils, monocytes, and macrophages to the injury site.

The number of neutrophils around the site increases to about 15,000/mm^3 to 25,000/mm^3, and they begin their role in

phagocytosis within a few hours. Monocytes become transient macrophages to augment the activity of the fixed macrophages; together they engulf dead cells, damaged tissue, nonfunctioning neutrophils, and invading bacteria.

Phagocytosis

Phagocytosis is a process by which a foreign agent or target cell is engulfed, destroyed, and digested. Neutrophils and macrophages, known as *phagocytes,* are the primary cells involved in phagocytosis. Once attracted to the inflammatory site, phagocytes select and engulf foreign material.

The following factors or processes help phagocytes differentiate foreign tissue from normal cells.

- *Smooth surface.* Normal tissue has a smooth surface that is resistant to phagocytosis, whereas the rough surface of a foreign agent or target cell promotes phagocytosis.
- *Surface charge.* Healthy body cells present an electronegative surface charge that repels phagocytes. Cellular debris and foreign agents, by contrast, have an electropositive charge that attracts them.
- *Opsonization.* This immune system process coats the surface of bacteria or target cells with a substance (an opsonin) as in the complement system (see Box 8–2). Opsonization enables the phagocyte to bind tightly with the foreign tissue, facilitating phagocytosis (Figure 8–5A■).

Phagocytes engulf the foreign agent or target cell by projecting pseudopodia ("false feet") in all directions around it (Figure 8–5B). This produces a chamber called a *phagosome* containing the antigen, which is ingested into the cytoplasm (Figure 8–5C). Once the phagosome has been engulfed, lysosomes fuse with the phagosome, killing any live organism and releasing digestive enzymes which destroy the antigen (Figure 8–5D).

Phagocytes—in particular, neutrophils and macrophages—contain bactericidal agents that kill most of the bacteria they in-

A Leukocytes in circulation

B Margination and pavementing

C Emigration

Figure 8–4 ■ The process of leukocyte emigration at the site of inflammation. *A,* Normal blood flow with free movement of formed elements. *B,* As blood flow slows, leukocytes move toward the periphery of stream and begin to cling to capillary endothelium, a process known as margination and pavementing. *C,* Leukocytes emigrate from the vessel into inflamed tissues.

gest before the bacteria can multiply and destroy the phagocyte itself. The phagocyte kills bacteria in a number of ways; for example, it alters the intracellular pH and produces bactericidal agents. Oxidizing agents, such as superoxide, hydrogen peroxide, and hydroxyl ions, are bactericidal. Two lysosomal substances that kill bacteria are lysozyme and phagocytin.

Some antigens, such as the tubercle bacterium, have coats or secrete substances that are resistant to lysosomal and bactericidal agents. To destroy such antigens, lysosomes release digestive enzymes into the phagosome. The lysosomes of neutrophils and macrophages contain an abundance of proteolytic (protein-destroying) enzymes that digest bacteria and other foreign protein components. The macrophage's lysosomes also contain lipases (fat-splitting enzymes) capable of digesting the

BOX 8–2   ■ The Complement System

The *complement system* consists of approximately 20 complex plasma proteins that are activated by a tissue injury or antigen-antibody reaction. The complement system is involved in both nonspecific and specific immune responses. Its activation results in the production of effector molecules that are involved in the processes of inflammation, phagocytosis, and cell lysis or destruction (Porth, 1998; Roitt, 1994). Specifically, complement activation leads to

■ *Mediation of the inflammatory response.* When the complement system is activated, chemical mediators such as histamine are released from mast cells and basophils, leading to smooth muscle contraction, increased vascular permeability and edema, and the attraction of leukocytes.
■ *Opsonization (or coating) of antigen-antibody complexes to facilitate phagocytosis.*
■ *Alteration of the cell membrane or viral capsule.* When the cell surface is altered, lysis results. Bacteria and viruses are destroyed; certain normal cells, such as RBCs, platelets, and lymphocytes, that are damaged or old may also be destroyed through this process.

The complement system has two "arms," or pathways, of protein and enzyme reactions. The *classic pathway* is activated by antibody-containing immunoglobulins and other substances such as DNA and C-reactive protein. The *alternate pathway* is activated by tissue injury, polysaccharides, or enzymes. When either pathway is activated, the results are mediation of the inflammatory process, attraction of phagocytes, facilitation of phagocytosis, and lysis of microbes.

A

B

C

D

Figure 8–5 ■ The process of phagocytosis. *A,* Opsonization coats the surface of the bacterium with IgG (an antibody) and complement. *B,* The bacterium is bound to and engulfed by the phagocyte. *C,* The phagosome is ingested into the cytoplasm of the phagocyte. *D,* Lysosomes fuse with the phagosome, releasing digestive enzymes and destroying the antigen.

thick lipid membranes of such bacteria as *Mycobacterium tuberculosis* and *Mycobacterium leprae.*

Once neutrophils have ingested toxic substances to their capacity, they in turn are killed. Neutrophils have the capacity to phagocytize 5 to 20 bacteria before they become inactive. Macrophages then digest the dead neutrophils. Monocytes or macrophages are capable of phagocytizing up to 100 bacteria. Because of their size, they can ingest larger particles than neutrophils can ingest, such as whole RBCs, necrotic tissue, cell fragments, malarial parasites, and dead neutrophils. Macrophages have the ability to extrude (release) the toxic substances and lysosomal enzymes within their phagosomes. As a result, they can continue to function for months and even years.

Healing

Inflammation is the first phase of the healing process. During the inflammatory process, particulate matter, bacteria, damaged cells, and inflammatory exudate are removed by phagocytosis. This process, called debridement, prepares the wound for healing.

The second phase of the healing process, known *as reconstruction,* may overlap the inflammatory phase. The ideal result of the healing process is *resolution,* the restoration of the original structure and function of the damaged tissue. Simple resolution occurs when there is no destruction of the normal tissue and the body is able to neutralize and remove the offending agent through the inflammatory process.

Resolution may also occur when the damaged tissue is capable of regeneration. The ability to regenerate, or replace lost parenchyma (functional tissue) with new, functional cells varies by tissue and cell type. *Labile cells* continue to regenerate throughout life. These cells are found in tissues where there is a daily turnover of cells—namely, bone marrow and the epithelial cells of the skin, mucous membranes, cervix, gastrointestinal tract, and genitourinary tract. *Stable cells* normally stop

Figure 8–6 ■ Antibody-mediated (humoral) immunity. On initial exposure to the antigen, B cells with appropriate receptor sites are activated to become plasma cells and produce antibodies or memory cells. This is known as the primary response. With subsequent exposures, memory cells respond rapidly with antibody production. This is known as the secondary response.

replicating when growth ceases, but are capable of regeneration when stimulated by an injury. Osteocytes (which are found in bone) and parenchymal cells of the kidneys, liver, and pancreas are stable cells. *Permanent* or *fixed cells* are unable to regenerate. When these cells are destroyed, they are replaced by fibrous scar tissue. Nerve cells, skeletal muscle cells, and cardiac muscle cells are fixed cells (Porth, 1998).

When regeneration and complete resolution is not possible, healing occurs by replacement of the destroyed tissue with collagen scar tissue. This process is known as *repair.* Although tissue that has undergone repair lacks the physiologic function of the destroyed tissue, the scar fills the lesion and provides tensile tissue strength. The healing process is discussed further in Chapter 7. ∞

Specific Immune Response

The introduction of antigens into the body causes a more specific reaction than the nonspecific inflammatory response. On the first exposure to an antigen, a change occurs in the host, resulting in a specific and rapid response following subsequent exposures. This specific response is known as the *immune response.*

The immune response to an antigen has the following distinctive properties:

- The immune response typically is directed against materials recognized as foreign (i.e., from outside the body) and is not usually directed against the self (i.e., cells or structures produced by the body). This property is known as self-recognition.
- The immune response is *specific.* It is initiated by and directed against particular antigens (such as a specific virus, bacterium, or transplanted tissue).
- Unlike a localized inflammatory response, the immune response is systemic. Immunity is generalized; it is not restricted to the initial site of infection or entry of foreign tissue.
- The immune response has memory. Repeated exposures to an antigen produce a more rapid response.

A client whose immune system is able to identify antigens and effectively destroy or remove them is said to be **immunocompetent.** Health problems may occur when the immune response is altered (see Chapter 9 for further discussion). ∞

Antibody-Mediated Immune Response

The antibody-mediated (humoral) immune response is produced by B lymphocytes (B cells). B cells are constantly replaced through cell division and proliferation in the bone marrow. It is believed that B cells mature in the bone marrow and then migrate to the spleen to await activation. They normally constitute 10% to 15% of circulating lymphocytes.

B cells are activated by contact with an antigen and by T cells (discussed in the next section). Each B cell has receptor sites for a specific antigen or antigens. When the antigen is encountered, the activated B cell proliferates and differentiates into antibody-producing plasma cells and memory cells (Figure 8–6 ■). Plasma cells are short-lived, lasting only about 1 day. While alive, however, they can produce thousands of antibody molecules per second. Memory cells retain antibody-producing information, allowing a rapid response if the antigen is again encountered.

An antibody is an **immunoglobulin (Ig)** molecule with the ability to bind to and inactivate a specific antigen. Immunoglobulins comprise the gamma globulin portion of the blood proteins. The immune system produces numerous antibodies, each active against a specific antigen. Antibodies fall into five classes of immunoglobulins: IgG, IgA, IgM, IgD, and IgE. Each has a slightly different structure and function. Their roles are summarized in Table 8–2.

TABLE 8–2 Immunoglobulin Characteristics and Functions

Class	Percentage of Total	Characteristics and Function
IgG	75%	Most abundant Ig; also known as gamma globulin; found in blood, lymph, and intestines Active against bacteria, bacterial toxins, and viruses Activates complement The only Ig to cross the placenta, providing immune protection to neonate
IgA	10% to 15%	Found in saliva, tears, and bronchial, gastrointestinal, prostatic, and vaginal secretions, as well as blood and lymph Provides local protection on exposed mucous membrane surfaces and potent antiviral activity by preventing binding of the virus to cells of the respiratory and gastrointestinal tracts Levels decrease during stress
IgM	5% to 10%	Found in blood and lymph First antibody produced with primary immune response High concentrations early in infection, decreases within about a week Mediates cytotoxic response and activates complement
IgD	<1%	Found in blood, lymph, and surfaces of B cells Exact function unknown; may be receptor-binding antigens to B-cell surface
IgE	<0.1%	Found on mast cells and basophils Involved in release of chemical mediators responsible for immediate hypersensitivity (allergic and anaphylactic) response

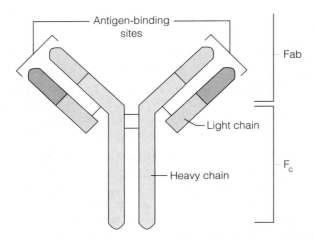

Figure 8–7 ■ An antibody molecule. The Fab section is unique, providing an antigen-specific binding site. The F$_c$ section is common to each class of immunoglobulin (IgG, IgA, IgM, IgD, IgE).

Antibodies are Y-shaped molecules of two light and two heavy polypeptide chains (Figure 8–7 ■). The top portion of the Y, called the *Fab* or *antigen-binding fragment,* is chemically variable and specific to the antigen. The lower portion, the *F$_c$,* or *crystallized fragment,* is constant for its class of immunoglobulin and directs the biologic activity of the immunoglobulin (the manner in which it functions). For example, the lower portion of immunoglobulin molecules produced against hepatitis A and hepatitis B are the same (IgG), but the upper portion is different and specific to the virus.

The antibodies produced by B cells (see Figure 8–7) link with the antigen (Figure 8–8 ■) and inactivate it through one of the following processes.

- Promoting phagocytosis of the antigen by neutrophils
- Precipitation: combining with soluble antigens to form an insoluble complex or precipitate

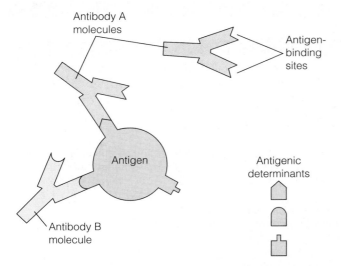

Figure 8–8 ■ Antigen-antibody binding. The unique Fab site on the antibody binds with specific receptor sites on the antigen. As shown, more than one kind of antibody may be produced to an antigen.

Figure 8–9 ■ Antibody production in the primary and secondary responses of the antibody-mediated immune response. Note the more rapid and effective production following subsequent exposure.

- Neutralization: combining with a toxin to neutralize its effects; the antigen-antibody complex is then destroyed by the process of phagocytosis
- Lysis of the antigen cell membrane caused by combination with antibodies and complement
- Agglutination (clumping) of antigens to form a noninvasive aggregate
- Opsonization: coating of the antigen with antibodies and complement, making them more susceptible to phagocytosis

The complete antibody-mediated response occurs in two phases. With initial exposure to an antigen, the primary response develops. B cells are activated to proliferate and begin producing antibodies. There is a latency period of 3 to 6 days before antibodies become detectable in the blood. Levels then continue to rise, peaking at 10 to 14 days after the initial exposure. With many illnesses (e.g., chickenpox), this peak correlates with recovery.

Subsequent exposure to the same antigen elicits a secondary response. Memory cells (Figure 8–6) formed during the primary response stimulate the production of plasma cells, and an almost immediate rise in antibody levels occurs (Figure 8–9 ■). This rapid secondary response is the basis of acquired immunity and is instrumental in preventing disease. It is also the mechanism through which vaccines provide protection from disease.

Cell-Mediated Immune Response

Many antigens cannot stimulate the antibody-mediated response or are "hidden" from it because they live inside the body's cells (viruses and mycobacteria are examples of such antigens). The immune response providing protection against these antigens is the cell-mediated immune response, also called *cellular immunity.* T lymphocytes (T cells) initiate this type of immune response.

Approximately 70% to 80% of circulating lymphocytes are T cells. T cells migrate to the thymus during fetal and early life, establishing the lifetime pool of cells. T cells have a life span measured in years, maintaining their numbers through proliferation, primarily in the lymph nodes.

T cells are much more complex than B cells. There are two major classes of T cells, *effector cells* and *regulator cells.* The main effector T cell is the *cytotoxic cell,* also called the *killer T cell.* Regulator T cells are further classified into two groups: *helper T cells* and *suppressor T cells.*

T cells are antigen specific; that is, each subset is activated by a particular antigen. The antigens that activate T cells must be presented on another cell surface, such as pieces of virus presented on the surface of an infected cell, or the histocompatibility locus antigen (HLA) on a cell of transplanted tissue. When activated, T cells divide and proliferate, forming antigen-specific clones (Figure 8–10 ■). (A clone is an exact copy of another cell.)

Cytotoxic T cells bind with cell surface antigens on virus-infected or foreign cells. Killer T cells destroy the antigen by combining with it and then either destroying its cell membrane or releasing cytotoxic substances into the cell. They are vital in the control of viral and bacterial infections.

Regulator T cells play a key role in controlling the immune response. The majority of regulator T cells are helper T cells. They stimulate the proliferation of other T cells, amplify the cytotoxic activity of killer T cells, and activate B cells to proliferate and differentiate. They interact directly with B cells to promote their multiplication and conversion into plasma cells capable of producing antibodies. The other regulatory T-cell group, suppressor T cells, provide negative feedback, making the immune response a self-limiting process.

On activation, both effector and regulator T cells synthesize and release lymphokines, a type of soluble protein. Lymphokines are a subgroup of nonspecific defense mechanisms known as **cytokines** (Box 8–3). Lymphokines secreted by cytotoxic and helper T cells are important in amplifying the im-

mune response and the nonspecific inflammatory response. They stimulate the following:

- B cells to become plasma cells and produce antibodies
- Macrophages to become activated macrophages (the most aggressive phagocyte)
- Proliferation of killer T cells

Figure 8–10 ■ Cellular immune response. *A,* An infected cell, abnormal cell, or phagocyte presents antigen on its surface that binds with a receptor site on a killer T or a helper T cell. The killer T cell is activated to proliferate into memory cells or mature cytotoxic cells. *B,* The helper T cell is activated to augment the cytotoxic response and stimulate the antibody-mediated immune response.

Viral antigen

Processed antigen presented on cell surface of infected tissue

A

B

Infected cell — Killer T cell

Helper T cell

Killer T memory cell

Augment activity of killer cells

Mature killer T cells

Mature helper T cells

Interact with B cells to promote antibody production

TABLE 8–3 Major Cytokines and Their Functions

Cytokine	Where Produced	Primary Functions
Interleukin-1 (IL-1)	Monocytes and macrophages; other cells	Activates T and B cells Induces fever and tissue catabolism Enhances NK activity Attracts neutrophils, macrophages, and lymphocytes Stimulates endothelial cell growth, collagen, and collagenases
Interleukin-2 (IL-2)	Helper T cells	Stimulates T and B cell proliferation Activates killer T and NK cells
Interleukin-3 (IL-3)	T cells	Stimulates growth and differentiation of bone marrow stem cells
Interleukin-4 (IL-4)	Activated helper T cells	Stimulates proliferation of T and B cells Increases IgE secretion by B cells
Interleukin-5 (IL-5)	T cells and activated mast cells	Promotes differentiation of B cells and eosinophils Stimulates production of IgA
Gamma interferon	T and NK cells	Stimulates phagocytosis by neutrophils and macrocytes Activates NK cells Augments B cell proliferation, enhancing both cellular and humoral immune responses
Alpha and beta interferons	Virus-infected cells; macrophages	Activate macrophages and endothelial cells Augment NK cell activity Act at gene level to protect neighboring cells from invasion by intracellular parasites, such as viruses, rickettsia, malaria
Tumor necrosis factor (TNF)	Activated macrophages, T cells, and NK cells	Major chemical mediator of inflammatory response Stimulates T-cell activation, antibody production, and accumulation of leukocytes at inflammatory site Directly cytotoxic to some tumor cells Induces fever

Suppressor T cells release lymphokines, which inhibit the activity of other T cells and B cells.

Although T cells can be activated only by specific antigens, much of the resulting effect is nonspecific—in other words, an enhanced inflammatory response. Like the antibody-mediated response, the cell-mediated response has memory. Subsequent exposures to an antigen result in a more rapid and effective inflammatory response and more effective phagocytosis by macrophages. This memory provides the basis for skin testing. A client previously exposed to tuberculosis, for example, develops a more pronounced inflammatory response when minute amounts are injected under the skin.

NORMAL IMMUNE RESPONSES

THE CLIENT WITH TISSUE INFLAMMATION AND HEALING

As noted, inflammation is a nonspecific response to injury that serves to destroy, dilute, or contain the injurious agent or damaged tissue. Inflammation may be either acute or chronic. Acute inflammation is a short-term reaction of the body to all types of tissue damage. It is immediate and aimed at protecting the body and preventing further invasion or injury. Acute inflammation usually lasts less than 1 to 2 weeks. Once the injurious agent is removed, the inflammation subsides. Healing with tissue repair or scar formation occurs, and the body functions in normal or near-normal capacity.

Chronic inflammation is slower in onset and may not have an acute phase. Its clinical manifestations occur over months or years. It involves cell proliferation and is debilitating, with long-term adverse effects. There is increased cellular exudate, necrosis, fibrosis, and sometimes tissue scarring, resulting in severe tissue damage.

PATHOPHYSIOLOGY OF TISSUE INFLAMMATION

The tissue damage that evokes an inflammatory response may be caused by specific or nonspecific agents. These agents may be *exogenous,* from outside the body, or *endogenous,* from within the body. Causes of inflammation include the following:

- Mechanical injuries, such as cuts or surgical incisions
- Physical damage, such as burns
- Chemical injury from toxins or poisons
- Microorganisms, such as bacteria, viruses, or fungi
- Extremes of heat or cold
- Immunologic responses, such as hypersensitivity reactions
- Ischemic damage or trauma, such as a stroke or myocardial infarction

TABLE 8–4	Major Chemical Mediators of Inflammation	
Factor	**Source**	**Effect**
Histamine	Mast cells, basophils, and platelets	Vasodilation and increased capillary permeability, producing tissue redness, warmth, and edema
Kinins (bradykinin and others)	Plasma protein factors	Histaminelike effects; chemotaxis and pain inducers
Prostaglandins	Metabolism of anachidonic acid from cell membranes	Histaminelike effects; chemotaxis, pain, and fever inducers
Leukotrienes	Anachidonic acid metabolism	Smooth muscle constriction (especially bronchoconstriction), increased vascular permeability, chemotaxis

Acute Inflammation

Regardless of the cause, location, or extent of the injury, the acute inflammatory response follows the previously outlined sequence of vascular response, cellular and phagocytic response, and healing.

Many of the manifestations of inflammation are produced by inflammatory mediators such as histamine and prostaglandins released when tissue is damaged (see Table 8–4 and Box 8–1 on inflammatory mediators).

The cardinal signs of inflammation include the following:

- Erythema (redness)
- Local heat caused by the increased blood flow to the injured area (hyperemia)
- Swelling due to accumulated fluid at the site
- Pain from tissue swelling and chemical irritation of nerve endings
- Loss of function caused by the swelling and pain

The degree of functional loss depends on the location and extent of the injury. With increased tissue damage, more fluid exudate is formed, resulting in more swelling, pain, and functional impairment. Pain may be immediate or delayed. Prostaglandins in-

tensify and prolong the pain. Kinins cause irritation to the nerve endings and contribute to the pain sensation.

Dead neutrophils, necrotic tissue, and digested bacteria accumulate as a result of inflammation and phagocytosis, forming *pus*. It usually forms and remains until after the infection subsides. Pus may push itself to the surface of the body or become internalized. In the latter case, pus is gradually autolyzed (self-digested) by enzymes over a period of days. The end product is then absorbed by the body. On occasion, pus may remain after the infection is resolved. Pockets of pus, called abscesses, may need to be artificially drained with a procedure called *incision and drainage (I&D)*. Ectopic calcifications are another possible result of residual collections of pus.

Systemic responses to inflammation include an increase in the size of lymph nodes due to the accumulation of bacteria, phagocytes, and destroyed lymph tissue. Enlarged lymph nodes are usually noted in the groin, axillae, and neck (Figure 8–11 ■). Fever, often precipitated by inflammatory mediators or bacterial toxins, inhibits the growth of many microorganisms and increases tissue repair functions. Loss of appetite and fatigue may occur in the effort to conserve energy during the inflammatory process. Leukocytosis occurs with increased WBC production to support inflammation and phagocytosis.

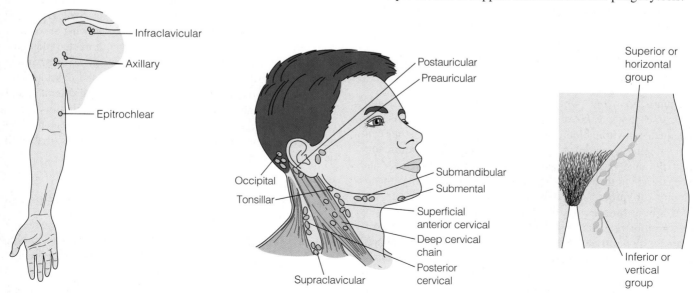

Figure 8–11 ■ Lymph nodes that may be assessed by palpation.

Manifestations of Inflammation

LOCAL MANIFESTATIONS

- Erythema
- Warmth
- Pain
- Edema
- Functional impairment

SYSTEMIC MANIFESTATIONS

- T >100.4°F (38°C) or <96.8°F (36°C)
- P >90/min
- R >20/min (tachypntea)
- WBC >12,000/mm³ or >10% bands

Local and systemic manifestations of inflammation are summarized in the box above.

Chronic Inflammation

Whereas acute inflammation is a self-limiting process lasting less than 2 weeks, chronic inflammation tends to be self-perpetuating, lasting weeks to months or years. Chronic inflammation may develop when the acute inflammatory process has been ineffective in removing the offending agent. For example, mycobacteria have cell walls with high lipid and wax content, making them resistant to phagocytosis. Chronic inflammation and granuloma formation is common with *Mycobacterium tuberculosis* infection. Persistent irritation by chemicals, particulate matter, or physical irritants such as talc, asbestos, or silica may also result in chronic inflammation.

The chronic inflammatory process is characterized by a dense infiltration of the site by lymphocytes and macrophages. The macrophages mass or coalesce to form a multinucleated giant cell surrounded by lymphocytes, in a lesion called a *granuloma*. The granuloma is effective in walling off the offending agent, isolating it from the rest of the body; however, the infectious agent or offending irritant may not be destroyed and can survive within the granuloma for a long period of time. The granuloma formed in tuberculosis is called a tubercle. *Mycobacterium tuberculosis* may survive for many years within the tubercle, emerging when the client's immune system is no longer able to contain it.

Complications

Inflammation and wound healing are highly metabolic processes that may be affected by a number of factors. Without adequate nutrition, blood supply, and oxygenation, tissues cannot effectively complete the process. Impaired inflammatory and immune processes can interfere with phagocytosis and preparation of the wound for healing. Infection prolongs the inflammatory process and delays healing.

Chronic diseases may also impair healing. Diabetes mellitus is a prominent example. With high blood glucose levels associated with poorly controlled diabetes, chemotaxic and phagocytic function is decreased. Collagen formation and tensile strength of the wound are also impaired. Small blood vessel disease is common in people with diabetes, a factor that further impairs the healing process.

TABLE 8–5 Factors That May Impair Healing

Factor	Effect
Malnutrition	
Protein deficit	Prolongs inflammation and impairs healing process
Carbohydrate and kilocalorie deficit	Impairs metabolic processes and promotes catabolism; proteins are used for energy rather than for healing
Fat deficit	Impairs cell membrane synthesis in tissue repair
Vitamin deficits	
Vitamin A	Limits epithelialization and capillary formation
B-Complex	Inhibits enzymatic reactions that contribute to wound healing
Vitamin C	Impairs collagen synthesis
Tissue hypoxia	Associated with an increased risk of infection and impaired healing, because oxygen is required to support cell function and collagen synthesis
Impaired blood supply	Inadequate delivery of oxygen and nutrients to healing tissues and removal of waste products
Impaired inflammatory and immune processes	Decreased phagocytosis and wound debridement; increased risk of infection; delayed healing

Drug therapy, particularly corticosteroid medications, may suppress the immune and inflammatory responses, delaying healing (Porth, 2002). Other external factors, such as exposure to ionizing radiation and wound cleansing agents, can also affect healing. Table 8–5 summarizes major factors that affect the inflammatory process and wound healing.

COLLABORATIVE CARE

Management of the client with inflamed tissue focuses on promoting healing. Care is generally supportive, allowing the client's own physiologic processes to remove foreign matter and damaged cells. Wound care may be minimal, involving only simple cleaning, or extensive, involving irrigations and debridement. The client is encouraged to rest, to increase fluid intake, and to eat a well-balanced, nutritious diet. Anti-inflammatory medications are administered only when the inflammatory process has become problematic. Antibiotics may also be prescribed to help eliminate infectious causes of inflammation.

Diagnostic Tests

The following diagnostic tests may be ordered to identify the source and extent of inflammation.

- *WBC with differential* provides information about the type and extent of inflammatory response. The differential count (the percentage of the total WBC made up by each type of leukocyte) provides further clues about inflammatory processes (Table 8–6).

TABLE 8-6 The White Blood Cell Count and Differential

Cell Type and Normal Value	Increased	Decreased
Total WBCs: 4000 to 10,000 per mm³	*Leukocytosis:* Infection or inflammation, leukemia, trauma or stress, tissue necrosis	*Leukopenia:* Bone marrow depression, overwhelming infection, viral infections, immunosuppression, autoimmune disease, dietary deficiency
Neutrophils (segs, PMNs, or polys): 55% to 70%	*Neutrophilia:* Acute infection or stress response, myelocytic leukemia, inflammatory or metabolic disorders	*Neutropenia:* Bone marrow depression, overwhelming bacterial infection, viral infection, Addison's disease
Eosinophils (eos): 1% to 4%	*Eosinophilia:* Parasitic infections, hypersensitivity reactions, autoimmune disorders	*Eosinopenia:* Cushing's syndrome, autoimmune disorders, stress, certain drugs
Basophils (basos): 0.5% to 1%	*Basophilia:* Hypersensitivity responses, chronic myelogenous leukemia, chickenpox or smallpox, splenectomy, hypothyroidism	*Basopenia:* Acute stress or hypersensitivity reactions, hyperthyroidism
Monocytes (monos): 2% to 8%	*Monocytosis:* Chronic inflammatory disorders, tuberculosis, viral infections, leukemia, Hodgkin's disease, multiple myeloma	*Monocytopenia:* Bone marrow depression, corticosteroid therapy
Lymphocytes (lymphs): 20% to 40%	*Lymphocytosis:* Chronic bacterial infection, viral infections, lymphocytic leukemia	*Lymphocytopenia:* Bone marrow depression, immunodeficiency, leukemia, Cushing's syndrome, Hodgkin's disease, renal failure

Note. Data are from Laboratory Tests and Diagnostic Procedures *(2nd ed.) by R. Chernecky and B. J. Berger, 1997, Philadelphia: W. B. Saunders; and* Mosby's Diagnostic and Laboratory Test Reference *(3rd ed.) by K. D. Pagana and T. J. Pagana, 1997, St. Louis: Mosby-Year Book.*

- *Erythrocyte sedimentation rate (ESR or sed rate)* is a nonspecific test to detect inflammation. The rate at which RBCs fall to the bottom of a vertical tube is an indicator of inflammation. An increased ESR may indicate acute or chronic inflammation, tuberculosis, autoimmune disorders, some malignancies, and nephritis. Decreased ESR is found in congestive heart failure, sickle cell anemia, and polycythemia vera.
- *C-reactive protein (CRP) test* is used to detect CRP. This abnormal glycoprotein is produced by the liver and is excreted into the bloodstream during the acute phase of an inflammatory process. The expected result of this test is negative for CRP. A positive result indicates an acute or chronic inflammatory process. It may also indicate the client's response to therapy, because it decreases when inflammation subsides (Kee, 2001).

In addition to the above diagnostic tests, cultures of the blood and other body fluids may be ordered to determine if infection is the cause of inflammation.

Medications

Medications may be prescribed for the client with an inflammatory response to help alleviate distressing symptoms or destroy infectious agents.

Acetaminophen (Tylenol) may be administered to reduce the fever and pain associated with inflammation. Acetaminophen has no anti-inflammatory effect; it will not reduce the inflammatory process but will relieve associated symptoms. Acetaminophen decreases fever by acting directly on the hypothalamus heat-regulating center. It also works on the central nervous system to relieve pain sensations.

Antibiotics may be used either prophylactically to prevent infection from interfering with the healing process of damaged tissue, or therapeutically to treat the infection. If infection is present, the organism and its response or sensitivity to various antibiotics are used to guide therapy. Antibiotic therapy is presented in greater depth in the section of this chapter on infectious diseases.

Although inflammation is a beneficial process to prepare acutely injured tissue for healing, it can have damaging effects as well. When these effects are a concern or the manifestations of inflammation are deleterious to the client, anti-inflammatory medications may be prescribed. Anti-inflammatory medications fall into three broad groups: salicylates, such as aspirin; other nonsteroidal anti-inflammatory drugs (NSAIDs); and corticosteroids.

Aspirin (also called acetylsalicylic acid, or ASA) is an NSAID that has antipyretic, analgesic, and antiplatelet effects. Its beneficial effects are largely dose related. Low doses (as little as 81 mg per day) inhibit platelet aggregation and normal blood clotting. Higher doses (650 to 1000 mg 4 to 5 times per day) are required to accomplish its anti-inflammatory effects. However, 650 mg of aspirin is an effective analgesic and antipyretic dosage. To relieve pain, aspirin acts primarily on peripheral sensory nerves by inhibiting the synthesis of prostaglandins and kinins, which are chemical stimuli of sensory nerves. As an antipyretic, aspirin acts both centrally and peripherally. It inhibits the formation of pyrogenic substances that raise the hypothalamic thermostat. It also dilates peripheral blood vessels and promotes diaphoresis, increasing the dissipation of heat (Shannon, Wilson, & Stang, 2001).

In therapeutic doses, aspirin mediates the inflammatory process by inhibiting the synthesis of prostaglandins and acting on the mobility and activation of leukocytes. Inflammation is reduced, along with the swelling, redness, and impaired function that accompanies it.

The other NSAIDs have activity similar to that of aspirin. They inhibit prostaglandin synthesis, reducing the inflammatory and pain response. NSAIDs fall into the following classifications.

- *Salicylates,* which include aspirin and related compounds
- *Acetic acids,* including indomethacin (Indocin), ketorolac (Toradol), sulindac (Clinoril), and tolmetin (Tolectin)
- *Propionic acids,* including ibuprofen (Motrin and numerous nonprescription preparations), fenoprofen (Nalfon), and naproxen (Naprosyn)
- *Fenamates,* including meclofenamate (Meclomen)
- *Pyrazoles,* including phenylbutazone (Butazolidin)
- *Oxicams,* including piroxicam (Feldene)

Each group has a slightly different mode of action for prostaglandin inhibition. Clients may have varying degrees of relief with different NSAIDs; sometimes, several different agents must be tried before the most effective is identified. Side effects also differ to a certain extent; however, all have a potential cross-sensitivity with aspirin, all irritate the gastrointestinal tract, and all cause some degree of sodium and water retention. They also are more costly than aspirin, but they have a longer duration of action; therefore, fewer daily doses are required to achieve the desired effect. Indomethacin and phenylbutazone are the most toxic of the NSAIDs. Their use is limited to short-term therapy. (See Chapter 4 for further information on NSAIDs.)

For acute hypersensitivity reactions, such as reactions to poison oak, or for inflammation that cannot be managed by aspirin or NSAID therapy, corticosteroid therapy may be prescribed. The glucocorticoids are hormones produced by the adrenal cortex that have widespread effects on body metabolism and the immune response. Glucocorticoids inhibit inflammation and may be lifesaving in acute fulminating or chronic progressive inflammation. They do not cure disease; they are palliative to manage the inflammatory process.

When glucocorticoids are prescribed to manage inflammation, the following principles are used to guide therapy.

- The smallest possible effective dose is used.
- If a local-acting preparation such as a topical agent or intra-articular injection will be effective, it is prescribed.
- To minimize suppression of adrenal gland activity, an alternate-day dose schedule is used when possible.
- High-dose corticosteroid therapy is never stopped abruptly, but tapered, allowing the client's adrenal glands to resume normal function.

The incidence of potentially harmful side effects increases with higher doses and prolonged therapy.

The nursing implications of caring for a client receiving corticosteroid medications are discussed in Chapter 23. ⊙

Nutrition

Healing depends on cell replication, protein synthesis, and the function of specific organs—the liver, heart, and lungs in particular. Weight loss and protein depletion are risk factors for poor healing and wound complications. Even a few days of severely impaired nutritional intake can noticeably affect healing.

The client with an inflammatory process or healing wound requires a well-balanced diet of sufficient kilocalories to meet the metabolic needs of the body (see Table 8–5). Inflammation often produces *catabolism,* a state in which body tissues are broken down. Healing, by contrast, is a process of *anabolism,* or building up. Without sufficient kilocalories and nutrients, catabolism may predominate, impairing healing.

Carbohydrates are important to meet energy demands, as well as to support leukocyte function. Adequate protein is necessary for tissue healing and the production of antibodies and WBCs. Lack of adequate protein increases the risk of infection. Complete protein sources, those that provide the essential amino acids, are preferred. Dietary fats are used in the synthesis of cell membranes.

Vitamins A, B-complex, C, and K are also important to the healing process. Vitamin A is necessary for capillary formation and epithelialization. B-complex vitamins promote wound healing, and vitamin C is necessary for collagen synthesis. Vitamin K provides a vital component for the synthesis of clotting factors in the liver.

Although it has been established that minerals contribute to the inflammatory and healing processes, less is known about required amounts. Zinc appears to be important for tissue growth, skin integrity, cell-mediated immunity, and other general immune mechanisms (Lutz & Przytulski, 2001).

NURSING CARE

Acute inflammation may be self-limiting or extensive and require hospitalization. Nursing care includes teaching clients with acute and chronic inflammatory conditions self-management at home.

Health Promotion

Health promotion activities to prevent inflammation focus on reducing the risk for accidents and exposure to harmful agents that can result in subsequent injury. It is important to educate the public about potential hazards in both the work and home environments. In addition, safety education guidelines such as not drinking and driving, wearing a protective helmet when riding a bicycle, and using a safety belt in the car are important areas for discussion. Because most injuries occur at home, it is also important to discuss ways to make the home safer.

Assessment

The following data are collected through the health history and physical examination. Further focused assessments are described with nursing interventions in the next section.

- Health history: risk factors, nutrition, medication use (anti-inflammatory and corticosteroids), location, duration, and type (redness, heat, pain, swelling, and impaired function) of symptoms
- Physical assessment: movement of injured area, circulation, wounds, lymph nodes

Nursing Diagnoses and Interventions

The nursing care needs of the client with an inflammatory process are related to the manifestations of inflammation (pain in particular) and altered tissue integrity. Priority nursing diagnoses include *pain, impaired tissue integrity,* and *risk for infection.*

Pain

Along with redness, warmth, swelling, and impaired function, pain is one of the cardinal manifestations of inflammation. Depending on the cause, affected area, and degree of inflammation, pain may be acute and immobilizing or chronic and demoralizing. It is important to remember that pain is a subjective experience and that client responses to pain vary. (Refer to Chapter 4 for more information about pain and its management.) 🔗

- Assess pain using a scale of 0 to 10, with 0 being no pain and 10 being the worst pain; note the character and location of the pain. *Because pain is subjective, the client provides the most accurate information regarding his or her pain experience.*
- Use physical and nonverbal cues to further assess the level of pain. *This intervention is especially important if the client is nonverbal or tends to underreport pain.*
- Administer anti-inflammatory medications as prescribed. *These medications help reduce the pain resulting from acute inflammation.*
- Administer analgesic medications as prescribed. *Although most analgesics do little to reduce inflammation, they provide additional pain relief by reducing the perception of pain.*
- Monitor effectiveness of interventions. *Results may call for modifications in the regimen.*
- Provide comfort measures, such as back rubs, position changes, or relaxation techniques. *These measures reduce muscle tension, relieve areas of pressure, and provide distraction.*
- Encourage activities such as reading, watching television, and taking part in social interactions. *Such activities provide distraction from the pain experience.*
- Encourage rest. *Strenuous activity or exercising an inflamed body part may increase discomfort and tissue damage.*
- Provide cold or heat as pain-relief measures, as ordered. *For an acute injury, cold reduces swelling and relieves pain; after the initial stage, heat increases blood flow to the affected tissue and relieves pain and swelling by promoting absorption of edema. Either heat or cold may be contraindicated with some inflammatory processes; for example, if the appendix is acutely inflamed, applying heat to the abdomen may prompt the appendix to rupture, increasing the risk of peritonitis. If unsure, check with the client's primary care provider.*

PRACTICE ALERT *Use heat or cold application cautiously in older clients who have fragile skin and are at risk for tissue injury.* ■

- Elevate the inflamed area if possible. *Elevation promotes venous return and reduces swelling.*
- Teach about the appropriate use and expected effects of anti-inflammatory medications. *If the client's pain continues after the initial doses of anti-inflammatory medication, he or she may become discouraged and stop taking the medication before it becomes fully effective.*

Impaired Tissue Integrity

The inflammatory response can either precipitate or result from an impairment in the integrity of skin, support, or other tissues. Whatever the cause of the tissue alteration, it is vital that the nurse consider this alteration in delivering care.

- Assess general health and nutritional status. *Poor general health or chronic diseases such as diabetes mellitus or renal failure interfere with the healing processes and increase the risk of infection.*
- Assess circulation to the affected area. *Adequate tissue perfusion and oxygenation are necessary for healing.*
- Monitor the skin and surrounding tissue for increased signs of inflammation. *Inflammation can spread to adjacent tissues leading to conditions such as cellulitis.*
- Provide protection and support for inflamed tissue. *This reduces discomfort and decreases the risk of further tissue damage.*
- Clean inflamed tissue gently; if possible, use water, normal saline, or nontoxic wound cleansers such as Comfeel (Coloplast Corporation) only. *Soap and harsh cleansers such as povidone-iodine (Betadine) and hydrogen peroxide can cause further drying and tissue damage. Granulation tissue in a healing wound is fragile and easily damaged.* (See Chapter 7 for further discussion of wound care.) 🔗
- Keep the inflamed area dry, and expose it to air as much as possible. *This promotes healing and helps prevent infection.*
- Balance rest with the tolerable degree of mobility. *Rest decreases metabolic demands and allows for cell regeneration while mobility helps to promote oxygenation and perfusion of the tissues.*
- Provide supplemental oxygen as ordered. *Supplemental oxygen improves tissue oxygenation and reduces hypoxia.*
- Provide a well-balanced diet with adequate kilocalories to meet the body's metabolic and healing needs. If the client is allowed nothing by mouth (NPO), suggest parenteral or enteral nutrition. For the client who is unable to consume an adequate diet, consult with a dietitian for between-meal supplements, and/or multivitamin supplements. *Careful attention to diet and nutrient intake is important to provide the nutrients necessary for immune function and healing and to prevent catabolism.*

Risk for Infection

The inflammatory response often indicates that body defense mechanisms have been set in motion to protect against invading microorganisms. Wounds, whether traumatic or surgical in nature, are typically contaminated, as attested to by subsequent wound infections. The client with a healing wound is at particular risk for infection.

- Assess the wound for specific signs of infection, including purulent drainage, odor, and poor healing. *The normal inflammatory response can indicate infection and, on occasion, mask its presence.*

- Monitor temperature, pulse, and respirations at least every 4 hours. *In response to the inflammatory process the temperature rises, usually in the range of 99°F (37.2°C) to 100.9°F (38.2°C). A temperature of 101.0°F (38.3°C) or above indicates infection. Fever is usually accompanied by increased heart and respiratory rates.*
- Culture purulent or odorous wound drainage. *Wound culture is used to determine the infectious organism and to direct antibiotic therapy.*
- Apply dry or moist heat to the affected area for no longer than 20 minutes several times a day. *Heat increases the circulation of blood to and from the inflamed tissue. Time is limited to prevent burns.*
- Provide fluid intake of 2500 mL per day. *Adequate hydration promotes blood flow and nutrient supply to the tissues as well as dilutes and removes waste products from the body.*
- Assure adequate nutrition. *Adequate nutrition enhances the function and production of T cells and B cells, which are important in the immune response.*
- Use good handwashing techniques. *Handwashing removes transient microorganisms and is the best mechanism to prevent the spread of infection to a susceptible person.*
- Wear sterile gloves when providing wound care. *Using sterile gloves helps prevent further contamination of the wound and the spread of infection to other clients.*

Using NANDA, NIC, and NOC

Chart 8–1 shows links between NANDA, NIC, and NOC when caring for the client with inflammation.

Home Care

Client and family teaching enhances understanding of the inflammatory process, its cause, and its management. Teaching is also important to prevent further compromise that could result in infection.

Instructions, verbal and written, should include the following:

- Increase fluid intake to 2500 mL (approximately 2.5 quarts) per day.
- Eat a well-balanced diet high in vitamins and minerals and with adequate protein and kilocalories for healing.
- Use good handwashing techniques, particularly when caring for wounds or inflamed tissue and after using the bathroom.
- Elevate the inflamed area to reduce swelling and pain.
- Apply heat or cold for no longer than 20 minutes at a time to reduce the risk of tissue damage from burns or frostbite.
- Take all medications as prescribed, notifying the physician if adverse effects or hypersensitivity responses are noted.
- Rest acutely inflamed tissue; do not engage in strenuous activity until the inflammation has subsided.

THE CLIENT WITH NATURAL OR ACQUIRED IMMUNITY

Immunity refers to the protection of the body from disease. Immunity to disease may be either natural or acquired, active or passive (see Table 8–7).

CHART 8–1   NANDA, NIC, AND NOC LINKAGES

The Client with Tissue Inflammation and Healing

NURSING DIAGNOSES	NURSING INTERVENTIONS	NURSING OUTCOMES
• Activity Intolerance • Imbalanced Nutrition: Less than Body Requirements	• Energy Management • Fluid Monitoring • Nutrition Monitoring	• Energy Conservation • Self-Care: Activities of Daily Living • Nutritional Status: Food & Fluid Intake

Note. Data from Nursing Outcomes Classification (NOC) by M. Johnson & M. Maas (Eds.), 1997, St. Louis: Mosby; Nursing Diagnoses: Definitions & Classification 2001–2002 by North American Nursing Diagnosis Association, 2001, Philadelphia: NANDA; Nursing Interventions Classification (NIC) by J.C. McCloskey & G. M. Bulechek (Eds.), 2000, St. Louis: Mosby. Reprinted by permission.

TABLE 8–7   Types of Acquired Immunity

Type of Immunity		How Developed	Examples
Active Immunity	Natural	Acquired by infection with an antigen, resulting in the production of antibodies	Chickenpox, hepatitis A
	Artificial	Acquired by immunization with an antigen, such as attenuated live virus vaccine	MMR, polio, DPT, hepatitis B vaccines
Passive Immunity	Natural	Acquired by transfer of maternal antibodies to the fetus or neonate via the placenta or breast milk	Neonate initially protected against MMR if mother immune
	Artificial	Acquired by administration of antibodies or antitoxins in immune globulin	Gamma globulin injection following hepatitis A exposure

Immunity develops from the activation of the body's immune response. Depending on the antigen, antibody-mediated or cell-mediated responses are activated. The immune response typically involves components of both. In the immunocompetent client, these responses inactivate and remove the antigen, allowing recovery to occur or preventing the development of disease.

PATHOPHYSIOLOGY

The processes of antibody-mediated and cell-mediated immunity result in the development of **acquired immunity** or **active immunity.** Active immunity occurs when the body produces antibodies or develops immune lymphocytes against specific antigens. Memory cells, which can produce an immediate immune response on reexposure to the antigen, provide long-term immunity.

Active immunity can be naturally acquired, resulting from contact with the disease-producing antigen and subsequent development of the disease. Naturally acquired immunity is common for diseases such as chickenpox and hepatitis A, making the risk of developing the disease a second time very low.

For many diseases, the potential consequences of a single disease episode on the individual and society make prevention desirable, especially for highly contagious diseases capable of causing epidemics. In these instances, immunization or vaccination is used to provide artificially acquired immunity. The purpose of vaccination is to establish adequate levels of antibody and/or memory cells to provide effective immunity (Roitt, 1994). Vaccination introduces the disease-producing antigen into the body in a manner that will stimulate the immune system to form antibodies and memory cells but will not produce disease. Vaccines may be made of killed organisms or of live organisms that have been attenuated or modified to reduce their disease-producing capability. Typhoid is an example of a killed organism vaccine; measles-mumps-rubella (MMR) vaccine, by contrast, is made from attenuated organisms. Many newer vaccines use subunits of the antigen; these are portions of the organism that have antigenic properties but are unable to produce disease.

Passive immunity provides temporary protection against disease-producing antigens. Passive immunity is provided by antibodies produced by other people or animals. These acquired antibodies are used up; they either combine with the antigen or are naturally degraded by the body, and their protection is gradually lost. Naturally acquired passive immunity is provided by the transfer of maternal antibodies via the placenta and breast milk to the infant. Rabies human immune globulin and hepatitis B immune globulin (HBIG) are examples of immunizations used to provide artificially acquired passive immunity. The types of active and passive immunity are summarized in Table 8–7.

COLLABORATIVE CARE

Collaborative care focuses primarily on assessing the client's immune status and ensuring acquired immunity to prevent disease.

Diagnostic Tests

A number of diagnostic tests can be performed to assess the client's immune status.

- *Serum protein* measures the total protein in the blood including albumin and globulins. Normal levels for the adult are 6 to 8 g/dL; albumin is approximately 60% (3.2 to 4.5 g/dL) of the total serum protein; and globulins are normally 2.3 to 3.4 g/dL. Total protein levels, albumin, and globulin are decreased in malnutrition and liver disease. Decreased globulin levels are noted with immunologic deficiencies.

- *Protein electrophoresis* analyzes protein content especially for albumin and gamma globulin and is used to assess immune function. Gamma globulins subjected to further electrophoresis separate into immunoglobulins: IgA, IgD, IgE, IgG, and IgM (see Table 8–3.) Analysis of specific levels of each provides clues about the immune status of the client. IgG levels are increased during acute infection. Decreased levels of IgG, IgA, and IgM are found in malignancies.

- *Antibody testing* is ordered to determine if a client has developed antibodies in response to an infection or immunization. Antibodies for hepatitis, HIV, rubella, toxoplasmosis, and *Treponema pallidum* (the organism causing syphilis) can be identified. An elevated titer level for hepatitis and rubella indicates immunity. For the other disorders and hepatitis, it may also be used to determine if the client has the disease.

- *Skin testing* can assess cell-mediated immunity. A known antigen such as streptokinase, tuberculin purified protein derivative (PPD), or candida is injected intradermally. The site is then observed for induration and erythema, which typically peaks at 24 to 48 hours. An induration of at least 10 mm in diameter is a positive reaction indicating previous exposure and sensitization to the antigen. (See Chapter 9 for further information on skin testing for hypersensitivity reactions.) ∞ No reaction, or **anergy,** indicates depressed cell-mediated immunity.

Immunizations

Vaccines are suspensions of whole or fractionated bacteria or viruses that have been treated to make them nonpathogenic. Vaccines are given to induce an immune response and subsequent immunity. Although vaccine development has been a major factor in improving public health, no vaccine is completely effective or entirely safe. Table 8–8 outlines the vaccines recommended for the adult client to maintain optimal health and immune status.

Adults born before 1956 are generally considered to be immune to measles, mumps, and rubella by prior infection. For persons born after 1956 whose immunologic status is unclear or who are at significant risk of exposure to these diseases (e.g., persons entering health care careers), reimmunization is recommended.

Tetanus and diphtheria toxoids are combined in a single immunization. The pediatric form of the vaccine is known as DT; the adult form is Td. The vaccine stimulates active immunity by inducing the production of antibodies and antitoxins. After

TABLE 8-8   Recommended Immunizations for Adults

Vaccine	Type	Dose	Indications	Precautions and Nursing Implications
Measles / mumps / rubella (MMR)	Live virus	0.5 mL SC	All adults born after 1956, particularly those who are at risk for infection, such as college students and military recruits. Measles and mumps vaccination particularly recommended for males without history of previous infection; rubella vaccination recommended for all seronegative females.	As a live virus vaccine, should not be administered to pregnant women or immunocompromised clients. Do not administer to clients with a history of anaphylactic reaction to egg protein or neomycin.
Tetanus and diphtheria toxoids (Td)	Inactivated toxins	0.5 mL IM	Initial series of 3 injections (2 doses, 4 to 6 weeks apart; third dose 6 to 12 months after dose 2) if never immunized; booster every 10 years; following a major or contaminated wound if more than 5 years since last booster	Do not give in first trimester of pregnancy or to clients with a history of anaphylactic reaction to horse serum; administer deep IM in deltoid of dominant arm.
Hepatitis B (HB)	Inactive viral antigen	1.0 mL IM	Series of 3 doses: initial and at 1 and 6 months. Recommended for anyone at risk for exposure and for postexposure prophylaxis	Use with caution in pregnant or lactating females, older clients, and clients with active infection; have epinephrine 1:1000 available on unit in case of anaphylaxis and laryngospasm.
Influenza	Inactivated virus or viral components	0.5 mL IM	Yearly for all clients over age 65 and those at risk for complications, including debilitated clients and clients with chronic disease	Do not administer to acutely ill clients or clients with history of anaphylactic reaction to egg protein.
Pneumococcal	Bacterial polysaccharides	0.5 mL IM or SC	One dose for clients over age 65 and those at risk for pneumococcal pneumonia, including clients with chronic lung disease or other chronic diseases	Do not administer to pregnant women.

an initial series of three immunizations, an intramuscular (IM) booster injection of 0.5 mL is recommended every 10 years to maintain protection. Older clients, particularly those who never entered the workforce (e.g., older female adults), may have never received the initial series of DT vaccine.

Hepatitis B (HB) vaccine is given as a series of three or four immunizations to promote active immunity to hepatitis B. This vaccine is recommended for everyone at high risk for exposure through blood or other body fluids. It is mandated by the Occupational Health and Safety Administration (OSHA) for all health care workers at risk. Other high-risk populations include intravenous drug users, sexual partners of infected individuals, clients on hemodialysis, prison guards, and athletic coaches.

Influenza vaccine is recommended for persons at high risk for serious sequelae of influenza, including older adults, persons with lung disease or other chronic illness, and immunosuppressed individuals. The antigenic strain included in influenza vaccine varies each year according to the predicted predominant strains affecting the population. Yearly reimmunization is therefore required.

Pneumococcal vaccine is generally recommended for the same populations as influenza vaccine. A single dose of this vaccine confers lifetime immunity, although repeating immunization every 6 years may be considered for high-risk clients.

In addition to routine immunizations, people traveling outside the United States and Canada should receive vaccines against diseases that are endemic in certain regions of the world.

Other immunologic substances may be administered as indicated. Immune globulins provide passive immunity as protection against a known or potential exposure to an antigen. Standard immune globulin is given to household contacts of clients with hepatitis A and persons traveling to areas in which it is endemic. Hepatitis B immune globulin (HBIG) contains higher titers of antibody to hepatitis B virus and is used for persons exposed by blood or sexual contact. Following confirmed or suspected contact with a pathogen, selected vaccines may be administered to stimulate an immediate immune response (Table 8–9).

For most vaccines, a sensitivity test should be performed prior to administration to detect sensitivity to substances such as horse serum or eggs. The substance is injected intradermally; if after 20 minutes there is no evidence of a reaction, the selected vaccine can be administered.

Moderate to severe local reactions may occur following administration of an immunization. Common reactions include redness, swelling, tenderness, and muscle ache. Administering the vaccine in the dominant arm of the client helps minimize local reactions, because use and movement of the arm facilitates absorption of the solution. Applying heat to the site is

TABLE 8–9 Preparations for Postexposure Prophylaxis

Disease	Preparation and Dose	Indications
Hepatitis A	Human immune globulin (IG), 0.02 mL/kg IM	Contacts in day care centers, households, custodial institutions; patrons of eating establishments known to have been exposed by infected food worker
Hepatitis B	Hepatitis B immune globulin (HBIG), 0.06 mL/kg IM	Possible percutaneous or sexual contact with blood or body fluids of an infected individual; usually given concurrently with hepatitis B vaccine
Varicella	Varicella-zoster immune globulin (VZIG), 12.5 units/kg; minimum dose 125 units, maximum 625 units	Susceptible adults exposed to varicella virus (e.g., chickenpox or shingles)
Tetanus	Tetanus immune globulin (TIG), 500 to 3000 units IM (part infiltrated around wound)	Clients with major or contaminated wounds who have no history of tetanus immunization or an unclear one that is not up-to-date; Td usually given as well
Rabies	Human rabies immune globulin (HRIG), 20 IU/kg, half IM, half infiltrated around wound	Persons with a significant exposure to a rabid or potentially rabid animal; followed with 5-dose course of rabies vaccine
Measles	Human immune globulin (IG), 0.25 mL/kg IM	Susceptible close contacts, especially people who are immunosuppressed; postpone immunization with measles vaccine until 3 months after IG
Rubella	Human immune globulin (IG), 0.55 mL/kg IM	Pregnant women exposed in first trimester when termination of pregnancy is not an option; does not ensure protection of fetus

Note. Table adapted from Harrison's Principles of Internal Medicine (14th ed.) by A. S. Fauci et al. (Eds.), 1998, New York: McGraw-Hill.

also beneficial. Occasionally local ulcerations occur; when they do, warm, wet pack, or sterile wet-to-dry dressings may be prescribed.

NURSING CARE

Maintaining a population that is fully immunized against common, potentially epidemic, and devastating diseases is a major public health task for nursing. Nurses not only recommend and administer vaccines to individual clients and their families, but also plan and implement preventive care for whole communities.

Although this process may appear to be straightforward, multiple issues affect society's ability to immunize the entire population. For some people, for example, religious beliefs may preclude the use of immunizations to prevent disease. Also, people who are not citizens and the medically indigent population have difficulty accessing immunization services. Lack of immunization not only puts the individual at increased risk for infectious disease, but also increases the cost of medical services and the possibility of exposing immunocompromised people to disease.

Health Promotion

In the public health setting, the nurse looks at the immunization needs and illness risk for an entire community. Communities include not only cities and localities but also groups of people, such as college populations and employees in a workplace. Public education needs may be met through presentations to groups of people, feature articles in newspapers and other local publications, advertising, radio presentations and public service announcements, and one-to-one discussion and teaching.

Assessment

Collect the following data through the health history and physical examination. Further focused assessments are described with nursing interventions in the next section.

- Health history: age, medication use (corticosteroids and antibiotics) and blood transfusion, nutrition, allergies, infection, immunizations, autoimmune disorders, chronic diseases such as diabetes mellitus, cancer
- Physical assessment: skin lesions or rashes, breath sounds, respiratory rate

Nursing Diagnoses and Interventions

Nursing care focuses on preventing injury from the immunization and educating the client.

Health-Seeking Behaviors: Immunization

For individual clients and their families, nurses promote immunocompetence by assessing immune status, recommending appropriate immunizations, and administering vaccines as ordered or indicated. Once a person reaches adulthood, routine immunizations often become a neglected part of health care.

- Determine knowledge level, understanding, attitudes, and religious beliefs about immunization. *This provides a basis for further education and determines if religious beliefs may contraindicate immunization.*
- Discuss the value and reasons for recommended immunizations. *Understanding promotes adherence.*

- Reinforce positive health-seeking behaviors. *This will help promote future health maintenance activities.*
- Using recommended immunization schedules, develop a plan to attain optimal immunization status. *Adherence with recommended schedules for immunization is important in preventing disease and disability.*
- Do not administer MMR or influenza vaccine if allergic to eggs or tetanus antitoxin if sensitive to horse serum. *Vaccines prepared from chicken or duck embryos are contraindicated in clients who are allergic to eggs. Tetanus antitoxin is prepared from horse serum. Both will cause a severe allergic reaction.*
- Withhold administration of active immunologic products in the presence of an upper respiratory infection (URI) or other infection. *Active immunizations can cause a greater inflammatory reaction in the presence of infections.*
- Do not administer oral polio vaccine (OPV), MMR, or any live virus vaccine to immunosuppressed clients or to clients who are in close household contact with an immunosuppressed person. *Live virus vaccines can cause disease in the immunosuppressed client. The virus may be transmitted from close household contacts during the initial postvaccination period.*
- Do not administer live attenuated virus vaccines and passive immunizations such as gamma globulin simultaneously. *Passive antibodies interfere with the response of the live attenuated virus.*
- Prior to administering prescribed vaccine, check expiration date and manufacturer's instructions. *Outdated vaccines cannot provide adequate immunization protection. Certain injection sites have better absorption than others.*
- Keep epinephrine 1:1000 readily available when administering immunizations. *Epinephrine causes vasoconstriction and reduces laryngospasm; in acute anaphylaxis, it can be lifesaving.*

PRACTICE ALERT   *Observe the client for 20 to 30 minutes following inoculation to monitor for possible adverse reactions.* ∎

Using NANDA, NIC, and NOC

Chart 8–2 shows links between NANDA, NIC, and NOC when caring for the client who is receiving an immunization.

Home Care

Educating individual clients, families, and the public about the maintenance of immune status is a significant nursing responsibility. For individual clients and their families, instructions focus on the following areas.

- Appropriate immunizations and recommended schedules for initial vaccination and boosters
- How and where to obtain immunizations
- The need to observe the client for up to 30 minutes following a vaccine for possible adverse reactions
- Possible side effects and adverse effects of the immunization administered
- Self-care measures for side effects and postvaccination discomfort
- Responses to immunization that should be reported immediately to the primary care provider
- Maintenance of a permanent immunization record
- Beneficial resources:
  - County or public health departments
  - Centers for Disease Control and Prevention National Immunization Program
  - National Institute of Allergy and Infectious Diseases

THE CLIENT WITH AN INFECTION

In an effort to find a suitable environment in which to grow and reproduce, microorganisms—including bacteria, viruses, fungi, and parasites—often invade the human body. In most cases, contact between humans and microorganisms is incidental and may even be beneficial to both organisms. Resident bacteria of the skin, mucous membranes, and gastrointestinal tract are an important part of the body's defense system. However, many microorganisms are virulent; that is, they have the ability to cause disease. **Pathogens** are virulent organisms rarely found in the absence of disease. Some microorganisms known as opportunistic pathogens rarely, if ever, cause harm to persons with intact immune systems, but are capable of producing infectious disease in the immunocompromised host (Porth, 2002).

Infectious disease has been pervasive throughout history. Modern medicine, antibiotic therapy, immunizations, and

CHART 8–2   NANDA, NIC, AND NOC LINKAGES

The Client with Acquired Immunity

NURSING DIAGNOSIS	NURSING INTERVENTIONS	NURSING OUTCOMES
• Risk for Injury	• Health Screening • Immunization/Vaccination Management • Health Education • Health Beliefs	• Immune Status • Immunization Behaviors

Note. Data from Nursing Outcomes Classification (NOC) by M. Johnson & M. Maas (Eds.), 1997, St. Louis: Mosby; Nursing Diagnoses: Definitions & Classification 2001–2002 by North American Nursing Diagnosis Association, 2001, Philadelphia: NANDA; Nursing Interventions Classification (NIC) by J.C. McCloskey & G. M. Bulechek (Eds.), 2000, St. Louis: Mosby. Reprinted by permission.

Nursing Care Plan
A Client with Acquired Immunity

Terry Adams is a 48-year-old executive who is planning a trip to central Africa. In preparation, he contacts his local health care provider to obtain the necessary immunizations. Jane Wong, the registered nurse in the clinic, obtains a nursing history on Mr. Adams.

ASSESSMENT

Mr. Adams's history reveals that he has always been very healthy and active, apart from a mild case of asthma. As an adult, he has had little problem with his asthma, "except for those rare occasions on which I am dumb enough to smoke more than one cigarette!" He is divorced and is not currently in a continuing relationship. He has two grown daughters with whom his relationship is good. Since contracting hepatitis A several years ago, he drinks alcohol only rarely, and never more than one or two drinks at any one time. He confesses to little organized exercise but plays golf two or three times a week and states that he is such a hyperactive workaholic that he rarely sits for any length of time. Mr. Adams has not seen a physician since recovering from the hepatitis and is unsure when he last received any immunizations. He does know if he had all recommended childhood immunizations, but recalls getting both Salk and Sabin polio vaccines when they became available. His physical examination reveals an alert and healthy individual with no abnormalities noted. His vital signs are as follows: T 97.4°F, P 64, R 14, and BP 142/82.

The physician orders the following immunizations for Mr. Adams:

- Measles-mumps-rubella (MMR)
- Combined tetanus and diphtheria toxoids (Td)
- Yellow fever vaccine
- Typhoid vaccine
- Meningococcal meningitis vaccine

DIAGNOSES

- *Health-seeking behaviors: immunization* related to impending international travel
- *Altered health maintenance* related to apparent lapse in immunization status
- *Risk for injury* related to adverse response to immunization

EXPECTED OUTCOMES

- Obtain necessary immunizations.
- Verbalize a schedule for maintaining up-to-date immunization status.
- Experience no significant adverse effects from immunization.

PLANNING AND IMPLEMENTATION

- Administer MMR, Td, and meningococcal meningitis vaccines prior to discharge from clinic.
- Observe closely for 30 minutes following immunization for potential adverse responses.
- Schedule return visit in 1 week for typhoid vaccine.
- Provide referral to a registered vaccination center for yellow fever vaccine and documentation of vaccination.
- Provide instructions for comfort measures to relieve local and systemic adverse effects of vaccines. Provide written instructions on manifestations that should be reported to the physician.
- Document immunizations on a permanent record at the clinic and for the client.

EVALUATION

Terry Adams completes his prescribed immunizations without major adverse effects, although he does complain of fever, malaise, and general achiness for several days following the typhoid vaccination. His trip to Africa is successful, and he returns to the United States without contracting any infectious diseases.

Critical Thinking in the Nursing Process

1. Explain why it is important for adults to continue receiving immunizations throughout their life span.
2. If a client says said to you, "I don't believe in immunizations. I hear they are dangerous," how would you respond?
3. When should a client contact the primary caregiver after receiving an immunization?

See Evaluating Your Responses in Appendix C.

---

other public health measures to protect food and water supplies have significantly reduced the prevalence of infectious diseases in many parts of the world. In spite of these advances, many infections, including malaria, typhoid, and tuberculosis, remain prevalent in developing nations. Sexually transmitted infections (STIs) rage through modern cities and industrialized populations. New varieties and strains of pathogens, such as human immunodeficiency virus (HIV), evolve to cause disease.

To a certain extent, modern medicine has contributed to the development of infectious diseases caused by antibiotic-resistant strains of microorganisms. Tuberculosis is on the rise in the United States, partially because organisms have become resistant to standard therapies. Clients receive immunosuppressive therapy following organ or tissue transplant or in the treatment of neoplasms, making them more susceptible to infection. Metal and plastic prosthetic devices are implanted, providing potential sites for colonization by disease-producing organisms (Fauci et al., 1998). It has also become apparent that many diseases long considered unrelated to microorganisms may actually be infectious; for example, colonization of the gastric mucosa with *Helicobacter pylori* may be the predominant cause of peptic ulcer disease, and oncogenic viruses have the ability to transform normal cells into malignant cells.

PATHOPHYSIOLOGY

Infection occurs when an organism is able to colonize and multiply within a host. The host can be any organism capable of supporting the nutritional and physical growth requirements of the microorganism—for example, humans. When the host experiences injury, pathologic changes, inflammation, or organ dysfunction in response to an infection or from intoxication

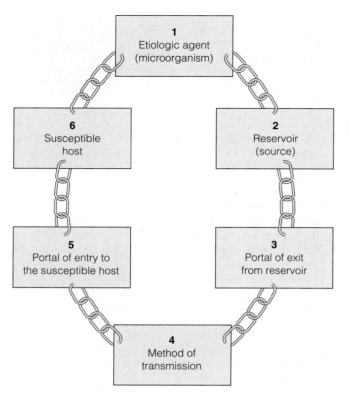

Figure 8–12 ■ The chain of infection.

by cellular poisons produced by a pathogen, it is called an infectious disease.

For a microorganism to cause infection, it must have disease-causing potential (virulence), be transmitted from its reservoir, and gain entry into a susceptible host. This is known as the chain of infection (Figure 8–12 ■).

Pathogens

Pathogens capable of infecting and causing disease in a susceptible host include bacteria, viruses, mycoplasma, rickettsia, chlamydia, fungi, and parasites such as protozoa, helminths (worms), and arthropods (Box 8–4). Each organism causes a different specific reaction in the host.

A number of different mechanisms have evolved in pathogens to facilitate their transmission and increase their ability to invade the host and cause disease. Factors influencing the transmission of an organism include its resistance to drying and to variations in environmental temperature. For example, spore-forming organisms are extremely resistant to drying.

Many microorganisms are capable of producing toxins or enzymes to facilitate their invasion of the host, increase their resistance to host defenses, and increase their ability to cause disease. Adhesion factors produced by or incorporated into the cell wall or membrane of the pathogen improve its ability to attach and colonize the host. Pathogens may also produce enzymes to enhance their spread to local tissues, chemicals to block specific

---

BOX 8–4   ■ Pathogenic Organisms

BACTERIA

Bacteria are single-celled organisms capable of autonomous reproduction. Relatively small and simple organisms, they contain a single chromosome: A flexible cell membrane and rigid cell wall surrounds their cytoplasm, giving them a distinctive shape; some also have an extracellular capsule for additional protection. Bacteria have different characteristics and growth requirements: *aerobes* require oxygen for survival, whereas *anaerobes* cannot survive in the presence of oxygen; *gram-positive* bacteria stain purple when subjected to crystal violet stain, whereas *gram-negative* bacteria do not stain with crystal violet but turn red when subjected to safranin stain; the colonies formed by replicating bacteria differ from one another.

VIRUSES

Viruses are obligate intracellular parasites that are incapable of reproducing outside of a living cell. Viruses consist of a protein coat around a core of either DNA or RNA. Some viruses are shed continuously from infected cell surfaces; others, after inserting their genetic material into that of the infected cell, remain latent until they are stimulated to replicate. Viruses may or may not cause lysis and death of the host cell during replication. Oncogenic viruses are able to transform normal cells into malignant cells.

MYCOPLASMA

Although similar to bacteria, mycoplasma are smaller and have no cell wall, making them resistant to antibiotics that inhibit cell wall synthesis (e.g., penicillins).

RICKETTSIA AND CHLAMYDIA

As obligate intracellular parasites with a rigid cell wall, rickettsia and *Chlamydia* have some features of both bacteria and viruses. Rather than depending on the host cell for reproduction, they use vitamins, nutrients, or products of metabolism (e.g., ATP) from the host. *Chlamydia* are transmitted by direct contact, whereas many rickettsiae infect the cells of arthropods (e.g., fleas, ticks, and lice) and are transmitted from these vectors to humans.

FUNGI

Fungi are prevalent throughout the world, but few are capable of causing disease in humans. Most fungal infections are self-limited, affecting the skin and subcutaneous tissue. Some fungi, such as *Pneumocystis carinii,* can cause life-threatening opportunistic infections in the immunocompromised host.

PARASITES

The term *parasite* is typically applied to members of the animal kingdom that infect and cause disease in other animals. Protozoa, helminths, and arthropods are considered parasites. Protozoa are single-celled organisms transmitted via direct or indirect contact or an arthropod vector. Helminths are wormlike parasites: roundworms, tapeworms, and flukes are examples. They gain entry into humans primarily through ingestion of fertilized eggs or penetration of larvae through the skin or mucous membranes. Arthropod parasites, such as scabies (mites), lice, and fleas, typically infest external body surfaces, causing localized tissue damage and inflammation. Transmission is by direct contact with the arthropod or its eggs.

Note. Data summarized from Pathophysiology: Concepts of Altered Health States *(6th ed.) by C. M. Porth, 2002, Philadelphia: Lippincott.*

immune processes or deplete neutrophils and macrophages, or extracellular capsules to discourage phagocytosis.

Pathogens are often capable of producing toxins that alter or destroy the normal function of host cells and promote colonization, proliferation, and invasion by the pathogen. Toxins often increase the disease-producing capability of the pathogen and, in some cases, are totally responsible for it; for example, cholera, tetanus, and botulism result from bacterial toxins, not from the direct effects of the infection. **Exotoxins** are soluble proteins secreted into surrounding tissue by the microorganism. Exotoxins are highly poisonous, causing cell death or dysfunction. **Endotoxins** are found in the cell wall of gram-negative bacteria and are released only when the cell is disrupted. Endotoxins have less specific effects than exotoxins, but they act as activators of many human regulatory systems, producing fever, inflammation, and potentially clotting, bleeding, or hypotension when released in large quantities.

Reservoir and Transmission

The reservoir or source, where the pathogen lives and multiplies, may be either endogenous or exogenous. Organisms that reside on skin or mucosal surfaces of the host are endogenous. Exogenous sources can include other humans, animals, soil, water, intravenous fluid, or equipment. Infectious diseases are usually transmitted from human sources, that is, persons who have clinical disease or carriers with subclinical infection. Carriers harbor the pathogen without showing evidence of clinical disease. Pathogens exit human hosts via respiratory secretions, body fluids from the gastrointestinal and genitourinary tracts, skin or mucous membrane lesions, the placenta, and blood.

Organisms may be transmitted from the source to the susceptible host by direct or indirect contact, droplet or airborne transmission, or a vector. Direct contact includes person-to-person spread or contact with infected body fluids, as well as transmission from contaminated food or water. Indirect contact occurs when the infectious agent is contracted by use of inanimate objects, such as dirty eating utensils. Sneezing, talking, and coughing allow transmission by droplet contact when the host is within 2 to 3 feet of the source. Smaller respiratory particles that stay suspended in air and are carried via air currents allow airborne transmission. Vectors are insects and animals such as flies, mosquitoes, or rodents that act as intermediate hosts between the source and host. Microorganisms usually first colonize the portal of entry: nonintact skin, wounds, mucous membranes, and the respiratory, gastrointestinal, or genitourinary tracts.

Host Factors

The susceptible host is the final link in the chain of infection. Exposure to pathogens does not automatically cause infection or infectious disease. The outcome of contact with a pathogenic microorganism is determined by the balance of microbial virulence and host resistance. Factors that can enable the host to resist infection include the following:

- Physical barriers, such as the skin and mucous membranes
- The hostile environment created by acid stomach secretions, urine, and vaginal secretions

- Antimicrobial factors in saliva, tears, and prostatic fluid
- Respiratory defenses, including humidification, filtration, the mucociliary escalator, cough reflex, and alveolar macrophages
- Specific and nonspecific immune responses to pathogenic invasion

Stages of the Infectious Process

When infectious disease develops in the host, it typically follows a predictable course with stages based on the progression and intensity of manifestations.

The initial stage is the incubation period, during which the pathogen begins active replication but does not yet cause symptoms. Depending on the organism and host factors, the incubation period may last from hours, as with salmonella, to years, as with HIV infection.

The prodromal stage follows, during which symptoms first begin to appear. At this stage, symptoms are often nonspecific and include general malaise, fever, myalgias, headache, and fatigue.

Maximal impact of the infectious process is felt during the acute phase as the pathogen proliferates and disseminates rapidly. Toxic by-products of microorganism metabolism and cell lysis, along with the immune response, produce tissue damage and inflammation during this stage (Porth, 2002). Manifestations are more pronounced and specific to the infecting organism and site during the acute stage. Fever and chills may be significant during this phase. However, alcoholic clients and the very old may respond to severe infection by becoming hypothermic. The client is often tachycardic and tachypneic because of increased metabolic demands. Localized manifestations include redness, heat, swelling, pain, and impaired function. When the infectious disease affects an internal organ, manifestations are related to inflammatory changes in that organ and surrounding tissue. The client may experience tenderness to palpation over the site or show signs of impaired function, such as the hematuria and proteinuria characteristic of renal infections.

If the infectious process is prolonged, manifestations of the continuing immune response may become apparent. Catabolic and anorexic effects of the infection can lead to loss of body fat and muscle wasting. Immune complexes may be deposited at sites other than the primary infection, resulting in an inflammatory process. Glomerulonephritis (e.g., following strep throat) and vasculitis are possible results. Another possible consequence of prolonged infection and immune response is the triggering of an autoimmune disease process (discussed in Chapter 9), such as rheumatic cardiomyopathy or celiac disease. Juvenile-onset diabetes mellitus is thought to be the result of such a response (Fauci et al., 1998).

As the infection is contained and the pathogen eliminated, the convalescent stage of the disease occurs. During this stage, affected tissues are repaired and manifestations resolve. Resolution of the infection is total elimination of the pathogen from the body without residual manifestations. If a balance between organism and host factors occurs with neither predominating, chronic disease may develop or the organism may be driven into a protected site, such as an abscess. A carrier state develops when host defenses eliminate the infectious disease but the organism continues to multiply on mucosal sites (Fauci et al., 1998).

Complications

Multiple and varied complications are associated with infectious diseases. They are typically specific to the infecting organism and the body system affected.

Acute invasion of the blood by certain microorganisms or their toxins can result in septicemia and septic shock. Whereas bacteremia, the presence of bacteria in the blood, may not have serious effects, septicemia refers to systemic disease associated with their presence or toxins. Septic shock indicates a state of hypotension and impaired organ perfusion resulting from sepsis. Unless treated aggressively, septic shock leads to diffuse cell and tissue injury, and potentially to organ failure. See Chapter 6 for an in-depth discussion of septic shock, other shock syndromes, and their management. ⊘⊘

Nosocomial Infections

Nosocomial infections are acquired in a health care setting, such as a hospital or nursing home. Currently, 5% of clients acquire a nosocomial infection while hospitalized, but this rate may rise to 10% in larger institutions (Wenzel and Edmond, 2001). Hospital-acquired infections add over 7.5 million hospital days, directly result in approximately 20,000 deaths, and contribute to 60,000 more deaths yearly in the United States (Fauci et al., 1998).

Clients entering hospitals are often the least able to mount immune defenses to infection. Immunologic responses may be compromised and normal defenses impaired in clients with, for example, cancer or chronic diseases, pressure ulcers, or organ transplants (Tierney et al., 2001). Nosocomial infections also occur when antibiotic therapy has altered natural defenses and impaired resistance to harmful microorganisms. Endogenous organisms outside their normal habitats (such as in *Escherichia coli* in the urinary tract) become a threat to the client. Other pharmacologic and therapeutic procedures such as chemotherapy, the use of corticosteroids, or radiation therapy also contribute to nosocomial infections. Gram-negative enteric bacteria and gram-positive *Staphylococcus aureus* are the most common bacteria responsible.

Invasive procedures and altered immune defenses are the main factors contributing to infection. Urinary catheterization is the number-one cause; cardiac catheterization, peripheral and central intravenous lines, respiratory care procedures, and surgical procedures are also closely linked to nosocomial infection (Box 8–5). Consequently, the urinary tract, surgical wounds, the respiratory tract, and invasive catheter sites on the skin are most often affected by hospital-acquired infection. The American Hospital Association (2001) reports that hospital-acquired pneumonia is the second most common nosocomial infection, and has the highest morbidity and mortality. Organisms causing the infection are often resistant to many drugs, not responding to antibiotics usually effective in treating infections acquired outside the hospital.

> ### BOX 8–5 ■ Nosocomial Infections
>
> - Nosocomial infections typically manifest after 48 hours of hospitalization.
> - Urinary tract infection is the most common type, accounting for about 45% of all nosocomial infections.
> - Pneumonia accounts for 15% of all nosocomial infections related to endotracheal or nasogastric intubation.
> - Surgical wounds account for 30% of all nosocomial infections.
> - Bacteremia accounts for 7% of all nosocomial infections related to invasive devices (e.g., intravenous catheters, arterial lines).
> - Antibiotic-associated diarrhea accounts for less than 3% of all nosocomial infections related to prophylactic antibiotic doses.

Prevention is the most important control measure for nosocomial infections. The pathogens causing these infections are transmitted primarily by contact with hospital personnel. **Effective hand washing is the single most important measure in infection control.** Although infections may also be transmitted by the airborne route, contaminated equipment, or from the environment, these are less significant causes. Invasive procedures and equipment should be used only when absolutely necessary; for example, it is not appropriate to insert an indwelling catheter when the only indication is incontinence. Peripheral intravenous equipment and sites must be changed regularly: intravenous bags and bottles every 24 hours, tubing every 24 to 72 hours, and sites every 2 to 3 days according to agency policy (Smith, Duell, & Martin, 2000).

Antibiotic-Resistant Microorganisms

Antibiotic-resistant microorganisms are increasing at an alarming rate primarily due to prolonged or inappropriate use of antibiotic therapy. Although antibiotic therapy is expected to eradicate all targeted microorganisms, sometimes a few bacteria survive, leading to bacteria that reproduce with antibiotic resistance already encoded into their genetic makeup (Glover, 2000). Other bacteria produce enzymes that inactivate drugs, change drug binding sites, or alter their cell membrane to prevent drug absorption.

Some of the current resistant strains include:

- Methicillin-resistant *Staphylococcus aureus* (MRSA)
- Multidrug-resistant tuberculosis (MDR-TB)
- Penicillin-resistant *Streptococcus pneumoniae* (PRSP)
- Vancomycin-resistant *Enterococci* (VRE)
- Vancomycin intermediate-resistant *Staphylococcus aureus* (VISA)

Methicillin-resistant *Staphylococcus aureus* (MRSA) exists not only in hospitals but also is becoming more prevalent in nonhospital settings. MRSA colonizes in the nares and skin; health care personnel often transmit *S. aureus* unknowingly on their hands. Most *S. aureus* strains resist treatment by methicillin and other similar drugs, the treatment of choice for *S. aureus* infections. Vancomycin has been the only uniformly effective drug for MRSA; however, in 1997, a new form of

S. aureus emerged with intermediate resistance to vancomycin, known as **vancomycin intermediate-resistant *Staphylococcus aureus* (VISA).** Clients with MRSA and VISA are isolated in a private room using contact precautions.

Enterococci are part of the normal flora of the gastrointestinal and female genital tracts. Frequent use of vancomycin caused *Enterococci* to develop resistance, leading to **vancomycin-resistant *Enterococci* (VRE).** Direct transmission occurs on the hands of health care personnel or contact with contaminated equipment. Stringent infection control measures are instituted; care is provided using contact precautions and clients are placed either alone or with other VRE-infected clients.

Streptococcus pneumoniae, the most common cause of community-acquired pneumonia, has developed into its resistant form, **penicillin-resistant *Streptococcus pneumoniae* (PRSP).** Unlike MRSA and VRE, PRSP is transmitted by droplets from the respiratory tract and requires transmission-based droplet precautions.

Biological Threat Infections

Following the terrorist attacks on September 11, 2001, and the development of anthrax cases in the United States, concern has arisen about the possible use of biological weapons. The most likely pathogens to be used for this purpose include anthrax, smallpox, botulism, pneumonic plague, and viral hemorrhagic fevers.

Anthrax is an acute bacterial infection caused by *Bacillus anthracis,* a gram-positive, spore-producing organism that occurs in inhaled, cutaneous, and gastrointestinal forms. The spores are impervious to temperature and sunlight, and remain viable for years.

Inhalation anthrax carries the highest mortality rate because spores of 1 to 5 microns are easily inhaled and deposited in the alveoli (Coleman, 2001). The client initially exhibits influenzalike symptoms such as fever, nonproductive cough, headache, and malaise that advances to respiratory failure and hemodynamic collapse. Untreated clients die in 2 to 3 days. The characteristic lesion of cutaneous anthrax progresses from an itching papule to a painless, serosanguinous-filled vesicle that forms a black necrotic center. Clients who ingest the anthrax bacillus develop nausea, vomiting, severe abdominal pain, and bloody diarrhea. Diagnosis is confirmed by a positive blood culture, polymerase chain reaction, and serology. On confirmation of anthrax exposure, prophylaxis is initiated with oral ciprofloxacin (Cipro) or doxycycline (Doxylin) for 60 days; whereas people with confirmed systemic anthrax cases must receive anti-infectives intravenously.

In 1980, the World Health Organization certified that *smallpox* was eradicated. Routine smallpox vaccination was discontinued in 1972, leaving people under the age of 30 at risk for this disease if it reappears or is used as a weapon. Smallpox spreads by direct contact or by inhalation of respiratory droplets. Symptoms include a high fever, headache, and malaise, followed by a vesicular/pustular rash appearing simultaneously on the face and extremities. Once the pustules become scabs, people are highly contagious and should be placed in negative-pressure rooms. Anyone exposed to the client should

be vaccinated and monitored closely. Vaccination within 2 to 3 days of exposure provides almost complete protection.

Health care providers should be alert to illness patterns that could indicate an unusual infectious disease outbreak. Indicators of a biological agent release include increased disease incidence among people in the same geographic area (e.g., people who attended the same event); the disease pattern is inconsistent with client age, such as chickenpox among adults; and a client presents with symptoms of a rare disease (Centers for Disease Control and Prevention [CDC], 2001). Presence of one or more of these indicators should be reported to public health authorities to determine the infectious disease source and to prevent further exposure.

Infectious Process in Older Adults

Older adults, particularly those over the age of 75 years, are at greater risk of acquiring an infection. Although the incidence of septicemia in the United States is increasing in all age groups, the greatest increase is among people over the age of 65 years (Schlossberg, 2001). Physiologic changes of aging that put the elderly at an increased risk for infection include the following:

- Cardiovascular changes: decreased cardiac output, loss of capillaries, and decreased tissue perfusion delaying inflammatory response and healing
- Respiratory system changes: decreased mucociliary escalator, decreased elastic recoil, and a diminished cough reflex leading to decreased clearance of respiratory secretions
- Genitourinary changes: loss of muscle tone, reduced bladder contractility, altered bladder reflexes, and prostatic hypertrophy in men leading to reduced bladder capacity and incomplete emptying
- Gastrointestinal system changes: impaired swallow reflex, decreased gastric acidity, and delayed gastric emptying thus increasing the risk of aspiration
- Skin and subcutaneous tissue changes: thinning of skin, decreased cushioning, and decreased sensation leading to increased risk of injury and ulceration
- Immune changes: decreased phagocytosis, reduced inflammatory response, slowed or impaired healing processes leading to reduced immunity

In addition to the previous physiologic changes, other factors that may contribute to the older adult's increased risk for infectious disease are as follows:

- Decreased activity level related to musculoskeletal, neurologic, or balance problems
- Poor nutrition and an increased risk of dehydration (see the Nursing Research box on page 220)
- Chronic diseases, such as diabetes mellitus, cardiac disease, and renal disease
- Chronic medication use
- Lack of recent immunizations against preventable infectious diseases
- Altered mentation and dementias
- Hospitalization or residence in a long-term care facility
- Presence of invasive devices, such as indwelling urinary catheters and gastric tubes

Nursing Research

Evidence-Based Practice for Meeting Nutritional Needs in Older Adults

Inadequate nutrition decreases normal functioning of the immune system. Older adults with declining immunity and often poor dietary habits have an increased risk for developing infections. Family members who provide nutritional assistance to older clients are challenged to provide an adequate nutritional intake.

A pilot project conducted to determine what family caregivers know about older adults' nutritional needs, the judgments and decisions they make regarding the nutritional needs of their elderly family members, and their actions in providing appropriate food intake (Biggs & Freed, 2000). Family caregivers assume a key role in promoting the nutritional status of their elderly family members; yet they often provide such assistance with minimal knowledge of sound nutritional principles. For instance, they may supply smaller, low-calorie meals mistakenly believing that the elderly need less food regardless of their medical condition. However, when provided with appropriate nutrition information, family caregivers can make correct nutritional decisions and meet the dependent older person's needs.

IMPLICATIONS FOR NURSING

Nurses in community health settings assume an important role in assessing the nutritional status and potential risk factors of dependent elderly persons. Equally important is determining the nutritional knowledge base of both the elderly client and the family caregiver. Because caregiver assistance may range from buying groceries to feeding the older adult, the nurse must identify the caregiver's level of involvement.

Therefore, the nurse needs to include the family caregiver in all nutritional teaching sessions and evaluate the caregiver's level of understanding and adherence to the guidelines provided. If older clients are malnourished and have an infection, their risk for prolonged recovery increases. An increased balanced nutritional intake should improve immune system function, shorten recovery time, and reduce the risk of future infections.

Critical Thinking in Client Care

1. Develop strategies that a family caregiver can use to improve the nutritional intake of an elderly family member who has no interest in eating.
2. An 86-year-old woman is being discharged to her home following repair of a broken hip. Identify the nutritional factors you would assess before she is discharged.
3. Discuss how prescription and over-the-counter medications affect the nutritional needs of the older adult.
4. Discuss the interrelationship between malnutrition and immune system function.

In addition, the thymus gland atrophies and by age 50 to 60 years thymic hormone levels are undetectable. Although the exact relationship of these events to T-cell function is unclear, some T-cell populations decrease or decline in function as the person ages. The ability of T cells to proliferate following activation also declines with advancing age; in addition, a portion of T cells cannot be activated in the elderly (Hazzard, Bierman, Blass, Ettinger, & Halter, 1994). With these changes, cell-mediated immune function declines. The client has reduced resistance to antigens such as *Mycobacterium tuberculosis,* influenza and varicella-zoster viruses, malignant cells, and tissue grafts.

Immunoglobulin levels remain relatively stable, but primary and secondary antibody responses decline with aging. This diminished antibody production has clinical implications in that immunizations (single-dose and booster) may not produce the expected protective immune response.

The older adult is not only at increased risk for infection, but also may not exhibit the classic manifestations of inflammation and infection. Older adults are more likely to take nonsteroidal anti-inflammatory agents and corticosteroids that interfere with inflammation and healing. The cardinal signs of inflammation—redness, heat, and swelling—tend to be diminished or absent in older adults. The classic signs of infection—fever and chills—may be absent altogether because of age-related changes in the immune system, loss of central temperature control mechanisms, decreased muscle mass, and loss of shivering ability. The older adult may have only subtle signs of sepsis, including changes in mental status, disorientation, and tachypnea (Hazzard et al., 1994). Infectious diseases commonly seen in the elderly client are outlined on page 221.

COLLABORATIVE CARE

The goals of care for the client with an infection are to identify the organ system affected by the infection, to identify the causative agent, and to achieve a cure by the least toxic, least expensive, and most effective means. Fortunately, most infectious diseases are self-limiting and will resolve with little or no medical care. However, medical treatment can be lifesaving in an overwhelming infection or immunocompromised host.

The body part or organ system affected by the infection is often obvious from the client's history and presenting signs and symptoms. Identifying the system allows the range of possible infecting organisms to be narrowed to those known to affect that system. The manner of presentation provides further cues as to the diagnosis. For example, pneumococcal pneumonia typically presents with an acute onset of chills, fever, and cough in a previously healthy adult, whereas the client with viral pneumonia relates a gradual onset of symptoms, with systemic manifestations such as muscle aches and headache often predominant. A history of recent activities also provides clues. Family members who all vomit and have diarrhea within 12 hours after a picnic probably do not have the flu.

Once the infecting agent has been identified, either positively or by probability, therapy can be specifically tailored to the client's needs. Viral infections often resolve without treatment other than supportive care, such as providing rest and fluids. Skin infections may respond to a topical agent, avoiding the potential adverse effects of one administered systemically.

Nursing Care of the Older Adult

INFECTION

Because immune function declines with aging, older adults are more susceptible to infections. In fact, infections are among the top 10 causes for hospitalization and 1 of the 5 leading causes of death among people over 65 years of age.

Age-related changes may obscure the presentation of infection in older adults. Rather than an elevated temperature to signal an infection, confusion and subtle changes in behavior such as restlessness may be observed. The white blood cell count may be slightly elevated.

In addition to monitoring for changes in the client's mental status or behavior, the nurse should collect data on the amount of fluids consumed, urinary output, activity levels, complaints of fatigue, and respiratory status. A thorough assessment is necessary to facilitate an early diagnosis and prompt treatment that will improve outcomes for the older adult. Delay in treating infection may prolong the client's immobility and reduce the ability to perform activities of daily living.

URINARY TRACT INFECTIONS

Urinary tract infection (UTI) is not only the most common infection but also the leading cause of bacteremia and sepsis in older adults. Factors that contribute to UTI include poor hygiene, incomplete bladder emptying, inadequate fluid intake, and long-term indwelling catheters. In addition, chronic conditions and medications may contribute to retention, which can result in urinary tract infection.

RESPIRATORY TRACT INFECTIONS

The leading causes of pneumonia in older adults include *Streptococcus pneumoniae, Hemophilus influenzae, Klebsiella pneumoniae, Staphylococcus aureus,* and pneumococci. As a result of physiological changes, the older adult with pneumonia may not present with cough or sputum production. Influenza A and B are prevalent in the aged; however, strain A accounts for greater illness severity and death (Eliopoulus, 2000). Both pneumonia and influenza cause high mortality rates in the older person.

Frail older adults, especially those with chronic respiratory conditions such as emphysema, are at risk for developing pneumonia as a complication of influenza. To prevent this complication, all persons over 65 should receive an annual immunization for influenza. In addition, pneumonia caused by pneumococcus bacteria can be deadly for older adults. Therefore, it is recommended that individuals over 65 also receive the pneumococcal immunization.

Tuberculosis has a relatively high incidence in older adults, especially those living in long-term care facilities. It often occurs as reactivation or secondary tuberculosis when the immune system can no longer contain the bacteria.

OTHER INFECTIONS

Older adults have the highest incidence of gangrene of the appendix and gallbladder. Diverticulitis increases due to chronic constipation and changes in the intestinal wall. Postoperative wound infections and decubitus ulcers are also most prevalent in older adults.

NOSOCOMIAL INFECTIONS

Nosocomial infections are more common in older adults. Nursing interventions should focus on prevention strategies such as (1) avoiding prolonged bed rest unless the medical condition contraindicates mobilization, (2) encouraging clients to take deep breaths, (3) providing adequate fluids, and (4) providing regular toileting schedules with good hygiene. The nurse must steadfastly adhere to principles of infection control.

HOME CARE

To prevent infection, the older adult should be taught to:
- Eat a well-balanced diet.
- Drink adequate fluids.
- Get adequate rest.
- Obtain an annual influenza immunization.
- Use good handwashing techniques.

Older adults and families should be taught to seek medical attention if they:

- Develop a fever or other signs and symptoms of infection.
- Exhibit changes in mental status and/or behavior.
- Experience fatigue or changes in activity levels.

Diagnostic Tests

To assess the client's response to infection, identify the infecting organism, and monitor the progress of therapy, the following diagnostic tests may be ordered.

- *WBC count* provides clues about the infecting organism and the body's immune response to it (see Table 8–6).
- *WBC differential* is also ordered (see Table 8–6). Neutrophilia, increased numbers of circulating neutrophils (or PMNs), is a common response with infection as the bone marrow responds to an increased need for phagocytes. Along with neutrophilia, a shift to the left is common in acute infection. This means that there are more immature neutrophils in circulation than normal (Figure 8–13 ■), indicating an appropriate bone marrow response.
- *Cultures of the wound, blood, or other infected body fluids* are used to identify probable microorganisms by their char-

acteristics, such as shape, growth patterns, and Gram-staining qualities. After the organism is cultured, it is subjected to various antibiotics known to be effective against its particular strain to determine which antibiotic is likely to be most effective. This is known as sensitivity testing. Generally 24 to 48 hours are required to grow the organism, potentially delaying the institution of therapy. Because antibiotics (and possibly oxygen therapy) can alter the ability to culture an organism, specimens should be obtained before instituting therapy.

- *Serologic testing* provides an indirect means of identifying infecting agents by detecting antibodies to the suspected organism. When the antibody titer against a specific organism rises during the acute phase of an infectious disease and begins to fall during convalescence, the diagnosis is supported. Although it is not as accurate as culture, serology is particularly useful for organisms that cannot easily be cultured, such as hepatitis B or HIV (Porth, 2002).

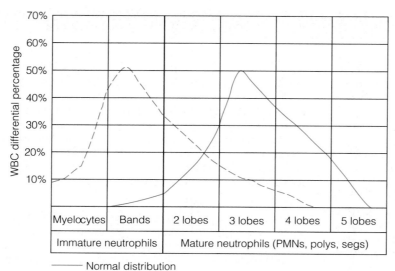

Type of WBC	Normal differential	Shift to left
Myelocytes	0%	Present
Band neutrophils (bands)	3% to 5%	Increased
Segmented neutrophils (segs, polys, PMNs)	50% to 65%	May be stable, increased, or decreased

Figure 8–13 ■ Neutrophils by stage of maturity and normal distribution in the blood.

- *Direct antigen detection methods* are in the process of being developed. These tests use monoclonal antibodies, which are purified antibody forms, to detect antigens in specimens from the diseased host (Porth, 2002). See Box 8–6. These tests offer rapid and accurate identification of the offending microorganism.
- *Antibiotic peak and trough levels* monitor therapeutic blood levels of the prescribed medication(s). The therapeutic range, that is, the minimum and maximum blood levels at which the drug is effective, is known for a given drug. By measuring blood levels at the predicted peak (1 to 2 hours after oral administration, 1 hour after intramuscular administration, and 30 minutes after intravenous administration) and trough (lowest level, usually a few minutes before the next scheduled dose), health care personnel can determine that the client is maintaining a level within the therapeutic range at all times, ensuring maximal effect from the drug. It is also possible to determine whether the drug is reaching a toxic or harmful level during therapy, increasing the likelihood of adverse effects.
- *Radiologic examination of the chest, abdomen, or urinary system* may be ordered to detect organ abnormalities indicating an inflammatory response or tissue damage.
- *Lumbar puncture* is performed to obtain cerebrospinal fluid (CSF) for examination and culture if a central nervous system (CNS) infection, such as meningitis or encephalitis, is suspected.
- *Ultrasonic examination* is a noninvasive diagnostic test to evaluate organ function such as an echocardiogram or renal ultrasonography.

Medications

Once the infecting organism and affected body system have been identified, specific therapy to cure the infectious disease can be instituted. The number of antimicrobial agents available makes choosing the appropriate one seem overwhelming. The perfect anti-infective agent would destroy pathogens while preserving host cells, would be effective against many different organisms while not promoting the development of resistance, would distribute to necessary tissues, and would remain in the body for relatively long periods.

Because no currently available antimicrobial meets all the above criteria, physicians look for the agent that will be effective, has little toxicity, can be administered with relative convenience, and is cost-effective. Characteristics of both the host and the infecting organism are considered in making the selection. The following host factors are considered in choosing an antimicrobial agent.

- *History of hypersensitivity.* Previous hypersensitivity responses to an antimicrobial contraindicate the use of that agent or one of its class.
- *Age and childbearing status of the client.* Sulfonamides and tetracyclines as well as some less common agents are contraindicated for pregnant women due to their possible effects on the fetus.
- *Renal function.* Because most antimicrobials are excreted through the kidneys, renal function is important. Impaired renal function may contraindicate a specific drug, such as an aminoglycoside, because of its nephrotoxicity, or it may call for a reduced dosage.
- *Hepatic function.* Because hepatic function may alter the metabolism of a particular antimicrobial, the risk of toxicity increases. Again, certain drugs are avoided with impaired hepatic function; others may dictate a reduced dosage.
- *Site of the infection.* The infection site is critical in choosing both the antimicrobial to be used and the route by which it is administered. Antimicrobials can be applied topically or administered by oral, intramuscular, intravenous, interperitoneal, intrathecal, or intramedullary routes. Oral and intravenous routes are most commonly used.
- *Other host factors.* Chronic diseases or other medications in the treatment regimen are also considered.

BOX 8–6   ■ Monoclonal Antibodies

Antigens typically have numerous antigenic determinant sites, each capable of stimulating a different subset of B cells. Each clone secretes a slightly different antibody from the others. The immunoglobulin produced as a result is therefore *polyclonal,* with multiple different antibodies. In 1975, researchers devised a technique for making a single clone of "immortal" B cells that could be maintained indefinitely in a laboratory and would produce a single antibody to a specific antigen (see figure below). This pure antibody, known as a *monoclonal* antibody, offers the following advantages:

- It can target specific antigens.
- It has a single, constant binding affinity for the antigen.
- It can be diluted to a specific titer or concentration, because it is not mixed with other antibodies.
- It can be purified to avoid adverse responses (McCance & Huether, 1998).

In addition to their use in providing passive protection from disease, multiple other uses are being identified for monoclonal antibodies, including the diagnosis and treatment of cancer, immunosuppression to prevent rejection of transplanted tissue or organs, immune response analysis, imaging techniques for diagnostic uses, and the early detection of viral infections (McCance & Huether, 1998, Roitt, 1994).

Antigen injected into mouse

Spleen removed

Suspension of B lymphocytes

Combine myeloma cells (immortal in culture)

Antibody producing cells from mouse spleen (limited life in culture)

Cell fusion

Hybridoma cells

B-cell clone for individual cells

Desired monoclonal antibodies secreted into culture fluid

Test for desired monoclonal antibody and grow additional antibodies

Note. Figure adapted from The World of the Cell *by W. Becker & D. Deane, 1986, Redwood City, CA: Benjamin Cummings;* Textbook of Diagnostic Microbiology *by C. R. Mahon & G. Manuselis Jr., 1995, Philadelphia: W.B. Saunders. Reprinted by permission.*

Antimicrobial preparations are broadly classified as bacteriostatic or bactericidal. **Bacteriostatic** agents inhibit the growth of the microorganism, leaving its destruction to the host's immune system. These agents are generally not indicated for the immunocompromised host. Tetracyclines, erythromycin, and chloramphenicol are bacteriostatic preparations. **Bactericidal** agents are capable of killing the organism without immune system intervention. These include the penicillins, cephalosporins, and aminoglycoside antibiotics.

The activity of antimicrobial agents on bacteria, fungi, and viruses falls under five basic mechanisms:

- Impairing cell wall synthesis, leading to lysis and cell destruction
- Inhibiting protein synthesis, causing impaired microbial function
- Altering cell membrane permeability, causing intracellular contents to leak
- Inhibiting the synthesis of nucleic acids
- Inhibiting cell metabolism and growth

Obviously, agents that work on the cell wall will not be effective against organisms that have no cell wall, such as mycoplasma and viruses. The antimicrobial's spectrum of activity is also considered in making a selection. Therapy is often initiated with a broad-spectrum antimicrobial until the specific organism is identified.

Finally, many microorganisms have the ability to develop resistance to an anti-infective agent; that is, the pathogen continues to live and grow in the presence of the anti-infective. Resistance develops as a result of a chance mutation by the pathogen, allowing a subpopulation of cells to survive. The chance of an organism's becoming resistant to an agent is partially related to the dose delivered. Resistance is less likely to occur when a lethal dose is administered; therefore, it is vital that clients understand the need to take all doses of the prescribed drug as ordered.

Antimicrobial medications are generally classified as antibacterial or antibiotic, antiviral, antifungal, and antiparasitic.

Antibiotics

Medications used to treat bacterial infections are generally known as antibiotics. Their development and use began before World War II and has proliferated rapidly since. Most antibiotics are biologic substances, that is, substances produced by other microorganisms. Antibiotics fall into classes of drugs with related chemical structure and activity. Some are effective against only gram-positive bacteria, and others are effective against only gram-negative organisms. Newer broad-spectrum antibiotics have activity against a wide variety of bacteria, including both gram-positive and gram-negative forms. No antibiotic is totally safe. Hypersensitivity responses occur, and some drugs are toxic to organ systems, exhibiting hepatotoxicity, nephrotoxicity, ototoxicity, or bone marrow suppression. Therefore, always check for allergies before administering the first dose. Antibiotics are presented in the box below.

Medication Administration

Antibiotic Therapy

PENICILLINS

Penicillin G	Dicloxacillin (Dynapen)
Penicillin V	Methicillin (Staphcillin)
Amoxicillin (Amoxil)	Mezlocillin (Mezlin)
Amoxicillin and potassium clavulanate (Augmentin)	Nafcillin (Unipen) Oxacillin (Prostaphlin)
Ampicillin (Polycillin)	Piperacillin (Pipracil)
Carbenicillin (Geopen, Geocillin)	Ticarcillin (Ticar)

Penicillins are bactericidal and interfere with cell wall synthesis and the enzymes involved in cell division and synthesis. They are more effective on gram-positive than gram-negative organisms. Resistance is now more common among *Streptococci* and *Staphylococci*. They are considered to be safe, effective, and of low toxicity.

Nursing Responsibilities

- Monitor for hypersensitivity responses such as local erythema and itching at the site of injection, skin rashes, urticaria (hives), itching, fever, chills, and anaphylaxis.
- Observe clients receiving parenteral penicillin for at least 30 minutes.
- Discontinue the drug immediately if any hypersensitivity response occurs. Be prepared to administer antihistamines or corticosteroids for a mild reaction. Anaphylaxis is treated with epinephrine subcutaneously or intravenously and airway support.
- Do not administer penicillin to anyone with a history of a severe allergic reaction to any form of the drug; a cross-reactivity may occur in clients allergic to cephalosporin antibiotics.
- Assess for superinfection (vaginitis, stomatitis, or diarrhea) due to elimination of resident bacteria.
- Monitor for therapeutic response.

Client and Family Teaching

- Notify the physician if you see white patches are noted on the oral mucosa or if vaginitis develops. An antifungal drug may be prescribed and the antibiotic continued.
- Consuming yogurt or buttermilk may prevent superinfection. Do not take these products within 1 hour of taking the drug.

CEPHALOSPORINS

1st Generation	**3rd Generation**
Cephalexin (Keflex)	Cefoperazone (Cefobid)
Cefazolin (Ancef)	Ceftazidime (Fortaz)
2nd Generation	Ceftriaxone (Rocephin)
Cefaclor (Ceclor)	**4th Generation**
Cefuroxime (Zinacef)	Cefepime (Moxapime)

Cephalosporins are structurally similar to the penicillins and also inhibit cell wall synthesis. They are divided into four groups, or generations. First-generation cephalosporins act primarily against gram-positive organisms. Second- and third-generation drugs are more effective against gram-negative organisms than against gram-positive ones. Fourth-generation cephalosporins act effectively against both gram-positive and gram-negative organisms.

Nursing Responsibilities

- Monitor for previous hypersensitivity response to cephalosporins or penicillins.
- Assess intravenous site for phlebitis; intramuscular site may cause local pain.
- Monitor laboratory results for adverse response, such as leukopenia and thrombocytopenia, nephrotoxicity (elevated BUN and serum creatinine), or hepatotoxicity (elevated bilirubin, LDH, ALT, AST, and alkaline phosphatase).
- Assess for signs of superinfections.

Client and Family Teaching

- Take the medication on an empty stomach, 1 hour before or 2 hours after meals.
- Space doses of the medication relatively evenly throughout the day and evening hours.
- Increase consumption of buttermilk or yogurt to prevent intestinal superinfection.

AMINOGLYCOSIDES

Amikacin (Amikin)	Netilmicin (Netromycin)
Gentamicin (Garamycin)	Streptomycin (Stepolin)
Kanamycin (Kantrex)	Tobramycin (Nebcin)

Medication Administration

Antibiotic Therapy (continued)

Aminoglycosides are bactericidal, interfering with protein synthesis in the pathogen. They are especially effective against gram-negative organisms. To provide a broader spectrum of activity, they are often combined with other antibiotics, especially penicillins. Aminoglycosides can be administered in multiple or single daily doses. They are ototoxic and nephrotoxic; the risk is highest for older adults, clients with preexisting renal disease, and persons receiving other ototoxic or nephrotoxic drugs.

Nursing Responsibilities

- Assess renal function before and during aminoglycoside therapy. Monitor intake and output, daily weight, BUN, and serum creatinine.
- Assess for adverse effects on hearing such as loss of perception of high tones, tinnitus, and vertigo.
- Notify the physician if the client is receiving other nephrotoxic or ototoxic drugs such as furosemide (Lasix) and ethacrynic acid (Edecrin).
- Administer intravenous preparations separately from other drugs; flush tubing before and after administration.

Client and Family Teaching

- Monitor for a sudden weight gain that may indicate adverse effects on the kidney and report it to the physician.

FLUOROQUINOLONES

Ciprofloxacin (Cipro)   Levofloxacin (Levaquin)
Gatifloxacin (Tequin)

Fluoroquinolones are bactericidal and especially active against gram-negative and some gram-positive organisms. They are used to manage infections of the respiratory, gastrointestinal, and genitourinary tracts.

Nursing Responsibilities

- Increase fluid intake to 2000 to 3000 mL per day unless contraindicated to prevent crystalluria.
- Monitor laboratory results for hepatotoxicity (elevated ALT, AST).

Client and Family Teaching

- Drink six to eight glasses of water per day.
- Avoid exposure to sunlight while taking these drugs.

TETRACYCLINES

Tetracycline HCl   Minocycline HCl (Minocin)
Doxycycline (Vibramycin)   Oxytetracycline (Terramycin)

Tetracyclines are active against many gram-positive and gram-negative bacteria, such as Mycoplasma, Rickettsia, and Chlamydia. They are bacteriostatic, interfering with microbial protein synthesis. Tetracycline binds readily with metal and solid elements in the bowel, limiting its absorption when administered with food; the other preparations are highly soluble in lipids and can be administered with food.

Nursing Responsibilities

- Schedule doses 1 hour before or 2 hours after meals. Do not give with milk or milk products or antacids.
- Monitor for signs of superinfection.
- If the client is taking an anticoagulant, monitor prothrombin time, and for signs of bleeding.

Client and Family Teaching

Avoid excessive sun exposure to reduce the risk of photosensitivity reactions.

MACROLIDES

Erythromycin (E-Mycin)   Erythromycin salts (Ilosone,
Azithromycin (Zithromax)   E.E.S., Erythrocin)

Macrolides are bacteriostatic and act effectively against gram-positive and gram-negative organisms. Erythromycin is used to treat streptococcal pharyngitis in clients who are allergic to penicillin. Azithromycin is ordered more frequently because the client takes the drug for 5 days, increasing client adherence.

Nursing Responsibilities

- Administer erythromycin on an empty stomach or immediately before meals.
- Give the drug with a full glass of water. Do not administer with acidic fruit juice.

Client and Family Teaching

- Gastric distress is a common side effect with erythromycin.

SULFONAMIDES AND TRIMETHOPRIM

Sulfamethizole (Thiosulfil Forte)
Sulfamethoxazole (Gantanol; in combination with Trimethoprim, TMP-SMZ, Bactrim, Septra)
Sulfisoxazole (Gantrisin)

Sulfonamides are bacteriostatic. Trimethoprim is an antibiotic effective against most gram-positive and many gram-negative organisms. It is often combined with sulfamethoxazole to manage urinary tract infections, *Pneumocystis carinii* pneumonia (PCP), and otitis media. Skin rashes and pruritus are the most common hypersensitivity reactions. Severe reactions include exfoliative dermatitis and Stevens-Johnson syndrome. *(continued)*

Nursing Responsibilities

- Assess for history of hypersensitivity to sulfonamides and related medications, such as thiazide diuretics and hypoglycemic preparations.
- Monitor intake and output. Maintain a fluid intake of at least 1500 mL per day.
- Assess for evidence of bleeding, easy bruising, or systemic infection, and monitor blood count for possible bone marrow depression.

Client and Family Teaching

- Take medication on an empty stomach with a full glass of water. Maintain a fluid intake of at least 2 quarts per day.
- Protect the skin from excessive sun exposure with clothing and sunscreens to reduce the risk of photosensitivity.

METRONIDAZOLE (FLAGYL)

Metronidazole is effective against anaerobic gram-negative bacteria and protozoan infections caused by amebiasis, giardiasis, and trichomoniasis. It is commonly used to prevent and treat infections following intestinal surgery.

(continued on page 226)

Medication Administration
Antibiotic Therapy (continued)

Nursing Responsibilities
- Monitor for central nervous system effects of dizziness, headache, ataxia, confusion, depression, and peripheral neuropathy.
- Administer with food to minimize gastric distress and metallic taste. Infuse intravenous metronidazole over 60 minutes.
- Discontinue the medication and notify the physician if neurologic reactions occur.
- Increase fluid intake to 2500 mL per day to minimize the risk of nephrotoxicity.

Client and Family Teaching
- This medication may turn urine reddish brown; caution client that this is expected and not harmful.
- Discontinue the drug and notify the physician if hypersensitivity reaction or adverse effects occur, such as changes in mentation or coordination, painful or frequent urination, painful or difficult intercourse, impotence.
- Do not drink alcohol while taking this medication; an Antabuse-type reaction (flushing, sweating, headache, vomiting, and abdominal cramps) may occur.
- Maintain a fluid intake of 2.5 to 3 quarts per day.
- When the drug is prescribed for Trichomonas infections, treatment of both partners is necessary.
- While taking metronidazole, use condoms to prevent cross-contamination during intercourse.

Antivirals

Antiviral therapy is a relatively new phenomenon. Most antibiotics have little effect on viruses, because the virus has no cell wall and no cytoplasm, produces no enzymes, and sequesters itself in a host cell to reproduce. Antiviral agents must be very selective in differentiating normal cellular activity from viral activity. In addition, the immune function of the host is a vital component in fighting viral infections; antiviral therapy may be relatively ineffective in the severely immunocompromised host. Making a timely diagnosis to allow institution of antiviral therapy can be an additional problem, because viruses are less easily identified using laboratory techniques. Antiviral agents in common use are summarized in the box to the right. Antiretroviral agents used in the management of HIV and AIDS are presented in Chapter 9. 🔗

Antifungals

Antifungal agents are available in both topical and systemic forms. They act by interfering with the cytoplasmic membrane of the fungus. Topical agents include preparations for cutaneous use to treat candidiasis, tineas, and ringworm. Vaginal preparations to treat vulvovaginal candidiasis are also available, as are several nonprescription topical and vaginal antifungal agents.

Amphotericin B (Fungizone) is a systemic antifungal agent for parenteral administration. It is used to treat severe, life-threatening fungal infections including histoplasmosis, blastomycosis, and candidiasis. Another systemic antifungal in current use is flucytosine (Ancobon). Unlike amphotericin B, flucytosine

can be administered orally. It is used to treat severe candidiasis infections such as candidae septicemia, endocarditis, pulmonary or urinary tract infections, and *Cryptococcus* meningitis.

Fluconazole (Diflucan) has the broadest use as an antifungal agent. It can be administered either orally or parenterally and is used to treat candidiasis infections as well as *Cryptococcus* meningitis. It is generally better tolerated than other systemic antifungal medications.

Antiparasitics

Drugs used to treat parasitic infections are as varied as the organisms that cause them. Generally, agents classified as antiparasitic are both expensive and likely to be toxic. Quinine was one

Medication Administration
Antiviral Agents

AMANTADINE (SYMMETREL)
Amantadine is used to prevent and treat influenza A. It has been shown to be 55% to 80% or more effective in preventing the disease. When administered within 24 to 72 hours after the onset of symptoms, it reduces common manifestations of influenza. It is generally well tolerated; minimal central nervous system side effects, such as dizziness, anxiety, insomnia, and difficulty concentrating, may occur.

ACYCLOVIR (ZOVIRAX) AND GANCICLOVIR (CYTOVENE)
Acyclovir and ganciclovir are related compounds used primarily in the treatment of herpesviruses. Acyclovir is prescribed mainly in the treatment of genital herpes simplex infections. Although it does not kill the virus, acyclovir is effective in reducing the severity, duration, and frequency of recurrence of symptoms. Ganciclovir is indicated primarily in the treatment of cytomegalovirus infection. Although acyclovir is generally well tolerated with little toxicity, ganciclovir may profoundly suppress bone marrow function, and its use is therefore limited.

ZIDOVUDINE (AZT, RETROVIR)
Zidovudine inhibits replication of HIV, although it does not kill it. Zidovudine's use is limited to clients with symptomatic HIV infection or CD4 cell counts of less than 200/mm³. Zidovudine may be administered either orally or parenterally. Many clients are unable to tolerate recommended doses because of the drug's adverse effects, including nausea, anorexia, malaise, severe anemia, and granulocytopenia. Zidovudine is usually administered in combination with other antiretroviral medications.

VIDARABINE (VIRA-A)
Vidarabine inhibits viral DNA synthesis and is effective against many herpesvirus infections. Its primary use is in treatment of herpes simplex encephalitis.

INTERFERONS
Interferons are naturally produced cytokines whose use as antiviral agents is being explored. When administered intranasally, interferons have been shown to be effective in preventing rhinovirus upper respiratory infections. Other uses being explored include treatment of human papillomavirus (genital warts) and preventing or reducing Kaposi's sarcoma in clients with AIDS.

of the first antiparasitic drugs developed in the treatment of malaria. Quinine is highly toxic, but newer forms such as chloroquine (Aralen, Chlorocon) and hydroxychloroquine (Plaquenil) are widely used as antimalarial drugs. Metronidazole (e.g., Flagyl) is used to treat infections of protozoan parasites (see the Medication Administration box on pages 225–226).

Isolation Techniques

Controlling the spread of infectious diseases in the hospital or long-term care setting is particularly important to preventing nosocomial infection. Handwashing remains the single most important factor in preventing the transmission of infections. Not all infectious diseases spread readily, necessitating special techniques or procedures. However, diseases such as chickenpox (varicella) and pulmonary tuberculosis are highly contagious and are spread by the airborne route, requiring special precautions to protect other hospitalized clients.

In determining the need for isolation precautions, health care personnel consider the usual reservoir or source of the microorganism, the mode of transmission, and susceptibility of hospital staff and other clients. For example, clients with *Pneumocystis carinii* pneumonia do not require isolation, because immunocompetent persons are not susceptible to this infection.

The Centers for Disease Control and Prevention (CDC) has published guidelines for isolation precautions to be used in health care facilities. These guidelines include both *standard precautions* and *category-specific isolation precautions*.

Standard Precautions

Standard Precautions, published by the Hospital Infection Control Practices Advisory Committee of the Centers for Disease Control in 1996, provides guidelines for the handling of blood and other body fluids. These guidelines are used with all clients, regardless if they have a known infectious disease. The guidelines were developed in light of the realization that many clients with an infectious disease such as HIV or hepatitis B have no apparent symptoms, but can transmit the disease to others. Standard precautions are used by all health care workers who have direct contact with clients or with their body fluids or have indirect contact, such as by emptying trash, changing linens, or cleaning the room.

Standard precautions apply to the following:

- Blood
- All body fluids, secretions, and excretions, regardless if they contain visible blood
- Nonintact skin
- Mucous membranes

Barrier protection is used to prevent exposing skin and mucous membrane surfaces to blood and body fluids. Barrier protection involves using gloves for touching or handling body fluids, and adding other protection such as gowns, masks, and goggles if splashing or spraying is likely. Needles and other sharp objects are not recapped or bent, but disposed of in puncture-proof containers to prevent inadvertent percutaneous (needle-stick) exposure. Standard precautions are presented in Appendix A. ⊂⊃

Transmission-Based Precautions

In addition to handwashing and standard precautions, the nature and spread of some infectious diseases require that special techniques be used to protect uninfected clients and workers. The CDC identifies three types of transmission-based precautions: airborne, droplet, and contact precautions. Transmission-based precautions may be combined for diseases that have multiple routes of transmission. Indications for the use of transmission-based isolation precautions and the specific measures to be taken are outlined in Table 8–10.

NURSING CARE

Nursing management related to infectious disease has two foci: (1) *prevention* and (2) *health promotion and maintenance*. Prevention focuses on assessing the client's risk for infection based on underlying conditions, immune response, and prophylactic measures such as immunizations.

Health Promotion

Preventing infection requires education of not only health care personnel but also the general public. Part of an education program includes understanding the importance of immunizations, the guidelines for using antibiotics to prevent drug-resistant microorganisms, and the ways to prevent the spread of infection. Check immunization records for all family members and encourage them to keep immunizations up to date. Increase public awareness regarding appropriate antibiotic use. Guidelines for preventing the spread of infection to others include the following:

- Avoid crowds and contact with susceptible persons, especially those who are immunosuppressed (e.g., persons who have HIV infection, who are undergoing therapy for cancer, or who have had an organ transplant).
- Use disposable tissues to contain respiratory secretions when coughing or sneezing.
- Use appropriate food-handling precautions for diseases spread via the fecal-oral route, such as hepatitis A.
- Avoid contact with or sharing of body fluids. For example, do not share needles or razors; use a condom during sexual activity, or abstain; have each person clean their own blood spills or wounds if possible.

Assessment

The following data are collected through the health history and physical examination. Further focused assessments are described with nursing interventions in the next section.

- Health history: age, medication use (antipyretics and anti-infectives), nutrition, exposure to infectious persons, immunizations, invasive procedures and therapies, chronic diseases such as diabetes mellitus, cancer
- Physical assessment: vital signs, body system(s) where infection is suspected, lymph node enlargement, and tenderness

TABLE 8-10 Transmission-Based Precautions

Category	Infectious Diseases	Purpose	Precautions
Airborne precautions	Pulmonary tuberculosis, chickenpox (with contact precautions), measles, respiratory infections (pneumonia)	Reduce risk of airborne transmission of infectious agents. Airborne transmission occurs by dissemination of either airborne droplet nuclei or dust particles containing the infectious agent.	Private room with handwashing, toilet facilities, and special ventilation that does not allow air to circulate to general hospital ventilation; mask or special filter respirator for everyone entering room.
Droplet precautions	Meningitis, pertussis	Reduce risk of droplet transmission of infectious agents. Droplet transmission involves contact of conjunctivae of the eyes or mucous membranes of the nose or mouth with large-particle droplets generated during coughing, sneezing, talking, or procedures such as suctioning.	Private room with handwashing and toilet facilities; mask, eye protection, and/or face shields worn by everyone entering room.
Contact precautions	Acute diarrhea, chickenpox, (with airborne precautions), respiratory syncytial virus (RSV); skin, wound, or urinary tract infection with multidrug-resistant organisms; *Staphylococcus aureus* infections	Reduce risk of transmission by direct or indirect contact. Direct contact transmission involves skin-to-skin contact and physical transfer of organisms. It may occur between clients or during direct care activities such as bathing or turning clients. Indirect contact involves contact with a contaminated object.	Private room with handwashing and toilet facilities; gowns and protective apparel to provide barrier protection; disposable supplies or decontamination of all articles leaving room.

Nursing Diagnoses and Interventions

Clients with an infection may be managed in the hospital or at home. During the acute phase, nursing care includes administering prescribed antibiotics, implementing and maintaining aseptic technique and infection control measures, and encouraging a balance of rest and activity, good nutritional intake, and other general health measures to support immunologic function and healing. The key nursing diagnoses are *risk for infection, anxiety,* and *hyperthermia.*

Risk for Infection

The spread of infection is a risk in any facility that houses many people. It is a particular risk in hospitals, where many clients have at least some degree of immunosuppression and many drug-resistant strains of pathogens are prevalent. It is vital that nurses use good handwashing techniques at all times, employ standard precautions with all clients, and use category-specific isolation techniques as indicated to prevent infectious spread to other clients, themselves, and their families.

- Admit clients with known or suspected infections to a private room. *This is important to minimize the risk to other clients.*
- Wash hands on entering and leaving the client's room, using a 10- to 15-second vigorous scrub with soap or antibacterial scrub solution. *A 10- to 15-second scrub removes transient microorganisms from the skin and helps prevent transmission of infection to or from the client.*
- Use standard precautions and personal protective devices to reduce the risk of transmission. *Gloves, gowns, and masks are to be worn whenever there is a risk of skin or mucous membrane contamination by direct contact with infectious material, airborne spread of organisms, or droplet nuclei.*
- Explain the reasons for and importance of isolation procedures during hospitalization. *Clients with isolation precautions may feel neglected, dirty, or shunned. Explanation of reasons and procedures can enhance the client's and family's understanding and acceptance.*
- Place a mask on the client and/or cover all infectious lesions or wounds completely when transporting the client to other parts of the facility for diagnostic or treatment procedures. *These measures help minimize air contamination and the risk to visitors and personnel.*
- Collect a culture and sensitivity (C&S) specimen as ordered or indicated by purulent drainage, pyuria, or other manifestations of infection. *C&S is performed to determine the presence and type of infectious organisms as well as antibiotics most likely to be effective in eradicating it.*

PRACTICE ALERT *Collect the specimen before the first dose of antibiotics is administered to ensure adequate organisms for culture.* ■

- Administer prescribed anti-infective agents. *Anti-infectives are used to destroy the invading microorganism.*
- Inform all personnel having contact with the client of the diagnosis. *This is particularly important for a client with a disease requiring category-specific isolation so that personnel can take appropriate precautions.*

- Ensure that visitors don appropriate protective wear before they enter the client's room. *Protective wear reduces their risk of infection.*
- Use appropriate measures for disposing of contaminated tissues, dressings, or other material and for removing soiled linens and equipment from the client's room. *Check hospital policy or published guidelines for category-specific isolation.*
- Teach the importance of complying with prescribed treatment for the entire course of the regimen. *Because anti-infective agents kill only a portion of the pathogen population with each dose, completion of the entire course of therapy is necessary to reduce the risk of relapse and of creating drug-resistant organisms.*

Anxiety

The client with an infectious disease may experience anxiety related to his or her manifestations, treatment measures, the prognosis, and expected outcome of the disease. The diagnosis of an infection can be traumatic, causing feelings of uneasiness, isolation, guilt (e.g., in regard to sexually transmitted diseases), apprehension, or depression.

- Assess level of anxiety. *The level of anxiety influences the client's response to and interpretation of the situation and degree of threat it poses.*
- Discuss the infection, treatments, prognosis, and outcomes. *Discussions help to allay fears and misconceptions.*
- Support and enhance the client's coping strategies. *A person uses intrapersonal and interpersonal mechanisms to reduce or relieve anxiety.*
- Include significant others in the plan of care. *Inclusion of the client and family members provides assurance and confidence, and promotes understanding of the unknown.*
- Explain isolation procedures, and answer any concerns. *Isolation may be necessary to prevent the spread of infection but can cause great anxiety for the client and family members.*
- Provide referrals as needed for continuing care, for example, to home health agencies, for dressing changes or periodic assessment. *Referrals are often necessary to provide ongoing interventions and maintain continuity of care.*

Hyperthermia

Hyperthermia is an expected consequence of the infectious disease process. Fever may produce mild, short-term effects or, when prolonged, may cause serious life-threatening effects.

- *Monitor temperature especially during episodes of chills; note heart rate and rhythm. Chills indicate a rising temperature. Hyperthermia can cause dysrhythmias.*

> **PRACTICE ALERT**   *Monitor temperature between 5 P.M. and 7 P.M. as the body's daily temperature cycle peaks at this point.* ∎

- Administer prescribed antipyretic as indicated for elevated temperature. *Although antipyretics lower the temperature and enhance comfort for the client, this benefit must be weighed against the possible beneficial effect of an elevated temperature in the immune response. Fever increases the motility and activity of WBCs, stimulates the production of interferon, and activates T cells. In addition, temperatures above the normal range inhibit the growth of many microorganisms* (Porth, 2002).
- Promote body cooling through lowering room temperature. *Rapid cooling stimulates the hypothalamus to increase the body's temperature; this increases both shivering and metabolic rate.*

> **PRACTICE ALERT**   *Use ice packs, cool/tepid baths, or hypothermia blanket with caution to prevent unnecessary shivering.* ∎

- Monitor fluid loss; encourage increased fluid and electrolyte intake either orally or intravenously. *Hyperthermia causes fluid loss from evaporation and may result in dehydration and electrolyte imbalance.*
- If diaphoretic, bathe and provide dry clothing and bedding. *These measures increase client comfort and decrease further water evaporation.*
- Promote rest periods. *Rest increases energy reserve that is depleted by an increased metabolic, heart, and respiratory rate.*

Using NANDA, NIC, and NOC

Chart 8–3 shows links between NANDA, NIC, and NOC when caring for the client with an infection.

CHART 8–3 NANDA, NIC, AND NOC LINKAGES

The Client with an Infection

NURSING DIAGNOSES	NURSING INTERVENTIONS	NURSING OUTCOMES
• Risk for Deficient Fluid Volume • Risk for Activity Intolerance • Ineffective Health Maintenance	• Fluid Management • Fluid Monitoring • Energy Management • Health Education • Teaching Individual	• Fluid Balance • Hydration • Endurance • Health-Promoting Behavior • Health-Seeking Behavior

Note. Data from *Nursing Outcomes Classification (NOC)* by M. Johnson & M. Maas (Eds.), 1997, St. Louis: Mosby; *Nursing Diagnoses: Definitions & Classification 2001–2002* by North American Nursing Diagnosis Association, 2001, Philadelphia: NANDA; *Nursing Interventions Classification (NIC)* by J.C. McCloskey & G. M. Bulechek (Eds.), 2000, St. Louis: Mosby. Reprinted by permission.

Home Care

Client and family teaching is directed toward helping the client recover from the infection or disease, preventing its spread to others, and preventing life-threatening complications. Instructions should include the following points.

- Use good handwashing techniques, particularly after touching infected wounds or lesions, coughing, sneezing, blowing the nose, or using the bathroom. Wash hands thoroughly before eating or performing any procedures such as dressing changes.
- Take all prescribed antibiotics as ordered even after symptoms have subsided. Notify your health care provider if:
  - Symptoms do not improve within 24 to 48 hours after antibiotic therapy is instituted.
    - Signs of antibiotic allergy (itching, rash, difficulty breathing) occur.
    - Adverse responses, such as gastrointestinal distress, interfere with completion of the prescription.
    - Signs of superinfection (vaginitis, oral candidiasis, or diarrhea) occur.
    - Manifestations of infection recur after completing prescribed antibiotic.
- Report redness, swelling, or drainage around wounds or persistent high fever.
- Increase fluid intake to at least 2500 mL (2.5 quarts) per day.
- In addition, suggest the following resources:
  - County or public health department
  - Centers for Disease Prevention and Control

 EXPLORE MediaLink

NCLEX review questions, case studies, care plan activities, MediaLink applications, and other interactive resources for this chapter can be found on the Companion Website at www.prenhall.com/lemone.

Click on Chapter 8 to select the activities for this chapter. For animations, video clips, more NCLEX review questions, and an audio glossary, access the Student CD-ROM accompanying this textbook.

TEST YOURSELF

1. When a client receives gamma globulin following exposure to hepatitis A, the nurse expects the client to develop:
   a. Natural passive immunity
   b. Natural active immunity
   c. Acquired passive immunity
   d. Acquired active immunity

2. When performing a physical assessment of a client, the nurse should expect which of these findings related to a systemic infection?
   a. Erythema
   b. Enlarged lymph nodes
   c. Pain
   d. Decreased heart rate

3. Which one of the following medications is known to inhibit prostaglandin synthesis?
   a. Acetaminophen (Tylenol)
   b. Prednisone
   c. Penicillin
   d. Aspirin

4. The client with an acute infection shows a shift to the left on the WBC differential count. The nurse recognizes a shift to the left because of which laboratory finding?
   a. Increased band neutrophils
   b. Increased eosinophils
   c. Decreased leukocytes
   d. Decreased monocytes

5. A client is admitted with methicillin-resistant *Staphylococcus aureus* in a draining sacral wound. The client should be placed in which type of isolation precautions?
   a. Droplet precautions
   b. Contact precautions
   c. Airborne precautions
   d. Protective precautions

See Test Yourself answers in Appendix C.

BIBLIOGRAPHY

Ackley, B. J., & Ladwig, G. B. (2002). *Nursing diagnosis handbook* (5th ed.). St. Louis: Mosby.

American Hospital Association. (2001). ATS: Hospital-acquired pneumonia remains a serious problem. Available http://www.ahanews.com

Andreoli, T., Bennett, J., Carpenter, C., & Plum, F. (Eds.). (1997). *Cecil essentials of medicine* (4th ed.). Philadelphia: Saunders.

Biggs, A. J., & Freed, P. E. (2000). Nutrition and older adults What do family caregivers know and do? *Journal of Gerontological Nursing, 26*(8), 6–14.

Bullock, B. L., & Henze, R. L. (2000). *Focus on pathophysiology.* Philadelphia: Lippincott.

Burggraf, V., & Weinstein, B. F. (2000). Don't miss this opportunity: Promote adult immunizations. *MEDSURG Nursing, 9*(6), 198–200.

Centers for Disease Control. (1996). Guidelines for isolation precautions in hospitals. *American Journal of Infection Control, 24* (1), 32–52.

_____ . (2000a). *Preventing emerging infectious diseases. A strategy for the 21st century.* Atlanta: CDC.

_____ . (2002). *Recommended adult immunization schedule, United States, 2002–2003.* Atlanta: CDC.

_____ . (2000b). *Vaccine-preventable adult diseases.* Atlanta: CDC.

_____ . (2001, October). Update: Investigation of anthrax associated with intentional exposure and interim public health guidelines. *MMWR, 50*(41), 889–897.

Coleman, E. A. (2001). Anthrax. *American Journal of Nursing, 101*(12), 48–52.

Copstead, L. C., & Banasik, J. L. (2000). *Pathophysiology, biological, and behavioral responses* (2nd ed.). Philadelphia: W.B. Saunders.

Eliopoulous, C. (2000). *Gerontological nursing* (5th ed.). Philadelphia: Lippincott.

Fauci, A., et al. (1998). *Harrison's principles of internal medicine* (14th ed.). New York: McGraw-Hill.

Fraser, D. (1997). Assessing the elderly for infections. *Journal of Gerontological Nursing, 23*(11), 5–10, 52–58.

Glover, T. L. (2000). How drug-resistant microorganisms affect nursing. *Orthopaedic Nursing, 19*(2), 19–27.

Gylys, K. H. (1999). Antimicrobial resistance. *Journal of Cardiovascular Nursing, 13*(2), 66–69.

Hazzard, W., Bierman, E., Blass, J., Ettinger, W., & Halter, J. (Eds.). (1994). *Principles of geriatric medicine and gerontology* (3rd ed.). New York: McGraw-Hill.

Inman, W. B. (2000). Pathogens invade 21st century. *Nursing 2000, 30*(8), 22–23.

Jackson, M. M., Rickman, L. S., & Pugliese, G. (1999). Pathogens, old and new: An update for cardiovascular nurses. *Journal of Cardiovascular Nursing, 13*(2), 1–22.

Johnson, M., Maas, M., & Moorhead, S. (2000). *Iowa outcomes project: Nursing outcomes classification (NOC)* (2nd ed.). St. Louis: Mosby.

Kee, J. (2001). *Handbook of laboratory & diagnostic tests with nursing implications* (4th ed.). Upper Saddle River, NJ: Prentice Hall.

Lueckenotte, A. G. (2000). *Gerontologic nursing* (2nd ed.). St. Louis: Mosby.

Lutz, C., & Przytulski, K. (2001). *Nutrition and diet therapy* (3rd ed.) Philadelphia: F.A. Davis.

Markis, A. T., Morgan, L., Gaber, D. J., Richter, A., & Rubino, J. R. (2000). Effect of comprehensive infection control program on the incidence of infections in long-term care facilities. *American Journal of Infection Control, 28*(1), 3–7.

McCance, K., & Huether, S. (1998). *Pathophysiology: The biologic basis for disease in adults and children.* St. Louis: Mosby.

McCloskey, J., & Bulechek, G. (2000). *Iowa intervention project: Nursing interventions classification (NIC)* (3rd ed.). St. Louis: Mosby.

Miller, J. M., Walton, J. C., & Tordicella, L. L. (1998). Recognizing and managing *Clostridium difficile*–associated diarrhea. *MEDSURG Nursing, 7*(6), 348–356.

Miller, N. C., & Rudoy, R. C. (2000). Vancomycin intermediate-resistant *Staphylococcus aureus* (VISA). *Orthopaedic Nursing, 19*(6), 45–50.

National Institute of Allergy and Infectious Diseases. (2000). *Antimicrobial resistance.* Bethesda: National Institutes of Health.

Porth, C. (2002). *Pathophysiology: Concepts of altered health states* (6th ed.). Philadelphia: Lippincott.

Price, S., & Wilson, L. (2003). *Pathophysiology: Clinical concepts of disease processes* (6th ed.). St. Louis: Mosby.

Reece, S. M. (1999). The emerging threat of antimicrobial resistance: Strategies for change. *The Nurse Practitioner, 24*(11), 70, 73, 77–80, 85–86.

Roitt, I. (1994). *Essential immunology* (8th ed.). London: Blackwell.

Rowsey, P. J. (1997a). Pathophysiology of fever. Part 1: The role of cytokines. *Dimensions of Critical Care Nursing, 16*(4), 202–207.

_____ . (1997b). Pathophysiology of fever. Part 2: Relooking at cooling interventions. *Dimensions of Critical Care Nursing, 16*(5), 251–256.

Sandhu, S. K., & Mossad, S. B. (2001). Influenza in the older adult. *Geriatrics, 56*(1), 43–44, 47–48, 51.

Schlossberg, D. (2001). *Current therapy of infectious disease* (2nd ed.). St. Louis: Mosby.

Shannon, M., Wilson, B., & Stang, C. (2001). *Nursing drug guide 2001.* Upper Saddle River, NJ: Prentice Hall.

Sheff, B. (1998). VRE & MRSA: Putting bad bugs out of business. *Nursing 98, 28*(3), 40–45.

_____ . (1999). Minimizing the threat of *C. difficile. Nursing 99, 29*(2), 33–39.

Silverblatt, F. J., Tibert, C., Mikolich, D., Blazek-D'Arezzo, J., Alves, J., Tack, M., & Agatiello, P. (2000). Preventing the spread of vancomycin-resistant enterococci in a long-term care facility. *Journal of the American Geriatrics Society, 48*(10), 1211–1214.

Smith, S. F., Duell, D. J., & Martin, B. C. (2000). *Clinical nursing skills* (5th ed.). Upper Saddle River: Prentice Hall.

Tenover, F. C., & McGownan, J. E. (1997). Antimicrobial resistance. *Infectious Disease Clinics of North America, 11*(4), 813–928.

Tierney, L., McPhee, S., & Papadakis, M. (Eds). (2001). *Current medical diagnosis & treatment* (40th ed.). Stamford, CT: Appleton & Lange.

Wenzel, R. P., & Edmond, M. B. (2001). The impact of hospital-acquired bloodstream infections. *Emerging Infectious Diseases, 7*(2), 174–177.

Nursing Care of Clients with Altered Immunity

MediaLink

www.prenhall.com/lemone

Additional resources for this chapter can be found on the Student CD-ROM accompanying this textbook, and on the Companion Website at www. prenhall.com/lemone. Click on Chapter 9 to select the activities for this chapter.

CD-ROM
- Audio Glossary
- NCLEX Review

Animations
- Histamine
- T-Cell Destruction of HIV

Companion Website
- More NCLEX Review
- Case Study
  HIV Prevention
- Care Plan Activity
  A Clients with AIDS
- MediaLink Application
  At Risk for HIV/AIDS

LEARNING OUTCOMES

After completing this chapter, you will be able to:

- Review normal anatomy and physiology of the immune system and the immune response (see Chapter 8).

- Describe the four types of hypersensitivity reactions.

- Discuss the pathophysiology of autoimmune disorders and tissue transplant rejection.

- Discuss the characteristics of immunodeficiencies.

- Identify laboratory and diagnostic tests used to diagnose and monitor immune response.

- Describe pharmacologic and other collaborative therapies used in treating clients with altered immunity.

- Provide teaching for clients with altered immune responses and their families.

- Correlate the pathophysiological alterations with the manifestations of HIV/AIDS infection.

- Use the nursing process as a framework to provide individualized care to clients with altered immune responses.

Recent years have seen the emergence of new diseases affecting the immune system. These diseases include human immunodeficiency virus (HIV) infection and altered strains of familiar diseases such as multidrug-resistant tuberculosis. At the same time, understanding of the components of the immune system and specific immune responses is increasing. It is therefore vital that today's nurses understand the foundations of the immune system and the immune response.

OVERVIEW OF THE IMMUNE SYSTEM

The immune system functions to protect the body from invasion by foreign antigens, to identify and destroy potentially harmful cells, and to remove cellular debris. This realm is accomplished by the lymphoid organs and specifically designed lymphocytes through the processes of antibody-mediated immune response and cell-mediated immune response.

The effectiveness of the immune system depends on its ability to differentiate normal host tissue from abnormal or foreign tissue. Body cells, tissues, and fluids have unique antigenic properties recognized by the immune system as "self." External agents, such as microorganisms, cells and tissues from other humans or animals, and some inorganic substances, have antigenic properties recognized by the immune system as "nonself."

Each body cell displays specific cell surface characteristics, or markers, that are unique to each person. These are known as human leukocyte antigens (HLA). A person's HLA characteristics are coded within a large cluster of genes known as the major histocompatibility complex (MHC) located on chromosome 6. Recall that chromosomes are paired; each person inherits one member of the pair from each parent. A chromosome pair contains multiple genes, each carrying instructions for production of one polypeptide chain. The number of genes in the MHC results in a multitude of HLA combinations. As a result, the possibility of two people having the same HLA type is extremely remote. Identical twins may be the exception, and some siblings have very similar HLA patterns. In tissue grafting and organ transplants, matching the HLA type as closely as possible tends to decrease rejection.

Immunocompetent clients have an immune system that identifies antigens and effectively destroys or removes them. When the immune system functions improperly, the result may be an overreaction or deficiency resulting in health problems. Overreaction of the immune system leads to hypersensitivity disorders, such as allergies. When the immune system loses the ability to recognize self, autoimmune disorders may ensue (see Table 9–1). Immunodeficiency diseases or malignancies can develop when the immune system is incompetent or unable to respond effectively, as is the case with acquired immunodeficiency disorder. These alterations in immunity are discussed later in this chapter.

As discussed previously in Chapter 8, the *antibody-mediated immune response* is accomplished by B lymphocytes (B cells) that are further divided into memory cells and plasma cells. They are activated by contact with an antigen and by T cells. B cells produce antibodies, also known as immunoglobulins (see Table 8–2), and serve to inactivate an invading antigen. One immunoglobulin in particular, IgM, forms natural antibodies, such as those for ABO blood group antigens, and is an important component of the immune system complexes seen in autoimmune disorders. Memory cells "remember" an antigen and when exposed to it a second time, immediately initiate the immune response. This action provides the foundation of acquired immunity.

In contrast, *cell-mediated immunity* acts at the cellular level by attacking antigens directly and by activating B cells. T lymphocytes comprise the cell-mediated immune response and are subdivided into effector cells and regulator cells. The cytotoxic cell or killer T cell is the primary effector cell. Regulator T cells are divided into two subsets known as helper T cells and suppressor T cells.

Proteins on the surface of the T cell help define its function and also provide a marker that can be used to identify the cell class. These proteins are known as the cluster of differentiation antigen or *CD antigen.* The two primary CD proteins are CD4 and CD8. Both cytotoxic and suppressor T cells carry the CD8 antigen. Helper T cells have the CD4 antigen and are often called CD4 cells. CD4 cells are the most numerous of the T lymphocytes, making up 70% of the circulating population.

Helper T cells initiate the immune response, whereas suppressor T cells limit it. Helper T cells accomplish their role by promoting growth of additional T cells, by stimulating proliferation of B cells, and by activating killer T cells. It is believed that suppressor T cells are important in preventing autoimmune disorders. Proper immune system function depends on the correct balance between helper and suppressor T cells.

In addition to destroying viruses and bacteria, cytotoxic T lymphocytes also attack malignant cells. They also are responsible for the rejection of transplanted organs and grafted tissues.

CHANGES IN IMMUNE FUNCTION IN THE OLDER ADULT

Immune function declines with aging, although many of the mechanisms leading to this decline are not clear. External factors, such as nutritional status and the effects of chemical exposure, ultraviolet radiation, and environmental pollution, affect the older adult's immune status. Internal factors affect it as well, including genetics, the function of the neurologic and endocrine systems, chronic and prior illnesses, and individual anatomic and physiologic variations. These myriad influences make it difficult to determine the effect of aging on the immune system. In some older individuals, the immune system is as effective as that of younger persons.

Whereas the antibody response to foreign antigens is diminished, autoantibodies (antibodies that react to the client's own tissues) are more common in older persons. The presence of autoantibodies suggests impaired regulation of the immune system, but it is not associated with an increased incidence of autoimmune disorders (discussed later in this chapter). There is also reduced or delayed hypersensitivity response.

ASSESSMENT OF ALTERED IMMUNE SYSTEM FUNCTION

Unlike body systems that are composed of a few closely related organs, the immune system is diverse and scattered. Optimal immune function depends on intact skin and mucous membrane barriers, adequate blood cell production and differentiation, a functional system of lymphatics and the spleen, and the ability to differentiate foreign tissue and pathogens from normal body tissue and flora. Because of this diversity of organs and function, assessment of the immune system is often integrated throughout the history and physical examination.

Health History

Prior to interviewing the client, review the biographic data, including age, sex, race, and ethnic background. This information can provide valuable clues about possible immunologic disorders. For example, many autoimmune disorders are more prevalent in women than in men. Family history is also important, because there is a genetic component in the etiology of many disorders affecting the immune system.

Many interview questions related to the immune system and disorders that affect it are of a sensitive nature. Be sure to provide for privacy prior to the interview. If family members are present, request that they leave as well. Establish a trusting relationship with the client prior to asking the most sensitive questions (e.g., those related to the use of illicit drugs or sexual activity).

Physical Assessment

The techniques of inspection and palpation are especially important in assessing a client's immune system.

- *Assess the general appearance.* Note whether the client's stated and apparent age coincide. Evident fatigue or weakness may indicate acute or chronic illness or immunodeficiency. Assess height, weight, and body type for apparent weight loss or wasting. Observe ease of movement and note any evident stiffness or difficulty moving. Check vital signs. An elevated temperature may indicate an infection or inflammatory response.
- *Assess skin color, temperature, and moisture.* Pale or jaundiced skin may indicate a hemolytic reaction. Pallor may also indicate bone marrow suppression with accompanying immunodeficiency. Inspect the skin for evidence of rashes or lesions, such as petechiae, numerous bruises, purple or blue patches or lesions indicative of Kaposi's sarcoma, and wounds that are infected, inflamed, or unhealed. Note the location and distribution of any rashes or lesions.
- *Inspect the mucous membranes of the nose and mouth for color and condition.* Pale, boggy (edematous) nasal mucosa is often associated with chronic allergies. Note petechiae, white patches, or lacy white plaques in the oral mucosa; they may indicate hemolysis or immunodeficiency.
- *Inspect and palpate the cervical lymph nodes for evidence of lymphadenopathy (swelling) or tenderness.* Palpate the nodes of the axillae and groin as well (see Figure 8–11).
- *Assess the musculoskeletal system by inspecting and palpating the joints for redness, swelling, tenderness, or deformity.* Such changes may indicate an autoimmune disorder such as rheumatoid arthritis or systemic lupus erythematosus (SLE). Check joint range of motion as well, including that of the spine.

ALTERED IMMUNE RESPONSES

Considering the complexity of the immune system, it is not surprising that abnormal or harmful responses occur. Altered immune system responses include those characterized by hyperresponsiveness of the immune system and those characterized by an impaired immune response. Allergies, autoimmune disorders, and reactions to organ or tissue transplants are all examples of hyperresponsive immune function. AIDS and other immunodeficiency disorders result from impairment of the immune system.

THE CLIENT WITH A HYPERSENSITIVITY REACTION

Hypersensitivity is an altered immune response to an antigen that results in harm to the client. When the antigen is environmental or exogenous, it is called an **allergy,** and the antigen is referred to as an *allergen.* The tissue response to a hypersensitivity reaction may be simply irritating or bothersome, causing a runny nose or itchy eyes, or it may be life threatening, leading to blood cell hemolysis or laryngospasm.

Hypersensitivity reactions are primarily classified by the type of immune response that occurs on contact with the allergen. They may also be classified as immediate or delayed hypersensitivity responses. Anaphylaxis and transfusion reactions are examples of immediate hypersensitivity reactions; contact dermatitis is a typical delayed response. Allergies are sometimes referred to by the affected organ system (e.g., allergic rhinitis) or the allergen involved, as in hay fever. Classification by immunologic response is the most accurate and preferred means of studying allergies (Tierney, McPhee, & Papadakis, 2001).

PATHOPHYSIOLOGY

In a hypersensitivity reaction, an antigen-antibody or antigen-lymphocyte interaction causes a response that is damaging to body tissues. Antigen-antibody responses characterize types I, II, and III, also known as immediate hypersensitivity responses. Type IV hypersensitivity is an antigen-lymphocyte reaction, resulting in a delayed hypersensitivity response.

Type I IgE-Mediated Hypersensitivity

Common hypersensitivity reactions, such as allergic asthma, allergic rhinitis (hay fever), allergic conjunctivitis, hives, and anaphylactic shock, are typical of type I or IgE-mediated hypersensitivity. This type of hypersensitivity response is triggered when an allergen interacts with IgE bound to mast cells and basophils. The antigen-antibody complex prompts release of histamine and other chemical mediators, complement, acetylcholine, kinins, and chemotactic factors (Figure 9–1 ■).

When a potent allergen such as bee or wasp venom or a drug is injected, resulting in widespread antibody-antigen reaction and response to these chemical mediators, a systemic response such as anaphylaxis, urticaria, or angioedema results.

Anaphylaxis is an acute systemic type I response that occurs in highly sensitive persons following injection of a specific antigen. Substances known to trigger anaphylaxis are summarized in Box 9–1. Anaphylaxis rarely follows oral ingestion, although this is possible. The reaction begins within minutes of exposure to the allergen and may be almost instantaneous. The release of histamine and other mediators causes vasodilation and increased capillary permeability, smooth muscle contraction, and bronchial constriction. These chemical mediators

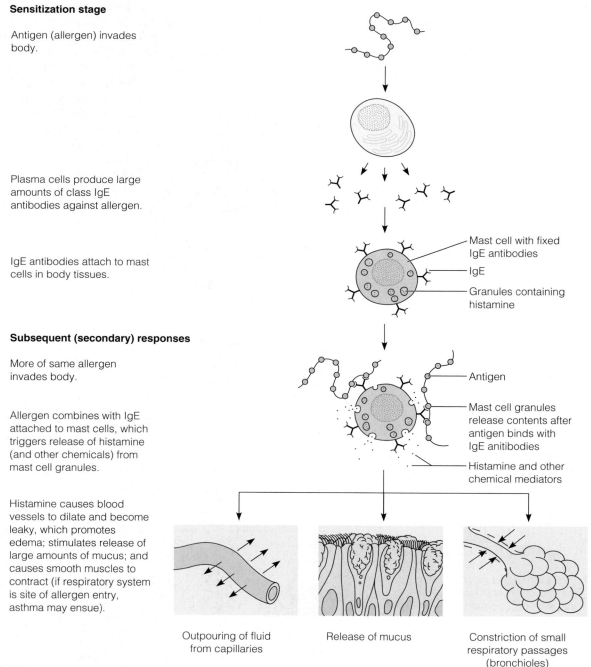

Sensitization stage

Antigen (allergen) invades body.

Plasma cells produce large amounts of class IgE antibodies against allergen.

IgE antibodies attach to mast cells in body tissues.

Subsequent (secondary) responses

More of same allergen invades body.

Allergen combines with IgE attached to mast cells, which triggers release of histamine (and other chemicals) from mast cell granules.

Histamine causes blood vessels to dilate and become leaky, which promotes edema; stimulates release of large amounts of mucus; and causes smooth muscles to contract (if respiratory system is site of allergen entry, asthma may ensue).

Mast cell with fixed IgE antibodies

IgE

Granules containing histamine

Antigen

Mast cell granules release contents after antigen binds with IgE anitbodies

Histamine and other chemical mediators

Outpouring of fluid from capillaries

Release of mucus

Constriction of small respiratory passages (bronchioles)

Figure 9–1 ■ Type I IgE-mediated hypersensitivity response.

BOX 9–1 ■ Substances Known to Trigger Anaphylaxis in Sensitized Persons

Hormones
- Insulin
- Vasopressin
- Parathormone

Enzymes
- Trypsin
- Chymotrypsin
- Penicillinase

Pollens
- Ragweed
- Grass
- Trees

Foods
- Eggs
- Seafoods
- Nuts
- Grains
- Beans
- Cottonseed oil
- Chocolate

Vitamins
- Thiamine
- Folic acid

Insect Venom
- Yellow jacket
- Hornet
- Paper wasp
- Honey bee

Occupational Agents
- Rubber products
- Industrial chemicals (ethylenes)

Antibiotics
- Penicillins
- Cephalosporins
- Amphotericin B
- Nitrofurantoin

Local Anesthetics
- Procaine
- Lidocaine

Medical Diagnostic Agents
- Sodium dehydrocholate
- Sulfobromophthalein

Antiserum
- Antilymphocyte gamma globulin

cause the client to experience the typical manifestations of anaphylaxis. Initially, a sense of foreboding or uneasiness, lightheadedness, and itching palms and scalp may be noted. Hives may develop, along with angioedema (localized tissue swelling) of the eyelids, lips, tongue, hands, feet, and genitals. Swelling can also affect the uvula and larynx, impairing breathing. This is further complicated by the bronchial constriction. The client exhibits air hunger, stridor and wheezing, and a barking cough. These respiratory effects can be lethal if the reaction is severe and intervention is not immediately available. Vasodilation and fluid loss from the vascular system can lead to impaired tissue perfusion and hypotension, a condition known as anaphylactic shock.

Fortunately, localized responses are more common manifestations of type I hypersensitivity. These are typically atopic responses; that is, they have a strong genetic predisposition. Atopic reactions are the result of localized, rather than systemic, IgE-mediated responses to an allergen. They are prompted by contact of the allergen with cell-bound IgE in the bronchial tree, nasal mucosa, and conjunctival tissues. Chemical mediators are released locally, producing symptoms such as asthma, allergic rhinitis (hay fever), conjunctivitis, or atopic dermatitis. Allergens commonly associated with atopic reactions of this type include pollens, fungal spores, house dust mites, animal dander, and feathers (Porth, 2002). Food allergens can also cause localized responses such as diarrhea or vomiting. If the gastrointestinal mucosa is altered by a local

Antigen attaches to foreign cell or tissue.

Antigen

Plasma cells produce IgG or IgM antibodies, which bind to antigens.

Plasma cell

Antibody

Binding of antigens with antibodies stimulates complement activation.

Complement activation results in destruction of the target cell by lysis, phagocytosis, or activation of killer T cells.

Cell lysis

Phagocyte

Killer T cell

Figure 9–2 ■ Type II cytotoxic hypersensitivity response.

allergic response, then the allergen may be absorbed, leading to a systemic reaction. Urticaria (hives) is the most common systemic response to food allergies.

Type II Cytotoxic Hypersensitivity

A hemolytic transfusion reaction to blood of an incompatible type is characteristic of a type II or cytotoxic hypersensitivity reaction. IgG or IgM type antibodies are formed to a cell-bound antigen such as the ABO or Rh antigen. When these antibodies bind with the antigen, the complement cascade is activated, resulting in destruction of the target cell (Figure 9–2 ■).

Type II reactions may be stimulated by an exogenous antigen, such as foreign tissue or cells, or a drug reaction, in which the drug forms an antigenic complex on the surface of a blood cell, stimulating the production of antibodies. The affected cell is then destroyed in the resulting antigen-antibody reaction; for example, hemolytic anemia is sometimes associated with the administration of chlorpromazine (Thorazine). Withdrawal of the drug stops the reaction and cell destruction (Roitt, 1994).

Endogenous antigens can also stimulate a type II reaction, resulting in an autoimmune disorder such as Goodpasture's syndrome, in which antigens are formed to specific tissues in the lungs and kidneys. Hashimoto's thyroiditis and autoimmune hemolytic anemia are additional examples of autoimmune type II reactions.

Type III Immune Complex–Mediated Hypersensitivity

Type III hypersensitivity reactions result from the formation of IgG or IgM antibody-antigen immune complexes in the circulation. When these complexes are deposited in vessel walls and extravascular tissues, complement is activated and chemical mediators of inflammation such as histamine are released. Chemotactic factors attract neutrophils to the site of inflammation. When neutrophils attempt to phagocytize the immune complexes, lysosomal enzymes are released, increasing tissue damage (Figure 9–3 ■).

Antigens invade body and bind to antibodies in circulation. Antigen-antibody complexes are formed.

Antigen-antibody complexes are deposited in the basement membrane of vessel walls and other body tissues, activating complement.

Complement activation leads to release of inflammatory chemical mediators. Infiltration of polymorphonuclear leukocytes (PMNs) is followed by release of lysozymes. Tissue damage may be extensive.

Antigen
Antibody
Antigen-antibody complex
Basement membrane
Polymorphonuclear leukocyte
Lysosome
Chemical mediators
Release of lysosomal granules

Figure 9–3 ■ Type III immune complex–mediated hypersensitivity response.

Either systemic or local responses may be seen with type III reactions. For example, serum sickness is a systemic response, so named because it was first identified after administration of foreign serum (e.g., horse antitetanus toxin). Although foreign serums are no longer administered, serum sickness occurs in response to some drugs, such as penicillin and sulfonamides. Immune complexes are deposited in walls of small blood vessels, the kidneys, and joints. Manifestations of serum sickness include fever, urticaria or rash, arthralgias, myalgias, and lymphadenopathy.

Localized responses may occur at a number of different sites. As immune complexes accumulate in the glomerular basement membrane of the kidneys—for example, following a streptococcal infection or with systemic lupus erythematosus—glomerulonephritis develops. When an antigen such as dust from moldy hay is inhaled, an acute alveolar inflammatory response can occur. This condition can develop in agricultural workers.

Type IV Delayed Hypersensitivity

Type IV reactions differ from other hypersensitivity responses in two ways. First, these reactions are cell mediated rather than antibody mediated, involving T cells of the immune system. Second, type IV reactions are delayed rather than immediate, developing 24 to 48 hours after exposure to the antigen. Type IV hypersensitivity responses result from an exaggerated interaction between an antigen and normal cell-mediated mechanisms. This exaggerated interaction results in the release of soluble inflammatory and immune mediators (from the lysozymes within the macrophages) and recruitment of killer T cells, causing local tissue destruction (Figure 9–4 ■).

Contact dermatitis is a classic example of a type IV reaction. Intense redness, itching, and thickening affect the skin in the area exposed to the antigen. Fragile vesicles are often present as well. Many antigens can provoke this response; poison ivy is a prime perpetrator. In the health care setting, an allergic response to latex can also produce contact dermatitis. An estimated 8% to 12% of health care workers are allergic to latex (National Institute of Occupational Safety and Health [NIOSH], 1997). Other examples of cell-mediated responses include a positive tuberculin test and graft rejection episodes.

Antigen-presenting cell encounters cytotoxic T cell.

Antigen-presenting cell

T cell

Interaction causes release of lympho-kines, which attract macrophages.

Lymphokines

Lysozymes

Macrophage

Macrophages release lysozymes, resulting in local tissue damage.

Figure 9–4 ■ Type IV delayed hypersensitivity response.

COLLABORATIVE CARE

The focus of care for clients with allergic responses is on the following:

- Minimize exposure to the allergen.
- Prevent a hypersensitivity response.
- Provide prompt, effective interventions for allergic responses when they occur.

Identifying allergens for the individual to reduce the likelihood of exposure is a key aspect of management. A complete history of the client's allergies is obtained, including medications, foods, animals, plants, and other materials. The type of hypersensitivity response is documented, as is its onset, manifestations, and usual treatment.

When a documented or suspected hypersensitivity reaction occurs, the allergen (e.g., intravenous medication or transfusion) is withdrawn immediately. With a type I hypersensitivity response, managing the client's airway takes highest priority, followed by maintaining cardiac output. Type II hypersensitivity responses may necessitate aggressive management of bleeding or renal failure. Type III (immune complex) reaction is treated by removing the offending antigen and interrupting the inflammatory response.

With a hypersensitivity response, supportive care is important to relieve discomfort. This often involves the administration of selected antihistamine or anti-inflammatory medications. Other therapies, such as plasmapheresis, may be prescribed in selected instances.

Diagnostic Tests

To identify possible allergens or hypersensitivity reactions, the following laboratory tests may be ordered.

- *WBC count with differential* can detect high levels of circulating eosinophils. Normally, eosinophils constitute a very small percentage (1% to 4%) of the total WBCs. Eosinophilia, however, is often present in clients with type I hypersensitivities.
- *Radioallergosorbent test (RAST)* measures the amount of IgE directed toward specific allergens. Test results are compared with control values and used to identify hypersensitivities. RAST poses no risk for an anaphylactic reaction. It is particularly useful in detecting allergies to some occupational chemicals and toxic allergens (Tierney et al., 2001).
- *Blood type and crossmatch* are ordered prior to any anticipated transfusions. The client's ABO blood group and Rh status are determined. Two major antigens, designated A and B, may be present on RBCs. Clients with the A antigen are designated as blood type A; those with blood type B have the B antigen. When neither antigen is found on the RBCs, the person is identified as type O. A third major RBC antigen is the Rh antigen. Persons with this antigen are called Rh positive; those without are Rh negative. Because a blood transfusion is actually a transplant of living tissue, antigen matching is vital to prevent significant hypersensitivity reactions. Once blood type is determined, a sample of the client's blood

is mixed with a sample of matching donor blood and observed for antigen-antibody reactions in the crossmatch portion of this test. Although this procedure greatly reduces the risk of a hemolytic transfusion reaction (type II hypersensitivity), it does not totally eliminate it.

- *Indirect Coombs' test* detects the presence of circulating antibodies (other than ABO antibodies) against RBCs. The client's serum is mixed with the donor's RBCs. If the client's serum contains antibodies to an RBC antigen, agglutination (clumping together) will occur. This is called a positive response. The normal value is negative, or no agglutination. This test is also part of the crossmatch of a blood type and crossmatch.
- *Direct Coombs' test* detects antibodies on the client's RBCs that damage and destroy the cells. This is used following a suspected transfusion reaction to detect antibodies coating the transfused RBCs. It can also identify hemolytic anemia when the cause is unknown. In the direct Coombs' test, the client's RBCs are mixed with Coombs' serum, which contains antibodies to IgG and several complement components. Agglutination will occur if the client's RBCs are coated with antibodies, resulting in a positive test. As with the indirect Coombs' test, the normal test result is negative.
- *Immune complex assays* may be performed to detect the presence of circulating immune complexes in suspected type III hypersensitivity responses. The assays are particularly useful in diagnosing suspected autoimmune disorders. Nonspecific assays of IgG-, IgM-, and IgA-containing immune complexes, which do not detect specific antibodies, as well as specific antibody assays may be done. The normal result is a test negative for circulating immune complexes. A negative test does not, however, rule out an immune complex hypersensitivity response. In some cases, a negative result may indicate that the disease process has reached a later stage, in which complexes are no longer circulating but have initiated extensive tissue damage, such as glomerulonephritis (Braunwald et al., 2001).
- *Complement assay* is also useful in detecting immune complex disorders. In these disorders, complement is, in effect, used up by the development of antigen-antibody complexes. Decreased levels are seen on examination. Both total complement level and amounts of individual components of the complement cascade can be determined.

Skin tests are also used to determine causes of hypersensitivity reactions. These tests are used to identify specific allergens to which a person may be sensitive. Allergens for testing are selected according to the client's history. Test solutions made from extracts of inhaled, ingested, or injected materials, such as pollens, mites, venoms, or some drugs, are used for the prick test and intradermal testing. Epicutaneous testing (prick testing) is generally done first to avoid a systemic reaction; it is followed by intradermal testing of allergens with a negative response to prick testing (Tierney et al., 2001).

- *Prick (epicutaneous or puncture) test:* A drop of diluted allergenic extract is placed on the skin, and the skin is then pricked or punctured through the drop. With a positive test,

Figure 9–5 ■ Skin testing on the forearm showing induration and erythema typical of a positive response to an antigen.

Source: Southern Illinois University/Photo Researchers, Inc.

a localized pruritic wheal and erythema occurs. The response is maximal at 15 to 20 minutes.

- *Intradermal:* A small amount (just enough to create a wheal) of allergen extract at a 1:500 or 1:1000 dilution is injected on the forearm or intrascapular area. If several allergens are being tested, injections are spaced 0.25 to 0.5 inches apart. As control measures, plain diluent (negative control) and histamine (positive control) are also injected. If there is no response to a particular allergen at 15 to 20 minutes, the test is negative. The appearance of a wheal and erythema, with a wheal diameter at least 5 mm greater than that produced by the control, indicates a positive response (Figure 9–5 ■).
- *Patch:* A 1-inch patch impregnated with the allergen (e.g., perfume, cosmetics, detergents, or clothing fibers) is applied to the skin for 48 hours. Absence of a response indicates a negative test result. Positive responses are graded from mild (erythema in the exposed area) to severe (erythema, papules, vesicles, or ulceration).
- *Food allergy testing* is done when a food allergy is suspected but the source or implicated food item has not been clearly identified. Food allergy symptoms are typically demonstrated within hours of eating. Initially, the client is asked to keep a diary of foods consumed and allergic responses for a week. An elimination diet is then prescribed. The diet excludes most common food allergens and all suspected foods for 1 week. Any foods that may contain allergens in combination, such as breads, are also eliminated. If symptoms do not improve, a different variation of the elimination diet is prescribed. If symptoms are relieved, foods are reintroduced to the diet one at a time until symptoms recur, indicating allergy to that food.

Medications

When it is impossible to avoid the offending allergen and allergic manifestations are severe or disrupt the client's activities of daily living (ADLs), pharmacologic intervention is prescribed. *Immunotherapy,* also called hyposensitization or desensitization, consists of injecting an extract of the allergen(s) in gradually increasing doses. Immunotherapy is used primarily for allergic rhinitis or asthma related to inhaled allergens. It has also been shown to be effective in preventing anaphylactic responses to insect venom. With weekly or biweekly subcutaneous injections of the allergen, the client develops IgG antibodies to the allergen that appear to block effectively the allergic IgE-mediated response. Once a therapy plateau is reached, injections are continued indefinitely either monthly or bimonthly.

Antihistamines are the major class of drugs used in treating the symptoms of hypersensitivity responses, type I in particular. They are also useful to some extent in relieving manifestations (such as urticaria) of some type II and type III reactions.

Antihistamines block H1-histamine receptors, acting as a competitive antagonist to histamine, but they do not affect the production or release of histamine. The prototype antihistamine is diphenhydramine (Benadryl). It and other antihistamines alleviate the systemic effects of histamine such as urticaria and angioedema. They are also useful in relieving allergic rhinitis, although they are not effective in all clients. Antihistamines are available in both prescription and nonprescription preparations. The preferred route of administration is oral, although diphenhydramine and others can be given parenterally, particularly when immediate action is needed, as in anaphylaxis. They also dry respiratory secretions through an anticholinergic effect. Their use is limited by their side effects, especially drowsiness and dry mouth. Antihistamines are not effective in relieving asthmatic responses to allergens and may actually worsen symptoms by their drying effect on respiratory secretions.

Antihistamines are often combined with a sympathomimetic agent such as pseudoephedrine to improve their decongestant activity and counteract their sedative effect. Antihistamines are discussed further in Chapter 35. ⌐⌐

The immediate treatment for anaphylaxis is parenteral epinephrine, an adrenergic agonist (sympathomimetic) drug that has both vasoconstricting and bronchodilating effects. These qualities, combined with its rapid action, make epinephrine ideal for treating an anaphylactic reaction. For mild reactions with wheezing, pruritus, urticaria, and angioedema, a subcutaneous injection of 0.3 to 0.5 mL of 1:1000 epinephrine is generally sufficient. For clients with an injected toxin such as a bee sting, an additional amount equivalent to one-half the above may be injected directly into the site of the sting and a tourniquet applied above it to prevent further systemic absorption. Intravenous epinephrine using a 1:100,000 concentration may be used in the client with a more severe anaphylactic reaction.

Clients who have experienced an anaphylactic reaction to insect venom or other potentially unavoidable allergen should carry a kit (commonly called a bee sting kit) for immediate treatment of future exposures. This kit typically includes a prefilled syringe of epinephrine and an epinephrine nebulizer, allowing prompt self-treatment.

Cromolyn sodium (Intal, Nasalcrom) is a drug used to treat allergic rhinitis and asthma. Cromolyn sodium acts by stabilizing the mast cell membrane, thus preventing chemical mediator release (Shannon, Wilson, & Stang, 2001). Because it is effective only when applied directly to involved tissue, it is delivered by inhaler or nasal spray. It has few side effects and a wide margin of safety, making it a good choice for clients in whom it is effective (Tierney et al., 2001).

Glucocorticoids (corticosteroids) are used in both systemic and topical forms for many types of hypersensitivity responses. Their anti-inflammatory effects, rather than their immunosuppressive effects, are of most benefit. A short course of corticosteroid therapy is often used for severe asthma, allergic contact dermatitis, and some immune-complex disorders (Tierney et al., 2001). Corticosteroids in topical forms or delivered by inhaler may be used for longer periods of time with few side effects; however, systemic absorption can occur.

Other Therapies

Other treatments used for hypersensitivity responses are generally dictated by the severity of the response and the organ system affected. Airway management takes highest priority for the client with an acute anaphylactic reaction. Insertion of an endotracheal tube or emergency tracheostomy may be required to maintain airway patency with severe laryngospasm. Because anaphylaxis places the person at risk for vasomotor collapse and significant hypotension, it is necessary to insert an intravenous line and initiate fluid resuscitation with an isotonic solution such as Ringer's lactate.

Plasmapheresis, removal of harmful components in the plasma, may be used to treat immune complex responses such as glomerulonephritis and Goodpasture's syndrome. Plasma and the glomerular-damaging antibody-antigen complexes are removed by passing the client's blood through a blood cell separator. The RBCs are then returned to the client along with an equal amount of albumin or human plasma. This procedure is usually done in a series rather than as a one-time treatment. It is not without risk, and informed consent is required. Potential complications of plasmapheresis include those associated with intravenous catheters, shifts in fluid balance, and alteration of blood clotting.

NURSING CARE

Nursing care related to hypersensitivity reactions is primarily directed toward prevention, early identification, and providing prompt, effective treatment.

Health Promotion

Health promotion activities include helping clients to identify possible allergens that prompt a hypersensitivity response and discussing possible strategies to avoid these allergens. Anyone with severe food allergies may need assistance from a dietitian to discuss necessary dietary changes and ways to continue meeting nutrient needs. It is important that persons with hypersensitivities inform health care personnel of all allergens. People who experience anaphylactic reactions should wear a bracelet or tag at all times to identify the substance(s) that provokes this response.

Assessment

Collect the following data through the health history and physical examination. Further focused assessments are described with nursing interventions in the next section.

- Health history: risk factors, hypersensitivities (medications, household dust, bee stings, etc.), reaction (rash, hives, difficulty breathing), type of treatment for hypersensitivity reactions; allergy skin testing; asthma, hay fever, or dermatitis
- Physical assessment: mucous membranes of nose and mouth, skin for lesions or rashes, eyes (tearing and redness), respiratory rate, and adventitious breath sounds

Nursing Diagnoses and Interventions

Priority nursing diagnoses will vary according to the type of hypersensitivity reaction experienced by the client. Because nurses are most likely to become involved with a client experiencing a type I or type II response, this section focuses on diagnoses for these clients. Airway, breathing, and circulation (the ABCs) are of greatest importance for the client with an anaphylactic reaction. When a hemolytic reaction to an incompatible blood transfusion occurs, the client is at risk for injury.

Ineffective Airway Clearance

In anaphylactic reactions, the airway may be obstructed due to facial angioedema, bronchospasm, or laryngeal edema. Establishing and maintaining a patent airway is of highest priority.

- Administer oxygen per nasal cannula at a rate of 2 to 4 L/min. *This increases the alveolar oxygen and its availability to cells of the body.*

PRACTICE ALERT *Placing in Fowler's to high-Fowler's position allows optimal lung expansion and ease of breathing.* ■

- Assess respiratory rate and pattern, level of consciousness and anxiety, nasal flaring, use of accessory muscles of respiration, chest wall movement, audible stridor; palpate for respiratory excursion; auscultate lung sounds and any adventitious sounds, such as wheezes. *Extreme anxiety or agitation, nasal flaring, stridor, and diminished lung sounds indicate air hunger and possible airway obstruction, necessitating immediate intervention.*
- Insert a nasopharyngeal or oropharyngeal airway, and arrange for immediate intubation as indicated. *Assuring an adequate airway is vital to preserve life.*
- Administer subcutaneous epinephrine 1:1000, 0.3 to 0.5 mL as prescribed. This may be repeated in 20 to 30 minutes if necessary. Administer parenteral diphenhydramine (deep intramuscular or intravenous) as prescribed. *Epinephrine is a potent vasoconstrictor and bronchodilator, counteracting the effects of histamine. Diphenhydramine is an antihistamine that blocks histamine receptors and its effect. These medications can be effective in rapidly reversing manifestations of anaphylaxis.*
- Provide calm reassurance. *Hypoxemia and air hunger are terrifying for the client. Anxiety can impair the client's ability to cooperate with treatment and increase the respiratory rate, making breathing less effective.*

Decreased Cardiac Output

Peripheral vasodilation and increased capillary permeability from the release of histamine can significantly impair cardiac output. When it falls to the degree that tissue perfusion becomes impaired and hypoxia results, a state of anaphylactic shock exists.

- Monitor vital signs frequently, noting fall in blood pressure, decreasing pulse pressure, tachycardia, and tachypnea. *These vital sign changes may indicate shock.*
- Assess skin color, temperature, capillary refill, edema, and other indicators of peripheral perfusion. *As cardiac output falls, peripheral vessels constrict and tissue perfusion is impaired.*
- Monitor level of consciousness. *A change in level of consciousness (lethargy, apprehension, or agitation) is often the first indicator of decreased cardiac output.*
- Insert one or more large-bore (18-gauge or larger) intravenous catheters. *It is important to insert intravenous catheters as soon as possible to provide sites for rapid fluid replacement.*
- Administer warmed intravenous solutions of lactated Ringer's or normal saline, as prescribed. *These isotonic solutions help maintain intravascular volume. Warmed solutions are used to prevent hypothermia from the rapid administration of large amounts of fluid at room temperature (about 70°F, or 21.1°C).*
- Insert an indwelling catheter, and monitor urinary output frequently. *As the cardiac output drops, the glomerular filtration rate (GFR) falls. With an output of less than 30 mL per hour, the client is at risk for acute renal failure from ischemia.*
- Place a tourniquet above the site of an injected venom (such as a bee sting), and infiltrate the site with epinephrine as prescribed. *Use of a tourniquet and the vasoconstriction resulting from epinephrine infiltration reduce further absorption of the allergen.*
- Once breathing is established, place the client flat with the legs elevated. *This position enhances perfusion of the central organs, such as the brain, heart, and kidneys.*

PRACTICE ALERT *Aggressive fluid therapy may lead to hypervolemia and pulmonary edema; assess for shortness of breath and crackles in the lungs.* ■

Risk for Injury
As noted, the potential for hypersensitivity responses is high in clients subjected to medical treatments. Because a blood transfusion is a transplant of living tissue, the risk for adverse immunologic response and injury is particularly significant.

- Obtain and record a thorough history of previous blood transfusions and any reactions experienced, *no matter how mild.* Alert the physician if previous transfusion reactions have occurred. *The client who has received prior blood transfusions is at increased risk for a hypersensitivity reaction, because antibody production may have been stimulated by prior exposure to antigens.*
- Check for a signed informed consent to administer blood or blood products. *It is important to obtain informed consent for this invasive and risky procedure.*
- Using two licensed health care professionals, double-check the type, Rh factor, crossmatch, and expiration date for all

blood and blood components received from the blood bank with the client's data. *This is an important safety measure to reduce the risk of a hemolytic transfusion reaction due to incompatible blood types.*

PRACTICE ALERT *Begin a blood transfusion within 30 minutes of its delivery from the blood bank to reduce bacterial contamination.* ■

- Take and record vital signs within 15 minutes prior to initiating the blood infusion. *This provides a baseline for evaluating any changes related to the blood transfusion.*
- Infuse blood into a site separate from any other intravenous infusion. Use at least an 18-gauge catheter for the infusion. *This reduces the risk of damage to the blood cells due to incompatibility with other intravenous solutions or physical trauma. When blood is administered with dextrose solutions (e.g., D5W, D5NS), blood cell hemolysis and aggregation occurs; administration with lactated Ringer's can cause agglutination of cells.*
- Administer 50 mL of blood during the first 15 minutes of the transfusion. *Reactions generally occur within the first 15 minutes.*
- During transfusion, monitor for complaints of back or chest pain, an increase in the temperature of more than 1.8°F, chills, tachycardia, tachypnea, wheezing, hypotension, hives, rashes, or cyanosis. *These signs may indicate an adverse reaction to the blood transfusion.*
- Stop the blood transfusion immediately if a reaction occurs, no matter how mild, keeping the intravenous line open with normal saline. Notify the physician and the blood bank.
- If a reaction is suspected, send the blood and administration set to the laboratory with a freshly drawn blood sample and urine specimen from the client. *These will be used to identify the cause of the reaction as well as its effect on the client.*
- If no adverse reaction occurs, administer the transfusion over 2 to 4 hours. *This time frame is important to limit the risk of bacterial growth.*

Using NANDA, NIC, and NOC
Chart 9–1 shows links between NANDA, NIC, and NOC when caring for the client with hypersensitivities.

Home Care
The vast majority of hypersensitivity responses are appropriately treated by the client and/or family members with little or no medical intervention. Teaching, therefore, is a vital component of care. If the client is at risk for anaphylaxis, involving the family in teaching is essential because the response may occur with such rapidity that the client will be unable to provide self-care.

Include the following points in teaching the client and family about managing hypersensitivities.

- When and how to use an anaphylaxis kit containing epinephrine and antihistamines in injectable, inhaler, and oral forms
- When to seek medical attention

CHART 9–1 NANDA, NIC, AND NOC LINKAGES

The Client with a Hypersensitivity Reaction

NURSING DIAGNOSES	NURSING INTERVENTIONS	NURSING OUTCOMES
• Ineffective Health Maintenance • Risk for Latex Allergy Response	• Health Education • Teaching: Individual • Allergy Management • Latex Precautions	• Health-Promoting Behavior • Health-Seeking Behavior • Immune Hypersensitivity Control • Risk Detection

Note. Data from Nursing Outcomes Classification (NOC) *by M. Johnson & M. Maas (Eds.), 1997, St. Louis: Mosby;* Nursing Diagnoses: Definitions & Classification 2001–2002 *by North American Nursing Diagnosis Association, 2001, Philadelphia: NANDA;* Nursing Interventions Classification (NIC) *by J.C. McCloskey & G. M. Bulechek (Eds.), 2000, St. Louis: Mosby. Reprinted by permission.*

- Use and adverse reactions of prescription and nonprescription antihistamines and decongestants
- Advantages of autologous blood transfusion if future surgery is scheduled
- Preventing an immune complex reaction such as glomerulonephritis
- Skin care to prevent contact dermatitis, including:
  Expose affected areas to air and sun as much as possible.
  Avoid direct contact with people who have an infection.
  Wear cool, light, nonrestrictive clothing of natural fibers, such as cotton, to avoid irritating affected areas.
  Avoid exposure to extremes of heat or cold.
  Use bath oils or plain water instead of soaps and detergents.
  Take tub baths in cool to lukewarm water rather than showers.
  To decrease pruritus, maintain a cool environment and avoid exercising.
  Trim fingernails to reduce the risk of skin damage.
- Helpful resources:
  - ALERT, Inc., Allergy to Latex Education and Resource Team
  - Food Allergy Network

THE CLIENT WITH AN AUTOIMMUNE DISORDER

Maintaining optimal health and preventing disease depend not only on the immune system's ability to recognize and destroy foreign tissues and other antigens, but also on the immune system's ability to recognize self. When this self-recognition is impaired and immune defenses are directed against normal host tissue, the result is an **autoimmune disorder.**

Autoimmune disorders can affect any tissue in the body. Some are tissue or organ specific, affecting particular tissue or a particular organ. Hashimoto's thyroiditis is an example of an organ-specific autoimmune disorder. Circulating antibodies are formed to certain thyroid components, resulting ultimately in destruction of the gland. In other disorders, autoantibodies are formed that are not tissue specific, but tend to accumulate and cause an inflammatory response in certain tissue, for example, the renal glomerulus or the hepatic small bile ductules.

Autoimmune disorders may also be systemic, with neither antibodies nor the resulting inflammatory lesions confined to any one organ. Rheumatologic disorders, such as rheumatoid arthritis and systemic lupus erythematosus (SLE), are characteristic of systemic autoimmune disorders (Roitt, 1994). A list of selected autoimmune disorders is included in Table 9–1.

PATHOPHYSIOLOGY

The mechanism that causes the immune system to recognize host tissue as a foreign antigen is not clear. The following factors are under study as possible contributors to the development of autoimmune disorders.

- The release of previously "hidden" antigens into the circulation, such as DNA or other components of the cell nucleus, which elicits an immune response
- Chemical, physical, or biologic changes in host tissue that cause self-antigens to stimulate the production of autoantibodies
- The introduction of an antigen, such as a bacteria or virus, whose antigenic properties closely resemble those of host tissue, resulting in the production of antibodies which target not only the foreign antigen but also normal tissue
- A defect in normal cellular immune function that allows B cells to produce autoantibodies unchecked
- Initiation of the autoimmune response by very slow-growing mycobacteria

Although the exact mechanism producing autoimmunity is unclear, several characteristics of autoimmune diseases are known. It is apparent that genetics plays a role, because a higher incidence is seen in family members of people with autoimmune disorders. Autoimmune disorders are far more prevalent in females than in males. The disorders tend to overlap, so that the client with one autoimmune disorder may develop another or some manifestations of another. The onset of an autoimmune disorder is frequently associated with an abnormal stressor, either physical or psychologic. Autoimmune disorders are frequently progressive relapsing-remitting disorders characterized by periods of exacerbation and remission.

Specific autoimmune disorders are discussed in the sections of this textbook related to the affected organ systems or functional disruption.

TABLE 9–1   Selected Autoimmune Disorders

More organ specific	Hashimoto's thyroiditis	A chronic progressive inflammatory disease of the thyroid with lymphocyte infiltration and gradual destruction of the gland. See Chapter 17.
	Primary myxedema	Thyroid deficiency resulting from destruction of the thyroid gland due to an autoimmune process, often Hashimoto's thyroiditis. See Chapter 17.
	Thyrotoxicosis	Hyperthyroidism resulting from thyroid-stimulating immunoglobulins that stimulate activity of the gland. See Chapter 17.
	Pernicious anemia	Anemia resulting from absence of intrinsic factor associated with loss of parietal cells; most clients have antibodies to parietal cells. See Chapter 32.
	Addison's disease	Atrophy and hypofunction of the adrenal cortex, probably autoimmune in origin. See Chapter 17.
	Myasthenia gravis	A disease characterized by episodic muscle weakness caused by antibodies to the acetylcholine receptor of the neuromuscular junction. See Chapter 43.
	Insulin-dependent diabetes mellitus	Impaired insulin secretion, often the result of islet cell destruction by antibodies directed at the cell surface or cytoplasm. See Chapter 18.
	Goodpasture's syndrome	A type II hypersensitivity disorder with pulmonary hemorrhage and progressive glomerulonephritis characterized by circulating antiglomerular basement membrane antibodies. See Chapter 27.
	Multiple sclerosis	A probable autoimmune process resulting in disseminated patches of demyelination in the brain and spinal cord and varied neurologic manifestations. See Chapter 43.
	Idiopathic thrombocytopenic purpura	A chronic disorder characterized by petechiae, purpura, mucosal bleeding, and antibodies against platelets. See Chapter 32.
	Primary biliary cirrhosis	Inflammation and fibrosis of the bile ducts, probably of autoimmune origin. See Chapter 22.
	Active chronic hepatitis	A serious liver disease often resulting in hepatic failure and/or cirrhosis; may be autoimmune with infiltration by T cells and plasma cells. See Chapter 22.
Less organ specific	Ulcerative colitis	A chronic inflammatory disease of colon mucosa, possibly of autoimmune origin. See Chapter 21.
	Sjogren's syndrome	A systemic inflammatory disorder characterized by dryness of the mouth, eye, and other mucous membranes with lymphocyte infiltration of affected tissues. See Chapter 39.
	Rheumatoid arthritis	A chronic syndrome with inflammation of peripheral joints and generalized manifestations, characterized by infiltration of synovium by lymphocytes and plasma cells. See Chapter 39.
	Scleroderma	Diffuse fibrosis, degenerative changes, and vascular abnormalities of skin, joint structures, and internal organs; probably of autoimmune origin. See Chapter 39.
Non–organ specific	Systemic lupus erythematosus	An inflammatory connective tissue disorder characterized the presence of antinuclear antibodies. See Chapter 39.

COLLABORATIVE CARE

For the most part, the diagnosis of an autoimmune disorder is based on the client's clinical manifestations. Serum assays are useful to identify autoantibodies. Other diagnostic tests are generally specific to the suspected disorder and to identifying the degree of tissue damage and destruction. Although the manifestations of these disorders can often be managed, a cure typically is not possible unless the affected target tissue is removed (e.g., colectomy for the client with ulcerative colitis).

Diagnostic Tests

Serologic assays are used to identify and measure antibodies directed toward host tissue antigens or normal cellular components. Many detectable autoantibodies are not specific to a single autoimmune disorder and are used to establish the au-

toimmune process rather than the specific disorder. Although healthy people often have low levels of autoantibodies, levels are much higher in clients affected by an autoimmune disorder. The following serologic assays may be ordered.

- *Antinuclear antibody (ANA)* detects antibodies produced to DNA and other nuclear material. These antibodies can cause tissue damage characteristic of autoimmune disorders, such as SLE. The client's serum is combined with nuclear material and tagged antihuman antibody to detect ANA-antihuman antibody complexes. A negative, or normal, result is a titer <1:20. When complexes are detected at higher titer levels (>1:20), the test is positive for ANA. This test is not specific for SLE, because high levels of ANA may be present in rheumatoid arthritis and cirrhosis of the liver; nevertheless, 95% of clients with SLE have a positive ANA titer.
- *Lupus erythematosus (LE) cell test* is also used to detect SLE and monitor its treatment. Neutrophils that contain

large masses of phagocytized DNA from the nuclei of PMNs are called LE cells. Like the ANA, the LE cell prep is nonspecific for SLE. A positive result may also be seen in rheumatoid arthritis or with medications such as isoniazid, penicillin, phenytoin, procainamide, streptomycin, or sulfonamide drugs.

- *Rheumatoid factor (RF)* is an immunoglobulin present in the serum of approximately 80% of clients with rheumatoid arthritis. Low titer levels (<1:20) may be present in the elderly. An RF titer 1:80 or higher indicates rheumatoid arthritis. A titer between 1:20 and 1:80 could indicate SLE, scleroderma, or liver cirrhosis (Kee, 1999).
- *Complement assay* may also be useful in identifying autoimmune disorders. In these disorders, complement may be consumed in the development of antigen-antibody complexes. Decreased levels are seen on examination. Both total complement level and amounts of individual components of the complement cascade can be determined.

Medications

Various approaches are used in the treatment of autoimmune disorders. Anti-inflammatory medications such as aspirin, NSAIDs, and corticosteroids may be prescribed to reduce the inflammatory response and minimize tissue damage. (Refer to Chapter 4 for additional detail on these drugs.) When these agents are not effective or well tolerated by the client, slow-acting anti-inflammatory medications may be prescribed. Slow-acting or antirheumatic drugs include such medications as gold salts, hydroxychloroquine (Plaquenil), and penicillamine. Their use is further detailed in Chapter 39. Cytotoxic drugs may be used in combination with plasmapheresis in treating many autoimmune disorders. Cytotoxic drugs are discussed in further detail in the next section of this chapter.

NURSING CARE

Nursing care measures for the client with an autoimmune disorder are individualized and tailored to needs dictated by manifestations of the disorder. Nurses often will be involved with the client in an outpatient setting such as an office or home, evaluating the client's response to therapy and self-care management.

Consider the following nursing diagnoses in planning care for the client with an autoimmune disorder.

- *Activity intolerance* related to inflammatory effects of autoimmune disorder
- *Ineffective coping* related to chronic disease process
- *Interrupted family processes* related to lack of understanding about autoimmune disorder and its effects
- *Ineffective protection* related to disordered immune function
- *Risk for ineffective therapeutic regimen management* related to lack of understanding

Home Care

Because many autoimmune disorders are chronic, teaching the client and family about the disorder and its management is a key nursing care component. The client may be taking drugs with multiple side effects or long-term effects, necessitating effective teaching. Clients with autoimmune disorders often do not appear to be ill, making it difficult for friends and families to understand their care needs. The chronicity of these disorders also puts the client at high risk for unproven remedies and quackery. Provide psychologic support, listening, and teaching. In addition, suggest resources such as local support groups and the American Autoimmune Related Diseases Association.

THE CLIENT WITH A TISSUE TRANSPLANT

Since the first kidney transplant performed from one identical twin to the other in 1954, organ and tissue transplantation has become an increasingly popular and viable treatment option. The transplantation of avascular tissues, such as skin, cornea, bone, and heart valves, is considered routine, with little need for tissue matching and immunosuppression. Transplants of organs (e.g., the kidney, heart, heart and lung, liver, and bone marrow) are increasingly common and are no longer considered experimental or extraordinary procedures. Common organ transplants are outlined in Table 9–2.

Transplant success is closely tied to obtaining an organ with tissue antigens as close to those of the recipient as possible. As noted earlier in this chapter, every body cell has cell surface antigens known as human leukocyte antigens that are unique to the individual. Although identical twins may have the same HLA type, the chance is reduced to 1 in 4 for siblings, and less than 1 in several thousand for unrelated individuals (Tierney et al., 2001). Matching the HLA type of the donor and recipient as closely as possible decreases the potential for rejection of the transplanted organ or tissue but does not eliminate it.

PATHOPHYSIOLOGY

An **autograft,** a transplant of the client's own tissue, is the most successful type of tissue transplant. Skin grafts are the most common examples of autografts. Increasingly, autologous bone marrow transplants and blood transfusions are being used to reduce immunologic responses. When the donor and recipient are identical twins, the term **isograft** is used. Because of the high likelihood of an HLA match, the success of these grafts is good and rejection episodes are mild. Few people, however, have an identical twin to provide tissue for donation; and when the need is for an organ such as the heart, liver, or lungs, a living-donor transplantation is not possible. Most often, organ and tissue transplants are **allografts,** which are grafts between members of the same species but who have different genotypes and HLA. Allografts may come from living donors; examples are bone marrow, blood, and a kidney. Most often, however, organs for transplantation are obtained from a cadaver. Donors are typically people who meet the criteria for brain death; are less than 65 years old; and are free of systemic disease, malignancy, or infection, including HIV, hepatitis B, or hepatitis C. The organ is removed immediately

TABLE 9-2 Organ Transplants

Organ	Graft Type	Indications for Transplant	Success Rate
Kidney	Allograft; may be isograft	End-stage renal disease	80% to 90% at 1 year
Heart	Allograft	End-stage cardiac disease refractory to medical management	74% at 5 years
Lung	Allograft	Pulmonary hypertension, cystic fibrosis, pulmonary fibrosis, chronic obstructive pulmonary disease	70% at 1 year for combined heart-lung; 60% for single lung
Liver	Allograft	Severe liver dysfunction due to chronic active hepatitis, primary biliary cirrhosis, sclerosing cholangitis	70% to 90% 1-year survival
Bone marrow	Autograft or allograft	Leukemia, aplastic anemia, congenital immunologic defects	40% to 75% at 1 year
Skin	Autograft, allograft, or xenograft	Severe burns, plastic surgery	>95% at 5 years
Cornea	Allograft	Corneal ulceration and opacification	>95% at 5 years
Pancreas	Allograft	Pancreatic insufficiency, diabetes	65% at 1 year

Note. Summarized from Current Medical Diagnosis and Treatment *(40th ed.) by L. M. Tierney, S. J. McPhee, and M. A. Papadakis, 2001, New York: Lange Medical Books / McGraw-Hill.*

before or after cardiac arrest and preserved until it is transplanted into the waiting recipient. Finally, **xenograft** is a transplant from an animal species to a human. These transplants are the least successful but may be used in selected instances, such as the use of pig skin as a temporary covering for a massive burn.

Tissue typing is used to determine the **histocompatibility,** the ability of cells and tissues to survive transplantation without immunologic interference by the recipient. Tissue typing is performed in an attempt to match the donor and recipient as closely as possible for HLA type and blood type (ABO, Rh) and to identify preformed antibodies to the donor's HLA.

Both antibody-mediated and cell-mediated immune responses are involved in the complex process of transplant rejection. Host macrophages process donor antigen, presenting it to T and B lymphocytes. Activated lymphocytes produce both antibody- and cell-mediated effects. Killer T cells bind with cells of the transplanted organ, resulting in cell lysis.

Helper T cells stimulate the multiplication and differentiation of B cells, and antibodies are produced to graft endothelium. Complement activation or antibody-dependent cell-mediated cytotoxicity leads to transplant cell destruction. Rejection typically begins after the first 24 hours of the transplant, although it may present immediately. Rejection episodes are characterized as hyperacute, acute, or chronic, as summarized in Table 9–3.

Hyperacute tissue rejection occurs immediately to 2 to 3 days after the transplant of new tissue. Hyperacute rejection is due to preformed antibodies and sensitized T cells to antigens in the donor organ. Hyperacute rejection is most likely to occur in clients who have had a previous organ or tissue transplant, such as a blood transfusion. Hyperacute rejection may be evident even before the transplant procedure is completed. The grafted organ initially appears pink and healthy, but soon becomes soft and cyanotic as blood flow is impaired. Organ function deteriorates rapidly, and symptoms of organ failure develop.

TABLE 9-3 Transplant Rejection Episodes

Type	Cause	Presentation	Treatment
Hyperacute	Preexisting antibodies to donor ABO or HLA antigens	Occurs within minutes to hours or days of the transplant. Rapid deterioration of organ function	The transplant usually cannot be saved; prevent with crossmatch, and use antimetabolites or anti-inflammatory drugs before surgery.
Acute	Primarily a cell-mediated immune response to HLA antigens; antibody-mediated response may also contribute	Occurs within days to months after the transplant. Signs of inflammation and impaired organ function	Increase immunosuppression using steroids, cyclosporine, monoclonal antibodies, or antilymphocyte globulins.
Chronic	Probably antibody-mediated response; may also involve inflammatory damage to vessel endothelium	Occurs 4 months to years after the transplant. Gradual deterioration of organ function	None; loss of graft will occur, requiring retransplant.

Acute tissue rejection is the most common and treatable type of rejection episode. It occurs between 4 days and 3 months after the transplant. Acute rejection is mediated primarily by the cellular immune response, resulting in transplant cell destruction. The client experiencing acute rejection demonstrates manifestations of the inflammatory process, with fever, redness, swelling, and tenderness over the graft site. Signs of impaired function of the transplanted organ may be noted (e.g., elevated BUN and creatinine, liver enzyme and bilirubin elevations, or elevated cardiac enzymes and signs of cardiac failure).

Chronic tissue rejection occurs from 4 months to years after transplant of new tissue. Chronic rejection is most likely the result of antibody-mediated immune responses. Antibodies and complement are deposited in transplant vessel walls, causing narrowing and decreased function of the organ due to ischemia. The gradual deterioration of transplanted organ function is seen with chronic tissue rejection.

Graft-versus-host disease (GVHD) is a frequent and potentially fatal complication of bone marrow transplant. When there is no close match between donor and recipient HLA, immunocompetent cells in the grafted tissue recognize host tissue as foreign and mount a cell-mediated immune response. If the host is immunocompromised, as is often the case when a bone marrow transplant is performed, host cells are unable to destroy the graft and instead become the targets of destruction. Of clients with very closely matched bone marrow, 30% to 60% nevertheless develop GVHD. Acute GVHD occurs within the first 100 days following a transplant and primarily affects the skin, liver, and gastrointestinal tract. The client develops a maculopapular pruritic rash beginning on the palms of the hands and soles of the feet. The rash may spread to involve the entire body and lead to desquamation. Gastrointestinal manifestations include abdominal pain, nausea, and bloody diarrhea. GVHD that lasts longer than 100 days is said to be chronic. If it is limited to the skin and liver, the prognosis is good. If multiple organs are involved, the prognosis is poor (Porth, 2002; Roitt, 1994).

COLLABORATIVE CARE

Pretransplant care and posttransplant care are directed toward reducing the risk that transplanted tissue will be rejected or result in GVHD. Diagnostic studies are directed first at identifying a suitable donor, then at monitoring the immune response to the transplant. Immunosuppressive therapy with medications is a vital part of posttransplant care. Indeed, the development of effective immunosuppressive drugs is responsible for the success of organ transplants using allografts.

Diagnostic Tests

The following diagnostic tests may be ordered prior to organ or tissue transplantation.

- *Blood type and Rh factor* of both the donor and recipient are determined. Although there is some question about the benefit of histocompatibility testing prior to transplant of a cadaver organ, there is no question about the need for ABO blood group compatibility.

- *Crossmatching* of the client's serum against the donor's lymphocytes is performed to identify any preformed antibodies against antigens on donor tissues. If present, these antibodies would likely result in an immediate or hyperacute graft rejection with probable loss of the transplant.

- *HLA histocompatibility testing* identifyies donors with an HLA type close to that of the recipient. It is used primarily to identify living donors for bone marrow and kidney transplant. Because of GVHD, histocompatibility tests to identify an identical or very close HLA match are particularly important in bone marrow transplant. HLA tests are performed using lymphocytes from a blood sample. The sample should not be obtained within 72 hours of a blood transfusion, because this will interfere with results.

- *Mixed lymphocyte culture (MLC) assay tests* also are used to determine histocompatibility between the donor and the recipient. This test identifies whether mononuclear cells of the recipient will react against the potential donor's leukocyte antigens. The disadvantage of this test is that results cannot be obtained until 7 to 10 days later (Chernecky & Berger, 1997). Factors that could interfere with the results of this test include use of oral contraceptives, a radioisotope scan within 1 week prior to the test, and chemotherapy.

- *Ultrasonography* or *magnetic resonance imaging (MRI)* of the transplanted organ may be performed to evaluate its size, perfusion, and function.

- *Tissue biopsies* of the transplanted organ are performed routinely to assess for evidence of tissue rejection.

Medications

Prior to transplantation, several antibiotic and antiviral drugs may be prescribed, including the following:

- Trimethoprim-sulfamethoxazole (Septra, Bactrim), which decreases the incidence of gram-negative bacterial infections
- Acyclovir (Zovirax), which prevents the development of herpes simplex virus (HSV) pneumonia in bone marrow transplant recipients
- Ganciclovir (Cytovene), which prevents the development of cytomegalovirus (CMV) pneumonia with bone marrow transplant recipients

The mainstays of drug therapy for clients following a tissue or organ transplant are immunosuppressive agents. Varying regimens of these drugs are used, depending on the transplanted tissue and the medical center; however, a combination of corticosteroids and cyclosporine is common for maintenance therapy. Antilymphocyte therapy and the use of monoclonal antibodies are increasingly common in the immediate posttransplant period and for treating steroid-resistant rejection episodes.

Corticosteroids, primarily prednisone (Deltasone, others) and methylprednisolone (Solu-Medrol, others) were among the first medications used to prevent transplant rejection, and they remain important agents today. Although the exact anti-inflammatory and immunosuppressive activity of corticosteroids is unknown, they are known to suppress production of interleukin 1 and 2, decrease monocyte migration, and suppress proliferative and cytotoxic T-cell activity. Although they are very effective, large doses of corticosteroids used posttransplant are associated with significant adverse effects. Wound healing is impaired, and the metabolism of fats, proteins, and carbohydrates is altered. Fat distribution changes, producing a cushingoid appearance with moon facies, increased truncal fat, and "buffalo hump." Fluid retention and hypertension are potential problems, as are osteoporosis, gastrointestinal bleeding, and emotional disturbances.

Azathioprine (Imuran) has been in use as an immunosuppressant for more than 25 years and continues to be a component of many regimens. Azathioprine inhibits both cell-mediated and antibody-mediated immunity, although its activity is more specific for T cells than B cells. Because it is rapidly metabolized by the liver, azathioprine can be given to clients with impaired renal function but may not be effective in clients with impaired hepatic function. Bone marrow suppression is the most common adverse effect of this drug, necessitating frequent evaluation of the CBC. Hepatotoxicity, pancreatitis, and increased risk of neoplasm are also associated with azathioprine administration. Nursing responsibilities related to azathioprine are included in the box below. Clients who cannot tolerate azathioprine may receive a newer immunosuppressant, mycophenolate mofetil (CellCept). Primarily, it is prescribed following renal and cardiac transplants.

Medication Administration

Immunosuppressive Agents

CYTOTOXIC AGENTS
- Azathioprine (Imuran)
- Cyclophosphamide (Cytoxan)
- Mycophenolate (CellCept)
- Cyclosporine (Sandimmune, Neoral)

Certain drugs that are identified as cytotoxic or antineoplastic agents are effective as immunosuppressive agents. They act by decreasing the proliferation of cells within the immune system and are widely used to prevent rejection following a tissue or organ transplant. They are usually administered concurrently with corticosteroid therapy, allowing lower doses of both preparations and resulting in fewer side effects.

Nursing Responsibilities
- Monitor blood count, with particular attention to the WBC and platelet counts. Notify the physician if WBCs fall below 4000 or platelets below 75,000.
- Monitor renal and liver function studies, including creatinine, BUN, creatinine clearance, and liver enzymes. Report abnormal levels to the physician.
- Administer the drug as ordered. Administer oral preparations with food to minimize gastrointestinal effects. Antacids may be ordered.
- Increase fluids to maintain good hydration and urinary output.
- Monitor intake and output.
- Monitor for signs of abnormal bleeding bleeding gums, bruising, petechiae, joint pain, hematuria, and black or tarry stools.
- Use meticulous handwashing and other appropriate measures to protect the client from infection. Assess for signs of infection.
- Pulmonary fibrosis is a potential adverse effect of cyclophosphamides. Therefore, monitor respiratory function using pulmonary function studies and clinical signs of dyspnea or cough.

Client and Family Teaching
- Avoid large crowds and situations where exposure to infection is probable.
- Report signs of infection, such as chills, fever, sore throat, fatigue, or malaise, to the physician.
- Use contraceptive measures to prevent pregnancy while on immunosuppressive therapy; these drugs are teratogenic.
- Avoid the use of aspirin or ibuprofen while taking these drugs. Report any signs of bleeding to the physician.

- With cyclophosphamide, amenorrhea may occur. The menses will resume after the drug is discontinued.
- If taking cyclophosphamide, report difficulty breathing or cough to the physician.

MONOCLONAL ANTIBODY
Muromonab-CD3 or OKT3 (Orthoclone)

This monoclonal antibody against T cells is formed by immunizing a mouse with an antigen to produce a specific antibody. Lymphocytes producing the antibody, OKT3, are cloned, and the antibody is harvested. When injected into humans, OKT3 binds with a surface antigen on T cells, removing them from circulation and inactivating those bound to allograft cells. Due to the high incidence of adverse effects, the first two doses of OKT3 are administered by a physician and the client closely observed for 2 hours following each dose.

Nursing Responsibilities
- Be sure a chest X-ray has been performed within 24 hours preceding initiation of OKT3 therapy and that no congestion is present. The risk of anaphylaxis is greater in the client with fluid overload.
- Premedicate as ordered with hydrocortisone, acetaminophen, and diphenhydramine to reduce potential adverse effects.
- Position a crash cart or code cart with emergency medications in the client's room or in close proximity to it.
- After each of the first two doses, monitor vital signs every 15 minutes for 2 hours, then every 30 minutes for 2 hours.
- After the first two doses, administer a 2.5- to 10-mg dose by intravenous push over 1 to 2 minutes.
- Observe closely for potential adverse effects, including chills and fever; tachycardia; headache and tremor; hypertension or hypotension; nausea, vomiting, and diarrhea; chest pain, dyspnea, and wheezing.
- OKT3 can also cause anaphylaxis; observe for evidence of urticaria, angioedema, laryngeal edema, wheezing, or other signs of anaphylactic reaction.
- Monitor CBC for evidence of leukopenia or pancytopenia.
- Assess for infection. Remember that typical signs of infection, including symptoms such as fever and inflammation, may be masked or reduced by immunosuppressive therapy.

Cyclosporine has contributed significantly to the success of organ transplantation since its introduction in the 1970s. Cyclosporine inhibits T-cell function and the normal cell-mediated immune response. The incidence of cyclosporine toxicity and side effects is related to blood levels, so blood levels are monitored closely. Cyclosporine is both nephrotoxic and hepatotoxic, especially at high doses. Observable toxic effects include hypertension and CNS symptoms such as flushing or tingling of the extremities, confusion, visual disturbances, and seizures or coma.

Muromonab-CD3, also known as OKT3 or Orthoclone, is the first monoclonal antibody produced for therapeutic use in humans. As a monoclonal antibody, OKT3 is specific to T cells, blocking their generation and function. It binds with a surface antigen on T cells, inactivating and removing them from circulation. It also blocks killer T cells attached to the graft. Because of significant side effects, the use of OKT3 is limited primarily to treatment of steroid-resistant rejection. Two newer monoclonal antibodies, basiliximab (Simulect) and daclizumab

Medication Administration

Immunosuppressive Agents (continued)

Client and Family Teaching
- Teach about the drug and its purpose.
- Discuss potential adverse and side effects, and emphasize the need to report symptoms promptly.
- Inform the client that adverse effects are most likely to occur following the first two doses, necessitating close observation at that time. Reassure the client that this is standard protocol for this medication.

ANTILYMPHOCYTE GLOBULINS
- Antithymocyte globulin or ATG (ATGAM)
- Antilymphocyte globulin or ALG

These globulins containing antilymphocyte antibodies are produced by immunizing horses (the main source), rabbits, or sheep with human lymphocytes to stimulate production of antibodies (see figure at right). Serum from the animal is then recovered, and the active IgG fraction is isolated, purified, and administered parenterally to the client. It binds with periheral lymphocytes and mononuclear cells, removing them from circulation.

ATG or ALG is used both to induce immunosuppression immediately following a transplant and to treat steroid-resistant rejection episodes. As with monoclonal antibody, multiple side effects are associated with ATG or ALG.

Nursing Responsibilities
- Perform a skin test for sensitivity to horse serum prior to initial dose. Report any positive reaction to the physician and hold administration until desensitization therapy has been completed.
- Premedicate as ordered with acetaminophen and diphenhydramine prior to each dose. Steroids may also be administered before the initial dose. Have epinephrine and hydrocortisone injections available at the bedside in case of anaphylactic reaction.
- Administer by intravenous infusion into a central line over 4 to 6 hours.
- Monitor vital signs hourly while medication is infusing.
- Assess for adverse effects, including chills and fever, erythema, and pruritus. Notify the physician, these may be treated symptomatically.
- Monitor CBC daily, notify the physician if WBC falls to less than 3000/mm^3 or platelet count to less than 100,000/mm^3. The medication may be stopped or reduced.
- Assess renal function studies to monitor for serum sickness. Report complaints of joint pain.
- Monitor for signs of infection, and report any signs promptly.

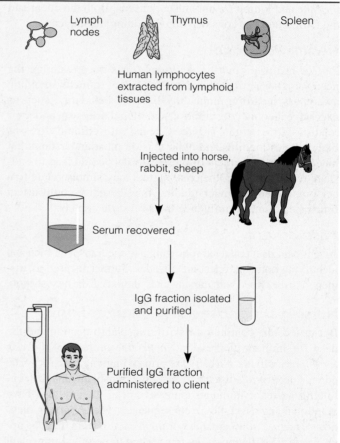

A horse is inoculated with washed human lymphocytes, stimulating the production of immunoglobulin with polyclonal antilymphocyte antibodies. These are then extracted from horse serum, purified, and administered intravenously to the client.

Client and Family Teaching
- Explain the need for special precautions and close monitoring while this drug is being administered.
- Instruct the client to report any adverse effects, including malaise or joint pain, promptly.
- Ask the client to report any evidence of easy bruising, bleeding gums, or black stools.
- Teach family members about the importance of not exposing the client to persons with infectious diseases.

(Zenapax), are a combination of mouse and human antibodies and cause fewer side effects.

Polyclonal antilymphocyte antibodies are also used as adjunctive immunosuppressant therapy. These are administered as antilymphocyte globulin (ALG) or antithymocyte globulin (ATG). These globulins contain antibodies against both T and B cells, as well as other mononuclear leukocytes. When administered, they deplete circulating lymphocytes, platelets, and granulocytes.

NURSING CARE

The client who has an organ or tissue transplant has both immediate and long-term nursing care needs. Both the client and the family must be considered in providing nursing care.

Health Promotion

Part of health promotion activities focus on preventing the need for a tissue transplant. It is important to increase public awareness regarding unhealthy lifestyle behaviors, such as excessive alcohol consumption and illegal drug use, and their relationship to organ failure. Clients with chronic diseases like diabetes mellitus and hypertension must understand that inadequate management of these disorders could lead to end-stage renal disease. Other risk factors may simply relate to a person's heredity; understanding how heredity could affect future health might influence their lifestyle choices.

Assessment

Assessment data collected following a tissue transplant focus on identifying potential rejection episodes. Further focused assessments are described with nursing interventions in the next section.

Nursing Diagnoses and Interventions

Because of the continuing risk of transplant rejection and the need for immunosuppression, *ineffective protection* and *risk for impaired tissue integrity* are priority nursing care foci. The client's underlying disease process, the transplant, and the continuing need for immunosuppressive drug therapy also have emotional and psychologic consequences. Many nursing diagnoses, such as *powerlessness* or *ineffective coping,* may be appropriate. The diagnosis *anxiety* related to potential transplant rejection is considered in this section.

Ineffective Protection

Altered protection is a problem for the transplant client at all stages. Before the transplant occurs, failure of the affected organ may put the client at risk for infection and other multisystemic problems. Incisions and invasive perioperative procedures impair skin and mucous membrane protection from infectious organisms and other antigens. Immunosuppressive drugs given postoperatively to prevent graft rejection disarm the immune response to a certain extent, increasing the risk of infections and neoplastic growths.

- Wash hands on entering room and before providing direct care. *Handwashing removes transient organisms from the skin, reducing the risk of transmission to the client.*

PRACTICE ALERT *Use strict aseptic technique in changing dressings and caring for invasive catheters such as intravenous lines and indwelling urinary catheters to protect against external and resident host microorganisms.* ■

- Assess frequently for signs and symptoms of infection. Monitor the temperature and vital signs every 4 hours. Assess for evidence of inflammation, abnormal wound drainage, changes in urine or other body secretions, complaints of pain, or behavior changes that may indicate infection. Culture abnormal wound drainage. *The client on immunosuppressive therapy is more susceptible to infection, and usual signs and symptoms may not be evident. Both the temperature and inflammatory response can be suppressed by therapy. Prompt identification and intervention for infection is important in the immunosuppressed client.*
- Monitor laboratory values, including CBC and tests of organ function; report changes to the physician. *An elevation in the WBC count with increased numbers of immature cells (bands) or a decline in function of the transplanted organ (e.g., a rising BUN and creatinine in the renal transplant client) may be early indications of infection or transplant failure.*
- Initiate reverse or protective isolation procedures as indicated by the client's immune status. *These procedures further protect the severely immunocompromised client from infection.*
- Instruct ill family members and visitors to avoid contact with the client. *A "minor" upper respiratory infection can be a significant illness in the immunocompromised host.*
- Help ensure adequate nutrient intake, offering supplementary feedings as indicated or maintaining parenteral nutrition if necessary. *Adequate nutrition is important for healing and immune system function.*
- Change intravenous bags and tubing at least every 24 hours, and change peripheral intravenous sites every 48 to 72 hours, unless contraindicated. Remove invasive catheters and lines as soon as they are no longer necessary. *Changing lines and sites is important to reduce bacterial contamination. Fewer invasive lines provide fewer sites for bacterial invasion of the body.*
- Emphasize the importance of washing hands thoroughly after using the bathroom and before eating. *This reduces the risk of infection with endogenous organisms.*
- Provide good mouth care. *Good mouth care reduces the population of oral microorganisms and helps maintain an intact mucous membrane lining.*
- Monitor for potential adverse effects of medications:
  Thrombocytopenia and possible bleeding
  Fluid retention with edema and possible hypertension
  Loss of bone density, osteoporosis, and possible pathologic fractures
  Renal or hepatic toxicity
  Cardiac effects, particularly in the presence of fluid retention and hypervolemia
  Medications used to maintain immunosuppression and preserve the allograft have many potential adverse effects that can alter normal protective and homeostatic mechanisms.

Risk for Impaired Tissue Integrity: Allograft

As noted, the risk for transplant rejection is highest in the initial postoperative period, but it is never completely eliminated for the client who has had an allograft. The client who has had a bone marrow transplant has the additional risk of developing GVHD, which can affect the integrity of skin, mucous membranes, and other organs.

- Administer immunosuppressive therapy as prescribed. *Suppression of the immune response is necessary to reduce the risk of graft destruction by normal immune responses and to preserve its function.*
- Assess for evidence of graft rejection, including tenderness, erythema, and swelling over the site; sudden weight gain, edema, and hypertension; chills and fever; malaise; and an increased WBC count and sedimentation rate. Report any changes immediately. *Early identification of rejection allows adjustment of medication regimens and, possibly, preservation of the graft.*
- Monitor results of laboratory studies for function of the transplanted organ. *With a functional graft, results (e.g., renal or liver function studies) will improve; a functional decline may be an early indicator of rejection.*
- Assess for and report signs of GVHD immediately, including maculopapular rash, erythema of the skin and possible desquamation, hair loss, abdominal cramping and diarrhea, jaundice with elevated bilirubin and liver enzymes (AST, ALT). *GVHD is a potentially lethal complication in the immunosuppressed client and necessitates immediate intervention.*
- Stress the importance of maintaining immunosuppressive therapy and reporting signs of graft rejection promptly to the physician. *Continued immunosuppression and prompt treatment of rejection are vital to preserving graft function.*

Anxiety

The client who undergoes an organ or tissue transplantation often faces the unwelcome choices of death from organ failure or receiving an organ that his or her body will likely attempt to reject. In most cases, the client understands that to receive this transplant, someone else must die and be willing to give up an organ. When the transplant comes from a living donor (bone marrow or kidney), the client may worry not only about himself or herself, but also about the condition of the donor. Fear of rejection and guilt may be even greater in this instance.

- Assess level of anxiety by noting such cues as expressions of apprehension, fear, or inadequacy; facial expression, tension, or shakiness; difficulty focusing; helplessness; poor eye contact; and restlessness. *Clients may have difficulty identifying or verbalizing feelings of fear and anxiety. Nonverbal cues are often useful in recognizing states of anxiety.*
- Provide opportunities to express feelings. Use opening statements such as, "Facing an organ transplant must be very stressful." Listen attentively. *Encouragement and active listening allow the client to express feelings of anxiety or fear.*
- Arrange tasks to allow as much time with the client as possible. When leaving, tell the client when you will return. *Time spent with the client facilitates the development of trust.*
- Provide clear, concise directions. *Highly anxious clients have difficulty focusing and retaining information.*
- Encourage involvement in care but do not request unnecessary decisions. *The client needs to feel a sense of control but may become irritated if asked to make decisions unrelated to the situation.*
- Encourage family members to remain with the client as much as possible. *This can help reduce the client's anxiety.*
- Encourage the use of coping behaviors that have been effective for the client in the past. *Coping mechanisms and behaviors help lower anxiety to a more acceptable level.*
- Reduce or eliminate environmental stressors to the extent possible. *This gives the client a better sense of control.*
- Assist with stress-reduction and relaxation techniques, such as guided imagery, meditation, and muscle relaxation. *These techniques help the client gain control over physical responses to anxiety.*
- Arrange for a counselor or mental health specialist to work with the client. *Counseling can help the client identify and deal with his or her feelings.*

Using NANDA, NIC, and NOC Linkages

Chart 9–2 shows links between NANDA, NIC, and NOC when caring for a client posttransplant.

CHART 9–2 NANDA, NIC, AND NOC LINKAGES

The Client with a Tissue Transplant

NURSING DIAGNOSES	NURSING INTERVENTIONS	NURSING OUTCOMES
• Ineffective Protection	• Infection Protection	• Immune Status
		• Infection Status
• Disturbed Body Image	• Body Image Enhancement	• Self-Esteem
		• Psychosocial Adjustment: Life Change
• Anxiety	• Anxiety Reduction	• Anxiety Control
		• Coping
• Ineffective Health Maintenance	• Health Education	• Health-Promoting Behavior
	• Teaching: Individual	• Health-Seeking Behavior

Note. Data from Nursing Outcomes Classification (NOC) by M. Johnson & M. Maas (Eds.), 1997, St. Louis: Mosby; Nursing Diagnoses: Definitions & Classification 2001–2002 by North American Nursing Diagnosis Association, 2001, Philadelphia: NANDA; Nursing Interventions Classification (NIC) by J.C. McCloskey & G. M. Bulechek (Eds.), 2000, St. Louis: Mosby. Reprinted by permission.

Home Care

Teaching of the client and family regarding an organ or tissue transplant begins well before the transplant and continues throughout hospitalization and follow-up treatment.

Initial teaching focuses on the options, risks, and potential benefits of the transplant itself. Include the procedure by which the organ is selected and obtained, as well as the procedure by which it is transplanted into the client. If a living related donor is an option, discuss the risks and benefits for both the client and the donor. Outline the posttransplant treatment regimen, including any lifestyle changes that may be necessary.

Following the transplant, provide verbal and written instructions, including the following:

- Manifestations of transplant rejection and the importance of notifying the physician
- Immunosuppressive drug regimen and side effects
- Wound care
- Avoiding exposure to infectious diseases, particularly respiratory infections, and wearing a mask when going outside
- Meticulous personal hygiene, handwashing technique, and frequent mouth care
- Wearing a medical alert bracelet or tag
- Follow-up visits to the physician or clinic
- Helpful resources:
  - American Council on Transplantation
  - Local and state support groups related to specific organ transplant, such as the National Kidney Foundation

IMPAIRED IMMUNE RESPONSES

Disorders of impaired immune system responses may be either congenital or acquired. Often the function of either T or B cells is impaired, reducing the body's ability to defend against foreign antigens or abnormal host tissue.

No matter what the cause, clients with immunodeficiency disorders demonstrate an unusual susceptibility to infection. When the antibody-mediated response is primarily affected, the client is at particular risk for severe and chronic bacterial infections. These clients also do not develop long-lasting immunity to such diseases as chickenpox and are prone to recurrent cases. Clients with a defect of cell-mediated immunity tend to develop disseminated viral infections such as herpes simplex and CMV. Candidiasis and other fungal infections are also common. Because T cells are involved with activating antibody-mediated immune responses as well, overwhelming bacterial infections may occur. Immunodeficiency in its most severe form occurs when both antibody-mediated and cell-mediated responses are impaired. Clients with combined immunodeficiency are susceptible to all varieties of infectious organisms, including those not normally considered to be pathogens.

Most immunodeficiency diseases are genetically determined and rare. They affect children more than adults. The noted exception is AIDS, an infectious disease caused by a virus.

THE CLIENT WITH HIV INFECTION

In 1981, five cases of *Pneumocystis carinii* pneumonia (PCP) and 26 cases of a rare cancer, Kaposi's sarcoma, were diagnosed in young, previously healthy homosexual males in Los Angeles and New York City. The term **acquired immunodeficiency syndrome (AIDS)** was ascribed to this new phenomenon to describe the immune system deficits associated with these opportunistic disorders. Prior to this time, both PCP and Kaposi's had been seen only in elderly, debilitated, or severely immunodeficient people. Other groups at risk for

AIDS were soon identified: injection drug users, persons with hemophilia, recipients of blood transfusions, and immigrants from Haiti.

Research to identify the cause of this apparently new disease progressed feverishly, and in 1983, a common antibody was identified in clients with AIDS. The **human immunodeficiency virus (HIV)** was isolated in 1984. It then became apparent that AIDS was the final, fatal stage of HIV infection.

> It began, like so many epidemics, with a few isolated cases, a whisper that caught the ear of only a few in medical research. Today, that whisper has become a roar heard around the world. AIDS—acquired immunodeficiency syndrome—is now the epidemic of our generation, invading our lives in ways we never imagined—testing our scientific knowledge, probing our private values, and sapping our strength. AIDS no longer attracts our attention—it commands it. (Novello, 1993)

INCIDENCE AND PREVALENCE

As of December 2000, the CDC estimated that 800,000 to 900,000 persons in the United States were infected with HIV, with AIDS as the fifth leading cause of death among adults age 25 to 44. As many as one-third of those infected are unaware of their HIV infection. By the end of June 2000, a cumulative total of 753,907 cases of AIDS had been reported. By 1999, death rates among people with AIDS had decreased (Bihari, Levin, Malebranche, & Valdez, 2000), the result of a slowing of the epidemic and improved treatments.

Among men with new HIV infection, 60% were men who have sex with men, 25% were those injecting drugs, and 15% were people having heterosexual contact (primarily with injecting drug users). The majority (75%) of women were infected through heterosexual contact, with the remaining 25% through injection drug use. Among risk groups, the most rapid increases are noted in young gay and bisexual men, women, and inner-city intravenous drug users, especially African Americans and Hispanics (Bihari et al., 2000). In the United States, the reported rate of adult/adolescent AIDS cases (per 100,000 population) reported was 84.2 among African Americans, 34.6 among Hispanics, 11.3 among American Indians/Alaska Natives, 9.0 among whites, and 4.3 among Asians/Pacific Islanders (National Institute of Allergy and Infectious Diseases [NIAID], 2001). The rapid increase of AIDS cases among women is of special concern; those numbers increased from 7% of cases in 1985 to 23% of newly reported cases in 2000 (NIAID, 2000).

In addition, AIDS in the adult over age 50 accounts for 10% of all reported cases in the United States. Declining immune system function in older adults significantly increases their risk for contracting HIV/AIDS, along with the belief that they cannot be affected by it. Just as younger persons with HIV/AIDS contract the diseases primarily through sexual intercourse, so does the elderly population. Because older adults are beyond childbearing years, they often fail to use condoms when engaging in sexual activity. Manifestations may be overlooked by health care professionals, leading to a delayed diagnosis and increased severity of the disease.

There are an estimated 36.2 million people infected with AIDS worldwide, with virtually every country in the world reporting cases of AIDS (Joint United Nations Programme on HIV/AIDS [UNAIDS], 2000). The highest incidence is found in sub-Saharan Africa, South and Southeast Asia, the United States, western Europe, South America, and Canada. Approximately 70% of all people infected with HIV or who have AIDS live in sub-Saharan Africa, and another 16% live in South and Southeast Asia, especially in Thailand and India. The most common mode of transmission is heterosexual intercourse. The cofactors of general health status, the presence of genital ulcers, and the number of sexual partners correlate with incidence (Tierney et al., 2001).

HIV is a retrovirus transmitted by direct contact with infected blood and body fluids. Significant concentrations of the virus are present in blood, semen, vaginal and cervical secretions, and cerebrospinal fluid (CSF) of infected individuals. It is also found in breast milk and saliva. Sexual contact is the primary mode of transmission. HIV is also transmitted through contact with infected blood via needle sharing during injection drug use or by transfusion. Approximately 15% to 30% of infants born to HIV-positive mothers are infected perinatally.

The risk factors for HIV infection are behavioral. Among adults in the United States, 60% of reported cases are in men who have sex with other men, including homosexuals, bisexuals, and such groups as prison populations. Unprotected anal intercourse is the major route of transmission in this group. Injection drug use is the second leading risk factor, accounting for approximately 25% of cases. Sharing of needles and other drug paraphernalia is the primary route of transmission in this group. Heterosexual intercourse with an infected drug user and exchanging sex for drugs are major risk factors for women. Hemophiliacs who require large amounts of intravenous clotting factors and people infected through blood transfusion account for a small number of cases, approximately 2% to 3%.

Among the general population of the United States, the prevalence of HIV infection is very low. Less than 0.04% of people voluntarily donating blood (a process that generally excludes people with high-risk behavior) are found to be HIV positive. HIV is not transmitted by casual contact, nor is there any evidence of its transmission by vectors such as mosquitoes. Blood donation also poses no risk of contracting HIV to the donor, because only new sterile equipment is used. A small but real occupational risk exists for health care workers. Percutaneous exposure to infected blood or body fluids through a needle-stick injury or nonintact skin is the primary route of transmission. Documented evidence indicates that parenteral exposure poses a 0.3% risk of becoming HIV positive (Carrico, 2001). Mucosal exposures, such as splashing in the eyes or mouth, pose a much smaller risk.

PATHOPHYSIOLOGY AND MANIFESTATIONS

HIV is a retrovirus, meaning it carries its genetic information in RNA. On entry into the body, the virus infects cells which have the CD4 antigen. Once inside the cell, the virus sheds its protein coat and uses an enzyme called *reverse transcriptase* to convert the RNA to DNA (Figure 9–6 ■). This viral DNA is then integrated into host cell DNA and duplicated during normal processes of cell division. Within the cell, the virus may remain latent or become activated to produce new RNA and to form virions. The virus then buds from the cell surface, disrupting its cell membrane and leading to destruction of the host cell.

Although the virus may remain inactive in infected cells for years, antibodies are produced to its proteins, a process known as **seroconversion.** These antibodies are usually detectable 6 weeks to 6 months after the initial infection. Helper T or CD4 cells are the primary cells infected by HIV. It also infects macrophages and certain cells of the CNS. Helper T cells play a vital role in normal immune system function, recognizing foreign antigens and infected cells and activating antibody-producing B cells. They also direct cell-mediated immune activity and influence the phagocytic activity of monocytes and macrophages. The loss of these helper T cells leads to the immunodeficiencies seen with HIV infection (Porth, 2002). Figure 9–7 ■ illustrates the typical course of HIV infection.

Pathologic changes are also noted in the CNS of many infected individuals. Although the mechanism of neurologic dysfunction is unclear, neurologic manifestations of HIV infection may be seen in clients who have no apparent immune deficiency (Porth, 2002; Tierney et al., 2001). The clinical manifestations of HIV infection range from no symptoms to severe immunodeficiency with multiple opportunistic infections and cancers (see the Manifestations box on page 255). It appears that the majority of clients develop an acute mononucleosis-type illness within days to weeks after contracting the virus. Typical manifestations include fever, sore throat, arthralgias and myalgias, headache, rash, and lymphadenopathy. The client may also experience nausea, vomiting, and abdominal cramping. The client often attributes this initial manifestation of HIV infection to a common viral illness such as influenza, upper respiratory infection, or stomach virus.

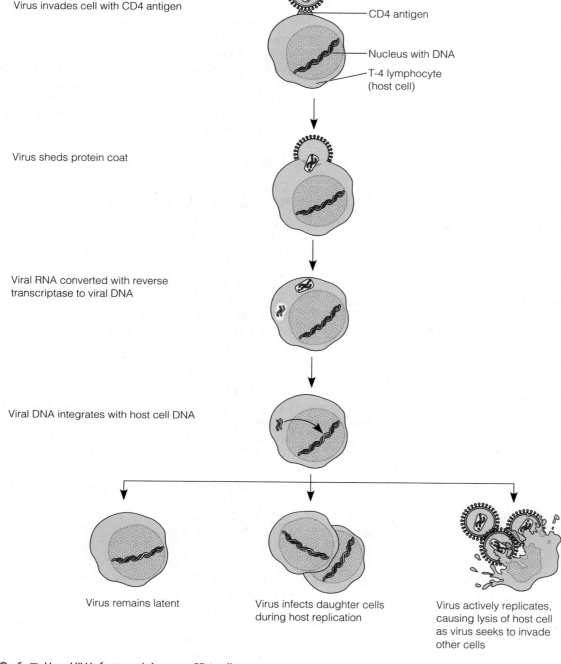

Virus invades cell with CD4 antigen

HIV

CD4 antigen

Nucleus with DNA

T-4 lymphocyte (host cell)

Virus sheds protein coat

Viral RNA converted with reverse transcriptase to viral DNA

Viral DNA integrates with host cell DNA

Virus remains latent

Virus infects daughter cells during host replication

Virus actively replicates, causing lysis of host cell as virus seeks to invade other cells

Figure 9–6 ■ How HIV infects and destroys CD4 cells.

Following this acute illness, clients enter a long-lasting asymptomatic period. Although the virus is present and can be transmitted to others, the infected host has few or no symptoms. Clearly, the majority of HIV-infected persons are in this stage of the disease. The length of the asymptomatic period varies widely, but its mean length is estimated to be 8 to 10 years.

Some clients with few other symptoms develop persistent generalized lymphadenopathy. This is defined as enlargement of two or more lymph nodes outside the inguinal chain with no other illness or condition to account for the lymphadenopathy.

The move from asymptomatic disease or persistent lymphadenopathy to AIDS is often not clearly defined. The client may complain of general malaise, fever, fatigue, night sweats, and involuntary weight loss. Persistent skin dryness and rash may be a problem. Diarrhea is common, as are oral lesions such as hairy leukoplakia, candidiasis, and gingival inflammation and ulceration.

With the development of significant constitutional disease, neurologic manifestations, or opportunistic infections or cancers, the client has manifestations that are characteristic of

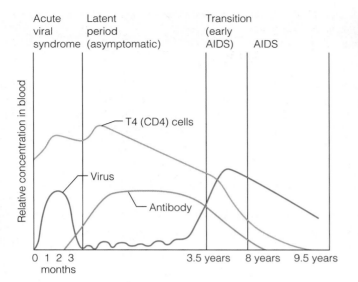

Figure 9–7 ■ The progression of HIV infection. Acute illness develops shortly after the virus is contracted, corresponding with a rapid rise in viral levels. Antibodies are formed and remain present throughout the course of infection. Late in the disease, viral activation results in a marked increase in virus while CD4 (T4) cells diminish as they are destroyed with viral replication. Antibody levels gradually decrease as immune function is impaired.

AIDS and a very poor prognosis. HIV infection and AIDS may be classified by using the CDC's matrix classification system. Under this system, HIV disease is determined by the presence of clinical symptoms (clinical categories A, B, and C) and by T4 cell counts (categories 1, 2, and 3) (see Box 9–2).

When clinical manifestations develop, the outcome varies. With improvements in therapy, many clients are living longer after being diagnosed with AIDS. For example, in San Francisco, mean survival after a first bout with PCP is 18 to 24 months. The time of survival has increased from about 12 months at the start of the epidemic; however, survival after diagnosis of HIV-related lymphomas still averages less than 8 months.

AIDS Dementia Complex and Neurologic Effects

Neurologic manifestations of HIV are common, affecting 40% to 60% of clients with AIDS. They result from both the direct effects of the virus on the nervous system and opportunistic infections.

AIDS dementia complex is the most common cause of mental status changes for clients with HIV infection. This dementia results from a direct effect of the virus on the brain and affects cognitive, motor, and behavioral functioning. Fluctuating memory loss, confusion, difficulty concentrating, lethargy, and diminished motor speed are typical manifestations of AIDS dementia complex. Clients become apathetic, losing interest in work and social and recreational activities. As the complex progresses, the client develops severe dementia with motor disturbances such as ataxia, tremor, spasticity, incontinence, and paraplegia (Porth, 2002; Braunwald et al., 2001).

Manifestations of HIV Infection and AIDS

I. Acute Retroviral Syndrome (ARS) or Primary HIV Infection
   • Fever
   • Sore throat
   • Arthralgias and myalgias
   • Headache
   • Rash
   • Nausea, vomiting, and abdominal cramping
II. Asymptomatic Infection
   • None; converts to seropositive status
III. Persistent Generalized Lymphadenopathy
   • Enlargement of two or more extrainguinal sites for more than 3 months
IV. Other Acute Disease Symptoms
   • General malaise, fatigue
   • Low grade fever
   • Night sweats
   • Involuntary weight loss
   • Skin dryness, or rashes
V. Other Diseases and AIDS
   A. *AIDS Dementia Complex*
   B. *Secondary Infectious Diseases*
      • *Pneumocystis carinii* pneumonia
      • *Mycobacterium* tuberculosis
      • *Mycobacterium avium* complex
      • Candidiasis
      • Cryptosporidiosis
      • Cryptococcosis
      • Toxoplasmosis
      • Herpes simplex or herpes zoster
      • Cytomegalovirus
   C. *Secondary Cancers*
      • Kaposi's sarcoma
      • Non-Hodgkin's lymphoma
      • Cervical dysplasia and cervical cancer
   D. *Other Conditions*
      • Pelvic inflammatory disease
      • Human papillomavirus

Infections and lesions common with AIDS may also affect the CNS. Toxoplasmosis and non-Hodgkin's lymphoma are space-occupying lesions that may cause headache, altered mental status, and neurologic deficits. Cryptococcal meningitis and CMV infection also are common in people with AIDS.

Peripheral nervous system manifestations are also common in HIV-infected clients. Sensory neuropathies with manifestations of numbness, tingling, and pain in the lower extremities affect about 30% of clients with AIDS. A Guillain-Barré type of inflammatory demyelinating polyneuropathy can also occur, resulting in progressive weakness and paralysis.

Opportunistic Infections

Opportunistic infections are the most common manifestations of AIDS, often occurring simultaneously. The risk of opportunistic infections is predictable by the T4 or CD4 cell count. The normal CD4 cell count is greater than $1000/mm^3$. When the CD4 count falls to less than $500/mm^3$, manifestations of

BOX 9–2 ■ Classification System for HIV Infection and Expanded AIDS Surveillance Case Definition for Adolescents and Adults

	Diagnostic Categories		Clinical Categories	
CD4 + T-cell Categories	A Asymptomatic, Acute (Primary) HIV or PGL		B Symptomatic, Not (A) or (C) Conditions	C AIDS-Indicator Conditions
(1) ≥500/mm³	A1		B1	C1
(2) 200–499/mm³	A2		B2	C2
(3) <200/mm³	A3		B3	C3

As of January 1, 1993, people with AIDS-indicator conditions (clinical category C) and those in categories A3 or B3 were considered to have AIDS.

CLINICAL CATEGORY A
One or more of the following conditions in an adolescent or adult with documented HIV infection and without conditions in categories B and C:

- Asymptomatic HIV infection
- Persistent generalized lymphadenopathy
- Acute HIV infection with accompanying illness or history of acute HIV infection

CLINICAL CATEGORY B
Examples of conditions but are not limited to:

- Candidiasis, oral (thrush), or vulvovaginal (persistent, frequent, or poorly responsive to therapy)
- Cervical dysplasia / cervical carcinoma in situ
- Constitutional symptoms, such as fever (38.5°C) or diarrhea exceeding 1 month duration
- Hairy leukoplakia
- Herpes zoster involving at least two distinct episodes
- Pelvic inflammatory disease
- Peripheral neuropathy

CLINICAL CATEGORY C
- Candidiasis of bronchi, trachea, or lungs; esophagus
- Coccidioidomycosis
- Cryptococcosis
- Cryptosporidiosis with persistant diarrhea
- Cytomegalovirus infection (other than of liver, spleen, or lymph nodes)
- CMV retinitis
- HIV encephalopathy
- Herpes simplex: chronic ulcers or bronchitis, pneumonitis, or esophagitis
- *Mycobacterium avium* complex or disseminated
- *Mycobacterium* tuberculosis
- *Pneumocystis carinii* pneumonia
- Progressive multifocal leukoencephalopathy
- *Salmonella* septicemia
- Toxoplasmosis of the brain
- Kaposi's sarcoma
- Cervical cancer, invasive
- Lymphoma
- HIV wasting syndrome

Note. Adapted from "Revised Classification System for HIV Infection and Expanded Case Definition for AIDS Among Adolescents and Adults," 1993, MMWR, CDC Recommendations and Reports, 41(RR 17), pp. 1–19.

immunodeficiency are seen. With a count of less than 200/mm³, opportunistic infections and cancers are likely.

Pneumocystis Carinii Pneumonia
Pneumocystis carinii pneumonia (PCP) is the most common opportunistic infection affecting clients with AIDS. Approximately 75% to 80% of clients develop PCP at some point in their disease (Tierney et al., 2001). It tends to be recurrent, and is the cause of death in about 20% of clients with AIDS. PCP is caused by a common environmental fungus that is not pathogenic in clients with intact immune systems.

Unlike many pneumonias, the manifestations of PCP are nonspecific and may progress insidiously. Clients often present with fever, cough, shortness of breath, tachypnea, and tachycardia. Complaints of mild chest pain and sputum may also be present. Breath sounds may initially be normal. With severe disease, the client may present with cyanosis and significant respiratory distress.

Tuberculosis
An estimated 4% of clients with AIDS develop tuberculosis, contributing significantly to the rise in incidence of this disease in the United States. In some clients, active tuberculosis results from reactivation of a prior infection. In other clients, it is a new, primary disease facilitated by impaired immune function. Rapid progression, diffuse pulmonary infiltrates, and disseminated disease occur more commonly in clients with AIDS. Multidrug-resistant strains of tuberculosis present a significant problem (Tierney et al., 2001).

Clients with pulmonary tuberculosis present with a cough productive of purulent sputum, fever, fatigue, weight loss, and lymphadenopathy. Disseminated disease affects the bone marrow, bone, joints, liver, spleen, CSF, skin, kidneys, gastrointestinal tract, lymph nodes, brain, and other sites.

Candidiasis
Candida albicans infection is a common opportunistic infection in clients with AIDS. It is usually manifested as oral thrush or esophagitis. In women, vaginal candidiasis is frequent and often recurrent. Oral thrush presents as white, friable plaques on the buccal mucosa or tongue and, in the HIV-infected client, is often the first indication of progression to AIDS. Clients with esophagitis have difficulty swallowing and substernal pain or burning which increases with swallowing.

Figure 9–8 ■ Wasting syndrome in a client with AIDS.

Figure 9–9 ■ Kaposi's sarcoma lesions.

Source: Zeva Oelbaum/Peter Arnold, Inc.

Mycobacterium Avium Complex

Mycobacterium avium complex (MAC) affects up to 25% of clients with AIDS, typically occurring late in the course of the disease when CD4 cell counts are less than $50/mm^3$. MAC is more common in women than men. MAC is caused by organisms commonly found in food, water, and soil. It is a major cause of "wasting syndrome" in persons with AIDS (Figure 9–8 ■). Manifestations of MAC include chills and fever, weakness, night sweats, abdominal pain and diarrhea, and weight loss. Nearly every organ can be infected, and most people with MAC develop disseminated disease.

Other Infections

Herpes virus infections are common in clients with AIDS and may be severe. CMV can affect the retina, the gastrointestinal tract, or lungs. Disseminated herpes simplex or herpes zoster may occur, although severe mucocutaneous manifestations are more common.

Parasitic infections with *Toxoplasma gondii* and *Cryptococcus neoformans* commonly affect the CNS. Toxoplasmosis occurs as encephalitis or an intracerebral mass lesion. Changes in mental status, focal neurologic signs, and seizures may result. *Cryptococcus* infection may present as either meningitis or disseminated disease, primarily affecting the lungs. *Cryptosporidium,* a protozoon affecting the gastrointestinal tract, is an important cause of prolonged diarrhea in AIDS clients. Bacterial salmonella infections are also a relatively common cause of diarrhea.

Women with AIDS have a high incidence of pelvic inflammatory disease (PID). Although the pathogens appear to be the same as those in PID affecting non-HIV-infected women, the disease is more severe. Inpatient treatment with intravenous antibiotics is often necessary.

Secondary Cancers

As cell-mediated immune function declines, the risk of malignancy increases. The CDC classification of AIDS currently includes four cancers: Kaposi's sarcoma, non-Hodgkin's lymphoma, primary lymphoma of the brain, and invasive cervical carcinoma.

Kaposi's Sarcoma

Kaposi's sarcoma (KS) is often the presenting symptom of AIDS. It remains the most common cancer associated with the disease. KS affects homosexual males with AIDS predominantly, occurring much less commonly in injection drug users and heterosexuals. At this time, the reason for the discrepancy is unknown.

A tumor of the endothelial cells lining small blood vessels, KS presents as vascular macules, papules, or violet lesions affecting the skin and viscera (Figure 9–9 ■). The face is a common site for skin lesions, especially the tip of the nose and pinnae of the ears. Common sites for visceral disease include the gastrointestinal tract, lungs, and lymphatic system.

The lesions of KS are usually painless initially, but may become painful as the disease progresses. Internally, the tumors may obstruct organ function or cause bleeding. When the lungs are involved, gas exchange may be severely impaired, resulting in pulmonary hemorrhage. This disease may progress slowly or rapidly. KS is an indicator of late-stage HIV disease, with an average survival time of 18 months after diagnosis.

Lymphomas

Lymphomas are malignancies of the lymphoid tissue, including lymphocytes, lymph nodes, and the lymphoid organs such as the spleen and bone marrow. In AIDS, two lymphomas are common, non-Hodgkin's lymphoma and primary lymphoma of the brain. Hodgkin's disease also occurs 5 times more frequently in clients with HIV infection. The CNS is the usual site for these lymphomas, although they may be found in the bone marrow, gastrointestinal tract, liver, skin, and mucous membranes. They are aggressive tumors, growing and spreading rapidly. Headache and changes in mental status are common early symptoms of lymphomas affecting the CNS.

Cervical Cancer

Of women with HIV infection, 40% have cervical dysplasia. Cervical cancer develops frequently and tends to be aggressive. Women with concurrent HIV infection and cervical cancer usually die of the cervical cancer, not AIDS. Because of this, it is recommended that women with HIV infection have Papanicolaou

(Pap) smears every 6 months and aggressive treatment of cervical dysplasia with colposcopic examination and cone biopsy.

COLLABORATIVE CARE

Although multiple research studies to identify a cure for HIV infection and AIDS are underway, no cure is currently available. This fact, plus the apparent universally fatal nature of the disease, make prevention a vital strategy in HIV care. New treatments are under investigation (see Box 9–3 below).

The goals of care for the client with HIV disease are as follows:

- Early identification of the infection
- Promoting health-maintenance activities to prolong the asymptomatic period as long as possible
- Prevention of opportunistic infections
- Treatment of disease complications, such as cancers
- Providing emotional and psychosocial support

Diagnostic Tests

Diagnostic testing is used to screen and identify the infection, as well as to monitor the client's disease and immune status. The following diagnostic tests may be ordered.

- *Enzyme-linked immunosorbent assay (ELISA)* is the most widely used screening test for HIV infection. The ELISA test was developed in 1985 to screen blood donors. ELISA tests for HIV antibodies; it does not detect the virus. Therefore, a client may have a negative ELISA test early in the course of infection, before detectable antibodies have developed. The test has a 99.5% or higher sensitivity when performed at least 12 weeks after infection. This means that more than 99.5% of tests performed on blood containing HIV antibodies will show a positive result. False positives can occur; therefore, an initial positive result is always tested repeatedly and confirmed using a different method of antibody detection, usually the Western blot.

- *Western blot antibody testing* is more reliable but more time consuming and more expensive than ELISA. When combined with ELISA, however, a specificity of greater than 99.9% is achieved. Specificity is a measure of the probability that a negative test result indicates that no antibodies are present. In this test, the client's serum is mixed with HIV proteins to detect reaction. If antibodies to HIV are present, a detectable antigen-antibody response will occur.

- *HIV viral load tests* measure the amount of actively replicating HIV. Levels correlate with disease progression and response to antiretroviral medications. Levels greater than 5000 to 10,000 copies/mL indicate the need for treatment.

- *CBC* is performed to detect anemia, leukopenia, and thrombocytopenia, which are often present in HIV infection. Lymphopenia (or low levels of lymphocytes) is especially common in this disease.

- *CD4 cell count* is the most widely used test to monitor the progress of the disease and guide therapy. The CD4 cell count correlates so closely with the immunodeficiency disorders seen in AIDS. AIDS is now defined not only by the presence of opportunistic infections and other diseases indicative of immunodeficiency, but also by HIV-seropositive status and a CD4 count of less than $200/mm^3$ or a percentage of CD4 lymphocytes of less than 14%. CD4 counts are recommended every 3 to 6 months for all people with HIV disease.

BOX 9–3 ■ Investigational Immune-Based Treatment for HIV

HIV infection progressively alters the function of and destroys CD4+ lymphocytes. CD4+ cells are essential to the function of the immune system, including the body's ability to respond to infections. These cells initiate, direct, and regulate immune responses and may also directly attack infected cells. They also are a source of cytokines, the chemical messengers of the immune system. Destruction of CD4+ cells by HIV devastates the immune system, facilitating the development of fatal infections and neoplasms in the infected person. Immune-based treatments indirectly affect the HIV by improving the function of the immune system through actions that inhibit cytokines, replenish cytokines, or restore immune function. These treatments, used alone or in combination with antiretroviral drugs, are being investigated for use in the treatment of HIV.

INHIBITING CYTOKINES

Tumor necrosis factor alpha (TNF-alpha) is a cytokine secreted by activated monocytes and macrophages in response to infection, infestation, or tumor growth. It causes a proliferation of B cells and T cells. However, high levels of this cytokine may actually facilitate the development of disease by blocking the normal inflammatory response. It is believed that blocking the effect of TNF-alpha can suppress HIV production, although caution must be used.

REPLENISHING CYTOKINES

Some cytokines (interleukin-2 [IL-2], interleukin-12 [IL-12], and interferon alpha [IFN-alpha]) may be helpful in treating HIV by stimulating the production of killer cells as well as increasing the function of lymphocytes. The interferons are part of the body's first line of defense against viruses. All of these agents have toxic side effects, requiring careful nursing assessment and care.

RESTORING IMMUNE SYSTEM FUNCTION

HIV infection not only destroys CD4+ cells, but also eventually destroys the lymphoid organs, such as bone marrow and the thymus gland. Lymphocytes, including the CD4+ cells, are derived from stem cells in bone marrow and mature in the thymus. Two investigational treatments to restore the immune system are bone marrow transplant and thymus transplant. Bone marrow transplants have been used to correct other types of immune disorders (such as leukemia or lymphoma) but have yet to be effective in persons with HIV. A few thymus transplants have been done in HIV-infected persons, but have provided only temporary benefits.

In addition to these widely used tests, several other diagnostic tests may be performed:

- *Blood culture for HIV* provides the most specific diagnosis but is an expensive and cumbersome test that is not widely available in the United States.
- *Immune-complex-dissociated p24 assay* is a test for p24 (HIV) antigen in the blood. This antigen indicates active reproduction of HIV and tends to be positive prior to seroconversion and with advanced disease. It is most useful in monitoring disease progress and the antiviral activity of medications (Tierney et al., 2001).

Other diagnostic tests are used primarily to detect secondary cancers and opportunistic infections in the client with HIV. Tests ordered are both general and specific to the client's manifestations and may include the following:

- *Tuberculin skin testing* to detect possible tuberculosis infection
- *Magnetic resonance imaging (MRI)* of the brain to identify lymphomas
- *Specific cultures and serology examinations for opportunistic infections* such as PCP, toxoplasmosis, and others
- *Pap smears* every 6 months for early detection of cervical cancer in women

Medications

Pharmacologic management of the client with HIV disease has two primary foci: (1) *to suppress the infection itself,* decreasing symptoms and prolonging life, and (2) *to treat opportunistic infections and malignancies.* Effectiveness of treatment is monitored by viral load and CD4 cell counts; positive results are indicated by a reduction in viral load along with preserving the CD4 count above 500 mm^3.

Three classes of drugs used in antiretroviral treatment include nucleoside reverse transcriptase inhibitors (NRTIs), nonnucleoside reverse transcriptase inhibitors (NNRTIs), and protease inhibitors. The new treatment protocol, highly active antiretroviral therapy (HAART), combines three or four antiretroviral drugs to reduce the incidence of drug resistance. However, when clients with AIDS at earlier stages or at lower risk of rapid progression are treated, combination therapies may burden them with complicated and expensive medication schedules and increase the potential of developing drug toxicities and drug resistance (Tierney et al., 2001). Clients beginning the HAART protocol must understand the benefits, risks, costs, and affects on daily life. HAART medications are expensive, costing more than $15,000 per year, and this does not include medications to prevent or treat opportunistic infections or cancer. Medications are scheduled for specific times throughout the day; therefore, leading a normal life becomes a challenge. In addition, all HAART medications cause major adverse reactions. Adherence to the treatment regimen is less than perfect, as with most chronic diseases, but in this case, the outcome could be fatal.

Nucleoside Reverse Transcriptase Inhibitors

The NRTIs (also called nucleoside analogs) inhibit the action of viral reverse transcriptase, a retroviral enzyme that catalyzes the substrates for conversion and copying of viral RNA to DNA sequences. This enzyme is necessary for viral integration into cellular DNA and replication. The nucleoside analogs act as a chemical decoy for building blocks of the formation of the DNA copy, preventing the RNA from being copied into DNA. Each drug substitutes for a particular nucleoside base at different points on the chain. Medication administration guidelines for this group of drugs are discussed in the box below.

Medication Administration

Antiretroviral Nucleoside Analogs

ZIDOVUDINE (AZT, RETROVIR, ZDT)

Zidovudine is the first antiretroviral agent developed to treat HIV infection. It interferes with reverse transcriptase, thus inhibiting replication of the virus. Zidovudine is used for clients with CD4 cell counts of less than 500/µL. The usual dose is 500 to 600 mg per day in divided doses. It is administered orally.

Nursing Responsibilities

- Assess for possible contraindications to therapy including allergic response or a CD4 count of greater than 500/mm^3.
- Administer by mouth, instructing the client to swallow capsules whole.
- Assess for adverse effects. Nausea and headache are common. They may be self-limiting, decreasing with time, or significant and continuing, necessitating a change of therapy. Other adverse effects include insomnia, malaise, and confusion.
- Assess CBC and differential. Notify the physician of significant changes.

Client and Family Teaching

- Zidovudine will not cure HIV infection but slows its progress and reduces significant symptoms.
- Take the drug as prescribed every 4 to 6 hours to maintain an effective blood level.
- Take the drug at least 1/2 hour before or 1 hour after meals if tolerated.
- With this and all antiretroviral drugs, it is important to emphasize that the client is still infective and can pass the infection to others. Use safer sex practices and other measures to prevent transmission to partners. Do not donate blood.
- Notify the physician if signs of an infection or adverse response to zidovudine develop: sore throat, swollen lymph glands, fever; unusual fatigue or weakness; easy bruising, bleeding gums, or an injury that will not heal; persistent or intractable nausea; muscle pain or wasting.
- Continue all scheduled follow-up visits and laboratory studies to monitor for drug toxicity.

(continued on page 260)

Medication Administration

Antiretroviral Nucleoside Analogs (continued)

- Check with the physician before taking any prescription or over-the-counter drug containing aspirin or other NSAID.

DIDANOSINE (DDI, VIDEX)

As with zidovudine, didanosine does not kill HIV but inhibits its replication within the cells. Its activity is similar to that of zidovudine. Didanosine has been shown to increase CD4 cell counts and lower p24 antigen levels (Tierney et al., 2001). Didanosine is used alone for clients who are intolerant or resistant to zidovudine. It is also being used with zidovudine in combination therapy regimens. Didanosine does not cause the anemia associated with zidovudine, but it may cause granulocytopenia. Didanosine is also associated with an increased risk of pancreatitis, peripheral neuritis, and dry mouth.

Nursing Responsibilities

- Assess for possible contraindications to didanosine therapy, including previous episodes of pancreatitis and impaired renal or liver function.
- Administer as directed. Tablets are to be chewed thoroughly or dissolved in 1 ounce of water at room temperature. The powder form is dissolved in water prior to administration.
- Administer with caution to clients taking vincristine, rifampin, pentamidine, ethambutol, or metronidazole; the action of both drugs may be affected by concurrent administration. Intravenous pentamidine and trimethoprim-sulfamethoxazole taken concurrently may increase the risk of acute and fatal pancreatitis.
- Didanosine interferes with the absorption of ketoconazole and dapsone. Doses of these drugs should be scheduled at least 2 hours apart from didanosine doses.
- Evaluate for therapeutic response and possible adverse effects. Notify the physician if manifestations of peripheral neuropathy, diarrhea, depression, or other adverse effects develop.
- Stop the drug and notify the physician immediately if the client develops manifestations of pancreatitis or hepatic failure, including nausea and vomiting, severe abdominal pain, elevated bilirubin, or elevated serum enzymes (e.g., amylase, AST, ALT).

Client and Family Teaching

- Take the drug as directed. The prescribed two-tablet dose must always be taken to get the required amount of antacid to prevent the drug from being destroyed by stomach acid.
- Take on an empty stomach, at least 1 hour before or 2 hours after meals.
- Do not use alcohol while taking didanosine; alcohol may increase the risk of pancreatitis.

- Stop the drug and call the doctor immediately if nausea, vomiting, abdominal pain, or diarrhea develops. These may indicate pancreatitis.
- Call the doctor if extremity pain, weakness, numbness, or tingling occurs. These side effects usually disappear when didanosine is discontinued.
- Other side effects to report to the physician include unusual bleeding or bruising, fatigue, weakness, fever, or persistent sore throat.

ZALCITABINE (DDC, HIVID)

Another inhibitor of retroviral replication, zalcitabine is generally used in combination therapy regimens with zidovudine. It may also be used alone in clients who have become resistant to zidovudine. Unlike zidovudine and didanosine, zalcitabine is not toxic to the bone marrow, is inexpensive, and easy to administer (Tierney et al., 2001). It is, however, associated with severe peripheral neuropathy and an increased risk of pancreatitis. Other adverse effects include stomatitis, rash, fever, and arthritis.

Nursing Responsibilities

- Assess for possible contraindications to zalcitabine: history of pancreatitis or evidence of impaired hepatic function.
- Check with the physician prior to administering the drug concurrently with vincristine, rifampin, intravenous pentamidine, ethambutol, pyrimethamine, dapsone, acyclovir, or metronidazole.
- Administer as prescribed, generally every 8 hours.
- Evaluate for desired effect of increased CD4 counts and lower blood levels of p24 antigen.
- Notify the physician if the client develops evidence of pancreatitis, impaired hepatic function, or painful peripheral neuropathy.

Client and Family Teaching

- Take the medication on an empty stomach, 1 hour before or 2 hours after meals.
- Check with the physican before taking any other prescription or over-the-counter medication.
- Do not consume alcohol while taking this medication; alcohol increases the risk of pancreatitis.
- Notify the physician immediately if symptoms of peripheral neuropathy (see above section on didanosine) or pancreatitis develops.
- Report to the physician signs of infection or changes in condition.

- Zidovudine (Retrovir, AZT) was the first antiretroviral agent approved for use with HIV infection. It remains in widespread use and has been shown to decrease symptoms and prolong the lives of clients with AIDS. Zidovudine is often given to clients with a CD4 cell count of less than 500 because of evidence that it slows the progression to severe disease (Tierney et al., 2001). Zidovudine may also be used prophylactically following a documented parenteral exposure to HIV. AZT is used in combination with ddI, ddC, or 3TC.

- Didanosine (ddI, Videx) also inhibits reverse transcriptase and viral replication. It is used in combination therapy with AZT.
- Zalcitabine (ddC, Hivid) is also a retroviral inhibitor that interferes with the reproduction of HIV. It provides a valuable combination agent with AZT.
- Stavudine (d4T, Zerit) is a retroviral inhibitor that has been shown to increase CD4 cell counts and decrease serum p24 antigen levels. Current use is for clients who are intolerant of AZT.

- Lamivudine (3-TC, Epivir) is used for low CD4 cell counts or symptomatic disease as a first-line treatment in combination with AZT.
- Abacavir (Ziagen) is a potent inhibitor of reverse transcriptase; however, it may cause serious hypersensitivity reactions.
- Zidovudine plus lamivudine (Combivir) is the first combination drug and currently decreases HIV zidovudine-resistant strains.

Protease Inhibitors

Protease is a viral enzyme necessary for the formation of specific viral protein needs for viral assembly and maturation. Protease inhibitors bond chemically with protease to block the function of the enzyme and result in the production of immature, noninfectious viral particles. When combined with other antiviral drugs, these chemicals increase the chance of eliminating the virus by interfering with different stages of its life cycle. However, viral resistance occurs rather quickly.

- Saquinavir (Invirase) is used in combination with nucleoside analogs to treat progression of the disease.
- Ritonavir (Norvir) is used in combination with nucleoside analogs to treat progression of the disease.
- Indinavir (Crixivan) is used in combination with nucleoside analogs to treat progression of the disease.

- Nelfinavir (Viracept) is used in cases of failure of or intolerance to other protease inhibitors.
- Amprenavir (Agenerase) is the newest protease inhibitor.
- Lopinavir/Ritonavir (Kaletra) is the first combination of protease inhibitors active against some HIV strains resistant to other protease inhibitors.

Nonnucleoside Reverse Transcriptase Inhibitors

Nevirapine (Viramune), Delavirdine (Rescriptor), and Efavirenz (Sustiva) are NNRTIs that may be used in combination with nucleoside analogs and protease inhibitors. However, one limitation to NNRTIs is the high incidence of cross-resistance to NRTIs. Some studies have shown that Nevirapine and Efavirenz may significantly reduce serum levels of the protease inhibitors. Optimal combinations of these agents have not been established.

Other agents may also be administered in combination with antiretroviral therapy. Interferons, which are naturally occurring lymphokines, have been used alone and in combination. Alpha-interferon may be used to treat KS and in combination with zidovudine to slow disease progression. Gamma-interferon is also used.

A number of pharmacologic agents are used to prevent and treat opportunistic infections and malignancies in the client with HIV. These agents are outlined in Table 9–4.

TABLE 9–4 Pharmacologic Treatment of Common Opportunistic Infections and Malignancies in HIV Disease

Condition	Treatment	Potential Adverse Effects
Infections		
Pneumocystis carinii pneumonia	Trimethoprim/sulfamethoxazole	Rash, neutropenia, anemia, thrombocytopenia, Stevens-Johnson syndrome
	Pentamidine	Hypotension, altered blood glucose levels, hypocalcemia, anemia and leukopenia, liver and renal toxicity, pancreatitis
Tuberculosis	Combination drug therapy using isoniazid, rifampin, ethambutol, pyrazinamide, or streptomycin	Multiple; see Chapter 36
Candidiasis		
Oral thrush	Clotrimazole troches	Few toxic responses noted for either medication
	Nystatin suspension	
Esophagitis or recurrent vaginitis	Ketoconazole	Hepatitis, adrenal insufficiency
	Fluconazole	Hepatitis
	Amphotericin B	Bone marrow toxicity, acute renal or hepatic failure; nausea, vomiting; chills, fever, headache
Mycobacterium avium complex	Combination therapy using	
	• Clarithromycin, plus	• Hepatitis, nausea, diarrhea
	• Clofazimine	• Diarrhea, nausea, vomiting; skin discoloration, pruritus, rash
	• Ethambutol	• Thrombocytopenia, hepatitis, optic neuritis
	• Rifampin	• Bone marrow depression, renal failure, hepatitis
	• Ciprofloxacin	• Nausea, rash
	• Amikacin	• Bone marrow depression, renal failure, ototoxicity, hepatitis
Cytomegalovirus	Ganciclovir	Bone marrow depression, fever
	Foscarnet	Renal failure, electrolyte imbalances, seizures
Herpes simplex or herpes zoster	Acyclovir	Nausea, vomiting, diarrhea; CNS effects; renal failure
Toxoplasmosis	Pyrimethamine, plus	Bone marrow depression, rash; respiratory failure; nausea, vomiting,
	Sulfadiazine or clindamycin and folinic acid	abdominal pain; hematuria
Malignancies		
Kaposi's sarcoma	Intralesional vinblastine	Inflammation and pain at injection site
Lymphoma	Combination chemotherapy	Nausea, vomiting; bone marrow toxicity; alopecia

Many clients at some point require an implanted venous access device, such as a Groshong catheter, to facilitate blood sampling, intravenous medication administration, transfusions, and parenteral nutrition. See Chapter 10 for nursing care of the client with an intravenous access device implant. ⌘

It is recommended that all HIV-infected clients receive pneumococcal, influenza, hepatitis B, and *Haemophilus influenzae b* vaccines. Persons with a positive PPD and negative chest X-ray are given prophylactic isoniazid (INH). When the client's CD4 cell count falls to less than 200, prophylactic treatment for PCP is begun, usually with trimethoprim-sulfamethoxazole. Clients with a CD4 count of less than 100 are started on prophylactic treatment for MAC.

NURSING CARE

The client with HIV and AIDS has many care needs, including both physical and psychosocial support (see the Nursing Research box below). Because there is as yet no cure or effective treatment for HIV disease, many of these needs fall within the realm of nursing to promote knowledge and understanding, self-care, comfort, and quality of life. As with many diseases that have an ultimately fatal outcome, the course of HIV infection may well be affected by the client's social support systems, control, perceived self-efficacy in management, and coping mechanisms.

As the epidemic spreads, nurses are providing care for increasing numbers of clients with HIV infection. These clients are not only in special care settings, but also on general units, maternal-child units, hospice, and home settings. As clients with HIV disease live longer, nurses will increasingly encounter clients in whom HIV disease is a secondary diagnosis, with another primary diagnosis, for example, heart disease, diabetes mellitus, or an operative procedure.

Prevention

To date, no safe immunization to protect against HIV infection has been developed. Education, counseling, and behavior modification are the primary tools for AIDS prevention. The benefit of education and behavior modification is evident in the homosexual male population. The incidence of new HIV infections in this population has declined dramatically in high-prevalence cities such as San Francisco. Nurses play a vital role in providing education about this epidemic and infection prevention for individuals and communities.

All sexually active individuals need to know how HIV is spread. Following are the only *totally* safe sex practices:

- No sex
- Long-term mutually monogamous sexual relations between two uninfected people
- Mutual masturbation without direct contact

Clients who do engage in sexual activity need to know and practice safer sex (see Box 9–4). Reducing the number of sexual partners—for example, by entering into and remaining in a long-term mutually monogamous relationship with an unin-

Nursing Research

Evidence-Based Practice and Nurses' Willingness to Care for People with AIDS

As reported by the Centers for Disease Control, the number of deaths from AIDS has declined. This is believed to be the result of both the slowing of the epidemic and of improved treatment, which has lengthened the life span of people with AIDS. However, as treatment continues to improve survival, a key challenge will be the increasing number of people living with HIV and AIDS—and the additional resources needed for services, treatment, and care.

Several studies have found that some professional nurses and students are resistant to caring for clients with AIDS. The willingness to provide care for clients with this illness involves moral choices about one's own mortality (death anxiety), spirituality, and social support. Sherman (1996) conducted a descriptive study to examine relationships among these choices and nurses' willingness to care for clients with AIDS. In a survey of 220 registered nurses employed in eight hospitals in the New York Metropolitan area, she found that willingness to care for AIDS patients was positively correlated with spirituality and perceived social support and negatively correlated with death anxiety. It is suggested that nurses' willingness to care for people with AIDS may be related not only to nurses' personal values and beliefs (expressed in spirituality) but also to their professional identity and role expectations.

Implications for Nursing
Standards of professional nursing clearly state that nurses will care for people with AIDS. To increase nurses' willingness to do so, students need to be better socialized into their roles and respon-

sibilities. Discussions within the classroom and clinical settings provide a safe means of bringing fears into the open and sharing experiences, one means of increasing self-awareness and developing a spiritual frame of reference. Student groups can thus serve as support groups, improving communications, decreasing isolation and anxiety, and improving self-esteem and morale. Within the work setting, perceived support from colleagues and administrators as well as increased contact with people with AIDS are important factors in making caring a rewarding and positive experience.

Critical Thinking in Client Care
1. This study was of registered nurses. What differences do you think might have been found if the study had been of student nurses in their first clinical course?
2. Carefully consider each of the following clients with AIDS and write a brief paragraph about how you would feel if you were assigned to care for them:
   a. A heterosexual female, age 25
   b. A homosexual male, age 35
   c. A newborn baby girl
   d. A 40-year-old single mother of three teenagers
   e. A 30-year-old homeless drug user
   f. A 17-year-old male with hemophilia, infected by blood transfusions

BOX 9–4	■ Guidelines for Safer Sex

- Practice mutual monogamy; if you are not in a mutually monogamous relationship, limit the number of sexual partners.
- Do not engage in unprotected sex, especially if HIV status of partner is unknown (remember that a person may be infected and infective for up to 6 months before converting to seropositive status).
- When entering into a new monogamous relationship, both partners should undergo HIV testing initially. If both are negative, practice abstinence or safer sex for 6 months, followed by retesting. If results still indicate that both partners are negative, sexual activity can probably be considered safe.
- Use latex condoms for oral, vaginal, or anal intercourse; avoid natural or animal skin condoms, which allow passage of HIV.
- For vaginal or anal sex, lubricate the condom with the spermicidal agent nonoxynol-9 for additional protection.
- Do not use an oil-based lubricant such as petroleum jelly, which can result in condom damage; water-based lubricants are acceptable.
- Women should carry and use a female condom.

- Remember that use of other means of birth control, such as oral contraceptives, provide no protection against HIV; barrier protection with a condom is necessary.
- Engage in safer sexual practices that are less damaging to sensitive tissues (e.g., mutual masturbation, avoiding anal or oral sex).
- Do not use drugs or alcohol.
- Do not share needles, razors, toothbrushes, sexual toys, or other items that may be contaminated with blood or body fluids.
- If HIV positive:
  a. Do not engage in unprotected sexual activity.
  b. Inform all current and former sexual partners of HIV status.
  c. Inform all health care personnel—primary care providers, physicians and dentists in particular—of HIV status.
  d. Do not donate blood, plasma, blood products, sperm, organs, or tissue.
  e. If female, do not become pregnant.

fected partner—reduces the risk. Clients should not engage in unprotected sex, especially if the HIV status of the partner is unknown. Latex condoms have been shown to reduce the risk of transmitting HIV. Their effectiveness is improved when nonoxynol-9, a spermicide, is used for lubrication; however, it may cause genital ulcers which can facilitate HIV transmission. To be effective, condoms must be used with every sexual encounter involving vaginal, oral, or anal intercourse. They also need to be applied and removed properly. A female condom is also available for use.

The most difficult group of high-risk people to reach and educate has been injection drug users. People in this group should never share needles, syringes, or other drug paraphernalia. Many cities have initiated needle-exchange programs, providing a sterile needle and syringe in exchange for a used one. A fresh solution of household bleach and water in a 1:10 ratio is effective to clean "works" when sterile supplies are not available. It is important to also teach people in this population about safer sex practices, because most heterosexual HIV transmission occurs between injection drug users and their partners.

Screening of voluntary blood donors and donated blood supplies has reduced the risk of transmission by transfusion to 1 in 100,000. Because current blood-screening methods use antibody testing, receiving donated blood continues to carry a small risk. Clients in the *window period* between contraction of the virus and the development of detectable antibodies are able to transmit the virus to others, even though they do not yet test positive for HIV. This window period usually lasts from 6 weeks to 6 months; rarely, it lasts up to 1 year. When possible, encourage clients to use autologous transfusion, donating their own blood prior to an anticipated surgery. Seeking donations from family members is not encouraged for several reasons. Family members may have engaged in high-risk behaviors but lie about their risk because of embarrass-

ment or fear of discovery. Furthermore, the family member may have a different blood type or have other contraindications to donating.

Encourage HIV-positive clients to abstain from donating blood, organs, or sperm. They should understand tactics to avoid exchange of body fluids by not sharing needles or other drug paraphernalia, not sharing razors, and not obtaining a tattoo. Stress the importance of informing all medical personnel providing direct care (especially anyone performing a dental, surgical, or obstetric procedure) about the diagnosis.

Health care workers can prevent most exposures to HIV by using standard precautions (refer to Appendix and see Figure 9–10 ■). Testing to determine HIV status remains voluntary and relies on the use of antibody-screening methods. It is therefore impossible to identify every client who is HIV positive. With standard precautions, all clients are treated alike, eliminating the need to know the client's HIV status. All high-risk body fluids are treated as if they are infectious, and barrier precautions are used to prevent skin, mucous membrane, or percutaneous exposure to them. Counseling and testing are provided to health care workers with a documented needle-stick exposure. Some clinicians and facilities recommend prophylactic AZT therapy after needle-stick or splash exposure; however, it must be initiated immediately, and its effectiveness has yet to be established.

Assessment

Collect the following data through health history and physical examination. Further focused assessments are described with nursing interventions below.

- Health history: risk factors (transfusion, unprotected sex, needle exposure), infections (sexually transmitted diseases, hepatitis, TB), medications, recreational drug use, foreign travel, pets

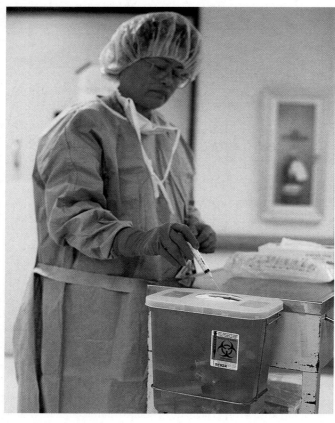

Figure 9–10 ■ This nurse is disposing of a needle and syringe in a special container, a necessary practice to avoid the transmission of HIV through needle sticks with contaminated needles.

- Physical assessment: height, weight, nutrition, skin and mucous membranes, vision, lymph nodes, breath sounds, abdominal tenderness, motor strength, coordination, cranial nerves, gait, deep tendon reflexes, genitourinary examination, mental status

Nursing Diagnoses and Interventions

Nursing care needs for the client with HIV infection change over the course of the disease. Preventive health care measures, health maintenance activities, education, and support of coping mechanisms are important in the early stages of the disease. Counseling the client with a new diagnosis of HIV infection is vital. HIV infection and AIDS continue to carry a social stigma that may interfere with the client's usual support systems and coping mechanisms. As the disease progresses and the client experiences more physical symptoms, direct care needs become more important while the need for psychosocial support continues. Acute exacerbation of opportunistic infections may necessitate hospitalization, but typically the client is managed at home.

Ineffective Coping

On receiving the test results indicating HIV seropositive status, the person with HIV infection is faced with multiple issues rarely affecting other clients. First and foremost, HIV is a disease for which there is no known cure and which is, at this time,

thought to be almost universally fatal. Social support systems, family relationships, and the ability to obtain and retain useful work and health insurance may be disrupted by the disease. The client may experience guilt about his or her lifestyle and how the disease was contracted. As the disease progresses, social isolation, fatigue, body image changes, medication side effects, and multiple other issues affect the client's abilities to cope.

- Assess social support network and usual methods of coping. *This will help both the nurse and the client identify people and mechanisms that can help the client cope more effectively with the disease.*
- If possible, assign a primary nurse, whether the setting is home health, hospice, or acute care. *This helps promote the development of a therapeutic and trusting relationship and provides for continuity of care.*
- Plan for consistent, uninterrupted time with the client. *Time and a consistent presence encourage the client to express feelings and work through issues related to HIV infection.*
- Interact at every opportunity outside of providing specific nursing care treatments. *This purposeful interaction communicates caring and acceptance without fear of HIV disease.*
- Support the client's social network. *Nontraditional families may offer more support than the traditional family. This in turn may necessitate a liberal interpretation of the term* family *if unit policy is* immediate family only.
- Promote interaction between the client, significant others, and family. *Hospitalization and manifestations of HIV disease may bring about isolation from others and decrease the client's ability to cope.*
- Encourage involvement in making care decisions. *This gives the client a greater sense of self-worth and control over the situation, increasing coping abilities.*
- Set and maintain limits on manipulative and other destructive behaviors. *The client who is unable to limit inappropriate behaviors needs the external control established by setting limits.*
- Assist to accept responsibility for actions without blaming others. *Effective coping cannot occur without accepting responsibility for one's actions.*
- Support positive coping behaviors, decisions, actions, and achievements. *As self-esteem is enhanced, coping improves.*

Impaired Skin Integrity

Dryness, malnutrition, immobility from fatigue, and skin lesions on pressure sites contribute to impaired integrity of the skin for the client with HIV disease. Maintaining skin integrity is important because of the progressive and debilitating nature of the disease. It is also a consideration both as the first line of defense against infection in an immunosuppressed client and as a site for secondary manifestations such as KS and herpes.

- Monitor the skin frequently for lesions and areas of breakdown. *Early identification of impaired skin integrity allows prompt intervention.*
- Monitor lesions for signs of infection or impaired healing. *Infection or poor tissue perfusion not only impairs healing but may lead to further skin breakdown.*

- Turn at least every 2 hours, more frequently if necessary. *Turning decreases unrelieved pressure on bony prominences and improves circulation to the tissues.*
- Use pressure-relieving devices, such as pressure and egg crate mattresses, or sheep skin pads for elbows and heels. *These devices provide prophylactic relief of pressure.*
- Keep skin clean and dry using mild, nondrying soaps or oils for cleansing. *Night sweats and diarrhea, if present, can cause breakdown and damage to the skin. Frequent cleansing with nondrying products discourages bacterial growth, thus reducing the risk of infection.*

PRACTICE ALERT *Applying protective creams to reddened areas in the rectal area protects skin from the caustic effects of diarrhea.* ■

- Massage around but not over affected pressure sites to increase circulation to the surrounding tissue. *Massaging over the affected area can cause skin breakdown.*
- If blisters are noted, leave intact, and dress with a hydrocolloid (Duoderm) dressing. *Blisters provide natural sterile coverings for damaged tissue, improving healing and preventing bacterial invasion.*
- Caution against scratching. If confused, trim fingernails and use mitts or soft restraints to prevent scratching. Check for circulation of hands and fingers frequently if mitts or restraints are used. *Scratching and skin damage allow bacteria to be introduced into lesions, increasing the risk of infection. Tight or restrictive restraints or mitts may compromise circulation.*
- Avoid the use of heat or occlusive dressings. *Heat can further dry and damage the skin; occlusive dressings may impair circulation and lead to ulceration.*
- Prevent skin shearing by using a turnsheet and adequate personnel when repositioning. *Shearing causes tissue trauma that can lead to decubitus ulcers.*
- Encourage ambulation if possible; if the client is confined to bed, encourage active or passive range-of-motion exercises. *Activity increases circulation, decreases pressure and skin breakdown, and helps maintain muscle tone.*
- Monitor nutritional intake and albumin levels. *Maintenance of optimal nutrition decreases the risk of tissue breakdown and improves resistance to infection.*

Imbalanced Nutrition: Less Than Body Requirements

Many factors associated with HIV disease, including manifestations of the disease itself, put the client at risk for altered nutrition and weight loss. Nausea and anorexia may be manifestations of the disease or the result of antiretroviral therapy. Chronic diarrhea is a common manifestation of constitutional HIV disease. Wasting syndrome is also common. It is manifested by involuntary weight loss of greater than 10% to 15% of baseline weight, severe diarrhea, fever, and chronic fatigue and weakness. The exact cause of wasting syndrome is unclear, but the diarrhea and fatigue contribute, as does the increased metabolic rate associated with fever. Oral and esophageal candidiasis and KS of the gastrointestinal tract may cause painful

swallowing, making eating difficult and thereby contributing to anorexia. Poor nutritional status in the client with HIV can ultimately result in altered comfort, a change in body image, muscle wasting, increased risk of infection, and higher mortality and morbidity.

- Assess nutritional status, including weight; body mass; caloric intake; and laboratory studies, such as total protein and albumin levels, hemoglobin, and hematocrit. *These factors provide a baseline to determine the effectiveness of interventions.*
- Identify possible causes of altered nutrition. *Identification of causes provides direction for planned interventions.*
- Administer prescribed medications for candidiasis and other manifestations as ordered. *Eliminating this opportunistic infection improves comfort and facilitates food intake. Topical viscous anesthetic can help reduce pain and improve oral intake.*
- Administer antidiarrheal medications after stools and antiemetics prior to meals. Provide antipyretics as needed to control fever. *Reducing diarrhea will improve nutrient absorption; preprandial medication with an antiemetic reduces nausea and improves food intake. Reduction of fever lowers the body's metabolic demands.*

PRACTICE ALERT *High-fiber foods can increase intestinal motility and the incidence of diarrhea.* ■

- Provide a diet high in protein and kilocalories. *A high-protein, high-kilocalorie diet provides the necessary nutrients to meet metabolic and tissue healing needs.*
- Offer soft foods and serve small portions. *Soft foods are easily digested. Small portions are more appealing to the anorectic or nauseated client.*
- Involve in meal planning and encourage significant others to bring favorite foods from home. *The client is more likely to consume adequate amounts of preferred foods. Allowing food choices enhances the client's sense of control.*
- Assist with eating as needed. *Fatigue and weakness can prevent the client from eating an adequate amount of food.*
- Provide supplementary vitamins and enteral feedings, such as Ensure. *This improves nutritional status and caloric intake.*
- Provide or assist with frequent oral hygiene. *Oral hygiene improves comfort and appetite, and reduces the risk of mucosal lesions.*
- Administer appetite stimulants, such as megestrol (Megace) and dronabinol (Marinol) as ordered. *Both drugs may increase appetite and promote weight gain.*

Ineffective Sexuality Patterns

The diagnosis of HIV infection can significantly alter the client's expressions of sexuality. Guilt over the diagnosis may interfere with libido. The client may be angry with a significant other or partner if that person was the probable source of infection. The client may fear spreading the disease to others via sexual relations. As the disease progresses, its manifestations can affect body image and self-esteem, impairing sexuality. Other symptoms, such as nausea, fatigue, and weakness, may also interfere with libido and sexual satisfaction.

- Examine your feelings about sexuality, your role in dealing with a client's sexuality, the client's lifestyle, and sexual preferences. *To deal effectively with the client's concerns, it is vital that the nurse be comfortable with his or her own feelings of sexuality and be able to accept the client's lifestyle. Referring the client to another nurse or counselor may be necessary.*
- Establish a trusting, therapeutic relationship through the use of time, active listening, caring, and self-disclosure. Maintain a nonthreatening, nonjudgmental attitude toward the client. *Sexuality is a private issue that will be uncomfortable or impossible for the nurse and client to discuss without a mutually trusting relationship.*
- Provide factual information about HIV infection and its effects. *This helps the client separate fears and myths from reality.*
- Discuss safer sex practices, including hugging, cuddling, nonsexual contact, the use of latex condoms and spermicidal lubricant, and mutual masturbation. *Alternative forms of sexual activity and expressing affection can allow the client and significant other to remain close throughout the course of the disease.*
- Encourage discussion of fears and concerns with significant other. *Open communication helps them to deal with issues related to sexuality.*
- For the client without a significant other, stress the need to continue to meet people and develop social relationships while practicing safer sex. *The risk of isolation is high in the client with HIV infection, and relationships with others help the client to cope with the disease.*
- Refer the client and significant other to local support groups for people and partners of people with HIV. *Support groups provide a social and support network of people facing the same issues.*

Using NANDA, NIC, and NOC

Chart 9–3 shows links between NANDA, NIC, and NOC when caring for the client with AIDS.

Home Care

Teaching needs for both the client and significant other are extensive. The primary need is information about the disease, its spread, and its expected course. The client and family need current factual information to plan realistically and to combat myths, misperceptions, and prejudices. At the same time, it is important to include information about current research and progress in treating the disease to maintain a sense of hopefulness.

The following topics should be discussed with the client and family to prepare for home care.

- Guidelines for safer sex practices
- Nutrition, rest and exercise, stress reduction, lifestyle changes, and maintaining a positive outlook
- Infection prevention and transmission including handwashing and wearing gloves when handling client's secretions or excretions
- Importance of regular medical follow-up and monitoring of immune status
- Signs and symptoms of opportunistic infections and malignancies, as well as other symptoms that should be reported
- Medications and adverse effects
- Use and care of implanted venous access devices, total parenteral nutrition, intravenous pumps and continuous medication delivery systems, and intravenous or aerosolized medications
- Cessation of smoking, alcohol, and recreational or illicit drug use
- Home health services
- Hospice and respite care services
- Community resources, such as support groups, social agencies, and counselors
- Helpful resources:
  - CDC National AIDS Hotline
  - Gay Men's Health Crisis Network
  - National Association of People with AIDS
  - National Organization for HIV over Fifty

MediaLink | AIDS/HIV RESOURCES

CHART 9–3   NANDA, NIC, AND NOC LINKAGES

The Client with HIV Infection

NURSING DIAGNOSES	NURSING INTERVENTIONS	NURSING OUTCOMES
• Disturbed Body Image • Caregiver Role Strain	• Body Image Enhancement • Caregiver Support	• Self-Esteem • Caregiver Emotional Health • Caregiver Performance: Direct Care
• Diarrhea	• Diarrhea Management	• Electrolyte and Acid-Base Balance • Fluid Balance
• Fatigue	• Energy Management	• Endurance • Nutritional Status: Energy
• Ineffective Airway Clearance • Risk for Disturbed Thought Processes	• Airway Management • Dementia Management	• Respiratory Status: Gas Exchange • Cognitive Orientation

Note. Data from Nursing Outcomes Classification (NOC) by M. Johnson & M. Maas (Eds.), 1997, St. Louis: Mosby; Nursing Diagnoses: Definitions & Classification 2001–2002 by North American Nursing Diagnosis Association, 2001, Philadelphia: NANDA; Nursing Interventions Classification (NIC) by J.C. McCloskey & G. M. Bulechek (Eds.), 2000, St. Louis: Mosby. Reprinted by permission.

Nursing Care Plan
A Client with HIV Infection

Sara Lu is a 26-year-old elementary school teacher who lives with her parents and two younger sisters. Ms. Lu is very close to her parents and sisters; they share everything with each other. During the required physical for admission to graduate school, Ms. Lu tells her physician that lately she has felt fatigued. She also states that she has had a persistent sore throat, intermittent bouts of diarrhea, and mild shortness of breath for about a month. She takes no routine medications other than a daily multivitamin and an occasional acetaminophen tablet for a headache. She is active in a drama club in her community, and she jogs 3 miles three to four times a week. She is engaged to be married; her wedding date is 6 months away. Her fiancé is the only person with whom she has had sexual relations. Her sexual activity has been unprotected. Ms. Lu has a history of open heart surgery 7 years ago to correct a congenital valve defect. She has been physically healthy since that time, until about a month or two ago. The physician orders a mononucleosis test, enzyme-linked immunosorbent assay (ELISA), Western blot analysis, CD4 T-cell count, a p24 antigen test, and an erythrocyte sedimentation rate (ESR). She has been asked to return in 1 week for follow-up.

ASSESSMENT

On Ms. Lu's follow-up visit, Carole Kee, RN, obtains her nursing history. Ms. Lu continues to have flulike symptoms but has improved somewhat. She states that she just has not been as active as usual and is worried about her health. Her appetite has decreased because of soreness in her mouth, and she has noted some whitish patches on her tongue and cheeks.

A chest X-ray film reveals no abnormality. The results of her laboratory tests are as follows:

- ELISA: positive for antibodies against HIV
- Western blot analysis: positive for antibodies against HIV
- p24 antigen test: positive for circulating HIV antigens
- ESR: increased to 25 mm/h (normal for women is 15 to 20 mm/h; normal for men is 10 to 15 mm/h)
- CD4 T-cell count: 599/mm^3 (normal range is 600 to 1200 mm^3)

Ms. Lu's physical examination reveals that she has enlarged lymph nodes in her neck and white patches on her oral mucosa. Her skin is warm to the touch. Her vital signs are as follows: T 99.9°F (37.7°C), P 84, R 20, and BP 120/78.

Ms. Lu is told of the results of her laboratory tests and the medical diagnosis of HIV infection. Ms. Lu is obviously distressed and wants to know how this happened, its meaning, whether she has infected her loved ones, and whether she will get better.

DIAGNOSIS

- *Imbalanced nutrition: Less than body requirements* related to soreness in mouth
- *Risk for deficient fluid volume* related to decreased fluid intake and diarrhea
- *Risk for infection* related to altered immune protection
- *Anxiety* related to diagnosis and fear
- *Deficient knowledge* about the HIV disease process

EXPECTED OUTCOMES

- Maintain adequate nutrition for optimal body and cellular function.

- Consume at least 2500 mL of fluid per day.
- Remain free of infections and their complications.
- Verbalize anxiety and use appropriate coping mechanisms.
- Verbalize and demonstrate knowledge of HIV disease.
- Verbalize measures to prevent HIV transmission to others, including safer sex practices.

PLANNING AND IMPLEMENTATION

- Monitor daily weight and intake and output.
- Monitor dietary habits and serum albumin levels.
- Teach Ms. Lu the importance of consuming a nutritionally balanced diet and maintaining adequate fluid intake.
- Suggest strategies for coping with anorexia and nausea.
- Provide dietary consultation referral.
- Encourage oral care before and after meals.
- Assess bowel sounds and monitor elimination pattern.
- Administer antiemetic and antimotility medications as ordered.
- Monitor for signs of dehydration, such as poor skin turgor, oliguria, and orthostatic hypotension.
- Increase fluid to 2500 mL daily.
- Use strict aseptic technique for all invasive procedures.
- Teach Ms. Lu to avoid exposure to infection and people with known illnesses.
- Administer antiretroviral medications and antibiotics as prescribed, and monitor response.
- Encourage maintenance of regular physical exercise.
- Provide opportunities for Ms. Lu to verbalize her feelings.
- Avoid false reassurances.
- Provide appropriate and adequate information about HIV/AIDS.
- Teach safer sex practices and other measures to prevent HIV transmission.
- Teach anxiety-controlling techniques, such as deep breathing and meditation.

EVALUATION

Ms. Lu is eager to learn about her illness and wants her family to come with her for further explanation. She states that she is sure her fiancé will be available as well. Ms. Lu is taking home antifungal medication, diet plans, and a schedule for increased exercise. She will return in 1 week for counseling and in 1 month for a follow-up physical.

Critical Thinking in the Nursing Process

1. How does age effect the body's response to fighting HIV? What other factors affect the risk of HIV infection and its progression?
2. Are the laboratory results for Ms. Lu a true indication that she is HIV positive? What additional tests might be ordered?
3. What is the most likely source of Ms. Lu's infection? What measures are used to reduce this risk, and how did she contract HIV? What is another possible source of Ms. Lu's HIV infection?
4. Ms. Lu says that her fiancé would like to have a child. How will you counsel her regarding pregnancy and childbearing?

See Evaluating Your Response in Appendix C.

EXPLORE MediaLink

NCLEX review questions, case studies, care plan activities, MediaLink applications, and other interactive resources for this chapter can be found on the Companion Website at www.prenhall.com/lemone.

Click on Chapter 9 to select the activities for this chapter. For animations, video clips, more NCLEX review questions, and an audio glossary, access the Student CD-ROM accompanying this textbook.

TEST YOURSELF

1. Which one of the following conditions is caused by a type I IgE-mediated hypersensitivity reaction?

   a. Autoimmune hemolytic anemia
   b. Systemic lupus erythematosus
   c. Graft rejection
   d. Anaphylaxis

2. A client received a liver transplant 1 day ago. If the client were to develop an acute transplant rejection episode, when should the nurse expect to see the manifestations?

   a. Approximately 4 days to 3 months later
   b. Approximately 2 days later
   c. Within the first 24 hours
   d. Within the first 8 hours

3. The nurse notes a cough, shortness of breath, and tachypnea in a client with AIDS. Which opportunistic infection is probably causing these manifestations?

   a. *Toxoplasma gondii*
   b. *Cytomegalovirus*
   c. *Pneumocystis carinii*
   d. *Cryptococcus neoformans*

4. Which of the following explanations should the nurse give to a client who has tested positive for HIV?

   a. "You have been diagnosed with AIDS."
   b. "At this point, AIDS is not active in your blood."
   c. "This means that you will not develop AIDS in the future."
   d. "Antibodies to the AIDS virus are present in the blood."

5. Clients taking zidovudine (Retrovir) should be monitored for which of the following adverse reactions?

   a. Cardiotoxicity
   b. Leukopenia
   c. Nephrotoxicity
   d. Polycythemia

See Test Yourself answers in Appendix C.

BIBLIOGRAPHY

Abramowicz, M. (Ed.). (2000). *Drugs for HIV infection.* New Rochelle, NY: The Medical Letter, Inc.

Abrams, A. C. (2001). *Clinical drug therapy: Rationales for practice* (6th ed.). Philadelphia: Lippincott.

Ackley, B. J., & Ladwig, G. B. (2002). *Nursing diagnosis handbook* (5th ed.). St. Louis: Mosby.

American Nurses Association. (1997). *Position statement: Needle exchange and HIV.* Washington, DC: ANA.

Bihari, B., Levin, S., Malebranche, D., & Valdez, H. (2000). Caring for diverse populations: Identifying HIV infection. *Patient Care, 34*(9), 55–56, 58, 60–62, 65–66, 68, 73, 76–77.

Braunwald, E., Fauci, A. S., Kasper, D. L., Hauser, S. L., Longo, D. L., & Jameson, J. L. (2001). *Harrison's Principles of internal medicine* (15th ed.). New York: McGraw-Hill.

Bullock, B. A., & Henze, R. L. (2000). *Focus on pathophysiology.* Philadelphia: Lippincott.

Carrico, R.M. (2001). What to do if you're exposed to a bloodborne pathogen. *Home Health-care Nurse, 19*(6), 362–368.

Centers for Disease Control. (1992). 1993 Revised classification system for HIV infection and expanded case definition for AIDS among adolescents and adults. *MMWR, CDC Recommendations and Reports, 41*(RR-17), 1–19.

———. (1996). Update: Provisional public health recommendations for chemoprophylaxis after occupational exposure to HIV. *MMWR, 45,* 468–472.

Cheng, C., & Umland, E.M. (2001). A practical update on antiretroviral therapy. *Patient Care, 35*(10), 99–106.

Chernecky, R., & Berger, B. (1997). *Laboratory tests and diagnostic procedures* (2nd ed.). Philadelphia: Saunders.

Cournoyer, S. (1997). How much do you know about the opportunistic diseases of AIDS? *Nursing97, 27*(6), 1–2, 4, 6.

Early HIV Infection Guideline Panel. (1994). *Evaluation and management of early HIV infection: Clinical practice guidelines* (AHCPR Publication No. 94-0572). Rockville, MD: AHCPR Public Health Service, USDHHS.

Esch, J.F., & Frank, S.V. (2001). HIV drug resistance and nursing practice. *American Journal of Nursing, 101*(6), 30–36.

Fryback, P., & Reinert, B. (1997). Alternative therapies and control for health in cancer and AIDS. *Clinical Nurse Specialist, 11*(2), 64–69.

Joint United Nations Programme on HIV/AIDS. (2000). Men make a difference. Press kit: world AIDS day. HIV/AIDS in Africa. Available http://www.unaids.org/wac/2000/wad00/files/FS_Africa.htm

Kee, J. (1999). *Laboratory & diagnostic tests with nursing implications* (5th ed.). Upper Saddle River, NJ: Prentice Hall.

Kirton, C.A., Ferri, R.S., & Eleftherakis, V. (1999). Primary care and case management of persons with HIV/AIDS. *Nursing Clinics of North America, 34*(1), 71–94.

Johnson, M., Maas, M., & Moorhead, S. (2000). *Iowa outcomes project: Nursing outcomes classification (NOC)* (2nd ed.). Upper Saddle River, NJ: Prentice Hall.

Lueckenotte, A.G. (2000). *Gerontologic nursing* (2nd ed.). St. Louis: Mosby.

Lutz, C., & Przytulski, K. (2001). *Nutrition and diet therapy* (3rd ed.). Philadelphia: F.A. Davis.

Lyon, D.E., & Munro, C. (2001). Disease severity and symptoms of depression in black Americans infected with HIV. *Applied Nursing Research, 14*(1), 3–10.

McCloskey, J.C., & Bulechek, G. M. (2000). *Iowa interventions project: Nursing interventions classifications (NIC)* (3rd ed.). Upper Saddle River, NJ: Prentice Hall.

Muehlbauer, P., & White, R. (1998). Are you prepared for interleukin-2? *RN, 61*(2), 34, 36–38.

National Institute of Allergy and Infectious Diseases. (2000). *HIV infection in women.* Bethesda, MD: National Institutes of Health.

_____ . (2001). HIV/AIDS statistics (fact sheet). Available, http://www.niaid.nih.gov/factsheets/aidstat.htm

National Institute of Occupational Safety and Health. (1997). *Preventing allergic reactions to natural rubber latex in the workplace.* Washington, DC: USDHHS.

Novello, A. (1993, June). *Surgeon General's report to the American public on HIV infection and AIDS—extracts.* Rockville, MD: CDC National AIDS Clearinghouse.

Panel on Clinical Practices for Treatment of HIV Infection. (2000). Guidelines for the use of antiretroviral agents in HIV-infected adults and adolescents. Available http://www.hivatis.org

Porche, D.J. (1999). State of the art: Antiretroviral and prophylactic treatments in HIV/AIDS. *Nursing Clinics of North America, 34*(1), 95–112.

Porth, C. (2002). *Pathophysiology: Concepts of altered health states* (6th ed.). Philadelphia: Lippincott.

Roitt, I. (1994). *Essential immunology* (8th ed.). London: Blackwell.

Shannon, M.T., Wilson, B.A., & Stang, C.L. (2001). *Nursing drug guide 2001.* Upper Saddle River, NJ: Prentice Hall.

Sherman, D. (1996). Nurses' willingness to care for AIDS patients and spirituality, social support, and death anxiety. *Image: Journal of Nursing Scholarship, 28*(3), 205–213.

Sowell, R.L., Moneyham, L., & Aranda-Naranjo, B. (1999). The care of women with AIDS. *Nursing Clinics of North America, 34*(1), 179–199.

Swenson, M.R. (2000). Autoimmunity and immunotherapy. *Journal of Intravenous Nursing, 23*(5S), S8–S13.

Szirony, T.A. (1999). Infection with HIV in the elderly population. *Journal of Gerontological Nursing, 25*(10), 25–31.

Thurlow, K.L. (2001). Latex allergies: Management and clinical responsibilities. *Home Healthcare Nurse, 19*(6), 369–376.

Tierney, L., McPhee, S., & Papadakis, M. (Eds). (2001). *Current medical diagnosis & treatment* (40th ed.). New York: Lange Medical Books/McGrawHill.

Trzcianowska, H., & Mortensen, E. (2001). HIV and AIDS: Separating fact from fiction. *American Journal of Nursing, 101*(6), 53, 55, 57, 59.

Ungvarski, P. (1996). Waging war on HIV wasting. *RN, 59*(2), 26–32.

_____ . (2001). The past 20 years of AIDS. *American Journal of Nursing, 101*(6), 26–29.

Valdez, M.R. (2001). A metaphor for HIV-positive Mexican and Puerto Rican women. *Western Journal of Nursing Research, 23*(5), 517–535.

Williams, A.B. (2001). Adherence to HIV regimens: 10 vital lessons. *American Journal of Nursing, 101*(6), 37–44.

Nursing Care of Clients with Cancer

MediaLink

www.prenhall.com/lemone
Additional resources for this chapter can be found on the Student CD-ROM accompanying this textbook, and on the Companion Website at www.prenhall.com/lemone. Click on Chapter 10 to select the activities for this chapter.

CD-ROM
- Audio Glossary
- NCLEX Review

Companion Website
- More NCLEX Review
- Case Study
  Pain Management
- Care Plan Activity
  Weight Loss and Chemotherapy
- MediaLink Application
  Terminal Cancer Support Groups

LEARNING OUTCOMES

After completing this chapter, you will be able to:

- Define cancer and differentiate benign from malignant neoplasms.
- Discuss the theories of carcinogenesis, known carcinogens, and risk factors for cancer.
- Compare the mechanisms and characteristics of normal cells with those of malignant cells.
- Describe the effects of cancer on the body.
- Describe the laboratory and diagnostic tests used to diagnose cancer.
- Discuss the role of chemotherapy in cancer treatment.
- Discuss the use of surgery, radiation therapy, and biotherapy in the treatment of cancer.
- Describe the nursing interventions required for selected oncologic emergencies.
- Provide teaching to the client and family experiencing cancer.
- Use the nursing process as a framework for providing individualized care to the client with cancer.

Cancer is a family of complex diseases with manifestations that vary according to the body system affected and the type of tumor cells involved. This disease can affect people of any age, gender, ethnicity, or geographic region. Although the incidence and mortality rates of cancer have continued to decline since 1990, it remains one of the most feared diseases. The fear engendered by even the suggestion of a cancer diagnosis often brings forth feelings of dread and helplessness.

This chapter looks at the general pathogenesis, pathophysiology, and etiology of cancer; identifies current diagnostic and treatment modalities; and discusses nursing care appropriate for most clients with cancer. Discussions of cancers that affect specific body systems (e.g., leukemia, lung cancer) can be found in corresponding body system chapters in the text.

Cancer results when normal cells mutate into abnormal, deviant cells that then perpetuate within the body. Cancer can affect any body tissue. Providing cancer care is a potentially complex process, reflecting cancer's many different types and manifestations.

Nursing focuses on cancer not as one disease, but as many diseases. The nurse recognizes that cancer is a disruptive process that affects the whole person and that person's significant others. Nursing interventions reflect the fact that cancer is a chronic disease that has acute episodes, that the client is often treated in the home, and that the client is usually treated with a combination of therapeutic modalities. Equally important, the nurse recognizes that caring for the client with cancer involves prevention, detection, rehabilitation, long-term follow-up, and terminal care (Oncology Nursing Society [ONS], 1997).

Oncology is the study of cancer. The term is derived from the Greek word *oncoma* ("bulk"). Oncologists specialize in caring for clients with cancer; they may be medical doctors, surgeons, radiologists, immunologists, or researchers. Another significant member of the oncology team is the oncology nurse, who has received specialized training in such cancer treatment modalities as chemotherapy. Oncology nurses also have special skills in assisting the client and family with the psychosocial issues associated with cancer and terminal illness. Often the client with cancer has the benefit of a team of physicians, nurses, and other health care professionals who collaborate to provide the most effective treatment.

INCIDENCE AND PREVALENCE

Only heart disease has a higher mortality rate than cancer. Despite continuing research, the rates of death from some forms of cancer continue to rise. Statistics from the American Cancer Society (ACS) show that approximately 25% of all deaths were attributable to cancer in the year 2001. It was estimated that 1.28 million new cases of cancer would occur in that year, with a projected death rate of 555,500 (ACS, 2002).

In 1994, prostate cancer surpassed lung and colon cancer for the position of highest incidence. Despite remaining the most frequently occurring cancer in men (189,000 new cases in 2002), the incidence of prostate cancer has begun to decline, due to the effects of prostate-specific antigen screening that allowed for diagnosis of cases earlier. Breast cancer is the most frequently occurring cancer in women, with an incidence of 203,500 in 2002. Lung and bronchial cancer (169,400 cases in 2002) and colorectal cancer (148,300 cases in 2002) rank second and third for both men and women. One of the most rapidly increasing cancers is melanoma (53,600 new cases in 2002) which has increased an average of 3% per year since 1981. The mortality rates for different cancers vary. In 2002, lung cancer is predicted to have the highest mortality rate with 154,900 estimated deaths, followed by colorectal (56,600), breast (40,000), and prostate cancer (30,2500). Information about the most recent cancer cases and mortality rates are available on the World Wide Web at www.cancer.org. The number of new cancer cases and cancer deaths is declining in the United States, and the 5-year survival rate for individual cancers continues to improve. Still, the gains are not equal for men and women nor for European Americans versus African Americans. The 5-year survival rate for all cancers is 62%, but African Americans are 33% more likely to die of cancer than whites (ACS, 2002). For example, although breast cancer occurs more commonly in white women than in black women, the survival rate is 86% for white women compared to only 71% for African Americans. Similar disparities are seen in survival rates for colorectal, prostate, and endometrial cancers in these ethnic groups. For information about diversity and cancer risk and incidence see the Focus on Diversity box below.

Cancer is a disease associated with aging; 80% of cancer diagnoses occur after age 55. The mortality rate for adults over 65 with cancer is 70%. These data are significant for health care as our elderly population increases.

RISK FACTORS

Risk factors make an individual or a population vulnerable to a specific disease or other unhealthy outcome. Risk factors can be divided into those that are controllable and those that are not controllable. Knowledge and assessment of risk factors are especially important in counseling clients and families about measures to prevent cancer.

Focus on Diversity

RISK AND INCIDENCE OF CANCER

- The incidence and mortality rates for all types of cancer are 35% to 39% lower in Hispanics.
- The incidence of cervical, stomach, and liver cancer is almost twice as high in Hispanics.
- Blacks are more likely to develop cancer than any other ethnic or racial group in the United States.
- Blacks have the highest incidence and mortality for colorectal and lung cancers.
- Breast cancer occurrence is about 13% lower in black women than in white women, but the mortality rate is approximately 28% higher.
- Black men are at least 50% more likely to develop prostate cancer than men of any other ethnic or racial group.
- Cancer incidence and mortality are lower in American Indian men and women than in any other ethnic or racial group.

Heredity

It is estimated that 5% to 10% of cancers may have a hereditary component. The familial pattern of some breast and colon cancers has been well documented. Lung, ovarian, and prostate cancers have also shown some familial relationships. The Human Genome Project has identified new cancer-linked genes (Futreal et al., 2001). For most cancers, research has yet to distinguish true genetic transfer from environmental causes. So although further research is needed to identify cancers that are due to the inheritance of defective genes, familial predisposition to malignancies should be counted among risk factors so that people at risk can reduce behaviors that promote cancer. For example, a client with a family history of lung cancer should be counseled to avoid smoking, to avoid areas where smoking is allowed, and to avoid working in an occupation that may expose the client to inhaled carcinogens.

Age

Approximately 70% of all cancers occur in people over age 65. A number of factors are associated with this increased risk in older adults. One possible factor is that at least five cycles of genetic mutations seem necessary to cause permanent damage to the afflicted cells. In addition, long-term exposure to high doses of promotional agents is usually necessary to allow the cancer to take hold. Evidence indicates that the immune response alters with aging; its actions become more generalized and less specific. Another problem is that free radicals (molecules resulting from the body's metabolic and oxidative processes) tend to accumulate in the cells over time, causing damage and mutation.

Hormonal changes that occur with aging can be associated with cancer. Postmenopausal women receiving exogenous estrogen have an increased risk for breast and uterine cancers. Older men are at risk for prostate cancer, possibly due to breakdown of testosterone into carcinogenic forms. See the box below for a discussion about older adults and cancer.

Severe and/or cumulative losses also are implicated in promoting cancer. These losses, which are common to older adults, include the death of a spouse or friends, loss of position and status in society, and a decline in physical abilities (Selye, 1984). These repeated stressors are related to changes in the immune system that may lead to the development of cancer.

Gender

Gender is a risk factor for certain types of cancer, rather than for acquiring cancer in general. For example, thyroid cancer occurs more commonly among females, whereas bladder cancer is seen more often among male clients. Chapters 47 and 48 provide more information on gender-specific cancers. ⬯

Poverty

The poor are at higher risk for cancer than the population in general. Inadequate access to health care, especially preventive

Meeting Individualized Needs

OLDER ADULTS WITH CANCER

Nurses need to be aware of how cancer and cancer treatments affect older adults. Cancer is the second leading cause of death in people over age 65. The incidence of cancer increases with advancing age, probably as a result of the accumulated exposure to carcinogens and to age-related declines in the action of the immune system. The most commonly seen cancers in older women are colorectal, breast, lung, pancreatic, and ovarian. In older men, lung, colorectal, prostate, pancreatic, and gastric cancers occur most frequently.

The importance of screening and early detection of cancer does not diminish with age. Unfortunately, many older adults do not receive adequate cancer screening. Because the older adult is closer to the end of life, some health care providers may believe that cancer screening is not as important as it is for the younger client. This attitude may result in delayed diagnosis and treatment.

Older adults may not participate in screening programs or seek treatment for cancer due to fear, depression, cognitive impairments, poor access to health care, or financial constraints. Some older adults (and health care providers) mistake cancer symptoms for normal age-related changes. Believing that little can be done, they do not seek health care for their symptoms. Fear of the cancer diagnosis also keeps older adults from seeking appropriate health care. When they do seek treatment, chronic conditions frequently seen in older adults may make the diagnosis of cancer more difficult by masking or confounding the usual symptoms associated with cancer.

Older adults are at greater risk for side effects associated with cancer treatment because of age-related physiologic changes and chronic conditions associated with aging. This is particularly true for the side effects of chemotherapeutic agents. Older adults have increased incidence of cardiotoxicity and toxicity of the central nervous system when undergoing chemotherapy than younger adults. The side effects of chemotherapy can contribute to fatigue and cause problems related to immobility and functional decline. Alterations in the function of the immune system are also more frequent in older adults, which increases their risk for developing infection.

The problems associated with chemotherapy do not rule out its use, but the nurse must be aware of potential problems and monitor the client closely for the development of side effects. The nurse must consider how the aging process will alter the response to the disease and treatment plan when planning care for older adults.

Client and Family Teaching

- Discuss the warning signs of cancer.
- Stress the importance of seeking health care if any of the warning signs develop.
- Get an annual physical examination.
- For women, learn how to perform a breast self-exam and perform the exam every month.
- For men, undergo prostate-specific antigen (PSA) screening for prostate cancer.

screening and counseling, may be a major factor. Although other factors that may be involved, such as diet and stress, usually come under the category of controllable risks, these risks are frequently uncontrollable in this population.

Stress

Continuous unmanaged stress that keeps hormones such as epinephrine and cortisol at high levels can result in systematic "fatigue" and impaired immunologic surveillance. When the body attempts to adapt to physiologic and psychologic stressors, it goes through a series of stages called the general adaptation syndrome (GAS) (Selye, 1984). First, the "alarm reaction" occurs, in which adrenal hormones increase, allowing the body to cope with the stressor. Eventually, the body reaches the "stage of resistance," in which the stress hormones are significantly reduced, indicating that adaptation has occurred. If the physiologic adaptation is supported by appropriate coping strategies, the stressor is considered managed and body systems return to the prealarm functioning. However, if adaptation continues and the stress hormones remain elevated, the "stage of exhaustion" sets in. This stage will maintain life, but at great expense to body systems, resulting in general wear-and-tear and depression of the immune system (Selye, 1984).

The literature mentions a type C, or "cancer personality," describing people who have unhealthy coping behaviors for life stressors. Type C people are identified as those who tend to others' needs to the exclusion of their own and who rarely ask for help or support, even in personal crises. These people tend to be emotionally, and sometimes even physically, isolated and have a great deal of buried, unexpressed anger. It is thought that this kind of behavior pattern harms the immune system over time, promoting vulnerability to cancer. Depression is also considered a major risk factor, especially depression that is chronic or related to multiple or major losses. It is thought that depression and hopelessness tend to shut down the energizing chemicals in the body and depress immune responses (Kaye, Morton, Bowcutt, & Maupin, 2000).

Diet

Some foods are considered genotoxic, such as the nitrosamines and nitrosindoles found in preserved meats and pickled, salted foods. Migrant workers have been found to have a high incidence of esophageal and gastric cancers related to their excessive consumption of these items. Other foods, such as high-fat, low-fiber foods—the mainstay of many American diets—promote colon, breast, and sex hormone–dependent tumors. When fish and meat are excessively fried or broiled, potent carcinogenic compounds can form that may cause tumors in the mammary glands, colon, liver, pancreas, and bladder. Also, repeatedly using fat to fry foods at high temperatures produces high levels of polycyclic hydrocarbons, which increase cancer risk considerably. Although many people profess to have changed their dietary habits, one only has to observe the large number of people who still lunch on cheeseburgers and french fries (and who teach their children to do the same) to realize that much more educational and motivational work is needed in this area. Other food-related substances believed to increase cancer risk include sodium saccharine, red food dyes, and both regular and decaffeinated coffee.

Occupation

Occupational risk might be considered to be either controllable or uncontrollable. For many people, both education and ability limit their choice of occupation; during times of high unemployment, moreover, changing one's occupation because it poses risk factors may not be a viable option. Federal standards are designed to protect workers from hazardous substances, but many believe that these standards are not strict enough and that inspections are not frequent enough to prevent violations.

Specific risks vary according to the occupation. For example, outdoor workers such as farmers and construction workers are exposed to solar radiation; health care workers such as X-ray technicians and biomedical researchers are exposed to ionizing radiation and carcinogenic substances; and exposure to asbestos is a problem for people who work in old buildings with asbestos insulation in the walls. Table 10–1 correlates known carcinogens and occupations.

TABLE 10–1 Chemical Carcinogens and Relationship to Occupation

Chemical Agent	Action	Occupation Affected
Polycyclic hydrocarbons (smoke, soot, tobacco, smoked foods) Benzopyrene	Genotoxic	Miners, coal/gas workers, chimney sweeps, migrant workers, workers in offices where smoking is allowed in closed areas
Arsenic	Genotoxic	Pesticide manufacturers, mining
Vinyl chloride polymers	Promotional	Plastics workers Artists
Methylaminobenzine	Genotoxic	Fabric workers Rubber and glue workers
Asbestos	Promotional	Construction workers, workers in old, run-down buildings with asbestos insulation, insulation makers
Wood and leather dust	Promotional	Woodworkers, carpenters, leather toolers
Chemotherapy drugs	Genotoxic	Drug manufacturers, pharmacists, nurses

Infection

Because a number of viruses have been linked to some cancers, avoiding those specific infections will decrease risk. Although some infections may be unavoidable (Epstein-Barr, for example), others, such as genital herpes and papillomavirus-induced genital warts, can often be avoided by following safe sex practices (e.g., the use of condoms).

Tobacco Use

Lung cancer is considered highly preventable because of its relationship to smoking. The genotoxic carcinogenic substances in tobacco are considered weak; therefore, stopping smoking can reverse the damage it causes. However, many other substances in tobacco are highly promotional, so that the larger the dose and longer the use, the higher the risk for developing cancer. Research has shown a significantly lower lung cancer death risk for former smokers compared to current smokers. Smokers who quit before middle age avoid more than 90% of the risk of lung cancer that can be attributed to tobacco (Peto et al., 2000).

Tobacco is also related to other forms of cancer. Smokers face an increased risk for oropharyngeal, esophageal, laryngeal, gastric, pancreatic, and bladder cancers. Pipe and cigar smokers are especially susceptible to oropharyngeal and laryngeal cancers. Oral and esophageal cancers are more common among those who chew tobacco or use snuff. Smokers who have a genetic decrease in alpha-1 antitripsin (an enzyme that protects lung tissue) that results in emphysema face an even higher cancer risk than smokers without this defect.

Additional research has documented the deleterious effects of secondhand tobacco smoke (Williams & Sandler, 2001). Tobacco-specific nitrosamines were recovered in the urine of children living with smokers. It is now accepted that nonsmokers exposed to tobacco smoke over long periods of time, whether in the workplace or the home, have an increased risk for lung or bladder cancers.

Alcohol Use

Alcohol promotes cancer by modifying the metabolism of carcinogens in the liver and esophagus, thus increasing the effectiveness of the carcinogens in some tissues. People who both smoke and drink a considerable amount of alcohol daily have an increased risk for oral, esophageal, and laryngeal cancers.

Recreational Drug Use

Recreational drug use often promotes an unhealthy lifestyle that increases general cancer risk; for example, drug users often do not maintain adequate nutrition. Furthermore, recreational drugs are implicated as promoters because of their suppressive effect on the immune system. Although it has not been directly implicated in cancer development, marijuana has been demonstrated to cause chromosomal damage that may over time also result in cancer-causing DNA damage and genetic mutations. Marijuana smoke is also much more injurious to lung tissue than tobacco smoke.

Obesity

Excessive body fat has been linked to an increased risk of hormone-dependent cancers. Because sex hormones are synthesized from fat, obese people often have excessive amounts of the hormones that feed hormone-dependent malignancies of the breast, bowel, ovary, endometrium, and prostate.

Sun Exposure

As the protective ozone layer thins, more of the sun's damaging ultraviolet radiation reaches the earth. As a consequence, the rate of skin cancers has increased. Sun-related skin cancers are now considered to be a problem for all people, regardless of skin color, but people of Northern European extraction with very fair skin, blue or green eyes, and light-colored hair are most vulnerable. Elderly people with decreased pigment are also more at risk, even those with darker skin.

Figure 10–1 ■ summarizes the interaction of factors that promote cancer.

PATHOPHYSIOLOGY

Cancer is a complex disease with hundreds of agents that can contribute to its pathogenesis. Advances in research have greatly increased the understanding of how cancer develops. It is now known that the development of cancer is a process in which normal cells are changed and acquire malignant properties. Before a discussion of the various theories of the causes of cancer, it is useful to review how normal cells divide and adapt to changing conditions.

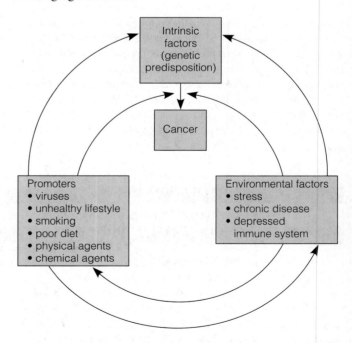

Figure 10–1 ■ Interaction of factors that promote cancer. Most people have immune systems that are competent enough to resist the establishment of cancer from an initiated cell. Cancer takes hold when a number of promotional factors occur together and over enough time to weaken immune resistance. Like factors are grouped together for ease of presentation but may occur in any combination.

BOX 10–1 ■ Functions of DNA

■ Orders production of enzymes.
■ Instructs cells to produce specific chemicals.
■ Instructs cells to develop specific structures.
■ Determines individual traits and characteristics.
■ Controls other DNA by telling a cell to "switch on" and use some portion of the genetic information stored in it.

Normal Cell Growth

Mature normal cells are uniform in size and have nuclei that are characteristic of the tissue to which the cells belong. Within the nucleus of normal cells, chromosomes containing deoxyribonucleic acid (DNA) molecules carry the genetic information that controls the synthesis of polypeptides (proteins). Genes are subunits of chromosomes and consist of portions of DNA that specify the production of particular sets of proteins. Thus, genes control the development of specific traits. The genetic code in the DNA of every gene is translated into protein structures that determine the type, maturity, and function of a cell. Any change or disruption in a gene can result in an inaccurate "blueprint" that can produce an aberrant cell, which may then become cancerous. Box 10–1 lists some of the functions of DNA.

The Cell Cycle

Two coordinated events are responsible for cellular reproduction. Reproduction occurs as the result of replication of cellular DNA and mitosis, when the cell divides into two daughter cells with identical DNA.

The cell cycle consists of four phases. In the gap 1 or G_1 phase, the cell enlarges and synthesizes proteins to prepare for DNA replication. During this phase the cell prepares to replicate and enter into the synthesis phase. During the synthesis (S) phase, DNA is replicated and the chromosomes in the cell are duplicated. During the next phase, gap 2 (G_2), the cell prepares itself for mitosis. Finally, with all preparation complete, the cell begins mitosis (M). This phase culminates in the division of the parent cell into two exact copies called daughter cells, each having identical genetic material. The cells then immediately enter G_1 where they begin the cell cycle again, or divert into a resting phase called G_0. The cell cycle is controlled by cyclins, which combine with and activate enzymes called cyclin-dependent kinases (CDKs). Some cyclins cause a "braking" action and prevent the cycle from proceeding (Dunlop & Campbell, 2000). Checkpoints in the cell cycle ensure that it proceeds in the correct order.

A malfunction of any of these regulators of cell growth and division can result in the rapid proliferation of immature cells. In some cases, these cells are considered cancerous (malignant). Knowledge of cell cycle events is used in the development of chemotherapeutic drugs, which are designed to disrupt the cancer cells during different stages of their cell cycle. These drugs and their use are discussed later in the chapter.

Differentiation

Differentiation is a normal process occurring over many cell cycles that allows cells to specialize in certain tasks. For ex-

ample, some epithelial cells lining the lungs develop into tall columnar cells with cilia. These columnar cells sweep potentially dangerous debris out of the lungs. When adverse conditions occur in body tissues during differentiation, protective adaptations can produce alterations in cells. Some of these alterations are helpful, but in other cases the cells mutate beyond usefulness and become liabilities (Porth, 1998). Following are potentially unproductive cellular alterations occurring during cell differentiation.

- **Hyperplasia** is an increase in the number or density of normal cells. Hyperplasia occurs in response to stress, increased metabolic demands, or elevated levels of hormones. Examples include the hyperplasia of myocardial cells in response to a prolonged increase in the body's demand for oxygen, and hyperplasia of uterine cells in response to rising levels of estrogen during pregnancy. Hyperplastic cells are under normal DNA control.
- **Metaplasia** is a change in the normal pattern of differentiation such that dividing cells differentiate into cell types not normally found in that location in the body. The metaplastic cell is normal for its particular type, but it is not in its normal location. Some metaplastic cells are less functional than the cells they replace. Metaplasia is a protective response to adverse conditions. Metaplastic cells are under normal DNA control and are reversible when the stressor or other disruptive condition ceases.
- **Dysplasia** represents a loss of DNA control over differentiation occurring in response to adverse conditions. Dysplastic cells show abnormal variation in size, shape, and appearance and a disturbance in their usual arrangement. Examples of dysplasia include changes in the cervix in response to continued irritation, such as from the human papillomavirus (HPV), or leukoplakia on oral mucous membranes in response to chronic irritation from smoking.
- **Anaplasia** is the regression of a cell to an immature or undifferentiated cell type. Anaplastic cell division is no longer under DNA control. Anaplasia usually occurs when a damaging or transforming event takes place inside the dividing, still undifferentiated cell, leading to loss of useful function. Anaplasia may occur in response to overwhelmingly destructive conditions inside the cell or in surrounding tissue (Porth, 2002).

Although hyperplasia, metaplasia, and dysplasia often reverse after the irritating factor is eliminated, they can lead to malignancy under certain conditions. This is especially true of dysplasia, which represents a loss of DNA control. Anaplasia is not reversible, but the degree of anaplasia determines the potential risk for cancer.

Etiology

Intensive research efforts during the past several decades have led to an increased understanding of how cancer develops. The Human Genome Project, begun in 1990, has provided critical information about the development of cancer. Continuing research will provide information that will be key in the detection and prevention of cancer.

Cancer research has brought new options for cancer treatment and improved clients' overall survival rate. Almost daily, people hear of research studies indicating that certain foods, habits, or environmental factors may cause cancer. Although much of this is true and is inspiring a welcome preventive focus to health care, it is not true that one can determine the specific factors that cause cancer in any individual. Although taking responsibility for one's own health is a positive step, the emphasis on prevention may have a negative result if clients feel so guilty and blameworthy that they fail to seek out early and appropriate health care. Also, clients who feel that their bodies have failed them may become depressed, and such feelings can impair the functioning of an already stressed immune system.

Factors that cause cancer are both external (chemicals, radiation, and viruses) and internal (hormones, immune conditions, and inherited mutations). Causal factors may act together or in sequence to initiate or promote carcinogenesis. Ten or more years often pass between exposures or mutations and detectable cancer.

Theories of Carcinogenesis

Cellular Mutation

The theory of cellular mutation suggests that carcinogens cause mutations in cellular DNA. It is believed that the carcinogenic process has three stages: initiation, promotion, and progression. The initiation stage involves permanent damage in the cellular DNA as a result of exposure to a carcinogen (e.g., radiation, chemicals) that was not repaired or had a defective repair. Promotion may last for years and includes conditions, such as smoking or alcohol use, that act repeatedly on the already affected cells. In the progression stage further inherited changes acquired during the cell replication develop into a cancer.

Oncogenes

Oncogenes are genes that promote cell proliferation and are capable of triggering cancerous characteristics. Oncogenes can be classified according to their overall function. Several oncogenes and their relationship to human cancers have been identified. For example, BRCA-1 and BRCA-2 are associated with breast cancer (Surbone, 2001).

A decrease in the body's immune surveillance may allow the expression of oncogenes; this can occur during times of stress or in response to certain carcinogens. For example, clients with AIDS, who have a decreased number of helper T lymphocytes, have a much higher than normal incidence of certain cancers, including non-Hodgkin's lymphoma and Kaposi's sarcoma (Donahue, Wernz, & Cooper, 2000).

Tumor Suppressor Genes

Tumor suppressor genes normally suppress oncogenes. They can become inactive by deletion or mutation. Inherited cancers have been associated with tumor suppressor genes. An example is p53, a suppressor gene that has been associated with sarcoma and cancer of the breast and brain.

Central to these theories are two important concepts about the etiology of cancer. First, damaged DNA, whether inherited or from external sources, sets up the necessary initial step for cancer to occur. Second, impairment of the human immune system, from whatever cause, lessens its ability to destroy abnormal cells.

Known Carcinogens

A number of agents are known to cause cancer, or at least are strongly linked to certain kinds of cancers. These known carcinogens include viruses, drugs, hormones, and chemical and physical agents.

Carcinogens can be categorized in two groups: Genotoxic carcinogens directly alter DNA and cause mutations, and promoter substances cause other adverse biologic effects, such as cytotoxicity, hormonal imbalances, altered immunity, or chronic tissue damage. Promoter substances do not cause cancer in the absence of previous cell damage (initiation) and often require high-level and long-term contact with the altered cells (see Table 10–1).

Note also that although everyone comes into contact with a vast number of substances that are considered carcinogenic, not everyone develops cancer. Other factors, such as genetic predisposition, impairment of the immune response, and repeated exposure to the carcinogen, are necessary for a cancer to develop.

Viruses

Several viruses have been associated with the development of cancer. They damage cells and induce hyperplastic cell growth. Viral infection may play a role in cell mutation that can progress to malignant cells. Most people are able to suppress this progression (Spitalnick & diSant'Angnese, 2001). Box 10–2 identifies these viruses and the cancers with which they are associated.

BOX 10–2	■ Cancers Associated with Different Viruses

HERPES SIMPLEX VIRUS TYPES I AND II (HSV-1 AND HSV-2)
■ Carcinoma of the lip
■ Cervical carcinoma
■ Kaposi's sarcoma

HUMAN CYTOMEGALOVIRUS (HCMV)
■ Kaposi's sarcoma
■ Prostate cancer

EPSTEIN-BARR VIRUS (EBV)
■ Burkitt's lymphoma

HUMAN HERPESVIRUS-6 (HHV-6)
■ Lymphoma

HEPATITIS B VIRUS (HBV)
■ Primary hepatocellular cancer

PAPILLOMAVIRUS
■ Malignant melanoma
■ Cervical, penile, and laryngeal cancers

HUMAN T-LYMPHOTROPIC VIRUSES (HTLV)
■ Adult T-cell leukemia and lymphoma
■ T-cell variant of hairy-cell leukemia
■ Kaposi's sarcoma

In addition, viruses play a significant role in weakening immunologic defenses against neoplasms. For example, HIV, which infects helper T lymphocytes and monocytes, impairs the person's protection against certain cancers such as lymphoma and Kaposi's sarcoma.

Other viruses have also been associated with human malignancies. Hepatitis B virus (HBV) integrates its DNA with liver cell DNA and is believed to cause primary hepatocellular carcinoma. Papillomaviruses cause plantar, common, and flat warts, which are benign and usually regress spontaneously; however, they also cause genital warts and laryngeal papillomas, which are associated with malignant melanoma and cervical, penile, and laryngeal cancers. Retroviruses have been found to cause cancer in animals. Adult T-cell leukemia is the only human cancer known to be associated with a retrovirus (Hill, 2001).

Vaccines to prevent virus-induced cancers are being investigated. Preliminary results of the use of vaccines to treat malignancies, such as melanoma, have been encouraging (Berd, 2001).

Drugs and Hormones

Certain drugs can be either genotoxic or promotional. For example, chemotherapeutic drugs used to disrupt the cell cycle of malignant cells can be genotoxic for normal cells. They can also be promotional: By drastically reducing the number of leukocytes, they impair immune function. Examples of these chemotherapeutic drugs include busulfan, chlorambucil, and cycloposphamide. Some recreational drugs also are implicated as carcinogens. These include the genotoxic betel nut chewed by many Pacific Islanders and the immunosuppressant promoters heroin and cocaine.

Hormones are also potential genotoxic carcinogens or promoters. Gonadotropic hormones often mediate cancers of the reproductive organs. Estrogen, both natural and synthetic, and diethylstilbestrol (DES) have been linked to cervical, endometrial, and breast cancers. Estrogen-containing contraceptive pills have been implicated in breast cancer, but they also have been shown to decrease the risk of ovarian cancer. Investigators have not reached a final conclusion about the cancer risk posed by contraceptives. Newer research suggests that alterations in the molecular structure of testosterone in older men may promote the development of prostate cancer. Also, glucocorticosteroids (cortisone) and anabolic steroids may act as promoters by altering the immune response or endocrine balance (Chapman & Goodman, 2000; Held-Warmkessel, 2000; Rubin, Williams, Okunieff, Rosenblatt, & Sitzmann, 2001).

Chemical Agents

Many chemicals have been demonstrated to be both genotoxic and promotional. Because many of these substances are encountered in the workplace, they constitute occupational hazards, which will be discussed more thoroughly. Examples of industrial and environmental carcinogens include polycyclic hydrocarbons, found in soot; benzopyrene, found in cigarette smoke; and arsenic, found in pesticides. These chemicals have some genotoxic action; some alter DNA replication. Other industrial and environmental chemicals are considered promotional agents. These include wood and leather dust, polymer esters (used in plastics and paints), carbon tetrachloride, asbestos, and phenol.

Natural substances in the body may also be carcinogenic or promotional. For example, end products of metabolism that are produced in excess amounts or are ineffectively eliminated, such as bile acids from a high-fat diet, may promote cancer.

Some foods contain carcinogens added during preparation or preservation. Examples include the sugar substitute sodium saccharine and nitrosamines and nitrosindoles, which are found in pickled, salted foods. In some cases, food contaminants produce carcinogenic chemicals. The Aspergillus fungi produce aflatoxin, a highly potent carcinogen. These organisms grow on improperly stored vegetable products, such as grains and peanuts.

Polycyclic aromatic hydrocarbons, nitrosamines, phenols, and other chemicals in tobacco act as either carcinogens or promoters of cancer (see Table 10–1).

Physical Agents

It has been well documented that excessive exposure to radiation causes increased rates of cancer by damaging the DNA in cells, by activating other oncogenetic factors, or by suppressing antitumor activity (protein inhibitors). Both solar radiation from ultraviolet rays and ionizing radiation from industrial or medical sources are carcinogenic. This fact has implications for workers exposed to these agents and for the population in general. Radon, a naturally formed radioactive gas found in the basements of many homes, is also a known carcinogen. People who have lived in areas where nuclear weapons have been tested or whose groundwater has been polluted by nuclear wastes are at risk for developing cancers. The effects of high-dose radiation exposure and subsequent cancer development have been demonstrated in the survivors of the atomic bomb at Nagasaki and Hiroshima and workers exposed to radiation during the cleanup of nuclear disasters such as Chernobyl.

Types of Neoplasms

A **neoplasm** is a mass of new tissue (a collection of cells) that grows independently of its surrounding structures and has no physiologic purpose. The term *neoplasm* is often used interchangeably with *tumor*, from the Latin word meaning "swelling." Neoplasms are said to be autonomous because of the following:

- They grow at a rate uncoordinated with the needs of the body.
- They function independently of usual homeostatic controls.
- They share some of the properties of the parent cells but with altered size and shape.
- They do not benefit the host and in some cases are actively harmful.

Neoplasms are not completely autonomous, however, because they require a blood supply with nutrients and oxygen to sustain their growth. Neoplasms typically are classified as benign or malignant on the basis of their potential to damage the body and on their growth characteristics.

Benign Neoplasms

Benign neoplasms are localized growths. They form a solid mass, have well-defined borders, and frequently are encapsulated. Benign neoplasms tend to respond to the body's homeostatic controls. Thus, they often stop growing when they reach the boundaries of another tissue (a process called contact inhibition). They grow slowly and often remain stable in size. Because they are usually encapsulated, benign neoplasms often are easily removed and tend not to recur.

Although typically harmless, benign neoplasms nevertheless can be destructive if they crowd surrounding tissue and obstruct the function of organs. For example, a benign meningioma (from the meninges of the brain and spinal cord) can cause severely increased intracranial pressure (ICP), which progressively impairs the person's cerebral function. Unless the meningioma can be successfully removed, the steadily rising ICP will eventually lead to coma and death.

Malignant Neoplasms

In contrast to benign neoplasms, malignant neoplasms grow aggressively and do not respond to the body's homeostatic controls. Malignant neoplasms are not cohesive, and present with an irregular shape. Instead of slowly crowding other tissues aside, malignant neoplasms cut through surrounding tissues, causing bleeding, inflammation, and necrosis (tissue death) as they grow. This invasive quality of malignant neoplasms is reflected in the word origin of *cancer,* from the Greek *karkinos,* meaning "crab." Health care professionals are referring to a malignant neoplasm when they use the term *cancer.*

Malignant cells from the primary tumor may travel through the blood or lymph to invade other tissues and organs of the body and form a secondary tumor called a metastasis. This term also refers to the process by which such spreading of malignant neoplasms—perhaps their most destructive trait—occurs. Malignant neoplasms can recur after surgical removal of the primary and secondary tumors and after other treatments. Table 10–2 compares benign and malignant neoplasms.

Malignant neoplasms vary in their degree of differentiation from the parent tissue. Highly differentiated cancer cells try to mimic the specialized function of the parent tissue, but undifferentiated cancers, consisting of immature cells, have almost no resemblance to the parent tissue and so perform no useful function. To make matters worse, undifferentiated cancers rob the body of its energy and nutrition as they grow. Undifferentiated anaplastic cells have little structural or functional relationship to the parent cells and are the basis of many malignant neoplasms. The degree of differentiation of anaplastic cells is a consideration in the classification and staging of neoplasms, discussed later in this chapter.

Characteristics of Malignant Cells

Malignant neoplasms may be identified by the following predictable cellular characteristics.

- *Loss of regulation of the rate of mitosis.* This results in rapid cell division and growth of the neoplasm.
- *Loss of specialization and differentiation.* Malignant cells do not perform typical cellular functions. Many produce hormones and enzymes similar to those of the parent tissue, but usually in excessive amounts, possibly revealing their presence.
- *Loss of contact inhibition.* Malignant cells do not respect other cellular boundaries. They easily invade and destroy other tissues.
- *Progressive acquisition of a cancerous phenotype.* Cellular mutation seems to be a sequential process involving successive generations of cells, each generation becoming more deviant than the previous one. Additionally, malignant cells seem to be "immortal"; that is, they do not stop growing and die, as do normal cells, which have a genetically determined life span.
- *Irreversibility.* The transformation into a malignant cell is irreversible. Rarely does a malignant neoplasm revert to a benign state.
- *Altered cell structure.* Cytologic examination of malignant cells reveals distinct differences in the cell nucleus and cytoplasm as well as an overall cell shape that differs from that of normal cells of the particular tissue type.
- *Simplified metabolic activities.* The work of malignant cells is simpler than that of normal cells; they show an increased synthesis of substances needed for cell division, and they have no need to create proteins for the specialized functions of the tissues they invade.
- *Transplantability.* Malignant cells often break away from the primary tissue site and travel to other locations in the body, where they establish new growths.
- *Ability to promote their own survival.* Malignant cells may create ectopic sites to produce the hormones they need for their growth. By their very presence and their ability to initiate vascular permeability, malignant cells promote the development of nonneoplastic stroma, a connective tissue framework consisting of collagen and other components, which then supports the neoplasm. They may also create their own blood supply. Through a process called angiogenesis, tumor cells secrete a polypeptide angiogenic growth factor that stimulates blood vessels from surrounding normal tissue to grow into the tumor. Finally, malignant cells divert nutrition from the host to meet their own needs, by diffusion when the tumor is less than 1 mm and thereafter by means of the newly formed blood vessels. If unchecked, malignant cells eventually destroy their host.

TABLE 10–2	Comparison of Benign and Malignant Neoplasms
Benign	**Malignant**
Local	Invasive
Cohesive	Noncohesive
Well-defined borders	Does not stop at tissue border
Pushes other tissues out of the way	Invades and destroys surrounding tissues
Slow growth	Rapid growth
Encapsulated	Metastasizes to distant sites
Easily removed	Not always easy to remove
Does not recur	Can recur

BOX 10-3 ■ Characteristics of Malignant Cells

- Loss of regulation of mitotic rate
- Loss of cell specialization
- Loss of contact inhibition
- Progressive acquisition of the cancerous phenotype and immortality
- Irreversibility of cancerous phenotype to greater aggressiveness
- Altered cell structure: differences in cell nucleus and cytoplasm
- Simplified metabolic activity
- Transplantability (metastasis)
- Ability to promote own survival

The characteristics of malignant cells are summarized in Box 10–3.

Tumor Invasion and Metastasis

The ability of cancer cells to invade adjacent tissues and travel to distant organs is considered their most ominous characteristic. This quality makes treatment a considerable challenge (Hawkins, 2001).

Invasion

Aggressive tumors possess several qualities that facilitate invasion (Figure 10–2 ■):

- *Ability to cause pressure atrophy.* The pressure of a growing tumor can cause atrophy and necrosis of adjacent tissues. The malignancy then moves into the vacated space.
- *Ability to disrupt the basement membrane of normal cells.* Many cancer cells can bind to elements of the basement membrane and secrete enzymes that degrade that physical barrier, thus facilitating their movement into normal tissues, lymph, and blood circulation.
- *Motility.* Because malignant cells are less tightly bound to each other than normal cells (reduced adhesiveness), they easily separate from the neoplasm and move into surrounding body fluids and tissues.
- *Response to chemical signals from adjacent tissues.* Chemotaxis (the movement of cells in response to a chemical stimulus) calls the tumor cells into the normal tissues, possibly as a result of the degrading of the basement membranes of the normal cells. This breakdown of normal cellular membranes releases the chemical stimulus physiologically designed to draw normal phagocytic cells to clean up the debris. (See Chapter 8 on the inflammatory response for more information on chemotaxis. ⌾) Malignant cells are also known to respond chemotactically to the end product of cellular metabolism. Some cancer cells even produce a substance called autocrine motility factor, which calls other malignant cells to a normal tissue. The first invading cells produce this substance, which then actively draws other malignant cells from the primary tumor into the invaded normal tissue.

Metastasis

The factors that favor invasion also contribute to the process of metastasis. **Metastasis** can occur by means of one or more mechanisms including embolism in the blood or lymph or spread by way of body cavities.

A blood- or lymph-borne metastasis allows a new tumor to be established in a distant organ. Figure 10–3 ■ shows metastasis through the bloodstream. A tumor's ability to metastasize in this manner requires the following steps:

1. Intravasation of malignant cells through blood or lymphatic vessel walls and into the circulation

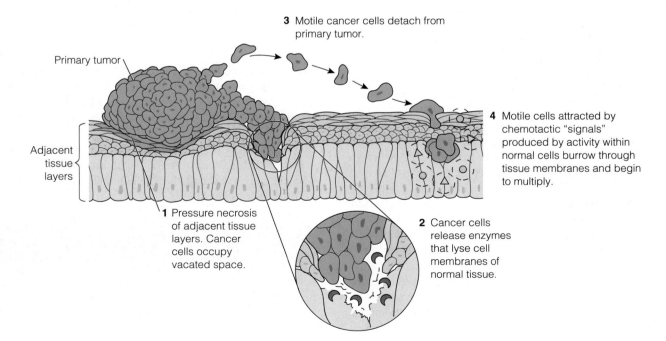

3 Motile cancer cells detach from primary tumor.

Primary tumor

4 Motile cells attracted by chemotactic "signals" produced by activity within normal cells burrow through tissue membranes and begin to multiply.

Adjacent tissue layers

1 Pressure necrosis of adjacent tissue layers. Cancer cells occupy vacated space.

2 Cancer cells release enzymes that lyse cell membranes of normal tissue.

Figure 10–2 ■ How cancer cells invade normal tissue.

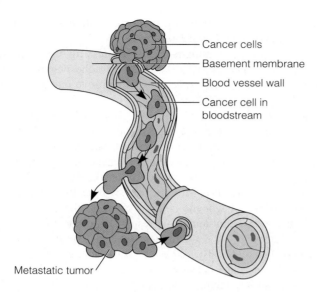

Figure 10–3 ■ Metastasis through the bloodstream. Cancer cells secrete enzymes and a motility factor that disrupt the basement membrane in the blood vessel. In this way, the cancer cells gain access into the circulation. Once in the blood, only about 1 cell in 1000 escapes immune detection, but that can be enough. Undetected cells move out of the blood, again secreting enzymes and cutting through the vessel wall into new tissue. The tissue selected for establishing a new tumor may be downstream from the original tumor, or a chemical attraction may cause the malignant cells to target a specific site. Once in the new site, the malignant cells multiply and establish a metastatic tumor.

2. Survival of the malignant cells in the blood (To survive, the cells must escape the notice of the body's immune surveillance; only about 1 in 1000 cells does so.)
3. Extravasation from the circulation and implantation in a new tissue

The tumor cells tend to clump together, forming an embolus, and continue growing until their size prevents further travel in the vessel or lymph channel. The growing neoplastic mass then uses its invasive abilities (secreting enzymes and motility factor) to move into the nearest organ.

About 60% of metastatic lesions tend to occur in a schema reflecting the pattern of blood or lymph circulation. However, it has been demonstrated that some malignant cells defy a bloodborne pattern and actually target specific organs to which they prefer to metastasize. For example, lung cancer frequently metastasizes to the adrenal glands and breast cancer frequently metastasizes to bone.

Malignant cells that gain access to the lymph channels may travel to a preferred organ and then move into it the same way they emigrate through blood vessels. Alternatively, the malignant cells may become trapped in the lymph node and continue to grow. Eventually, the malignant cells replace the node's tissues. At this point, emboli from the cancerous node disseminate to other nodes, creating a cascade reaction. The malignant cascade causes widespread transfer of the tumor to uncharacteristic sites.

TABLE 10–3	Various Cancers and Sites of or Metastases
Primary Tumor	**Common Metastatic Sites**
Bronchogenic (lung)	Spinal cord, brain, liver, bone
Breast	Regional lymph nodes, vertebrae, brain, liver, lung, bone
Colon	Liver, lung, brain, ovary, bone
Prostate	Bladder, bone (especially vertebrae), liver
Malignant melanoma	Lung, liver, spleen, regional lymph nodes, brain

A malignant tumor may break through the walls of the organ in which it is primarily housed, shedding cells into the nearby body cavity. The cells then are free to establish new tumors in a distant area of that cavity. For example, malignant cells from a colon cancer may be seeded into the peritoneal cavity, establishing a new tumor in the mesenteric epithelium.

Metastatic lesions are differentiated from primary neoplasms by cell morphology: Metastatic cells do not resemble the tissue in which they reside. The most common sites of metastasis are the lymph nodes, liver, lungs, bones, and brain. Table 10–3 lists different cancers and common sites of metastasis.

For metastasis to occur, the cancerous cells must avoid detection by the immune system. Thus, impairment of the immune system is a major factor in the establishment of metastatic lesions. Cells may escape detection in several different ways:

• Aggressive cancer cells may compile a large mass (greater than 1 cm) so rapidly that the immune system is unable to overcome the tumor before it takes hold in a new tissue.
• For tumor cells to be recognized as foreign by the immune system, they must display on their surface a special antigen called tumor-associated antigen (TAA). TAA marks tumor cells for destruction by the lymphocytes. Some oncogenic viruses depress the expression of TAA on infected cells. Also, some tumors in advanced stages of growth no longer display TAA. Thus, such tumor cells escape detection as they travel through the blood or lymph.
• If the person's immune response is weakened or altered, then a metastatic tumor may take hold with little opposition. Factors that may weaken or alter the immune response are listed in Box 10–4.

BOX 10–4	■ Factors That May Weaken or Alter the Immune Response

■ Accumulated stress
■ Depression
■ Increased age
■ Pregnancy
■ Chronic disease
■ Chemotherapy treatment for the primary cancer

An estimated 50% to 60% of all cancers have already metastasized by the time the primary tumor is identified. This may account for the current 50% death rate and certainly supports the need for client education to facilitate early diagnosis. The time it takes for metastasis to occur is extremely variable and often difficult to predict. Some cancers, such as basal cell carcinomas, do not metastasize. The aggressiveness and location of the tumor, and the state of the person's immune system, determine whether and how rapidly metastasis takes place.

Physiologic and Psychologic Effects of Cancer

Much of the nursing care for clients with cancer is related to the generalized effects of cancer on the body and the side effects of the treatments used to remove or destroy the cancer. Although pathophysiologic effects of the cancer vary with the type and location of the cancer, the following effects usually are observed.

Disruption of Function

Physiologic functioning can be upset by obstruction or pressure. For example, a large tumor in the bowel can stop intestinal motility, resulting in a bowel obstruction. Prostatic tumors can obstruct the bladder neck or urethra, resulting in urine retention. Intracranial pressure can be dangerously increased by a glioma.

Obstruction or pressure can cause anoxia and necrosis of surrounding tissues, which in turn cause a loss of function of the involved organ or tissue. For example, a kidney tumor may progress to renal failure. Pressure against the superior vena cava from an adjacent lung tumor or tumor-infiltrated lymph nodes can interrupt the blood flow to the heart.

In the liver, either a primary hepatocellular cancer or metastatic lesion can have several significant effects:

- In liver parenchymal tissue, it impairs the multiple life-sustaining functions of the liver, such as carbohydrate metabolism, synthesis of plasma proteins, detoxification, and immunologic functions. These functional impairments result in severe nutritional, hormonal, hematologic, and immunologic problems. (See Chapter 19 for a more complete discussion of liver functions and effects of disruption. ⊙⊙)
- Because more than 1 L of blood per minute passes through the liver via the portal vein, obstruction to this flow by a tumor can cause portal hypertension. This results in backup of fluid and increased pressure in the splanchnic circulation. The end result is ascites (third-spaced fluid in the peritoneal cavity) and varices (friable, overdistended blood vessels) of the esophageal, gastric, mesenteric, and hemorrhoidal vessels.

Hematologic Alterations

Hematologic alterations can impair the normal function of blood cells. For example, in leukemia, a malignant proliferative disease of the hematopoietic (blood cell–producing) system, the immature leukocytes cannot perform the normal protective phagocytic functions and immunity is compromised. Additionally, the excessive numbers of immature leukocytes in the bone marrow diminish erythrocyte and thrombocyte (platelet) production, resulting in secondary anemia and clotting disorders (Scigliano, Vlachos, Najfeld, & Shank, 2001).

Other examples of hematologic alteration include the following:

- Gastrointestinal tumors disrupt the absorption of vitamin B_{12} and iron.
- Growing tumors need purines and folate and have a unique ability to accumulate and store these substances. Thus, the tumor deprives the bone marrow of these substances, which are needed for erythropoiesis (red blood cell production).
- Renal cell carcinoma produces its own erythropoietin hormone, which causes an excessively large number of red blood cells to be produced and dumped into the bloodstream. The resulting polycythemia causes viscous blood, which impairs circulation, plugs small capillaries, and promotes thrombus formation.

Infection

If the tumor invades and connects two incompatible organs, such as the bowel and bladder, and thus creates a fistula, infection becomes a serious problem. As they destroy viable tissue and thus their source of nutrition, tumors may become necrotic and septicemia may result. Some tumors are less efficient in creating capillaries; as a consequence, the center of the tumor may become necrotic and infected. When a tumor grows near the surface of the body, it may erode through to the surface, thus breaking down the natural defenses of intact skin and mucous membranes and providing a site for the entry of microorganisms. Any malignant involvement of the organs or tissues of immunity—such as the liver, bone marrow, Peyer's patches in the small intestine, spleen, or lymph nodes—can seriously impair the immune response, allowing infections to develop in vulnerable tissues.

Hemorrhage

Tumor erosion through blood vessels can cause extensive bleeding, giving rise to severe anemia. Hemorrhage can be serious enough to cause life-threatening hypovolemic shock.

Anorexia-Cachexia Syndrome

A characteristic feature of cancer is the wasted appearance of its victims, called **cachexia**. In many cases, unexplained rapid weight loss is the first symptom that brings the client to a health care provider. This can be due to a variety of problems associated with cancer, such as pain, infection, depression, or the side effects of chemotherapy and radiation. Usually, however, the emaciation, malnutrition, and loss of energy are attributed to the anorexia-cachexia syndrome.

This syndrome is specific to cancer because of the effect of cancer cells on the host's metabolism. The neoplastic cells divert nutrition to their own use while causing changes that reduce the client's appetite. Early in the disease, glucose metabolism is altered, causing an increase in serum glucose levels. Through the process of negative feedback, anorexia (loss of appetite) results. In addition, the tumor secretes substances that decrease appetite by altering taste and smell and producing early satiety. Pain, infection, and depression also contribute to anorexia. Some types of cancers cause specific food aversions, such as to red meat, coffee, or chocolate.

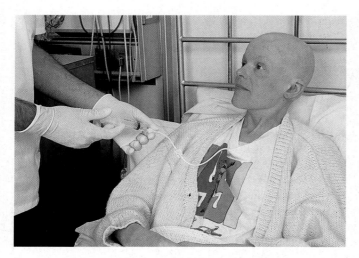

Figure 10–4 ■ Cachexic person. Cancer robs its host of nutrients and increases body catabolism of fat and muscle to meet its metabolic needs.

Source: Photo Researchers, Inc.

TABLE 10–4	Laboratory Indicators of Ectopic Functioning
Hormone	**Specific Laboratory Test**
Antidiuretic hormone (ADH)	Serum and urine osmolality
Adrenocorticotropic hormone (ACTH)	Plasma ACTH ACTH suppression test ACTH stimulation test Urine catecholamines
Calcitonin	Serum calcitonin
Insulin	Serum glucose Glucose tolerance test
Parathyroid hormone (PTH)	Serum PTH Serum calcium
Thyroxine	Serum thyroid-stimulating hormone (TSH), T_3, T_4

Avaricious cancer cells support their growth through widespread catabolism of the body's tissue and muscle proteins. This catabolism, coupled with inadequate nutrient intake, results in the typical cachexia. Normally, a starvation state reduces the body's basal metabolic rate. However, in many people with cancer, the metabolic rate is increased, probably because of the hyperactive metabolic and reproductive activities of the malignant cells. One theory suggests that cytokinins the body produces in response to the tumor are responsible for both early satiety and cachexia. One specific cytokine, called tumor necrosis factor-alpha or cachectin, is believed to enhance the increased metabolic consumption of nutrients. Cancers of the gastrointestinal system further promote anorexia-cachexia by decreasing absorption and use of nutrients; the side effects of some treatment modalities enhance this effect. Figure 10–4 ■ shows the characteristic appearance of a cachexic person.

Paraneoplastic Syndromes

Paraneoplastic syndromes are indirect effects of cancer. They may be early warning signs of cancer or indicate complications or return of a malignancy. The most frequently occurring paraneoplastic syndromes are endocrine, occurring when cancers set up ectopic sites of hormone production (Haapoja, 2000). Table 10–4 lists laboratory indicators of ectopic funtioning. These ectopic sites produce excessive amounts of the hormone, which harm the host. Consider the following examples.

- Breast, ovarian, and renal cancers may set up ectopic parathyroid hormone sites, causing severe hypercalcemia.
- Oat cell and other lung cancers may produce ectopic secretions of insulin (causing hypoglycemia), parathyroid hormone (PTH), antidiuretic hormone (ADH, which causes excessive fluid retention, hypertension, and peripheral edema), and adrenocorticotropic hormone (ACTH). See Chapter 20 for the description of the multiple problems caused by excessive secretions of cortisone. ⊖⊖

Other paraneoplastic syndromes include hematological abnormalities such as anemia, thrombocytopenia, and coagulation abnormalities; nephrotic syndrome; cutaneous syndromes; and neurological syndromes, such as distant tumors that produce increased intracranial pressure (Haapoja, 2000).

Pain

Pain is ranked as one of the most serious concerns of clients, families, and oncology health care professionals. Because pain management for people with cancer has a reputation for being ineffective, the anticipation of pain may engender fear in even the most stoic people. Most persons fear pain and suffering even more than possible death, although pain management strategies have improved tremendously. The findings from a 10-year study of over 2000 patients in a palliative care program are encouraging. Following the World Health Organization Guidelines for cancer pain relief, 88% of patients reported good to satisfactory pain relief (Zech, Grond, Lynch, Hertel, & Lehmann, 1995). Research on pain with its devastating statistics has led to great improvement in the pain management strategies.

TYPES OF CANCER PAIN. Cancer pain can be divided into two main categories, acute and chronic, with subgroupings. These classifications serve to indicate appropriate therapeutic approaches. Acute pain has a well-defined pattern of onset, exhibits common signs and symptoms, and is often identified with hyperactivity of the autonomic system. Chronic pain, which lasts more than 6 months, frequently lacks the objective manifestations of acute pain, primarily because the autonomic nervous system adapts to this chronic stress. Unfortunately, chronic pain often results in personality changes, alterations in functional abilities, and lifestyle disruptions that can seriously affect compliance with treatment and the quality of life.

Most cancer clients who cite acute pain as the primary symptom that led to the diagnosis tend to associate pain with the introduction to their disease. If these clients experience pain during the illness or after therapy, they often perceive the pain as introducing another cancer or as a recurrence of the original cancer. Other clients report experiencing pain as a component of cancer therapy. These clients often are able to endure the pain in anticipation of a successful outcome of treatment.

Chronic pain may be related to treatment or may indicate progression of the disease. Identifying the pain as treatment related rather than tumor related is extremely important because it has a definite effect on the client's psychologic outlook. For the client whose pain is due to the advancement of the disease, psychologic factors play an even more important role. Hopelessness and fear of impending death intensify physiologic pain and contribute to overall suffering (which goes well beyond just physical pain).

Three other categories used to classify clients with cancer pain are worth mentioning: clients with preexisting pain, those with a history of drug abuse, and dying clients with cancer-related pain. The first two groups may have altered perceptions of pain and may not have the anticipated response to pain medication. For the dying client, pain is strongly associated with both the client's and family's confrontation of issues of hopelessness and death. Confronting these issues can intensify the perception of pain (see Chapter 4). ⌘

CAUSES OF CANCER PAIN. Direct tumor involvement is the primary cause of the pain experienced by people with cancer. This includes metastatic bone disease, nerve compression, and involvement of visceral organs. The pain from tumor involvement is believed to be mechanical, resulting from stretching of tissues and compression. Chemicals from ischemia or tumor metabolites and toxins that activate and sensitize nociceptors and mechanoreceptors are also responsible for tumor pain. See Chapter 4 for a more complete discussion of the mechanics of pain.

Side effects or toxic effects of cancer therapies (e.g., surgery, radiation, and chemotherapy) may also cause cancer pain. These are usually the result of traumatized tissue; one example of this is the oropharyngeal ulcerations that occur with some types of chemotherapy. However, these therapies may also be used to manage pain, such as radiation to decrease pain associated with bone metastasis.

Physical Stress

When the immune system discovers a neoplasm, it tries to destroy it using the resources of the body. The body mounts an all-out assault on the foreign invader, calling on many resources:

- Chemical mediators
- Hormones and enzymes
- Blood cells
- Antibodies
- Proteins
- Inflammatory and immune responses

These protective responses also mobilize fluid, electrolytes, and nutritional systems. This massive effort requires tremendous energy. See Chapters 5 and 19 for specific information on these systems. ⌘ If the neoplasm is small enough (i.e., microscopic), the immune system can destroy it, and a tumor will never manifest. A neoplasm of 1 cm is large enough to overwhelm most immune systems; however, the body will continue

to try to fight it until it reaches the stage of exhaustion and is no longer capable (Selye, 1984). Thus, many clients with cancer present with fatigue, weight loss, anemia, dehydration, and altered blood chemistries (e.g., decreases in electrolytes).

Psychologic Stress

People confronted with the diagnosis of cancer exhibit a variety of psychologic and emotional responses. Some people see cancer as a death sentence and experience overwhelming grief, often giving up. Others may feel guilt, considering the cancer a punishment for past behaviors, such as smoking, unhealthy eating habits, or for delaying diagnosis or treatment. The person may experience anger, especially if the person believes that he or she had been practicing a healthful lifestyle; beneath that anger may reside feelings of powerlessness. Fear is common: fear of the outcome of the illness, fear of the

---

BOX 10–5 ■ Physiologic and Psychosocial Effects of Cancer

- Disruption of function (due to obstruction or pressure)
- Hematologic alterations
  - a. Decreased leukocytes, erythrocytes, and thrombocytes
  - b. Altered erythropoiesis
- Infections
  - a. Fistula between noncompatible organs
  - b. Necrosis of tumor center
  - c. Malignant involvement of organs of immunity
- Hemorrhage (caused by erosion of neoplasm through blood vessels or surface of skin)
- Anorexia-cachexia syndrome
  - a. Hyperglycemia
  - b. Catabolism of tissue and muscle proteins
  - c. Altered taste and smell
- Creation of ectopic sites of hormones
  - a. PTH   c. ADH
  - b. Insulin   d. ACTH
- Paraneoplastic syndromes
  - a. Deep-vein thrombosis
  - b. Peripheral nerve problems
  - c. Increased intracranial pressure
  - d. Anorexia-cachexia syndrome
  - e. Nephritic syndrome
- Pain
  - a. Acute and chronic
  - b. Caused by direct tumor involvement or side effects of therapy
- Physical stress
  - a. Increased general adaptation syndrome activity
  - b. Increased immunologic activity
  - c. Increased inflammatory response activity
  - d. Nutritional, fluid, and electrolyte alterations
- Psychologic stress
  - a. Grief   e. Fear
  - b. Hopelessness   f. Isolation
  - c. Guilt   g. Body image concerns
  - d. Anger   h. Sexual dysfunction

Note. Manifestations depend on the type and location of the cancer.

effects of treatment, fear of pain, fear of death. Some people feel isolated because of the stigma of cancer and old beliefs of contagion. Body image concerns and sexual dysfunction may be present but often unexpressed, especially if the cancer is of the breast or sexual organs or causes visible body changes. Box 10–5 summarizes the physiologic and psychosocial effects of cancer.

COLLABORATIVE CARE

Collaborative care begins with a variety of specialized laboratory and diagnostic tests. Once cancer is diagnosed, the initial focus is on medical treatment. The goals of treatment are:

- Eliminating the tumor or malignant cells.
- Preventing metastasis.
- Reducing cellular growth and the tumor burden.
- Promoting functional abilities and providing pain relief to those whose disease has not responded to treatment.

Laboratory and Diagnostic Tests

Diagnosis
Several procedures are used to diagnose cancer. X-ray imaging, computed tomography, ultrasonography, and magnetic resonance imaging can locate abnormal tissues or tumors. However, only microscopic histologic examination of the tissue reveals the type of cell and its structural difference from the parent tissue. Tissue samples are acquired through biopsy, shedded cells (e.g., Papanicolaou smear), or collections of secretions (e.g., sputum). Lymph nodes are also biopsied to determine whether metastasis has begun. Simple screening procedures can be used to pick up substances secreted by the tumor, such as the prostatic-specific antigen (PSA) blood test now being used to identify early prostatic cancers. Increases in enzymes or hormones released by normal tissues when they are damaged can also contribute to the diagnosis. Increased alkaline phosphatase noted in bone metastases and osteosarcoma is one example of an enzyme increase associated with cancer. Recent research has identified tumor markers; they are used for early diagnosis, tracking response to therapy, and for devising immunologic treatments.

Some investigators studying chemical mediators of the immune system have noted that there seems to be communication between the chemical mediators and the emotional centers of the brain. A person who states, "I feel I have cancer," should be listened to, and the complaint investigated thoroughly.

Classification
To help standardize diagnosis and treatment protocols, an elaborate identification system has been developed. This consists of naming the tumor (classification) and describing its aggressiveness (grading) and spread within or beyond the tissue of origin (staging).

Tumors are classified and named by the tissue or cell of origin. Tumor nomenclature often incorporates the Latin stem identifying the tissue from which the tumor arises. For example, a carcinoma arises from epithelial tissue; adjectives are added to further specify the location. A glandular malignancy arising from epithelial tissue is classified as an adenocarcinoma. A tumor arising from supportive tissues is called a sarcoma; the specific type of tissue is added as a prefix. For example, a cancer of fibrous connective tissue is called fibrosarcoma, and a smooth muscle cancer is a leiomyosarcoma. A tumor from seminal or germ tissue is called a seminoma. Table 10–5 compares the nomenclature of benign and malignant neoplasms.

Other names for tumors incorporate the name of the discoverer of that particular cancer, such as Burkitt's lymphoma or Hodgkin's disease. Hematopoietic malignancies (also known as "liquid tumors") are usually named by the type of immature blood cell that predominates. An example is myelocytic leukemia, named for the immature form of the granulocyte that is predominant in this malignancy.

Grading and Staging
Grading evaluates the amount of differentiation (level of functional maturity) of the cell and estimates the rate of growth based on the mitotic rate. Cells which are the most differentiated—that is, most like the parent tissue and therefore the least malignant—are classified as grade 1 and are associated with a better prognosis. Grade 4 is reserved for the least differentiated and most aggressively malignant cells. Because of the differences inherent in tumor appearance and biologic behavior, grading criteria may vary with different locations and types of tumors.

Staging is used to classify solid tumors and refers to the relative size of the tumor and extent of the disease. The TNM classification system is an internationally agreed upon staging system: The T stands for the relative tumor size, depth of invasion, and surface spread; N indicates the presence and extent of lymph node involvement; and M denotes the presence or absence of distant metastases. Table 10–6 shows the basic outline of the TNM system; however, there are other systems used to differentiate types and locations of tumors (e.g., melanomas, cervical cancer, Hodgkin's disease).

Cytologic Examination
For the malignant tissues to be identified by name, grade, and stage, they must first be subjected to histologic and cytologic examination by light or electron microscope. Specimens are collected by three basic methods:

1. *Exfoliation from an epithelial surface.* Examples include scraping cells from the cervix (Pap smear) or bronchial washings.
2. *Aspiration of fluid from body cavities or blood.* Examples include white blood cells for evaluation of hematopoietic cancers, pleural fluid, and cerebral spinal fluid.
3. *Needle aspiration of solid tumors.* This could include the breast, lung, or prostate.

Cytologic examination is also carried out on specimens from biopsied tissues or tumors and on collected body secretions, such as sputum or urine.

TABLE 10-5 Nomenclature for Benign and Malignant Neoplasms

	Tissue of Origin	Benign	Malignant
Ectoderm/Endoderm	Epithelium	Papilloma	Carcinoma
	Gland	Adenoma	Adenocarcinoma
	Liver cells	Hepatocellular adenoma	Hepatocellular carcinoma
	Neuroglia	Glioma	Glioma
	Melanocytes	Melanoma	Malignant melanoma
	Basal cells		Basal cell carcinoma
	Germ cells	Tetroma	Seminoma
Mesoderm	Connective tissue		
	Adipose tissue	Lipoma	Liposarcoma
	Fibrous tissue	Fibroma	Fibrosarcoma
	Bone tissue	Osteoma	Osteosarcoma
	Cartilage	Chondroma	Chondrosarcoma
	Muscle		
	Smooth muscle	Leiomyoma	Leiomyosarcoma
	Striated muscle	Rhabdomyoma	Rhabdomyosarcoma
	Neural tissue		
	Nerve cells	Ganglioneuroma	Neuroblastoma
	Endothelial tissues		
	Blood vessels	Hemangioma	Angiosarcoma
			Kaposi's sarcoma
	Meninges	Meningioma	Malignant meningioma
Hematopoietic Tissues	Granulocytes	Granulocytosis	Leukemia
	Plasma cells		Multiple myeloma
	Lymphocytes		Lymphomas

After collection, specimens are spread on a glass slide, fixed, and stained if necessary. The morphologic features of the cells are examined, with special attention to the nucleus and cytoplasm. Other special pathologic procedures can be carried out on the specimen, but they must be ordered ahead of time if special preparations of the specimen are necessary.

Several special diagnostic cytologic procedures, such as cytogenetics, are proving useful in diagnosing and monitoring client response to treatment.

TABLE 10-6 TNM Staging Classification System

	Stage	Manifestations
Tumor	T_0	No evidence of primary tumor.
	T_{IS}	Tumor in situ.
	T_1, T_2, T_3, T_4	Ascending degrees of tumor size and involvement.
Nodes	N_0	No abnormal regional nodes.
	N_{1a}, N_{2a}	Regional nodes—no metastasis.
	N_{1b}, N_{2b}, N_{3b}	Regional lymph nodes— metastasis suspected.
	N_x	Regional nodes cannot be assessed clinically.
Metastasis	M_0	No evidence of distant metastasis.
	M_1, M_2, M_3	Ascending degrees of metastatic involvement of the host including distant nodes.

Tumor Markers

A tumor marker is a protein molecule detectable in serum or other body fluids. This marker is used as a biochemical indicator of the presence of a malignancy. Small amounts of tumor marker proteins are found in normal body tissues or benign tumors and are not specific for malignancy. However, high levels are suspicious and mandate follow-up diagnostic studies. Tumor marker tests are in the developmental and investigational phase and are most useful for monitoring the client's response to therapy and for detecting residual disease. However, one marker, prostatic-specific antigen (PSA) has received a great deal of media attention as a detector of prostate cancer. As a result, many health care practitioners recommend screening for it in men over 40, much as Pap smears and mammograms are recommended for women.

Tumor markers fall into two general categories: those derived from the tumor itself and those associated with host (immune) response to the tumor. Examples of tumor markers include the following:

- *Antigens.* These are present in fetal tissue but normally are suppressed after birth. Thus, their presence in large amounts may reflect an anaplastic process in tumor cells. Alpha-fetoprotein (AFP) and carcinoembryonic antigen (CEA) are oncofetal antigens.
- *Hormones.* Hormones are, of course, present in considerable amounts in human blood and tissues, but very high levels not related to other conditions may signify the presence

TABLE 10-7   Tumor-Derived Markers Associated with Specific Neoplasms

	Tumor Marker	Associated Neoplasm
Oncofetal Antigens	Carcinoembryonic antigen (CEA) Alpha-fetoprotein (AFP)	Adenocarcinomas of colon, lung, breast, ovary, stomach, pancreas Hepatocellular carcinoma, gonadal germ cell tumors (seminoma)
Hormones	Human chorionic gonadotropin (HCG) Calcitonin Catecholamines/metabolites	Gonadal germ cell tumors Medullary cancer of thyroid Pheochromocytoma
Isoenzymes	Prostatic acid phosphatase (PAP) Neuron-specific enolase	Adenocarcinoma of prostate Small-cell lung carcinoma, neuroblastoma
Specific Proteins	Prostate-specific antigen (PSA) Immunoglobin CA 125 CA 19-9 CA 15-3	Adenocarcinoma of prostate Multiple myeloma Epithelial ovarian cancer Adenocarcinoma of pancreas, colon Breast cancer

Note. Adapted from "The Pathologic Evaluation of Neoplastic Disease" by J. D. Pfeifer and M. R. Wick, in American Cancer Society Textbook of Clinical Oncology (pp. 75–95) by A. I. Holleb, D. J. Fink, and G. P. Murphy, Eds., 1995, Atlanta: American Cancer Society.

of a hormone-secreting malignancy. Some common hormones seen as tumor markers include human chorionic gonadotropin (HCG), antidiuretic hormone (ADH), parathyroid hormone (PTH), calcitonin, and catecholamines.

- *Proteins.* These narrow down the type of tissue that may be malignant, although they can also be increased in hyperplastic disorders. Examples of tissue-specific proteins include serum immunoglobin and beta-2 microglobulin.
- *Enzymes.* Rapid, excessive growth of a tissue may cause some of the enzymes and isoenzymes normally present in that particular tissue to spill into the bloodstream. Elevated levels can point to either hyperplasia of the tissue or cancer. Prostatic acid phosphatase (PAP) and neuron-specific enolase (NSE) are examples. Table 10–7 compares selected tumor-derived markers with their presence in neoplasms and other conditions.

Oncologic Imaging

Because physical assessment usually cannot detect cancer until the tumor has reached a size that poses a major risk for metastasis, radiologic examination is extremely important in early diagnosis. This diagnostic process may involve routine X-ray imaging (usually for screening only), computed tomography, magnetic resonance imaging, ultrasonography, nuclear imaging, angiography, positron emission tomography, and tagged antibodies.

X-RAY IMAGING. Considered the least expensive and least invasive diagnostic procedure, film screen imaging (standard X-ray imaging) is the method of choice for screening such body areas as the breast (mammography), lung, and bone to identify changes in tissue density that may indicate malignancies. X-ray studies are limited in that they do not easily distinguish among calcifications, benign cystic growths, and true malignancies. However, as a screening tool, X-ray imaging can usually reas-sure the client if findings are negative or encourage follow-up studies if findings are suspicious. X-ray imaging is still the method of choice for lung cancer. Unfortunately, it does not usually reveal tumors until they have reached about 1 cm in size, which is late in their development.

COMPUTED TOMOGRAPHY. Computed tomography (CT) has vastly advanced the effectiveness of traditional X-ray methods. By applying computers and mathematics to diagnostic imaging, CT allows the visualization of cross sections of the anatomy. Because CT scans reveal subtle differences in tissue densities, they provide much greater accuracy in tumor diagnosis. This procedure, although more expensive than X-ray imaging, is useful in the screening for some cancers such as renal cell and most gastrointestinal tumors. CT scans are especially useful to evaluate possible lymph node involvement.

MAGNETIC RESONANCE IMAGING. Like CT, magnetic resonance imaging (MRI) involves computerized mathematical technology. The patient is placed within a strong magnetic field, pulsed radio waves are directed at the patient, and transmitted signals based on tissue characteristics are analyzed by a computer. Related diagnostic imaging procedures—positron emission tomography (PET) and single photon emission computed tomography (SPECT)—create visible images by measuring electrical impulses from different body structures. Although MRI is relatively expensive, it is the diagnostic tool of choice for both screening and follow-up of cranial and head and neck tumors.

Some clients become claustrophobic during the MRI procedure because they must be placed inside the diagnostic imaging machine, an experience that has been likened to being encased in a small tube. In addition, some machines make loud thumping sounds that can be frightening if the client is not informed beforehand that this is normal.

ULTRASONOGRAPHY. Ultrasonography is relatively safe and noninvasive. It measures sound waves as they bounce off various body structures, giving an image of normal anatomy as well as revealing abnormalities that indicate tumors. Ultrasonography has been adapted for diagnosing some specific tumors. For example, transrectal ultrasonography has provided excellent imaging of early prostate cancers and is used to guide needle biopsy. Ultrasound imaging is also more useful for detecting masses in the denser breast tissue of young women.

NUCLEAR IMAGING. Nuclear imaging involves the use of a special scintillation scanner in conjunction with the ingestion or injection of specific radioactive isotopes. This is an invasive but usually safe diagnostic method for identifying tumors in various body tissues. For the client with a newly diagnosed cancer, the procedure is often used to check for possible bone or other organ metastases. This evaluation helps the health care provider determine appropriate treatment.

The principle underlying the technology is that certain isotopes have an affinity for specific tissues; for example, radioactive iodine (I 131) has an affinity for the thyroid gland. Malignancies in these tissues sequester an abnormally large amount of the isotope, which then can be traced and measured by the scintillation scanner. This procedure is considered safe because the amount of isotope used is small enough not to damage normal cells.

The procedure is usually minimally distressing for clients. Drinking the isotope solution is not pleasant but is tolerable; some anxious clients may have difficulty lying still during the scan. Antianxiety medication may help. Some clients may experience nausea from drinking the isotope and require antiemetic drugs to complete the procedure. Client preparation may include allowing nothing by mouth or clear fluids only after midnight.

ANGIOGRAPHY. An expensive and invasive procedure, angiography is used infrequently for tumor diagnosis. Angiography is performed when the precise location of the tumor cannot be identified or there is a need to visualize the tumor's extent prior to surgery. The procedure involves injecting a radiopaque dye into a major blood vessel proximal to the organ or tissue to be examined. The movement of the dye through the vasculature of the organ or tissue is then traced by means of fluoroscopy or serial X-ray films. In some cases, small catheters are threaded through the vein under fluoroscopy to ensure the specific placement of the dye. Blockage to the flow of the dye indicates the tumor's location. Dye may also be used to identify blood vessels supplying a tumor, allowing the surgeon to know where to safely ligate vessels. Angiography requires preparation similar to that for minor surgery. This includes ensuring that the client takes in only fluids on the day of the examination, performing skin preparation at the insertion site, and administering sedative drugs prior to the procedure. Clients should be informed that injection of the dye used to enhance imaging may cause a hot, flushing sensation or nausea and vomiting. Although angiography is usually done on an outpatient basis, the client will be kept in a short-stay unit for several hours and monitored for such complications as bleeding at the catheter insertion site.

Direct Visualization

Direct visualization procedures are invasive but do not require the use of radiography. Examples include the following:

- Sigmoidoscopy (viewing the sigmoid colon with a fiberoptic flexible sigmoidoscope)
- Cystoscopy (viewing the urethra and bladder)
- Endoscopy (viewing the upper gastrointestinal tract)
- Bronchoscopy (inspecting the tracheobronchial tree)

These methods allow the visual identification of the organs within the limits of the scope and usually permit biopsy of suspicious lesions or masses. Flexible fiberoptic scopes may be more useful, because they allow deeper penetration than do traditional scopes. These procedures all require some client preparation, cause moderate to considerable discomfort, and may require sedation or even anesthesia, as in the case of bronchoscopy. Some procedures, such as sigmoidoscopy and cystoscopy, may be performed in the physician's office and therefore cost less, making them more accessible screening procedures.

Client preparation includes a thorough bowel cleansing prior to the sigmoidoscopy and cystoscopy; the client may ingest only liquids the morning of the procedure. Because anesthesia may be required, clients undergoing bronchoscopy and endoscopy may be instructed to have nothing by mouth from midnight until the procedure. These procedures are discussed in greater detail in later chapters of this textbook. A more radical method of direct visualization for suspected malignancies is exploratory surgery with biopsy. The client undergoes the usual preoperative preparation (see Chapter 7 ⊙) for the type of surgery anticipated. When the tumor is exposed, a sample of tissue (biopsy) is sent to the pathology laboratory for a "frozen-section" histologic examination. This can be done rapidly while the client remains on the operating table under anesthesia. If the initial report is negative, the benign mass is usually removed to prevent further symptoms. If the report is positive for cancer, the tumor and, often, adjacent lymph nodes are resected, along with any other suspicious tissue. The tumor, nodes, and any other specimens are sent to the pathology laboratory for more in-depth analysis. The client then receives the usual postoperative care.

Laboratory Tests

Most laboratory tests of blood, urine, and other body fluids are used to rule out nutritional disorders and other noncancerous conditions that may be causing the client's symptoms. For example, a complete blood count (CBC) helps screen for such problems as anemia, infection, and impaired immunity. Blood chemistries can point out nutritional disturbances and electrolyte imbalances. However, in conjunction with other diagnostic studies, some laboratory tests can be quite useful either in screening for other pathologic conditions or for validating the cancer diagnosis (Kee, 2002). These

TABLE 10–8   Laboratory Tests Used for Cancer Diagnosis*

Test	Reference Value	Abnormality Indicated
Acid phosphatase (ACP)	0.0 to 0.8 U/L	Elevated in prostate, breast, and bone cancer and in multiple myeloma
Adrenocorticotropic hormone (ACTH)	8 to 80 pg/mL	Decreased in adrenal cancer Elevated in pituitary cancer or with tumor that secretes ACTH (bronchiogenic cancer)
Alanine aminotransferase (ALT)	5 to 35 U/mL (Frankel)	Moderate elevation in liver cancer
Albumin	3.5 to 5.0 g/dL	Decreased in malnutrition, metastatic liver cancer
Alkaline phosphatase (ALP)	20 to 90 U/L	Elevated in cancer of liver, bone, breast, and prostate, in leukemia, and in multiple myeloma
Alpha fetoprotein (AFP)	Male and nonpregnant female: <15 ng/mL	Elevated in germ cell tumors (e.g., seminoma), testicular cancer
Aspartate aminotransferase (AST)	5 to 40 U/mL (Frankel)	Elevated in liver cancer
Bilirubin	Total: 0.1 to1.2 mg/dL Direct: 0.0 to 0.3 mg/dL	Elevated in liver and gallbladder cancer
Bleeding time	Ivy method: 3 to 7 minutes	Prolonged in leukemia and metastatic liver cancer
Blood urea nitrogen (BUN)	5 to 25 mg/dL	Decreased in malnutrition; increased in renal cancer
Calcitonin	Male: <40 pg/mL Female: <20 pg/mL	Elevated to >500 pg/mL in thyroid medullary cancer, breast cancer, and lung cancer
Calcium (Ca)	4.5 to 5.5 mEq/L 9.0 to 11.0 mg/dL	Elevated in bone cancer and ectopic parathyroid hormone production (paraplastic syndrome)
Carcinoembryonic antigen (CEA)	2.5 ng/mL in nonsmokers 5 ng/mL in smokers; >12 ng/mL neoplasms	Elevated with GI cancers, lung, breast, bladder, kidney, cervical, leukemias Used to evaluate effectiveness of cancer treatment
Chloride (Cl)	95 to 105 mEq/L	Decreased in vomiting, diarrhea, syndrome of inappropriate antidiuretic hormone (SIADH)
C-reactive protein	>1:2 titer is positive	Elevated in metastatic cancer and Burkitt's lymphoma
Creatinine	0.5 to 1.5 mg/dL	Decreased in malnutrition; elevated in most cancers
Dexamethasone suppression test	>50% reduction in plasma cortisol	Nonsuppression in adrenal cancer and ACTH-producing tumors, severe stress
Estradiol-Serum	Female: 20 to 300 pg/mL Menopausal female: <20 pg/mL Male: 15 to 50 pg/mL	Elevated in estrogen-producing tumors and testicular tumors
Fibrinogen	200 to 400 mg/dL	Decreased in leukemia and as a side effect of chemotherapy
Gamma glutamyltransferase (GGT)	Male: 10 to 80 IU/L Female: 5 to 25 IU/L	Elevated in cancer of liver, pancreas, prostate, breast, kidney, lung, and brain
Fasting blood sugar	70 to 110 mg/dL	Decreased in malnutrition, cancer of stomach, liver, and lung
Haptoglobin	20 to 240 mg/dL	Elevated in Hodgkin's disease and cancer of lung, large intestine, stomach, breast, and liver
Hematocrit (Hct)	Male: 40% to 54% Female: 36% to 46%	Decreased in anemia, leukemia, Hodgkin's disease, lymphosarcoma, multiple myeloma, and malnutrition and as a side effect of chemotherapy
Hemoglobin (Hgb)	Male: 13.5 to 18 g/dL Female: 12 to 16 g/dL 1:3 ratio of Hgb:Hct	Decreased in anemia, many cancers, Hodgkin's disease, leukemia, and malnutrition and as a side effect of chemotherapy
Human chorionic gonadotropin (HCG)	Nonpregnant female <0.01 IU/L	Elevated in choriocarcinoma
Insulin	5 to 25 µU/mL	Elevated in insulinoma (islet cell tumor) and insulin-secreting cancers (e.g., lung cancer)
Lactic dehydrogenase (LDH)	100 to 190 IU/L	Elevated in liver, brain, kidney, muscle cancers, acute leukemia, anemia

*All values refer to serum values unless otherwise indicated. Values are approximate; check the reference standards specified by your own agency's laboratory.

TABLE 10–8   Laboratory Tests Used for Cancer Diagnosis* (continued)

Test	Reference Value	Abnormality Indicated
Occult blood	Negative	Positive in gastric and colon cancers
Serum osmolality	280 to 300 mOsm/kg H_2O	Decreased in SIADH
Urine osmolality	50 to 1200 mOsm/kg H_2O	Increased in SIADH
Parathyroid hormone (PTH)	400 to 900 pg/mL	Increased in PTH-secreting tumors
Platelet (thrombocyte) count	150,000/mm^3 to 400,000/mm^3	Decreased in bone, gastric, and brain cancer, in leukemia, and as a side effect of chemotherapy
Potassium (K)	3.5 to 5.0 mEq/L	Decreased in vomiting and diarrhea and in malnutrition
Prostate-specific antigen (PSA)	0 to 4 ng/mL	Elevated from 10 to 120+ in prostate cancer
Total protein	6.0 to 8.0 g/dL	Decreased in malnutrition, gastrointestinal cancer, Hodgkin's disease; elevated in vomiting, diarrhea, multiple myeloma
Red blood cells (RBCs)	Male: 4.6 to 6.0 million/mm^3 Female: 4.0 to 5.0 million/mm^3	Decreased in anemia, leukemia, infection, multiple myeloma
Sodium (Na)	135 to 145 mEq/L	Decreased in SIADH, vomiting; elevated in dehydration
Uric acid	Male: 3.5 to 8.0 mg/dL Female: 2.8 to 6.8 mg/dL	Increased in leukemia, metastatic cancer, multiple myeloma, Burkitt's lymphoma, after vigorous chemotherapy
White blood cells (WBC) Total leukocytes	4,500/mm^3 to 10,000/mm^3	Elevated in acute infection, leukemias, tissue necrosis; decreased as a side effect of chemotherapy
Neutrophils	50% to 70%	Elevated in bacterial infection Hodgkin's disease; decreased in leukemia and malnutrition and as a side effect of chemotherapy
Eosinophils	1% to 3%	Elevated in cancer of bone, ovary, testes, and brain
Basophils	0.4% to 1.0%	Elevated in leukemia and healing stage of infection
Monocytes	4% to 6%	Elevated in infection, monocytic leukemia and cancer; decreased in lymphocytic leukemia and as a side effect of chemotherapy
Lymphocytes	25% to 35%	Elevated in lymphocytic leukemia, Hodgkin's disease, multiple myeloma, viral infections, and chronic infections; decreased in malnutrition, cancer, and other leukemias and as a side effect of chemotherapy

tests include evaluating levels of enzymes such as alanine aminotransferase (ALT), aspartate aminotransferase (AST), and lactic dehydrogenase (LDH) for liver metastases. Special protein tumor markers such as PSA for prostate cancer and CEA for colon cancer are also used. Table 10–8 identifies some useful laboratory tests, their normal values, and their possible indications.

Psychologic Support During Diagnosis

Preparing for and awaiting the results of diagnostic tests can create extreme anxiety. Many clients compare the experience to that of a prisoner awaiting trial and sentencing: After they know what the "sentence" is, then they can prepare for the future. In addition to coping with the possibility of a life-threatening disease, or at least a life-altering one, clients often also face the prospect of uncomfortable, even painful, diagnostic procedures. They have important decisions to make that depend on the outcome of those tests. Many unspoken questions may exist, including the following:

- Do I have cancer?
- If so, what kind, and how serious?
- Has it spread?
- Will I survive?
- What kind of treatment is needed?
- How will this affect my lifestyle?
- How will this affect family members and friends?

Denial or intellectualization serve some clients well, but others display signs of anxiety and stress as they attempt to cope with this perceived menace. The nurse can provide valuable support during this very difficult stage by helping clients become actively involved in managing their life and disease. Talk with clients as soon as they enter the health care system, asking what they know already about what is going to happen and soliciting questions from them. Taking this approach and encouraging clients to share what knowledge and experience they have allows them to maintain control. From there, the nurse can provide the information needed.

It is essential that clients thoroughly understand the preparation required for their tests, especially if they will be preparing at home. They also need to be informed of any unusual effects that may occur as a result of the procedure, such as nausea from radioactive dye. If possible, a phone call the evening before to verify the client's understanding of the procedure and to answer questions can be helpful and supportive.

As clients begin to feel more comfortable with the nurse, they may express concerns, fears, and other emotions. The nurse should actively listen and be supportive, but avoid giving advice and false reassurance, providing appropriate information when needed. For clients who are not ready to discuss concerns or for those who appear angry, being nonjudgmental and providing nonverbal support may facilitate more open communication. An atmosphere of calmness, warmth, caring, and respect can ease the tension and often unspoken terror of this initial period.

Support of and communication with the client's significant others is extremely important. Often they try to be strong for the client but have many fears and emotional concerns that they do not feel comfortable expressing. The nurse needs to be available to the family while the client is undergoing diagnostic procedures. Allowing them to talk without the need to edit for the client's benefit can help them manage their own difficulties in coping with their loved one's potential cancer diagnosis.

Chemotherapy

The goals of cancer treatment are aimed at cure, control, or palliation of symptoms. These goals may overlap. Cancer may be treated through chemotherapy, surgery, radiation therapy, or biotherapy. **Chemotherapy** involves the use of cytotoxic medications to cure some cancers, such as leukemias, lymphomas, and some solid tumors; to decrease tumor size, adjunctive to surgery or radiation therapy; or to prevent or treat suspected metastases. Chemotherapy may also be used in conjunction with biotherapy. All chemotherapy has side effects or toxic effects. The type and severity depend upon the drugs used.

Chemotherapy disrupts the cell cycle in various phases by interrupting cell metabolism and replication. It also works by interfering with the ability of the malignant cell to synthesize vital enzymes and chemicals. Phase-specific drugs work during only some phases of the cell cycle; non-phase-specific drugs work through the entire cell cycle. Figure 10–5 ■ lists some of the drugs useful in each phase of the cell cycle.

Most chemical treatment involves combinations of drugs in specific protocols given over varying periods of time. For example, one protocol for adult acute lymphocytic leukemia (ALL) uses the acronym DVPA: daunorubicin given on days 1 through 3; vincristine given on days 1, 8, 15, and 22; prednisone given on days 1 through 28, and asparaginase given on days 17 through 28. The treatment regimen is given in cycles with rest periods allowed, especially if toxic effects such as liver dysfunction or severe neutropenia occur. The treatment is continued until the disease goes into remission. If the disease progresses, the particular protocol is abandoned and a new one may be tried.

Researchers have examined the possibility of basing chemotherapy administration on the body's circadian rhythms. Some drugs work better if they follow the normal cyclic fluctuations of body hormones during the night, whereas others are more effective when given during daytime hours. Chemotherapy administration that follows circadian rhythms appears to be

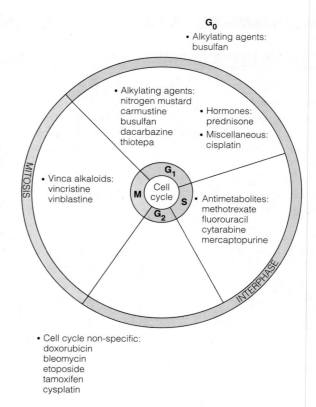

Figure 10–5 ■ Chemotherapeutic drugs useful in each phase of the cell cycle. Based on their chemical makeup and biologic activity, different drugs used for cancer treatment act in specific phases and subphases of the cell cycle. Some drugs, called non-phase-specific drugs, are generalized and act throughout the cycle. Chemotherapy often involves combinations of drugs designed to attack the cancer cells at many different times in the cycle and thus to enhance effectiveness.

more effective and causes fewer side effects with some types of cancer. A study of people with advanced colon cancer who were treated in this cyclic fashion (circadian rhythmic delivery, or CRD) demonstrated a 51% shrinkage in their tumors, compared with a shrinkage of only 28% in people who received chemotherapy in a steady dosage over 24 hours. In addition, the frequency and severity of side effects was decreased in the CRD group (Misset & Levi, 1995).

The cell-kill hypothesis explains why several courses of chemotherapy are necessary. A 1 cm tumor contains about 10^9 (10 billion) total cells, most of which are viable. During each cell cycle, the chemotherapy kills a fixed percentage of cells, always leaving some behind. With each reduction, the tumor burden of cells decreases until the number of viable, clonogenic cells (i.e., those that are able to clone daughter cells) becomes small enough to allow the body's immune system to finish the job. For this reason, oncologists usually give the maximum amount of chemotherapy tolerated by the client. High-dose chemotherapy (HDCT) remains controversial (Weiss et al., 2000). In a randomized study of 525 women with high-risk early breast cancer, individually tailored chemotherapy was compared with standard chemotherapy followed by HDCT. Women in the tailored chemotherapy group had significantly improved relapse-free survival and fewer severe side effects compared to women in the HDCT group (Bergh et al., 2000). Another study examined outcomes of women with metastatic breast cancer who were eligible for HDCT, but who were treated with standard-dose chemotherapy. The findings that progression-free survival and overall survival were higher for the HDCT group could be due in part to selection of subjects with better prognoses. The researchers concluded that the findings emphasize the importance of completing ongoing studies with randomized comparison groups (Rahman et al., 1997).

Classes of Chemotherapy Drugs

Chemotherapeutic agents fall basically into six major classes: alkylating agents, antimetabolites, antitumor antibiotics, mitotic inhibitors, hormones and hormone antagonists, and miscellaneous agents.

ALKYLATING AGENTS. Alkylating agents are non-phase specific and basically act on preformed nucleic acids by creating defects in tumor DNA. They cause cross linking of DNA strands, which can permanently interfere with replication and transcription.

Alkylating agents work with both proliferating and nonproliferating cells (those in G_0 phase). Their toxicity relates to their ability to kill slowly cycling stem cells and manifests in delayed, prolonged, or permanent bone marrow failure. Toxicity can also cause a mutagenic effect on bone marrow stem cells, culminating in a treatment-resistant form of acute myelogenous leukemia. Because of the alkylating agents' effect on stem cells, they also cause irreversible infertility. Other common adverse effects include nephrotoxicity and hemorrhagic cystitis.

The several subclasses of alkylating agents include nitrogen mustard (mechlorethamine), nitrosoureas (carmustine), alkyl sulfonates (busulfan), triazines (dacarbazine), ethylenimines (thiotepa), and cisplatin. Cisplatin is an alkylating agent containing platinum and chlorine atoms. It is most active in the G_1 subphase, but it is also non-phase specific. Cisplatin binds to DNA and acts much like alkylating agents by forming intrastrand DNA cross links (gluing strands of DNA together so that they cannot separate). Its major toxic effect is reversible renal tubular necrosis. Cisplatin may be used alone or in combination with other chemotherapeutic drugs for testicular and ovarian cancers.

ANTIMETABOLITES. Antimetabolites, a group of somewhat diverse drugs, are phase specific, working best in the S phase and having little effect in G_0. They interfere with nucleic acid synthesis by either displacing normal metabolites at the regulatory site of a key enzyme or by substituting for a metabolite that is incorporated into DNA or RNA molecules.

Toxic effects usually do not occur until very high levels of the drug are administered. Toxicity is also more likely when the drugs accumulate in third-spaced fluid, such as pleural fluid (a characteristic that also makes them useful in treating malignant pleural effusions). Because the drug diffuses out slowly from the third-spaced fluid, exposure of the tissue to the drug is prolonged. Most toxic effects relate to rapidly proliferating cells, such as cells in the gastrointestinal tract, hair, and skin and WBCs. Signs and symptoms include the following:

- Nausea and vomiting
- Stomatitis
- Diarrhea
- Alopecia
- Leukopenia

Some of the drugs can also cause liver and pulmonary toxicity.

The different types of antimetabolites include folic acid analogues (methotrexate), pyrimidine analogues (5-fluorouracil), cytosine arabinoside (ARA-C), and purine analogues (6-mercaptopurine).

ANTITUMOR ANTIBIOTICS. Antitumor antibiotics are originally derived from natural sources that are generally too toxic to be used as antibacterial agents. They are non-phase specific and act in several ways: They disrupt DNA replication and RNA transcription; create free radicals, which generate breaks in DNA and other forms of damage; and interfere with DNA repair. In addition, these drugs bind to cells and kill them, probably by damaging the cell membrane. Their main toxic effect is damage to the cardiac muscle. This limits the amount and duration of treatment. Examples of these antibiotics include actinomycin D, doxorubicin, bleomycin, mitomycin-C, and mithramycin.

MITOTIC INHIBITORS. Mitotic inhibitors are drugs that act to prevent cell division during the M phase. Mitotic inhibitors include the plant alkaloids and taxoids. Plant alkaloids consist of medications extracted from plant sources: Vinca alkaloids (e.g., vincristine and vinblastine) and etoposide (also called VP-16). The Vinca alkaloids are phase specific, acting during mitosis. They bind to a specific protein in tumor cells that promotes chromosome migration during mitosis and serves as a conduit for neurotransmitter transport along axons. The toxicity of these drugs is characterized by depression of deep-tendon reflexes, paresthesias (pain and altered sensation), motor weakness, cranial nerve disruptions, and paralytic ileus. Etoposide acts in all phases of the cell cycle, causing breaks in DNA and metaphase arrest. Although etoposide may cause bone marrow suppression and nausea and vomiting, the most common toxic effect is hypotension resulting from too rapid intravenous administration.

The taxoids act during the G_2 phase to inhibit cell division. Paclitaxel is used for the treatment of Kaposi's sarcoma and metastatic breast and ovarian cancer. Taxotere is used for breast cancer. Toxicities associated with these drugs include alopecia, bone marrow depression, and severe hypersensitivity reactions (e.g., hypotension, dyspnea, and urticaria).

HORMONES AND HORMONE ANTAGONISTS. The main hormones used in cancer therapy are the corticosteroids (e.g., prednisone), which are phase specific (G_1). These act by binding to specific intracellular receptors, repressing transcription of mRNA and thereby altering cellular function and growth. Corticosteroids have multiple side effects such as impaired healing, hyperglycemia, hypertension, osteoporosis, and hirsutism.

Hormone antagonists work with hormone-binding tumors, usually those of the breast, prostate, and endometrium. They block the hormone's receptor site on the tumor and prevent it from receiving normal hormonal growth stimulation. These drugs do not cure, but do cause regression of the tumor in about 40% of breast and endometrial tumors and 80% of prostate tumors. Tamoxifen competes with estradiol receptors in breast tumors. Raloxifene blocks estrogen in the breast. Diethylstilbestrol competes with hormone receptors in endometrial and prostate tumors. Antiandrogen (flutamide) and luteinizing hormone–releasing hormone (LHRH) block testosterone synthesis in prostate cancers. The main side effects of these drugs are alterations of the secondary sexual characteristics.

MISCELLANEOUS AGENTS. Several miscellaneous agents act at different phases in the cell cycle. L-asparaginase and hydroxyurea are examples of miscellaneous agents.

Effects of Chemotherapeutic Drugs

As described, the side effects and toxic effects of chemotherapy vary with the drug used and the length of treatment. Because most of these drugs act on fast-growing cells, the side effects are manifestations of damage to normal rapidly dividing somatic cells. The side effects of hormones express the action of the hormone used or suppression of the normal hormone,

such as the masculinizing effects of male hormones administered for ovarian cancers.

Tissues usually affected by cytotoxic drugs include the following:

- Mucous membranes of the mouth, tongue, esophagus, stomach, intestine, and rectum. This may result in anorexia, loss of taste, aversion to food, erythema and painful ulcerations in any portion of the gastrointestinal tract, nausea, vomiting, and diarrhea.
- Hair cells, resulting in alopecia.
- Bone marrow depression affecting most blood cells (e.g., granulocytes, lymphocytes, thrombocytes, and erythrocytes). This results in an impaired ability to respond to infection, a diminished ability to clot blood, and severe anemia.
- Organs, such as heart, lungs, bladder, kidneys. This kind of damage is related to specific agents, such as cardiac toxicity with doxorubicin or pneumonitis with bleomycin.
- Reproductive organs, resulting in impaired reproductive ability or altered fetal development.

Table 10–9 gives the classifications of chemotherapeutic drugs, common examples, target malignancies, adverse effects and side effects, and nursing implications. Consult current pharmacology textbooks for additional drugs and for new combination therapies as they are developed.

TABLE 10–9 Classifications of Chemotherapeutic Drugs

Drug Classification	Common Drugs	Target Malignancies	Adverse Effects or Side Effects	Nursing Implications
Alkylating agents	Mechlorethamine (Mustargen)	Hodgkin's disease Lymphosarcoma Lung cancer Chronic leukemia	Nausea and vomiting Leukopenia Thrombocytopenia Hyperuricemia	Maintain good hydration. Alkalinize urine. Administer antiemetics prior to chemotherapy. Monitor WBC, uric acid. Assess for infection.
	Busulfan (Myleran)	Chronic myelogenous leukemia	Leukopenia Thrombocytopenia Renal failure Pulmonary fibrosis	Monitor WBCs, BUN. Maintain adequate fluid intake. Assess for infection. Assess lungs for fibrotic (coarse, loud) rales.
	Cyclophosphamide (Cytoxan)	Lymphomas Multiple myeloma Leukemias Adenocarcinoma of lung and breast	Hemorrhagic cystitis Renal failure Alopecia Stomatitis Liver dysfunction	Encourage daily fluid intake of 2 to 3 L during treatment. Monitor WBCs, BUN, liver enzymes. Teach ways to manage hair loss.
Antimetabolites	Methotrexate	Acute lymphoblastic leukemia Osteosarcoma Gestational trophoblastic carcinoma	Oral and gastrointestinal ulcerations Anorexia and nausea Leukopenia Thrombocytopenia Pancytopenia	Monitor CBC, WBC differential, BUN, uric acid, creatinine. Assess oral mucous membranes; treat ulcers prn. Assess for infection, bleeding.

TABLE 10–9	Classifications of Chemotherapeutic Drugs (continued)			
Drug Classification	**Common Drugs**	**Target Malignancies**	**Adverse Effects or Side Effects**	**Nursing Implications**
	5-Fluorouracil (5-FU)	Colon carcinoma Rectal carcinoma Breast carcinoma Gastric carcinoma Pancreatic cancer	Stomatitis Alopecia Nausea and vomiting Gastritis Enteritis Diarrhea Anemia Leukopenia Thrombocytopenia	Monitor CBC with differential, BUN, uric acid. Administer antiemetics prn. Assess for bleeding; check stool occult blood. Evaluate hydration and nutrition status. Teach oral care for stomatitis. Assess for infection. Teach care for hair loss.
Antitumor antibiotics	Doxorubicin (Adriamycin)	Acute lymphoblastic leukemia (ALL) Acute myeloblastic leukemia Neuroblastoma Wilms' tumor Breast, ovarian, thyroid, lung cancer	Stomatitis Alopecia Nausea and vomiting Gastritis Enteritis Diarrhea Anemia Leukopenia Thrombocytopenia Cardiac toxicity	Monitor ECG; assess for arrythmias, gallops, and congestive heart failure (CHF). Monitor CBC with differential, BUN, uric acid. Administer antiemetics prn. Assess for bleeding; check stool for occult blood. Evaluate hydration and nutrition status. Teach oral care for stomatitis. Assess for infection. Teach care for hair loss.
	Bleomycin (Blenoxane)	Squamous cell carcinoma Lymphosarcoma Reticulum cell sarcoma Testicular carcinoma Hodgkin's disease	Mucocutaneous ulcerations Alopecia Nausea and vomiting Chills and fever Pneumonitis and pulmonary fibrosis	Check for fever 3 to 6 hours after administration. Have chest X-ray films taken every 2 to 3 weeks. Assess respiratory status, and check for coarse rales. Evaluate hydration and nutrition status. Teach oral care for stomatitis. Assess for infection. Teach care for hair loss.
Plant alkaloids	Vincristine (Oncovin)	Combination therapy for acute leukemia, Hodgkin's and non-Hodgkin's lymphomas, rhabdomyosarcoma, neuroblastoma, Wilm's tumor	Areflexia Muscle weakness Peripheral neuritis Constipation Paralytic ileus Mild bone marrow Depression	Assess neuromuscular function. Monitor CBC with differential. Evaluate gastrointestinal function. Manage constipation.
	Vinblastine (Velban)	Combination therapy for Hodgkin's disease, lymphocytic and histocytic lymphoma. Kaposi's sarcoma, advanced testicular carcinoma, unresponsive breast cancer	Areflexia Alopecia Nausea and vomiting Bone marrow depression	Assess neuromuscular function. Monitor CBC with differential. Administer antiemetics prn. Teach ways to manage hair loss.

(continued on page 294)

TABLE 10-9	Classifications of Chemotherapeutic Drugs (continued)			
Drug Classification	Common Drugs	Target Malignancies	Adverse Effects or Side Effects	Nursing Implications
Plant alkaloids *continued*	Etoposide, also called VP-16 (VePesid)	Nonresponsive testicular tumors Small-cell lung cancer	Alopecia Hypotension with rapid infusion	Hydrate adequately before administration. Administer for 60 minutes. Monitor vital signs every 15 minutes during administration and every 2 to 4 hours thereafter. Teach ways to manage hair loss.
	Prednisone	Combination therapy for many tumors Leukemia Lymphoma	Fluid retention Hypertension Steroid diabetes Emotional lability Silent bleeding ulcers Increased risk for infection	Monitor vital signs. Administer diuretics prn. Check blood glucose regularly. Evaluate mental status. Administer oral medications with food. Administer hydrogen ion antagonist drugs (antacids) as ordered. Monitor WBC with differential. Check for signs of systemic infection.
	Diethylstilbestrol (DES)	Advanced breast and prostrate cancers	Fluid retention Feminization Uterine bleeding	Monitor vital signs. Administer diuretics prn as ordered. Explain reason for feminization to men, bleeding to women. Monitor for excessive bleeding.
	Tamoxifen (Nolvadex)	Breast cancer	Hot flashes Nausea and vomiting	Teach ways to manage hot flashes. Explain reason for hot flashes. Administer antiemetics as ordered.
Miscellaneous drugs	Cisplatin (CDDP) (Platinol)	Combination and single therapy for metastatic testicular and ovarian cancers, advanced bladder cancer, head and neck tumors, non-small-cell lung carcinoma, osteogenic sarcoma, neuroblastoma	Bone marrow depression: leukopenia and thrombocytopenia Renal tubular damage Deafness	Monitor WBC with differential and platelets, BUN, creatinine, uric acid. Watch for bleeding. Monitor for signs of infection. Evaluate hearing; check for tinnitus. Ensure that client is well hydrated before drug is administered. Encourage 2 to 3 L of fluid intake daily.

Preparation and Administration

Many states and individual hospitals require that personnel be trained and certified to administer chemotherapy. Pharmacists in large hospitals and independent home care agencies usually prepare chemotherapeutic drugs for parenteral administration under specific safety guidelines established by the federal government or the Oncology Nursing Society. In some agencies, nurses both prepare and administer these drugs. Because of the potential carcinogenic effects, it is usually recommended that the health care professional wear gloves, a mask, and gown while preparing and administering the drug and disposing of equipment. The nurse must use care when handling excretory products of clients undergoing chemotherapy and teach clients to dispose of their own body fluids safely. Oral medications pose a lesser risk of exposure, but a risk nonetheless, primarily through excretion in the urine.

Chemotherapeutic drugs can be administered orally, such as cyclophosphamide (Cytoxan) and chlorambucil (Leukeran). Other drugs, such as hormones or hormone-blocking agents, may also be given intramuscularly. However, many drugs require intravenous infusion or direct injection into intraperitoneal or intrapleural body cavities. Intravenous preparations can be given through large peripheral veins, but the risk of extravasation or irritation to the vein may preclude this method for long-term therapy. Many clients now receive vascular access devices (VADs), especially if their treatment requires several cycles over weeks or months. VADs are also useful for adjunctive parenteral nutrition in the client who needs continuous intravenous infusions to manage pain or frequent blood drawing to monitor blood counts. Different types of VADs are available:

- Catheters that are inserted nonsurgically by threading them through a large peripheral vein into the vena cava. Called peripherally inserted central catheters (PICCs), they have multiple lumens that facilitate blood drawing. Placement is usually monitored by fluoroscopy.
- Catheters tunneled under the skin on the chest into a major vein, such as the subclavian vein. Hickman or Groshong catheters may be used.
- Surgically implanted ports, which are placed under the skin with a connected catheter inserted into a major vein. These are accessed by means of a special needle with a 90-degree angle inserted through the skin directly into the rubber dome of the port, which has a hard plastic back to prevent tissue damage.

Figure 10–6 ■ shows examples of different catheters and vascular access ports.

Risk of infection, catheter obstruction, and extravasation are the main problems associated with VADs. Nurses therefore must teach clients and family members to observe for redness, swelling, pain, or exudate at the insertion site, which may indicate infection; to observe for swelling of the neck or skin near the VAD for extravasation and infiltration; and to flush catheters and provide site care (cleaning and dressing changes) on a regular basis. During each encounter with the client, the nurse always inspects the site; observes for infection, infiltration, and catheter occlusion; and provides site care when necessary.

Management of Clients Receiving Chemotherapy

In addition to providing the above nursing interventions, nurses help identify and manage toxic effects or side effects of the drugs and provide psychosocial support. Careful assessment and monitoring of the client's signs and symptoms, including appropriate laboratory tests, alert the nurse to the onset of toxicity. Nausea and vomiting, diarrhea, inflammation and ulceration of oral mucous membranes, hair loss, skin changes, anorexia, and fatigue require specific medical and nursing

A

B

C

D

Figure 10–6 ■ Vascular access devices. *A*, Single-, double-, and triple-lumen catheters; *B*, single- and double-lumen Groshong catheters; *C*, Port-a-Cath Access System; *D*, Norport-SP, a side-entrance port.

actions. These actions are discussed later in this chapter under the appropriate nursing diagnoses. Indicators of organ toxicities, such as nephrotoxicity, neurotoxicity, or cardiac toxicity, must be reported immediately to the physician. Another aspect of managing clients undergoing chemotherapy is to teach them how to care for access sites and to dispose of used equipment and excretions safely. Nurses also teach clients to increase fluid intake to flush out the drugs; to get extra rest, which can both assist therapy and help the client avoid other illnesses; to identify major complications of their particular drug protocol; to know when to call the physician or emergency medical services; and, if their WBC count is low, to limit their exposure to other people, especially those with infections or children.

During chemotherapy, a number of psychologic issues that can cause moderate to severe emotional distress may arise. The need to plan activities around chemotherapy treatments and their side effects can impair the client's ability to work, manage a household or care for family members, function sexually, or participate in social and recreational activities. Weight loss and alopecia may prompt feelings of powerlessness and depression. The nurse can assist by carefully evaluating symptoms, providing specific interventions as indicated, and allowing clients opportunities to express their fears, concerns, and feelings. Clients should be encouraged to participate in their care and maintain control over their life as much as possible (McDaniel & Rhodes, 1998). Specific interventions will be discussed later in the chapter under the appropriate nursing diagnoses. Table 10–9 includes nursing implications for specific adverse effects of common chemotherapy drugs.

Surgery

Surgical resection is used for diagnosis and staging of more than 90% of all cancers and for primary treatment of more than 60% of cancers. When possible, the tumor is removed in its entirety. This sometimes necessitates mutilation of the body and the creation of new structures to assume function of the lost structures. For example, removal of the distal sigmoid colon and rectum requires a new means of bowel elimination, so the remaining healthy segment of the bowel is brought out through a created opening (stoma) in the abdominal wall, resulting in a permanent colostomy (see Chapter 24). In like manner, when the bladder is removed, the ureters are transplanted into a created pouch just under the abdominal wall. This serves as a continent ileostomy, a substitute reservoir for urine (see Chapter 26). Surgery can also destroy sensitive nerve plexes, resulting in alteration or loss of normal functioning; for example, prostate surgery may result in incontinence and impotence. ඟ

Not all surgery results in such radical changes in functioning. The following surgeries can eliminate cancer successfully with less distressing results.

- Removing a nonessential portion of the organ or tissue containing the tumor, such as in situ small bowel tumors
- Removing an organ whose function can be replaced chemically, such as the thyroid
- Resecting one of a pair of organs when the unaffected organ can take over the function of the missing one, such as a lung

Although the removal of any major body part has physiologic and psychologic consequences, the alternative—terminal disease—is usually less desirable.

If the tumor is in a nonresectable location or deeply invasive with metastases, surgery may be only a palliative measure to allow the involved organs to function as long as possible, to relieve pain, or to bypass an obstruction. Surgery may also be done to reduce the bulk of the tumor in advanced disease, both at primary and metastatic sites. Decreasing the tumor size enhances the ability to control the remaining disease through other modalities. Surgery is often used in conjunction with other treatments to effect a cure. For example, in cases when extensive removal of tissue is contraindicated (e.g., in surgical removal of a brain tumor), radiation may be used prior to surgery in an attempt to shrink the tumor before it is removed.

Surgical intervention may also be used for reconstruction and rehabilitation. One example is the construction of transabdominal mycocutaneous (TRAM) flaps in conjunction with or following modified radical mastectomy (see Chapter 48). For surgical interventions for cancers affecting specific body systems, refer to later chapters. ඟ

Surgical oncologists are working with researchers to identify premalignant disease earlier in high-risk populations and to conduct studies on ways to reverse oncogenic cell activity. Surgeons also work with molecular biologists using sophisticated techniques to develop monoclonal antibodies. Laser technology is being explored for use in different types of cancer surgery because it minimizes blood loss, reduces deformity, increases the accuracy of tissue resection, and enhances healing. Lasers are currently being used to treat radical prostectomy in order to preserve urinary continence and sexual functioning. Another collaborative strategy under development is intraoperative radiation therapy, in which radiosensitive, nondiseased organs that may be damaged by radiation therapy are moved away from the radiation field and shielded. Radiation is then administered while the patient is on the operating table. This technique allows more penetrating radiation to be directed to the malignant tumor with less trauma to normal, vulnerable tissues or organs.

Nursing responsibilities focus on preparing the client physically and psychologically for the specific surgery, as well as teaching routine postoperative care in which the client is expected to participate. For example, the nurse teaches the client about respiratory care and the use of the incentive spirometer to improve postoperative ventilation, early ambulation to prevent circulatory problems, and how the client will receive fluids and nutrition (intravenously or orally, depending on the type of surgery). In addition, the nurse explains the specific surgical procedure and any anticipated alterations to the client's body, especially those that require major lifestyle adjustments, such as a colostomy. Before surgery, the nurse should give the client the opportunity to ask questions and to discuss concerns and fears. In some cases, the client may want to discuss alternative treatment options. In the latter case, the nurse should avoid trying to persuade the client to accept any one option; rather, the nurse should contact the oncologist and the surgeon and set up a conference for the client before surgery.

Radiation Therapy

Still the treatment of choice for some tumors or by some oncologists, radiation may be used to kill the tumor, to reduce its size, to decrease pain, or to relieve obstruction. Lymph nodes and adjacent tissues are irradiated when beginning metastasis is suspected. Radiation therapy consists of delivering ionizing radiations of gamma and X-rays in one of two ways:

- **Teletherapy.** Also called external radiation, teletherapy involves delivery of radiation from a source at some distance from the client. A relatively uniform dosage is delivered to the tumor.
- **Brachytherapy.** In brachytherapy, the radioactive material is placed directly into or adjacent to the tumor, a technique that delivers a high dose to the tumor and a lower dose to the normal tissues. This allows delivery of high doses of radiation to the tumor while sparing adjacent tissue. Brachytherapy is also referred to as internal, interstitial, or intracavitary radiation.

For many common neoplasms, a combination of these two therapies is used.

Lethal injury to DNA is believed to be the primary mechanism by which radiation kills cells, especially cells in faster growing tumors and tissues. As a result, when given over time, radiation can destroy not only rapidly multiplying cancer cells but also rapidly dividing normal cells, such as those of the skin and mucous membranes. A malignant tumor is considered cured when there are no surviving tumor stem cells. The goal of radiation therapy is to achieve maximum tumor control with a minimum of damage to normal tissue.

Implanted or ingested radiation can be dangerous for those living with, taking care of, or treating the client. Caregivers must use protection by, for example, shielding themselves from the source of radiation, limiting the time of exposure to the client, increasing the distance from the client, and using specific safety procedures for handling secretions. Box 10–6 identifies safety principles to be followed by those caring for clients undergoing internal radiation.

Tumors have differing sensitivities to radiation. Tumors that have the greatest number of rapidly proliferating cancer cells usually exhibit the best early response to radiation. The decision to use radiation rather than other modalities is based on balancing the probability of controlling the tumor against the probability of causing complications, such as tissue damage. The decision is usually made by risk-benefit analysis. Planning for radiation therapy includes assessing the disease site, tumor size, and histologic findings. Treatment schedules vary based on these factors (Neal & Hoskin, 1997). Box 10–7 lists the degree of radiosensitivity for selected cancers.

The client receiving external radiation may experience skin changes such as blanching, erythema, desquamation, sloughing, or hemorrhage. Ulcerations of mucous membranes may cause severe pain; in addition, oral secretions can decrease, making the client more vulnerable to infection and dental caries. Gastrointestinal effects include nausea and vomiting, diarrhea, or bleeding. Lungs may develop interstitial exudate, a condition called radiation pneumonia. Occasionally, external

radiation therapy may cause fistulas or necrosis of adjacent tissues. Implanted radioactive materials can lead to similar problems; moreover, the excretory products of these clients are usually considered dangerous and need special disposal. See the Nursing Care box on page 298 for nursing implications for clients receiving radiation therapy.

BOX 10–6 ■ Safety Principles for Radiation

These recommendations apply to caregivers working with clients receiving internal radiation (brachytherapy).

- Maintain the greatest possible distance from the source of radiation.
- Spend the minimum amount of time close to the radiation source.
- Shield yourself from the radiation with lead gloves and aprons when possible.
- If pregnant, avoid contact with radiation sources.
- If you work routinely near radiation, wear a monitoring device to measure whole-body exposure.
- Avoid direct exposure with radioisotope containers; for example, do not touch the container.
- Keep clients with implanted radioisotopes in a private room with private bath and as far away from other hospitalized persons as possible.
- Dispose of body fluids of clients with unsealed implanted radioisotopes with special care and in specially marked containers.
- Handle bed linen and clothing with care and according to agency protocol.
- Use long-handled forceps to place any dislodged implants into a lead container.
- Consult with the radiation therapy department for any questions or problems in caring for clients with radioactive implants.

BOX 10–7 ■ Degree of Radiosensitivity for Selected Cancers

VERY RADIOSENSITIVE
- Neuroblastoma
- Lymphomas
- Chronic leukemia

MODERATELY RADIOSENSITIVE
- Bronchogenic carcinoma
- Esophageal carcinoma
- Squamous cell carcinoma
- Prostate carcinoma
- Cervical carcinoma
- Testicular carcinoma

NONRADIOSENSITIVE
- Many adenocarcinomas
- Fibrosarcoma
- Osteogenic carcinoma

NURSING CARE OF THE CLIENT RECEIVING RADIATION THERAPY

NURSING RESPONSIBILITIES FOR EITHER EXTERNAL OR INTERNAL RADIATION THERAPY

- Carefully assess and manage any complications, usually in collaboration with the radiation oncologist.
- Assist in documenting the results of the therapy; for example, clients receiving radiation for metastases to the spine will show improved neurologic functioning as tumor size diminishes.
- Provide emotional support, relief of physical and psychologic discomfort, and opportunities to talk about fears and concerns. For some clients, radiation therapy is a last chance for cure or even just for relief of physical discomfort.

EXTERNAL RADIATION

Prior to the start of treatments, the treatment area will be specifically located by the radiation oncologist and marked with colored semipermanent ink or tatoos. Treatment is usually given 5 days per week for 15 to 30 minutes per day over 2 to 7 weeks.

Nursing Responsibilities

- Monitor for adverse effects: skin changes, such as blanching, erythema, desquamation, sloughing, or hemorrhage; ulcerations of mucous membranes; nausea and vomiting, diarrhea, or gastrointestinal bleeding.
- Assess lungs for rales, which may indicate interstitial exudate. Observe for any dyspnea or changes in respiratory pattern.
- Identify and record any medications that the client will be taking during the radiation treatment.
- Monitor white blood cell counts and platelet counts for significant decreases.

Client and Family Teaching

- Wash the skin that is marked as the radiation site only with plain water, no soap; do not apply deodorant, lotions, medications, perfume, or talcum powder to the site during the treatment period. Take care not to wash off the treatment marks.
- Do not rub, scratch, or scrub treated skin areas. If necessary, use only an electric razor to shave the treated area.
- Apply neither heat nor cold (e.g., heating pad or ice pack) to the treatment site.
- Inspect the skin for damage or serious changes, and report these to the radiologist or physician.

- Wear loose, soft clothing over the treated area.
- Protect skin from sun exposure during treatment and for at least 1 year after radiation therapy is discontinued. Cover skin with protective clothing during treatment; once radiation is discontinued, use sun-blocking agents with a sun protection factor (SPF) of at least 15.
- External radiation poses no risk to other people for radiation exposure, even with intimate physical contact.
- Be sure to get plenty of rest and eat a balanced diet.

INTERNAL RADIATION

The radiation source, called an implant, is placed into the affected tissue or body cavity and is sealed in tubes, containers, wires, seeds, capsules, or needles. An implant may be temporary or permanent. Internal radiation may also be ingested or injected as a solution into the bloodstream or a body cavity or be introduced into the tumor through a catheter. The radioactive substance may transmit rays outside the body or be excreted in body fluids.

Nursing Responsibilities

- Place the client in a private room.
- Limit visits to 10 to 30 minutes, and have visitors sit at least 6 feet from the client.
- Monitor for side effects such as burning sensations, excessive perspiration, chills and fever, nausea and vomiting, or diarrhea.
- Assess for fistulas or necrosis of adjacent tissues.

Client and Family Teaching

- While a temporary implant is in place, stay in bed and rest quietly to avoid dislodging the implant.
- For outpatient treatments, avoid close contact with others until treatment has been discontinued.
- If the radiologist indicates the need for such measures, dispose of excretory materials in special containers or in a toilet not used by others.
- Carry out daily activities as able; get extra rest if feeling fatigued.
- Eat a balanced diet; frequent, small meals often are better tolerated.
- Contact the nurse or physician for any concerns or questions after discharge.

Biotherapy

Biotherapy modifies the biologic processes that result in malignant cells, primarily through enhancing the person's own immune responses. The development of this therapy was based on the immune surveillance hypothesis. Although it has been established that a competent immune system is the body's most important defense against any disease, the role that various immune cells play in combating different types of malignancies continues to be investigated. Currently, biotherapy is used for both hematological malignancies, such as lymphoma and hairy cell leukemia, and solid tumors, such as renal cancer and melanoma.

Tumor immunology has the following applications: detection screening in high-risk groups, differential diagnosis and classification of tumor cells, monitoring the course of the disease with early detection of recurrence, and active therapies to halt or limit the disease. The theory underlying tumor immunology is that most tumor cells have a structural appearance recognizable by the immune cells. Tumor-associated antigens (TAAs) exist on tumor cells but not on normal cells. TAAs elicit an immune response that, in a person with a competent immune system, destroys or inhibits tumor growth. Thus, TAAs can be isolated from serum and used for both diagnosis and various treatment modalities. The prostate-specific antigen (PSA) is one such TAA currently in successful diagnostic use.

Tumor cells are often in a stage of arrested development (i.e., in the differentiation stage) for the cell type they represent; thus, they express antigens characteristic of that particular stage of development. The immaturity of the cells provides the physician with information about the relative aggressiveness of the cancer.

Another aspect of immunotherapy is the development of monoclonal antibodies that enhance the immune system's ability to fight the cancer. Monoclonal antibodies are developed by inoculating an animal with the tumor antigen and recovering the specific antibodies produced. The antibodies are then given to the person with that cancer to assist in the destruction of the tumor. Monoclonal antibodies are also recreated, or cloned, in the genetic laboratory by recombining DNA to produce the specific antibody. Techniques involving recombinant DNA have been used to combine these antibodies with toxins and drugs that are then delivered selectively to the tumor sites.

A number of cytokines (normal growth-regulating molecules) with antitumor activity have been synthesized. Alpha interferon, bacillus Calmette-Guérin (BCG, which has been used for many years as an inoculation against tuberculosis), and interleukin-2 (IL-2) have shown some therapeutic benefit in eliciting increased immune responses. Combination strategies have also helped stimulate the function of macrophages.

A most promising discovery has been the recently identified natural killer (NK) cells. These cells are like large granular lymphocytes, but have a cell surface phenotype different from that of T lymphocytes or macrophages. They have demonstrated a spontaneous cytotoxic effect on some types of cancer cells. They also provide a strong resistance to metastasis and secrete cytokines. When augmented by biologic response modifiers such as IL-2, they show increased tumor destructive activity (Battiato & Wheeler, 2000).

The use of hematopoietic growth factors (HGF) has been one of the most successful in biotherapy. HGF, such as granu-locyte colony-stimulating factor (G-CSF) and erythropoietin, offset the suppression of granulocytes and erythrocytes that results from chemotherapy (Battiato & Wheeler, 2000).

As promising as these biotherapies are, they are accompanied by serious side effects and toxicities. IL-2 can cause acute alterations in renal, cardiac, liver, gastrointestinal, and mental functioning. Alpha interferon causes mental slowing, confusion, and lethargy and, when used in combination with 5-fluorouracil or IL-2, severe flulike symptoms—chills and fever of 103° to 106°F (39.4° to 41.1°C), nausea, vomiting, diarrhea, anorexia, severe fatigue, and stomatitis—may result. The toxic effects are probably exaggerations of the normal systemic effects that these substances cause when fighting infection. For example, IL-2 is known to raise body temperature substantially in an attempt to create a hostile environment for foreign invaders.

The box below discusses nursing implications for clients receiving immunotherapy. For nursing care of specific problems, refer to the appropriate nursing diagnoses later in this chapter.

Photodynamic Therapy

Photodynamic therapy is a method of treating certain kinds of superficial tumors. It is known by several different names: phototherapy, photoradiation, and photochemotherapy. Clients suffering from tumors growing on the surface of the bladder, peritoneal cavity, chest wall, pleura, bronchus, or head and neck are candidates for this treatment. The client is given an intravenous dose of a photosensitizing compound, Photofrin, which is selectively retained in higher concentrations in malignant tissue. This drug is activated by a laser treatment that is started 3 days after the drug injection and administered for 3 days. The drug interacts with oxygen molecules in the tissue to produce a cytotoxic oxygen molecule called singlet oxygen.

NURSING CARE   OF CLIENTS RECEIVING IMMUNOTHERAPY

Immunotherapy can consist of various substances used alone, such as interleukin-2, or combination biotherapy, such as alpha interferon with 5-fluorouracil. The nurse's role is to enhance the client's quality of life.

Nursing Responsibilities
- Monitor for side effects: Alpha interferon may cause mental slowing, confusion, and lethargy; combination therapy of 5-fluorouracil or interleukin-2 and alpha interferon may cause severe flulike symptoms, with chills and fever of 103° to 106°F (39.4° to 41.1°C), nausea, vomiting, diarrhea, anorexia, severe fatigue, and stomatitis; erythropoietin may cause acute hypertension.
- Monitor enzymes and other appropriate biochemical indicators for acute alterations in renal, cardiac, liver, or gastrointestinal functioning, which can be side effects of interleukin-2.
- Evaluate response to therapy by conducting a thorough evaluation of clients' symptoms.
- Assess clients' coping behaviors and teach new strategies as needed.

- Manage fatigue and depression.
- Encourage self-care and participation in decision making.
- Provide close supervision for clients with altered mental functioning, either by caretakers or frequent nursing visits to the client's home.
- If client is unable to manage alone, teach medication administration and care of equipment to caregivers.

Client and Family Teaching
- Minimize symptoms by managing fever and flulike symptoms: increase fluid intake, take analgesic and antipyretic medications, and maintain bed rest until symptoms abate.
- Seek help for serious problems not managed by usual means, such as dehydration from diarrhea.
- Use correct techniques for providing subcutaneous injections.
- Identify how to work and care for ambulatory pumps when medication is administered through an intercatheter or vascular access device.

At the time of the first intravenous injection, clients are observed for adverse hypersensitivity reactions, such as nausea, chills, and hives. Systemic or long-term toxicities are rare. The main side effects are local skin reactions and temporary photosensitivity, transiently elevated liver enzymes, and inflammatory responses of the tissues being treated, such as peritoneal or pleural tissues. This treatment has been used successfully with early-stage lung cancer with response rates as high as 90% (Bruce, 2001).

The major nursing responsibilities associated with photodynamic therapy are to address the client and family's anxiety about undergoing a relatively new treatment procedure and to educate them in managing side effects. The drug remains in the subcutaneous tissues for 4 to 6 weeks after injection. Any direct or indirect exposure to the sun activates the drug, resulting in a chemical sunburn. Clients are taught to protect themselves from sunlight (even on cloudy days) by covering themselves from head to toe in opaque clothing, including a wide-brimmed hat, gloves, shoes and stockings, and sunglasses with 100% ultraviolet block. Long-term care of treated skin includes moisturizing lotions and protection from trauma or irritation.

Bone Marrow and Peripheral Blood Stem Cell Transplantations

Bone marrow transplantation (BMT) is an accepted treatment to stimulate a nonfunctioning marrow or to replace marrow. BMT is given as an intravenous infusion of bone marrow cells from donor to client. Most commonly used in leukemias, this therapy is being expanded to include treatment of other cancers including melanoma and testicular cancer. Chapter 32 provides an in-depth discussion of this procedure. ⨂ Peripheral blood stem cell transplantation (PBSCT) is the process of removing circulating stem cells from the peripheral blood through apheresis and returning these cells to the patient after dose-intensive chemotherapy. PBSCT has fewer side effects, shorter hospitalization, and decreased cost compared to BMT.

Pain Management

Pain management is an important component of oncology care and is considered a crucial part of the collaborative treatment plan. It is estimated that 20% to 50% of clients with early-stage cancer and up to 95% of clients with advanced cancer experience pain that requires analgesia (Cady, 2001). There are three main categories of pain syndromes in clients with cancer, and the category influences the type of treatment.

- *Pain associated with direct tumor involvement.* The most common causes are metastatases to bone, nerve compression or infiltration, and involvement of hollow visceral organs.
- *Pain associated with treatment.* This may include postsurgical incisional or wound pain; peripheral neuropathy, ulceration of mucous membranes, and pain from herpes zoster outbreaks secondary to chemotherapy; and pain in nerve plexes, muscles, and peripheral nerves from radiation therapy.
- *Pain from a cause not related to either the cancer or therapy,* such as diabetic neuropathy.

The goal of pain therapy is to provide relief that allows clients to function as they wish and, in the case of terminally ill clients, to die relatively free of pain. Drug therapy with opioid and nonopioid analgesics as well as adjuvant medications (those that enhance the effect of the analgesic) is the basis of most physician-guided pain management. Other therapies include injection of anesthetic drugs into spinal cord or specific nerve plexes, surgical severing of nerves, radiation to reduce tumor size and pressure, and behavioral approaches. Pharmacologic pain management follows these steps:

1. Conduct careful initial and ongoing assessment of the pain.
2. Evaluate the client's functional goals.
3. Establish a plan with combinations of nonnarcotic drugs (such as aspirin or ibuprofen) with adjuvants (such as corticosteroids or antidepressants).
4. Evaluate the degree of pain relief.
5. Progress to stronger drugs as needed, from mild narcotics such as oxycodone (Percodan) or propoxyphene (Darvon) to strong narcotics such as morphine or hydromorphone (Dilaudid), and monitor side effects.
6. Continue to try combinations and escalate dosages until maximal pain relief balanced with client's need to function is achieved.

Medication usually is administered by the oral route as long as this route continues to be effective. Medication is given on a regular time schedule (e.g., every 4 hours) with additional medication prescribed to cover breakthrough pain. When the oral route alone becomes inadequate, the primary narcotic can be administered intramuscularly, subcutaneously, or rectally on an intermittent schedule or continuously by transdermal patches or intravenously by a continuous drip, usually controlled by an infusion pump. Some newer pumps are portable, deliver medication continuously, and allow clients to control their breakthrough pain with a limited number of boluses. When narcotic doses are increased gradually, there is no limit to the amount the client can receive, as long as adverse reactions can be managed. Clients have received up to 4800 mg daily (200 mg per hour) of morphine sulfate with up to six 200- to 400-mg breakthrough doses daily without major ill effects and with good pain control. The body develops tolerance to the sedative after a short period, and most clients are able to tolerate the level of medication needed to control the pain. Other side effects, such as constipation, nausea and vomiting, and itching, can be managed through the usual means and are discussed under the appropriate nursing diagnoses. If the client has persistent untoward side effects that do not respond to treatment, or if the client does not get adequate relief from the narcotic, different narcotics and combinations are tried. Morphine sulfate and transdermal fentanyl are the most commonly used drugs for relief of cancer pain (Ferrell & McCaffery, 1997).

Clients receiving high-dose narcotics should not have the medication abruptly stopped, because withdrawal symptoms will occur. If the drug needs to be stopped, it must be tapered gradually. For more information on pain management, and on alternative therapies in particular, see Chapter 4. ⨂

NURSING CARE

Nurses face a major challenge in educating clients about preventive measures and lifestyle changes to reduce the risk of cancer. At the same time, clients with cancer must be reassured that they are not responsible for having acquired cancer.

Once a cancer diagnosis is established, nurses help clients recover and support them during the rehabilitation phase. In cases of terminal cancer, nurses provide comfort and facilitate positive growth for the client and significant others.

Health Promotion

Early detection and treatment are considered the most important factors influencing the prognosis of those afflicted with cancer. However, many people do not seek early diagnosis and treatment because of denial, fear and anxiety, stigma, or the absence of specific early signs such as pain or weight loss (which usually are late signs). For this reason, screening procedures such as mammograms, PSA, occult blood stool tests, and sigmoidoscopy may be lifesaving.

The American Cancer Society (ACS) promotes early detection through public education using the CAUTION model (see Box 10–8). This model encourages people to seek medical attention when they discover signs and symptoms characteristic of cancer. For people without symptoms, the ACS recommends a cancer checkup every 3 years for those ages 20 to 39 and yearly for those over 40. If a person is at special risk due to heredity, environment, occupation, or lifestyle, special tests or more frequent examinations may be necessary. A routine cancer checkup should include counseling to improve health behaviors and physical examination with related tests of the breast, uterus, cervix, colon, rectum, testes, prostate, skin, thyroid, and lymph nodes. Box 10–9 lists the tests recommended for a cancer checkup. Nurses have a special role in public education and should encourage all with whom they come into contact to schedule their cancer checkup. Nurses must be familiar with the ACS guidelines so that they can advise clients, their families, and significant others.

Assessment

Focused Interview

During this initial phase of the nursing process, collect the following significant data about the client.

BOX 10–8 ■ American Cancer Society CAUTION Model

Change in bowel or bladder habits
A sore that does not heal
Unusual bleeding or discharge
Thickening or lump in breast or elsewhere
Indigestion or difficulty in swallowing
Obvious change in wart or mole
Nagging cough or hoarseness

If you have a warning signal, see your doctor!

Note. From the American Cancer Society.

BOX 10–9 ■ American Cancer Society Recommendations for Cancer Checkups

BREAST CANCER
- Routine monthly breast self-examination starting at age 20
- Breast examination by a health care professional every 3 years from age 20 to 39 and yearly thereafter
- Screening mammography every year from age 40

COLON AND RECTUM CANCER—FOR PEOPLE AT AVERAGE RISK
- Fecal occult blood test every year beginning at age 50
- Flexible sigmoidoscopy every 5 years with digital rectal exam
- Colonoscopy double-contrast barium enema every 10 years with digital rectal exam

CERVIX OR UTERINE CANCER
- Yearly pelvic examination and Pap test for sexually active girls and any women over 18; less often for women with three consecutive negative results
- An endometrial tissue sample at menopause for high-risk women with repeated samples at physician's discretion

PROSTATE CANCER
- Digital rectal exam yearly beginning at age 50 (higher risk begin at age 40)
- Prostate-specific antigen (PSA) test yearly beginning at age 50 (begin at age 45 for African American men and men with first-degree relative)

Note. From the American Cancer Society.

- History of the client's disease, including the signs and symptoms that led the client to seek health care
- Other concurrent diseases, such as diabetes
- Current physical or psychologic problems resulting from the cancer, such as pain or depression
- Understanding of the treatment plan
- Expectations of the treatment plan
- Functional limitations due to illness or treatment (see Box 10–10)
- Effect of the disease on current lifestyle
- Reliable support systems or caretakers for the client
- Coping strategies and how well they are working

INTERVIEW QUESTIONS. The following are appropriate questions to ask the client during the initial interview and at subsequent assessments.

- "What brought you in to see the doctor?" Asking this question allows clients to tell their story in their own way, which may elicit more information than asking specific questions. The answer should elicit not only data about the signs and symptoms but also fears or concerns. If the cancer was discovered during a routine physical examination or checkup, the client may have some difficulty accepting the disease, especially if there were no symptoms. For clients who offer insufficient information in response to this open-ended question, more specific questions may be necessary, such as "Did you have pain or any specific physical problems that caused you to seek health care?"

MediaLink | CANCER RESOURCES

BOX 10–10 ■ Two Scales of Functional Status for Cancer Clients

KARNOFSKY SCALE: CRITERIA OF PERFORMANCE STATUS (PS)

100   Normal; no complaints; no evidence of disease.

90   Able to carry on normal activity; minor signs or symptoms of disease.

80   Able to carry on normal activity with effort; some signs or symptoms of disease.

70   Cares for self; unable to carry on normal activity or to do active work.

60   Requires occasional assistance but is able to care for most of own needs.

50   Requires considerable assistance and frequent medical care.

40   Disabled; requires special care and assistance.

30   Severely disabled; hospitalization indicated, although death not imminent.

20   Very sick; hospitalization necessary; active supportive treatment necessary.

10   Moribund; fatal processes progressing rapidly.

0   Dead.

EASTERN COOPERATIVE ONCOLOGY GROUP SCALE (ECOG)

0   Fully active, able to carry on all predisease activities without restriction. (Karnofsky 90 to 100)

1   Restricted in physically strenuous activity, but ambulatory and able to carry out work of a light or sedentary nature, for example, light housework or office work. (Karnofsky 70 to 80)

2   Ambulatory and capable of all self-care, but unable to carry out work activities. Up and about more than 50% of waking hours. (Karnofsky 50 to 60)

3   Capable of only limited self-care, confined to bed or chair 50% or more of waking hours. (Karnofsky 30 to 40)

4   Completely disabled, cannot carry out any self-care, totally confined to bed or chair. (Karnofsky 10 to 20)

Note. "Nitrogen Mustards in the Palliative Treatment of Carcinoma" by D. A. Karnofsky, L. Craver, & J. Burchenal, 1948. Cancer 1, pp. 634–656. Copyright © American Cancer Society. Reprinted by permission of Wiley-CISS, Inc. a subsidiary of John Wiley & Sons.

- "Do you have any other medical conditions or problems that are troubling you at this time?" It may be necessary to ask about specific diseases to help the client focus. For example, "Do you have high blood pressure?" or "Are you having any problems with your lungs?" Information gained from these questions can help you anticipate problems and formulate potential nursing diagnoses related to other diseases that may interact with the cancer.

- "What kinds of physical problems are you having at this time? Do you have pain? Are you nauseated? Have you lost a great deal of weight? Are you so tired you have difficulty carrying on your daily activities? Are you feeling blue or discouraged because of your illness?" For each positive response, ask follow-up questions to narrow down or define the exact nature of the problem. Again, these data help identify what nursing diagnoses should be included in the care plan.

- "What options has your physician suggested for treating your cancer?" The answer will indicate clients' knowledge about their treatment and, possibly, their communication with the physician. Often, under the stress of a cancer diagnosis, clients do not hear or understand what the doctor is saying and are afraid to ask questions. Lack of knowledge indicates a need to collaborate with the physician to explain the information to the client so that the client can absorb and understand it. If the client has a good understanding of the treatment plan, discussing how he or she feels about it can be useful in exposing fears, concerns, and emotional responses.

- "What do you expect to happen as a result of this treatment?" The answer may reveal unrealistic expectations or lack of understanding of consequences of the treatment.

- "What effect is the disease and/or treatment having on your ability to carry on with your usual daily activities?" Additional questions may also be needed to pinpoint the types of limitations. The response to this question should provide information on the client's functional status such as those shown in Box 10–10. This information can also be used to identify the need to collaborate with professionals from other disciplines. For example, if the client is the sole financial support of the family and is unable to work, a social worker may be able to help with resources; if the client is extremely weak, referral to a physical therapist may help with energy conservation strategies and strengthening exercises.

- "Who is available to help you at home and run errands for you? Who can provide transportation for you to get to your appointments or treatments? Who can you rely on to be a good listener when you're sad or just to be a comfortable companion? Is there someone you would like to make health care decisions for you if there is a time that you are unable to make them for yourself?" It often seems that the person with cancer is the one who takes care of everyone else; asking for help may be difficult for this person. This information can identify how much support and help the client has access to. The last question introduces the concept of advanced directives and durable power of attorney regarding health care (see Chapter 11).

- "How do you manage your stress or your feelings of discomfort? What helps you feel better? Do you think these measures work well for you?" The responses to these questions provide information about the client's coping strategies and may identify maladaptive strategies such as alcohol or drug use. Lack of appropriate coping methods can interfere with the client's response to treatment and decrease overall quality of life.

Other assessment questions may be useful at different stages of the client's illness. For example, if the client is not expected to survive the cancer, it is important to ask whether the client has made decisions about last wishes (e.g., for a funeral and burial), whether these have been discussed with significant others, and whether the client has made out a will.

Physical Assessment

As soon as the client is admitted to the health care service or agency, conduct a complete physical assessment to establish a

TABLE 10–10 Signs of Nutritional Status

System	Good Nutrition	Poor Nutrition
General	Alert, energetic, good endurance, psychologically stable	Withdrawn, apathetic, easily fatigued, irritable
	Weight within range for height, age, body size	Over- or underweight
Integumentary	Skin glowing, good turgor, smooth, free of lesions	Skin dull, pasty, scaly-dry, bruises, multiple lesions
	Hair shiny, lustrous, minimal loss	Hair brittle, dull, falls out easily
Head, eyes, ears, nose, and throat	Eyes bright, clear, no fatigue circles	Eyes dull, conjunctiva pale, discoloration under eyes
	Oral mucous membranes pink-red and moist	Oral mucous membranes pale
	Gums pink, firm	Gums red, spongy, and bleed easily
	Tongue pink, moderately smooth, no swelling	Tongue bright to dark red, swollen
Abdomen	Abdomen flat, firm	Abdomen flaccid or distended (ascites)
Musculoskeletal	Firm, well-developed muscles	Flaccid muscles, wasted appearance
	Good posture	Stooped posture
	No skeletal changes	Skeletal malformations
Neurologic	Good attention span, good concentration, astute thought processes	Inattentive, easily distracted, impaired thought processes
	Good reflexes	Paresthesias, reflexes diminished or hyperactive

baseline against which to evaluate later changes. It is especially important to document the nutritional status of the client using anthropomorphic measurements (i.e., frame size, height, weight, body fat, and muscle mass), and to evaluate laboratory results and note any specific signs and symptoms. Table 10–10 compares the manifestations of good nutrition with those of malnutrition.

It is also important to assess the client's hydration status, especially if the client is not taking oral food and fluids well or is having bouts of vomiting. Box 10–11 lists specific assessments for hydration status. Other recommended assessments are discussed under the specific nursing diagnoses that follow. They can also be found in other chapters that address specific body systems affected by the cancer.

Nursing Diagnoses and Interventions

Nursing goals focus on supporting the whole person and managing specific problems such as pain, poor nutrition, dehydration, fatigue, adverse emotional responses, altered individual and family coping, and the side effects of medical treatment. Nursing also focuses on improving the quality of life by promoting rehabilitation for survivors of cancer and helping those who succumb to the disease maintain their dignity in the dying process. Because cancer affects the whole family, nursing care includes everyone involved with the client from the onset of diagnosis through the entire disease and treatment process and the ultimate outcome. Many diagnoses are pertinent to clients with cancer; this section addresses only the most common diagnoses. Diagnoses specific to individual diseases can be found in their respective chapters.

Anxiety

Early in the disease continuum, for example, during diagnosis and treatment, threats to or changes in health status, physical comfort, role functioning, or even socioeconomic status can cause anxiety. Later, anxiety may result from the anticipation of pain, disfigurement, or the threat of death. In particular, clients whose coping skills have been poor in the past (e.g., in managing anger) may find themselves at a loss to manage this current crisis. The client may manifest overt signs of anxiety: trembling, restlessness, irritability, hyperactivity, stimulation of the sympathetic nervous system (increased blood pressure, pulse, respiration, excessive perspiration, pallor), withdrawal, worried facial expressions, and poor eye contact. The client may report insomnia and feelings of tension and apprehension, or express concerns regarding perceived changes brought about by the disease and fear of future events.

- Carefully assess the client's level of anxiety (moderate anxiety, severe anxiety, or panic) and the reality of the threats represented in the client's current situation. The level of anxiety and the reality of the perceived threat influence the type of intervention that is appropriate for the client. *A client in panic may need medical intervention with appropriate medications, whereas those with moderate or severe anxiety are often managed by the nurse through counseling and teaching new coping skills.*
- Establish a therapeutic relationship by conveying warmth and empathy and listening nonjudgmentally. *A client who feels safe in the relationship with the nurse more easily expresses feelings and thoughts. The client will be able to trust*

BOX 10–11 ■ Factors to Consider in Assessing Hydration Status

- Intake and output
- Rapid weight changes
- Skin turgor and moisture
- Venous filling
- Vital sign changes
- Tongue furrows and moisture
- Eyeball softness
- Lung sounds
- Laboratory values

the nurse and perhaps be willing to try new behaviors as suggested. The amount of time this relationship may take to develop depends on the client's current emotional and mental state and the stage of the disease process.

- Encourage the client to acknowledge and express feelings, no matter how inappropriate they may seem to the client. *Just by expressing their feelings, clients often can significantly diminish anxiety. Expressing feelings also allows the client to direct energy toward healing and thus has a positive therapeutic effect. Moreover, by acknowledging feelings, especially those the client considers unacceptable, the client can lay a groundwork for new coping behaviors.*
- Review the coping strategies the client has used in the past and build on past successful behaviors, introducing new strategies as appropriate. Explain why inappropriate strategies, such as repressing anger or turning to alcohol, are not helpful. *The client will be more willing to make changes that build on what has already worked in the past. The client will also be more willing to reject inappropriate strategies if he or she is given a persuasive reason why they have not had the desired effect in managing previous crises.*
- Identify resources in the community, such as crisis hotlines and support groups, that can help the client manage anxiety-producing situations. *The client may not have support systems available, or the client's significant others may be having their own difficulties in dealing with the cancer diagnosis. Programs such as "I Can Cope," sponsored by the American Cancer Society in most communities, provide education, counseling, and support in a group setting with other cancer clients.*
- Provide specific information for the client about the disease, its treatment, and what may be expected, especially for those clients with obvious misinformation. *Knowing what is to come gives the client a sense of control and enables the client to make decisions. Also, knowing that every effort will be made to keep the client as free of pain as possible can do a great deal to relieve anxiety.*
- Provide a safe, calm, and quiet environment for the client in panic. Remain with the client and administer antianxiety medications as ordered. *Staying with the client and displaying calmness and confidence can protect the client from injury and prevent further panic. If the panic does not subside with the nurse's presence and support, referral to the physician for medication management may be necessary.*
- Use crisis intervention theory to promote growth in the client and significant others, regardless of the outcome of the disease. *During a major crisis, people can, with assistance, transform the experience from one that causes defeat and despair to one that enhances personal and spiritual growth.* If you are not skilled in this area, a referral to an appropriate mental health professional may be helpful to the client and family.

Disturbed Body Image

Cancer and cancer treatments frequently result in major physiologic and psychologic body image changes. See the box on this page for manifestations of cancer. Loss of a body part (e.g., amputation, prostatectomy, or mastectomy), skin changes and hair loss from chemotherapy or radiation therapy, or creation

Manifestations of Cancer

- Hair loss
- Depression
- Fever
- Bleeding gums
- Oropharyngeal ulcerations
- Stomatitis
- Anorexia
- Nausea and vomiting
- Diarrhea
- Emaciation
- General weakness
- Flaccid muscles
- Stooped posture
- Pallor
- Excessive bruising
- Radiation burns
- Visible tumor (abdomen)
- Odor of decay
- Hypotension

of unnatural openings on the body for elimination (e.g., colostomy or ileostomy) may have a major effect on the person's self-image. The gaunt, wasted appearance of the cachexic client or draining, malodorous lesions that result when cancer breaks through the skin are other significant etiologies of body image disturbance. This may also give rise to fear of rejection, which plays a major role in sexual dysfunction. In addition to all of the other afflictions the cancer brings about, the client may undergo major changes in appearance and function. The client may exhibit a visible physical alteration of some portion of the body, verbalize negative feelings about the body and/or fear of rejection by others, refuse to look at the affected site, and depersonalize the body change or lost part (e.g., by calling the colostomy "that thing").

- Discuss the meaning of the loss or change with the client. *Doing so helps the nurse discover the best approach for this particular client and involves the client more actively in interventions. A small, seemingly trivial loss may have a big impact, especially when viewed in light of the other changes that are occurring in the client's life. Likewise, a major loss may not be as important as the nurse might imagine. To ensure more appropriate and individualized care, evaluate each situation in terms of the reactions of the specific client.*
- Observe and evaluate interaction with significant others. *People who are important to the client may unintentionally reinforce negative feelings about body image; on the other hand, the client may perceive rejection where none exists.*
- Allow denial, but do not participate in the denial; for example, if a client does not want to look at the wound, the nurse may say, "I am going to change the dressing to your breast incision now." *During the initial stage of shock at the loss of a body part, denial is a protective mechanism and should not be challenged, nor should it be promoted. A matter-of-fact approach and an empathetic attitude will go far to facilitate the eventual acceptance of the change.*
- Assist the client and significant others to cope with the changes in appearance:
  a. Provide a supportive environment.
  b. Encourage the client and significant others to express feelings about the situation.
  c. Give matter-of-fact responses to questions and concerns.
  d. Identify new coping strategies to resolve feelings.

e. Enlist family and friends in reaffirming the client's worth. *A supportive, safe environment in which feelings are respected and new coping strategies can be tried promotes acceptance, as does reaffirming that the client's worth is not diminished by any physical changes.*

- Teach the client or significant others to participate in the care of the afflicted body area. Provide support and validation of their efforts. *Active involvement in providing care, such as changing a dressing or emptying a colostomy bag, empowers the client and/or significant others. This intimate involvement also desensitizes feelings about disfigurement and promotes acceptance. Involving significant others reduces the risk of their rejecting the client and can promote closeness. Positive reinforcement from the nurse encourages them to continue these behaviors.*

- Teach strategies for minimizing physical changes, such as providing skin care during radiation therapy and dressing to enhance appearance and minimize change in the body part. *Early intervention can limit the negative side effects of treatment and actually promote recovery. Involving the client provides an additional way for the client to be in control of a difficult situation.*

- Teach ways to reduce the alopecia that results from chemotherapy and to enhance appearance until the hair grows back:

  a. Discuss the pattern and timing of hair loss. *This allows the client to cope with changes and incorporate them into daily activities.*

  b. Encourage wearing cheerful, brightly colored head coverings; assist in color coordinating them with usual clothing. *Attractive head coverings protect the bald head while allowing the client to feel stylish and well dressed.*

  c. Refer to a good wig shop before hair loss is experienced. *Hair color and texture can be matched to minimize obvious changes in appearance.*

  d. Refer to support programs such as "Look Good . . . Feel Better," which is sponsored by the American Cancer Society and the Cosmetic, Toilet, and Fragrance Association Foundation. *A support group can diminish feelings of isolation and provide practical tips for managing problems. For a list of community resources available to clients with cancer, refer to a local phone book.*

  e. Reassure that hair will grow back after chemotherapy is discontinued, but also inform that the color and texture of the new hair may be different. Hair loss has been identified as the most distressing symptom by many clients (Ferrell, 2000; Williams, Wood, & Cunningham-Warburton, 1999). *Interventions to reduce that loss can have a significant impact on body image concerns. Moreover, knowing what to expect may decrease anxiety and distress.*

Anticipatory Grieving

Anticipatory grieving is a response to loss that has not yet occurred. Overall, only 50% of people with cancer fully recover, and certain types of cancer have a much higher death rate; thus, the client with cancer is often confronted with facing death and making preparations for it. This can be a healthy response that allows the client and family to work through the dying process and achieve growth in the final stage of life. Perceived changes in body image and lifestyle also can prompt anticipatory grieving. The client or significant others may show sorrow, anger, depression, or withdrawal, expressing distress at the potential loss or verbalizing concern about unfinished life business.

- Use the therapeutic communication skills of active listening, silence, and nonverbal support to provide an open environment for the client and significant others to discuss their feelings realistically and to express anger or other negative feelings appropriately. *This helps the client and family to get in touch with feelings and confront the possibility of the loss or death.*

- Answer questions about illness and prognosis honestly, but always encourage hope. *This allows for realistic appraisal of the situation and planning, and it also helps combat feelings of hopelessness and depression.*

- Encourage the dying client to make funeral and burial plans ahead of time and to be sure the will is in order. Make sure the necessary phone numbers can be easily located. *This gives a sense of control and relieves family members of these concerns at a time when the client is most in need of their support and when they themselves are extremely stressed.*

- Encourage the client to continue taking part in activities he or she enjoys, including maintaining employment as long as possible. *This gives a sense of continuity of life even in the face of severe losses.*

Risk for Infection

Malnutrition, impaired skin and mucous membrane integrity, tumor necrosis, and suppression of the white blood cells from chemotherapy or radiation may contribute to the risk for infection. Anorexia, as well as the disease itself, deprives the body of nutrients needed for healing, while impaired integrity of skin and mucous membranes (a result of chemotherapy and/or radiation therapy) compromise the first lines of defense against microbial invasion. Cells in the center of large or not very vascular tumors may die from malnutrition, eventually eroding through tissues to increase the risk of sepsis. Bone marrow depression resulting from the effects of certain types of cancers and from chemotherapy undermine the body's ability to respond to infection. The client may exhibit the classic signs of infection: lassitude, fever, anorexia, pain in the affected area, and physical evidence of infection, such as a purulent, draining lesion or wound. If the bone marrow is compromised, the usual signs and symptoms of infection may be absent or reduced.

- Monitor vital signs. *Fever and sympathetic nervous system responses, such as increased pulse and respiration, are usual early signs of infection. However, severely immunosuppressed clients may be unable to mount a fever; therefore, the absence of fever cannot rule out infection.*

- Monitor white blood cell counts frequently, especially if the client is receiving chemotherapy known to cause bone marrow suppression. *This allows the nurse to notify the physician at the first sign of diminishing white blood cell counts so that corrective action can be taken.*

- Teach the client to avoid crowds, small children, and people with infections when white blood cell count is at nadir (lowest point during chemotherapy) and to practice scrupulous personal hygiene. *During periods of leukopenia, the client may lose immunity to his or her own natural flora. Careful attention to hygiene reduces the risk of infection. Crowds, which promote contact with a greater variety of infectious agents, and friends with minor infections can be very dangerous for the immunosuppressed. Small children should be avoided because they often have microbes to which most people are usually immune but which the client may not be able to resist.*
- Protect skin and mucous membranes from injury. Teach appropriate skin care measures, such as good hygiene, use of a moisturizing lotion to prevent dryness and cracking, frequent changes of position for the bed-bound, and immediate attention to skin breaks or lesions. *Ensuring intact skin strengthens the first line of defense against infection.*
- Encourage the client to consume a diet high in protein, minerals, and vitamins, especially vitamin C. *Improving nutrition decreases the risk of infection. Vitamin C has been shown to help prevent certain types of infection, such as colds.*

Risk for Injury

In addition to infection, cancer can pose a risk for injury from, for example, obstruction by a large tumor or one located in a limited body space (e.g., in the brain, bowel, or bronchial airways). If the cancer is one that creates ectopic sites of hormones, elevated levels of hormones that are not under the control of the pituitary gland can injure the client in a variety of ways. Signs of obstruction depend on the organ involved: Bowel obstruction presents with pain, distention, and cessation of bowel activities; obstruction in the brain gives signs of increased intracranial pressure or personality/behavioral change; bronchial obstruction manifests as respiratory distress, cyanosis, and altered arterial blood gases. Ectopic production of parathyroid hormone manifests as high serum calcium levels as well as signs of hypercalcemia; ectopic production of antidiuretic hormone causes fluid retention and manifests as hypertension and peripheral and pulmonary edema.

- Assess frequently for signs and symptoms indicating problems with organ obstruction. *Early detection of major problems allows the nurse to seek medical help before the problem evolves into a physiologic crisis.*
- Teach to differentiate minor problems from those of a serious nature. Encourage the client to consult with the nurse or physician if in doubt or to call 911 if the client becomes very ill. Box 10–12 provides guidelines to help clients identify serious problems. *Having guidelines for when to call the doctor provides an anxiety-reducing safety net for the client and family and promotes early detection of complications.*
- Monitor laboratory values that may indicate the presence of ectopic functioning and report abnormal findings to physicians immediately. (See Table 10–4 for laboratory indicators of ectopic functions.) *Early detection promotes early medical intervention and prevents serious consequences from the ectopic secretion.* Refer to Chapters 5, 17, and 18 for

---

BOX 10–12 ■ When to Call for Help

Instruct the client or family member to call the nurse or physician if any of the following signs or symptoms occur:

- Oral temperature greater than 101.5°F (38.6°C)
- Severe headache; significant increase in pain at usual site, especially if the pain is not relieved by the medication regimen; or severe pain at a new site
- Difficulty breathing
- New bleeding from any site, such as rectal or vaginal bleeding
- Confusion, irritability, or restlessness
- Withdrawal, greatly decreased activity level, or frequent crying
- Verbalizations of deep sadness or a desire to end life
- Changes in body functioning, such as the inability to void or severe diarrhea or constipation
- Changes in eating patterns, such as refusal to eat, extreme hunger, or a significant increase in nausea and vomiting
- Appearance of edema in the extremities or significant increase in edema already present

Instruct the client or family member to call 911 if the client

- Is having much difficulty breathing or if the lips or face has a bluish tinge.
- Becomes unconscious or has a convulsion.
- Exhibits unmanageable behavior, such as being physically abusive, hurting self, or engaging in uncontrollable activity.

---

specific signs and symptoms of electrolyte imbalances and endocrine disorders. ⌒

Imbalanced Nutrition: Less Than Body Requirements

The anorexia-cachexia syndrome (described earlier in this chapter) is a common cause of malnutrition in cancer clients. Metabolism increases in response to increased cancer cell production while the cancer's parasitic activity reduces the nutrients available to the body. Loss of appetite, food aversion, nausea and vomiting, and painful oral lesions from chemotherapy or radiation may contribute to impaired nutrition. Tumors of the gastrointestinal tract that affect absorption also contribute to the problem. Manifestations include wasted appearance, considerable weight loss over a relatively short period of time, anthropometric measurements below 85% of standard for fat and muscle tissue, decreases in serum proteins, and negative responses to antigen testing.

- Assess current eating patterns, including usual likes and dislikes, and identify factors that impair food intake. *This allows for a more individualized plan based on needs and preferences.*
- Evaluate degree of malnutrition:
  a. Check laboratory values for total serum protein, serum albumin and globins, total lymphocyte count, serum transferrin, hemoglobin, and hematocrit. *These values represent the laboratory values that are most likely to decrease with malnutrition.*
  b. Calculate nitrogen balance and creatinine-height index. Calculate skeletal muscle mass, and compare findings to

normal ranges. *Urinary creatinine is an index of lean body mass and decreases in malnutrition. Lean muscle mass is catabolized for energy in clients with cancer.*

c. Take anthropometric measurements and compare them to standards: height, weight, elbow breadth, arm circumference, triceps skinfold thickness, and arm muscle mass. *This estimates the degree of wasting; findings below 85% of standard are considered malnutrition.*

- Teach the principles of maintaining good nutrition by using the food guide pyramid and adapting the diet to medical restrictions and current preferences. *This tailors the food plan to the client's needs and thereby promotes compliance.*

- Manage problems that interfere with eating:

  a. Encourage eating whatever is appealing and consider adding nutritional supplements such as Ensure or Isocal to diet. *It is better to eat something even if it is not nutritionally balanced.*

  b. Eat small, frequent meals. *These are more easily digested and absorbed and usually better tolerated by the client with anorexia.*

  c. Encourage to try icy cold foods (such as ice cream) or those that are more highly seasoned if food has no taste. *Chemotherapy and radiation therapy may harm taste buds and prevent distinguishing the taste of foods. Strong seasonings and coldness make food more enjoyable to the client with diminished taste.* However, spicy foods are not recommended for patients with stomatitis.

  d. Encourage cold and bland semisoft and liquid foods with painful oropharyngeal ulcers; use a nonalcohol anesthetic mouthwash prior to eating. *These foods are less irritating to sensitive mucous membranes; deadening the pain can make chewing and swallowing easier.*

  e. Manage nausea and vomiting by administering antiemetic drugs (around-the-clock medication may be an effective preventive measure). Encourage client to eat small, frequent, low-fat meals with dry foods such as crackers and toast, to avoid liquids with meals, and to sit upright for an hour after meals. Remove emesis basins, and encourage oral hygiene before eating. *Dry, low-fat foods are more readily tolerated when nauseated. Removing vomiting cues, such as odor and supplies associated with vomiting, can reduce nausea.*

- Teach to supplement meals with nutritional supplements such as Ensure Plus or Isocal and to take multivitamin and mineral tablets with meals. Suggest increasing calories by adding ice cream or frozen yogurt to the liquid supplement or commercial protein-carbohydrate powders to milk or fruit juice. *Because the food intake is usually less than that needed to maintain or gain weight, these supplements can add calories in a manner often tolerated.*

- Teach to keep a food diary to document daily intake. *If the client can see how little is being consumed, he or she may eat more. A food diary also helps the nurse keep a calorie count and alert the physician if more drastic nutritional measures, such as a feeding tool or parenteral nutrition, need to be instituted.*

- Teach to administer parenteral nutrition via a central line or other VAD. Teach safety measures and care of the VAD, and explain how the pump delivering the solution works. Provide an emergency phone number for help with administration problems. (See Chapter 20 for safety guidelines for administering parenteral nutrition.) ⊖ *The client with chronic or terminal cancer requiring parenteral nutrition is usually managed at home, so information on how to manage the entire process may be needed.*

Impaired Tissue Integrity

The most common impairment of tissue integrity occurs in the oral-pharyngeal-esophageal mucous membranes. It is secondary to the effects of some chemotherapeutic drugs and radiation treatment to the head and neck. The oral-pharyngeal-esophageal tissues are lined with cells with a high mitotic turnover rate and are therefore vulnerable to many chemotherapeutic drugs. Leukemias, bone marrow transplants, and herpes viral infections are other etiologic factors in the disruption of oral-pharyngeal-esophageal tissue. Manifestations of this problem may include the following:

- Small ulcers occur on the tongue and mucous membranes in the mouth and throat.
- Herpes simplex type I lesions or vesicles evolve into ulcerations.
- Fungal infections, such as thrush (due to Candida infections), are manifested by a white, yellow, or tan coating with dry, red, fissured tissue underneath.
- Red, swollen, friable gums bleed with minimal or no trauma.
- **Xerostomia** is excessive dryness of the mucous membranes (due to chemotherapy or radiation).

Manage such problems with the following interventions.

- Carefully assess and evaluate the type of tissue impairment present. Identify possible sources, such as chemotherapy or radiation therapy to head and neck. *This allows the nurse to implement corrective measures appropriate to the type of problem.*

- Implement and teach measures for preventing oropharyngeal infection:

  a. Observe for systemic signs of infection. Be suspicious of any fever that has no apparent cause. *This facilitates early identification of an infection before it spreads.*

  b. Encourage cleaning teeth gently and using a nonalcohol mouthwash several times a day. This can be done after waking up in the morning, after any oral intake, and before bedtime. Soak dentures nightly in hydrogen peroxide and floss gently with waxed floss after meals and bedtime; this measure may be contraindicated for people with leukemia or thrombocytopenia. *Disrupted mucous membranes allow the normal oral bacterial flora into the systemic circulation, which can result in sepsis in the immunocompromised person. Reducing the oral flora by frequent hygiene decreases the risk of infection.*

  c. Culture any oral lesions, and report the problem to the physician. Herpes lesions may not follow a typical pattern in immunosuppressed clients. *Identifying the cause of the infection, whether viral, fungal, or bacterial, allows the physician to prescribe the appropriate treatment.*

- Implement and teach measures for reducing trauma to delicate tissues:
  a. Counteract dry mouth (xerostomia) with lubricating and moisturizing agents, such as Gatoraid, sugarless gum, and Blistex. *This protects mucous membranes from infection and trauma.*
  b. Avoid putting sharp instruments in the mouth. Use smooth plastic spoons and forks for eating, especially with a bleeding disorder. Dental work should be done by dental oncologists.
  c. Brush teeth with a very soft toothbrush and obtain a new toothbrush monthly. If gums are friable and bleeding, clean teeth with a soft cloth or toothpaste over finger. Chlorhexidine mouthwash (Peridex) may be used. *This protects gums from trauma and decreases risk of hemorrhage.*
- Administer specific medications as ordered to control infection and/or pain:
  a. Acyclovir is often used to treat viral infections.
  b. Systemic antibiotics are used to treat bacterial infections.
  c. Nystatin or clotrimazole solution for "swish and swallow" or lozenges that dissolve slowly in the mouth are used for fungal infections.
  d. Use viscous xylocaine or various combination mouthwashes before meals and as needed. These agents reduce pain and inflammation. See Box 10–13 for the ingredients of combination mouthwashes. *Knowing the contents of each mouthwash can prevent hypersensitivity reactions (e.g., to lidocaine) and assist in client teaching.*

Nursing Interventions for Oncologic Emergencies

In caring for clients with cancer, nurses may encounter a number of emergency situations in which their role may be pivotal to the client's survival. Most of these emergencies require astute observations, accurate judgments, and rapid action once the problem has been identified. A brief description of the more common oncologic emergencies with nursing interventions follows. In all cases, immediate notification of the physician or emergency team is the first step.

Pericardial Effusions and Neoplastic Cardiac Tamponade

Malignant pericardial effusion is an accumulation of excess fluid in the pericardial sac that compresses the heart, restricts heart movement, and results in a cardiac tamponade. The signs of cardiac tamponade are caused by compression of the heart leading to decreased cardiac output and impaired cardiac function. Signs include hypotension, tachycardia, tachypnea, dyspnea, cyanosis, increased central venous pressure, anxiety, restlessness, and impaired consciousness.

Interventions include the following:

- Start oxygen and alert respiratory therapy for other respiratory support as needed.
- Insert an intravenous catheter if one is not already in place.
- Monitor vital signs and initiate hemodynamic monitoring.
- Prepare vasopressor drugs.
- Bring emergency to bedside.
- Set up for and assist physician with a pericardial tap (pericardiocentesis).
- Reassure the client.

Superior Vena Cava Syndrome

The superior vena cava can be compressed by mediastinal tumors or adjacent thoracic tumors. The most common cause is small-cell or squamous-cell lung cancers. Occasionally the problem is caused by thrombus around a central venous catheter that then plugs up the vena cava, resulting in obstruction and backup of the blood flowing into the superior vena cava.

Obstruction of the venous system causes increased venous pressure, venous stasis, and engorgement of veins that are drained by the superior vena cava. Signs and symptoms may develop slowly; facial, periorbital, and arm edema are early signs. As the problem progresses, respiratory distress, dyspnea, cyanosis, tachypnea, and altered consciousness and neurologic deficits may occur. Figure 10–7 ■ illustrates the superior venal cava syndrome.

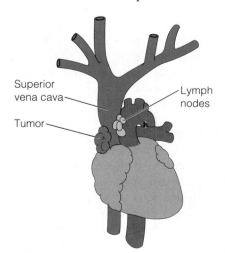

Superior vena cava

Lymph nodes

Tumor

Figure 10–7 ■ The superior vena cava syndrome. The enlargement of a tumor adjacent to the superior vena cava (usually in the lung or mediastinum) compresses that major blood vessel, which leads into the right atrium of the heart. As a result, blood backs up into the venous system behind the obstruction, diminishing blood flow into the heart.

BOX 10–13 ■ Combination Mouthwashes for Oropharyngeal Pain Control	
Kaiser Mouthwash	**Xyloxylin Suspension**
■ Nystatin	■ Benylin syrup
■ Hydrocortisone	■ Lidocaine
■ Tetracycline	■ Maalox suspension
Stanford Mouthwash	**Stomafate Suspension**
■ Nystatin	■ Sucralfate
■ Tetracycline	■ Sterile water
■ Lidocaine	■ Benylin syrup
■ Hydrocortisone	■ Maalox suspension

Emergency measures include the following:

- Provide respiratory support with oxygen, and prepare for tracheostomy.
- Monitor vital signs.
- Administer corticosteroids (e.g., dexamethasone) to reduce edema.
- If the disorder is due to a clot, administer antifibrinolytic or anticoagulant drugs.
- Provide a safe environment, including seizure precautions.

After the emergency is managed, the client often receives radiation or chemotherapy to reduce the tumor size.

Sepsis and Septic Shock

Tumor necrosis, immune deficiency, antineoplastic therapy, malnutrition, and comorbid conditions can lead to the development of sepsis. Bacteria gain entrance to the blood, grow rapidly, and produce septicemia. Because malignant tumors are more likely to use anaerobic metabolic pathways, the bacteria of tumor sepsis are usually gram negative and damage the body through a combination of bacterial endotoxins and an uncontrolled immune reaction. Gram-negative sepsis progresses to systemic shock and eventually results in multisystem failure. Signs and symptoms appear in two phases. The first phase is characterized by vasodilation with vascular dehydration, high fever, peripheral edema, hypotension, tachycardia, tachypnea, hot flushed skin with creeping mottling beginning in the lower extremities, and anxiety or restlessness. Without treatment, the shock progresses to the second phase which shows the more classic signs of shock: hypotension, rapid thready pulse, respiratory distress, cyanosis, subnormal temperature, cold clammy skin, decreased urinary output, and altered mentation. Identifying the problem while the client is still in the hyperdynamic state is crucial to the client's survival. See Chapter 6 for further discussion of septic shock. ∞

Spinal Cord Compression

Spinal cord compression is most commonly associated with pressure from expanding tumors of the breast, lung, or prostate; lymphoma; or metastatic disease. Spinal cord compression constitutes an emergency because of the potential for irreversible paraplegia. Back pain is the initial symptom in 95% of the cases of spinal cord compression. This may progress to leg pain, numbness, paresthesias, and coldness. Later, bowel and bladder dysfunction occur and, finally, neurologic dysfunction progressing from weakness to paralysis. Treatment often consists of radiation or surgical decompression, but early detection is essential. See Chapter 41 for further discussion of spinal cord compression. ∞

Obstructive Uropathy

Clients with intraabdominal, retroperitoneal, or pelvic malignancies, such as prostate, cervical, or bladder cancers, may experience obstruction of the bladder neck or the ureters. Bladder neck obstruction usually manifests as urinary retention, flank pain, hematuria, or persistent urinary tract infections, but ureteral obstruction is not often evident until the client is in

renal failure. See Chapters 26 and 47 for further discussion of obstructive uropathy.

Hypercalcemia

Hypercalcemia in clients with cancer results from the excessive ectopic production of parathyroid hormone and is most commonly associated with cancers of the breast, lung, esophagus, thyroid, head, and neck and with multiple myeloma. Bone metastases may also cause hypercalcemia. When the rate of calcium mobilization from the bone exceeds the renal threshold for excretion, serum calcium levels can become dangerously elevated. Clients with hypercalcemia often present with nonspecific symptoms of fatigue, anorexia, nausea, polyuria, and constipation. Neurologic symptoms include muscle weakness, lethargy, apathy, and diminished reflexes. Without treatment, hypercalcemia progresses to alterations in mental status, psychotic behavior, cardiac arrythmias, seizures, coma, and death (see Chapter 5). ∞

Hyperuricemia

Hyperuricemia usually is a complication of rapid necrosis of tumor cells after vigorous chemotherapy for lymphomas and leukemias. Hyperuricemia may be related to increased uric acid production or to the tumor lysis syndrome associated with Burkitt's lymphoma. Uric acid crystals are deposited in the urinary tract, causing renal failure and uremia. Clients with hyperuricemia manifest with nausea, vomiting, lethargy, and oliguria.

Syndrome of Inappropriate Antidiuretic Hormone Secretion

Occurring in only about 2% of cancer clients, syndrome of inappropriate antidiuretic hormone secretion (SIADH) is related to an ectopic secretion of antidiuretic hormone (ADH) that is usually associated with small-cell lung carcinoma, but also occasionally with prostate and adrenal cancers. The kidney secretes an excessive amount of sodium and conserves a disproportionate amount of free water, causing profound hyponatremia. Signs and symptoms include anorexia, nausea, muscle aches, and subtle neurologic symptoms that can progress to lethargy, confusion, seizures, and coma from cerebral edema (see Chapter 42). ∞

Using NANDA, NIC, and NOC

Chart 10–1 shows links between NANDA, NIC, and NOC when caring for the client with cancer.

Client and Family Teaching
Prevention

The ACS makes specific recommendations for cancer prevention in addition to the screening measures discussed earlier in this chapter. Based on these recommendations, nurses teach clients and families to decrease risk factors by:

- Avoiding tobacco and excessive alcohol use.
- Avoiding situations where secondhand smoke is abundant.
- Eating a low-fat, high-fiber diet.
- Consuming ample amounts of antioxidant foods, such as those containing beta carotene (a vitamin A precursor), vitamins E and C, and omega-3 oils.

CHART 10-1 NANDA, NIC, AND NOC LINKAGES

The Client with Cancer

NURSING DIAGNOSES	NURSING INTERVENTIONS	NURSING OUTCOMES
• Chronic Pain	• Analgesia Administration • Anxiety Reduction • Pain Management	• Pain Level • Symptom Severity
• Fatigue • Imbalanced Nutrition: Less than Body Requirements • Fear	• Energy Management • Nutrition Management • Nutritional Therapy • Anxiety Reduction • Emotional Support • Spiritual Support • Support Group	• Energy Conservation • Nutritional Status (Nutrient Intake, Body Mass, Energy) • Anxiety Control • Coping

Note. Data from Nursing Outcomes Classification (NOC) by M. Johnson & M. Maas (Eds.), 1997, St. Louis: Mosby; Nursing Diagnoses: Definitions & Classification 2001–2002, by North American Nursing Diagnosis Association, 2001, Philadelphia: NANDA; Nursing Interventions Classification (NIC) by J. C. McCloskey and G. M. Bulechek (Eds.), 2000, St. Louis: Mosby. Reprinted by permission.

BOX 10-14 ■ American Cancer Society Dietary Guidelines to Prevent Cancer

■ Avoid obesity.
■ Cut down on total fat intake.
■ Include a variety of vegetables and fruits in the daily diet.
■ Eat more high-fiber foods, such as whole-grain cereals, vegetables, and fruits.
■ Limit consumption of alcoholic beverages, if you drink at all.
■ Limit consumption of salt-cured, smoked, and nitrate-cured foods.

Note. From the American Cancer Society.

• Avoiding foods with carcinogenic additives, dyes, or chemicals used in processing. Box 10–14 lists the ACS dietary guidelines.
• Taking certain medications and hormones, such as estrogen or tamoxifen, only under close medical supervision.
• Limiting exposure to radiation, including sun exposure.
• Using extreme caution if employed in an industry that uses carcinogenic chemicals or airborne particles (smoke). Seek new employment if at risk for related cancers.
• Protecting self from viral diseases known to cause cancer.
• Improving immunity by maintaining a healthy lifestyle and managing stress.

In addition, encourage people to report to the public health department any known leaking of chemicals or radioactive materials into the water or air and any noted increase in the incidence of cancer, especially of one specific type, in their communities.

Rehabilitation and Survival

Rehabilitation from cancer not only involves regaining strength, recovering from surgery or chemotherapy, and learning to live with an altered body part or appliance, but also entails recovering from associated psychologic and emotional turmoil.

Rehabilitation centers provide physical therapy, occupational therapy, speech therapy, job retraining, and an opportunity to recuperate before resuming full responsibilities. In addition, many clients go home to convalesce and receive in-home support in the form of nursing supervision, direct care, and teaching. Hygiene and home maintenance can be provided by a certified home health aide. Physical and occupational therapists provide muscle strengthening and mobility training (especially with prostheses), and home safety teaching.

Psychologic rehabilitation of cancer survivors addresses quality of life issues. Three "seasons of cancer survival" have been described (Mullan, 1985). The first starts with diagnosis but is dominated by treatment. The second stage is one of extended survival, which occurs when treatment ends and the watchful waiting period begins. This period is characterized by fear of recurrence. Permanent survival is said to begin when the survival period has gone on long enough that the risk of recurrence is small. In this period, the client has to deal with secondary problems related to health and social issues resulting from the cancer experience. Employment may be a problem, health insurance may be cancelled, and life insurance may be difficult to get. Relationships may have suffered from the strain of the illness on significant others and the essential self-focusing required for recovery. However, both the client and significant others may have undergone a personal and spiritual growth that ushers in a new and enriching period of their lives.

New self-help groups are emerging in many communities to support others through their "seasons of survival." Many cancer survivors speak to groups about assisting other cancer survivors. Clients and families need to be informed about the many resources available through community agencies as well as the survivor support groups.

Home Care

Before the client is discharged, teach both the client and significant others or caregivers to manage the client at home. Discuss problems that may result from the type of cancer and the treatment received, and provide information on how to manage these problems and when to call the physician.

- Teach wound care to the client with an open wound or draining lesion, and provide a referral to a home health nurse to monitor progress.
- Explain special diets clearly, or refer the client to a dietitian before discharge.
- Carefully review the physician's instructions with the client and family, making sure they understand medications to be taken, any other treatments, and when to see the doctor for follow-up care.
- Provide or order equipment and supplies needed for home care, especially any specialized bed or equipment to aid mobility and ensure safety in the home.
- For the client who will need complex care, such as parenteral nutrition, provide a referral to a home health nurse before discharge.

Because the hospital stay is often short, the client and family will benefit from follow-up phone calls at home for several days. People do not learn well under the stress of going home; give the client and family a number to call if they have concerns or questions.

Hospice Care

More and more cancer clients with terminal disease are electing to die at home. This decision has been made easier by the increased availability of hospice programs. When a client and family or significant others elect hospice care, they are usually precluding additional hospitalizations other than those required to manage reversible problems. Hospice clients also refuse resuscitation measures (CPR and other extraordinary measures).

Hospice care involves a multidisciplinary team and is designed to give the client comfort and to assist in a peaceful death with support to caretakers. The team usually consists of a nurse case manager, a physician, an anesthesiologist or pharmacist, an infusion therapist, a social worker, a physical therapist, a home health aide, and volunteers.

Many hospice services are connected with an inpatient respite care unit, where the client can receive 24-hour care for up to several weeks. This source provides the necessary care to the client if a family member becomes ill or needs to be relieved temporarily of the tremendous burden of caring for a dying loved one. Veterans Administration medical centers are very good models for these programs.

Studies of families that have participated in hospice services have found that family members were very positive about the experience (Teno et al., 2001). The aspects of hospice they most appreciated were the 24-hour accessibility and availability of the health team and the quality of communication from all team members. Family members emphasized that "the nurses listened, answered questions honestly, and prepared us for changes in the patient's condition." Team members were rated as very professional, but more relaxed and friendly than hospital staff; they talked with the family and displayed accepting, nonjudgmental attitudes. Team members were also seen as well informed, knowledgeable, and competent with excellent problem-solving skills. Chapter 11 provides more information on hospice care. 🔗

Nursing Care Plan
A Client with Cancer

James Casey, age 72, is of Northern European heritage. He has been receiving medical care for chronic obstructive pulmonary disease, chronic bronchitis, status postmyocardial infarction, and type I diabetes mellitus for over 15 years. He reports that he lost his wife from lung cancer 5 years ago and still "misses her terribly." He describes his bad habits as smoking two packs of cigarettes a day for 52 years (104 packs/year), one to two six-packs of beer a week, one "bourbon and water" a night, and "a lot of sugar-free junk food, like french fries." He assures the nurse that he quit smoking 2 years ago, when he could no longer walk a block without considerable shortness of breath, and just quit drinking alcohol a few weeks ago at his physician's insistence. About a year ago, he had a basal-cell carcinoma removed from his right ear. Six months ago, cancerous tumors were discovered in his bladder, and he underwent two 6-week chemotherapy courses of bladder instillations of BCG. His latest report indicates that the tumors have grown back and no further chemotherapy would be useful. The urologist had considered surgery but believed that Mr. Casey's other medical problems would compromise his chances of survival. Mr. Casey decides to let the disease run its course and to be managed at home through hospice care. Because he lives alone in a modest home, he asks his daughter,

Mary, and her family to move in with him to provide care and support during his final months. The daughter accepts, saying she is glad to be able to spend this time with her father; she has been informed of the physical and emotional stress this will entail.

ASSESSMENT

Glynis Jackson, RN, the hospice nurse assigned as case manager for James Casey, completes a health history and physical examination during her first two visits in his home, 1 day apart. She gathers this information over 2 days to conserve his strength and allow more time for Mr. Casey and his daughter to talk about their concerns.

During the physical assessment, Glynis notes that Mr. Casey is pale with pink mucous membranes, thin with a wasted appearance and a strained, worried facial expression. He complains of severe back pain no longer adequately relieved by Percodan and Vicodin alternating every 2 to 4 hours. His blood pressure is 90/50, right arm in the reclining position with no significant orthostatic change; his apical pulse is 102, regular and strong; respiratory rate 24 and unlabored; breath sounds are clear but diminished in the bases; oral temperature is 96.8°F.

(continued on page 312)

Nursing Care Plan
A Client with Cancer *(continued)*

A tunnelled Groshong catheter as a VAD is present in the right anterior chest. There is no drainage, redness, or swelling at the site. The catheter was placed last week when the client was being evaluated at the anesthesiologist's office for pain management, but no medication is running via the VAD. Mary reports that his urinary output is adequate. Approximately 200 mL of yellow, cloudy, nonmalodorous urine is present in the urinal at the bedside from his last voiding.

Mr. Casey states that he spends most of his time either in bed or sitting up in a chair in his room. He reports that he has no energy any more and is unable to walk to the bathroom unassisted, dress himself, or take care of his own personal hygiene. Glynis rates Mr. Casey's functional level at ECOG level 4: capable of only limited self-care, confined to bed or chair 50% or more of waking hours (Karnofsky 10 to 20). He tells the nurse that his daughter "is working day and night to help me and is looking awfully tired."

Many reports that Mr. Casey is eating very poorly: He usually eats a small bowl of oatmeal with milk for breakfast and vegetable soup and crackers for lunch, but he tells her that he is too tired for dinner and wants only fruit juice. Mr. Casey tells the nurse that he has no appetite and eats just to please Mary. He does drink at least three to four glasses of water a day plus juice. His fingerstick blood sugars remain within normal range.

His current weight is 120 pounds at 67 inches tall, down from 180 pounds a year ago. He has lost about 30 pounds over the last 2 months.

Available laboratory values from his visit with the doctor show the following:

Total protein: 4.1 g/dL (normal range: 6.0 to 8.0 g/dL)
Albumin: 2.2 g/dL (normal range: 3.5 to 5.0 g/dL)
Hemoglobin: 10.2 g/dL (normal range: 13.5 to 18.0 g/dL)
Hematocrit: 30.5% (normal range: 40.0% to 54.0%)
BUN: 30 mg/dL (normal range: 5 to 25 mg/dL slightly higher in older people)
Creatinine: 2.2 mg/dL (normal range: 0.5 to 1.5 mg/dL)

DIAGNOSIS
- *Imbalanced nutrition: Less than body requirements* related to anorexia and fatigue
- *Risk for caregiver role strain* related to severity of her father's illness and lack of help from other family members
- *Chronic pain* related to progression of disease process
- *Impaired physical mobility* related to pain, fatigue, and beginning neuromuscular impairment
- *Risk for impaired skin integrity* related to impaired physical mobility and malnourished state

EXPECTED OUTCOMES
- Increase oral intake and show improvement in serum protein values.
- Daughter will be able to maintain supportive caretaking activities as long as Mr. Casey needs them.
- Minimal pain for the rest of his life.
- Able to continue his current activity level.
- Maintain intact skin.

PLANNING AND IMPLEMENTATION
- Ask about favorite foods, and ask Mary to offer a small portion of one of these foods each day.
- Encourage drinking up to four cans of liquid nutritional supplement with fiber a day, sipping them throughout the day.
- Talk with the physician about prescribing a medication to help stimulate the appetite.
- Plan to have a home health aide come to the home, give him a shower or bed bath daily, and assist his daughter with some of the household chores.
- Talk with Mary about having her adult son and daughter relieve her of the housework and stay with Mr. Casey so that she can get out of the house occasionally. Offer to talk with them if she is uncomfortable doing so.
- Request a volunteer to spend up to 4 hours a day, twice a week with Mr. Casey so that Mary can attend to outside activities and chores.
- Talk with the anesthesiologist, and work out a pain control program, using the VAD and a CADD-PCA infusion pump with a continuous morphine infusion.
- Call the infusion therapist to set up the equipment and supplies (including the medication) for the morphine infusion.
- Teach how to use the pump and about the side effects of the morphine infusion, including those that require a call to the nurse for assistance. Teach which untoward effects should be reported.
- Request a physical therapy consultation to evaluate current level of functioning and determine how to maintain current level.
- Instruct Mary to allow ample rest periods for James between activities.
- Order a hospital bed with electronic controls to be delivered to the house.
- Order a special foam pad for bed and chair and a bedside commode from the medical supply house.
- Instruct Mary and the home health aide to inspect skin daily, give good skin care with emollient lotion after bathing, and report any beginning lesions immediately to the nurse.

EVALUATION
James Casey did increase his oral intake a little, sometimes eating the special treats his daughter prepared and drinking one or two cans of liquid nutritional supplement a day. However, his weight did not increase; it stayed at about 120 pounds until his death 2 weeks later. His daughter was very grateful for the extra help from the home health aide and the volunteer, though she could not bring herself to ask her son and daughter for help and did not want the nurse to do so. She did become more rested and reported that "Dad and I had some wonderful 3:00 A.M. talks when he couldn't sleep."

Mr. Casey was started on 20 mg of morphine per hour with boluses of 10 mg 4 times a day, for breakthrough pain. This medication relieved his pain quite well; after 2 days he was alert enough most of the time to carry on a normal conversation and still walk to the bathroom with help up until 2 days before he died.

Nursing Care Plan
A Client with Cancer *(continued)*

The hospital bed simplified Mr. Casey's care and made it much easier for him to rest comfortably and change position. His skin remained intact and in good condition.

Mary reported that Mr. Casey died peacefully in his sleep, about 2 weeks after care was started. She said spending the last weeks of his life together was a healing experience for both of them.

Critical Thinking in the Nursing Process

1. What other tests could be done to evaluate James Casey's nutritional status?
2. Mr. Casey had severe back pain. What were the possible pathophysiologic reasons for his pain?
3. One of the specified interventions was to consult the physician regarding medication to increase Mr. Casey's appetite. What medications might fulfill that function? What side effects might they have that would contraindicate these medications for him?
4. If Mr. Casey had developed signs and symptoms of sepsis, what manifestations would you expect to see? As the nurse making the home visits, what would be your nursing actions, and in what order of priority?

See Evaluating Your Response in Appendix C.

EXPLORE MediaLink

NCLEX review questions, case studies, care plan activities, MediaLink applications, and other interactive resources for this chapter can be found on the Companion Website at www.prenhall.com/lemone.

Click on Chapter 10 to select the activities for this chapter. For animations, video clips, more NCLEX review questions, and an audio glossary, access the Student CD-ROM accompanying this textbook.

TEST YOURSELF

1. Mr. Lawrence has a history of colon cancer. Cells from the colon tumor have traveled to his liver. This process is called:
   a. Carcinogenesis
   b. Dysplasia
   c. Metastasis
   d. Mutation

2. A client diagnosed with lung cancer reports he is having difficulty sleeping and often feels tense. The most appropriate initial nursing intervention would be to:
   a. Encourage the client to express his feelings about the cancer diagnosis
   b. Document the client's report of difficulty sleeping and tenseness in the chart
   c. Obtain an order for medication for sleep from the physician
   d. Offer an antianxiety drug such as Ativan (Lorazepam)

3. Mr. Roberts is receiving external radiation for treatment of lung cancer. Client education for care of the skin in the marked area includes:
   a. Apply antibacterial ointment daily
   b. Avoid contact with others
   c. Avoid rubbing or scratching treated skin areas
   d. Cleanse the skin with mild soap and water

4. Ms. Smith complains of nausea and vomiting following her daily chemotherapy treatment. The *most* appropriate nursing intervention would be to:
   a. Keep Ms. Smith NPO until her daily chemotherapy is completed
   b. Provide antiemetic medication 30 to 40 minutes prior to each treatment
   c. Provide clear liquids until the chemotherapy is completed
   d. Schedule chemotherapy administration for bedtime

5. Mrs. Smith experiences bone marrow depression as a result of chemotherapy. Which of the following would the nurse expect to find?
   a. Alopecia
   b. Nausea and vomiting
   c. Platelet count 50,000
   d. Temperature 102°F

See Test Yourself answers in Appendix C.

BIBLIOGRAPHY

American Cancer Society. (2002). *Cancer facts and figures—2002*. Atlanta: Author.

Battiato, L. A., & Wheeler, V. S. (2000). Biotherapy. In C. H. Yarbro, M. H. Frogge, M. Goodman, & S. L. Groenwald (Eds.), *Cancer nursing: Principles and practice* (5th ed.) (pp. 543–579). Boston: Jones and Bartlett.

Berd, D. (2001). Autologous, hapten-modified vaccine as a treatment for human cancers. *Vaccine, 19*, 2565–2570.

Bergh, J., Wiklund, T., Erikstein, B., Lidbrink, E., Lindman, H., Malmström, P., et al. (2000). Tailored fluorouracil, epirubicin, and cyclophosphamide compared with marrow-supported high-dose chemotherapy as adjuvant treatment for high-risk breast cancer: A randomised trial. *Lancet, 356*, 1384–1391.

Bruce, S. (2001). Photodynamic therapy: Another option in cancer care. *Clinical Journal of Oncology Nursing, 5*, 95–99.

Cady, J. (2001). Understanding opioid tolerance in cancer pain. *Oncology Nursing Forum, 28*, 1561–1568.

Chapman, D., & Goodman, M. (2000). Breast cancer. In C. H. Yarbro, M. H. Frogge, M. Goodman, & S. L. Groenwald (Eds.), *Cancer nursing: Principles and practice* (5th ed.) (pp. 994–1047). Boston: Jones and Bartlett.

Donahue, B. R., Wernz, J. C., & Cooper, J. S. (2000). HIV-associated malignancies. In J. D. Roseblatt, P. Okunieff, & J. V. Sitzmann (Eds.), *Clinical oncology: A multidisciplinary approach for physicians and students* (8th ed.) (pp. 199–207). Philadelphia: W.B. Saunders.

Dunlop R. J., & Campbell C. W. (2000). Cytokines and advanced cancer. *Journal of Pain & Symptom Management, 20*(3), 214–232.

Ferrell, B. (2000). Article captures the essence and meaning of alopecia. *Oncology Nursing Forum, 27*, 17.

Ferrell, B., & McCaffery, M. (1997). Nurses' knowledge about equianalgesia and opioid dosing. *Cancer Nursing, 20*, 201–212.

Foltz, A. (2000). Nutritional disturbances. In C. H. Yarbro, M. H. Frogge, M. Goodman, & S. L. Groenwald (Eds.), *Cancer nursing: Principles and practice* (5th ed.) (pp. 754–775). Boston: Jones and Bartlett.

Futreal, P. A., Kasprzyk, A., Birney, E., Mullikin, J. C., Wooster, R., & Stratton, M. R. (2001). Cancer and genomics. *Nature, 409*(6822), 850–852.

Haapoja, I. (2000). Paraneoplastic syndromes. In C. H. Yarbro, M. H. Frogge, M. Goodman, & S. L. Groenwald (Eds.), *Cancer nursing: Principles and practice* (5th ed.) (pp. 792–812). Boston: Jones and Bartlett.

Hawkins, R. (2001). Mastering the intricate maze of metastasis. *Oncology Nursing Forum, 28*(6), 959–965.

Held-Warmkessel, J. (2000). Prostate cancer. In C. H. Yarbro, M. H. Frogge, M. Goodman, & S. L. Groenwald (Eds.), *Cancer nursing: Principles and practice* (5th ed.) (pp. 1427–1451). Boston: Jones and Bartlett.

Hill, R. P. (2001). The biology of cancer. In P. Rubin (Ed.), *Clinical oncology: A multidisciplinary approach for physicians and students* (pp. 32–45). Philadelphia: W. B. Saunders.

Holland, J. (2001). New treatment modalities in radiation therapy. *Journal of Intravenous Nursing, 24*, 95–101.

Karnofsky, D., Abelmann, W., Craver, L., & Burchenal, J. (1948). The use of nitrogen mustard in the palliative treatment of carcinoma. *Cancer, 1*, 634–656.

Kaye, J., Morton, J., Bowcutt, M., & Maupin, D. (2000). Stress, depression, and psychoneuroimmunology. *Journal of Neuroscience Nursing, 32*, 93–100.

LeFever Kee, J. (2002). *Laboratory and diagnostic tests with nursing implications* (6th ed.) Upper Saddle River, NJ: Prentice Hall.

McDaniel, R., & Rhodes, V. (1998). Development of a sensory information videotape for women receiving chemotherapy for breast cancer. *Cancer Nursing, 21*, 143–148.

Misset, J., & Levi, F. (1995). Chronomodulated chemotherapy combining 5-fluorouracil, folinic acid, and oxaliplatin in advanced colorectal cancer: An overview of seven years of experience (Meeting abstract). *Cancer Investigation, 13*(Suppl 1), 49–50.

Mullan, F. (1985). Seasons of survival: Reflections of a physician with cancer. *New England Journal of Medicine, 313*, 270–273.

Neal, A., & Hoskin, P. (1997). *Clinical oncology: Basic principles and practice* (2nd ed.). New York: Oxford University Press.

Oncology Nursing Society Board of Directors. (1997). Oncology Nursing Society position paper on quality cancer care. *Oncology Nursing Forum, 24*, 951–953.

Pace, J. C. (2000). AIDS-related malignancies. In C. H. Yarbro, M. H. Frogge, M. Goodman, & S. L. Groenwald (Eds.), *Cancer nursing: Principles and practice* (5th ed.) (pp. 933–949). Boston: Jones and Bartlett.

Peto, R., Darby, S., Deo, H., Silcocks, P., Whitley, E., & Doll, R. (2000). Smoking, smoking cessation, and lung cancer in the UK since 1950: Combination of national statistics with two case-control studies. *BMJ, 321*(7257), 323–329.

Porth, C. (2002). *Pathophysiology: Concepts of altered health states* (6th ed.). Philadelphia: Lippincott.

Rahman, Z., Frye, D., Buzdar, A., Smith, T., Asmar, L., Champlin, R., & Hortobagyi, G. (1997). Impact of selection process on response rate and long-term survival of potential high-dose chemotherapy candidates treated with standard-dose doxorubicin-containing chemotherapy in patients with metastatic breast cancer. *Journal of Clinical Oncology, 15*, 3171–3177.

Rosenthal, D. (1998). Changing trends. *A Cancer Journal for Clinicians, 48*(1), 3–4.

Rubin, P., Williams, J. P., Okunieff, P., Rosenblatt, J. D., & Sitzmann, J. V. (2001). Statement of the clinical oncologic problem. In P. Rubin (Ed.). *Clinical oncology: A multidisciplinary approach for physicians and students* (pp. 1–31). Philadelphia: W. B. Saunders.

Scigliano, E., Vlachos, A., Najfeld, V., & Shank, B. (2001). The leukemias. In P. Rubin (Ed.), *Clinical oncology: A multidisciplinary approach for physicians and students* (pp. 565–614). Philadelphia: W. B. Saunders.

Selye, H. (1984). *The stress of life* (rev. 2nd ed.). New York: McGraw-Hill.

Spitalnick, P. F., & diSant' Angnese, P. A. (2001). The pathology of cancer. In P. Rubin (Ed.), *Clinical oncology: A multidisciplinary approach for physicians and students* (pp. 47–61). Philadelphia: W. B. Saunders.

Surbone, A. (2001). Ethical implications of genetic testing for breast cancer susceptibility. *Critical Reviews in Oncology-Hematology, 40*(2), 149–157.

Teno, J. M., Clarridge, B., Casey, V., Edgman-Levitan, S., & Fowler, J. (2001). Validation of toolkit after-death bereaved family member interview. *Journal of Pain & Symptom Management, 22*, 752–758.

Weiss, R. B., Rifkin, R.M., Stewart, F. M., Theriault, R. L., Williams, L. A., Herman, A. A., & Beveridge, R. A. (2000). High dose chemotherapy for high-risk primary breast cancer: An on-site review of the Bezwoda study. *Lancet, 355*, 999–1003.

Williams, J., Wood, C., & Cunningham-Warburton, P. (1999). A narrative study of chemotherapy-induced alopecia. *Oncology Nursing Forum, 26*, 1463–1468.

Williams, M. D., & Sandler, A. B. (2001). The epidemiology of lung cancer. *Cancer Treatment & Research, 105*, 31–52.

Yarbro, J. (2000). Carcongenesis. In C. H. Yarbro, M. H. Frogge, M. Goodman, & S. L. Groenwald (Eds.), *Cancer nursing: Principles and practice* (5th ed.) (pp. 48–57). Boston: Jones and Bartlett.

Zech, D., Grond, S., Lynch, J., Hertel, D., & Lehmann, K. (1995). Validation of World Health Organization Guidelines for cancer pain relief: A 10-year prospective study. *Pain, 63*, 65–76.

Nursing Care of Clients Experiencing Loss, Grief, and Death

After completing this chapter, you will be able to:

- Describe theories of loss and grief.
- Discuss factors affecting responses to loss.
- Begin to assess own feelings and values related to loss, grief, and death.
- Discuss legal and ethical issues in end-of-life care.
- Describe the philosophy and activities of hospice.
- Identify physiological changes in the dying client.
- Provide nursing interventions to promote a comfortable death.
- Use the nursing process as a framework for providing individualized care for clients and families experiencing loss, grief, or death.

MediaLink

www.prenhall.com/lemone
Additional resources for this chapter can be found on the Student CD-ROM accompanying this textbook, and on the Companion Website at www.prenhall.com/lemone. Click on Chapter 11 to select the activities for this chapter.

CD-ROM
- Audio Glossary
- NCLEX Review

Companion Website
- More NCLEX Review
- Case Study
  Dysfunctional Grieving
- Care Plan Activity
  Anticipatory Grieving
- MediaLink Application
  Grief and Unexpected Death

BOX 11–1 ■ Types of Losses

- ■ Death
- ■ Health
- ■ Body part
- ■ Social status
- ■ Lifestyle
- ■ Marital relationship (i.e., through divorce)
- ■ Reproductive function
- ■ Sexual function

Loss may be defined as an actual or potential situation in which a valued object, person, body part, or emotion that was formerly present is lost or changed and can no longer be seen, felt, heard, known, or experienced. A loss may be temporary or permanent, complete or partial, objectively verifiable or perceived, physical or symbolic. Only the person who experiences the loss can determine the meaning of the loss. Although the order of importance varies with the person, people most commonly fear the losses listed in Box 11–1.

Loss always results in change. The stress associated with the loss may be the precipitating factor leading to physiologic or psychologic change in the person or family. The effective or ineffective resolution of feelings surrounding the loss determines the person's ability to deal with the resulting changes.

Grief is the emotional response to loss and its accompanying changes. Grief as a response to loss is an inevitable dimension of the human experience. The loss of a job, a role (e.g., the loss of the role of spouse, as occurs in divorce), a goal, body integrity, a loved one, or the impending loss of one's own life may trigger grief. Loss is also integral to death. Although death is the ultimate loss, losses that occur in any phase of the life cycle may produce grief responses as intensely painful as those observed in the death experience.

Grieving may be thought of as the internal process the person uses to work through the response to loss. *Bereavement,* a form of depression accompanied by anxiety, is a common reaction to the loss of a loved one. *Mourning* describes the actions or expressions of the bereaved, including the symbols, clothing, and ceremonies that make up the outward manifestations of grief. Both grieving and mourning are healthy responses to loss because they ultimately lead the person to invest energy in new relationships and to develop positive self-regard.

Death is defined in many ways. One commonly used definition of death is an irreversible cessation of circulatory and respiratory functions or irreversible cessation of all functions of the entire brain, including the brainstem. With the current life-support systems available, the most often used criterion for determining death is whole-brain death (permanent irreversible cessation of the functioning of all areas of the brain). The criteria for whole-brain death are listed in Chapter 6. ∞

Although death is an inevitable part of life, it is often an immensely difficult loss for the person who is dying and for his or her loved ones. Death may be accidental (such as from trauma) or the end of a long and painful struggle with a terminal illness

such as cancer or AIDS. It may also be purposeful, if a person commits suicide.

THEORIES OF LOSS, GRIEF, AND DYING

Medical-surgical nurses often care for clients exhibiting responses typical of various stages of the grieving process. Highly individual in quality and duration, the grief process may range from discomforting to debilitating, and it may last a day or a lifetime, depending on what the loss means to the person experiencing it. Although each person experiences loss in a different manner, knowledge of some of the major theories of loss, grief, and dying can give the nurse a framework for holistic care of the client and family anticipating or experiencing a loss. Table 11–1 summarizes these theories.

Freud: Psychoanalytic Theory

Freud (1917, 1957) wrote about grief and mourning as reactions to loss. Freud described the process of mourning as one in which the person gradually withdraws attachment from the lost object or person. He observed that with normal grieving, this

TABLE 11–1	Summary of Theories of Loss
Theorist	**Dynamics**
Freud	Grief and mourning are reactions to loss. Grieving is the inner labor of mourning a loss. Inability to grieve a loss results in depression.
Bowlby	The successful grieving process initiated by a loss or separation during childhood ends with feelings of emancipation from the lost person or object.
Engel	After the person perceives and evaluates the loss, the person adapts to it. Shock and disbelief, developing awareness, and restitution occur during the first year following the loss; in the months following, the person puts the lost relationship into perspective.
Lindemann	A sequence of responses is experienced following a catastrophic event; defined concepts of anticipatory grieving and morbid grief reactions.
Caplan	Periods of psychologic crisis are precipitated by hazardous circumstances; successful resolution of grief involves feelings of hope and engaging in activities of ordinary living.
Kübler-Ross	There are five stages defining the response to loss: denial, anger, bargaining, depression, and acceptance. Stages are not necessarily sequential.
Carter	Identified the quality of grief's changing character, the need to hold on to that which was good in the loved one's lost existence, expectations of how to react to the experience, and the ways in which personal history affects the quality and meaning of the loss.

withdrawal of attachment is followed by a readiness to make new attachments. In comparing melancholia (prolonged gloominess, depression) with the "normal" emotions of grief, and its expression in mourning, Freud observed that the "work of mourning" is a nonpathologic condition that reaches a state of completion after a period of inner labor.

Bowlby: Protest, Despair, and Detachment

Bowlby (1973, 1980) believed that the grieving process initiated by a loss or separation from a loved object or person successfully ends when the grieving person experiences feelings of emancipation from the lost object or person. He divided the grieving process into three phases and identified behaviors characteristic of each phase.

- *Protest.* The protest phase is marked by a lack of acceptance of the loss. All energy is directed toward protesting the loss. The person experiences feelings of anger toward self and others, and feelings of ambivalence toward the lost object or person. Crying and angry behaviors characterize this phase.
- *Despair.* The person's behavior becomes disorganized. Despair mounts as efforts to deny the loss compete with acceptance of permanent loss. Crying and sadness, coupled with a desire for the lost object or person to return, result in disorganized thoughts as the client recognizes the reality of the loss.
- *Detachment.* As the person realizes the permanence of the loss and gradually relinquishes attachment to the lost object, a reinvestment of energy occurs. Both the positive and negative aspects of the relationship are remembered. Expressions of hopefulness and readiness to move forward are characteristic of this phase.

Engel: Acute Grief, Restitution, and Long-Term Grief

Engel (1964) related the grief process to other methods of coping with stress: After the person perceives and evaluates the loss (the stressful event), the person adapts to it. Engel's recognition of the impact of cognitive factors on the grieving process was an important contribution to our understanding of grieving.

Engel described three main stages in the grief process: an acute stage, a restitution stage, and a long-term stage. The acute stage occurs in two phases. The first phase, shock and disbelief, begins immediately after the person receives the news of the loss. The initial response may be denial, which may help the person to cope with the overwhelming pain. Alternatively, the grieving person in this phase may appear to accept the loss, making statements such as, "It was for the best," while repressing his or her feelings. This phase of shock and disbelief normally lasts only a few hours; however, it may continue for 1 or 2 days.

As the shock and disbelief begin to fade, the second phase, developing awareness, follows. The finality of the loss becomes a reality, and pain, anguish, anger, guilt, and blame surface. The person feels a need to make someone responsible for the loss. "If only" and "why" frequently punctuate the expressed or inner dialogue of the bereaved. Crying is common. "It is during this time that the greatest degree of anguish or despair, within the limits imposed by cultural patterns, is experienced or expressed" (Engel, 1964, p. 93). Culturally patterned behaviors, such as maintaining a stoic pose in public or weeping openly, characterize this phase.

The acute stage is followed by a stage of restitution, in which the mourning is institutionalized. Friends and family gather to support the grieving person through rituals dictated by the culture. As time passes, the mourner continues to feel a painful void and is preoccupied with thoughts of the loss. The mourner may join a support group or seek other social support for coping with the loss.

After the restitution stage, which lasts at least a year, the mourner begins to come to terms with the loss. In this long-term stage, interest in people and activities is renewed. The person puts the lost relationship in perspective as he or she begins to form new relationships. Engel observed that this period might last another 1 to 2 years.

Lindemann: Categories of Symptoms

Lindemann (1944) interviewed people who had lost a loved one during the course of medical treatment, disaster victims, and relatives of members of the armed forces who had died. Lindemann's research led him to describe normal grief, anticipatory grieving, and morbid grief reactions. He described symptoms characteristic of normal grief into categories of somatic (physical symptoms without an organic cause) distress, preoccupation with the image of the deceased, feelings of guilt, hostile reactions, and loss of patterns of conduct

Anticipatory grieving was defined as a cluster of predictable responses to an anticipated loss. These responses include the range of feelings experienced by the person or family preoccupied with an anticipated loss. The term *morbid grief reaction* described delayed and dysfunctional reactions to loss; a variety of debilitating health problems were seen in people who displayed excessive or delayed responses to loss.

Caplan: Stress and Loss

Caplan's (1990) theory of stress and its relationship to loss is useful in understanding the grief process. He expanded the focus of the grief process to include not only bereavement but also other episodes of stress that people experience, such as may result from surgery or childbirth. Caplan described these periods as "psychological crises precipitated by hazardous circumstances that lead to a temporary upset in the normal homeostatic balance of forces that characterizes transactions between an individual and his environment" (p. 28). He believed these "hazardous circumstances" lead to psychologic disequilibrium in some people because their coping skills are inadequate in helping them gain mastery over their predicament.

Caplan described three factors that influence the person's ability to deal with a loss. He believed these factors might cause distress for a year or more following the loss.

- The psychic pain of the broken bond and the agony of coming to terms with the loss
- Living without the assets and guidance of the lost person or resource
- The reduced cognitive and problem-solving effectiveness associated with the distressing emotional arousal

Caplan described the process of building new attachments to replace those that have been lost. This process involves two elements: a feeling of hope and the assumption of regular activity as a form of participating in ordinary living.

Kübler-Ross: Stages of Coping with Loss

Kübler-Ross's (1969, 1978) research on death and dying provided a framework for gaining insight about the stages of coping with an impending or actual loss. According to Kübler-Ross, not all people dealing with a loss go through these stages, and those who do may not experience the stages in the sequence described. In identifying the stages of death and dying, Kübler-Ross (1978) repeatedly stressed the danger of prematurely labeling a "stage" and emphasized that her goal was to describe her observations of how people come to terms with situations of loss.

Some or all of the following reactions may occur during the grieving process and may reappear as the person experiences the loss:

- *Denial.* A person may react with shock and disbelief after receiving word of an actual or potential loss. After receiving a terminal diagnosis, notification of a death, or other serious loss, people may make such statements as "This can't be happening to me" or "This can't be true." This initial stage of denial serves as a buffer in helping the person or family mobilize defenses to cope with the situation.
- *Anger.* In the anger stage, the person resists the loss. The anger is often directed toward family and health care providers.
- *Bargaining.* The bargaining stage serves as an attempt to postpone the reality of the loss. The person makes a secret bargain with God, expressing a willingness to do anything to postpone the loss or change the prognosis. This is the individual's plea for an extension of life or the chance to "make everything right" with a dying family member or friend.
- *Depression.* The person enters a stage of depression as the full impact of the actual or perceived loss is realized. The person prepares for the impending loss by working through the struggle of separation. While grieving over "what cannot be," the person may either talk freely about the loss or withdraw from others.
- *Acceptance.* The person begins to come to terms with the loss and resumes activities with an air of hopefulness for the future. Some dying people reach a stage of acceptance in which they may appear to be almost devoid of emotion. The struggle is past, and the emotional pain is gone.

Carter: Themes of Bereavement

Carter (1989) focused on identifying themes of bereavement expressed by grieving persons. She identified themes disclosed by people who had experienced the death of a loved one as:

- Grief's changing character, including "waves" of intense pain that may be triggered years after the death by a photograph of the loved one, a favorite song, a fragrance, or anything that calls the loved one to mind.
- Holding, an individual process of preserving the fact and the meaning of the loved one's existence.

- Expectations, both social and personal, regarding how the bereaved should react to the experience.
- The critical importance of personal history in affecting the quality and meaning of individual bereavement.

FACTORS AFFECTING RESPONSES TO LOSS

A variety of factors affect a person's responses to loss. These include age, social support, families, spirituality, and rituals of mourning.

Age

The understanding of and reaction to loss is influenced by the age of the person experiencing the loss. In general, as people experience life transitions, their ability to understand and accept the losses associated with the transitions increases. From the age of 3 years, the development of the concept of death as a loss proceeds rapidly. Table 11–2 outlines the development of the concept of death throughout the life span.

TABLE 11–2	Development of the Concept of Death
Age	**Beliefs/Attitudes about Death**
3	Fears separation; lacks comprehension of permanent separation.
3 to 5	Believes death is like sleeping and is reversible. Expresses curiosity about what happens to the body.
6 to 10	Understands finality of death. Views own death as avoidable. Associates death with violence. Believes wishes can be responsible for death.
11 to 12	Reflects views of death expressed by parents. Expresses interest in afterlife as an understanding of mortality develops. Recognizes death as irreversible and inevitable.
13 to 21	Usually has a religious and philosophic view of death but seldom thinks about it. Views own death as distant or a challenge, acting out defiance through reckless behavior. Previously held developmental awareness of death may still be present.
22 to 45	Does not think about death unless confronted with it. Emotionally distances self from death. Attitude toward death influenced by religious and cultural beliefs.
46 to 65	Experiences the death of parents or friends. Accepts own mortality. Experiences waves of death anxiety. Puts life in order to prepare for death and decrease anxiety.
66 and older	Fears lingering, incapacitating illness. Views death as inevitable but from a philosophical viewpoint: that is, as freedom from pain and illness or as a spiritual reunion with deceased friends and loved ones.

Social Support

Grieving is painful and lonely. One's social support system is important because of its potentially positive influence on the successful resolution of grief. Some losses may lead to social isolation, placing clients at high risk for dysfunctional grief reactions. For example, survivors of people with AIDS often report feeling excluded by the deceased person's family and by health care providers. Characteristic factors that can interfere with successful grieving include the following:

- Perceived inability to share the loss
- Lack of social recognition of the loss
- Ambivalent relationships prior to the loss
- Traumatic circumstances of the loss

A move, a divorce, or even the death of a pet can cause a person to feel extremely isolated, yet the person experiencing these types of loss does not ordinarily receive the same social support offered to the person mourning the death of a loved one. A woman having an abortion or giving up a child for adoption seldom receives the same social support as the mother of a child who died at birth. It is therefore especially important that the nurse does not place a value on the client's loss when assessing the need for support.

The painful nature of grief can cause the client to withdraw from a previously established social support system, thereby increasing the feelings of loneliness caused by the loss. A recently widowed woman, for example, may refuse invitations involving married couples with whom she had socialized while her husband was alive. The client's needs for social interaction remain similar to those established before the loss.

Families

A well-functioning family usually rallies after the initial shock and disbelief and provides support for each other during all phases of the grieving process. After a loss, the functional family is able to shift roles, levels of responsibility, and ways of communicating.

The family may have negative as well as positive effects. For example, the dying client may request that someone the family perceives as an outsider be near, and the family may respond with anger to the perceived "intrusion." Similarly, certain family members may express hurt feelings or anger if the client is unresponsive to other family members. Well-meaning family members also may try to shield the client from the pain of grieving. It is rare for the family and the client to experience anger, denial, and acceptance in unison. While one member is in denial, another may be angry because "not enough is being done."

Spirituality

Spirituality is at the core of human existence, integrating and transcending the physical, emotional, intellectual, and social dimensions (Reed, 1996). The principles, values, personal philosophy, and meaning of life by which the client has pursued goals and self-actualization, however, may be called into question when the client responds to an actual or perceived loss. Because of a fear of intruding on the personal spiritual beliefs and practices of the client, the nurse often feels at a loss in implementing interventions that would be helpful to the client responding to a loss.

Rituals of Mourning

Through the participation in religious ceremonies such as baptism, confirmation, and Bat or Bar Mitzvah, people joyously celebrate progression to a new stage of life and loss of a former way of being. The funeral ceremony serves many of the same purposes in meeting the needs of the bereaved as people gather to share loss. Through the ceremony, people symbolically express triumph over death and deny the fear of death. Culture is the primary factor that dictates the rituals of mourning. See the Focus on Diversity box on page 320 for examples of values and rituals for death in selected cultures.

NURSES' SELF-ASSESSMENT

Nurses care for clients and families at various stages of the grief process and may feel that crisis situations are not the time for self-reflection. However, because the nurse's conscious or unconscious reactions to the client's responses to the loss will influence the outcome of any interventions, nurses need to take time to analyze their own feelings and values related to loss and the expression of grief. The nurse can promote self-awareness by reflecting on the following questions.

- What are my personal feelings about how grief should be expressed?
- Am I making judgments about the meaning of this loss to the client?
- Are unresolved losses in my own life preventing me from relating therapeutically to the client?

END-OF-LIFE CONSIDERATIONS

Nurses care for the dying client in intensive care units, emergency rooms, hospital units, long-term care facilities, and the home. Regardless of the setting, the client's wishes about death should be respected. The Dying Person's Bill of Rights states that each person has "the right to be cared for by caring, sensitive, knowledgeable people who will attempt to understand my needs and will be able to gain some satisfaction in helping me face my death" (Barbus, 1975).

Legal and Ethical Issues

Issues such as those involved in advance directives and living wills, euthanasia, and quality of life are especially important to nurses in upholding the specific care requests of their clients.

Advance Directives and Living Wills

Advance directives are legal documents that allow a person to plan for health care and/or financial affairs in the event of incapacity. A **durable power of attorney for health care** (or health care proxy) is a legal document written by a competent (mentally healthy) adult that gives another competent adult the

Focus on Diversity

CULTURAL ASPECTS OF DYING AND DEATH

Culture/Ethnicity	Nursing Interventions
American Indian	Some tribes prefer not to openly discuss terminal prognosis and DNR decisions, as negative thoughts may make inevitable loss occur sooner. Suggest a family meeting to discuss care and end-of-life issues. If the family feels comfortable, all members of the family and close friends may remain 24 hours a day (eating, joking, singing). Mourning is done in private, away from the dying person. After death, the family may hug, touch, sing, and stay close to the deceased.
Black/African American	Suggest that the family have a family meeting or talk with a minister or family elder. Client may decide to have older family member disclose a poor prognosis. Care for the dying family member is often done at home until death is imminent.
Chinese American	Ensure the head of the family is present when terminal illness is discussed. The client may not want to discuss approaching death. Special amulets or cloths may be brought from home. Family members may prefer to bathe the body after death.
Iranian	Information about a terminal illness should be presented by a trusted member of the health care team to the family, and never to the client when he or she is alone. Most Iranians believe in *tagdir* (will of God) in life and death as a predestined journey. When death occurs, notify the head of the family first. DNR decisions are often made by the family. The family may want to bathe the body.
Mexican American	Based on the belief that worry may make health worse, the family may want to protect the client from seriousness of illness. The information is often handled by an older daughter or son. Extended family members are obligated to pay respects to the sick and dying, although pregnant women do not care for dying persons or attend funerals. May prefer the client die at home. Prayers, amulets, and rosary beads are used, and the priest should be notified. Death is seen as an important spiritual event. The family may bathe the body and spend time with the body.
Vietnamese	Consult head of family before telling client about a terminal illness. Entire family will make DNR decision, often with assistance from a priest or monk. Clients often prefer to die at home. Family should have extra time with the body, and may cry loudly and uncontrollably. Spiritual/religious rites are often conducted in the room.

Note. Adapted from Culture & Nursing Care: A Pocket Guide *by J.G. Lipson, S. L. Dibble, & P. A. Minarik (Eds.), 1996, San Francisco: UCSF Nursing Press.*

right to make health care decisions on his or her behalf if he or she cannot. The legal authority is limited to decisions about health care.

A **living will** is a legal document that formally expresses a person's wishes regarding life-sustaining treatment in the event of terminal illness or permanent unconsciousness (Figure 11–1 ■). It is not a type of durable power of attorney and usually does not designate a substitute decision maker. It is the responsibility of the nurse as client advocate to request and record the client's preference for care and include it in the plan of care. The nurse's documentation helps communicate these preferences to the other members of the health care team.

All facilities that receive Medicare and Medicaid funds are required to provide all clients with written information and counseling about advance directives and the institution's policies governing them (see the Nursing Research box on page 322). The specific terms of this requirement are found in the Patient Self-Determination Act (PSDA). A copy of the signed advance directive must be kept in the client's medical record, but clients do not have to sign it in order to be treated. Nurses are the ones in close contact with clients, so they are often left with unresolved feelings about the moral, ethical, and legal aspects of their actions. Although advance directives do not ease the pain of seeing clients die, they do help nurses provide clients with the care that the clients have chosen.

Do-Not-Resuscitate Orders

A **do-not-resuscitate (DNR, or "no-code") order** is written by the physician for the client who is near death. This order is usually based on the wishes of the client and family that no cardiopulmonary resuscitation be performed for respiratory or cardiac arrest. A **comfort measures only order** indicates that

Directive

I,_____ recognize that the best health care is based on a partnership of trust and communication with my physician. My physician and I will make health care decisions together as long as I am of sound mind and able to make my wishes known. If there comes a time that I am unable to make medical decisions about myself because of illness or injury, I direct that the following treatment preferences be honored:

If, in the judgment of my physician, I am suffering with a terminal condition from which I am expected to die within six months, even with available life-sustaining treatment provided in accordance with prevailing standards of medical care:

_____ I request that all treatment other than those needed to keep me comfortable be discontinued or withheld and my physician allow me to die as gently as possible; OR

_____ I request that I be kept alive in this terminal condition using available life-sustaining treatment. (This Selection Does Not Apply To Hospice Care)

If, in the judgment of my physician, I am suffering with an irreversible condition so that I cannot care for myself or make decisions for myself and am expected to die without life-sustaining treatment provided in accordance with prevailing standards of care:

_____ I request that all treatment other than those needed to keep me comfortable be discontinued or withheld and my physician allow me to die as gently as possible; OR

_____ I request that I be kept alive in this irreversible condition using available life-sustaining treatment. (This Section Does Not Apply to Hospice Care)

Addition request:

_____

_____

After signing this directive, if my representative or I elect hospice care, I understand and agree that only those treatments needed to keep me comfortable would be provided and I would not be given available life-sustaining treatment.

If I do not have a Medical Power of Attorney, and I am unable to make my wishes known, I designate the following person(s) to make treatment decisions with my physician compatible with my personal values:

1. _____
      (name of person)

2. _____
      (name of second person)

SIGNED _____ DATE _____
         (your name)   (date)

City, County, State of Residence

_____ , _____ , _____
     (city)   (county)   (state)

WITNESS #1: _____

WITNESS #2: _____

Excerpted. *Texas Directive to Physicians and Family or Surrogates.* Courtesy of Partnership for Caring Inc., Washington, DC 800-989-9455

Figure 11–1 ■ Sample living will. For more information and a complete document, contact Concern for Dying or the Society for the Right to Die.

Excerpted. *Texas Directive to Physicians and Family or Surrogates.* Courtesy of Partnership for Caring, Inc., 1620 Eye Street, NW, Suite 2002, Washington, DC.

Nursing Research

Evidence-Based Practice for Advance Directives

In accordance with the Patient Self-Determination Act (PSDA), passed in 1990, all health care institutions that receive any government funding are required to have written policies and procedures concerning the formulation and execution of advance directives. The PSDA requires institutions to ask clients upon admission whether they have an advance directive already prepared and then to provide them with information regarding advance directives, including any applicable state laws and the institution's policies. Public education is a major responsibility defined in the PSDA.

Although advance directives have been mandated for a decade, a noticeably small percentage of patients have completed them. One study (Ott & Hardie, 1997) suggested that a client's inability to understand advance directives may explain why this is true. It is known that many people read below the level of their completed education and that older adult clients often read at a 4th- to 8th-grade level. Teaching-learning guidelines recommend that written materials given to clients not be above the 6th-grade reading level, but studies have shown the mean client readability level for health-related materials to range from grades 11.2 to 17.5. The purpose of this study was to assess the readability of 10 advance directive documents from various sources. The estimated readability for all documents was at levels much more difficult than recommended reading levels. Based on these findings, the authors advised that any document used to document client decisions about future treatment decisions be readable by clients. Poor readability prevents understanding and adversely affects choices about advance directives.

IMPLICATIONS FOR NURSING

The American Nurses Association (1992) has stated that nurses have a responsibility to ensure that clients have the knowledge necessary to make informed decisions about treatment. There is a need for documents and supporting materials designed for clients with low reading levels. The following suggestions may help.

1. Use a readability formula as a screening device to determine whether documents are written at appropriate reading levels.
2. Increase collaboration and documentation of communications about treatment decisions among all health care providers and clients.
3. Provide client education about advance directives in community-based settings if at all possible, so that decisions are made before a client is seriously ill.
4. Encourage consumer and advocacy groups to develop documents and other supporting materials that have good readability.
5. Evaluate client education materials used in client education and print the readability level on each document. Use larger print for older adults.
6. Include considerations about cultural, ethnic, religious, and illness-related variables in all printed materials.

Critical Thinking in Client Care

1. Which factors may influence clients to prepare an advance directive?
2. What members of the health care team should be included in a discussion about end-of-life decisions?
3. What are the responsibilities of the hospital to ensure that clients receive accurate and compassionate information regarding advance directives?

---

no further life-sustaining interventions are necessary and that the goal of care is a comfortable, dignified death. Confusing or conflicting DNR orders create dilemmas, because nurses are involved in resuscitation and either begin CPR or ensure that unwanted attempts do not occur. The ANA has made specific recommendations related to a DNR order (see Box 11–2).

The ANA further recommends that guidelines and policies be developed to help resolve conflicts between clients and their families, between clients and health care professionals, and among health care professionals.

Euthanasia

Euthanasia (from the Greek for painless, easy, gentle, or good death) is now commonly used to signify a killing prompted by some humanitarian motive. There are many arguments for and against euthanasia, and nurses have often found themselves at the center of the debate. As a result, nurses have pushed for the development of appropriate guidelines and procedures for DNR orders. When no such orders exist, the nurse faces a dilemma. Certainly, there are situations in which the nurse's role is clear. For example, it is considered malpractice to participate in "slow codes" (in which the nurse does not hurry to

alert the emergency team when a terminally ill client who does not have a DNR order stops breathing).

The natural death laws seek to preserve the notion of voluntary versus involuntary euthanasia. In *voluntary euthanasia,* the competent adult client and a physician, nurse, or adult friend or relative make the decision to terminate life. *Involuntary euthanasia* ("mercy killing") is performed without the client's consent. Because care settings offer many complex and technologic interventions, it is not likely that the ethical aspects of euthanasia will soon be resolved. However, advance directives do give clients a much more active role in decisions about their own care.

Hospice

Hospice is a model of care (rather than a place of care) for clients and their families when faced with a limited life expectancy. Hospice care is initiated for clients as they near the end of life, emphasizing quality rather than quantity of life. Emotional, spiritual, and practical support is provided based on the wishes of the client and the needs of the family. Hospice regards dying as a normal part of life and provides support for a dignified and peaceful death.

BOX 11–2 ■ The ANA Position on Nursing Care and Do-Not-Resuscitate Decisions

■ The choices and values of the competent patient should always be given highest priority, even when these wishes conflict with those of health care providers and families.

■ In the case of the incompetent or never competent patient, any existing advance directives or the decisions of surrogate decision makers acting in the patient's best interest should be determinative.

■ The DNR decision should always be a subject of explicit discussion among the patient, the family, any designated surrogate decision maker acting in the patient's best interest, and the health care team. The decision should include consideration of the efficacy and desirability of CPR, a balancing of benefits and burdens to patients, and therapeutic goals.

■ DNR orders must be clearly documented, reviewed, and updated periodically to reflect changes in the patient's condition.

■ Nurses have a responsibility to educate patients and their families about various forms of advance directives such as living wills and durable power of attorney.

■ If it is the nurse's personal belief that his or her moral integrity is compromised by professional responsibility to carry out a particular DNR order, the nurse should transfer the responsibility for the patient's care to another nurse.

Note. From Task Force on the Nurse's Role in End of Life Decisions by ANA Board of Directors, 1992, new position statement.

The American hospice movement was originally led by volunteers (many of whom were nurses) who wanted to make life better for those who were dying. These devoted volunteers promoted the dignity of patients during their death and decreased their institutionalization. In 1986, Congress passed the Medicare Hospice Benefit and also gave states the option of including hospice services in their Medicaid programs. Since then, patients dying of cancer or any other terminal illness may receive hospice care in the comfort of their homes with their families.

Hospice care usually begins when the patient has 6 months or less to live and ends with the family 1 year after the death. Nurses providing hospice care work with an interdisciplinary team of other health professionals such as social workers, pastoral counselors, home health aides, and volunteers to provide comprehensive palliative care. The hospice nurse must combine all of the skills of the home care nurse with the ability to provide daily emotional support to dying patients and their families. Hospice nurses are especially skilled in pain and symptom management. Their focus is on improving quality of life and preserving dignity for the patient in death.

End-of-Life Care

End-of-life nursing care that ensures a peaceful death was mandated by the International Council of Nurses' (1997) and further supported by the American Association of Colleges of Nursing (AACN) (1999). The principles of hospice care are basic to end-of-life care: that people live until the moment they die; that care until death may be offered by a variety of health care professionals; and that such care is coordinated, is sensitive to diversity, offered around the clock, and incorporates the physical, psychological, social, and spiritual concerns of the patient and the patient's family. Following are selected competencies necessary for nurses to provide high-quality end-of-life care as defined by the AACN (1999).

• Promote the provision of comfort care to the dying as an active, desirable, and important skill, and an integral component of nursing care (Figure 11–2 ■).

• Communicate effectively and compassionately with the patient, family, and health care team members about end-of-life issues.

• Recognize one's own attitudes, feelings, values, and expectations about death and the individual, cultural, and spiritual diversity existing in those beliefs and customs.

• Demonstrate respect for the patient's views and wishes during end-of-life care.

• Use scientifically based standardized tools to assess symptoms (e.g., pain, dyspnea, constipation, anxiety, fatigue, nausea/vomiting, and altered cognition) experienced by patients at the end of life.

• Use data from symptom assessment to plan and intervene in symptom management using state-of-the-art traditional and complementary approaches.

• Assist the patient, family, colleagues, and one's self to cope with suffering, grief, loss, and bereavement in end-of-life care.

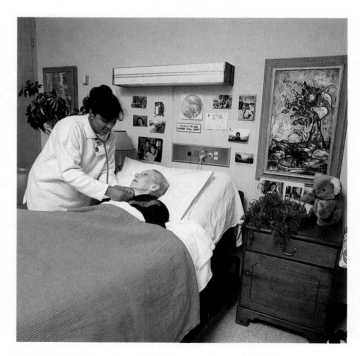

Figure 11–2 ■ The nurse helps the client visualize the hospital room as a safe, comfortable place to die by surrounding the client with familiar articles brought from the client's home.

Manifestations of Impending Death

- Difficulty talking or swallowing
- Nausea, flatus, abdominal distention
- Urinary and/or bowel incontinence, constipation
- Decreased sensation, taste, and smell
- Weak, slow, and/or irregular pulse
- Decreasing blood pressure
- Decreased, irregular, or Cheyne-Stokes respirations
- Changes in level of consciousness
- Restlessness, agitation
- Coolness, mottling, and cyanosis of the extremities

Physiological Changes in the Dying Client

Death may occur rapidly or slowly. Physiological changes are a part of the dying process. These changes result in any or all of the manifestations listed in the box above as death nears.

- *Weakness and fatigue.* Weakness and fatigue cause discomfort, especially in joints, and contribute to an increased risk for pressure ulcers.
- *Anorexia and decreased food intake.* Although anorexia and a decrease in food intake are normal in the dying client, the family often views this as "giving up." Anorexia may be a protective mechanism; the breakdown of body fats results in ketosis, which leads to a sense of well-being and helps decrease pain. Parenteral or enteral feedings do not improve symptoms or prolong life and may actually cause discomfort. As weakness and difficulty swallowing progress, the gag reflex is decreased and clients are at increased risk for aspiration if oral foods are given.
- *Fluid and electrolyte imbalances.* Decreased oral fluid intake is normal at the end of life and does not cause distress. Parenteral fluids are sometimes given to decrease delirium, but they may cause increased edema, breathlessness, cough, and respiratory secretions. If the client has edema or *ascites* (a collection of fluid in the abdominal cavity), excess body water is present so dehydration is not a problem.
- *Hypotension and renal failure.* As cardiac output decreases, so does intravascular blood volume. As a result, renal perfusion decreases and the kidneys cease to function. Urinary output is scanty. The client will have tachycardia, hypotension, cool extremities, and cyanosis with skin mottling.
- *Neurologic dysfunction.* Neurologic dysfunction results from any or all of the following: decreased cerebral perfusion, hypoxemia, metabolic acidosis, sepsis, an accumulation of toxins from liver and renal failure, the effects of medications, and disease-related factors. These changes may result in decreased level of consciousness or agitated delirium. Clients with terminal delirium may be confused, restless, or agitated. Moaning, groaning, and grimacing often accompany the agitation and are often misinterpreted as pain. Level of consciousness often decreases to the point where the client cannot be aroused. Although decreased consciousness and agitation are both normal states at the end of life, they are very distressing to the client's family. A client near death often has altered cerebral function, so the nurse must

BOX 11-3 ■ Providing Comfort for the Client Nearing Death

- Maintain clean skin and bed linens.
- Use a draw sheet to turn the client as often as possible so the client is comfortable.
- Position the client to promote comfort and protect bony areas with padding. Reposition the client and raise the head of the bed if fluids accumulate in the upper airways and back of the throat.
- Use bed pads or insert a Foley catheter (if ordered) for urinary incontinence.
- Use gentle massage to improve circulation and shift edema.
- Provide small, frequent sips of fluids, ice chips, or popsicles.
- Provide oral care, using a soft moist brush or glycerin swab.
- Clean secretions from the eyes and nose.
- Administer ordered pain medications as needed to maintain comfort.
- Administer oxygen as prescribed to relieve dyspnea.

stand near the bedside and speak clearly. Hearing is thought to be the last sense a dying client loses; the nurse should never whisper or engage in conversation with the family as if the client were not there.

- *Respiratory changes.* Respiratory changes are normal at this time. The client may have dyspnea, apnea, or Cheyne-Stokes respirations, and may use accessory muscles to breathe. Fluids accumulated in the lungs and oropharynx may lead to what is sometimes called "the death rattle." Oxygen may not relieve these manifestations.
- *Bowel and/or bladder incontinence.* Loss of sphincter control may lead to incontinence of feces or urine.
- *Pain.* A common problem for clients at the end of life, pain is what people often say they fear the most. It is of utmost importance to keep the client comfortable through general comfort measures (see Box 11–3) and by administering ordered medications for pain and anxiety.

PRACTICE ALERT *There is no maximum allowable dose for opioids such as morphine sulfate; the dose should be increased to whatever is necessary to relieve pain (Tierney, McPhee, & Papadakis, 2001).* ■

Support for the Client and Family

As the client's condition deteriorates, the nurse's knowledge of the client and family guides the care provided. It may be necessary to provide opportunities for clients to express personal preferences about where they want to die and about funeral and burial arrangements. If the family feels that this is morbid, the nurse explains that it helps clients to keep a sense of control as they approach death.

The client needs the opportunity to say goodbye to others. The nurse encourages and supports the client and family as they terminate relationships as a necessary part of the grief process. The nurse acknowledges that termination is painful and, if the client or family desires, stays with them during this

Manifestations of Death

- Absence of respirations, pulse, and heartbeat
- Fixed and dilated pupils; eyes may stay open
- Release of stool and urine
- Waxen color (pallor) as blood settles to dependent areas
- Body temperature drops
- Lack of reflexes
- Flat encephalogram

time. Family members are often afraid to be present at the moment of death, yet dying alone is the greatest fear expressed by clients.

DEATH

The manifestations listed in the box above are seen after death occurs, and are the basis for pronouncing death. They appear gradually and not in any special order. Pronouncement of death is legally required by a physician or other health care provider to confirm death. The time of death, with any related data, is documented in the client's chart.

The nurse may also fear being present at the moment of the client's death. In fact, Kübler-Ross (1969) noted that the nurse's fear of death frequently interferes with the ability to provide support for the dying client and family. Thoughts such as, "Please, God, don't let him die on my shift," are common, and they express the nurse's emotional turmoil in dealing with the task. Nurses who have worked through their own feelings about death and dying are more at ease in assisting the dying client toward a peaceful death.

After the death, the family is encouraged to acknowledge the pain of loss. The nurse's presence and support as the bereaved express their sorrow, anger, or guilt can help them resolve their grief. It is important for the bereaved not to suppress the pain of grieving with drugs. By accepting variations in the expression of grief, the nurse supports the family's grief reactions and helps prevent dysfunctional grieving. Dysfunctional grieving is an extended and unsuccessful resolution of grief.

Resolution of grief begins with acceptance of the loss. The nurse can encourage this acceptance by maintaining open, honest dialogue and by providing the family with the opportunity to view, touch, hold, and kiss the person's body (Carpenito, 2000). As family members realize the finality of the death, they are often comforted by the presence of the nurse who cared for the client during the final days.

Postmortem Care

The nurse documents the time of death (required for the death certificate and all official records), notifies the physician, and assists the family (if needed) in choice of a funeral home. If the client dies at home, death must be pronounced before the body is removed. In some states and in some situations, nurses can pronounce death; for specifics, consult state practice acts, laws, and agency policy. All jewelry is removed and given to the family unless they ask that it be left on. The body is kept in place until the family is ready and gives permission. If an au-

topsy is required or requested, the body must be left undisturbed (e.g., do not remove any tubes) for transportation to the medical examiner.

Documentation of the death is completed by sending a completed death certificate to the funeral home (for a death in the home), or by completing the required paperwork and sending the body to the morgue or funeral home (for a death in the hospital or long-term care setting).

Nurses' Grief

The nurse who has developed a close relationship with the client who has died may experience strong feelings of grief. Sharing grief with the family after the death of a loved one helps both the nurse and family to cope with their feelings about the loss. Taking time to grieve after the death of a client provides a release that can help prevent "blunting" of feelings, a problem often experienced by nurses who care for clients who are terminally ill.

PRACTICE ALERT *Crying with families (at one time considered unprofessional) is now recognized as simply an expression of empathy and caring.* ■

Nurses working with critically or terminally ill clients should be aware that witnessing a client's death and the family's grief may reactivate feelings about some unresolved grief in their own lives. In these cases, nurses may need to reflect on their responses to their own losses. Also, nurses who work with dying clients need support from peers and other professionals to work through the often overwhelming feelings that result from dealing with death, grief, and loss (Figure 11–3 ■).

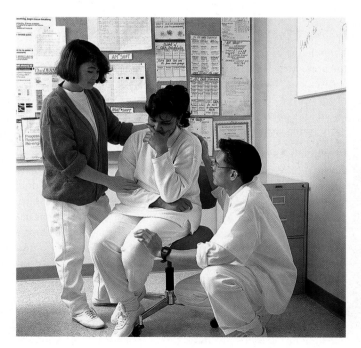

Figure 11–3 ■ Nurses who work with dying clients need support from their colleagues to work through their often overwhelming feelings of grief.

COLLABORATIVE CARE

Interventions for loss and grief may be planned and implemented by any or all members of the health care team. Nurses and social workers provide interventions to help clients or families adapt to a loss. They also make referrals to mental health professionals (grief counselors, social services), support groups, chaplains, or legal or financial assistance agencies.

Grieving clients frequently enter the health care system with significant somatic symptoms. In some cases, the symptoms of grief and loss are overlooked until the client reaches a crisis state requiring psychiatric medical intervention. Collaborative care by the physician and the nurse early in the normal grieving process can help the client achieve an early and effective resolution of grief and avoid physical or psychiatric health problems.

NURSING CARE

Nurses practicing in all types of settings care for clients who are in various stages of the grieving process. Grief is highly individual. The grief process may range from uncomfortable to debilitating, and it may last for a day or a lifetime, depending on what the loss means to the person experiencing it.

Health Promotion

In planning and implementing nursing care for the client experiencing a loss, the nurse considers the individual responses, which may vary greatly. In an era of short acute care stays for clients, nurses may feel that an elaborate grief assessment is impossible or, at the least, impractical. But research and clinical experience suggest that clients who delay the grieving process after a loss are prone to have health problems that may last a lifetime.

Assessment

Knowledge of the expected physical reactions to loss provides the nurse with a basis for identifying reactions requiring further assessment. To assess the extent of somatic distress, the nurse observes for changes in sensory processes and asks questions about the client's sleeping and eating patterns, activities of daily living, general health status, and pain.

Physical Assessment

Clients may experience one or more predictable somatic symptoms as they become aware of a loss. Gastrointestinal symptoms occur frequently. They may include indigestion, nausea or vomiting, anorexia, weight gain or loss, constipation, or diarrhea. The shock and disbelief that accompany a loss may cause shortness of breath, a choking sensation, hyperventilation, or loss of strength. Some clients also report insomnia, preoccupation with sleep, fatigue, and decreased or increased activity level.

Crying and sadness are observed during normal grief states. Crying may make the client feel exhausted and interfere with carrying out activities of daily living. However, a person who is unable to cry may have difficulty completing the mourning process. If the client does not express feelings of grief, somatic symptoms may increase.

It is imperative that the client's concerns about pain be assessed, especially if the client has cancer or another painful illness. Knowledge of pain theories and pain assessment can help the nurse assess the need for pain medication (see Chapter 4). During the last stages of dying, the client usually becomes very weak, and sensations and reflexes decrease; these changes call for careful assessment of the client's physical needs.

Reactions to loss are not always obvious. For example, in clients who experience an illness following a serious loss, assessment may reveal somatic complaints related to the grief state as well as the illness. When a person who has been healthy begins to develop patterns of increased illness, the nurse should be aware that this may signal dysfunctional grieving. This is especially common in the loss and grieving associated with a change in body image. In addition to making a physical assessment, assess the client's perception of the alteration in body image. The loss of a body part, weight gain or loss, and scars from surgery or trauma can be difficult for the client to accept. Some clients may grieve hair loss that accompanies chemotherapy used in cancer treatment.

Spiritual Assessment

Because spiritual beliefs and practices greatly influence people's reaction to loss, it is important to explore them with the client when assessing a loss. The spiritually healthy client has inner resources that help work through the grief process. Faith, prayer, trust in God or a superior being, perception of a purpose in life, or belief in immortality are examples of the inner resources that may sustain the client during an actual or perceived loss (Reed, 1996).

Assessing the client's spiritual life and its significance to the client and family helps identify spiritual support systems. Some nurses are uncomfortable with assessing the client's spiritual needs; the following questions may be helpful.

- What are the spiritual aspects of the client's philosophy about life? Death?
- Are the values and beliefs about life and death congruent with those of people who are important to the client?
- Which spiritual resources and rituals have significance for the client?

Belief systems that are incompatible with those of family members can be an additional source of stress for clients dealing with a loss. The anger and resentment often observed among families faced with decisions concerning dying members may be avoided if the nurse assesses the potential impact of differing beliefs.

Clients coping with a loss often perceive that it is a punishment from God for their wrongdoing or for their failure to remain faithful to their religious practices. Therefore, it is important to assess the level of guilt the client or family expresses. Assessing the client's comments regarding feelings of responsibility for the loss helps determine whether these feelings are an expected phase of grieving or indicate dysfunctional grieving.

Clients who had not considered themselves religious before the actual or perceived loss often turn to religion to seek comfort or to cope with feelings of despair, helplessness, hopelessness, or guilt. They may utter anguished statements such as "Why, God?" or "Please help me, God." The nurse continues to assess the client's verbalization of such feelings to determine the best interventions to help the client cope with the loss.

Psychosocial Assessment

When working through the grief process, clients can be overwhelmed by the fears associated with the loss and the changes it will produce. The client responding to an actual or perceived loss commonly expresses anxiety (fear of the unknown). An extreme level of anxiety can threaten the client's well-being. Assessment includes helping clients openly acknowledge their fears. Some clients may fear the feelings they experience while proceeding through the grief process more than the loss itself. The most common fear expressed by clients facing a loss is that of losing self-control.

Focusing on the meaning of the loss to the client is more important than attempting to place the client in a sequence or phase of grief. The degree of caring and sensitivity shown when asking questions about the meaning of the loss influences the amount of information the client will be willing to reveal. Asking such questions as, "Why do you feel this way?" or "What does this loss mean to you?" is less helpful than making a statement such as, "This must be difficult for you." The latter more effectively conveys a genuine interest in hearing how the client feels about the loss.

Awareness of the altered sensorium observed during the stage of shock and disbelief provides parameters for assessment. The nurse may note in the client feelings of numbness, unreality, emotional distance, intense preoccupation with the lost object, helplessness, loneliness, and disorganization. As awareness of the loss begins to develop, preoccupation with the lost person or object may increase, and self-accusation and ambivalence toward the lost person or object may follow.

Nursing Diagnoses and Interventions

A variety of nursing diagnoses may be appropriate for the client experiencing loss and grief, as well as for the client who is nearing death. Nurses practicing medical-surgical nursing will most often provide interventions for anticipatory grieving, chronic sorrow, and death anxiety.

Anticipatory Grieving

Anticipatory grieving is a combination of intellectual and emotional responses and behaviors by which people adjust their self-concept in the face of a potential loss. Anticipatory grieving may be a response to one's own future death; to potential loss of body parts or functions; to potential loss of a significant person, animal, or possession; or to potential loss of a social role. Nursing interventions are designed to assist with grief resolution.

- Assess for factors causing or contributing to the grief. Ask about support systems, how many losses have occurred, relationship with the lost person, significance of the body part, and previous experiences with loss and grief. *Grief and mourning occur when a person experiences any type of loss.*

- Use open-ended questions to encourage the person to share concerns and the possible effect on the family. *Grief resolution cannot occur until the client acknowledges the loss.*

- Promote a trusting nurse-client relationship: Allow enough time for communications; speak clearly, simply, and concisely; listen; be honest in responses to questions; do not give unrealistic hope; offer support; and demonstrate respect for the person's age, culture, religion, race, and values. *An effective nurse-client relationship begins with acceptance of the client's feelings, attitudes, and values related to the loss. If the client is ready to talk, listening and being present are the most appropriate interventions.*

- Ask about strengths and weakness in coping with the anticipated loss. *Current responses are influenced by past experiences with loss, illness, and death. Socioeconomic and cultural background, as well as cultural and spiritual beliefs and values, affect a person's ability to adapt to loss.*

- Teach the client and family the stages of grief. *This helps them to be aware of their emotions in each stage and reassures them that their reactions are normal.*

- Provide time for decision making. *In periods of stress, people may need extra time to make informed decisions.*

- Provide information about appropriate resources, including support from family, friends, and support groups, community resources, and legal/financial aides. *Support from others decreases feelings of loneliness and isolation and facilitates grief work.*

Chronic Sorrow

Chronic sorrow is a cyclical, recurring, and potentially progressive pattern of pervasive sadness experienced in response to continual loss, throughout the trajectory of an illness or disability. It is triggered by situations that bring to mind the person's losses, disappointments, or fears. It may be experienced by a client, parent or caregiver, or person with chronic illness or disability.

- Explain the difference between chronic sorrow and chronic grieving. *Grieving is time-limited and ends in adaptation to the loss. Chronic sorrow may vary in intensity, but it persists as long as the person with the disability or chronic sorrow condition lives.*

- Encourage verbalization of feelings about the loss, and about the personal relevance of the changes to hopes for the future. *Expressing feelings is normal and necessary to decrease the emotional pain.*

- Help identify triggers that intensify the sorrow, such as birthdays, anniversaries, and holidays. *When triggers have been identified, role-playing may make the events less painful.*

- Refer to appropriate community support groups. *Participating in support groups with others experiencing grief is helpful in coping with loss.*

- Encourage use of personal, family, significant other, and spiritual support systems *to facilitate coping with loss.*

Death Anxiety

Death anxiety is worry or fear related to death or dying. It may be present in clients who have an acute life-threatening illness, who have a terminal illness, who have experienced the death of a family member or friend, or who have experienced multiple deaths in the same family.

- Explore the client's knowledge of the situation. For example, ask, "What has your doctor told you about your condition?" *This informs you of the client's knowledge base about the condition and about his or her ability to make informed decisions.*
- Ask the client to identify specific fears about death. *This provides data about any unrealistic expectations or misperceptions.*
- Determine the client's perceptions of strengths and weakness in coping with death. *Identifying past strengths can help the client cope with loss, illness, and death.*
- Ask the client to identify needed help. *This determines whether available resources are adequate.*
- Encourage independence and control in decisions about treatment and care. *This promotes self-esteem, decreases feelings of powerlessness, and allows the client to retain dignity in dying.*
- Facilitate access to culturally appropriate spiritual rituals and practices. *This provides spiritual comfort.*
- Explain advance directives and assist with them if necessary. *Advance directives help ensure that the client's wishes for end-of-life care are carried out.*
- Encourage life review and reminiscence. *Life review is self-affirming.*
- Encourage activities such as listening to music, aromatherapy, massage, or relaxation exercises. *These activities decrease anxiety.*
- Suggest keeping a journal or leaving a written legacy. *A written document provides continuing support to others after death.*

Using NANDA, NIC, and NOC

Chart 11–1 shows linkages between NANDA, NIC, and NOC when caring for the client experiencing loss, grief, and death.

Home Care

In addition to teaching clients and families to carry out the physical skills that are necessary to the client's care, nurses also provide information on identifying signs of deterioration and additional sources of support. General guidelines for teaching clients and families about grief include those suggested in the box below. In addition, suggest the following resources:

- Hospice
- Support groups
- Home health care agencies
- Public health departments

Meeting Individualized Needs

TEACHING FOR CLIENTS EXPERIENCING A LOSS

- Encourage both children and adults to discuss expected or impending loss and to express feelings.
- Teach problem-solving skills: Define what the possible changes and problems are related to the predicted loss, develop potential strategies for dealing with problems, list pros and cons of each strategy, and decide which strategies might be most useful to try first to solve potential problems associated with loss.
- Teach individuals and families how to support a person who is dealing with an impending loss.
- Explain what to expect with a loss: sadness, fear, rejection, anger, guilt, loneliness.
- Teach signs of grief resolution:
  - No longer living in the past, becoming future oriented
  - Breaking ties with the lost object or person (Acute stage often shows signs of resolving in 6 to 12 months.)
  - The possibility of having painful "waves" of grief years after the loss, especially on the anniversary of the loss and in response to "triggers" such as pictures, events, songs, or memories

CHART 11–1 NANDA, NIC, AND NOC LINKAGES

The Client Experiencing Loss

NURSING DIAGNOSES	NURSING INTERVENTIONS	NURSING OUTCOMES
• Anticipatory Grieving	• Grief Work Facilitation • Emotional Support • Family Support • Hope Instillation	• Grief Resolution • Coping
• Dysfunctional Grieving	• Coping Enhancement • Counseling • Emotional Support • Spiritual Support	• Coping • Self-Esteem
• Death Anxiety	• Dying Care • Spiritual Support • Forgiveness Facilitation • Simple Guided Imagery • Medication Management	• Dignified Dying • Spiritual Well-Being • Acceptance: Health Status • Quality of Life • Knowledge: Medication

Note. Data from Nursing Outcomes Classification (NOC) by M. Johnson & M. Maas (Eds.), 1997, St. Louis: Mosby; Nursing Diagnoses: Definitions & Classification 2001–2002, by North American Nursing Diagnosis Association, 2001, Philadelphia: NANDA; Nursing Interventions Classification (NIC) by J. C. McCloskey and G. M. Bulechek (Eds.), 2000, St. Louis: Mosby. Reprinted by permission.

Nursing Care Plan
A Client Experiencing Loss and Grief

Pearl Rogers is a 79-year-old African American woman who is admitted to the Methodist Home Nursing Center. Mrs. Rogers lived with her husband of 58 years until his death 9 months ago. She had one son who died in an auto accident 2 years ago, and she has one daughter who lives nearby. After her husband's death, Mrs. Rogers lived with her daughter until her admission to the nursing center. Mrs. Rogers has become increasingly agitated and helpless, complaining constantly of pain. Her daughter states that Mrs. Rogers is chronically constipated, has difficulty sleeping, and has stopped engaging in all social activities, including weekly church services. She cries frequently. Extensive medical testing prior to her admission to the nursing center revealed Mrs. Rogers has arthritis but no other pathologic disorder.

ASSESSMENT

On admission to the nursing center, Mrs. Rogers says, "I'm a sick woman, and no one will listen to me! I can't walk, I'm so weak. My head hurts, and I'm always sick at my stomach. I haven't had a bowel movement in a week, and I never sleep more than 3 hours a night." Physical assessment finding include swollen knees and ankles, with limited mobility of the lower extremities.

DIAGNOSES

- *Dysfunctional grieving* related to stress of husband's death
- *Sleep pattern disturbance* related to grieving
- *Constipation* related to inactivity

EXPECTED OUTCOMES

- Engage in normal grief work: Work through grief process, discuss reality of losses, use nondestructive coping mechanisms, and discuss positive and negative aspects of the loss.
- Experience adequate and restful sleep: Fall asleep 20 to 30 minutes after retiring and awaken feeling rested after 7 to 8 hours of sleep.
- Have a bowel movement with soft formed stools at least every other day.

PLANNING AND IMPLEMENTATION

- Promote trust: Show empathy and caring, demonstrate respect for her culture and values, offer support and reassurance, be honest, engage in active listening.

- Assist in labeling her feelings: anger, fear, loneliness, guilt, isolation.
- Explore previous losses and the ways in which the client has coped.
- Encourage review of her relationship with her dead husband.
- Reinforce expressions of behaviors associated with normal grieving.
- Encourage participation in usual spiritual practices.
- Encourage participation in a grief group that meets at the facility.
- Consult with the physical and recreational therapist to help the nursing staff provide afternoon activities.
- Provide measures that assist in bowel evacuation: Encourage exercise as tolerated, including walks and rocking in a rocking chair. Offer foods that stimulate bowel movements. Offer privacy: Close the door, ensuring that the emergency call bell is within reach, and do not interrupt.
- Administer a mild laxative and/or stool softener, if necessary, but discontinue as soon as possible.

EVALUATION

After 4 weeks at the nursing center, Mrs. Rogers states, "I don't feel any better, but I know I have to accept my situation." Although Mrs. Rogers states that she doesn't feel better, she is walking the length of the hall, sleeping better, and having regular bowel movements. Mrs. Rogers is also less withdrawn and has openly discussed her feelings related to her husband's death, including her anger at the loss of her son and her husband less than 2 years apart. She has attended the grief group once and has attended chapel services on Sunday for the past 2 weeks. Her daughter visits her each Saturday and takes her in a wheelchair to the shopping mall.

Critical Thinking in the Nursing Process

1. What common physical manifestations of grief did Mrs. Rogers experience?
2. How might Mrs. Rogers's daughter be more involved in developing and implementing her mother's plan of care?
3. Suppose Mrs. Rogers says that she does not want any help, that she just wants to be left alone to die. How would you respond?

See Evaluating Your Response in Appendix C.

EXPLORE MediaLink

NCLEX Review questions, case studies, care plan activities, MediaLink applications, and other interactive resources for this chapter can be found on the Companion Website at www.prenhall.com/lemone.

Click on Chapter 11 to select the activities for this chapter. For animations, video clips, more NCLEX review questions, and an audio glossary, access the Student CD-ROM accompanying this textbook.

TEST YOURSELF

1. Which of the following statements *best* describes loss?
   a. It is determined by one's cultural values
   b. It is largely dependent on support of family and friends
   c. It can be determined only by the person who experiences it
   d. It is the same as grief and mourning

2. Kübler-Ross believed that one usually first responds to a situation of loss with:
   a. Anger
   b. Bargaining
   c. Depression
   d. Denial

3. What document expresses a person's wishes for life-sustaining treatment in the event of terminal illness or permanent unconsciousness?
   a. Durable power of attorney for health care
   b. Living will
   c. Physician's no-code order
   d. Patient Self-Determination Act

4. Which of the senses is believed to be the last one lost as a person nears death?
   a. Hearing
   b. Vision
   c. Touch
   d. Smell

5. Which of the following statements best describes the treatment of pain at the end of life?
   a. As client nears death, no pain is perceived and no medications are necessary
   b. It is important to withhold pain medications if the client has respiratory changes
   c. There is no maximum allowable dose for opioids during end-of-life care
   d. Nurses should not administer opioids to the dying client

See Test Yourself answers in Appendix C.

BIBLIOGRAPHY

American Association of Colleges of Nursing. (1999). *Peaceful death: Recommended competencies and curricular guidelines for end-of-life nursing care.* Washington, DC: AACN.

American Nurses Association. (1992). *Position statement on nursing and the Patient Self-Determination Act.* Kansas City: ANA.

_____. (1992). *Report from the task force on the nurse's role in end of life decisions.* Kansas City: ANA.

Barbus, A. J. (1975). The dying person's bill of rights. *The American Journal of Nursing, 75* (1), 99.

Bowlby, J. (1973). Attachment and loss, *Separation, anxiety, and anger* (Vol. 2). New York: Basic Books.

_____. (1980). Attachment and loss, *Loss, sadness, and depression* (Vol. 3). New York: Basic Books.

Caplan, G. (1990). Loss, stress, and mental health. *Community Mental Health Journal, 26*(1), 27–48.

Carpenito, L. (2000). *Nursing diagnoses: Application to clinical practice* (8th ed.). Philadelphia: Lippincott.

Carter, S. (1989). Themes of grief. *Nursing Research, 36*(6), 354–358.

Collins, D. (2001). Grief and loss experienced by patients with Alzheimer's disease and their caregivers. *Geriaction, 19*(1), 17–20.

Duffield, P. (1998). Advance directives in primary care. *American Journal of Nursing, 61*(4), 16CCC–16DDD.

Durham, E., & Weiss, L. (1997). How patients die. *American Journal of Nursing, 97*(12), 41–46.

Engel, G. (1964). Grief and grieving. *American Journal of Nursing, 64,* 93.

Freud, S. (1917/1957). Mourning and melancholia. In J. Strachey & A. Tyson (Eds.), *The complete psychological works of Sigmund Freud* (Vol. 14). London: Hogarth Press.

Goetschius, S. (1997). Families and end-of-life care: How do we meet their needs? *Journal of Gerontological Nursing, 23*(3), 43–49.

International Council of Nurses. (1997). *Basic principles of nursing care.* Washington, DC: American Nurses Publishing.

Johnson, M., & Maas, M. (Eds.). (1997). *Nursing outcomes classification (NOC).* St. Louis: Mosby.

Kaunonen, M., Tarkka, M., Paunonen, M., & Laippala, P. (1999). Grief and social support after the death of a spouse. *Journal of Advanced Nursing, 30*(6), 1304–1311.

Kübler-Ross, E. (1969). *On death and dying.* New York: Macmillan.

_____. (1978). *To live until we say goodbye.* Englewood Cliffs, NJ: Prentice Hall.

Libson, J., Dibble, S., & Minarik, P. (1996). *Culture & nursing care: A pocket guide.* San Francisco: UCSF Nursing Press.

Lindemann, E. (1944). Symptomatology and management of acute grief . *American Journal of Psychiatry, 32,* 141.

Matzo, P. L., & Sherman, D. W. (Eds.). (2001). *Palliative care nursing: Quality care to the end of life.* New York: Springer.

McCloskey, J.C., & Bulechek, G. M. (Eds.). (2000). *Nursing interventions classification (NIC)* (3rd ed.). St. Louis: Mosby.

McCorkle, R., Robinson, L., Nuamah, I., Lev, E., & Benoliel, J. (1998). The effects of home nursing care for patients during terminal illness on the bereaved's psychological distress. *Nursing Research, 47*(1), 2–10.

Ott, B., & Hardie, T. (1997). Readability of advance directive documents. *Image: Journal of Nursing Scholarship, 29*(1), 53–57.

Perrin, K. (1997). Giving voice to the wishes of elders for end-of-life care. *Journal of Gerontological Nursing, 23*(3), 18–27.

Poor, B., & Poirrier, G. (2001). *End of life nursing care.* Boston: Jones & Bartlett.

Reed, P. G. (1996). Transcendence: Formulating nursing perspectives. *Nursing Science Quarterly, 9*(1), 2–4.

Rushton, C., & Scanlon, C. (1998). A road map for navigating end-of-life care. *MEDSURG Nursing, 7*(1), 57–59.

Tierney, L. M., McPhee, S. J., & Papadakis, M. A. (2001). *Current medical diagnosis & treatment* (40th ed.). New York: McGraw Hill.

Tipton, K. (1997). How to discuss death with patients and families. *Nursing97, 27*(32), 10–12.

Ufema, J. (2000). Terminal illness: Compassion and raspberry tea. *Nursing, 30*(12), 66–67.

Nursing Care of Clients with Problems of Substance Abuse

MediaLink

www.prenhall.com/lemone
Additional resources for this chapter can be found on the Student CD-ROM accompanying this textbook, and on the Companion Website at www.prenhall.com/lemone. Click on Chapter 12 to select the activities for this chapter.

CD-ROM
- Audio Glossary
- NCLEX Review

Animation
- Cocaine

Companion Website
- More NCLEX Review
- Case Study
    Alcohol Abuse
- Care Plan Activity
    Alcohol Withdrawal
- MediaLink Application
    Support in Recovery

LEARNING OUTCOMES

After completing this chapter, you will be able to:

- Discuss risk factors associated with substance abuse.

- Describe common characteristics of substance abusers.

- Identify major addictive substances.

- Explain the effects of addictive substances on physiological, cognitive, psychological, and social well-being.

- Discuss collaborative care for the client with substance abuse problems, including diagnostic tests, emergency care for overdose, and treatment of withdrawal.

- Use the nursing process as a framework for providing individualized nursing care for clients experiencing problems with substance abuse.

Substance abuse refers to the use of any chemical in a fashion inconsistent with medical or culturally defined social norms despite physical, psychological, or social adverse effects. Anxiety and depressive disorders frequently occur with substance abuse and more than 90% of people who commit suicide have a depressive or substance abuse disorder (National Institute of Mental Health [NIMH], 2001).

In a recent report of the surgeon general, 6% of the adult U.S. population are estimated to have an addictive disorder and 3% have both mental and addictive disorders (U.S. Department of Health and Human Services [USDHHS], 1999). Consequently, 9% of the population (15.4 million) have a substance abuse disorder. The costs of addictive disorders are exceedingly high. Direct costs of all mental health services in the United States totaled $69 billion with nearly 20% ($12.6 billion) spent on substance abuse treatment (USDHHS, 1999).

Alcohol is the most commonly used and abused substance in the United States. One of every 10 persons in America is alleged to be alcoholic (American Psychiatric Association [APA], 2000a). Two thirds of the nation's adult population consume alcohol regularly. When used in moderation, alcohol can have positive physiological effects by decreasing coronary artery disease and protecting against stroke; however, when consumed in excess, alcohol can severely diminish one's ability to function and will ultimately lead to life-threatening conditions.

The *Diagnostic and Statistical Manual of Mental Disorders,* fourth edition, text revision (DSM-IV-TR) (APA, 2000b) includes a classification scheme for distinguishing between substance abuse and substance dependence. **Substance dependence** refers to a severe condition occurring when the use of the chemical substance is no longer under an individual's control for at least 3 months. Continued use of the substance usually persists despite adverse effects on the person's physical condition, psychological health, and interpersonal relationships. The DSM-IV-TR criteria deals with the behavioral aspects and the maladaptive patterns of substance use, emphasizing the physical symptoms of **tolerance** and **withdrawal.** Tolerance is a cumulative state in which a particular dose of the chemical elicits a smaller response than before. With increased tolerance, the individual needs higher and higher doses to obtain the desired effect. When a person is physically addicted to the drug and stops taking it, **withdrawal symptoms** can occur within hours. Withdrawal is an uncomfortable state lasting several days, manifested by tremors, diaphoresis, anxiety, high blood pressure, tachycardia, and possibly convulsions. An overview of the DSM-IV-TR diagnostic criteria for substance abuse and substance dependence is shown in Box 12–1.

RISK FACTORS

Various risk factors help explain why one person becomes addicted while another does not. Biological, psychological, and sociocultural factors shed light on how a person may abuse or become dependent on a substance.

- *Biological factors* include an apparent hereditary factor, especially with alcohol. Studies have shown that children of alcoholic parents are more likely to develop alcoholism than children of nonalcoholic parents (Kutlenios, 1998). This is primarily true with male relatives. One type of alcoholism seen mostly in the sons of alcoholic fathers is thought to be connected with an early onset, inability to abstain, and an antisocial personality (Stuart & Laraia, 2001). Another type of alcoholism may be more environmentally influenced and is linked with onset after the age of 25, inability to stop after one drink, and a passive-dependent personality (Stuart & Laraia, 2001). More recent studies have demonstrated that alcohol and drug use has specific effects

---

BOX 12–1 ■ Substance Abuse versus Substance Dependence	
Substance Abuse	**Substance Dependence**
Maladaptive pattern of substance use leading to clinically significant impairment or distress, manifested by **one or more** of the following within a 12-month period:	Maladaptive pattern of substance use leading to clinically significant impairment or distress, manifested by **three or more** of the following within a 12-month period:
1. Failure to fulfill major role obligations at work, school, and home. 2. Involvement in physically hazardous situations while impaired (driving while intoxicated, operating a machine, exacerbation of physical symptoms such as ulcers). 3. Recurrent legal or interpersonal problems. 4. Continued use despite recurrent social and interpersonal problems.	1. Presence of tolerance to the drug. 2. Presence of withdrawal symptoms. 3. Substance is taken in larger amounts or for longer periods than is intended. 4. Unsuccessful or persistent desire to cut down or control substance use. 5. More time spent in getting, taking, and recovering from the substance. May withdraw from family or friends and spend more time using substance in private. 6. Decline in or absence of important social, occupational, or recreational activities. 7. Continued use of substance despite knowledge of adverse effects.

Note. Adapted from Diagnostic and Statistical Manual of Mental Disorders (4th ed., text rev.) (DSM-IV-TR) by American Psychiatric Association, 2000, Washington, DC: APA.

on selected biochemicals in the brain. Alcohol and other CNS depressants, such as benzodiazepines and barbiturates, act on gamma-aminobutyric acid (GABA). This may be why additive and cross-tolerance effects occur when alcohol and other CNS depressants are used in combination (Varcarolis, 2002).

- *Psychological factors* attempt to explain substance abuse through a combination of psychoanalytic, behavioral, and family system theories. Psychoanalytic theorists view substance abuse as a fixation at the oral stage of development, while behavioral theorists see addiction as a learned, maladaptive behavior. Family system theory focuses on the pattern of family relationships throughout several generations. No addictive personality type has been identified; however, several common factors seem to exist among alcoholics and drug users. Many substance abusers have experienced sexual or physical abuse in their childhood and as a result have low self-esteem and difficulty expressing emotions. A link also exists between substance abuse and psychiatric disorders such as depression, anxiety, and antisocial and dependent personalities. The habit of using a substance becomes a form of self-medication to cope with day-to-day problems, and over time develops into an addiction.

- *Sociocultural factors* often influence individuals' decisions as to when, what, and how they use substances. Many Asian people do not drink alcohol because of an uncomfortable physiological response characterized by flushing and tachycardia. About half of the Asian population have a deficiency of aldehyde dehydrogenase, the chemical that breaks down alcohol acetaldehyde (APA, 2000b). A buildup of acetaldehyde causes toxic symptoms and therefore keeps the prevalence rate of alcoholism lower in Asians. Europeans, on the other hand, have higher alcoholism rates. Religious background may also correlate with the likelihood that a person will abuse alcohol. Among major religions, people of Jewish faith have the lowest rate of alcoholism while Roman Catholics have the highest rate. Many people have a desire for social acceptance and initiate drug use to "fit in" with a peer group. Others may suffer from social anxiety and need drugs or alcohol to feel less inhibited while interacting with others.

Many factors place a person at risk for substance use, abuse, and dependence. No single cause can explain why one individual develops a pattern of drug use and another person does not. Thorough assessment of these factors is necessary to understand the whole person and plan appropriate interventions.

CHARACTERISTICS OF ABUSERS

As mentioned, no addictive personality type exists; however, many abusers have several characteristics in common. There is a tendency for drug users to indulge in impulsive, risk-taking behaviors. Abusers often have a low tolerance for frustration and pain. The human tendency to seek pleasure and avoid stress and pain is partially responsible for substance abuse. The reinforcing properties of drugs can create a pleasurable experience and reduce the intensity of unpleasant experiences. Often, drug users are rebellious against social norms and engage in antisocial behaviors such as stealing, promiscuity, driving while intoxicated, and violence against others.

There is also a tendency toward anxiety, anger, and low self-esteem in substance abusers. Although there is no greater prevalence of psychiatric illness in substance abusers than in the general population, dual diagnosis is often present. **Dual diagnosis,** or **dual disorder,** refers to the coexistence of substance abuse or dependence and a psychiatric disorder in one individual. One disorder can be an indication of another, such as the relationship with alcoholism and depression. A depressed person may use self-medication in the form of alcohol to treat the depression, or the alcoholic person may become depressed. One recent study described the prevalence and characteristics of co-occurring serious mental illness (SMI) and substance abuse or dependence (Virgo et al., 2001). Most dual diagnoses in adult mental health patients were (1) alcohol and/or cannabis abuse with psychoses and heroin and/or (2) alcohol abuse or dependence with depression. Compared with other SMI patients, those who were dually diagnosed were younger, more often male, in less stable accommodation, more likely to be unemployed, and more likely to have more than one psychiatric diagnosis and personality disorder. They also tended to have more crises and pose greater risk to themselves and others (Virgo et al., 2001). Box 12–2 lists terminology associated with substance abuse.

ADDICTIVE SUBSTANCES AND THEIR EFFECTS
Nicotine

Nicotine enters the system via the lungs (cigarettes and cigars) and oral mucous membranes (smokeless tobacco as well as smoking). In low doses, nicotine stimulates nicotinic receptors in the brain to release norepinephrine and epinephrine, causing vasoconstriction. As a result, the heart rate accelerates and the force of ventricular contractions increases. Gastrointestinal (GI) effects include an increase in gastric acid secretion, tone and motility of GI smooth muscle, and promotion of vomiting. Nicotine acts on the central nervous system (CNS) as a stimulant, increasing respiration and arousal. Nicotine also activates the pleasure system in the mesolimbic system (Lehne, 2001). Moderate doses of nicotine can cause tremors. With high doses, such as acute poisoning from insecticides, convulsions and death can occur.

Tolerance can develop to nausea and dizziness, but not to the cardiovascular effects. Nicotine dependence results from chronic use with withdrawal seen as craving, nervousness, restlessness, irritability, impatience, increased hostility, insomnia, impaired concentration, increased appetite, and weight gain. Gradual reduction in nicotine use seems to prolong suffering. Chronic toxicity from smoking has been well established in the form of vascular diseases; chronic lung disease; and cancers of the larynx, esophagus, oral cavity, lung, bladder, and pancreas (Lehne, 2001). In addition, secondhand effects from smoking have been demonstrated, especially to fetuses during pregnancy. Smoking during pregnancy leads to increased risks for infants such as low birth weight, spontaneous abortions, perinatal mortality, and sudden infant death.

BOX 12–2 ■ Terminology Associated with Substance Abuse

Term	Definition
Abstinence	Voluntarily going without drugs
Addiction	A disease process characterized by the continued use of a specific chemical substance despite physical, psychological, or social harm (used interchangeably with substance dependence)
Codependence	A cluster of maladaptive behaviors exhibited by significant others of a substance abusing individual that serves to enable and protect the abuse at the expense of living a full and satisfying life
Cross dependence	Ability of one drug to support physical dependence on another drug
Cross-tolerance	Tolerance to one drug confers tolerance to another
Delirium tremens	A medical emergency usually occurring 3 to 5 days following alcohol withdrawal and lasting 2 to 3 days. Characterized by paranoia, disorientation, delusions, visual hallucinations, elevated vital signs, vomiting, diarrhea, and diaphoresis
Detoxification	The process of helping an addicted individual safely through withdrawal
Dual diagnosis	The coexistence of substance abuse/dependence and a psychiatric disorder in one individual (used interchangeably with dual disorder)
Dual disorder	Concurrent diagnosis of a substance use disorder and a psychiatric disorder. One disorder can precede and cause the other, such as the relationship between alcoholism and depression.
Korsakoff's psychosis	Secondary dementia caused by thiamine (B_1) deficiency that may be associated with chronic alcoholism; characterized by progressive cognitive deterioration, confabulation, peripheral neuropathy, and myopathy
Physical dependence	A state in which withdrawal syndrome will occur if drug use is discontinued
Polysubstance abuse	The simultaneous use of many substances
Psychologic dependence	An intensive subjective need for a particular psychoactive drug
Substance abuse	Continued use of a chemical substance in a fashion inconsistent with medical or social norms, for at least 1 month, despite related problems
Substance dependence	A severe condition occurring when the use of the chemical substance is no longer under control, for at least 3 months; continued use persists despite adverse effects (used interchangeably with addiction)
Tolerance	State in which a particular dose elicits a smaller response than it formerly did. With increased tolerance the individual needs higher and higher doses to obtain the desired response.
Wernicke's encephalopathy	Caused by thiamine (B_1) deficiency, characterized by nystagmus, ptosis, ataxia, confusion, coma, and possible death. Thiamine deficiency is common in chronic alcoholism.
Withdrawal syndrome	Constellation of signs and symptoms that occurs in physically dependent individuals when they discontinue drug use

Cannabis

Cannabis sativa is the source of marijuana. Use of cannabis is on the rise in the United States, with 10% of children age 12 to 17 using marijuana (Lehne, 2001). One recent study revealed that lifetime use of marijuana in a sample of 918 adolescents aged 12 to 21 years was 59%, while 18.4% reported frequent weekly use (Siqueira, Diab, Bodian, & Rolnitzky, 2001). Contributing factors to marijuana use in this population were negative life events, anger, and less parental support. The greatest psychoactive substances are in the flowering tops of the cannabis plant. Marijuana (also know as grass, weed, pot, dope, joint, and reefer) and hashish are the most common derivatives. The psychoactive component of marijuana is an oily chemical known as delta-9-tetrahydrocannabinol (THC). THC activates specific cannabinoid receptors in the brain. Recent evidence suggests that marijuana may act like opioids and cocaine in producing a pleasurable sensation, probably by causing release of endogenous opioids and then dopamine (Lehne, 2001).

Physiologic effects of cannabis are dose related and can cause an increase in heart rate and bronchodilation in short-term use, but airway constriction with chronic use leading to bronchitis, sinusitis, asthma, and possibly cancer. The reproductive system is also affected by marijuana; it causes decreased spermatogenesis and testosterone levels in males and decreased levels of follicle-stimulating, luteinizing, and prolactin hormones in females. Birth defects may also be associated with cannabis use. Subjective effects of marijuana include euphoria, sedation, and hallucinations. In addition, chronic use of marijuana can result in amotivational behaviors such as apathy, dullness, poor grooming, reduced interest in achievement, and disinterest. At extremely high doses, tolerance and physical dependence result.

Alcohol

Alcohol acts as a CNS depressant and enhances the action of gamma aminobutyric acid (GABA). Chronic use of alcohol can cause severe neurologic and psychiatric disorders. Severe damage to the liver occurs with chronic alcohol abuse, and can progress from fatty liver to other liver diseases such as hepatitis or cirrhosis. Chronic alcoholism is the major cause of fatal cirrhosis. Alcohol causes damaging effects to many other systems; its effects include myocardial disease, erosive gastritis, acute and chronic pancreatitis, sexual dysfunction, and an increased risk of breast cancer.

Malnutrition is another serious complication of chronic alcoholism, especially thiamine (B_1) deficiency that can result in neurological impairments. Thiamine depletion is thought to cause the Wernicke-Korsakoff syndrome observed in chronic alcoholics (Stuart & Laraia, 2001). Severe cognitive impairment is a principal feature of **Wernicke's encephalopathy** and **Korsakoff's psychosis.** Although alcohol is a CNS depressant, it actually disrupts sleep, thus altering the sleep cycle, decreasing the quality of sleep, intensifying obstructive sleep apnea, and reducing total sleeping time. Heavy drinkers have a higher mortality rate and many fatalities occur from alcohol-related accidents. Blood alcohol levels (BALs) are highly predictive of CNS effects. Euphoria, reduced inhibitions, impaired judgment, and increased confidence are seen at 0.05% (Vacarolis, 2002). The legal level of intoxication in most states is 0.10%. Toxic levels in excess of 0.5% can cause coma, respiratory depression, peripheral collapse, and death (Vacarolis, 2002). Chronic consumption of alcohol produces tolerance and creates cross-tolerance to general anesthetics, barbiturates, benzodiazepines, and other CNS depressants. If alcohol is withdrawn abruptly, withdrawal symptoms such as tachycardia, hypertension, diaphoresis, nausea, vomiting, tremors, sleeplessness, irritability, **delirium tremens (DT),** seizures, and convulsions result.

CNS Depressants

Central nervous system depressants including barbiturates, benzodiazepines, paraldehyde, meprobamate, and chloral hydrate are also subject to abuse. Cross dependence exists among all CNS depressants and cross-tolerance can develop to alcohol and general anesthetics. Chronic users of barbiturates require progressively higher doses to achieve subjective effects as tolerance develops, but they develop little tolerance to respiratory depression. The depressant effects related to barbiturates are dose dependent and range from mild sedation to sleep to coma to death. With larger doses over time and a combination of alcohol and barbiturates, the risk of death increases greatly. Benzodiazepines alone are safer than barbiturates, because an overdose of oral benzodiazepines rarely results in death.

Psychostimulants

Psychostimulants such as cocaine and amphetamines have a high potential for abuse. Euphoria is the main subjective effect associated with cocaine and amphetamines, leading to addiction. Cocaine base (freebase, cocaine, or "crack") is heat stable and is usually smoked (freebasing). Cocaine hydrochloride (HCl) is diluted or cut before sale and the pure form ("rocks") is administered intranasally (snorted) or in-

jected intravenously. "Skin popping" is a method many substance abusers are using to administer drugs, perhaps leading to the formation of abscesses under the skin. The use of crack cocaine reached epidemic proportions especially in teens (who have a high risk of lethal overdose) in 1985, but has declined in use over the past few years (Lehne, 2001). Mild overdose of cocaine produces agitation, dizziness, tremor, and blurred vision. Severe overdose produces anxiety, hyperpyrexia, convulsions, ventricular dysrhythmias, severe hypertension, and hemorrhagic stroke with possible angina or myocardial infarction (MI). The use of cocaine during pregnancy is especially problematic, because the drug crosses the placenta and enters the fetal bloodstream. Spontaneous abortion, premature delivery, retardation of intrauterine growth, congenital abnormalities, and fetal addiction can result. Long-term intranasal use of cocaine can cause atrophy of the nasal mucosa, necrosis and perforation of the nasal septum, and lung damage.

Amphetamine use is on the rise in the United States and poses a severe health risk to society. Between 1993 and 1999, amphetamine treatment admission rates increased by 250% or more in 14 states and 100% to 249% in another 10 states (USDHHS, 2001). Dextroamphetamine, methamphetamine, and amphetamine can be taken orally or intravenously. Methamphetamine is the primary form of amphetamine seen in the United States, comprising 94% of all amphetamine treatment admissions in 1999 (USDHHS, 2001). A form of dextroamphetamine ("ice" or "crystal meth") can be smoked. Amphetamines cause arousal and an elevation of mood with a sense of increased strength, mental capacity, self-confidence, and a decreased need for food and sleep. A psychotic state with hallucinations and paranoia are common with long-term use, requiring treatment similar to other psychotic disorders. The cardiovascular effects of amphetamines are comparable to those of cocaine, including vasoconstriction, tachycardia, hypertension, angina, and dysrhythmias. Tolerance to mood elevation, appetite suppression, and cardiovascular effects develops with amphetamines; however, dependence is more psychological than physical. Withdrawal from amphetamines produces dysphoria and craving with fatigue, prolonged sleep, excessive eating, and depression.

Opiates

Opiates such as morphine and heroin have been abused for many centuries and are major drugs of abuse. The urban poor constitute the majority of abusers, although opiates are used and abused by people of all socioeconomic status. A small percentage of individuals are originally exposed to opiates in the context of pain management; however, most people use opiates under social or illicit circumstances. Heroin is usually the opiate of choice, except among health care workers, who usually select meperidine (Demerol). Health care professionals have a higher risk for opiate abuse than other professionals due to the high accessibility of opiates in their line of work. If colleagues are showing signs of a substance abuse problem, information about impaired nurse programs is available through state boards of nursing to help individual nurses.

MediaLink | COCAINE ANIMATION

Heroin is usually administered intravenously and induces a "rush" or "kick" that lasts less than a minute, followed by a sense of euphoria for an extended period. Tolerance develops to the euphoria, respiratory depression, and nausea but not to constipation and miosis. Physical dependence occurs with long-term use of opiates. Initial withdrawal symptoms such as drug craving, lacrimation, rhinorrhea, yawning, and diaphoresis usually take 10 days to run their course, with the second phase of opiate withdrawal lasting for months with insomnia, irritability, fatigue, and potential GI hyperactivity and premature ejaculation as problems.

Hallucinogens

Hallucinogens are also called psychedelics or psychotomimetics and include d-lysergic acid diethylamide (LSD), mescaline, dimethyltryptamine (DMT), and psilocin. Psychedelics bring on the same types of thoughts, perceptions, and feelings that occur in dreams. LSD was first used to simulate psychosis. It affects serotonin receptors at multiple sites in the brain and spinal cord. LSD is usually taken orally but can be injected or smoked. The individual's response to a "trip," the experience of being high on LSD, cannot be predicted and psychological effects and "flashbacks" are common. Ecstasy (3,4-methylenediosy-methamphetamine or MDMA) had high use in the 1980s as a popular recreational "rave" drug and has reappeared in recent years as a date or rape drug. Current research has revealed that women might be more susceptible to the neurotoxic effects on serotonin neurons when using MDMA (Reneman et al., 2001). Serotonin imbalance is thought to affect impulse control and may be responsible for uninhibited sexual responses in women who have been given the drug without their knowledge. Phencyclidine (PCP, also called angel dust and peace pill) was formerly an anesthetic similar to ketamine used for animals but caused emergence delirium in humans. Other hallucinogens are similar to LSD but with different potency and time course of action.

Inhalants

Inhalants are categorized into three types: anesthetics, volatile nitrites, and organic solvents. Nitrous oxide (laughing gas) and ether are the most abused anesthetics. Amyl nitrite, butyl nitrite, and isobutyl nitrite are volatile nitrites used especially by homosexual males to induce venodilation and anal sphincter relaxation. Amyl nitrite is manufactured for medical use, but butyl and isobutyl nitrites are sold for recreational use. Other names for butyl and isobutyl nitrites are climax, rush, and locker room. Street names for amyl nitrite are "poppers" or "snappers." (See Table 12–1.) Brain damage or sudden death can occur from the first, tenth, or hundredth time an individual uses an inhalant, resulting in "sudden sniffing death." This danger makes the use of inhalants more hazardous than some other substances.

Organic solvents are ingested in three different methods: bagging, huffing, or sniffing. *Bagging* involves pouring the solvent in a plastic bag and inhaling the vapor. *Huffing* refers to pouring the solvent on a rag and inhaling. *Sniffing* refers to inhaling the solvent directly from the container. Common or-

TABLE 12–1	Common Street Names for Abused Substances
Substance	**Street Name**
Alcohol	Booze, brew, spirits, juice
Amphetamines	Bennies, crystal, crystal meth, diet pills, dolls, eye-openers, ice, lid poppers, pep pills, purple hearts, speed, uppers
Barbiturates	Barbs, beans, black beauties, blue angels, candy, downers, goof balls, nebbies, reds, sleepers, yellow jackets, yellows
Cocaine	Bernice, bernies, big C, blow, charlie, coke, dust, girl, heaven, jay, lady, nose candy, nose powder, snow, sugar, white lady Crack: conan, freebase, rock, toke, white cloud, white tornado
Heroin	H, horse, harry, boy, scag, shit, smack, stuff, white junk, white stuff
Marijuana	Acapulco gold, aunt mary, broccoli, dope, grass, grunt, hay, hemp, herb, J, joint, joy stick, killer weed, maryjane, pot ragweed, reefer, smoke, weed
Hallucinogens	Acid, big D, blotter, blue heaven, cap D, deeda, flash, L, mellow yellows, microdots, paper acid, sugar, ticket, yello, Ecstasy

ganic solvents are toluene, gasoline, lighter fluid, paint thinner, nail polish remover, benzene, acetone, chloroform, and model airplane glue. The effects from inhaling organic solvents are similar to alcohol, with prolonged use leading to multiple toxicity. There are no antidotes for these inhalants; therefore, management of toxicity is supportive.

COLLABORATIVE CARE

Effective treatment of substance abuse and dependence results from the collaborative efforts of an interdisciplinary team specializing in the treatment of psychiatric and substance abuse disorders. Therapies may include detoxification, aversion therapy to maintain abstinence, group and/or individual psychotherapy, psychotropic medications, cognitive-behavioral strategies, family counseling, and self-help groups. Clients suffering from substance abuse can be treated in either inpatient or outpatient settings. A substance overdose is a life-threatening condition that requires emergency hospitalization to stabilize the client medically before implementing any of the above interventions. Several diagnostic tests can provide valuable information about the patients physical condition and set the course for treatment.

Diagnostic Tests

The body fluids most often tested for drug content are blood and urine. A urine drug screen (UDS) and/or blood alcohol level (BAL) are useful biological measures for assessment purposes. The length of time that drugs can be found in blood and urine varies according to dosage and metabolic properties of the drug. All traces of the drug may disappear within 24 hours or may still be detectable 30 days later. Knowledge of the

BAL is helpful in ascertaining the level of intoxication, the level of tolerance, and whether the person accurately reported recent drinking. At 0.10% (after 5 to 6 drinks in 1 to 2 hours), voluntary motor action becomes clumsy and reaction time is impaired. The degree of impairment varies with gender, weight, and food ingestion. Small women who drink alcohol on an empty stomach will experience intoxication more rapidly than large males who have eaten a full meal. At 0.20% (after 10 to 12 drinks in 2 to 4 hours), function of the motor area in the brain is depressed, causing staggering and ataxia (Vacarolis, 2002). A level above 0.10% without associated behavioral symptoms indicates the presence of tolerance. A BAL greater than 0.10% is considered legal intoxication in most states. High tolerance is a sign of physical dependence. Assessing for withdrawal symptoms is important when the BAL is high. Medications given for treatment of withdrawal from alcohol are usually not started until the BAL is below a set norm (usually below 0.10%) unless withdrawal symptoms become severe. BAL may be repeated several times, several hours apart, to determine the body's metabolism of alcohol

and when it is safe to give the patient medication to minimize the withdrawal symptoms.

Emergency Care for Overdose

The care of a patient who has overdosed on any substance is a serious medical emergency. Respiratory depression may require mechanical ventilation. The patient may become severely sedated and difficult to arouse. Every effort must be made to keep the patient awake; however, stupor and coma may often result. A seizure is another serious complication that requires emergency treatment. If the overdose was intentional, the patient must be constantly monitored for further signs of suicidal ideation. Never leave an actively suicidal patient alone. Signs of overdose and withdrawal from major substances are summarized in Table 12–2 along with their recommended treatments.

Treatment of Withdrawal

All CNS depressants, including alcohol, benzodiazepines, and barbiturates, have a potentially dangerous progression of

TABLE 12–2 Signs and Treatment of Overdose and Withdrawal

| Drug | Overdose | | Withdrawal | |
	Signs	Treatment	Signs	Treatment
CNS Depressants: Alcohol Barbiturates Benzodiazepines	Cardiovascular or respiratory depression or arrest (mostly with barbiturates) Coma Shock Convulsions Death	*If awake:* Keep awake Induce vomiting Activated charcoal to absorb drug VS q 15 minutes *Coma:* Clear airway, intubate IV fluids Gastric lavage Seizure precautions Possible hemo or peritoneal dialysis Frequent VS Assess for shock and cardiac arrest	Nausea and vomiting Tachycardia Diaphoresis Anxiety or agitation Tremors Marked insomnia Grand mal seizures Delirium (after 5–15 years of heavy use)	Carefully titrated detoxification with similar drug NOTE: Abrupt withdrawal can lead to death.
Stimulants: Cocaine-crack Amphetamines	Respiratory distress Ataxia Hyperpyrexia Convulsions Coma Stroke Myocardial infarction (MI) Death	Antipsychotics Management for: 1. Hyperpyrexia 2. Convulsions 3. Respiratory distress 4. Cardiovascular shock 5. Acidify urine (ammonium Cl for amphetamine)	Fatigue Depression Agitation Apathy Anxiety Sleepiness Disorientation Lethargy Craving	Antidepressants (desipramine) Dopamine agonist Bromocriptine
Opiates: Heroin Meperidine Morphine Methadone	Pupil dilation due to anoxia Respiratory depression-arrest Coma Shock Convulsions Death	Narcotic antagonist, (Narcan) quickly reverses CNS depression	Yawning, insomnia Irritability Rhinorrhea Panic Diaphoresis Cramps Nausea and vomiting Muscle aches Chills and fever Lacrimation Diarrhea	Methadone tapering Clonidine-naltrexone detoxification Buprenorphine substitution

(continued on page 338)

TABLE 12–2 Signs and Treatment of Overdose and Withdrawal (continued)

Drug	Overdose Signs	Overdose Treatment	Withdrawal Signs	Withdrawal Treatment
Hallucinogens: Lysergic acid diethylamide (LSD)	LSD: Psychosis Brain damage Death	Low stimuli with minimal light, sound, activity Have one person "talk down client," reassure Speak slowly and clearly Diazepam or chloral hydrate for anxiety	No pattern of withdrawal	
Phencyclidine piperidine (PCP)	Possible hypertensive crisis Respiratory arrest Hyperthermia Seizures	Acidify urine to help excrete drug (cranberry juice, ascorbic acid); in acute stage: ammonium chloride Minimal stimulis Do NOT attempt to talk down, speak slowly in low voice Diazepam or Haldol		
Inhalants: Volatile Solvents such as butane, paint thinner, airplane glue, or nail polish remover	Intoxication: 1. Excitation 2. Drowsiness 3. Disinhibition 4. Staggering 5. Lightheadedness 6. Agitation Side Effects: 1. Damage to nervous system 2. Death	Support affected systems	No pattern of withdrawal	
Nitrates	Enhance sexual pleasure	Neurological symptoms may respond to vitamin B_{12} and folate Chronic users may experience polyneuropathy and myelopathy		
Anesthetics such as nitrous oxide	Giggling, laughter Euphoria			

BOX 12–3 ■ Drugs Used in the Treatment of Substance Withdrawal/Abuse

Drug	Dose	Purpose
Benzodiazepines		
1. Clordiazepoxide (Librium)	15–100 mg	Diminishes anxiety and has anticonvulsant qualities to
2. Diazepam (Valium)	4–40 mg	provide safe withdrawal. May be ordered q4h or prn to
3. Oxazepam (Serax)	30–120 mg	manage adverse effects from withdrawal, then dose is
4. Lorazepam (Ativan)	2–6 mg	tapered to zero.
Vitamins		
1. Thiamine (Vitamin B_1)	100 mg/day	Prevents Wernicke's encephalopathy
2. Folic acid	1 mg/day	Corrects vitamin deficiency caused by heavy long-term alcohol
3. Multivitamins	I tab/cap daily	abuse
Anticonvulsants		
1. Phenobarbital	30–320 mg	For seizure control and sedation
2. Magnesium sulfate	1 g q6h	Reduces postwithdrawal seizures
Abstinence medications		
1. Disulfiram (Antabuse)	250 mg/day	Prevents breakdown of alcohol
2. Naltrexone (ReVia)	50 mg/day	Diminishes cravings for alcohol and opioids
3. Methadone	40 mg/day	Blocks craving for heroin
Antidepressants		
1. Fluoxetine (Prozac)	20–80 mg/day	Enhances and stabilizes mood and diminishes anxiety
2. Sertraline (Zoloft)	50–200 mg/day	

withdrawal. Alcohol and the entire class of CNS depressants share the same withdrawal syndrome. Early signs of withdrawal appear within a few hours following cessation of the drug, peak after 24 to 48 hours, and then rapidly disappear unless the withdrawal progresses to delirium tremens. Severe withdrawal or delirium tremens is a medical emergency that usually occurs 2 to 5 days following alcohol withdrawal and persists 2 to 3 days. The symptoms of severe withdrawal include disorientation, paranoid delusions, visual hallucinations, and marked withdrawal symptoms. Seizures may also occur, requiring the use of emergency equipment. Treatment of severe withdrawal during detoxification is mostly symptomatic through acetaminophen, vitamins, and medications to minimize discomfort. Withdrawal symptoms from opiates and stimulants can be very unpleasant but are generally not life threatening. The patient experiencing an acute phase of cocaine withdrawal may become suicidal. Common drugs used in the treatment of substance abuse and withdrawal are presented in Box 12–3.

NURSING CARE

Health Promotion

Nursing care of the client with substance abuse or dependence is challenging and requires a nonjudgmental atmosphere promoting trust and respect. Health promotion efforts are aimed at preventing drug use among children and adolescents and reducing the risks among adults. Adolescence is the most common phase for the first experience with drugs (Stuart & Laraia, 2001), therefore teenagers are a vulnerable population, often succumbing to peer pressure. Healthy lifestyles, parental support, stress management, good nutrition, and information about ways to steer clear of peer pressure are important topics for the nurse to provide in school programs.

Nurses should provide adults with information on healthy coping mechanisms, relaxation, and stress reduction techniques to decrease the risks of substance abuse. Nurses have a responsibility to educate their clients about the physiological effects of substances on the body as well as ways to manage stress and anxiety. Nurses must encourage and support periods of abstinence while assisting clients to make major changes in lifestyles, habits, relationships, and coping methods. See the box below for nursing research about older clients with substance abuse problems.

Assessment

A comprehensive approach to the assessment of substance use is essential to ensure adequate and appropriate intervention. Three important areas to be assessed are a history of the client's past substance use, medical and psychiatric history, and the presence of psychosocial concerns. Ask questions in a nonthreatening, matter-of-fact manner, phrased as to not imply wrongdoing (Henderson-Martin, 2000). For instance, a nonthreatening question such as, "How much alcohol do you drink?" is preferable to the judgmental question, "You don't drink too much alcohol, do you?" Open-ended questions that

Nursing Research

Evidence-Based Practice for the Older Client with a Substance Abuse Problem

People of any age can have substance abuse problems, but the consequences in older adults can be more critical. Falls and accidents can rob older adults of their independence, and substance abuse increases the risk of falls by affecting alertness, judgment, coordination, and reaction time. In addition, older adults are more likely than younger people to use prescription or over-the-counter medicines, which can be harmful when mixed with alcohol and/or illicit drugs. Alcohol and drug abuse also can make some medical problems hard to diagnose, for example, by dulling a pain sensation that might warn of a heart attack.

The purpose of this study (Blixen, McDougall, & Suen, 1997) was to examine the prevalence and correlates of dual diagnosis in older adults and compare the findings with studies of younger clients. The leading psychiatric diagnosis for hospitalized elders was depression. Over one-third (37.6%) had a substance abuse disorder in addition to a psychiatric disorder. Almost three-fourths (71%) of this dual diagnosis group abused alcohol and 29% abused both alcohol and other substances. Because affective disorders in conjunction with alcohol abuse are the most frequently found disorders in completed suicides, the authors' findings have important relevance for routinely using screening tools for both substance abuse and mental disorders in this population.

IMPLICATIONS FOR NURSING
Findings from this study support other research that substance abuse in older adults is likely to increase over subsequent decades as baby boomers reach retirement age. Estimates of alcohol abuse in the older adult population range from 4% to 20% in the community-dwelling elderly and approximately 25% among hospitalized older adults (Adams & Cox, 1995; Adams & Kinney, 1995; Beresford, Blow, & Brower, 1990).

Unfortunately, a substance abuse problem in an older adult can be difficult to detect because many of the symptoms of abuse (e.g., insomnia, depression, loss of memory, anxiety, musculoskeletal pain) may be confused with conditions commonly seen in older patients. Health care professionals frequently fail to recognize and address the misuse and abuse of alcohol and drugs in the elderly (Ondus, Hujer, Mann, & Mion, 1999).

Critical Thinking in Client Care
1. You are caring for an 85-year-old man who tells you that since his wife died 6 months ago, he only feels like drinking to dull the pain of her loss. How would you respond?

2. Why do you think nurses and other health care professionals often fail to recognize and address substance abuse problems in the older adult?

3. You are caring for an older adult who denies that alcohol has become a serious problem, even though this is the third hospitalization for this client in 6 months due to accidents, falls, and blackouts. What would you do?

<table>
<tr><td>

BOX 12–4 ■ Examples of Open-Ended Questions for Assessment

■ On average, how many days per week do you drink alcohol or use drugs?

■ On a typical day when you use drugs or alcohol, how many hits or drinks do you have?

■ What is the greatest number of drinks you've had at any one time during the past month?

■ What drug(s) did you take before coming to the hospital or clinic?

■ How long have you been using the substances?

■ How often and how much do you usually use?

■ What kinds of problems has substance use caused for you, your family, friends, finances, and health?

</td></tr>
</table>

elicit more than a simple yes or no answer help to determine the direction of future counseling. Examples of open-ended questions are provided in Box 12–4. Use therapeutic communication techniques to establish trust prior to the assessment process.

History of Past Substance Use

A thorough history of the client's past substance use is important to ascertain the possibility of tolerance, physical dependence, or withdrawal syndrome. The following questions are helpful in eliciting a pattern of substance use behavior.

• How many substances has the client used simultaneously (**polysubstance abuse** or simultaneous use of many substances) in the past?

• How often, how much, and when did the client first use the substance(s)?

• Is there a history of blackouts, delirium, or seizures?

• Is there a history of withdrawal syndrome, overdoses, and complications from previous substance use?

• Has the client ever been treated in an alcohol or drug abuse clinic?

• Has the client ever been arrested for driving under the influence (DUI) or charged with any criminal offense while using drugs or alcohol?

• Is there a family history of drug or alcohol use?

Medical and Psychiatric History

The client's medical history is another important area for assessment and should include the existence of any concomitant physical or mental condition (e.g., HIV, hepatitis, cirrhosis, esophageal varices, pancreatitis, gastritis, Wernicke-Korsakoff syndrome, depression, schizophrenia, anxiety, or personality disorder). Ask about prescribed and over-the-counter medications as well as any allergies or sensitivity to drugs. A brief overview of the client's current mental status is also significant.

• Is there a history of abuse (physical or sexual) or family violence?

• Has the client ever tried to commit suicide?

• Is the client currently having suicidal or homicidal ideation?

Psychosocial Issues

Information about the client's level of stress and other psychosocial concerns can help in the assessment of substance use problems.

• Has the client's substance use affected his or her ability to hold a job?

• Has the client's substance use affected relationships with spouse, family, friends, or coworkers?

• How does the client usually cope with stress?

• Does the client have a support system that helps in time of need?

• How does the client spend his or her leisure time?

Assessment Tools

Several screening tools such as the Michigan Alcohol Screening Test (MAST) (Pokorny, Miller, & Kaplan, 1972), Drug Abuse Screening Test (DAST) (Skinner, 1982), and the CAGE questionnaire (Ewing, 1984) may help the nurse determine the degree of severity of substance abuse or dependence (see Figure 12–1 ■). These screening tools provide a nonjudgmental, brief, and easy method to ascertain patterns of substance abuse behaviors.

• *Michigan Alcohol Screening Test (MAST) Brief Version* is a 10-question, dichotomous, self-administered questionnaire that takes 10 to 15 minutes to complete. An answer of yes to 3 or more questions indicates a potentially dangerous pattern of alcohol abuse.

• *CAGE questionnaire* is more useful when the client may not recognize he or she has an alcohol problem or is uncomfortable acknowledging it. This questionnaire is designed to be a self-report of drinking behavior or may be administered by a professional. One affirmative response indicates the need for further discussion and follow-up. Two or more yes answers signify a problem with alcohol that may require treatment.

Have you ever felt you should *cut* down on your drinking?
Have people *annoyed* you by criticizing your drinking?
Have you ever felt bad or *guilty* about your drinking?
Have you ever had a drink first thing in the morning (an "*eye-opener*") to steady your nerves or to get rid of a hangover?

• *Drug Abuse Screening Test (DAST)* is a yes/no self-administered questionnaire that is useful in identifying people who are possibly addicted to drugs other than alcohol. A positive response to one or more questions suggests significant drug abuse problems and warrants further evaluation. Because the tools can be incorrect if the client is not answering truthfully, all clients who are screened positive for drug addiction should be evaluated according to diagnostic criteria.

Nursing Diagnoses and Interventions

The primary nursing diagnoses and interventions for clients with substance abuse problems are listed below. Implications for nursing care in acute and home care settings are combined in this discussion.

Risk for Injury

• Assess client's level of disorientation to determine specific risks to safety. *Knowledge of the client's level of cognitive functioning is essential to the development of an appropriate plan of care.*

- Obtain a drug history as well as urine and blood samples for laboratory analysis of substance content. *Subjective history is often not accurate and knowledge regarding substance use is important for accurate assessment.*
- Place client in a quiet, private room to decrease excessive stimuli, but do not leave client alone if excessive hyperactivity or suicidal ideation is present. *Excessive stimuli increase client's agitation.*
- Frequently orient client to reality and the environment, ensuring that potentially harmful objects are stored outside the client's access. *Client may harm self or others if disoriented and confused.*
- Monitor vital signs every 15 minutes until stable and assess for signs of intoxication or withdrawal. *The most reliable information about withdrawal symptoms are vital signs; they provide information about the need for medication during detoxification.*

Ineffective Denial

- Be genuine, honest, and respectful of client. Keep all promises and convey an attitude of acceptance of the client. *The development of a nonjudgmental, therapeutic nurse-client relationship is essential to gain the client's trust.*
- Identify maladaptive behaviors or situations that have occurred in client's life and discuss how the use of substances may have been a contributing factor. *The first step in combating denial is for the client to recognize the relationship between substance use and personal problems.*
- Do not accept the use of defense mechanisms such as rationalization or projection as the client attempts to blame others or make excuses for his or her behavior. Use confrontation with caring to avoid placing client on the defensive. *Confrontation interferes with the client's ability to use denial.*
- Encourage client participation in therapeutic group activities such as dual diagnosis or Alcoholics Anonymous (AA)

Scoring Yes to 3 or more indicates alcoholism

1. Do you feel you are a normal drinker?
2. Do friends or relatives think you are a normal drinker?
3. Have you ever attended a meeting of Alcoholics Anonymous?
4. Have you ever gotten in trouble at work because of drinking?
5. Have you ever lost friends or girlfriends/boyfriends because of drinking?
6. Have you ever neglected your obligations, your family, or your work for 2 or more days in a row because of your drinking?
7. Have you ever had delirium tremens (DTs), severe shaking, or heard voices or seen things that were not there after heavy drinking?
8. Have you ever gone to anyone for help about your drinking?
9. Have you ever been in a hospital because of your drinking?
10. Have you ever been arrested for drunken driving or other drunken behavior?

The following questions concern information about your involvement with drugs *not including alcoholic beverages* during the past 12 months.

In the statements, "drug abuse" refers to (1) the use of prescribed or OTC drugs in excess of the directions and (2) any nonmedical use of drugs. The various classes of drugs may include cannabis, solvents, antianxiety drugs, sedative-hypnotics, cocaine, stimulants, hallucinogens, and narcotics. Remember that the questions *do not include alcoholic beverages.*

Have you used drugs other than those required for medical purposes?	Yes ___	No ___
Do you abuse more than one drug at a time?	Yes ___	No ___
Are you always able to stop using drugs when you want to?	Yes ___	No ___
Have you had "blackouts" or "flashbacks" as a result of drug use?	Yes ___	No ___
Do you ever feel bad about your drug abuse?	Yes ___	No ___
Does your spouse (or parents) ever complain about your involvement with drugs?	Yes ___	No ___
Have you neglected your family because of your use of drugs?	Yes ___	No ___
Have you engaged in illegal activities in order to obtain drugs?	Yes ___	No ___
Have you ever experienced withdrawal symptoms (felt sick) when you stopped taking drugs?	Yes ___	No ___
Have you had medical problems as a result of your drug use (e.g., memory loss, hepatitis, convulsions, bleeding, etc.)?	Yes ___	No ___
Scoring: one positive response warrants further evaluation	Yes ___	No ___

Figure 12–1 ■ Screening tools for alcohol and drug abuse.

From "The Brief MAST: A Shortened Version of the Michigan Alcohol Screening Test" by A. D. Porkorny, B. A. Miller, and H. B. Kaplan, 1972, American Journal of Psychiatry, 129, pp. 342–345. Copyright 1972 by the American Psychiatric Association; and Drug Abuse Screening Test (DAST) (p. 363) by H. A. Skinner, 1982, Langford Lance, England: Elsevier Science Ltd. Copyright 1982. Both reprinted by permission.

ALCOHOL WITHDRAWAL CARE PLAN MediaLink

meetings with other people who are experiencing or have experienced similar problems. *Peer feedback is often more accepted than feedback from authority figures.*

Ineffective Individual Coping

- Establish trusting relationship. *Trust is essential to the nurse-client relationship.*
- Set limits on manipulative behavior and maintain consistency in responses. *Client is unable to set own limits and must begin to accept responsibility without being manipulative.*
- Encourage client to verbalize feelings, fears, or anxieties. Use attentive listening and validate client's feelings with observations or statements that acknowledge feelings. *Verbalization of feelings helps client to develop insight into behaviors and long-standing problems.*
- Explore methods of dealing with stressful situations other than resorting to substance use. Provide encouragement for changing to a healthier lifestyle. Teach healthy coping mechanisms (e.g., physical exercise, progressive muscle relaxation, deep breathing exercises, meditation, and imagery). *Client needs knowledge about how to adapt to stress without resorting to drug use.*

Imbalanced Nutrition: Less Than Body Requirements

- Administer vitamins and dietary supplements as ordered by physician. *Vitamin B_1 is necessary to prevent complications from chronic alcoholism such as Wernicke's syndrome.*
- Monitor lab work (e.g., total albumin, complete blood count, urinalysis, electrolytes, and liver enzymes) and report significant changes to physician. *Objective laboratory tests provide necessary information to determine the extent of malnourishment.*
- Collaborate with dietitian to determine number of calories needed to provide adequate nutrition and realistic weight gain. Document intake, output, and calorie count. Weigh daily if condition warrants. *Weight loss or gain is important assessment information so that an appropriate plan of care can be developed.*
- Teach the importance of adequate nutrition by explaining the food guide pyramid and relating the physical effects of malnutrition on body systems. *Client may have inadequate knowledge of proper nutritional habits.*

Low Self-Esteem

- Spend time with client and convey an attitude of acceptance. Encourage client to accept responsibility for own behaviors and feelings. *An attitude of acceptance enhances self-worth.*
- Encourage client to focus on strengths and accomplishments rather than weaknesses and failures. *Minimize attention to negative ruminations.*
- Encourage participation in therapeutic group activities. Offer recognition and positive feedback for actual achievements. *Success and recognition increase self-esteem.*
- Teach assertiveness techniques and effective communication techniques such as the use of "I feel" rather than "You make me feel" statements. *Previous patterns of communication may have been aggressive and accusatory, causing barriers to interpersonal relationships.*

Deficient Knowledge

- Assess client's level of knowledge and readiness to learn the effects of drugs and alcohol on the body. *Baseline assessment is required to develop appropriate teaching material.*
- Develop teaching plan that includes measurable objectives. Include significant others, if possible. *Lifestyle changes often affect all family members.*
- Begin with simple concepts and progress to more complex issues. Use interactive teaching strategies and written materials appropriate to the client's educational level. Include information on physiological effects of substances, the propensity for physical and psychological dependence, and the risks to a fetus if the client is pregnant. *Active participation and handouts enhance retention of important concepts.*

Disturbed Sensory Perceptions

- Observe for withdrawal symptoms. Monitor vital signs. Provide adequate nutrition and hydration. Place on seizure precautions. *These actions provide supportive physical care during detoxification.*
- Assess level of orientation frequently. Orient and reassure client of safety in presence of hallucinations, delusions, or illusions. *Client may be frightened.*
- Explain all interventions before approaching client. Avoid loud noises and talk softly to client. Decrease external stimuli by dimming lights. *Excessive stimuli increase agitation.*
- Administer prn medications according to detoxification schedule. *Benzodiazepines help to minimize the discomfort of withdrawal symptoms.*

Disturbed Thought Processes

- Give positive reinforcement when thinking and behavior are appropriate or when client recognizes that delusions are not based in reality. *Drugs and alcohol can interfere with client's perception of reality.*
- Use simple, step-by-step instructions and face-to-face interaction when communicating with client. *Client may be confused or disoriented.*
- Express reasonable doubt if client relays suspicious or paranoid beliefs. Reinforce accurate perception of people or situations. *It is important to communicate that you do not share that false belief as reality.*
- Do not argue with delusions or hallucinations. Convey acceptance that the client believes a situation to be true, but that the nurse does not see or hear what is not there. *Arguing with the client or denying the belief serves no useful purpose, because delusions are not eliminated.*
- Talk to client about real events and real people. Respond to feelings and reassure client that he or she is safe from harm. *Discussions that focus on the delusions may aggravate the condition. Verbalization of feelings in a nonthreatening environment may help the client develop insight.*

Using NANDA, NIC, and NOC

Chart 12–1 shows links between NANDA, NIC, and NOC when caring for the client with a substance abuse problem.

CHART 12–1 NANDA, NIC, AND NOC LINKAGES

The Client with a Substance Abuse Problem

NURSING DIAGNOSES	NURSING INTERVENTIONS	NURSING OUTCOMES
• Risk for Injury	• Anger Control Assistance • Delusion Management • Environmental Management: Violence Prevention • Impulse Control Training • Referral	• Risk Control • Safety Behavior: Personal • Knowledge: Personal Safety
• Ineffective Denial	• Anxiety Reduction • Coping Enhancement • Counseling • Decision-Making Support	• Anxiety Control • Coping • Symptom Control Behavior
• Defensive Coping	• Self-Awareness Enhancement • Coping Enhancement • Patient Contracting • Counseling	• Self-Esteem • Coping • Risk Control: Alcohol Use, Drug Use, Tobacco Use
• Disturbed Thought Processes	• Behavior Management: Overactivity/Inattention • Delusion Management • Calming Technique • Surveillance: Safety	• Cognitive Orientation • Distorted Thought Control • Information Processing • Safety Behavior: Personal, Home Physical Environment
• Imbalanced Nutrition: Less Than Body Requirements	• Nutritional Counseling • Nutritional Monitoring • Weight Gain Assistance	• Nutritional Status
• Chronic Low Self-Esteem	• Self-Esteem Enhancement • Substance Use Prevention • Substance Use Treatment: Alcohol Withdrawal, Drug Withdrawal, Overdose • Support Group • Therapy Group	• Self-Esteem • Abuse Recovery
• Deficient Knowledge (Specify)	• Health Education • Teaching: Substance Abuse • Behavior Modification • Counseling • Support Group	• Substance Abuse Control

Note. Data from Nursing Outcomes Classification (NOC) by M. Johnson & M. Maas (Eds.), 1997, St. Louis: Mosby; Nursing Diagnoses: Definitions & Classification 2001–2002, by North American Nursing Diagnosis Association, 2001, Philadelphia: NANDA; Nursing Interventions Classification (NIC) by J. C. McCloskey and G. M. Bulechek (Eds.), 2000, St. Louis: Mosby. Reprinted by permission.

MediaLink | RECOVERY AND SUPPORT RESOURCES

Home Care

Teaching the client and family includes:

- The negative effects of substance abuse including physical and psychological complications of substance abuse.
- The signs of relapse and the importance of after care programs and self-help groups to prevent relapse. An acronym that can assist the client in recognizing behaviors that lead to relapse is HALT: **h**ungry, **a**ngry, **l**onely, and **t**ired. Stress the importance of adequate sleep and nutrition, healthy recreation activities, and a caring support system in managing stressful situations.
- Information about specific medications that help to reduce the craving for alcohol (naltrexone [ReVia]) and maintain abstinence (disulfiram [Antabuse]), including the potential side effects, possible drug interactions, and any special precautions to be taken (e.g., avoiding over-the-counter medications such as cough syrup that may have alcohol content).
- Stress management techniques such as progressive muscle relaxation, abdominal breathing techniques, imagery, meditation, and effective coping skills.

In addition, suggest the following resources:

- Self-help groups
- Employee assistance programs
- Individual, group, and/or family counseling
- Community rehabilitation programs
- National Alliance for the Mentally Ill

Nursing Care Plan
A Client Experiencing Withdrawal from Alcohol

George Russell, age 58, fell at home and broke his arm. His wife took him to the ER and an open reduction internal fixation (ORIF) of his right wrist was performed under general anesthetic in the operating room. He was admitted to the postoperative unit for observation following surgery because he required large amounts of anesthesia during the procedure.

Mr. Russell has a ruddy complexion and looks older than his stated age. He discloses that he was laid off from his factory job 2 years ago and has been working odd jobs until last week when he was hired by a local assembly plant. His father was a recovering alcoholic and his 30-year-old son has been treated for alcohol abuse in the past. Mr. Russell states that he knows alcoholism runs in the family, but he feels that he has his drinking under control. However, he cannot remember the events that led up to his fall and how he might have broken his arm.

ASSESSMENT

During the nursing assessment, Mr. Russell is hesitant to provide information and refuses to make eye contact. Prior to his operation, a BAL was drawn because the ER nurse detected alcohol on his breath. His BAL was 0.42 % which is 4 times the legal limit for intoxication in many states. His vital signs are within the upper limits of normal, but he is confused and disoriented with slurred speech and a slight tremor of the hands. He is 6 feet tall and weighs 140 pounds. His total albumin is 3.5 mg and he has elevated liver enzymes. His wife states that he rarely eats the meals she prepares because he is usually drinking and has no appetite for food.

DIAGNOSIS

- *Ineffective individual coping* related to possible hereditary factor and personal vulnerability

EXPECTED OUTCOMES

- Client will express his true feelings associated with using alcohol as a method of coping with stressful situations.
- Client will identify three adaptive coping mechanisms he can use as alternatives to alcohol in response to stress.

- Client will verbalize the negative effects of alcohol and agree to seek professional help with his drinking.

PLANNING AND IMPLEMENTATION

- Establish trusting relationship with client and spend time with him discussing his feelings, fears, and anxieties.
- Consult with a physician regarding a schedule for medications during detoxification and observe for signs of withdrawal syndrome.
- Explain the effects of alcohol abuse on the body and emphasize that prognosis is closely associated with abstinence.
- Teach a relaxation technique that is useful in the client's opinion.
- Provide information about self-help groups and, if receptive, a list of meeting times and phone numbers.

EVALUATION

Mr. Russell was discharged from the postoperative unit without complications. He successfully underwent detoxification and contacted the Employee Assistance Program (EAP) at his new place of employment. He was on medical leave while his arm completely healed and now attends Alcoholics Anonymous meetings 5 days a week. He reports that he enjoys taking long walks with his wife in the warm weather and that his appetite has returned. He has gained 10 pounds in the past 6 weeks and feels physically better than he has in many years.

Critical Thinking in the Nursing Process

1. Explain why it would be important to include questions about Mr. Russell's medication history and his use of other medications during the initial nursing assessment.
2. Mr. Russell asks you to explain the risks of taking disulfiram (Antabuse). What should you tell him?
3. Develop a care plan for Mr. Russell for the nursing diagnosis of *Alteration in nutrition: Less than body requirements*. Why is this necessary?

See Evaluating Your Response in Appendix C.

EXPLORE MediaLink

TEST YOURSELF

1. What is the minimum level of alcohol in the blood for an individual to be considered intoxicated in most states?

   a. 0.05%
   b. 0.10%
   c. 0.50%
   d. 1.00%

2. Which of the following questions is *most* appropriate when interviewing the client who is suspected of alcohol abuse problems?

   a. "Typically, how many days per week do you drink alcoholic beverages?"
   b. "Have you been drinking lately?"
   c. "You don't drink much alcohol, do you?"
   d. "Has your drinking caused a lot of problems between you and your spouse?"

3. What is the rationale behind ordering thiamine (vitamin B_1) for a person with a history of chronic alcoholism?

   a. To prevent acute pancreatitis
   b. To prevent cirrhosis of the liver
   c. To prevent hepatic encephalopathy
   d. To prevent Wernicke's encephalopathy

4. Which of the following substances present the highest medical danger during withdrawal?

   a. CNS stimulants and amphetamines
   b. Opiates and marijuana
   c. Alcohol and CNS depressants
   d. Amphetamines and hallucinogens

5. What is the rationale for prescribing naltrexone (Trexan, ReVia) for a person who suffers from substance abuse?

   a. To decrease the discomfort of withdrawal symptoms
   b. To decrease the pleasant, reinforcing effects of the drug
   c. To inhibit impulsive drinking
   d. To block the signs and symptoms of opioid withdrawal

See Test Yourself answers in Appendix C.

BIBLIOGRAPHY

Adams, W. L., & Cox, N. S. (1995). Epidemiology of problem drinking among elderly people. *International Journal of the Addictions, 30,* 1693–1716.

Adams, W. L., & Kinney, J. (1995). *The clinical manual of substance abuse.* St. Louis: Mosby.

American Psychiatric Association. (2000a). *Practice guidelines for the treatment of psychiatric disorders compendium 2000.* Washington, DC: APA.

_____ (2000b). *Diagnostic and statistical manual of mental disorders* (4th ed., text revision) (DSM-IV-TR). Washington, DC: APA.

Beresford, T. P, Blow, F. C., & Brower, K. J. (1990). Alcoholism in the elderly. *Comprehensive Therapeutics, 16,* 38–43.

Blixen, C. E., McDougall, G. J., & Suen, L. J. (1997). Dual diagnosis in elders discharged from a psychiatric hospital. *International Journal of Geriatric Psychiatry, 12*(3), 307–313.

Ewing, J. A. (1984). Detecting alcoholism: The CAGE questionnaire. *Journal of the American Medical Association, 252*(14), 1905–1907.

Henderson-Martin, B. (2000). No more surprises: Screening patients for alcohol abuse. *American Journal of Nursing, 100*(9), 26–32.

Johnson, M., & Maas, M. (Eds.). (1997). *Nursing outcomes classification (NOC).* St. Louis: Mosby.

Kutlenios, R.M. (1998). Genetics and alcoholism—implications for advance practice psychiatric/mental health nursing. *Archives of Psychiatric Nursing, 12*(3), 154.

Lehne, R. A. (2001). *Pharmacology for nursing care.* Philadelphia: W.B. Saunders.

McCloskey, J. C., & Bulechek, G. M. (Eds.). (2000). *Nursing interventions classification (NIC).* St. Louis: Mosby.

National Institute of Mental Health. (2001). *Mental disorders in America.* NIH Publication No. 01-4584. Bethesda, MD: NIMH. Available. http://www.nimh.nih.gov/publicat/numbers.cfm (accessed on 4/11/02).

North American Nursing Diagnosis Association. (2001). *Nursing diagnoses: Definitions & classification 2001–2002.* Philadelphia: NANDA.

Ondus, K. A., Hujer, M. E., Mann, A. E., & Mion, L. C. (1999). Substance abuse and the hospitalized elderly. *Orthopaedic Nursing, 18*(4), 27–36.

Pokorny, A. D., Miller, B. A., & Kaplan, H. B. (1972). The brief MAST: A shortened version of the Michigan Alcohol Screening Test. *American Journal of Psychiatry, 129*: 342–345.

Reneman, L., Booij, J., de Bruin, K., Reitsma, J. B., de Wolff, F. A., Gunning, W. B., den Heeten, G. J., & van den Brink, W. (2001). Effects of dose, sex, and long-term abstention from use on toxic effects of MDMA (ecstasy) on brain serotonin neurons. *Lancet, 358*(9296), 1864–1869.

Siqueira, L., Diab, M., Bodian, C., & Rolnitzky, L. (2001). The relationship of stress and coping methods to adolescent use. *Substance Abuse, 22*(3), 157–166.

Skinner, H. A. (1982). *Drug Abuse Screening Test (DAST)* (p. 363). Langford Lance, England: Elsevier Science Ltd.

Stuart, G. W., & Laraia, M. T. (2001). *Stuart & Sundeen's principles and practice of psychiatric nursing* (7th ed.). St. Louis: Mosby.

U.S. Department of Health and Human Services. (1999). *Mental health: A report of the surgeon general—Executive summary.* Rockville, MD: USDHHS, Substance Abuse and Mental Health Services Administration, Center for Mental Health Services, National Institutes of Health, National Institute of Mental Health. Available http://www.surgeongeneral.gov/Library/MentalHealth (accessed on 4/11/02).

_____ (2001). *The DASIS Report: Amphetamine treatment admission increase: 1993–1999.* Rockville, MD: USDHHS, Substance Abuse and Mental Health Services Administration, Center for Mental Health Services, National Institutes of Health, National Institute of Mental Health. Available http://www.samhsa.gov/oas/facts/speed.cfm (accessed on 4/23/02).

Varcarolis, E. (2002). *Foundations of psychiatric mental health nursing: A clinical approach* (4th ed). Philadelphia: W.B. Saunders.

Virgo, N., Bennett, G., Higgins, D., Bennett, L., & Thomas, P. (2001). The prevalence and characteristics of co-occurring serious mental illness (SMI) and substance abuse or dependence in the patients of Adult Mental Health and Addictions Services in eastern Dorset. *Journal of Mental Health, 10*(2), 175–188.

NUTRITION AND METABOLIC PATTERNS

Functional Health Patterns with Related Nursing Diagnoses

HEALTH PERCEPTION HEALTH MANAGEMENT
- Perceived health status
- Perceived health management
- Health care behaviors: health promotion and illness prevention activities, medical treatments, follow-up care

VALUE-BELIEF
- Values, goals, or beliefs (including spirituality) that guide choices or decisions
- Perceived conflicts in values, beliefs, or expectations that are health related

COPING-STRESS-TOLERANCE
- Capacity to resist challenges to self-integrity
- Methods of handling stress
- Support systems
- Perceived ability to control and manage situations

NUTRITIONAL-METABOLIC
- Daily consumption of food and fluids
- Favorite foods
- Use of dietary supplements
- Skin lesions and ability to heal
- Condition of the integument
- Weight, height, temperature

Part 2
Nutrition and Metabolic Patterns
NANDA Nursing Diagnoses
- Risk for Aspiration
- Risk for Imbalanced Body Temperature
- Impaired Dentition
- Feeding Self-Care Deficit
- Fluid Volume Deficit
- Fluid Volume Excess
- Risk for Deficient Fluid Volume
- Hyperthermia
- Hypothermia
- Risk for Infection
- Impaired Oral Mucous Membranes
- Nausea
- Imbalanced Nutrition: Less than Body Requirements
- Imbalanced Nutrition: More than Body Requirements
- Impaired Skin Integrity
- Risk for Impaired Skin Integrity
- Impaired Swallowing
- Ineffective Thermoregulation
- Impaired Tissue Integrity
- Risk For Trauma
- Adult Failure to Thrive

SEXUALITY-REPRODUCTIVE
- Satisfaction with sexuality or sexual relationships
- Reproductive pattern
- Female menstrual and perimeno-pausal history

ELIMINATION
- Patterns of bowel and urinary excretion
- Perceived regularity or irregularity of elimination
- Use of laxatives or routines
- Changes in time, modes, quality or quantity of excretions
- Use of devices for control

ROLE-RELATIONSHIP
- Perception of major roles, relationships, and responsibilities in current life situation
- Satisfaction with or disturbances in roles and relationships

ACTIVITY-EXERCISE
- Patterns of personally relevant exercise, activity, leisure, and recreation
- ADLs which require energy expenditure
- Factors that interfere with the desired pattern (e.g., illness or injury)

SELF-PERCEPTION–SELF-CONCEPT
- Attitudes about self
- Perceived abilities, worth, self-image, emotions
- Body posture and movement, eye contact, voice and speech patterns

SLEEP-REST
- Patterns of sleep and rest-/relaxation in a 24-hr period
- Perceptions of quality and quantity of sleep and rest
- Use of sleep aids and routines

COGNITIVE-PERCEPTUAL
- Adequacy of vision, hearing, taste, touch, smell
- Pain perception and management
- Language, judgment, memory, decisions

Reprinted from Nursing Diagnosis: Process and Application, 3rd ed., by M. Gordon, pp. 80–96, Copyright © 1994, with permission from Elsevier Science.

Assessing Clients with Integumentary Disorders

MediaLink

www.prenhall.com/lemone

Additional resources for this chapter can be found on the Student CD-ROM accompanying this textbook, and on the Companion Website at www.prenhall.com/lemone. Click on Chapter 13 to select the activities for this chapter.

CD-ROM
- Audio Glossary
- NCLEX Review

Animation
- Integumentary Repair

Companion Website
- More NCLEX Review
- Functional Health Pattern Assessment
- Case Study
  Assessing a Rash

LEARNING OUTCOMES

After completing this chapter, you will be able to:

- Review the anatomy and physiology of the skin, hair, and nails.

- Discuss factors that influence skin color.

- Identify specific topics for consideration during a health history interview of the client with problems involving the skin, hair, and nails.

- Describe techniques for assessing the skin, hair, and nails.

- Describe normal variations in assessment findings for the client with dark skin.

- Identify abnormal findings that may indicate impairment of the integumentary system.

The skin, the hair, and the nails make up the integumentary system. The skin provides an external covering for the body, separating the body's organs and tissues from the external environment. It is the largest organ of the body and has many functions, summarized in Table 13–1.

In addition, the integumentary system:

- Protects the body from injury from the external environment.
- Provides a barrier to the loss of body fluids and electrolytes.
- Maintains the integrity of the body surface through wound repair.
- Serves as a sense organ for touch, pressure, pain, and temperature.
- Provides a film over the body through the action of glandular secretions, which protects the body from bacterial and fungal invasion.
- Dissipates body heat through the evaporation of sweat.
- Participates in the production of vitamin D.
- Serves as an indicator of emotions and health or illness through color changes.

REVIEW OF ANATOMY AND PHYSIOLOGY

The Skin

The **skin** has a total surface area of 15 to 20 square feet and weighs about 9 pounds. It has been estimated that each square inch of skin contains 15 feet of blood vessels, 4 yards of nerves, 650 sweat glands, 100 oil glands, 1500 sensory receptors, and over 3 million cells that are constantly dying and being replaced. The skin is composed of two regions: the epidermis and the dermis (Figure 13–1 ■).

The Epidermis

The **epidermis,** which is the surface or outermost part of the skin, consists of epithelial cells. The epidermis has either four or five layers, depending on its location; there are five layers over the palms of the hands and the soles of the feet, and four layers over the rest of the body.

The stratum basale is the deepest layer of the epidermis. It contains melanocytes, cells that produce the pigment melanin, and keratinocytes, which produce keratin. **Melanin** forms a protective shield to protect the keratinocytes and the nerve endings in the dermis from the damaging effects of ultraviolet light. Melanocyte activity probably accounts for the difference in skin color in humans. **Keratin** is a fibrous, water-repellent protein that gives the epidermis its tough, protective quality. As keratinocytes mature, they move upward through the epidermal layers, eventually becoming dead cells at the surface of the skin. Millions of these cells are worn off by abrasion each day, but millions are simultaneously produced in the stratum basale. The next layer of the epidermis is the stratum spinosum. Several cells thick, this layer contains abundant Langerhans cells that arise from the bone marrow and migrate to the epidermis. Mitosis occurs at this layer, although not as abundantly as in the stratum basale.

The stratum granulosum is only two to three cells thick, and also contains Langerhans cells. The cells of the stratum granulosum contain a glycolipid that slows water loss across the epidermis. *Keratinization,* a thickening of the cells' plasma membranes, begins in the stratum granulosum. The stratum lucidum is present only in areas of thick skin. It is made up of flattened, dead keratinocytes.

The outermost layer of the epidermis, the stratum corneum, is also the thickest, making up about 75% of the epidermis's total thickness. It consists of about 20 to 30 sheets of dead cells filled with keratin fragments arranged in "shingles" that flake off as dry skin.

The Dermis

The **dermis** is the second, deeper layer of skin. Made of a flexible connective tissue, this layer is richly supplied with blood cells, nerve fibers, and lymphatic vessels. Most of the hair follicles, sebaceous glands, and sweat glands are located in the dermis. The dermis consists of a papillary and a reticular layer. The papillary layer contains ridges that indent the overlying epidermis. It also contains capillaries and receptors for pain and touch. The deeper, reticular layer contains blood vessels, sweat and sebaceous glands, deep pressure receptors, and dense bundles of collagen fibers. The regions between these

TABLE 13–1	Functions of the Skin and Its Appendages
Structure	**Functions**
Epidermis	Protects tissues from physical, chemical, and biologic damage.
	Prevents water loss and serves as a water-repellent layer.
	Stores melanin, which protects tissues from harmful effects of the ultraviolet radiation in sunlight.
	Converts cholesterol molecules to vitamin D when exposed to sunlight.
	Contains phagocytes, which prevent bacteria from penetrating the skin.
Dermis	Regulates body temperature by dilating and constricting capillaries.
	Transmits messages via nerve endings to the central nervous system.
Sebaceous (oil) glands	Secrete sebum, which lubricates skin and hair and plays a role in killing bacteria.
Eccrine sweat glands	Regulate body heat by excretion of perspiration.
Apocrine sweat glands	Unknown.
Hair	Cushions the scalp. Eyelashes and cilia protect the body from foreign particles. Provides insulation in cold weather.
Nails	Protect the fingers and toes, aid in grasping, and allow for various other activities, such as scratching the skin, picking up small items, peeling an orange, and so on.

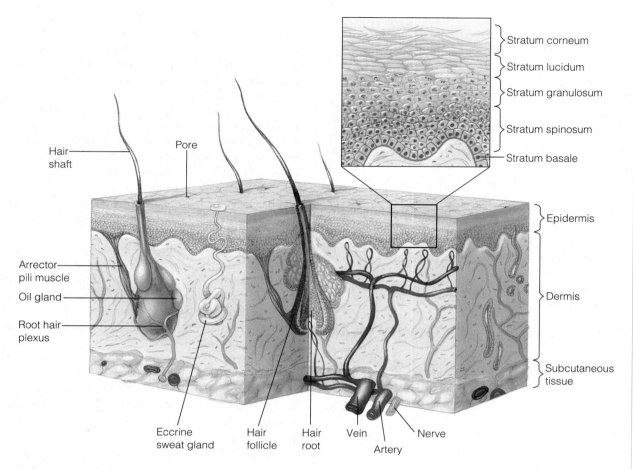

Figure 13–1 ■ Anatomy of the skin.

bundles form lines of cleavage in the skin. Surgical incisions parallel to these lines of cleavage heal more easily and with less scarring than incisions or traumatic wounds across cleavage lines.

Superficial Fascia

Underlying the skin is a layer of subcutaneous tissue called the **superficial fascia.** It consists primarily of adipose (fat) tissue, and helps the skin adhere to underlying structures.

Skin Color

The color of the skin is the result of varying levels of pigmentation. Melanin, a yellow-to-brown pigment, is darker and is produced in greater amounts in persons with dark skin color than in those with light skin. Exposure to the sun causes a buildup of melanin and a darkening or tanning of the skin in people with light skin. Carotene, a yellow-to-orange pigment, is found most in areas of the body where the stratum corneum is thickest, such as the palms of the hands. Carotene is more abundant in the skins of persons of Asian ancestry and, together with melanin, accounts for their golden skin tone. The epidermis in Caucasian skin has very little melanin and is almost transparent. Thus, the color of the hemoglobin found in red blood cells circulating through the dermis shows through, lending Caucasians a pinkish skin tone.

Skin color is influenced also by emotions and illnesses. **Erythema,** a reddening of the skin, may occur with embarrassment (blushing), fever, hypertension, or inflammation. It may also result from a drug reaction, sunburn, acne rosacea, or other factors. A bluish discoloration of the skin and mucous membranes, called **cyanosis,** results from poor oxygenation of hemoglobin. **Pallor,** or paleness of skin, may occur with shock, fear, or anger or in anemia and hypoxia. **Jaundice** is a yellow-to-orange color visible in the skin and mucous membranes; it is most often the result of a hepatic disorder.

Glands of the Skin

The skin contains sebaceous (oil) glands, sweat (sudoriferous) glands, and ceruminous glands. Each of these glands has a different function (see Table 13–1).

Sebaceous glands are found all over the body except on the palms and soles. These glands secrete an oily substance called sebum, which usually is ducted into a hair follicle. Sebum softens and lubricates the skin and hair and also decreases water loss from the skin in low humidity. Sebum also protects the body from infection by killing bacteria. The secretion of sebum is stimulated by hormones, especially androgens. If a sebaceous gland becomes blocked, a pimple or whitehead appears on the surface of the skin; as the material oxidizes and dries, it forms a blackhead. Acne vulgaris is an inflammation of the sebaceous glands.

There are two types of sweat glands: eccrine and apocrine. **Eccrine sweat glands** are more numerous on the forehead, palms, and soles. The gland itself is located in the dermis; the duct to the skin rises through the epidermis to open in a pore at the surface. **Sweat,** the secretion of the eccrine glands, is composed mostly of water but also contains sodium, antibodies, small amounts of metabolic wastes, lactic acid, and vitamin C. The production of sweat is regulated by the sympathetic nervous system and serves to maintain normal body temperature. Sweating also occurs in response to emotions. Most **apocrine sweat glands** are located in the axillary, anal, and genital areas. The secretions from apocrine glands are similar to those of sweat glands, but they also contain fatty acids and proteins. Their function is unknown.

Ceruminous glands are modified apocrine sweat glands. Located in the skin of the external ear canal, they secrete yellow-brown waxy cerumen. This substance provides a sticky trap for foreign materials.

The Hair

Hair is distributed all over the body, except the lips, nipples, parts of the external genitals, the palms of the hands, and the soles of the feet. Hair is produced by a hair bulb, and its root is enclosed in a hair follicle (Figure 13–2 ■). The exposed part, called the shaft, consists mainly of dead cells. Hair follicles extend into the dermis and in some places, such as the scalp, below the dermis. Many factors, including nutrition and hormones, influence hair growth.

Hair in various parts of the body has protective functions: The eyebrows and eyelashes protect the eyes; hair in the nose helps keep foreign materials out of the upper respiratory tract; and hair on the head protects the scalp from heat loss and sunlight. Table 13–1 summarizes the various functions of the hair.

The Nails

A **nail** is a modified scalelike epidermal structure. Like hair, nails consist mainly of dead cells. They arise from the stratum germinativum of the epidermis. The body of the nail rests on the nail bed (Figure 13–3 ■). The nail matrix is the active, growing part of the nail. The proximal visible end of the nail has a white crescent, called a lunula. The sides of the nail are overlapped by skin, called nail folds. The proximal nail fold is thickened and is called the eponychium or cuticle. Nails form a protective coating over the dorsum of each digit on the fingers and toes.

ASSESSING THE INTEGUMENTARY SYSTEM

The function of the integumentary system (skin, glands, hair, and nails) is assessed by both a health assessment interview to

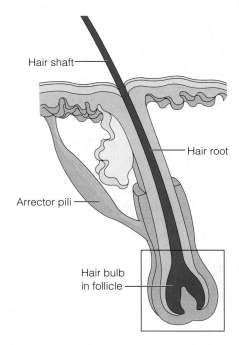

Figure 13–2 ■ Anatomy of a hair follicle.

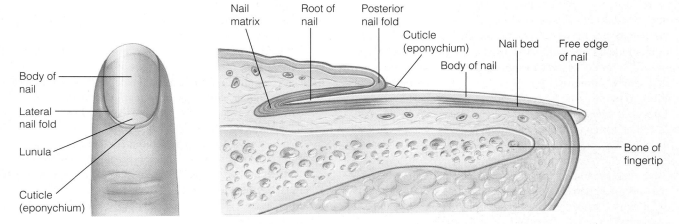

Figure 13–3 ■ Anatomy of a nail.

collect subjective data and a physical assessment to collect objective data.

The Health Assessment Interview

This section provides guidelines for collecting subjective data through a health assessment interview specific to the skin and its appendages. A health assessment interview to determine problems with the integumentary system may be conducted as part of a health screening or total health assessment, or it may focus on a chief complaint (such as itching or a rash). If the client has a skin problem, analyze its onset, characteristics and course, severity, precipitating and relieving factors, and any associated symptoms, noting the timing and circumstances. For example, ask the client:

- What type of itching have you experienced?
- When did you first notice a change in this mole?
- Did you change to any different kinds of shampoo or other hair products just before you started to lose your hair?

Ask about any change in health, rashes, itching, color changes, dryness or oiliness, growth of or changes in warts or moles, and the presence of lesions. Precipitating causes, such as medications, the use of new soaps, skin-care agents, cosmetics, pets, travel, stress, or dietary changes, must also be explored. In assessing hair problems, ask about any thinning or baldness, excessive hair loss, change in distribution of hair, use of hair-care products, diet, and dieting. When assessing nail problems, ask about nail splitting or breakage, discoloration, infection, diet, and exposure to chemicals.

The client's medical history is important. Questions focus on previous problems, allergies, and lesions. Skin problems may be manifestations of other disorders, such as cardiovascular disease, endocrine disorders, hepatic disease, and hematologic disorders. Occupational and social history may provide cues to skin problems; ask the client about travel, exposure to toxic substances at work, use of alcohol, and responses to stress.

Assess the presence of risk factors for skin cancer carefully. These include male gender; age over 50; family history of skin cancer; extended exposure to sunlight; tendency to sunburn; history of sunburn or other skin trauma; light-colored hair or eyes; residence in high altitudes or near the equator; and exposure to radiation, X-rays, coal, tar, or petroleum products.

Also explore the risk factors for malignant melanoma. These include a large number of moles, the presence of atypical moles, a family history of melanoma, prior melanoma, repeated severe sunburns, ease of freckling and sunburning, or inability to tan.

Interview questions categorized by functional health patterns can be found on the Companion Website.

Physical Assessment

Physical assessment of the skin, hair, and nails may be performed either as part of a total assessment or alone for clients with known or suspected problems. Conduct the physical examination of the skin, hair, and nails by inspection and pal-

pation. Assess the skin for color, presence of lesions (observable changes from normal skin structure), temperature, texture, moisture, turgor, and presence of edema. Characteristics of lesions to note include location and distribution, color, pattern, edges, size, elevation, and type of exudate (if present). Examine the hair for color, texture, quality, and scalp lesions. Determine the shape, color, contour, and condition of the nails.

The equipment necessary for assessment of the skin includes a ruler (to measure lesions), a flashlight (to illuminate lesions), and disposable rubber gloves to protect the examiner. Prior to the examination, collect all necessary equipment and explain techniques to the client to decrease anxiety.

The examination should be conducted in a warm, private room. The client removes all clothing and puts on a gown or drape. The areas to be examined should be fully exposed, but protect the client's modesty by keeping other areas covered. The client may be standing, sitting, or lying down at various times of the examination.

Integumentary Assessments with Abnormal Findings (✓)

- **Inspect skin color.**
  - ✓ Pallor and/or cyanosis are seen with exposure to cold and with decreased perfusion and oxygenation. In cyanotic dark-skinned clients, skin loses glow and appears ashen. Cyanosis may be more visible in the mucous membranes and nail beds of these clients.
  - ✓ In dark-skinned clients, jaundice may be most apparent in the sclera of the eyes.
  - ✓ Redness, swelling, and pain are seen with various rashes, inflammations, infections, and burns. First-degree burns cause areas of painful erythema and swelling. Red, painful blisters appear in second-degree burns, whereas white or blackened areas are common in third-degree burns.
  - ✓ **Vitiligo,** an abnormal loss of melanin in patches, typically occurs over the face, hands, or groin. Vitiligo is thought to be an autoimmune disorder.
- **Inspect the skin for lesions.** Primary, secondary, and vascular lesions are described and shown in Tables 13–2 through 13–4.
  - ✓ Pearly edged nodules with a central ulcer are seen in basal cell carcinoma.
  - ✓ Scaly, red, fast-growing papules are seen in squamous cell carcinoma.
  - ✓ Dark, asymmetric, multicolored patches (sometimes moles) with irregular edges appear in malignant melanoma.
  - ✓ Circular lesions are usually present in ringworm and in tinea versicolor.
  - ✓ Grouped vesicles may be seen in contact dermatitis.
  - ✓ Linear lesions appear in poison ivy and herpes zoster.
  - ✓ **Urticaria** (hives) appears as patches of pale, itchy wheals in an erythematous area.
  - ✓ In psoriasis, scaly red patches appear on the scalp, knees, back, and genitals.

✓ In herpes zoster, vesicles appear along sensory nerve paths, turn into pustules, and then crust over.

✓ Bruises are raised bluish or yellowish vascular lesions. Multiple bruises in various stages of healing suggest abuse.

- **Palpate skin temperature.**
  ✓ Skin is warm and red in inflammation and is generally warm with elevated body temperature.
  ✓ Decreased blood flow decreases the skin temperature; this may be generalized, as in shock, or localized, as in arteriosclerosis.

- **Palpate skin texture.**
  ✓ Changes in the texture of the skin may indicate irritation or trauma.
  ✓ The skin is soft and smooth in hyperthyroidism and coarse in hypothyroidism.

- **Palpate skin moisture.**
  ✓ Dry skin often is present in the elderly and clients with hypothyroidism.
  ✓ Oily skin is common in adolescents and young adults. Oily skin may be a normal finding, or it may accompany a skin disorder such as acne vulgaris.
  ✓ Excessive perspiration may be associated with shock, fever, increased activity, or anxiety.

- **Palpate skin turgor.**
  ✓ Pinch the client's skin gently over the collarbone. Tenting, in which the skin remains pinched for a few moments before resuming its normal position, is common in elderly clients who are thin (Figure 13–4 ■).
  ✓ Skin turgor is decreased in dehydration. It is increased in edema and scleroderma.

TABLE 13–2   Primary Skin Lesions

Macule, Patch	Flat, nonpalpable change in skin color. Macules are smaller than 1 cm, with a circumscribed border, and patches are larger than 1 cm and may have an irregular border. **Examples** Macules: freckles, measles, and petechiae. Patches: Mongolian spots, port-wine stains, vitiligo, and chloasma.	**Vesicle, Bulla**	Elevated, fluid-filled, round or oval shaped, palpable mass with thin, translucent walls and circumscribed borders. Vesicles are smaller than 0.5 cm; bullae are larger than 0.5 cm. **Examples** Vesicles: herpes simplex/ zoster, early chickenpox, poison ivy, and small burn blisters. Bullae: contact dermatitis, friction blisters, and large burn blisters.
Papule, Plaque	Elevated, solid, palpable mass with circumscribed border. Papules are smaller than 0.5 cm; plaques are groups of papules that form lesions larger than 0.5 cm. **Examples** Papules: elevated moles, warts, and lichen planus. Plaques: psoriasis, actinic keratosis, and also lichen planus.	**Wheal**	Elevated, often reddish area with irregular border caused by diffuse fluid in tissues rather than free fluid in a cavity, as in vesicles. Size varies. **Examples** Insect bites and hives (extensive wheals).
Nodule, Tumor	Elevated, solid, hard or soft palpable mass extending deeper into the dermis than a papule. Nodules have circumscribed borders and are 0.5 to 2 cm; tumors may have irregular borders and are larger than 2 cm. **Examples** Nodules: small lipoma, squamous cell carcinoma, fibroma, and intradermal nevi. Tumors: large lipoma, carcinoma, and hemangioma.	**Pustule**	Elevated, pus-filled vesicle or bulla with circumscribed border. Size varies. **Examples** Acne, impetigo, and carbuncles (large boils).
		Cyst	Elevated, encapsulated, fluid-filled or semisolid mass originating in the subcutaneous tissue or dermis, usually 1 cm or larger. **Examples** Varieties include sebaceous cysts and epidermoid cysts.

TABLE 13-3 Secondary Skin Lesions

Atrophy

A translucent, dry, paperlike, sometimes wrinkled skin surface resulting from thinning or wasting of the skin due to loss of collagen and elastin.

Examples Striae, aged skin.

Erosion

Wearing away of the superficial epidermis causing a moist, shallow depression. Because erosions do not extend into the dermis, they heal without scarring.

Examples Scratch marks, ruptured vesicles.

Lichenification

Rough, thickened, hardened area of epidermis resulting from chronic irritation such as scratching or rubbing.

Example Chronic dermatitis.

Scales

Shedding flakes of greasy, keratinized skin tissue. Color may be white, gray, or silver. Texture may vary from fine to thick.

Examples Dry skin, dandruff, psoriasis, and eczema.

Crust

Dry blood, serum, or pus left on the skin surface when vesicles or pustules burst. Can be red-brown, orange, or yellow. Large crusts that adhere to the skin surface are called scabs.

Examples Eczema, impetigo, herpes, or scabs following abrasion.

Ulcer

Deep, irregularly shaped area of skin loss extending into the dermis or subcutaneous tissue. May bleed. May leave scar.

Examples Decubitus ulcers (pressure sores), stasis ulcers, chancres.

Fissure

Linear crack with sharp edges, extending into the dermis.

Examples Cracks at the corners of the mouth or in the hands, athlete's foot.

Scar

Flat, irregular area of connective tissue left after a lesion or wound has healed. New scars may be red or purple; older scars may be silvery or white.

Examples Healed surgical wound or injury, healed acne.

Keloid

Elevated, irregular, darkened area of excess scar tissue caused by excessive collagen formation during healing. Extends beyond the site of the original injury. Higher incidence in people of African descent.

Examples Keloid from ear piercing or surgery.

TABLE 13-4 Vascular Skin Lesions

Port-Wine Stain

Source: Photo Researchers, Inc.

Flat, irregularly shaped lesion ranging in color from pale red to deep purple-red. Color deepens with exertion, emotional response, or exposure to extremes of temperature. It is present at birth and typically does not fade.

Cause A large, flat mass of blood vessels on the skin surface.

Localization/Distribution Most commonly appears on the face and head but may occur elsewhere.

Strawberry Mark

Source: NMSB/Custom Medical Stock Photo.

A bright red, raised lesion about 2 to 10 cm in diameter. It does not blanch with pressure. It is usually present at birth or within a few months of birth. Typically, it disappears by age 3. The lesion pictured here is located on the upper and lower lid of the left eye.

Cause A cluster of immature capillaries.

Localization/Distribution Can appear on any part of the body.

Spider Angioma

Source: Photo Researchers, Inc.

A flat, bright red dot with tiny radiating blood vessels ranging in size from a pinpoint to 2 cm. It blanches with pressure.

Cause A type of telangiectasis (vascular dilatation) caused by elevated estrogen levels, pregnancy, estrogen therapy, vitamin B deficiency, or liver disease, or may not be pathological.

Localization/Distribution Most commonly appear on the upper half of the body.

Venous Star

Source: Medichrome.

A flat blue lesion with radiating, cascading, or linear veins extending from the center. It ranges in size from 3 to 25 cm.

Cause A type of telangiectasis (vascular dilatation) caused by increased intravenous pressure in superficial veins.

Localization/Distribution Most commonly appear on the anterior chest and the lower legs near varicose veins.

Petechiae

Source: Custom Medical Stock.

Flat red or purple rounded "freckles" approximately 1 to 3 mm in diameter. Difficult to detect in dark skin. Do not blanch.

Cause Minute hemorrhages resulting from fragile capillaries, petechiae are caused by septicemias, liver disease, or vitamin C or K deficiency. They may also be caused by anticoagulant therapy.

Localization/Distribution Most commonly appear on the dependent surfaces of the body (e.g., back, buttocks). In the client with dark skin, look for them in the oral mucosa and conjunctivae.

(continued on page 358)

TABLE 13–4   Vascular Skin Lesions (continued)

Purpura

Flat, reddish blue, irregularly shaped extensive patches of varying size.

Cause Bleeding disorders, scurvy, and capillary fragility in the older adult (senile purpura).

Localization/Distribution May appear anywhere on the body, but are most noticeable on the legs, arms, and backs of hands.

Ecchymosis

Source: DeGrazia/Custom Medical Stock Photo.

A flat, irregularly shaped lesion of varying size with no pulsation. Does not blanch with pressure. In light skin, it begins as bluish purple mark that changes to greenish yellow. In brown skin, it varies from blue to deep purple. In black skin, it appears as a darkened area.

Cause Release of blood from superficial vessels into surrounding tissue due to trauma, hemophilia, liver disease, or deficiency of vitamin C or K.

Localization/Distribution Occurs anywhere on the body at the site of trauma or pressure.

Hematoma

Source: Science Photo/Custom Medical Stock.

A raised, irregularly shaped lesion similar to an ecchymosis except that it elevates the skin and looks like a swelling.

Cause A leakage of blood into the skin and subcutaneous tissue as a result of trauma or surgical incision.

Localization/Distribution May occur anywhere on the body at the site of trauma, pressure, or surgical incision.

Figure 13–4 ■ Tenting in an elderly client.

- **Assess for edema.**
  - ✓ Assess **edema** (accumulation of fluid in the body's tissues) by depressing the client's skin over the ankle (Figure 13–5 ■). Record findings as follows:

1+ Slight pitting, no obvious distortion
2+ Deeper pit, no obvious distortion
3+ Pit is obvious; extremities are swollen
4+ Pit remains with obvious distortion

- ✓ Edema is common in cardiovascular disorders, renal failure, and cirrhosis of the liver. It also may be a side effect of certain drugs.
- **Inspect distribution and quality of hair.**
  - ✓ A deviation in the normal hair distribution in the male or female genital area may indicate an endocrine disorder. **Hirsutism** (increased growth of coarse hair, usually on the face and trunk) is seen in Cushing's syndrome, acromegaly, and ovarian dysfunction. **Alopecia** (hair loss) may be related to changes in hormones, chemical or drug treatment, or radiation. In adult males whose hair loss follows the normal male pattern, the cause is usually genetic.

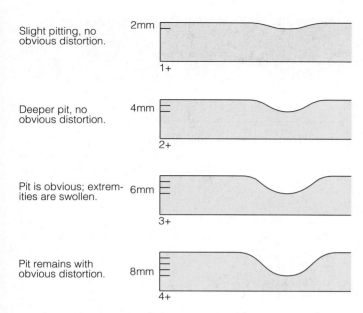

Slight pitting, no obvious distortion.

2mm

1+

Deeper pit, no obvious distortion.

4mm

2+

Pit is obvious; extremities are swollen.

6mm

3+

Pit remains with obvious distortion.

8mm

4+

Figure 13–5 ■ Degrees of pitting in edema.

- **Palpate hair texture.**
  - ✓ Some systemic diseases change the texture of the hair. For instance, hypothyroidism causes the hair to coarsen, whereas hyperthyroidism causes the hair to become fine.
- **Inspect the scalp for lesions.**
  - ✓ Mild dandruff is normal, but excessive, greasy flakes indicate seborrhea requiring treatment.
  - ✓ Hair loss, pustules, and scales appear on the scalp in tinea capitis (scalp ringworm).
  - ✓ Red, swollen pustules appear around infected hair follicles and are called furuncles.
  - ✓ Head lice may be seen as oval nits (eggs) adhering to the base of the hair shaft. Head lice are usually accompanied by itching.
- **Inspect nail curvature.**
  - ✓ Clubbing (Figure 13–6 ■), in which the angle of the nail base is greater than 180 degrees, is seen in respiratory disorders, cardiovascular disorders, cirrhosis of the liver, colitis, and thyroid disease. The nail becomes thick, hard, shiny, and curved at the free end.
- **Inspect the surface of the nails.**
  - ✓ The nail folds become inflamed and swollen and the nail loosens in paronychia, an infection of the nails.
  - ✓ Inflammation and transverse rippling of the nail is associated with chronic paronychia and/or eczema.

Flattened angle (180°)

Early clubbing

About 160°

Normal

Figure 13–6 ■ Assessing clubbing of the nails.

- ✓ The nail plate may separate from the nail bed in trauma, psoriasis, and Pseudomonas and Candida infections. This separation is called oncolysis.
- ✓ Nail grooves may be caused by inflammation, by planus, or by nail biting.
- ✓ Nail pitting may be seen with psoriasis.
- ✓ A transverse groove (Beau's line) may be seen in trachoma and/or acute diseases.
- ✓ Thin spoon-shaped nails (Figure 13–7 ■) may be seen in anemia.
- **Inspect nail color.**
  - ✓ The sudden appearance of a pigmented band may indicate melanoma. However, pigmented bands are normally found in over 90% of African Americans.
  - ✓ Yellowish nails are seen in psoriasis and fungal infections.
  - ✓ Dark nails occur with trauma, Candida infections, and hyperbilirubinemia.
  - ✓ Blackish-green nails are apparent in injury and in Pseudomonas infection.
  - ✓ Red splinter longitudinal hemorrhages may be seen in injury and/or psoriasis.
- **Inspect nail thickness.**
  - ✓ Trauma to the nails usually causes thickening. Other causes of thick nails include psoriasis, fungal infections, and decreased peripheral vascular blood supply.
  - ✓ Thinning of the nails is seen in nutritional deficiencies.

Figure 13–7 ■ Spoon-shaped nails.

EXPLORE MediaLink

NCLEX review questions, case studies, care plan activities, MediaLink applications, and other interactive resources for this chapter can be found on the Companion Website at www.prenhall.com/lemone.

Click on Chapter 13 to select the activities for this chapter. For animations, video clips, more NCLEX review questions, and an audio glossary, access the Student CD-ROM accompanying this textbook.

TEST YOURSELF

1. Which layer of the skin contains most of the hair follicles, sebaceous glands, and sweat glands?

   a. Epidermis
   b. Dermis
   c. Stratum basale
   d. Stratum spinosum

2. What pigment is responsible for skin tanning?

   a. Carotene
   b. Red blood cells
   c. Melanin
   d. Sebum

3. You are assessing the skin of an elderly client for dehydration. What finding would indicate this condition?

   a. Decreased turgor
   b. Increased moisture
   c. Presence of lesions
   d. Pallor

4. What part of the body would you palpate to assess edema?

   a. The scalp
   b. The fingers
   c. The clavicle
   d. The ankle

5. You note that your client with chronic dermatitis has rough, thickened areas of skin. You document these areas as:

   a. Ulcers
   b. Papules
   c. Atrophy
   d. Lichenification

See Test Yourself answers in Appendix C.

BIBLIOGRAPHY

Andresen, G. (1998). Assessing the older patient. *RN, 61*(3), 46–56.

Lawton, S. (2001). Assessing the patient with a skin condition. *Journal of Tissue Viability, 11*(3), 113–115.

McConnell, E. (1996). Assessing pruritus. *Nursing 96, 26*(12), 32.

Rupp, J., & Kaplan, D. (1999). Scratching the surface of pruritic disorders. *Consultant, 39*(11), 3161–3164, 3167.

Talbot, L., & Curtis, L. (1996). The challenge of assessing skin indicators in people of color. *Home Healthcare Nurse,14*(3), 167–173.

Weber, J., & Kelley, J. (2002). *Health assessment in nursing* (2nd ed). Philadelphia: Lippincott-Raven.

Wilson, S., & Giddens, J. (2001). *Health assessment for nursing practice* (2nd ed.). St. Louis: Mosby.

Young, T. (1997). Skin assessment and usual presentations. *Community Nurse, 3*(5), 33–36.

Nursing Care of Clients with Integumentary Disorders

MediaLink

www.prenhall.com/lemone
Additional resources for this chapter can be found on the Student CD-ROM accompanying this textbook, and on the Companion Website at www. prenhall.com/lemone. Click on Chapter 14 to select the activities for this chapter.

CD-ROM
• Audio Glossary
• NCLEX Review

Companion Website
• More NCLEX Review
• Case Study
  Lesions and Pruritis
• Care Plan Activity
  Pressure Ulcers

LEARNING OUTCOMES

After completing this chapter, you will be able to:

- Apply knowledge of normal anatomy, physiology, and assessments of the integument when providing nursing care for clients with disorders of the skin, hair, and nails (see Chapter 13).

- Describe the manifestations and nursing care of common skin problems and lesions.

- Compare and contrast the pathophysiology and collaborative care of clients with infections and infestations of the skin.

- Discuss the etiology, pathophysiology, and collaborative care of inflammatory disorders of the skin.

- Describe the pathophysiology and collaborative care of clients with malignant skin neoplasms.

- Explain the risk factors for, pathophysiology of, and nursing interventions to prevent and care for pressure ulcers.

- Discuss surgical options for excision of neoplasms, reconstruction of facial or body structures, and cosmetic procedures.

- Explain the pathophysiology of selected disorders of the hair and nails.

- Discuss nursing implications for pharmacologic agents used to treat disorders of the integument.

- Provide teaching appropriate for prevention and self-care of disorders of the integumentary system.

- Use the nursing process as a framework for providing individualized care to clients with disorders of the integument.

The skin and its accessory structures (the integumentary system) enclose the body, providing protection by serving as a barrier between the internal and external environments. The skin contains receptors for touch and sensation, helps regulate body temperature, and maintains fluid and electrolyte balance. The skin also provides cues to racial and ethnic background, and plays a major role in determining self-concept, roles, and relationships.

There are many disorders of the integument. The client with minor or benign disorders is usually treated in a health care provider's office or outpatient setting; but the client with disorders that involve large areas of the body, are chronic, or are malignant may require inpatient care. This chapter discusses disorders of the skin, hair, and nails; Chapter 15 discusses the client with burns. Primary and secondary skin lesions are described and illustrated in Tables 13–2 and 13–3. These terms are used throughout this and the next chapter.

COMMON SKIN PROBLEMS AND LESIONS

The disorders discussed in this section of the chapter are those experienced by a large number of people. Although they are considered minor health problems in terms of health care, they may cause major problems for the person experiencing a high level of discomfort and/or chronicity.

THE CLIENT WITH COMMON SKIN PROBLEMS AND LESIONS

PRURITUS

Pruritus is a subjective itching sensation producing an urge to scratch. Pruritus may occur in a small, circumscribed area, or it may involve a widespread area; it may or may not be associated with a rash. Pruritus is believed to result from either stimulation of itch receptors in the skin or as a response to the stimulation of skin receptors for pain and touch. The CNS interprets these stimuli as an itch through central summation (Porth, 2002).

Almost anything in the internal or external environment can cause pruritus. Insects, animals, plants, fabrics, metals, medications, allergies, and even emotional distress are among the most common causes. Pruritus also may occur as a secondary manifestation of systemic disorders, such as certain types of cancer, diabetes mellitus, hepatic disease, and renal failure. Although the exact physiology is unknown, it is known that heat and prostaglandins trigger pruritus and that histamine and morphine increase it.

The pathophysiologic response of pruritus to stimulation or irritation follows a similar pathway, regardless of cause. The irritating agent stimulates receptors in the junction between the epidermis and dermis, and may also trigger the release of histamine and other chemical mediators that either further stimulate or mediate the itch response. The response of the person experiencing the itch is to scratch or rub the affected area. This may irritate the skin and cause further inflammation, which in turn sets off a cycle of increasingly intense itching and scratching, called the *itch-scratch-itch cycle*.

Secondary effects of pruritus include skin excoriation, erythema (redness of the skin), wheals, changes in pigmentation, and infections. Persistent pruritus may interrupt sleep patterns,

because the itching sensation is often more intense at night. Long-term pruritus may be debilitating and increases the risk of infection as excoriation occurs.

Management of pruritus focuses on identifying and eliminating the cause and providing medications to relieve the itch. Antihistamines may relieve pruritus in some clients. Tranquilizers provide sedation, which may in turn relieve the emotional stress associated with pruritus; however, eliminating the stressors produces a more successful result. Systemic antibiotics are used to treat the infection resulting from the scratching and excoriation. Topical medications that contain corticosteroids are often used to relieve the pruritus and inflammation. Topical medications may also be administered through therapeutic baths or soaks with agents that relieve pruritus, such as cornstarch and baking soda or coal tar concentrates. Creams containing a topical anesthetic or antibiotic may also be used. Therapeutic baths are discussed in the Medication Administration box on page 363. Table 14–1 lists examples of topical agents used to treat skin disorders.

TABLE 14–1	Medications Used to Treat Skin Disorders	
Type	**Use**	**Examples**
Creams	Moisturize the skin	Aquacare Curel Nutraderm
Ointments	Lubricate the skin Retard water loss	Aquaphor Vaseline
Lotions	Moisturize the skin Lubricate the skin	Alpha-Keri Dermassage Lubriderm
Anesthetics	Relieve itching	Xylocaine
Antibiotics	Treat infection	Bacitracin Polysporin Gentamicin Silvadene
Corticosteroids	Suppress inflammation Relieve itching	Dexamethasone Hydrocortisone Clocortolone Desonide

Medication Administration

Therapeutic Baths

AGENTS USED IN THERAPEUTIC BATHS

Saline or tap water

Antibacterial agents: Potassium permanganate, acetic acid, hexachlorophene

Colloid substances: Oatmeal (Aveeno), cornstarch, sodium bicarbonate

Coal tar derivatives: Balnetar, Zetar, Polytar

Potassium permanganate

Emollients: Alpha-Keri, Lubath, mineral oil

Therapeutic baths have a variety of uses in treating skin disorders. Depending on the agent used, therapeutic baths soothe the skin, lower the skin bacteria count, clean and hydrate the skin, loosen scales, and relieve itching.

Nursing Responsibilities

- Ensure that the bath water is at a comfortable temperature that is neither too hot nor too cool (usually 110° to 115°F [45° to 46℃]).
- Fill the tub one-third to one-half full.

- Mix the agent well with the water.
- Assist the client into and out of the tub to prevent falls.
- Dry the client by blotting with the towel.

Client and Family Teaching

- Use a bath mat in the tub, the medications may cause the tub to become slippery.
- Keep the bathroom warm but adequately ventilated.
- Follow directions carefully for the amount of medication to use in the bath.
- Fill the bath one-third to one-half full of water that is at a comfortable temperature.
- Stay in the bath for 20 to 30 minutes, and immerse the areas to be treated.
- Do not get the bathwater in your eyes.
- Dry by blotting (not rubbing) with the towel.
- If the medications cause staining, use old towels or linens.
- If the itching is not relieved or the skin becomes excessively dry, call your health care provider.

DRY SKIN (XEROSIS)

Dry skin, also called **xerosis,** is most often a problem in the older adult (Figure 14–1 ■). Xerosis commonly results, especially in the older adult, from a decrease in the activity of sebaceous and sweat glands, which reduces the skin's lubrication and moisture retention. However, dry skin may occur at any age from exposure to environmental heat and low humidity, sunlight, excessive bathing, and a decreased intake of liquids.

Two types of severe dry skin are xeroderma and ichthyosis. **Xeroderma** is a chronic skin condition characterized by dry, rough skin. **Ichthyosis** is an inherited dermatological condition in which the skin is dry, fissured, and hyperkeratotic; the surface of the skin has the appearance of fish scales.

The primary manifestation of dry skin is pruritus. Other manifestations include visible flaking of surface skin and an observable pattern of fine lines over the area. If the skin has been excessively dry and pruritic for a long period, the client may have secondary skin lesions and *lichenification* (thickening).

NURSING CARE

Nursing care focuses on teaching the client and family how to reduce the dry skin and relieve the pruritus:

- Wash clothing in a mild detergent and rinse twice; do not use fabric softeners.
- Avoid using perfumes and lotions containing alcohol.
- Apply skin lubricants after a bath to help retain moisture.
- Soaps and hot water are drying. Clean the skin with tepid water and either a mild soap or cleansing creams. If soap is used, rinse it off carefully.
- It is not necessary to take a bath every day.
- If bath oils are used, add them to the bath water at the end of the bath (the moist skin is more likely to retain the oil). Use care not to slip in the tub.
- Use a humidifier to humidify the air.
- Apply creams and lotions when the skin is slightly damp after bathing.
- Increase fluid intake.
- Keep nails trimmed short, wear loose clothing, and keep the environment cool.
- A brief application of pressure or cold may relieve pruritus.
- Cotton gloves may be worn at night if scratching during sleep causes skin excoriation.
- Distraction or relaxation techniques may prove helpful.

Figure 14–1 ■ Severe xerosis, or dry skin, produces dry, rough skin with visible flaking of the skin surface.

Source: Camera M. D. Studios. Carroll H. Weiss, Director. 8290 N. W. 26th Place. Sunrise, FL 33322.

Medialink | www LESIONS AND PRURITIS CASE STUDY

BENIGN SKIN LESIONS

The skin is subject to many different types and kinds of benign skin lesions, including cysts, keloids, nevi, angiomas, skin tags, and keratoses. Although these benign lesions are often considered more of a nuisance than an illness, they do require monitoring for an increase in size that interferes with the skin's appearance or function.

Cysts

Cysts of the skin are benign closed sacs in or under the skin surface that are lined with epithelium and contain fluid or a semisolid material. Epidermal inclusion cysts and pilar cysts are the most common types.

Epidermal inclusion cysts may occur anywhere on the body but are most often found on the head and trunk. Although they are painless, they may grow so large that they become irritated by contact with clothing (e.g., if located on the back of the neck) or cause obstruction (e.g., if located on the nose). The cysts contain a semisolid material mainly of keratin. Pilar cysts are found on the scalp and originate from sebaceous glands. They are also painless. Both types of cysts rarely require treatment unless they become large and bothersome.

Keloids

Keloids are elevated, irregularly shaped, progressively enlarging scars. They arise from excessive amounts of collagen in the stratum corneum during scar formation in connective tissue repair. These lesions are more common in young adults and appear within 1 year of the initial trauma.

This abnormal response most often occurs in people of African and Asian descent who sustain burns of the skin, although, even seemingly minor trauma can result in keloid formation. There is a familial tendency to develop keloids. Other risk factors for keloid formation include excessive tension on a wound and poor alignment of skin edges following accidental or intentional skin trauma. Certain skin surfaces are also more likely to develop keloids: the chin, ears, shoulders, back, and lower legs.

The excessive scar formation is associated with increased metabolic activity of fibroplasts and increased type III collagen. The principal cells of the keloids are myofibroblasts, which have characteristics of both fibroblasts and smooth muscle cells. The swollen appearance of the keloids is the result of an excess of extracellular material.

The keloids first appear as red, firm, rubbery plaques that persist for several months after the initial trauma (Figure 14–2 ■). Uncontrolled overgrowth over time causes the keloids to extend beyond the original scar. Eventually, the keloid becomes smooth and hyperpigmented.

Nevi

Nevi, more commonly called *moles,* are flat or raised macules or papules with rounded, well-defined borders (Figure 14–3 ■). Nevi arise from melanocytes during early childhood, with the cells initially accumulating at the junction of the dermis and epidermis. Over time, the cluster of cells moves into the dermis, and the lesion becomes visible. Almost all adults have nevi.

Figure 14–2 ■ Keloids form from the deposit of excessive amounts of collagen during scar formation.

Source: Camera M. D. Studios. Carroll H. Weiss, Director. 8290 N. W. 26th Place. Sunrise, FL 33322.

Figure 14–3 ■ Nevi, more commonly called moles, arise from melanocytes and are common in all adults.

Source: Camera M. D. Studios. Carroll H. Weiss, Director. 8290 N. W. 26th Place. Sunrise, FL 33322.

Nevi range from flesh colored to black and occasionally contain hair. They can occur on any skin surface of the body and may arise as single lesions or in groups. Some pigmented nevi can transform into malignant lesions. Although the average adult has about 20 nevi, only 4 people out of 100,000 develop a malignant melanoma (Porth, 2002). However, it is important to monitor nevi for changes in size, thickness, color, bleeding, or itching. If any of these changes occur, the person should seek immediate professional assessment.

Angiomas

Angiomas, also called **hemangiomas,** are benign vascular tumors. They appear in the adult in different forms:

- Nevus flammeus (port-wine stain) is a congenital vascular lesion that involves the capillaries. The lesions tend to occur on the upper body or face as macular patches that range from light red to dark purple. These lesions are present at birth and grow proportionately with the child into adulthood.

- Cherry angiomas are small, rounded papules that may occur at any age, but they most commonly arise in the 40s and gradually increase in number. The lesions range in color from bright red to purple. These lesions are often found on the trunk.
- Spider angiomas are dilated superficial arteries. They are common in pregnant women and in clients with hepatic disease. Spider angiomas occur most often on the face, neck, and upper chest. The lesions are usually small, bright red papules with radiating lines.
- Telangiectases are single dilated capillaries or terminal arteries that appear often on the cheeks and nose. These lesions are most common in older adults and result from photoaged skin. The lesions look like broken veins.
- Venous lakes are small, flat, blue blood vessels. They are seen on the exposed skin of the older adult: the ears, lips, and backs of the hands.

Skin Tags

Skin tags are soft papules on a pedicle. They can be as small as a pinhead or as large as a pea and are most often found on the front or side of the neck and in the axillae, as well as in areas where clothing (such as underwear) rubs the skin. These lesions have normal skin color and texture.

Seborrheic Keratoses

A **keratosis** is any skin condition in which there is a benign overgrowth and thickening of the cornified epithelium. These lesions most often appear in adults after age 50. *Seborrheic keratoses* are lesions that appear as superficial flat, smooth, or warty-surfaced growths, 5 to 20 mm in diameter, most often on the face and trunk. The lesions may be tan, waxy yellow, dark brown, or flesh colored, and they often appear greasy. These lesions are most often seen in the older adult and do not appear to be related to damage from sun exposure.

COLLABORATIVE CARE

Most benign skin lesions do not require treatment, although excision or laser surgery may sometimes be necessary. Cysts may enlarge, skin tags may become irritated and bleed, nevi may change in appearance, or any of the lesions may cause discomfort with appearance.

THE CLIENT WITH PSORIASIS

Psoriasis is a chronic skin disorder characterized by raised, reddened, round circumscribed plaques covered by silvery white scales (Figure 14–4 ■). The size of these lesions varies. The lesions may appear anywhere on the body; but they are most commonly found on the scalp, extensor surfaces of the arms and legs, elbows, knees, sacrum, and around the nails.

Figure 14–4 ■ The characteristic lesions of psoriasis are raised, red, round plaques covered with thick, silvery scales.

Source: NMSB/Custom Medical Stock Photo.

The characteristic lesions in psoriasis are well-demarcated regions of erythematous plaques that shed thick gray flakes. As with any chronic illness, the skin manifestations may occur and disappear throughout life, with no discernible pattern to the recurrence.

PATHOPHYSIOLOGY

Psoriasis affects about 1% of the U.S. population. The incidence is lower in warm, sunny climates. Onset usually occurs in the 20s, but it may occur at any age. Psoriasis occurs more often in Caucasians, but men and women are affected equally.

Sunlight, stress, seasonal changes, hormone fluctuations, steroid withdrawal, and certain drugs (such as alcohol, corticosteroids, lithium, and chloroquine) appear to exacerbate the disorder. About one-third of clients have a family history of psoriasis. Trauma to the skin from such events as surgery, sunburn, or excoriation is also a common precipitating factor; lesions that result from trauma are called Koebner's reaction (Porth, 2002).

Normally, the keratinocyte (an epidermal cell making up 95% of the epidermis) migrates from the basal cell to the stratum corneum (the outer skin layer) in about 14 days and is sloughed off 14 days later. Psoriatic skin cells, by contrast, have a shorter cycle of growth, completing the journey to the stratum corneum in only 4 to 7 days, a condition called *hyperkeratosis*. These immature cells produce an abnormal keratin that forms thick, flaky scales at the surface of the skin. The increased cell metabolism stimulates increased vascularity, which contributes to the erythema of the lesions.

Psoriasis vulgaris is the most common form of psoriasis. The lesions can be found anywhere on the skin but most commonly involve the skin over the elbows, knees, and scalp. Initially, the lesions are papules that form into well-defined erythematous plaques with thick, silvery scales. The plaques in darker-skinned persons may appear purple.

Permanent remission of psoriasis is rare. The prognosis depends on the type, extent, and severity of the initial attack. The age of onset is also a factor; early-onset disease is usually more severe.

MANIFESTATIONS AND COMPLICATIONS

Pruritus is common over the psoriatic lesions. If the lesions are located in an intertriginous zone, such as between the toes, under the breasts, or in the perianal region, the psoriatic scales may soften, allowing painful fissures to form. When psoriasis affects the nails, pitting and a yellow or brown discoloration results. The nail may separate from the nail bed, thicken, and crumble. The involved nails, which are more often fingernails than toenails, are at high risk for infection.

COLLABORATIVE CARE

Treatment is based on the type of psoriasis, the extent and location of the lesions, the age of the client, and the degree of disfigurement or disability.

Diagnostic Tests

- *Skin biopsy* may be done if the client presents with atypical manifestations, or to differentiate psoriasis from other inflammatory or infectious skin disorders.
- *Ultrasonography* may be performed to measure skin thickness; results reveal typical psoriatic changes in the stratum corneum and dermal inflammation.

Medications

A variety of medications and treatments may be prescribed, including topical medications and photochemotherapy. Although there is no cure, treatment decreases the severity and pain of the lesions.

Topical medications are administered to decrease inflammation, prolong the maturity time of keratinocytes, and increase remission time. Corticosteroids, tar preparations, anthralin, and the retinoids are typically used. Box 14–1 outlines general guidelines for teaching clients to apply topical medications.

Topical corticosteroids decrease inflammation, suppress mitotic activity of psoriatic cells, and delay the movement of keratinocytes to the surface of the skin (thus giving them time to mature and decreasing hyperkeratinosis). Tazarotene gel, a topical retinoid, is useful in treating clients with mild to moderate cases. The most effective topical corticosteroids are potent preparations that are well absorbed through the skin and are used under an occlusive dressing. Corticosteroids may also be taken systemically or injected directly into the lesions.

Tar preparations (such as Estar, Psorigel, and Fototar) suppress mitotic activity and are also anti-inflammatory. Their exact mechanism of action is unknown, but they are effective in removing scales and increasing remission time. Preparations made of coal tar are messy, cause staining, and have an unpleasant odor, but they are an effective form of treatment.

Topical anthralin (dithranol) inhibits the mitotic activity of epidermal cells and is effective in some cases of chronic, localized psoriasis that do not respond to other topical agents. The medication is applied to the plaque patches at bedtime and left in place for 8 to 12 hours. Clients should be tested for sensitivity to the drug before use, and it should not be applied to inflamed or open areas of skin.

Calcipotriene (Dovonex) has been shown to be effective and safe in both the short-term and long-term treatment of psoriasis. It inhibits cell proliferation in the epidermis and facilitates cell differentiation. Although a derivative of topical vitamin D, calcipotriene does not seem to affect bone or calcium metabolism.

Treatments

Photochemotherapy

Photochemotherapy is the preferred treatment modality for severe psoriasis (Porth, 2002). A light-activated form of the drug methoxsalen is used. This drug is an antimetabolite that inhibits DNA synthesis and thereby prevents cell mitosis, decreasing hyperkeratosis. Exposure to ultraviolet-A (UVA) rays activates methoxsalen; it is administered orally, and the client is exposed to UVA 2 hours later. Treatments are administered 2 to 3 times a week; usually 10 to 20 total treatments are given over 1 to 2 months. The eyes are covered by dark glasses during the treatment. Treatment causes tanning, and direct sunlight must be avoided for

---

BOX 14–1 ■ General Guidelines for Applying Topical Medications

Each time a medication is applied, the skin surface must be clean and dry. Remove the medication from the previous application: Remove creams by washing the skin with tap water; remove ointments by washing the skin first with mineral oil and then with a mild soap and water.

- To apply gels, creams, and pastes: Squeeze about 1/2 to 1 inch of the gel or cream into the palm of the hand. Rub the hands together until they are covered. Apply gels and creams to the affected areas with long strokes until the skin is thinly covered. Differences from these general guidelines follow:
  a. Corticosteroids are usually applied two to three times a day in small amounts and rubbed directly onto the lesions. Apply the medication after a bath and cover with an occlusive dressing.
  b. Apply medications containing tar in the direction of hair growth. Do not apply these medications to the face, to the genitals, or in skinfolds. If the tar is water based or oil based, it will stain clothing.
  c. Wear gloves when applying anthralin stains.
- To apply lotions: Shake the bottle of lotion well. Pour a small amount into the palm of the hand, and pat the medication onto the skin. If the lotion is thin, apply it with a gauze pad.
- To apply sprays: Hold the container about 6 inches from the skin, and apply the medication in a short spray.
- To apply medicated shampoo: Rinse out medication from the previous application. Apply the shampoo, massage into the hair and over the scalp carefully, and allow it to remain for the prescribed time. Rinse.
- To apply pastes: Use enough paste on an applicator (such as a wooden tongue depressor) to cover the lesion thinly.

8 to 12 hours thereafter. If the client exhibits erythema, the treatments are stopped until the redness and swelling resolve.

Photochemotherapy has had a high success rate in achieving remission of psoriasis, but it can accelerate aging of exposed skin, induce cataract development, alter immune function, and increase the risk of melanoma.

Ultraviolet Light Therapy

Ultraviolet-B (UVB) light is often used to treat psoriasis. UVB light decreases the growth rate of epidermal cells, thereby decreasing hyperkeratosis. Mercury vapor lights or fluorescent UV tubes provide the UVB light; the latter are often arranged in a cabinet so the client can stand and expose psoriatic lesions more easily. These units may be purchased or constructed to be used in the client's home.

The light therapy is administered in gradually increasing exposure times, until the client experiences a mild erythema, like a mild sunburn. Treatments are given daily and are measured in seconds of exposure. The eyes are shielded during the treatment. The erythema response occurs in about 8 hours. Careful assessment is necessary to prevent more severe burning, which could exacerbate the psoriasis. In clients with extensive psoriasis, UVB treatments may be combined with tar preparations, which increase the photosensitivity of the skin.

NURSING CARE

The client with psoriasis requires nursing care to meet physical and psychologic responses to the illness. The nursing interventions discussed in this section focus on common problems of the client with psoriasis: risk for impaired skin integrity and body image disturbance.

Nursing Diagnoses and Interventions

Impaired Skin Integrity

Psoriatic lesions range from several scales to large, open areas. Typical psoriatic skin lesions increase the risk of infection, which can further compromise healing. In addition, certain treatments (e.g., the use of UVA or retinoids) may cause erythema or peeling of the skin, further altering skin integrity.

- Demonstrate methods to reduce injury to the skin when taking therapeutic baths or treatments:
  - Use warm, not hot, water.
  - Gently rub lesions with a soft washcloth, using a circular motion.
  - Dry the skin with a soft towel, using a blotting or patting motion.
  - Keep the skin lubricated at all times.

Hot water and dry skin increase pruritus, further stimulating the itch-scratch-itch cycle. Dry skin also worsens psoriasis. Washing or drying the skin with rough linens or pressure may excoriate the skin over the psoriatic lesions.

- Demonstrate application of topical medications:
  - Apply the medication as prescribed in a thin layer, using hands (gloved, if appropriate), wooden tongue depressors, or a gauze pad.
  - Avoid getting medications in the eyes, on mucous membranes, or in skinfolds.
  - Apply a covering (occlusive dressing) over the medicated areas as prescribed, especially when using corticosteroids. Usually, the covering is applied for only 12 hours, often during the evening and night hours. Choose some type of plastic wrap that covers the area well.

Applying a thin layer of medication more frequently is often more effective than applying a single thick layer of medication. The medications used to treat psoriasis may irritate the eyes and mucous membranes; when applied in skinfolds, they may also cause maceration (skin breakdown due to prolonged exposure to moisture). Topical corticosteroids are often covered with occlusive dressing to increase absorption and thus facilitate treatment. However, constant occlusion may increase the effects of the medications to undesired levels and also increases the risk for infections.

- Teach manifestations of infection and how to contact the health care provider if these occur: elevated temperature, increased swelling, redness, pain, increase in drainage, and any change in the color of the drainage. *The client with skin lesions is at high risk for infection, as the skin is the body's first line of defense.*

- Teach manifestations of the complications of treatment: excoriation, increased erythema, increased peeling, and blister formation. *The medications or treatments may damage cells through chemical burns or excessive exposure to ultraviolet light. Times and methods of treatment need to be adjusted if these manifestations occur.*

Disturbed Body Image

The obvious skin lesions that accompany psoriasis often cause clients to isolate themselves from social contacts, withdraw from normal roles and responsibilities, and feel helpless or powerless.

- Establish a trusting relationship by expressing acceptance of the client, both verbally and nonverbally. For example, touch the client during social communications, demonstrating that the lesions are not contagious or offensive. *One's body image is affected not only by self-perception but also by the responses of others. Nonjudgmental acceptance helps the client adapt to the change in body image. By touching the client during interactions, the nurse demonstrates that acceptance.*

- Encourage to verbalize feelings about self-perception in view of the chronic nature of psoriasis and to ask questions about the disease and treatment. *The client adapts to a changed body image through a process of recognition, acceptance, and resolution. Each person responds individually to disfigurement and loss.*

- Promote social interaction through family involvement in care, and referral to support groups of people with psoriasis or other chronic skin conditions. *Acceptance by others is critical to acceptance of self. Psoriasis treatment is lifelong, time consuming, and often unappealing. By becoming involved in care, the family communicates acceptance. Sharing experiences with others who have the same health problem is a source of strength in adjusting to a visible, chronic illness.*

Home Care

Client and family teaching focuses on treatments and skin care needs. The following topics should be addressed:

- The chronic nature of the disease, factors that may precipitate an exacerbation, and methods to reduce stress
- Interventions for pruritus and dry skin, and specific care for psoriasis:
  - Expose the skin to sunlight, but avoid sunburn.

- Avoid trauma to the skin (e.g., do not scrub off scales, and use only an electric razor).
- Avoid exposure to contagious illnesses such as influenza and colds.
- Discuss current medications with the health care provider. Certain drugs (such as indomethacin (Indocin), lithium, and beta-adrenergic blocking agents) are known to precipitate exacerbations of psoriasis.
- In addition, suggest the National Psoriasis Foundation as a resource.

INFECTIONS AND INFESTATIONS OF THE SKIN

The skin's resistance to infections and infestations is provided by protective mechanisms, including skin flora, sebum, and the immune response. Although the skin is normally resistant to infections and infestations, these disorders may occur as a result of a break in the skin surface, a virulent agent, and/or decreased resistance due to a compromised immune system. This section discusses skin disorders resulting from bacterial infections, fungal infections, parasitic infestations, and viral infections.

THE CLIENT WITH A BACTERIAL INFECTION OF THE SKIN

A number of bacteria normally inhabit the skin and do not cause an infection. However, when a break in the skin allows invasion by pathogenic bacteria, an infection, called a **pyoderma,** may occur. The most common bacterial infections are caused by gram-positive *Staphylococcus aureus* and beta-hemolytic streptococci.

Bacterial infections of the skin may be primary or secondary. Primary infections are caused by a single pathogen and arise from normal skin; secondary infections develop in traumatized or diseased skin.

Most bacterial infections are treated by a primary care provider, and the client remains at home for care. If the infection becomes more serious, however, inpatient care is required. In addition, nosocomial infections of wounds or open lesions in hospitalized clients are often the result of bacterial infections, especially by methicillin-resistant *Staphylococcus aureus (MRSA)*.

PATHOPHYSIOLOGY

Bacterial infections of the skin arise from the hair follicle, where bacteria can accumulate and grow and cause a localized infection. However, the bacteria also can invade deeper tissues and cause a systemic infection, a potentially life-threatening disorder. Various types of bacterial infections involve the skin, including folliculitis, furuncles, carbuncles, cellulitis, erysipelas, and impetigo.

Figure 14–5 ■ The lesions of folliculitis are pustules surrounded by areas of erythema.

Folliculitis

Folliculitis is a bacterial infection of the hair follicle, most commonly caused by *Staphylococcus aureus*. The infection begins at the follicle opening and extends down into the follicle. The bacteria release enzymes and chemical agents that cause an inflammation. The lesions appear as pustules surrounded by an area of erythema on the surface of the skin (Figure 14–5 ■). Folliculitis is found most often on the scalp and extremities. It is also often seen on the face of bearded men (called sycosis barbae), on the legs of women who shave, and on the eyelids (called a *stye*). Although folliculitis may appear without any apparent cause, contributing factors include poor hygiene, poor nutrition, prolonged skin moisture, and trauma to the skin.

Furuncles

Furuncles, often called boils, are also inflammations of the hair follicle. They often begin as folliculitis, but the infection spreads down the hair shaft, through the wall of the follicle, and into the dermis. The causative organism is commonly *Staphylococcus aureus*. A furuncle is initially a deep, firm, red, painful nodule from 1 to 5 cm in diameter (Figure 14–6 ■). After a few

Figure 14–6 ■ A furuncle (or boil) is a deep, firm, red, painful nodule.

Source: Camera M. D. Studios. Carroll H. Weiss, Director. 8290 N. W. 26th Place. Sunrise, FL 33322.

days, the nodule changes into a large, tender cystic nodule. The cysts may drain substantial amounts of purulent drainage.

One or more furuncles may occur on any part of the body that has hair. Contributing factors include poor hygiene, trauma to the skin, areas of excessive moisture (including perspiration), and systemic diseases such as diabetes mellitus and hematologic malignancies.

Carbuncles

A **carbuncle** is a group of infected hair follicles. The lesion begins as a firm mass located in the subcutaneous tissue and the lower dermis. This mass becomes swollen and painful and has multiple openings to the skin surface. Carbuncles are most frequently found on the back of the neck, the upper back, and the lateral thighs. In addition to the local manifestations, the client may experience chills, fever, and malaise. The contributing factors for carbuncles are the same as for furuncles. Both infections are more common in hot, humid climates.

Cellulitis

Cellulitis is a localized infection of the dermis and subcutaneous tissue. Cellulitis can occur following a wound or skin ulcer or as an extension of furuncles or carbuncles. The infection spreads as a result of a substance produced by the causative organism, called spreading factor (hyaluronidase). This factor breaks down the fibrin network and other barriers that normally localize the infection. The area of cellulitis is red, swollen, and painful (Figure 14–7 ■). In some cases, vesicles may form over the area of cellulitis. The client may also experience fever, chills, malaise, headache, and swollen lymph glands.

Erysipelas

Erysipelas is an infection of the skin most often caused by group A streptococci. Chills, fever, and malaise are prodromal symptoms, occurring from 4 hours to 20 days before the skin lesion appears. The initial infection appears as firm red spots

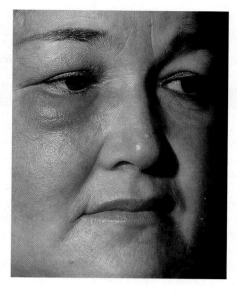

Figure 14–7 ■ Cellulitis is a bacterial infection localized in the dermis and subcutaneous tissue. The involved area is red, swollen, and painful.

Source: Camera M. D. Studios. Carroll H. Weiss, Director. 8290 N. W. 26th Place. Sunrise, FL 33322.

that enlarge and join to form a circumscribed, bright red, raised, hot lesion. Vesicles may form over the surface of the erysipelas lesion. The area usually is painful, itches, and burns. Erysipelas most commonly appears on the face, ears, and lower legs.

Impetigo

Impetigo is an infection of the skin caused by either *Staphylococcus aureus* or beta-hemolytic streptococci. Impetigo typically begins with a vesicle or pustule. This lesion ruptures, leaving an open area that discharges a honey-colored serous liquid that hardens into a crust (Figure 14–8 ■). Within

Figure 14–8 ■ Impetigo is characterized by red, macular lesions as well as broken, crusted vesicles.

Source: NMSB/Custom Medical Stock Photography.

hours, more vesicles form. The pruritus that accompanies the eruptions causes scratching and excoriation, which spreads the infection. This disease occasionally occurs in adults but is much more common in children.

COLLABORATIVE CARE

The diagnosis of a bacterial infection of the skin is made by assessing the appearance of the lesion and by identifying the causative organism. Antibiotics specific to the organism are used in treatment.

Diagnostic Tests

- Culture and sensitivity of the drainage from the lesion may be ordered to identify the organism and to target the most effective antibiotics.
- If the infection is systemic, a blood culture may be ordered to identify a causative organism.
- People who experience repeated bacterial skin infections, or who provide care for others who exhibit infections, may have a culture taken from the external nares to determine whether they are carriers of bacteria (e.g., MSRA) and are reinfecting themselves or others.

Medications

The primary treatment for bacterial infections of the skin is an antibiotic specific to the organism. The antibiotic is usually taken orally, and may also be applied topically. Multiple furuncles and carbuncles may be treated with cloxacillin (a penicillinase-resistant penicillin); the cephalosporins also are often effective.

NURSING CARE

Nursing care focuses on preventing the spread of infection and restoring normal skin integrity. Most clients provide self-care at home, but the incidence of secondary bacterial infections in the inpatient population is great enough to warrant their inclusion in planning and implementing care. Nursing interventions for inpatient and long-term care clients include the following:

- Practice good handwashing and teach its importance. Careful handwashing is one of the most effective methods to reduce the spread of infection both in and out of the hospital setting. Health care providers must wash their hands with soap and water before and after client care and between each client contact. All clients, family members, and visitors (both in the home and hospital setting) should be taught the importance of handwashing, but it is even more important for the client with a bacterial infection.
- Assess the client for any increase in infection, which may be manifested systemically by fever, tachycardia, chills, and malaise. Local manifestations of the spread of the infection include an increase in erythema, the size of the lesion, and drainage. This assessment is especially important for older, debilitated, or immunosuppressed clients, and for those who have large or dirty wounds.

- Place the client on isolation precautions to limit the spread of the organisms to other patients. All health care providers and visitors follow the procedures and protocols of the institution exactly to prevent cross-contamination.
- Cover draining lesions with a sterile dressing, and handle soiled dressings or linens according to standard precautions. When changing dressings, always wear disposable rubber gloves and masks.

Home Care

Client and family teaching focuses on facilitating tissue healing and eliminating the infection. Address the following topics:

- The importance of maintaining good nutrition
- The importance of maintaining cleanliness through careful handwashing and proper handling and disposal of dressings
- Preventing the spread of infection in the home by not sharing linens and towels and washing clothing and linens in hot water
- The importance of not squeezing or trying to open a bacterial lesion
- Avoiding the plucking of nasal hair or picking the nose
- The importance of taking the full course of prescribed antibiotics on a regular schedule until the prescribed supply is finished
- Bathing daily with an antibacterial soap (The client can gently wash off crusts during the bath. Warm compresses may be applied to the lesions two to three times a day to increase comfort and decrease swelling.)

THE CLIENT WITH A FUNGAL INFECTION

Fungi are free-living plantlike organisms that live in the soil, on animals, and on humans. The fungi that cause superficial skin infections are called **dermatophytes.** In humans, the dermatophytes live on keratin in the stratum corneum, hair, and nails. Fungal disorders are also called *mycoses.*

PATHOPHYSIOLOGY

Dermatophytoses (Tinea)

Superficial fungal infections of the skin are called **dermatophytoses** or, more commonly, *ringworm.* Fungal infections occur when a susceptible host comes in contact with the organism. The organism may be transmitted by direct contact with animals or other infected persons or by inanimate objects such as combs, pillowcases, towels, and hats. The most important factor in the development of the infection is moisture; the onset and spread of the fungal infection is greatest in areas where moisture content is high, such as within skinfolds, between the toes, and in the mouth. Other factors that increase the risk of a fungal infection include the use of broad-spectrum antibiotics that kill off normal flora and allow the fungi to grow, the presence of diabetes mellitus, immunodeficiencies, nutritional deficiencies, pregnancy, increasing age, and iron deficiency. Fungal infections of the skin are more common in

Figure 14–9 ■ Tinea pedis (athlete's foot) is a fungal infection that often occurs between the toes.

Source: Camera M. D. Studios. Carroll H. Weiss, Director. 8290 N.W. 26th Place. Sunrise, FL 33322.

Figure 14–11 ■ Tinea corporis commonly causes large, circular lesions with raised red borders.

Source: Custom Medical Stock, Inc.

warm, humid climates. The dermatophyte infections are named by the body part affected, as follows:

- **Tinea pedis** is a fungal infection of the soles of the feet, the space between the toes, and/or the toenail (Figure 14–9 ■). More often called *athlete's foot,* this is the most common tinea infection. The lesions vary from mild scaliness to painful fissures with drainage, and they are usually accompanied by pruritus and a foul odor. The infection is often chronic, reappearing in hot weather, when perspiring feet are encased in shoes.
- **Tinea capitis** is a fungal infection of the scalp. The primary lesions are gray, round, bald spots, often accompanied by erythema and crusting (Figure 14–10 ■). The hair loss is usually temporary. Tinea capitis is seen more often in children than in adults.

- **Tinea corporis** is a fungal infection of the body. It can be caused by several different fungi, and the lesions vary according to the causative organism. The most common lesions are large circular patches with raised red borders of vesicles, papules, or pustules (Figure 14–11 ■). Pruritus and erythema are also present.
- **Tinea versicolor** is a fungal infection of the upper chest, back, and sometimes the arms. The lesions are yellow, pink, or brown sheets of scaling skin. The patches do not have pigment and do not tan when exposed to ultraviolet light.
- **Tinea cruris** is a fungal infection of the groin that may extend to the inner thighs and buttocks (Figure 14–12 ■). Often called "jock itch," it is often associated with tinea pedis

Figure 14–10 ■ Tinea capitis is a fungal infection of the scalp that causes erythema, crusting, and hair loss.

Source: Camera M. D. Studios. Carroll H. Weiss, Director. 8290 N.W. 26th Place. Sunrise, FL 33322.

Figure 14–12 ■ Tinea cruris (jock itch) is a fungal infection of the groin and inner thighs.

Source: Camera M. D. Studios. Carroll H. Weiss, Director. 8290 N.W. 26th Place. Sunrise, FL 33322.

and is more common in people who are physically active, are obese, and/or wear tight underclothing.

Candidiasis

Candidiasis infections are caused by *Candida albicans*, a yeastlike fungus. This fungus is normally found on mucous membranes, on the skin, in the vagina, and in the gastrointestinal tract. The fungus becomes a pathogen when the following factors encourage its growth:

- A local environment of moisture, warmth, or altered skin integrity
- The administration of systemic antibiotics
- Pregnancy
- The use of birth control pills
- Poor nutrition
- The presence of diabetes mellitus, Cushing's disease, or other chronic debilitating illnesses
- Immunosuppression
- Some malignancies of the blood

Candidiasis affects the outer layers of the skin and mucous membranes of the mouth, vagina, uncircumcised penis, nails, and deep skinfolds. The first sign of infection is a pustule that extends under the stratum corneum. The pustule has an inflamed base and often burns and itches. As the infection spreads, the accumulation of inflammatory cells and shedding of surface cells produce a white to yellow curdlike substance that covers the infected area (Figure 14–13 ■). Satellite lesions (maculopapular areas found outside the clearly demarcated border of the original infection) are characteristic of candidiasis. The appearance of the infection differs by location, as summarized in Table 14–2.

Figure 14–13 ■ *Candida albicans,* a fungus, causes a skin infection characterized by erythema, pustules, and a typical white substance covering the area.

Source: Camera M. D. Studios. Carroll H. Weiss, Director. 8290 N.W. 26th Place. Sunrise, FL 33322.

TABLE 14–2	Characteristics of Candidiasis Infections by Location
Location	**Characteristics**
Skinfolds (under breasts, in groin, axillae, anus, umbilicus, and between toes or fingers)	Erythematous lesions that are either dry or moist. The lesions have clear borders, and satellite lesions are present.
Nails	Nail bed is red, swollen, and painful.
Mouth (thrush)	Mucous membranes are red and may be swollen; surface is covered with white, creamy material. Eroded areas may be present over the tongue and the oral cavity.
Penis (balanitis) (glans and shaft)	The penis is covered with small, red, clearly demarcated lesions that are painful and itch. The lesions may be covered with a white plaque.
Vagina	Red mucous membranes contain brighter red, demarcated, oozing lesions. The cervix may be covered with white plaque. A white, cheesy, foul-smelling vaginal discharge is present, accompanied by itching and burning. The vaginal and labial membranes may be swollen; the infection may extend to the anus and groin.

COLLABORATIVE CARE

Fungal infections are primarily diagnosed in outpatient settings and treated at home, but may also occur in hospitalized clients. The treatment is the same, regardless of the setting.

Diagnostic Tests

Diagnostic tests are conducted to determine the causative fungi and may include:

- Cultures of skin scrapings, nail scrapings, or hairs.
- Microscopic examination of scrapings from the lesions. The scrapings are prepared in a solution of 10% potassium hydroxide (KOH) to reveal more clearly the spores and filaments (hyphae) of each fungus.
- Observation of the skin under ultraviolet light (called a Wood's lamp). The fungal spores fluoresce blue-green.

Medications

Fungal infections of the skin are treated by topical or systemic antifungal medications. Nursing implications for the antifungal medications are described in the Medication Administration box on page 373.

Medication Administration

Treating Fungus Infections

ANTIFUNGAL AGENTS

Examples:

Butenafine (Mentax)
Clotrimazole (Mycelex)
Nystatin (Mycostatin, Nilstat)
Econazole (Spectazole)
Oxiconazole (Oxistat)
Miconazole (Monistat)

Undecylenic acid (Desenex)
Ketoconazole (Nizoral)
Fluconazole (Diflucan)
Amphotericin B (Fungizone)
Griseofulvin (Fulvicin)

Antifungal medications are prepared in a variety of forms, depending on the specific drug: powders, creams, shampoos, suspensions, troches, vaginal suppositories, and oral tablets. Some drugs interfere with the permeability of the fungal cell membrane; others interfere with DNA synthesis. Most of these medications are fungistatic but in large doses they may be fungicidal.

Nursing Responsibilities

- When taking the health history, ask about known hypersensitivity reactions to these agents; document carefully.
- Assess for side effects: skin rash, local irritation, gastrointestinal symptoms (if given PO), and mental status.
- Administer ketoconazole with food to minimize gastrointestinal irritation.
- Shake suspensions well before administration, and ask the client to swish them around the mouth before swallowing.
- Tell the client to allow oral tablets to dissolve in the mouth.

Client and Family Teaching

- Therapy usually continues over a long period of time, but regular use of medications for the recommended period is necessary. Do not miss doses, and complete the full treatment.
- For griseofulvin: Take with meals or foods high in fat (such as ice cream) to avoid stomach upset and help with absorption. Avoid alcohol (which may cause rapid pulse and flushing) and exposure to sunlight (this drug causes increased sensitivity).
- For nystatin: Dissolve lozenges completely in the mouth. Hold suspensions in the mouth and swish throughout the mouth as long as possible before swallowing. Insert intravaginal medication high in the vagina. Continue with intravaginal applications throughout the menses.
- For antifungal shampoo: Use two times a week for 4 weeks, allowing at least 3 days between each shampoo. Wet hair, apply shampoo to produce lather, leave in place for 1 minute, then rinse. Apply shampoo a second time, lather, leave in place for 3 minutes, then rinse thoroughly.
- For topical application: Rub well into the affected areas, but do not get the medication in your eyes.
- For vaginal candidiasis infections: During therapy, refrain from sexual intercourse or advise partner to use a condom.
- Your sexual partner will need to be treated at the same time so that you do not pass the infection back and forth to each other.

- Tinea capitis is treated by shampooing the hair two to three times a week, applying a topical antifungal to inactivate organisms on the hair, and taking griseofulvin (Fulvicin), an antifungal agent, orally.
- Tinea pedis is treated by soaking the feet in Burrow's solution, potassium permanganate solution, or saline solution to remove crusts and scales. Topical antifungals are applied to the infected areas for several weeks.
- Mild cases of tinea cruris are treated with topical medications for 3 to 4 weeks. More severe cases may require oral griseofulvin.

Candidiasis infections are treated, depending on the location, with oral medication or with powder or vaginal suppositories. Nystatin (Mycostatin) is an antibiotic effective in controlling the infection. Fluconazole (Diflucan), an oral antifungal agent, is also effective.

NURSING CARE

Many people treat themselves with over-the-counter antifungal medications. It is recommended, however, that the person be professionally diagnosed the first time the infection occurs. If symptoms reappear, self-treatment is usually satisfactory. The interventions discussed for nursing care of the client with a bacterial infection are also appropriate for the client with a fun-

gal infection. Teaching topics specific to fungal infections are as follows:

- Fungal diseases are contagious. Do not share linens or personal items with others.
- Use a clean towel and washcloth each day.
- Carefully dry all skinfolds, including those under the breasts, under the arms, and between the toes.
- Wear clean cotton underclothing each day.
- Fungi grow in moist environments, such as on sweaty feet. To prevent further infections:
  - Do not wear the same pair of shoes every day.
  - Wear socks that permit moisture to wick away from the skin surface.
  - Do not wear rubber- or plastic-soled shoes.
  - Use talcum powder or an over-the-counter antifungal powder twice a day.
- For vaginal *Candida albicans* infection:
  - Avoid tight clothing, such as jeans and pantyhose.
  - Wear cotton or cotton-crotch underwear.
  - Bathe more frequently, and dry the genital area well.
  - Have your sexual partner treated at the same time to avoid passing the infection back and forth to each other.

PRACTICE ALERT   *Recommend the client have a blood glucose test for repeated infections, as they may indicate diabetes mellitus.* ■

THE CLIENT WITH A PARASITIC INFESTATION

Infestations of the skin by parasites are more common in developing countries but may occur in any geographic area of the world. They affect people of all social classes but are associated with crowded or unsanitary living conditions.

PATHOPHYSIOLOGY

Two of the more common parasitic infestations of the skin are caused by lice and mites. These parasites do not normally live on the skin, but infest the skin through contact with an infested person or contact with clothing, linens, or objects infested with the parasites.

Pediculosis

Pediculosis is an infestation with lice. Lice are parasites that live on the blood of an animal or human host. The louse is a 2- to 4-mm oval organism with a stylet that pierces the skin; an anticoagulant in its saliva prevents host blood from clotting while it eats. The female louse lays its eggs (small pearl-gray or brown eggs, called nits) on hair shafts. The louse within the egg hatches, reaches the adult reproductive stage, and dies in 30 to 50 days (Porth, 2002).

There are three types of human pediculosis:

- **Pediculosis corporis** is an infestation with body lice. This type of infestation is more common in people who do not have access to facilities for bathing or washing clothes, such as the homeless. The lice live in clothing fibers and are transmitted primarily by contact with infested clothing and bed linens. The skin lesions occur at the site of a louse bite; macules appear initially, followed by wheals and papules. Pruritus is common, and scratching often results in linear excoriations. Secondary infections cause hyperpigmentation and scarring. The lesions are most often seen on the shoulders, trunk, and buttocks.
- **Pediculosis pubis** is an infestation with pubic lice (often called crabs). This infestation is spread through sexual activity with someone already infested or by contact with infested clothing or linens. The lice are found in the pubic region and occasionally spread to the axillae or men's beards. The lice cause skin irritation and intense itching.
- **Pediculosis capitis** is an infestation with head lice. This infestation primarily affects Caucasians and is more common in female children. The lice are most often found behind the ears and at the nape of the neck but may also spread to other hairy areas of the body: the eyebrows, pubic area, or beard. The lice are transmitted by contact with an infected person. Manifestations of head lice include pruritus, scratching, and erythema of the scalp. If untreated, the hair appears matted and crusted with a foul-smelling substance.

Scabies

Scabies is a parasitic infestation caused by a mite (Sarcoptes scabiei). The pregnant female mite burrows into the skin and lays two to three eggs each day for about a month. The eggs hatch in 3 to 5 days, and the larvae migrate to the surface of the skin but burrow into the skin for food or protection. The larvae develop, and the cycle repeats. Scabies infestation affects people of all socioeconomic classes. Formerly it was seen most often in times of war or famine, but it has become more common as a result of international travel and sexual activity. The infestation is found in webs between the fingers, the inner surfaces of the wrist and elbow, the axillae, the female nipple, the penis, the belt line, and the gluteal crease. The lesions are a small red-brown burrow, about 2 mm in length, sometimes covered with vesicles, which appears as a rash. Pruritus in response to the mite or its feces is common, especially at night, and excoriations may develop. The excoriations predispose the person to secondary bacterial infections.

COLLABORATIVE CARE

Parasitic infestations are diagnosed by identifying the organism and are treated with medications that kill the lice or mites.

Diagnostic Tests

- When a client exhibits manifestations of pediculosis, the hair shaft and the clothing are examined to identify the lice or the nits. Microscopic examination of the parasite provides a positive diagnosis.
- Scabies is diagnosed by skin scrapings and microscopic examination for the mites or their feces.

Medications

Lice are eradicated with agents that kill the parasite. Infestations of the body and pubic area are treated with topical medications that contain gamma benzene hexachloride, malathion (Prioderm lotion), or permethrin (NIX).

Infestations of the head are treated with shampoos containing lindane, such as Kwell. The shampoo is applied to dry hair and massaged in. A small amount of water is added to produce a lather, and the head is scrubbed for 4 minutes, then rinsed. The treatment may need to be repeated in a week to kill newly hatched lice. A fine-toothed comb can be used to comb the dead nits off the hair shaft. Infestations of the eyebrows are treated by applying a thick covering of petroleum jelly for several days.

Scabies may be eradicated by a single treatment of lindane lotion or Kwell applied to the entire skin surface for 12 hours.

The associated itching is treated with systemic or topical medications, including corticosteroids. Secondary bacterial infections are treated with the appropriate antibiotic.

NURSING CARE

Nursing care for clients with a parasite infestation most often focuses on teaching to prevent infestation or to eradicate an existing infestation. For a hospitalized client with pediculosis, isolation procedures are instituted until the client no longer has the infestation.

Client and family teaching is necessary to facilitate treatment at home, to prevent the spread of the infestation, and to dispel the myth that lice infest only people with poor hygiene or in dirty living conditions. Specific information includes the following:

- Wash clothing and linens in soap and hot water, or have them dry cleaned.
- Ironing the clothes kills any lice eggs.
- Personal care items, such as combs or brushes, may be boiled to kill the parasites.
- All family members and sexual partners must also be treated.
- Avoid using the combs, brushes, or hats of others.
- Lice and mites may infest anyone.

THE CLIENT WITH A VIRAL INFECTION OF THE SKIN

Viruses are pathogens that consist of an RNA or DNA core surrounded by a protein coat. They depend on live cells for reproduction and so are classified as intracellular pathogens. The viruses that cause skin lesions invade the keratinocyte, reproduce, and either increase cellular growth or cause cellular death.

An increase in the incidence of viral skin disorders has been attributed to a variety of causes. Some commonly used drugs, such as birth control medications and corticosteroids, are known to have immunosuppressive properties that allow the viruses to multiply. Other drugs, such as antibiotics, kill off normal skin bacteria that would otherwise serve as defense against viral infections.

PATHOPHYSIOLOGY

Viral infections cause many different kinds of skin disorders, including warts, herpes simplex infections, and herpes zoster infections.

Warts

Warts, or ***verrucae,*** are lesions of the skin caused by the human papillomavirus (HPV). Over 60 types of HPVs are found on the human skin and mucous membranes (Porth, 2002). Warts may be found on nongenital skin or genital skin and mucous membranes. Nongenital warts are benign lesions; genital warts may be precancerous. Warts are transmitted through skin contact. Wart lesions may be flat, fusiform (tapered at both ends), or round, but most are round and raised and have a rough, gray surface. There are many different types of warts; location and appearance of the warts depend on the causative virus. Those most common are as follows:

- A common wart (*verruca vulgaris*) may appear anywhere on the skin and mucous membranes of the body; most commonly appear on the fingers. Common warts grow above the skin surface and may be dome-shaped with ragged borders (Figure 14–14 ■).
- *Plantar warts* occur at pressure points on the soles of the feet. The pressure of shoes and walking prevents these warts

Figure 14–14 ■ The common wart is a lesion of the skin caused by a virus. It commonly appears as a raised, dome-shaped lesion.

Source: Camera M. D. Studios. Carroll H. Weiss, Director. 8290 N. W. 26th Place. Sunrise, FL 33322.

from growing outward, so they tend to extend deeper beneath the skin surface than do common warts. Plantar warts are often painful.
- A flat wart (*verruca plana*) is a small flat lesion, usually seen on the forehead or dorsum of the hand.
- *Condylomata acuminata,* also called venereal warts, occur in moist areas, along the glans of the penis, in the anal region, and on the vulva. They are usually cauliflowerlike in appearance and have a pink or purple color.

Warts resolve spontaneously when immunity to the virus develops. This response may take up to 5 years.

Herpes Simplex

Herpes simplex (also called a **fever blister** or **cold sore**) virus infections of the skin and mucous membranes are caused by two types of herpesvirus: HSV I and HSV II. Most infections above the waist are caused by HSV I, with herpes simplex lesions most often found on the lips, face, and mouth. (Genital herpes infections, which result from either HSV I or HSV II, are classified as sexually transmitted diseases and are discussed in Chapter 49.) ⊙ The virus may be transmitted by physical contact, oral sex, or kissing.

The infection begins with a burning or tingling sensation, followed by the development of erythema, vesicle formation, and pain (Figure 14–15 ■). The vesicles progress through pustules, ulcers, and crusting until healing occurs in 10 to 14 days.

The initial infection is often severe and accompanied by systemic manifestations, such as fever and sore throat; recurrences are more localized and less severe. The virus lives in nerve ganglia and may cause recurrent lesions in response to sunlight, menstruation, injury, or stress. Oral acyclovir may be used prophylactically to prevent reoccurrences and to treat recurrent outbreaks.

Figure 14–15 ■ Herpes simplex is a viral infection of the skin and mucous membranes. This client has lesions in the early stage, with erythema and vesicles.

Source: Camera M. D. Studios. Carroll H. Weiss, Director. 8290 N. W. 26th Place. Sunrise, FL 33322.

Figure 14–16 ■ Herpes zoster is a viral infection of a dermatome section of the skin. The typical lesions are painful vesicles lying along the path of the nerve.

Source: Custom Medical Stock, Inc.

Herpes Zoster

Herpes zoster, also called **shingles,** is a viral infection of a dermatome section of the skin caused by varicella zoster (the herpesvirus that also causes chickenpox). The infection is believed to result from reactivation of a varicella virus remaining in the sensory dorsal ganglia after a childhood infection of chickenpox. When reactivated, the virus travels from the ganglia to the corresponding skin dermatome area.

Herpes zoster affects an estimated 10% to 20% of the population, most often adults over the age of 50. Clients with Hodgkin's disease, certain types of leukemia, and lymphomas are more susceptible to an outbreak of the disease. Herpes zoster is more prevalent in immunocompromised people, such as those with HIV infections, those receiving radiation therapy or chemotherapy, and those who have had major organ transplants. The appearance of the lesions in people with HIV infections may be one of the first manifestations of immune compromise.

MANIFESTATIONS AND COMPLICATIONS

Herpes zoster lesions are vesicles with an erythematous base. The vesicles appear on the skin area supplied by the neurons of a single or associated group of dorsal root ganglia (although they may occur beyond this area in immunosuppressed people). The lesions usually appear unilaterally on the face, trunk, and thorax (Figure 14–16 ■). New lesions continue to erupt for 3 to 5 days, then crust and dry. Recovery occurs in 2 to 3 weeks. The client often experiences severe pain for up to 48 hours before and during eruption of the lesions. The pain may continue after the lesions have disappeared. The older adult is especially sensitive to the pain and often experiences more severe outbreaks of herpes zoster lesions.

Complications of herpes zoster include postherpetic neuralgia (a sharp, spasmodic pain along the course of one or more

nerves) and visual loss. The neuralgia, described as burning or stabbing, results from inflammation of the root ganglia. This complication is more common in clients over the age of 55 (Tierney, McPhee, & Papadakis, 2001). Permanent loss of vision may follow occurrence of lesions that arise from the ophthalmic division of the trigeminal nerve. The disease may disseminate in immunocompromised clients, causing lesions beyond the dermatome, visceral lesions, and encephalitis. This serious complication may cause death.

COLLABORATIVE CARE

The treatment for viral skin infections focuses on stopping viral replication and treating client responses, such as itching and pain.

Diagnostic Tests

Although diagnosis is usually based on manifestations and appearance of the lesions, laboratory tests may be necessary to differentiate herpes zoster from impetigo, contact dermatitis, and herpes simplex. The laboratory tests include the following:

- A Tzanck smear identifies the herpes virus, but it does not distinguish herpes zoster from herpes simplex. This is a microscopic examination of cells from the base of the lesion.
- Cultures of fluid from the vesicles and antibody tests are used to make the differential diagnosis of herpesvirus types.
- Immunofluorescent methods can identify varicella in skin cells.

Medications

Most viral skin disorders are treated with antiviral medications, and other types of medications are used to relieve pruritus and pain in clients with herpes zoster.

- *Warts.* Depending on their size, location, and any associated discomfort, warts may be treated with medications, cryotherapy, or electrodesiccation and curettage. A common method of wart removal is acid therapy, using a colloidal solution of 16% salicylic acid and 16% lactic acid. The solution is applied to the wart every 12 to 24 hours; the wart disappears in 2 to 3 weeks. Other methods of eradicating warts are cryosurgery, freezing with liquid nitrogen, and electrodesiccation of the wart with an electric current followed by excision of the dead tissue. Venereal warts are further described in Chapter 49.

- *Herpes simplex.* Herpes simplex lesions are treated with acyclovir (Zovirax), an antifungal agent. Acyclovir shortens the time of symptoms and speeds healing. Other antiviral mediations are discussed with herpes zoster.

- *Herpes zoster.* Antiviral drugs are used to treat herpes zoster infections. Acyclovir (Zovirax) interferes with viral synthesis and replication. Although it does not cure herpes infections, it does decrease the severity of the illness and also decreases pain. It may be administered topically, orally, or parenterally. It is more effective if administration begins within the first 1 to 2 days after the first vesicles appear. Acyclovir has little effect on postherpetic neuralgia. Famciclovir (Famvir) may have an advantage over acyclovir as it is more intracellularly stable in infected cells, inhibits DNA synthesis in infected cells, and has longer-lasting antiviral activity. Valacyclovir (Valtrex) is an antiviral agent that is hydrolyzed to acyclovir in the intestinal wall or liver, resulting in a higher plasma level that acyclovir when both are taken orally. Another antiviral drug that may be prescribed is vidarabine (Ara-A, Vira-A). This drug is given either by intravenous infusion or as an ophthalmic ointment.

Narcotic and nonnarcotic analgesics are prescribed for pain management, and antihistamines may be administered for relief of pruritus. Clients with eye involvement are treated with topical steroid ophthalmic ointments and mydriatics. Antivirals may sometimes be administered.

NURSING CARE

This section discusses care of the client with herpes zoster, focusing on the nursing diagnoses of acute pain, sleep pattern disturbance, and risk for infection.

Nursing Diagnoses and Interventions

Acute Pain

The client with herpes zoster often experiences severe pain over the entire dermatome supplied by the affected nerve root. The pain is described as burning, tearing, or stabbing. The client may avoid movement and does not want clothing or bed linens to touch the affected area.

- Monitor the location, duration, and intensity of the pain. *Each person experiences and expresses pain in his or her own manner. Pain tolerance is also individual. Accurate as-*sessment of the client's perception and tolerance of pain is essential in facilitating pain management.*

- Explain the rationale for taking prescribed medications on a regular schedule. *Delaying or withholding medications may allow the pain to reach an intensity at which the medication is less effective in promoting relief.*

- Teach measures to relieve pruritus:
  - Take prescribed antipruritic medications.
  - Apply calamine lotion or wet compresses, if prescribed.
  - Keep the room temperature cool.
  - Use a bed cradle to keep sheets off affected areas of the body.

Pruritus is a common problem for clients with herpes zoster; scratching may excoriate the skin and increase the risk for secondary infections. Pruritus may intensify the experience of pain. Lotions and cool, wet compresses are effective in decreasing the itch-scratch-itch cycle. Warmth and touch intensify pruritus.

- Encourage the use of distraction (such as music) or a specific relaxation technique (such as progressive muscle relaxation or deep breathing). *Noninvasive methods to relieve pain not only help the client manage the pain experience but also increase the effectiveness of pain medications.*

Disturbed Sleep Pattern

The pain and pruritus of herpes zoster interferes with normal sleep patterns. Those responses often are more intense at night, probably as a result of decreased distraction.

- Use appropriate measures to relieve pain and pruritus (as described above). *Pain and pruritus interfere with normal sleep. Analgesics and noninvasive methods of relief may be necessary before the client prepares for sleep.*

- Maintain a cool environment and avoid heavy bed covering. *Heat and touch intensify pruritus. Pruritus stimulates scratching, which awakens the client. The client may then perceive the pain more acutely. A cycle is established that interferes with sleep.*

Risk for Infection

Clients with herpes zoster have impaired skin integrity and pruritus with scratching and possible excoriation; moreover, they may be immunocompromised. All of these factors contribute to a high risk for secondary bacterial infection. In addition, the client is contagious to others who did not have chickenpox as children.

- Teach client the manifestations of infection:
  - Increased temperature
  - Increased redness, formation of pustules, and/or purulent drainage
  - Monitoring white blood cell count
  - Assessing for lymph gland enlargement

Secondary bacterial infections may occur in any client with impaired skin integrity; if the client is immunocompromised, the risk is even greater. Fever, changes in lesions or drainage, an increased white blood cell count, and lymph gland enlargement are manifestations of an infection.

- Teach interventions to decrease the itch-scratch-itch cycle, thereby decreasing the possibility of excoriation (see discussion about nursing care of clients with pruritus and psoriasis, earlier in this chapter). *Excoriation from scratching provides an avenue for bacterial invasion.*
- Institute infection control procedures for clients who are hospitalized:
  - Maintain strict isolation for immunocompromised clients.
  - Wear gloves and gown if contact with lesions is likely.
  - Instruct pregnant women to avoid exposure until lesions have crusted over.

Isolation procedures are instituted for the immunocompromised client to prevent client infection. Wear gloves and gown to prevent spreading the infection to self or others.

PRACTICE ALERT *Pregnant women must avoid exposure because the herpesvirus can cross the placental barrier.* ■

Using NANDA, NIC, and NOC

Chart 14-1 shows links between NANDA, NIC, and NOC when caring for the client with herpes zoster.

Home Care

Because most clients with viral infections provide self-care at home, the nurse focuses on teaching the client and family how to provide the necessary care. With herpes zoster increasing in incidence in clients who are older or have a serious chronic illness, it may also be necessary to make a referral to a community health provider for continued support. Provide the following information and instructions:

- The diseases are usually self-limiting and heal completely. Second occurrences of herpes zoster are rare.
- Do not have social contact with children or pregnant women until crusts have formed over the blistered areas with herpes zoster, as the disease is contagious to people who have not had chickenpox.
- Use pain medications regularly.
- Follow suggestions to help reduce itching, scratching, and pain: Use medications as prescribed, wear lightweight cotton clothing, keep room temperatures cool, wear cotton gloves at night if scratching is a problem, and practice relaxation and distraction activities.
- Report any increase in pain, fever, chills, drainage that smells bad and has pus, or a spread in the blisters to your health care provider.

CHART 14–1 NANDA, NIC, AND NOC LINKAGES

The Client with Herpes Zoster

NURSING DIAGNOSES	NURSING INTERVENTIONS	NURSING OUTCOMES
• Impaired Skin Integrity	• Skin Surveillance • Medication Administration • Infection Control	• Tissue Integrity: Skin and Mucous Membranes
• Disturbed Sleep Pattern	• Sleep Enhancement • Pain Management	• Pain Level • Pain Control Behavior
• Acute Pain	• Analgesia Administration • Environmental Management: Comfort	• Pain Level • Symptom Severity

Note. Data from Nursing Outcomes Classification (NOC) by M. Johnson & M. Maas (Eds.), 1997, St. Louis: Mosby; Nursing Diagnoses: Definitions & Classification 2001–2002 by North American Nursing Diagnosis Association, 2001, Philadelphia: NANDA; Nursing Interventions Classification (NIC) by J.C. McCloskey & G. M. Bulechek (Eds.), 2000, St. Louis: Mosby. Reprinted by permission.

INFLAMMATORY DISORDERS OF THE SKIN

Inflammatory skin disorders are rarely associated with systemic manifestations. The inflammatory skin disorders discussed in this section include dermatitis, acne, pemphigus, lichen planus, and toxic epidermal necrolysis.

THE CLIENT WITH DERMATITIS

Dermatitis is an inflammation of the skin characterized by erythema and pain or pruritus. Dermatitis may be acute or chronic.

PATHOPHYSIOLOGY

In dermatitis, various exogenous and endogenous agents cause an inflammatory response of the skin. Different types of skin eruptions occur, often specific to the causative allergen, infection, or disease. The initial skin responses to these agents or illnesses include erythema, formation of vesicles and scales, and pruritus (Figure 14–17 ■). Subsequently, irritation from scratching promotes edema, a serous discharge, and crusting. Long-term irritation in chronic dermatitis causes the

Nursing Care Plan
A Client with Herpes Zoster

Jesus Rivera is a 34-year-old migrant farm worker who currently lives in temporary housing in a rural area of the southwestern United States. His family includes his wife, Marta, who is 3 months' pregnant, and two children, ages 3 and 5. He takes his wife to a medical clinic staffed by volunteer nurses, physicians, and students from a nearby university for a prenatal checkup. The clinic is open only on Saturday and provides care on a sliding fee scale or for free if the family is unable to pay. While Mrs. Rivera is being examined, Mr. Rivera asks the nurse to have someone look at some very painful blisters on his chest that developed about a week ago. He is afraid that exposure to pesticides has caused the sores.

ASSESSMENT

Mr. Rivera speaks Spanish and is able to communicate only slightly in English. The initial assessment of Mr. Rivera is performed by Anita Mendez, a student nurse fluent in Spanish. Mr. Rivera's history reveals problems with lower back pain but no significant past medical illnesses. He is not aware of any allergies and cannot remember having had chickenpox as a child. Two years ago, both children were sick and had blisters on their bodies, and a friend told them it was chickenpox. Mrs. Rivera thinks she had chickenpox as a child.

Because Mr. Rivera has not had any medical care for several years, baseline laboratory tests are ordered to screen for any other illnesses; the complete blood count (CBC), blood chemistry, and urinalysis are all within normal limits.

Mr. Rivera says that he did not feel well for several days before the blisters appeared, having experienced chills and general achiness. He had not taken his temperature because the family does not own a thermometer. Current vital signs are as follows: T 99°F (37.2°C), p 74, R 22, and BP 148/88.

Physical examination of the trunk reveals a bandlike pattern of lesions across the left thorax. Some of the lesions are vesicles filled with serous fluid; others are darker in color and are oozing a light yellow drainage. The skin around the lesions is red and inflamed. Mr. Rivera complains of a severe, burning pain with itching across his chest. He is diagnosed with herpes zoster.

DIAGNOSIS

- *Risk for infection* related to open oozing areas on the left thorax
- *Acute pain* related to the presence of lesions and pruritus
- *Deficient knowledge* of the cause of the skin disorder and recommended treatment
- *Anxiety* related to need to work in areas of pesticide application
- *Altered health maintenance* related to limited access to health care, transitory work conditions, and cultural and language barriers

EXPECTED OUTCOMES

- Skin lesions will heal without evidence of a secondary infection.
- Limit exposure (as much as possible) to his wife and children and to persons with debilitating illnesses to prevent the spread of the virus.
- Obtain relief of pain and pruritus with the proper use of medications.
- Verbalize an understanding of the disease process and participate in the treatment plan.

- Obtain follow-up care.
- Make an appointment for a referral for information about occupational hazards.

PLANNING AND IMPLEMENTATION

- Provide verbal and written instructions (in Spanish) for self-care:
  - Wear a clean cotton undershirt each day.
  - Trim the fingernails short, and keep the hands clean.
  - Wash the hands each time the area is touched.
  - Wash any soiled clothes or linens in hot water and soap.
  - Do not allow other family members to use your towels.
  - Take medications as prescribed for itching and pain.
  - Take the medicine for your sores every 4 hours, even during nighttime hours, for 7 days.
  - As much as possible, do not touch your wife and children until the sores are covered with scabs. Do not have sex with your wife while you have these sores.
- Teach how to take care of skin lesions:
  - Wear the rubber gloves every time you do this treatment.
  - Wash the sores and the skin around them very gently with a soft washcloth and a mild soap.
  - Using your fingers, carefully rub the cream on the sores. Do this once every morning after breakfast and once every evening after supper.
  - Wash your hands carefully before and after each treatment.
- Make a follow-up appointment for the next week.
- Provide Mr. Rivera with the name and phone number of the Occupational Safety and Health Administration (OSHA) and recommend he call for an appointment to discuss his concerns about pesticides.

EVALUATION

Mrs. Rivera explains how she has taken care of her husband, and Mr. Rivera is careful to describe how he has followed the nurse's instructions. The skin lesions are dry and crusty, with no new blister formation. Mr. Rivera says he has not called OSHA and is not sure that he will, but he thanks Miss Mendez for the phone number. The nurses make an appointment in 1 month for a prenatal checkup for Mrs. Rivera and for follow-up of Mr. Rivera's herpes zoster. Mr. Rivera promises to return if they are still living close enough to keep the appointment.

Critical Thinking in the Nursing Process

1. Identify barriers to care present in this case study. How may nursing interventions promote health care delivery to disadvantaged populations?
2. Although most cases of herpes zoster are self-limiting, what further assessments and interventions might have been indicated had the lesions shown little improvement over time and/or the pain remained severe?
3. If Mr. Rivera is advised not to work until his lesions heal, the family may face economic and sociocultural hardships. Develop a plan of care for Mr. Rivera for the nursing diagnosis *Ineffective role performance*.

See Evaluating Your Response in Appendix C.

Figure 14–17 ■ Inflammation of the skin, or dermatitis, may be a response to allergens, infections, or chemicals. This client has contact dermatitis resulting from the metal salts in jewelry.

Source: Biophoto Associates/Photo Researchers, Inc.

skin to become thickened and leathery (a condition called *lichenification*) and darker in color.

Contact Dermatitis

Contact dermatitis is a type of dermatitis caused by a hypersensitivity response or chemical irritation. The major sources known to cause contact dermatitis are dyes, perfumes, poison plants (ivy, oak, sumac), chemicals, and metals (Box 14–2). A contact dermatitis common in the health care field is latex (glove) dermatitis.

Allergic contact dermatitis is a cell-mediated or delayed hypersensitivity to a wide variety of allergens. Sensitizing antigens include microorganisms, plants, chemicals, drugs, metals, or foreign proteins. On initial contact with the skin, the allergen binds to a carrier protein, forming a sensitizing antigen. The antigen is processed and carried to the T cells, which in turn become sensitized to the antigen. The first exposure is the sensitizing contact; skin manifestations occur with subsequent exposures. These manifestations include erythema, swelling, and pruritic

vesicles in the area of allergen contact. For example, a person hypersensitive to metal may have lesions under a ring or watch.

Irritant contact dermatitis is an inflammation of the skin from irritants; it is not a hypersensitivity response. Common sources of irritant contact dermatitis include chemicals (such as acids), soaps, and detergents. The skin lesions are similar to those seen in allergic contact dermatitis.

Atopic Dermatitis

Atopic dermatitis is an inflammatory skin disorder that is also called **eczema.** The exact cause is unknown, but related factors include depressed cell-mediated immunity, elevated IgE levels, and increased histamine sensitivity. The disorder is seen more often in children, but chronic forms persist throughout life.

Clients with atopic dermatitis have a family history of hypersensitivity reactions, such as dry skin, eczema, asthma, and allergic rhinitis. Although up to one-third of clients with atopic dermatitis also have food allergies, a positive correlation has not been found.

The dermatitis results when mast cells, T lymphocytes, monocytes, and other inflammatory cells are activated and release histamine, lymphokines, and other inflammatory mediators. The immune response interacts with the allergen to create a chronic inflammatory condition. In the adult form of atopic dermatitis, characteristic lesions include chronic lichenification, erythema, and scaling, the result of pruritus and scratching. The lesions are usually found on the hands, feet, or flexor surfaces of the arms and legs (Figure 14–18 ■). Scratching and excoriation increase the risk of secondary infections, as well as invasion of the skin by viruses such as herpes simplex.

Seborrheic Dermatitis

Seborrheic dermatitis is a chronic inflammatory disorder of the skin that involves the scalp, eyebrows, eyelids, ear canals, nasolabial folds, axillae, and trunk. The cause is unknown. This disorder is seen in all ages, from the very young (called "cradle cap") to the very old. Clients taking methyldopa (Aldomet) for hypertension occasionally develop this disorder, and it is a component of Parkinson's disease. Seborrheic dermatitis is also frequently seen in clients with AIDS.

BOX 14–2	■ Common Causes of Contact Dermatitis

- Acids
- Alkalis: soaps, detergents, household ammonia, lye, cleaners
- Bromide
- Chlorine
- Cosmetics: perfumes, dyes, oils
- Dusts of lime, arsenic, wood
- Hydrocarbons: crude petroleum, lubricating oil, mineral oil, paraffin, asphalt, tar
- Iodine
- Insecticides
- Fabrics: wool, polyester, dyes, sizing
- Metal salts: calcium chloride, zinc chloride, copper, mercury, nickel, silver
- Plants: ragweed, poison oak, poison sumac, poison ivy, pine
- Coloring agents
- Rubber products
- Soot

Figure 14–18 ■ Atopic dermatitis, or eczema, causes pruritus, resulting in lichenification, erythema, and scaling.

Source: NMSB/Custom Medical Stock Photo.

The lesions are yellow or white plaques with scales and crusts. The scales are often yellow or orange and have a greasy appearance. Mild pruritus is also present. Diffuse dandruff with erythema of the scalp often accompanies the skin lesions.

Exfoliative Dermatitis

Exfoliative dermatitis is an inflammatory skin disorder characterized by excessive peeling or shedding of skin. The cause is unknown in about half of all cases, but a preexisting skin disorder (such as psoriasis, atopic dermatitis, contact dermatitis, or seborrheic dermatitis) is found in about 40% of the cases (Tierney et al., 2001). Exfoliative dermatitis is also associated with leukemia and lymphoma.

Both systemic and localized manifestations may appear. Systemic manifestations include weakness, malaise, fever, chills, and weight loss. Scaling, erythema, and pruritus may be localized or involve the entire body (Figure 14–19 ■). In addition to peeling of skin, the client may lose the hair and nails.

Generalized exfoliative dermatitis may cause debility and dehydration. The impairment of skin integrity increases the risk for local and systemic infections.

COLLABORATIVE CARE

The client with dermatitis is treated primarily with topical medications and therapeutic baths. If the dermatitis is due to hypersensitivity to an allergen, the client avoids exposure to environmental irritants and suspected foods. The client also discontinues as many medications as possible to determine whether the dermatitis is the result of a drug allergy.

Diagnostic Tests

The diagnosis is often based on the manifestations of the disorder. Diagnostic tests may include the following:

- Scratch tests and intradermal tests are conducted to identify a specific allergen.
- Serum studies may find elevated eosinophil and IgE levels in atopic dermatitis.
- Skin biopsy may reveal specific changes in inflammatory dermatitis.

Medications

The medications used depend on the cause of the dermatitis and the severity of the manifestations. Minor cases are treated with antipruritic medications, whereas more severe cases are treated with oral antihistamines, oral and/or topical corticosteroids, and wet dressings. Topical anti-infectives may be prescribed if necessary.

NURSING CARE

Nursing care of the client with dermatitis focuses primarily on providing information for self-care at home. The client is responsible for managing skin problems and requires education and support. Address the following topics:

- Medications and treatments do not cure the disease; they only relieve the symptoms.
- Dry skin increases pruritus, which stimulates scratching. Scratching may in turn cause excoriation, and excoriation increases the risk of infection.
- It may be necessary to change the diet or environment to avoid contact with allergens.
- When using steroid preparations, apply only a thin layer to slightly damp skin (e.g., after taking a bath).
- If occlusive dressings are necessary, a plastic suit may be used.
- When using oral corticosteroids, never abruptly stop taking the medication. Rather, follow instructions to taper the dosage gradually.
- Antihistamines cause drowsiness. When using these medications, avoid alcohol and use caution when driving or working around machinery.

THE CLIENT WITH ACNE

Acne is a disorder of the pilosebaceous (hair and sebaceous gland) structure, which opens to the skin surface through a pore. The sebaceous glands, which empty directly into the hair follicle, produce sebum, a lipid substance. Sebaceous glands are present over the entire skin surface except the soles of the feet and the palms of the hands, but the largest

Figure 14–19 ■ Exfoliative dermatitis is an inflammatory skin disorder causing excessive skin peeling.

Source: Camera M. D. Studios. Carroll H. Weiss, Director. 8290 N. W. 26th Place. Sunrise, FL 33322.

glands are on the face, scalp, and scrotum. Sebum production is a response to direct hormonal stimulation by testicular androgens in men and adrenal and ovarian androgens in women.

PATHOPHYSIOLOGY

Acne may be noninflammatory or inflammatory. Noninflammatory acne lesions are primarily *comedones,* more commonly called pimples, whiteheads, and blackheads. Whiteheads are pale, slightly elevated papules categorized as closed comedones (Figure 14–20A ■). Blackheads are plugs of material that accumulate in the sebaceous glands. They are categorized as open comedones. The color is the result of the movement of melanin into the plug from surrounding epidermal cells. Inflammatory acne lesions include comedones, erythematous pustules, and cysts (Figure 14–20B). Inflammation close to the skin surface results in pustules; deeper inflammation results in cysts. The inflammation is believed to result from irritation from fatty acid constituents of the sebum and from substances produced by *Propionibacterium acnes* bacteria, both of which escape into the dermis when the follicular wall of closed comedones ruptures.

Several forms of acne occur at different periods of the life span. The most common are acne vulgaris, acne rosacea, and acne conglobata.

Acne Vulgaris

Acne vulgaris is the form of acne common in adolescents and young to middle adults. Although the lesions may persist longer in women, the incidence is greater in men. The actual cause of acne vulgaris is unknown. Possible causes include androgenic influence on the sebaceous glands, increased sebum

production, and proliferation of the organism *Propionibacterium acnes.* Many factors once thought to cause acne vulgaris, including high-fat diets, chocolate, infections, and cosmetics, have been disproved (Porth, 2002).

Mild cases may involve only a few scattered comedones, but severe cases are manifested by multiple lesions of all types. Most acne vulgaris lesions form on the face and neck, but they also occur on the back, chest, and shoulders. The lesions are usually mildly painful and may itch. The complications of acne vulgaris, especially in severe cases, are formation of cysts, pigment changes in persons with dark skin, severe scarring, and lowered self-concept from the obvious skin eruptions.

Acne Rosacea

Acne rosacea is a chronic type of facial acne that occurs more often in middle and older adults. The cause is unknown. The lesions of acne rosacea begin with erythema over the cheeks and nose. Other skin lesions may or may not appear. Over years of time, the skin color changes to dark red, and the pores over the area become enlarged (Figure 14–21 ■). The soft tissue of the nose may exhibit *rhinophyma,* an irregular bullous thickening that can be treated with plastic surgery.

Acne Conglobata

Acne conglobata is also a chronic type of acne of unknown cause that begins in middle adulthood. This type causes serious skin lesions: Comedones, papules, pustules, nodules, cysts, and scars occur primarily on the back, buttocks, and chest but may occur on other body surfaces. The comedones have multiple openings and a discharge that ranges from serous to purulent with a foul odor.

Figure 14–20 ■ Acne is a disorder of the hair and sebaceous skin structures. *A,* In noninflammatory forms of acne, the characteristic lesions are comedones (pimples). *B,* Inflammatory acne lesions include comedones, erythematous pustules, and cysts. These lesions often leave scars when they heal.

Figure 14–21 ■ Acne rosacea is more common in the middle to older adult. It causes changes in skin color, enlarged pores, and in some cases thickening of the soft tissues of the nose.

Source: Camera M. D. Studios. Carroll H. Weiss, Director. 8290 N. W. 26th Place. Sunrise, FL 33322.

COLLABORATIVE CARE

The management of acne is similar, regardless of type. Because acne vulgaris is most common, the discussions of collaborative and nursing care focus on that type.

Treatment is primarily by medications and continues for several weeks. Treatment is based on the type and severity of the lesions.

Diagnostic Tests

The disease is diagnosed by the typical location and appearance of lesions. If the client has pustules, a culture of the drainage is performed to differentiate viral or bacterial dermatitis from acne.

Medications

The treatment of acne is tailored to the individual and is based on the severity of the lesions. For acne with comedones, tretinoin (retinoic acid, Retin-A) or benzoyl peroxide preparations are prescribed. Azelaic acid (Azelex) may also be used. The administration of these vitamin A analogues is discussed in the Medication Administration box on this page. Benzoyl peroxide preparations are found in over-the-counter medications such as Fostex, Acne-Dome, Desquam-X, Benzagel, Clear By Design, and Xerac BP. These products are keratolytic and loosen the comedones.

Mild forms of papular inflammatory acne are treated with topical clindamycin (Cleocin T), a bacteriostatic agent that decreases the amount of fatty acids on the skin surface. This medication may be combined with tretinoin therapy.

Moderate forms of papular inflammatory acne are treated with oral or topical antibiotics, such as tetracycline, erythromycin, and minocycline. These antiacne antibiotics are admin-istered for 3 to 4 months; if the client's skin is clear, the dose is lowered gradually to a maintenance dose that will maintain clear skin.

Severe forms of papular inflammatory acne are treated with isotretinoin (Accutane). This drug is effective, but has serious side effects. Isotretinoin, with nursing responsibilities, is discussed below.

Medication Administration

Acne Medications

ANTIACNE RETINOIDS
Tretinoin (Retin-A)   Isotretinoin (Accutane)

Tretinoin is a vitamin A derivative classified as an acne agent. This topical agent acts as an irritant to decrease cohesiveness of follicular epithelial cells, thereby decreasing comedone formation while increasing the extrusion of comedones from the skin surface.

Isotretinoin is a vitamin A analogue classified as an acne product. It reduces the size of sebaceous glands, inhibits sebaceous gland differentiation to decrease sebum production, and alters sebum lipid composition.

Nursing Responsibilities
- Administer tretinoin with caution to pregnant women, the effects of absorption on the developing fetus are not clearly defined.
- Isotretinoin is absolutely contraindicated for pregnant women or for women who want to become pregnant. The medication poses a high risk of major deformities in the infant if pregnancy occurs during use, even use that continues only for short periods.
- Do not administer to clients with eczema or to those who are hypersensitive to the sun.

Client and Family Teaching
Tretinoin
- Use the cream in a test area twice at night to test for sensitivity; if no reaction occurs, increase applications gradually to the prescribed frequency.
- A pea-sized amount of the cream is enough to cover the entire face.
- Apply the cream to clean, dry skin.
- Do not apply the cream to the eyes, mouth, angles of the nose, or mucous membranes.
- Wash your face no more than two to three times a day, using a mild soap. Do not use skin preparations (such as aftershave lotion or perfumes) that contain alcohol, menthol, spice, or lime, they may irritate your skin.
- The medication may cause a temporary stinging or warm sensation but should not cause pain.
- The skin where you apply the cream will be mildly red and may peel; if you experience a more severe reaction, consult your health care provider.
- The medication may cause increased sensitivity to sunlight, use sunscreens and wear protective clothing when outdoors.
- Your acne may become worse during the first 2 weeks of treatment; this is an expected response.

(continued on page 384)

Medication Administration

Acne Medications (continued)

Isotretinoin
- Take the pills with food.
- Your acne may become worse during the initial period of treatment; this is an expected response.
- The medication causes dryness of the eyes, so you may have trouble wearing contact lenses during and after treatment.
- Do not take vitamin A supplements; they will increase the effects of the medication.
- Avoid prolonged exposure to sunlight; use sunscreen and protective clothing when in the sun.
- Notify the physician at once if you have abdominal pain, severe diarrhea, rectal bleeding, headache, nausea or vomiting, or visual disturbances.
- Do not drink alcohol while taking this medication (it causes an increase in triglycerides).
- Night vision may become worse; use caution when driving at night.
- Do not donate blood while or for 1 month after taking this medication.
- *(For female clients)* You must use two reliable forms of contraception simultaneously for at least 1 month before, during, and at least 1 month after therapy with this medication. The medication may cause deformities in a baby conceived at this time.

Treatments

Dermabrasion and Laser

Dermabrasion of inactive acne lesions can improve the client's appearance, especially if the scars are flat. (Dermabrasion is discussed in greater detail later in this chapter.) Laser excision of deep scars may also be used.

NURSING CARE

Nursing care is individualized to the client's developmental needs and is conducted primarily through teaching in clinics or the home setting. Regardless of the client's age or gender, it is important to remember that almost all clients with acne are embarrassed by and self-conscious of their appearance. Prior to teaching, establish rapport with the client and clarify beliefs; for example, the client may believe the lesions result from poor hygiene, masturbation, use of cosmetics, eating the wrong types of foods, or lack of sexual activity. It is critical to teach the client about the causes of and factors involved in acne prior to teaching self-care.

Home Care

The teaching plan for the client with acne includes general guidelines for skin care and health as well as specific guidelines for care of the acne lesions. The following topics should be addressed:

- Wash the skin with a mild soap and water at least twice a day to remove accumulated oils.
- Shampoo the hair often enough to prevent oiliness.

- Eat a regular, well-balanced diet. Foods do not cause or increase acne.
- Expose the skin to sunlight, but avoid sunburn.
- Get regular exercise and sleep.
- Try to avoid putting your hands on your face.
- Do not squeeze a pimple. Squeezing forces the material of the pimple deeper into the skin and usually causes the pimple to become larger and infected.
- The treatment for acne lasts months, in some cases for the rest of one's life. It is very important to take the medications each day for the prescribed length of time.

THE CLIENT WITH PEMPHIGUS VULGARIS

Pemphigus vulgaris is a chronic disorder of the skin and oral mucous membranes characterized by vesicle (blister) formation. The disease is caused by autoantibodies that cause *acantholysis* (the separation of epidermal cells from one another). The disorder is associated with IgG antibodies and HLA-A10 antigen. If untreated, the disease is usually fatal within 5 years (Tierney et al., 2001). However, better methods of diagnosis and treatment have improved the prognosis.

The disease occurs in middle and older adults of all races and ethnic backgrounds. The disorder has been associated with other autoimmune disorders and with the administration of certain drugs, such as penicillamine and captopril.

MANIFESTATIONS

The blisters that form in pemphigus vulgaris usually appear first in the mouth and scalp and then spread in crops or waves to involve large areas of the body, including the face, back, chest, umbilicus, and groin. Blisters in the mouth ulcerate. The blisters form in the epidermis and cause the epidermal cells to separate above the basal layer. These blisters rupture, leaving denuded skin, crusting, and oozing of fluid with a musty odor (Figure 14–22 ■). The lesions are painful. Pressure on a blister

Figure 14–22 ■ Pemphigus vulgaris is a chronic skin disorder characterized by vesicles that ooze fluid and form crusts.

causes it to spread to adjacent skin (Nikolsky's sign). The loss of fluid from the blisters may result in fluid and electrolyte imbalances. Secondary bacterial infections are a serious risk and a major cause of death.

COLLABORATIVE CARE

The goals of treatment are to control the severity of the disease, to prevent infection and loss of fluids, and to promote healing. Clients who experience severe attacks or secondary infections are usually hospitalized. Although the disease cannot be cured, the manifestations can be controlled.

Diagnostic Tests

Pemphigus vulgaris is diagnosed by clinical manifestations and laboratory and diagnostic tests. These tests may include the following:

- Immunofluorescence microscopy is done to identify the presence of IgG antibodies in the epidermis and serum.
- Skin biopsy may be performed to determine the presence of acantholysis.

Medications

Early lesions are treated with highly potent topical corticosteroids. As the disease becomes more severe, systemic corticosteroids or immunosuppressive agents (such as azathioprine or methotrexate) are prescribed. Secondary infections are treated with topical and/or systemic antibiotics.

Treatments

Plasmapheresis is occasionally used to treat pemphigus. In this procedure, the plasma is selectively removed from whole blood and reinfused into the client. This decreases the serum level of antibodies for a period of time. Plasmapheresis with related nursing care is discussed in Chapter 43. ⊙⊙

NURSING CARE

The hospitalized client with pemphigus requires careful assessment of skin lesions and monitoring for manifestations of infection. Provide skin care through bathing and applying dressings to denuded areas, using aseptic technique to prevent infection. The client may be placed on reverse isolation as a protective measure. Monitor the client's hydration status to prevent fluid volume deficit and incorporate pain medications and noninvasive pain management techniques in the plan of care. Oral lesions often make eating difficult; the client requires meticulous oral hygiene and nonirritating foods. The client often is depressed and fearful; establishing a therapeutic relationship is essential, and referrals for counseling may be necessary.

Home Care

Teaching the client and family how to provide care at home also involves skin care, oral care, diet, pain management, and prevention of infection. In addition, the nurse teaches the client and family how to take prescribed medications. A referral to a home health agency or local health department may be necessary.

THE CLIENT WITH LICHEN PLANUS

Lichen planus is an inflammatory disorder of the mucous membranes and skin. It has no known cause but has been associated with exposure to drugs or to film processing chemicals. The disease affects adults from 30 to 70 years of age.

The lesions first appear as violet papules, 2 to 10 mm in size, commonly occurring on the wrists, ankles, lower legs, and genitals (Figure 14–23 ■). The lesions are intensely pruritic. Over time, persistent lesions thicken and become dark red, forming hypertrophic lichen planus. Lesions on the oral mucous membranes appear as white lacey rings; lesions may also appear on the mucous membranes of the vaginal area and the penis. The nails become thin and may shed.

Lichen planus lesions are self-limiting but last for an average of 12 to 18 months. The disorder is diagnosed by clinical manifestations. Corticosteroids are used to control the inflammation, and antihistamines are used to control the pruritus. Lesions recur in about 20% of cases.

THE CLIENT WITH TOXIC EPIDERMAL NECROLYSIS

Toxic epidermal necrolysis (TEN) is a rare, life-threatening disease in which the epidermis peels off the dermis in sheets, leaving large areas of denuded skin. Conjunctivitis and mucositis of the mouth, upper airway, esophagus, and sometimes the genitourinary tract are often associated with TEN. The client

Figure 14–23 ■ These violet lesions are typical of lichen planus, a benign inflammatory disease of the skin and mucous membranes.

Source: Camera M. D. Studios. Carroll H. Weiss, Director. 8290 N. W. 26th Place. Sunrise, FL 33322.

usually requires critical care, often in a burn center. The incidence of TEN has not been documented, but it is seen more often in men and in people of African descent. The mortality rate ranges from 25% to 100% but is decreasing because of current methods of care. The cause of death is almost always sepsis.

Most cases result from a drug reaction, and others are associated with a serious concomitant illness, such as cancer or AIDS. In other cases, the disease has no known cause. Drugs that have been associated with TEN are the sulfonamides, barbiturates, NSAIDs, phenytoin, allopurinol, and penicillin.

The pathophysiologic process in TEN is not completely understood, but the triggering mechanism is believed to be a hypersensitivity or immune response. TEN begins with a painful, localized erythema of the face and extremities, accompanied by fever, chills, muscle aches, and generalized malaise. A macular rash develops, followed by the formation of large, flaccid blisters over the body surface during the next 24 to 96 hours. The skin begins to slough, leaving the dermal surface exposed. Even in areas without blistering, the skin may peel off in layers. The skin sloughing continues over several days and can expose 95% or more of the dermal surface (Figure 14–24 ■). Other manifestations include conjunctivitis, pharyngitis, stomatitis, and enlargement of lymph glands. Urethral slough is common, causing such painful voiding that the client voluntarily retains urine. The client is often disoriented, may be nearly comatose, and is seriously ill.

The loss of skin leads to fluid and electrolyte imbalances and secondary infections, as well as systemic effects on all other body systems. These complications may cause death. However, if the complications can be prevented, healing by epidermal regeneration occurs in about a month. The long-term

Figure 14–24 ■ Toxic epidermal necrolysis (TEN) is a life-threatening skin disease characterized by the sloughing of large skin surfaces.

Source: Camera M. D. Studios. Carroll H. Weiss, Director. 8290 N. W. 26th Place. Sunrise, FL 33322.

complications of TEN include blindness, lacrimal duct occlusion, scarring and contractures, loss of nails, esophageal strictures, and glomerulonephritis.

The client is hospitalized and requires rapid diagnosis and treatment. Any medication in use by the client is stopped immediately. Collaborative care involves fluid replacement, correction of electrolyte imbalances, prevention or management of infection, and pain control. The collaborative and nursing care are essentially the same as for the client with burns, discussed in Chapter 15.

MALIGNANT SKIN DISORDERS

The skin is a common site for malignant lesions. Many of these lesions are found on skin surfaces that have undergone long-term exposure to the sun or the environment. Malignant skin tumors are the most common of all cancers.

ACTINIC KERATOSIS

Actinic keratosis, also called senile or solar keratosis, is an epidermal skin lesion directly related to chronic sun exposure and photodamage. The prevalence is highest in people with light-colored skin; these lesions are rare in people with dark skin. Actinic keratosis may progress to squamous cell carcinoma. Fewer than 1% of early lesions become malignant, but many of those that persist progress to malignancy (Porth, 2002). Because of this tendency, the lesions are classified as premalignant.

The lesions are erythematous rough macules a few millimeters in diameter. They are often shiny but may be scaly; if the scales are removed, the underlying skin bleeds. They occur in multiple patches, primarily on the face, dorsa of the hands, the forearms, and sometimes on the upper trunk (Figure 14–25 ■).

Figure 14–25 ■ The effects of long-term sun exposure are illustrated in this epidermal skin lesion, called actinic keratosis.

Source: Camera M. D. Studios. Carroll H. Weiss, Director. 8290 N. W. 26th Place. Sunrise, FL 33322.

Enlargement or ulceration of the lesions suggests transformation to malignancy.

THE CLIENT WITH NONMELANOMA SKIN CANCER

The skin, despite its ability to protect the internal body from external damage, is a fragile organ and is subject to damage from ultraviolet radiation and chemicals. Over time, this damage results in alterations in cellular structure and function, and malignancies of the skin occur. The nonmelanoma skin cancers are basal cell cancer and squamous cell cancer.

INCIDENCE

Nonmelanoma skin cancer is the most common malignant neoplasm found in fair-skinned Americans. The American Cancer Society estimates that more than 1 million new cases of nonmelanoma skin cancer occur in the United States each year. Of that number 95% to 99% can be cured if detected and treated early. Men develop nonmelanoma skin cancer more often than do women, probably because of occupational exposures. Although nonmelanoma skin cancer may occur at any age, the incidence increases with each decade of life. Adults between the ages of 30 and 60 have the majority of these cancers.

PATHOPHYSIOLOGY AND MANIFESTATIONS

The two nonmelanoma skin cancers, basal cell cancer and squamous cell cancer, arise from epithelial tissue but have different pathophysiology, classifications, and manifestations.

Basal Cell Carcinoma

Basal cell carcinoma is an epithelial tumor believed to originate either from the basal layer of the epidermis or from cells in the surrounding dermal structures. These tumors are characterized by an impaired ability of the basal cells of the epidermis to mature into keratinocytes, with mitotic division beyond the basal layer. This results in a bulky neoplasm that grows by direct extension and destroys surrounding tissue, including healthy skin, nerves, blood vessels, lymphatic tissue, cartilage, and bone. Basal cell cancer is the most common but least aggressive type of skin cancer, rarely metastasizing.

Basal cell cancer is classified into different types: nodular, superficial, pigmented, morpheaform, and keratotic. These types are described below and are summarized in Table 14–3.

- Nodular basal cell cancer, the most common type of basal cell cancer, most often appears on the face, neck, and head. The tumor is made up of masses of cells that resemble epidermal basal cells and grow in a bulky, nodular form from lack of keratinization. In early stages, the tumor is a papule that looks like a smooth pimple. It is often pruritic and continues to grow at a steady rate, doubling in size every 6 to 12 months. As the tumor grows, the epidermis thins, but it remains intact. The skin over the tumor is shiny, and either pearly white, pink, or

TABLE 14–3	Types and Characteristics of Basal Cell Cancers	
Type	**Common Location**	**Manifestation**
Nodular	Face, neck, head	Small, firm papule; pearly, white, pink, or flesh colored; telangiectasis; enlarges; may ulcerate.
Superficial	Trunk, extremities	Papules or plaque that is flat, erythematous, or scaling; pink color; well-defined borders; may have shallow erosions and surface crusting.
Pigmented	Head, neck, face	Dark brown, blue, or black color; border is shiny and well defined.
Morpheaform	Head, neck	Looks like a flat scar; ivory or flesh colored.
Keratotic	Ear	Small, firm papule; pearly, white, pink, or flesh colored; may ulcerate.

skin colored. Telangiectasis may be visible over the area of the tumor. As the tumor continues to increase in size, the center or periphery may ulcerate, and the tumor develops well-circumscribed borders. It bleeds easily from mild injury.

- Superficial basal cell cancer, found most often on the trunk and extremities, is the second most common type of basal cell cancer. This tumor is a proliferating tissue that attaches to the undersurface of the epithelium. The tumor is a flat papule or plaque, often erythematous, with well-defined borders. The tumor may ulcerate and be covered with crusts or shallow erosions (Figure 14–26 ■).

- Pigmented basal cell cancer, found on the head, neck, and face, is less common. This tumor concentrates melanin pigment in the center of the basal cancer cells, giving it a dark brown, blue, or black appearance. The border of the tumor is shiny and well defined.

Figure 14–26 ■ A superficial basal cell cancer often is erythematous, has well-defined borders, and ulcerations.

- Morpheaform basal cell cancer, the rarest form of basal cell cancer, usually develops on the head and neck. The tumor forms fingerlike projections that extend in any direction along dermal tissue planes. The tumor resembles a flat ivory or flesh-colored scar. This form is more likely to extend into and destroy adjacent tissue, especially muscle, nerve, and bone. It is often more difficult to diagnose because of its appearance.
- Keratotic basal cell cancer (basosquamous) is found on the preauricular and postauricular groove. It contains both basal cells and squamoid-appearing cells that keratinize. Its appearance is much like that of nodular basal cell cancer. This type of basal cell cancer tends to recur locally and also is the type most likely to metastasize.

Basal cell cancers tend to recur. Tumors greater than 2 cm in diameter have a high recurrence rate. Predisposing factors for metastasis are the size of the tumor and the client's resistance to treatment with surgery or chemotherapy. Even though they rarely metastasize, untreated basal cell cancers invade surrounding tissue and may destroy body parts, such as the nose or eyelid.

Squamous Cell Cancer

Squamous cell cancer is a malignant tumor of the squamous epithelium of the skin or mucous membranes. It occurs most often on areas of skin exposed to ultraviolet rays and weather, such as the forehead, helix of the ear, top of the nose, lower lip, and back of the hands. Squamous cell cancer may also arise on skin that has been burned or has chronic inflammation. This is a much more aggressive cancer than basal cell cancer, with a faster growth rate and a much greater potential for metastasis if untreated.

The tumors arise when the keratinizing cells of the squamous epithelium proliferate, producing a growth that eventually fills the epidermis and invades the dermal tissue planes. Keratinization of some cells is present, and the formation of keratin "pearls" is common. The keratin formation diminishes as the tumor grows. As the tumor grows, the tumor cells increase in number and rate of mitosis, forming odd shapes.

Squamous cell cancer begins as a small, firm red nodule. The tumor may be crusted with keratin products. As it grows, it may ulcerate, bleed, and become painful. As the tumor extends into the surrounding tissue and becomes a nodule, the area around the nodule becomes indurated (hardened) (Figure 14–27 ■).

Figure 14–27 ■ As a squamous cell cancer grows, it tends to invade surrounding tissue. It also ulcerates, may bleed, and is painful.

Recurrent squamous cell cancer can be invasive, increasing the risk of metastasis. Invasive squamous cell cancer may arise from preexisting skin lesions, such as scars and actinic keratosis, and extend into the dermis (called intraepidermal squamous cell cancer). This form appears as a slightly raised erythematous plaque with well-defined borders. Metastasis occurs most often via the lymphatics. The degree of risk for metastasis depends on the size and depth of penetration of the tumor.

RISK FACTORS

There are multiple etiologic factors involved in the development of nonmelanoma skin cancer, including environmental factors and host factors.

Environmental Factors

The environmental factors implicated in the nonmelanoma skin cancers are ultraviolet radiation, pollutants, chemicals, ionizing radiation, viruses, and physical trauma.

Ultraviolet radiation (UVR) from the sun is believed to be the cause of most nonmelanoma skin cancers. Sunlight contains both short-length rays (UVB) and long-length rays (UVA). UVB rays are absorbed by the top layer of skin and cause sunburn. UVA rays penetrate deeper into the skin layers, causing tissue damage. Both types of rays are believed to cause DNA alterations and also suppress T-cell and B-cell immunity. The amount of ultraviolet radiation reaching the earth is increasing, most likely from depletion of the ozone layer surrounding the planet. The U.S. Environmental Protection Agency predicts that for every 1% decrease in the ozone layer, a corresponding 1% to 3% increase in nonmelanoma skin cancer per year will occur.

Geographic, environmental, and lifestyle factors affect the amount of exposure to the sun and the risk for nonmelanoma skin cancer. People who live in latitudes close to the equator and those who live at higher altitudes receive greater ultraviolet radiation exposure. The amount of clothing worn, the time of day, and amount of time in the sun also determine the amount of exposure. Exposure to ultraviolet radiation in tanning booths has also been implicated in the development of nonmelanoma skin cancer.

Certain chemicals have long been associated with nonmelanoma skin cancer. Polycyclic aromatic hydrocarbons, found in mixtures of coal, tar, asphalt, soot, and mineral oils, have been linked with skin cancers. Psoralens, used in conjunction with UVA for treatment of psoriasis and cutaneous T-cell lymphoma, increase the risk of squamous cell cancer.

Other factors associated with nonmelanoma skin cancer are the use of ionizing radiation, viruses, and physical trauma. X-ray therapy for tinea capitis and the use of radium to treat other malignancies are risk factors. Human papillomavirus is implicated in the development of squamous cell cancer, as is damage to the skin from burns.

Host Factors

Certain host factors increase the risk of nonmelanoma skin cancer. These include skin pigmentation as well as the presence of premalignant lesions.

Skin pigmentation is an important factor in the development of nonmelanoma skin cancer. The amount of melanin pigment produced by the melanocytes determines a person's skin color. The more melanin, the more the skin is protected from the damage produced by ultraviolet rays. Thus, African Americans, Asian Americans, and people of Mediterranean descent have a much lower incidence of nonmelanoma skin cancer than do people who have fair complexions and tend to freckle or sunburn easily, such as people of Irish, Scandinavian, or English ancestry.

Although most people have numerous pigmented lesions on their body, almost all of these are normal. However, a major risk factor in the development of nonmelanoma skin cancer is a change in an existing lesion or the presence of a premalignant lesion, such as actinic keratosis. Organ transplant recipients who undergo immunosuppression to prevent rejection are also at risk for the development of squamous cell cancer.

COLLABORATIVE CARE

Treatment of nonmelanoma skin cancer focuses on removal of all malignant tissue using such methods as surgery, curettage and electrodesiccation, cryotherapy, or radiotherapy. These modalities offer a greater than 90% cure rate. After the malignant tissue is removed, the client should have regular examinations for recurrence.

Diagnostic Tests

Nonmelanoma cancer is diagnosed by microscopic examination of tissue biopsied from the tumor. The biopsy is usually done as an office procedure under local anesthesia. The types of biopsy commonly conducted follow:

- Shave biopsy, in which the lesion is shaved with a scalpel to the level of the mid-dermis
- Punch biopsy, in which a circular punch removes a section of tissue in a "cookie cutter" fashion to a level of the reticular dermis or subcutaneous tissue
- Incisional biopsy, in which a part of the tumor is removed with a scalpel
- Excisional biopsy, in which the entire tumor is removed and analyzed

Treatments

Surgical Excision

Both basal cell and squamous cell cancers are excised surgically. The surgery may be minor or major, depending on the size and location of the tumor. Surgery for small tumors is most often performed in the outpatient surgery department or in the surgeon's office. Surgical excision allows rapid healing and yields good cosmetic results, but as does any surgery, carries the risk of infection.

The goal of surgical excision is to remove the tumor completely, so some surrounding tissue is excised along with the tumor. If the tumor is on the face, the incision is made along normal wrinkle or anatomic lines so that the scars will be less obvious. The incision is closed in layers to leave the smallest possible scar. A pressure dressing is usually applied over the incision to provide support.

If a large tumor is removed, a skin graft or skin flap may be performed to cover the excised area. If grafting is necessary, the client is hospitalized.

Mohs' ChemoSurgery Technique

In Mohs' chemosurgery technique, thin layers of the tumor are horizontally shaved off. A frozen section of the tissue is stained at each level to determine tumor margins. This method is the most accurate in assessing the extent of nonmelanoma skin cancer and the method that conserves the most normal tissue. It is often used in areas such as the nose, the nasolabial fold, the medial canthus, and the ear.

Curettage and Electrodesiccation

Curettage and electrodesiccation are used to treat basal cell cancers that are less than 2 cm in diameter, are superficial, or recur because of poor margin control. It may also be used for primary squamous cell cancers that are less than 1 cm in diameter and have distinct borders. This type of treatment is most successful for tumors on anatomic sites over a fixed underlying surface, such as the ear, chest, and temple.

Abnormal tissue is scraped away (curettage) within 1 to 2 mm of the margin and then a low-voltage electrode is used to abrade the tumor base (electrodesiccation). Tumor tissue is much softer and more friable than normal tissue. Therefore, curettage and electrodesiccation is not used for lesions where the dermis is thin (such as the eyelid) or where the tumor extends into the subcutaneous tissue.

Curettage and electrodesiccation provide good cosmetic results and preserve normal tissue. However, healing time is longer, and it is difficult to ensure that all tumor margins have been removed.

Instead of a low-voltage electrode, some physicians use a carbon dioxide laser to vaporize the tumor. When used in conjunction with curettage, this treatment is effective on superficial basal cell cancers. Carbon dioxide vaporization results in minimal thermal injury to adjacent cells, less pain, and quicker healing.

Radiation Therapy

Radiation is most often used for lesions that are inoperable because of their location (such as tumors on the corner of the nose, the eyelid, the canthus, and the lip) or size (between 1 cm and 8 cm). Radiotherapy is also used for clients who are older and of poor surgical risk. Radiation is painless and can be used to treat areas surrounding the tumor if necessary. However, the treatment is given over 3 to 4 weeks in a clinical facility, does not allow control of tumor margins, and may itself cause skin cancer.

NURSING CARE

The increasing number of people with skin cancer requires that nurses be involved in prevention and early detection, as well as provide nursing interventions. Nurses have the opportunity to teach preventive behaviors in all settings, including the hospital, home, community, school, and clinic.

Nursing care for the client with nonmelanoma skin cancer depends on the treatment employed. Surgical excision is the most common form of treatment; nursing care depends on the extent of the procedure. However, regardless of the type of treatment, the client will have impaired skin integrity, an increased risk for infection, and anxiety about the future following a diagnosis of cancer. Interventions with rationale for the client with any type of skin cancer are discussed in the section on malignant melanoma.

Health Promotion

It is well known that cumulative sun exposure positively correlates with nonmelanoma skin cancers. Many skin cancers can be prevented by limiting exposure to risk factors. Primary prevention behaviors recommended by the American Cancer Society and the Skin Cancer Foundation follow:

- Minimize exposure to the sun between the hours of 10 A.M. and 3 P.M., when ultraviolet rays are the strongest.
- Cover up with a wide-brimmed hat, sunglasses, long-sleeved shirt, and long pants made of tightly woven material when you are in the sun.
- Use a waterproof or water-resistant sunscreen with an SPF of 15 or more before every exposure to the sun. Apply sunscreen not only on sunny days but also on cloudy days, when ultraviolet rays can penetrate 70% to 80% of the cloud cover. Reapply the sunscreen before the protection time is up. See Box 14–3 for information about sunscreens.
- Use sunscreen and protective clothing when you are on or near sand, snow, concrete, or water, which can reflect more than half of the ultraviolet rays onto the skin.
- Avoid tanning booths; UVA radiation emitted by tanning booths damages the deep skin layers.

Nurses also provide client and family education for early detection of nonmelanoma skin cancer. Numerous brochures describing the types of skin cancers, photographs of lesions, and prevention behaviors are available from the American Cancer Society, health education and support agencies, and pharmaceutical companies that manufacture sunscreen. Most of this literature is free.

The client or family at risk for or diagnosed with a skin cancer must be taught how to conduct a self-examination of the skin as well as the importance of conducting the examination on the same day of each month. Family members can help with areas that are hard to examine, such as the ears, scalp, and back.

Home Care

Teach the client and family specific measures for self-care following surgery, including information about:

- How and when to change dressings.
- The use of aseptic technique and careful handwashing when caring for the wound.
- Symptoms to report (such as bleeding, fever, or signs of wound infection), and how to protect the operative site against trauma and irritations.

BOX 14–3 ■ Sunscreen Information

TYPES OF SUNSCREEN

Chemical
Chemical sunscreens absorb ultraviolet light and act as a radiation filter. Examples follow:

- *p*-aminobenzoic acid (PABA)
- Benzophenones
- Anthranilates
- Salicylates

Physical
Physical sunscreens reflect and scatter ultraviolet light. Examples follow:

- Zinc oxide
- Titanium dioxide
- Magnesium silicate
- Ferric chloride
- Kaolin
- Ichthyol

ADVERSE REACTIONS ASSOCIATED WITH SUNSCREENS

Adverse reactions associated with sunscreens include contact and photocontact dermatitis. People with previous hypersensitivity reactions to benzocaine, procaine, sulfonamides, or paraphenylenediamine may develop hypersensitivity responses to PABA. People who are also taking systemic thiazide diuretics or sulfonamides may develop eczematous dermatitis.

SUNSCREEN RATINGS

In the United States, the Food and Drug Administration (FDA) rates commercial sunscreens according to their "sun protection factor," or SPF. The SPF value is the ratio of the time required to produce minimal skin redness through a sunscreen product with the time required to produce the same degree of redness without the sunscreen. A person who can tolerate 1/2 hour of sun without a sunscreen should be able to tolerate 3 hours of sun when a sunscreen of SPF 6 is applied to the skin. SPF values of sunscreens range from 2 to 50.

THE CLIENT WITH MALIGNANT MELANOMA

Malignant melanoma arises from melanocytes. This serious skin cancer is increasing in incidence each year. At the current rate, it is predicted that 1 in 58 males and 1 in 82 females in the United States will develop melanoma in his or her lifetime (American Cancer Society, 2002).

INCIDENCE

This disease is over 10 times more common in fair-skinned people than in dark-skinned people. As with the nonmelanoma skin cancers, an increase in the incidence of malignant melanoma is believed to be related to the thinning ozone layer and increased exposure to ultraviolet rays. The incidence is highest in Caucasian upper-middle-class professionals who work indoors (Porth, 2002). This group of people often had severe sunburn with blistering during childhood and tend to vacation in areas of intense sun exposure. Malignant melanoma is also more common in people who live in sunny climates, burn easily, and patronize tanning parlors. However, malignant melanoma may arise from already present lesions or from skin normally covered with clothing.

PATHOPHYSIOLOGY AND MANIFESTATIONS

Melanocytes are located at or near the basal layer (the deepest epidermal layer). These cells produce melanin, the dark skin pigment. Melanin is made in granules and transferred to keratinocytes, where it accumulates on the superficial side of each keratinocyte and forms a shield of pigment over the nucleus as protection against ultraviolet rays. Malignant melanomas can develop wherever there is pigment, but about one-third of them originate in existing nevi.

Almost all malignant melanomas are more than 6 mm in diameter, are asymmetric, and initially develop within the epidermis over a long period. While they are still confined to the epidermis, the lesions (called *malignant melanoma in situ*) are flat and relatively benign. However, when they penetrate the dermis, they mingle with blood and lymph vessels and are capable of metastasizing. At this latter stage, the tumors develop a raised or nodular appearance and often have smaller nodules, called satellite lesions, around the periphery.

The prognosis for survival for people diagnosed with malignant melanoma is determined by several variables, including tumor thickness, ulceration, metastasis, site, age, and gender. Younger clients and women have a somewhat better chance of survival. Tumors on the hands, feet, and scalp have a poorer prognosis; tumors of the feet and scalp are less visible and may not be diagnosed until they grow into the dermis.

Precursor Lesions

The three specific precursor lesions for the development of malignant melanoma are congenital nevi, dysplastic nevi, and lentigo maligna. A precursor lesion is also called a premalignant lesion, a name that indicates that the lesion's risk of becoming malignant is greater than normal.

Congenital Nevi

Congenital nevi are present at birth. Some lesions are small; others are large enough to cover an entire body area. Their color can range from brown to black. They are often slightly raised, with an irregular surface and a fairly regular border.

Dysplastic Nevi

Dysplastic nevi are also called atypical moles. Although dysplastic nevi are not present at birth, they appear as normal nevi during childhood and become dysplastic (having abnormal development) after puberty. A client with classic dysplastic nevi has more than 100 nevi, at least one of which is larger than 8 mm in diameter, and at least one has the characteristics of malignant melanoma (asymmetry, irregular border, color variegation, and a diameter greater than 6 mm). A familial tendency to dysplastic nevi increases the risk for the development of malignant melanoma. However, it is not known whether people with dysplastic nevi and no family history of melanoma face a higher risk of melanoma.

Dysplastic nevi most often appear on the face, trunk, and arms but also are seen on the scalp, female breast, groin, and buttocks. The pigmentation of the nevi is irregular, with mixtures of tan, brown, black, red, and pink. An area of lighter pigmentation is surrounded by a papular area of deeper pigmentation (described as a "fried egg appearance"). The borders of the nevi are irregular.

Lentigo Maligna

Lentigo maligna, also called Hutchinson's freckle, is a tan or black patch on the skin that looks like a freckle. It grows slowly, becoming mottled, dark, thick, and nodular. It is usually seen on one side of the face of an older adult who has had a large amount of sun exposure.

Classification

Malignant melanomas are classified into different types. The major types are superficial spreading melanoma, lentigo maligna melanoma, nodular melanoma, and acral lentiginous melanoma. Each of these tumors is characterized by a radial and/or vertical growth phase. During the initial radial phase, which may last from 1 to 25 years (depending on the type), the melanoma grows parallel to the skin surface. During this phase, the tumor rarely metastasizes and is often curable by surgical excision. However, during the vertical growth phase, atypical melanocytes rapidly penetrate into the dermis and subcutaneous tissue, greatly increasing the risk for metastasis and death.

Superficial Spreading Melanoma

Superficial spreading melanoma is the most common type, comprising about 70% of all melanomas (Porth, 2002). The lesions are usually flat and scaly or crusty and are about 2 cm in diameter. They often arise from a preexisting nevus. This type of melanoma is found on the trunk and back of men and on the legs of women. Superficial spreading melanomas occur more often in women than in men. The median age of occurrence is the 50s.

The radial growth phase lasts from 1 to 5 or more years. When the lesion enters the vertical growth phase, it grows rapidly, and its color changes from a mixture of tan, brown, and black to a characteristic red, white, and blue. The lesion also develops irregular borders and often has raised nodules and ulcerations (Figure 14–28 ■).

Figure 14–28 ■ Malignant melanoma is a serious skin cancer that arises from melanocytes.

Source: L. Solomon/Custom Medical Stock Photography.

Lentigo Maligna Melanoma

Lentigo maligna melanoma often arises from the precursor lesion, lentigo maligna. The lesions are large and tan with different shades of brown. This type of melanoma makes up 4% to 10% of malignant melanomas and is the least serious form (Porth, 2002). It occurs on skin that has had long-term sun exposure, such as the face, neck, and sometimes the dorsal surface of the hands and lower extremities. Lentigo maligna melanoma affects women more than men. It is typically diagnosed in people in their 60s and 70s.

Lentigo maligna melanoma is characterized by a proliferation of atypical melanocytes parallel to the basal layer of the epidermis. The radial growth phase may last from 10 to 25 years, with the lesion growing to as large as 10 cm. The lesion becomes malignant as soon as the melanocytes invade the dermis. In the vertical growth phase, raised nodules may appear on the surface of the lesion. The lesion tends to acquire a freckled or mottled appearance.

Nodular Melanoma

Nodular melanoma lesions are raised, dome-shaped blue-black or red nodules on areas of the head, neck, and trunk that may or may not have been exposed to the sun. The lesions may look like a blood blister, or they may ulcerate and bleed. The lesions arise from unaffected skin rather than from a preexisting lesion. This type makes up 15% to 30% of malignant melanomas and is often diagnosed in people in their 50s (Porth, 2002).

Nodular melanoma has only a vertical growth phase, but it grows aggressively during that phase. However, the absence of a radial growth phase makes this type more difficult to diagnose before it metastasizes.

Acral Lentiginous Melanoma

Acral lentiginous melanoma, also called mucocutaneous melanoma, is less common in people with fair skin and more common in people with dark skin. The lesions progress from tan, brown, or black flat lesions to elevated nodules and are about 3 cm in diameter. The radial phase lasts from 2 to 5 years. They are found on the palms of the hands, soles of the feet, the mucous membranes, and the nailbeds. Acral lentiginous melanoma affects both men and women equally and is most often diagnosed in people in their 50s and 60s.

COLLABORATIVE CARE

The management of the client with malignant melanoma begins with identification, diagnosis, and tumor staging. If treatable, the tumor is removed through surgical excision. Malignant melanoma is also treated with chemotherapy, immunotherapy, and radiation therapy. Other therapies used with success include biological therapies with interleukin-2 and interferon and therapeutic vaccines containing melanoma antigens.

Identification

Malignant melanoma is most often found on the trunk of men and on the lower extremities of women. Nevertheless, it is important for the client to have a complete physical examination

and total skin assessment. In addition to a visual examination of all skin surfaces, palpation of regional lymph nodes, the liver, and the spleen is essential to assess for metastasis when a melanoma is suspected or found.

A change in the color or size of a nevus is reported in 70% of people diagnosed with a malignant melanoma. The ABCD rule is used to assess suspicious lesions:

A = asymmetry (one half of the nevus does not match the other half)
B = border irregularity (edges are ragged, blurred, or notched)
C = color variation or dark black color
D = diameter greater than 6 mm (size of a pencil eraser)

Diagnostic Tests

In addition to biopsy of any suspicious lesion, diagnostic tests are conducted to determine whether the tumor has metastasized. Because malignant melanoma may metastasize to any organ or tissue of the body, a variety of tests may be conducted.

- Epiluminescence microscopy helps identify lesions that require a biopsy.
- Biopsy of the lesion is the only definitive method of diagnosing a malignant melanoma. An excisional biopsy is the diagnostic procedure of choice because this allows the most complete histologic evaluation and microstaging.
- Prior to excision, lymphoscintigraphy may be performed to detect microscopic metastasis.
- If the client has manifestations indicating possible metastasis, diagnostic tests specific to the suspected site include liver function tests and CT scan of the liver, a complete blood count, serum blood chemistry profile, chest X-ray, bone scan, and CT scan or MRI of the brain.

Microstaging

The term *microstaging* describes the assessment of the level of invasion of a malignant melanoma and the maximum tumor thickness. In the Clark system of microstaging, the vertical growth of the lesion is measured from the epidermis to the subcutaneous tissue to determine the level of invasion (Figure 14–29 ■). However, variations in individual skin thicknesses

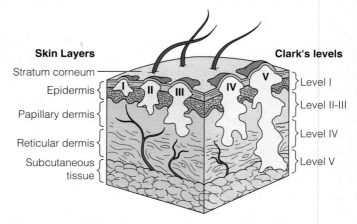

Figure 14–29 ■ Clark's levels for staging measure the invasion of a melanoma from the epidermis to the subcutaneous tissue.

and different anatomic sites can affect the accuracy of the measurement. In the Breslow system, an adaptation of the Clark system of assessment, the vertical thickness is measured from the granular level of the epidermis to the deepest level of tumor invasion. This determination is important, because as the thickness of the melanoma increases, survival rate decreases.

After the thickness and depth of the tumor are determined, a clinical stage is assigned. The traditional three-stage system is still used, although it does not include tumor thickness. The American Joint Committee on Cancer has adopted a four-stage system that includes tumor thickness, level of invasion, lymph node involvement, and evidence of metastasis.

Treatments

Surgical excision is the preferred treatment for malignant melanoma. Other methods are chemotherapy, immunotherapy, and radiation therapy.

Surgery

If a biopsy identifies the lesion as a melanoma, a wide excision is performed that includes the full thickness of the skin and subcutaneous tissue. Because the risk of local recurrence for thin melanomas (those less than 0.76 mm) is quite low, margins of 0.5 to 1.0 cm of normal skin are excised around the tumor. Thick tumors require a 1- to 3-cm margin excision because they are at risk for local recurrence or satellite lesions.

Regional lymph nodes are the most common sites for metastasis of malignant melanoma. Standard surgical treatment for clinically suspicious lymph node involvement includes excision of the primary lesions as well as surgical dissection of the involved lymph nodes. Elective lymph node dissection (ELND) in the treatment of localized malignant melanoma remains controversial. Advocates of ELND believe that the procedure benefits clients with intermediate-thickness tumors because approximately 20% of people whose lymph nodes were clinically negative at diagnosis show some metastasis on removal of the nodes. Those opposed to ELND believe the risks associated with the procedure are too high for the 80% of people who have no evidence of metastasis after removal of the nodes.

Surgery also is indicated for palliative management of isolated metastasis. Removal of metastatic tumors in the brain, liver, lung, gastrointestinal tract, or subcutaneous tissue may relieve symptoms and prolong life.

Immunotherapy

Immunotherapy is a relatively new treatment modality for malignant melanoma. The role of the immunologic response initially was recognized because of the numerous spontaneous remissions seen in clients with melanoma—a higher occurrence than with any other adult tumor. In addition, researchers have recently identified tumor-specific antigen-antibodies in clients with melanoma. This also has stimulated an interest in immunotherapeutic interventions for the treatment of malignant melanoma.

Agents such as interferons, interleukins, monoclonal antibodies, bacille Calmette-Guérin (BCG), levamisole, transfer factors, and tumor vaccines have shown activity in melanoma,

with varying response rates. The effectiveness of these agents, used either alone, in combination with chemotherapy, or in combination with each other, is under investigation. The use of immunotherapy in the treatment of melanoma is still new and requires further investigation.

Radiation Therapy

Melanoma responds to higher dose radiation, especially if the tumor is small. Response rates to radiation therapy depend on the site of the tumor, the thickness of the tumor, the type of melanoma, and the client's general health, but may range from 0% to 71%. Radiation frequently is used for palliation of symptoms resulting from metastasis to the brain, bone, lymph nodes, gastrointestinal tract, skin, or subcutaneous tissue. Liver and lung metastases are not treated with radiation therapy because a loss of organ function may result.

NURSING CARE

The nurse has the opportunity to assess the skin of clients requiring care for many different health problems and may be the first person to identify suspicious lesions. Wide excision and the high risk of metastasis from malignant melanoma usually requires inpatient surgical treatment, with the nurse providing care and teaching.

Health Promotion

The most important aspect of preventing malignant melanoma is a health history and skin assessment. The American Cancer Society recommends that people between the ages of 20 and 40 see a skin specialist every 3 years and those over 40 have annual skin checkups. People with actinic keratoses should also have their skin checked regularly for any signs of change. Clients at risk (those with precancerous lesions and with personal risk factors) should conduct a monthly skin self-examination (e.g., the first day of each month). Using a mirror to examine lesions on the back of the body and extremities, the client looks for a change in:

- Color, especially any lesion that becomes darker or variegated in shades of tan, brown, black, red, white, or blue.
- Size, especially any lesion that becomes larger or spreads out.
- Shape, especially any lesion that protrudes more from the skin or begins to have an irregular outline.
- Appearance of a lesion, especially bleeding, drainage, oozing, ulceration, crusting, scaliness, or development of a mushrooming outward growth.
- Consistency, especially any lesion that becomes softer or is more easily irritated.
- Skin around a lesion, such as redness, swelling, or leaking of color from a lesion into the surrounding skin.
- Sensation, such as itching or pain.

Assessment

Skin assessment is discussed in Chapter 13. Specific health history questions and assessments for skin cancer are outlined in Box 14–4.

BOX 14–4 ■ Nursing Assessment for Skin Cancer

INTERVIEW QUESTIONS

- Have any members of your family ever been treated for skin cancer?
- Have you had a skin cancer removed from any part of your body?
- Have you noticed any change in the size, shape, or color of a mole, wart, birthmark, or scar?
- Do you have any moles, warts, birthmarks, or scars that itch, are painful, have crusting, or bleed?
- In what parts of the country or world have you lived?
- Have you ever been badly sunburned?
- Do you visit tanning salons?
- Are you exposed to any hazardous chemicals in your job?
- Have you been taught how to examine your skin? If so, how do you do this examination? How often?

Physical Assessment

1. Ask the client to remove all clothing and put on an examination gown. Ensure good light; natural, bright light is best for inspection of lesions. The client may sit, stand, or lie down.
2. Inspect and palpate the skin. Stretching the skin tightly during assessment facilitates assessment of nodular and scaly lesions and lesions in the dermis. Assess for:
   a. Obvious lesions
   b. Visible swellings
   c. Alterations in normal contour and borders of nevi
   d. Enlarged lymph glands
   e. Skin or mucosal discolorations
   f. Areas of ulceration, scaling, crusting, or erosion
3. The order of assessment follows:
   a. Head and neck: entire scalp, eyelids, external ear, auditory canals, external surface of the nose, internal surface of the nose, the oral cavity, facial skin, the facial glands (parotid, submaxillary, sublingual)
   b. Thyroid and neck, including lymph glands
   c. Chest and abdomen, with special attention under pendulous breasts, in skinfolds, and in areas covered with hair
   d. Back and buttocks, with special attention to the area between the buttocks
   e. Extremities, with special attention to the axillae, nail beds, webs between the fingers and toes, and soles of the feet
   f. External genitals, with special attention to skinfolds, mucous membranes, and areas covered with hair
4. Measure and record a description of all skin lesions on an anatomic chart. Take photographs (if possible) of any suspicious lesion, and include them in the client's record for future reference.

Nursing Diagnoses and Interventions

Although many different nursing diagnoses may be appropriate for the client with a malignant melanoma, the most common responses are impaired skin integrity, hopelessness, and anxiety.

Impaired Skin Integrity

Impaired skin integrity is a common problem for the client with malignant melanoma. These cancers not only destroy skin layers but also invade body structures. Certain types of tumors may ulcerate prior to diagnosis, and treatment typically involves some type of surgical biopsy and excision. Any open lesion or incision increases the risk for secondary infection.

- Monitor for manifestations of infection: fever, tachycardia, malaise, incisional erythema, swelling, pain, or drainage that increases or becomes purulent. *Intact skin is the first line of defense against infection; impaired skin integrity increases the risk for infection. If infection is present, the client may have both systemic and local manifestations.*
- Keep the incision line clean and dry by changing dressings as necessary. *Moisture increases the risk of infection.*
- Follow principles of medical and surgical asepsis when caring for client's incision. Teach family members and visitors the importance of careful hand washing. Maintain standard precautions if drainage is present. Careful hand washing is essential in preventing the spread of infection. *Aseptic techniques are necessary when caring for any surgical incision to prevent infection.*

PRACTICE ALERT
Nurses must use standard precautions with blood and body fluids to protect themselves from exposure to HIV. ■

- Encourage and maintain adequate caloric and protein intake in the diet. Suggest a consultation with the dietitian if client does not want to eat. *Adequate kcalories and protein are necessary for proper healing. The client with cancer has increased metabolic needs; if these needs are not met, nutritional problems that impair healing may result.*

Hopelessness

Hopelessness is often described in the literature as a response to the diagnosis of cancer. It is an emotional state in which a person feels that there is no possibility that life will improve. Clients who experience hopelessness are often withdrawn, passive, and apathetic.

The diagnosis of malignant melanoma threatens the quality and quantity of life as the client faces the possibility or reality of metastasis; the possibility that the cancer may recur and cause death; and alterations in self-concept, roles, and relationships. Inspiring hope in clients during this health crisis is a legitimate nursing action.

- Provide an environment that encourages the client to identify and express feelings, concerns, and goals:
  - Use active listening, ask open-ended questions, and reflect on the client's statements.
  - Acknowledge and respect the client's feelings of apathy and/or anger as expressions of distress.
  - Convey an empathetic understanding of the client's fears and concerns.
  - Provide opportunities for the client to express positive emotions: hope, faith, a sense of purpose, and the will to live.

- Explore the client's perceptions, and modify or clarify them if necessary by providing information and correcting misconceptions.
- Encourage the client to identify support systems and sources of strength and coping in the past.

Verbalizing feelings, concerns, and goals allows others to validate or correct them, promotes a therapeutic nurse-client relationship, and fosters feelings of self-worth. Expressing positive emotions and calling on support systems and sources of strength that were effective in coping with past crises help the person resolve the crisis and develop hope.

- Encourage the client to participate actively in self-care as well as in mutual decision making and goal setting. *Meeting self-care needs and making decisions about care increase personal confidence in one's capacity for coping.*
- Encourage the client to focus not only on the present but also on the future: Review past occasions for hope, discuss the client's personal meaning of hope, establish and evaluate short-term goals with the client and family, and encourage them to express hope for the future. *The nurse mobilizes the client's resources to strengthen motivation, hope, and the will to live.*

Anxiety

Anxiety is aroused by a perceived threat; its intensity depends on the severity of the present situation and the client's ability to handle the threat. Anxiety is one of the most common psychosocial responses in clients with cancer. Anxiety increases at the time of diagnosis and remains a constant emotion throughout the course of treatment, regardless of treatment type or setting. Interventions center on helping the client recognize the manifestations of anxiety, determining whether the client wishes to do anything about the anxiety, and facilitating coping strategies (McCloskey & Bulechek, 2000).

- Provide reassurance and comfort:
  - Set aside time to sit quietly with the client.
  - Speak slowly and calmly.
  - Convey empathetic understanding by touch and supporting present coping mechanisms, such as crying and talking.
  - Do not make demands or expect the client to make decisions.

Coping behaviors differ from situation to situation and from person to person. Anxiety at moderate to severe levels narrows perceptions and the ability to function.

- Decrease sensory stimuli by using short, simple sentences; focusing on the here and now; and providing concise information. *Higher levels of anxiety result in a focus on the present, inability to concentrate, and difficulty in understanding verbal communications.*
- Provide interventions that decrease anxiety levels and increase coping:
  - Provide accurate information about the illness, treatment, and expected length of recovery.
  - Encourage discussion of expected physical changes and ways to minimize disfigurement through cosmetics and clothing.
  - Include family members in teaching sessions.
  - Provide the client with strategies for participating in the recovery process.

Although the prognosis and treatment of melanoma depend on various factors, the prognosis of complete cure is decreased with metastasis. Surgical incisions include excision with wide margins, which may cause disfigurement. Active participation in care give the client some control over the future and is often an effective means of coping with anxiety.

Using NANDA, NIC, and NOC

Chart 14–2 shows links between NANDA, NIC, and NOC when caring for the client with malignant melanoma.

CHART 14–2 NANDA, NIC, AND NOC LINKAGES

The Client with Malignant Melanoma

NURSING DIAGNOSES	NURSING INTERVENTIONS	NURSING OUTCOMES
• Impaired Skin Integrity	• Skin Surveillance • Medication Administration • Infection Control	• Tissue Integrity: Skin and Mucous Membranes
• Impaired Tissue Integrity	• Incision Site Care • Infection Protection • Wound Care	• Wound Healing • Tissue Integrity: Skin and Mucous Membranes
• Risk for Infection	• Infection Control • Wound Care	• Risk Control
• Hopelessness	• Hope Instillation • Sleep Enhancement • Spiritual Support	• Hope • Sleep • Spiritual Well-Being

Note. Data from Nursing Outcomes Classification (NOC) *by M. Johnson & M. Maas (Eds.), 1997, St. Louis: Mosby;* Nursing Diagnoses: Definitions & Classification 2001–2002 *by North American Nursing Diagnosis Association, 2001, Philadelphia: NANDA;* Nursing Interventions Classification (NIC) *by J.C. McCloskey & G. M. Bulechek (Eds.), 2000, St. Louis: Mosby. Reprinted by permission.*

Home Care

Teaching the client and family experiencing the diagnosis and treatment of malignant melanoma involves self-care and ongoing self-monitoring. Education for the client and family is specific to the type of treatment. In addition to wound care, clients who have had a lymph node dissection need instructions in how to protect the extremity from bleeding, trauma, and infection. In addition, address the following topics.

- Clients should schedule regular medical checkups every 3 months for the first 2 years, every 6 months for the next 5 years, and yearly thereafter.
- Emphasize that proper self-care combined with regular medical care can help the client lead a fairly normal life.
- If assistance for home care is necessary, provide referrals to a community health agency or a home care agency. In addition, refer the client to a local cancer support group if the client believes this will be helpful.

Nursing Care Plan
A Client with Malignant Melanoma

Geoff Sanders, age 69, is retired from the postal service. He has always been an avid participant in outdoor sports: When he was younger he played baseball and tennis, and for the last 10 years he has played golf at least twice a week. He now lives in Connecticut, but as a younger man he lived in Florida for almost 15 years. Mr. Sanders has a variety of warts and moles and rarely pays attention to them. However, after taking a shower one day he noticed that a mole on his left lower leg looked bigger and darker. Mr. Sanders had just seen a public announcement on television about the dangers of changes in moles, and he immediately called his primary HMO physician for an appointment at the dermatology clinic.

ASSESSMENT

On arriving at the clinic, Mr. Sanders is interviewed and examined by Tom Hall, a clinical nurse specialist. Following the assessment, Tom documents the following information.

Mr. Sanders has a family history of skin cancer; his father had several squamous cell cancers removed from his face. He has numerous nevi on his body; the one causing concern is located on the medial anterior left leg, 2 inches below the patella. Mr. Sanders states that the mole has been present for years but that he noticed just yesterday that it has become larger and darker. On further questioning, he states that the mole itches sometimes but has never hurt or bled. Mr. Sanders lived in Florida for 15 years and now experiences a sunburn early each summer before he tans. The sunburn involves the lower legs because Mr. Sanders wears shorts during his twice-weekly golf game.

A complete skin assessment reveals various freckles, warts, and nevi. With the exception of the nevus that prompted Mr. Sanders to come to the clinic, all lesions appear normal. The nevus in question is raised, 3 cm in diameter, with irregular borders and a nodular surface. It is variegated in color, with various shades of brown. The skin surrounding the nevus is slightly erythematous. Inguinal lymph nodes are not enlarged or painful. Tom Hall takes a photograph of the lesion with Mr. Sanders's permission.

Following the assessment, Mr. Sanders discusses the lesion with a surgeon, who recommends excision. They discuss the possibility of skin cancer and the importance of early detection and treatment. Mr. Sanders is scheduled for a biopsy of the nevus under a local anesthetic the following morning. Following the biopsy, histologic examination reveals lentigo maligna melanoma. Staging of the tumor reveals that it is a melanoma in situ, with no metastasis to regional lymph nodes. Mr. Sanders undergoes a wide excision of the lesion the following afternoon.

DIAGNOSIS

- *Impaired skin integrity* related to excision of melanoma from the left lower leg
- *Risk for infection* related to surgical wound on left lower leg
- *Acute pain* related to wide excision of melanoma on left lower leg
- *Anxiety* related to diagnosis of skin cancer

EXPECTED OUTCOMES

- Demonstrate complete healing of the incision without manifestations of infection.
- Verbalize relief of pain by the time the incision is healed.
- Verbalize fears and concerns about his diagnosis.

PLANNING AND IMPLEMENTATION

- Make the first dressing change, but ensure that Mr. Sanders can safely change the dressing himself prior to discharge the day after surgery.
- On discharge, provide adequate dressings and tape for the first home dressing change; include in discharge instructions necessary information about where to buy supplies and how many dressing supplies will be needed.
- Review and provide written instructions for prescribed systemic antibiotic and pain medication.
- Provide written instructions for dressing change, manifestations of infection, and phone number of clinic; stress importance of calling if any abnormal symptoms occur.
- Teach how to protect the incision from bumps and to protect the site from irritants.
- Discuss diagnosis, positive outlook for treatment of melanoma in situ, and the client's concerns.
- Stress importance of lifelong regular health care evaluations to identify any recurrence or metastasis.

EVALUATION

Mr. Sanders returned to the dermatology clinic 1 week after his surgical incision. His incision is well approximated and shows no signs of infection. He is taking his antibiotic 4 times a day as prescribed and reports that his need for pain medications is decreasing. During his clinic visit the following week, Tom Hall removes the sutures and assesses the wound as healed. Mr. Sanders completed his antibiotics and no longer requires pain medications. He says he is still "scared to death" about having cancer, but he has decided to join a local cancer support group. He also says he had gotten a list of skin safety rules from the American Cancer

(continued on page 397)

Nursing Care Plan
A Client with Malignant Melanoma (continued)

Society and will be sure to cover up and use sunscreens when he plays golf. Mr. Sanders makes an appointment for follow-up care in 3 months.

Critical Thinking in the Nursing Process
1. Consider reasons why people who notice a change in a skin lesion put off seeking health care. What can nurses do to effect change?
2. Design a teaching plan for young adults for preventing skin cancers.

3. What would you say to Mr. Sanders if he called the clinic and said that the antibiotics were making him sick and he didn't think he needed them anyway?
4. Design a nursing care plan for Mr. Sanders for the diagnosis *Powerlessness*.

See Evaluating Your Response in Appendix C.

SKIN TRAUMA

Trauma to the skin can be unintentional or intentional (as in the case of surgery). Chemicals, radiation, pressure, or thermal changes cause skin trauma. This section discusses pressure ulcers and frostbite, as well as intentional trauma from cutaneous and plastic surgery or treatment. Thermal injury, or burns, is discussed in Chapter 15.

THE CLIENT WITH A PRESSURE ULCER

Pressure ulcers are ischemic lesions of the skin and underlying tissue caused by external pressure that impairs the flow of blood and lymph (Porth, 2002). The ischemia causes tissue necrosis and eventual ulceration. These ulcers, also called bed sores or decubitus ulcers, tend to develop over a bony prominence (such as the heels, greater trochanter, sacrum, and ischia), but they may appear on the skin of any part of the body subjected to external pressure, friction, or shearing forces.

INCIDENCE

The incidence of pressure ulcers in hospitals, long-term care facilities, and home settings is high enough to warrant concern for health care providers. The incidence in hospitals has been reported as ranging from 3.5% to 29%, whereas the incidence in long-term care facilities is reported to be around 23%. Little research has been done to determine the extent of the problem in the home setting. However, with increasing numbers of clients (and especially older adult clients) being cared for in the home, it is probable that the incidence is great enough to warrant plans of care to prevent their occurrence.

PATHOPHYSIOLOGY

Pressure ulcers develop from external pressure that compresses blood vessels or from friction and shearing forces that tear and injure vessels. Both types of pressure cause traumatic injury and initiate the process of pressure ulcer development.

External pressure that is greater than capillary pressure and arteriolar pressure interrupts blood flow in capillary beds. When pressure is applied to skin over a bony prominence for 2 hours, tissue ischemia and hypoxia from external pressure cause irreversible tissue damage. For example, when the body is in the supine position, the body's weight applies pressure to the sacrum. The same amount of pressure causes more damage when it is applied to a small area than when it is distributed over a large surface.

Shearing forces result when one tissue layer slides over another. The stretching and bending of blood vessels cause injury and thrombosis. Clients in hospital beds are subject to shearing forces when the head of the bed is elevated and the torso slides down toward the foot of the bed. Pulling the client up in bed also subjects the client to shearing forces. (For this reason, always lift clients up in bed). In both cases, friction and moisture cause the skin and superficial fascia to remain fixed to the bed sheet, while the deep fascia and bony skeleton slides in the direction of body movement.

When a person lies or sits in one position for an extended length of time without moving, pressure on the tissue between a bony prominence and the external surface of the body distorts capillaries and interferes with normal blood flow. If the pressure is relieved, blood flow to the area increases, and a brief period of reactive hyperemia occurs without permanent damage. However, if the pressure continues, platelets aggregate in the endothelial cells surrounding the capillaries and form microthrombi. These microthrombi impede blood flow, resulting in ischemia and hypoxia of tissues. Eventually, the cells and tissues of the immediate area of pressure and of the surrounding area die and become necrotic.

Alterations in the involved tissue depend on the depth of the injury. Injury to superficial layers of skin results in blister formation, whereas injury to deeper structures causes the pressure ulcer area to appear dark reddish-blue. As the tissues die, the ulcer becomes an open wound that may be deep enough to expose the bone. The necrotic tissue elicits an inflammatory

BOX 14–5 ■ Pressure Ulcer Staging

STAGE I

Nonblanchable erythema of intact skin; the heralding lesion of skin ulceration. Identification of stage I pressure ulcers may be difficult in clients with darkly pigmented skin. *Note:* Reactive hyperemia can normally be expected to be present for one-half to three-fourths as long as the pressure occluded blood flow to the area. This should not be confused with stage I pressure ulcer.

STAGE II

Partial-thickness skin loss involving epidermis and/or dermis. The ulcer is superficial and presents clinically as an abrasion, blister, or shallow crater.

STAGE III

Full-thickness skin loss involving damage or necrosis of subcutaneous tissue that may extend down to, but not through, underlying fascia. The ulcer presents clinically as a deep crater with or without undermining of adjacent tissue.

STAGE IV

Full-thickness skin loss with extensive destruction, tissue necrosis, or damage to muscle, bone, or supporting structures (for example, tendon or joint capsule). Sinus tracts may also be associated with stage IV ulcers.

Note: When eschar is present, accurate staging of the pressure ulcer is not possible until the eschar has sloughed or the wound has been debrided.

Note. Text is from Pressure Ulcers in Adults: Prediction and Prevention *by the Agency for Health Care Policy and Research, 1992, Rockville, MD: U.S. Department of Health and Human Services. Photos courtesy of Karen Lou Kennedy, RN, FPN.*

response, and the client experiences increases in temperature, pain, and white blood cell count. Secondary bacterial invasion is common. Enzymes from bacteria and macrophages dissolve necrotic tissue, resulting in a foul-smelling drainage.

Pressure ulcers are graded or staged to classify the degree of damage. The stages are listed in Box 14–5.

RISK FACTORS

Although a pressure ulcer may develop in an adult of any age who has an impairment in mobility, those most at risk are older adults with limited mobility (see page 399), people with quadriplegia, and clients in the critical care setting (Porth, 2002).

Other clients prone to develop pressure ulcers are those with fractures of large bones (e.g., hip or femur) or who have undergone orthopedic surgery or sustained spinal cord injury. In addition to deficits in mobility and activity, incontinence and nutritional deficit also increase the risk of pressure ulcer development. Clients with chronic illnesses, such as renal failure and anemia, and those with edema or infection are also at increased risk.

Because of age-related skin changes, the older adult is at increased risk for the development of pressure ulcers. The skin of the older adult has a thicker epidermis, a thinner dermis with decreased vascularity, decreased sebaceous gland activity, and

Meeting Individualized Needs

PRESSURE ULCER PREVENTION IN OLDER ADULTS

Older adults are at a greater risk for developing pressure ulcers because of age-related changes in the integumentary system. Cell renewal slows, resulting in skin that has decreased elasticity. The margin between the epidermis and the dermis separates more easily, making the skin more prone to tearing. In addition, thinning subcutaneous tissue provides less cushioning over bony prominences. Water content decreases, and the skin becomes drier. These changes increase the older adult's susceptibility to skin trauma and prolong wound healing.

Chronic conditions associated with immobility and self-care deficit place older adults at risk of developing pressure ulcers. For example, bowel or bladder incontinence can produce regions of wet skin that are prone to infections and breakdown. Furthermore, sensory-perceptual alterations and impaired cognitive functioning may reduce the frequency in which the older adult shifts position when sitting or lying in bed. Finally, undernutrition, which is often seen in older adults, heightens the risk for developing pressure ulcers.

To prevent pressure ulcers, the skin of older adults should be kept clean, dry, and well hydrated. Moisturizers are recommended to keep the skin free of excessive dryness. Older adults should be taught to avoid bumping into furniture and to wear long skirts or pants to help protect the lower extremities from trauma.

When hospitalized, older adults should have a validated risk assessment for pressure ulcers completed on admission and as often as the tool suggests. A daily systematic skin inspection with particular attention to bony prominences should be completed.

Once pressure ulcers develop in older adults, the treatment is the same as for younger clients. However, there are additional steps that may need to be taken. Because local perfusion to tissues is compromised, steps should be taken to prevent under or over hydration. It is essential that optimal nutritional status be maintained. Also, keep in mind that it may take a longer time for the pressure ulcer to heal.

decreased strength and elasticity. As a result, the more fragile and less nourished dermal layer is more prone to shear and friction problems. In addition, the skin of the older adult responds more slowly to inflammation, and wounds heal more slowly; when pressure ulcers occur, they are more difficult to reverse.

COLLABORATIVE CARE

For the client at risk for pressure ulcers, the goal is prevention. Existing ulcers require collaborative treatment to promote healing and restore skin integrity.

Diagnostic tests are conducted to determine the presence of a secondary infection and to differentiate the cause of the ulcer.

If the ulcer is deep or appears infected, drainage or biopsied tissue is cultured to determine the causative organism.

Topical and systemic antibiotics specific to the infectious organism eradicate any infection present. Additionally, a variety of topical products promote healing. Examples are listed in Table 14–4.

Surgical debridement may be necessary if the pressure ulcer is deep; if subcutaneous tissues are involved; or if an eschar (a scab or dry crust that forms over skin damaged by burns, infections, or excoriations) has formed over the ulcer, preventing healing by granulation. Large wounds may require skin grafting for complete closure.

TABLE 14–4 Products Used to Treat Pressure Ulcers

Stage	Product	Purpose
I	Skin Prep	Toughens intact skin and preserves skin integrity.
	Granulex	Prevents skin breakdown, increases blood supply, adds moisture, contains trypsin to aid in removal of necrotic tissue.
	Hydrocolloid dressing (e.g., DuoDerm)	Prevents skin breakdown and promotes healing without the formation of a crust over the ulcer. Is permeable to air and water vapor; prevents the growth of anaerobic organisms.
	Transparent dressing (e.g., Tegaderm)	Prevents skin breakdown; prevents entrance of moisture and bacteria but allows oxygen and moisture vapor permeability.
II	Transparent dressing	Enhances healing (see above).
	Hydrocolloid dressing	Enhances healing (see above). Note: If infection is present, these types of dressings are contraindicated. A sterile dressing should be applied instead.
III	Wet-to-dry gauze dressing with sterile normal saline	Allows necrotic material to soften and adhere to the gauze, so that the wound is debrided.
	Hydrocolloid dressing	Enhances healing (see above).
	Proteolytic enzymes (such as Elase)	Proteolytic enzymes serve as a debriding agent in inflamed and infected lesions.
IV	Wet-to-dry gauze dressing with sterile normal saline	Enhances healing (see above). Note: Transparent or hydrocolloid dressings or skin barriers are contraindicated.
	Vacuum-assisted closure (V.A.C.)	Creates a negative pressure to help reduce edema, increase blood supply and oxygenation, and decrease bacterial colonization. Also helps promote moist wound healing and the formation of granulation tissue.

Nursing Research

Evidence-Based Practice for Preventing Pressure Ulcers in Acute Care and Home Care Settings

Chronic wounds treated in the United States are a growing and costly health care problem. It is estimated that 5.6 million chronic wounds are treated each year, and that the cost for pressure ulcers alone is $1.3 billion. One way to decrease the human and economic cost is to prevent pressure ulcers from forming in the first place. Pieper et al. (1997a, 1997b) have studied this problem extensively, examining the presence of pressure ulcer methods for at-risk clients (those with more medical diagnoses and longer hospitalizations) as compared to not-at-risk clients in hospital, acute rehabilitation, and home settings. Findings from these studies were that at-risk clients were more likely to have the head of the bed in a low position, a pressure-reducing bed surface, a positioning wedge, incontinence cleanser and ointment, heel protection, a trapeze, and a posted turning schedule. At-risk clients were also more likely to have a prevention care plan and documentation of prevention methods. It is important to implement these preventive methods as soon as possible, as ulcers develop quickly.

IMPLICATIONS FOR NURSING
The design and implementation of a pressure ulcer care plan is essential for any person who is at risk, including the older adult, those with disorders limiting mobility, and those with debilitating or multiple illnesses. Nursing care is critical to the prevention of this problem. As documented in these studies, the percentage of clients placed on a pressure ulcer–prevention program was low for those considered both at-risk and not-at-risk. Health care providers and institutions must continue to explore this critical area affecting client outcomes.

Critical Thinking in Client Care
1. Describe the differences and similarities in a pressure ulcer–prevention plan of care you would develop for two clients: a 76-year-old man in a nursing home who has had a stroke that paralyzed the left side of his body, and a 36-year-old man with spinal cord damage from a motorcycle accident who cannot walk and lives at home.
2. Consider the activities necessary to prevent pressure ulcers. If you were managing a client's care, what would you do about the following:
   a. What level of health care provider would you assign to care for the client?
   b. How much time in an 8-hour period would be needed for nursing care?
   c. What would you teach family caregivers about providing activities at home?

NURSING CARE

The client with one or more pressure ulcers not only has impaired skin integrity but also is at increased risk for infection, pain, and decreased mobility. Pressure ulcers also prolong treatment for other conditions, increase health care costs, and diminish the client's quality of life (see the box above).

Nursing Diagnoses and Interventions

The following interventions and rationales are adapted from the clinical guidelines developed by the Agency for Health Care Policy and Research (1992, 1994) in identifying adults at risk and treating those with stage I pressure ulcers.

Risk for Impaired Skin Integrity
- Identify at-risk individuals needing prevention and the specific factors placing them at risk.
- Assess bed- and chair-bound clients, as well as those who are unable to reposition themselves, for additional risk factors: immobility, incontinence, nutritional factors (such as inadequate dietary intake and impaired nutritional status), and altered level of consciousness.
- Assess clients on admission to acute care and rehabilitation hospitals, nursing homes, home care programs, and other health care facilities.
- Use a systematic risk assessment by using a validated risk assessment tool (such as the Braden scale).
- Document all assessments of risk.

Individuals at risk for pressure ulcers must be identified so that risk factors can be reduced through intervention. The primary risk factors for pressure ulcers are immobility and limited activity; therefore, assess clients who cannot reposition themselves or whose activity is limited to bed or chair. Validated tools ensure systematic evaluation of individual risk factors. The client requires periodic reassessment for pressure ulcers. Accurate and complete documentation of all risk assessments ensures continuity of care and may be used as a foundation for the skin care plan.

- Conduct a systematic skin inspection at least once a day, paying particular attention to the bony prominences. Systematic, comprehensive, and routine skin care may decrease pressure ulcer incidence (although the exact role is unknown. Inspect the following to assess a pressure ulcer:
  - Location of any lesion or ulcer
  - Estimation of the stage
  - Dimensions of the ulcer: length, width, depth
  - Presence of any abnormal pathways in the wound
    - Sinus tract: a cavity or channel underneath the wound
    - Tunneling: a passageway or opening that may be visible at skin level, but with most of the tunnel under the surface of the skin
    - Undermining: areas of tissue destruction underneath intact skin along wound margins
  - Visible necrotic tissue (Slough is necrotic tissue that is in the process of separating from viable tissue.)
  - Presence of an exudate
  - Presence or absence of granulation tissue

Skin inspection provides data the nurse uses in designing interventions to reduce risk and in evaluating outcomes of those interventions.

- Clean the skin at the time of soiling and at routine intervals, as frequently as the client's need or preference dictates. Avoid hot water, use a mild cleansing agent, and clean the skin gently, applying as little force and friction as possible. *Metabolic wastes and environmental contaminants accumulate on the skin; these potentially irritating substances should be removed frequently. Feces and urine cause chemical irritation and should be removed as soon as possible. Hot water may cause skin injury. Mild cleansing agents are less likely to remove the skin's natural barrier.*

- Minimize environmental factors leading to skin drying, such as low humidity and exposure to cold. Treat dry skin with moisturizers. *Well-hydrated skin resists mechanical trauma. Hydration decreases as the ambient air temperature decreases, especially when the air humidity is low. Poorly hydrated skin is less pliable, and severe dryness is associated with fissuring and cracking of the stratum corneum. Moisturizers reduce dry skin.*

- Avoid massage over bony prominences. *Although massage has been practiced for years, evidence now suggests that massage over bony prominences may lead to deep tissue trauma in clients at risk for or with beginning skin manifestations of a pressure ulcer.*

- Minimize skin exposure to moisture due to incontinence, perspiration, or wound drainage. When these sources of moisture cannot be controlled, use underpads or briefs made of materials that absorb moisture and present a quick-drying surface to the skin. Change underpads and briefs frequently. Do not place plastic directly against the skin. *Moisture from incontinence, perspiration, or wound drainage may contain factors that irritate the skin; moisture alone can increase the susceptibility of the skin to injury.*

- To minimize skin injury due to friction and shearing forces, use proper positioning, transferring, and turning techniques. Lubricants (such as cornstarch or creams), protective films (such as transparent dressings and skin sealants), protective dressings (such as hydrocolloids), and protective padding may also reduce friction injuries. *Shear injury occurs when skin remains stationary and the underlying tissue shifts. This shift diminishes the blood supply to the skin and results in ischemia and tissue damage. Proper positioning, however, can eliminate most shear injuries. Friction injuries to the skin occur when it moves across a coarse surface, such as bed linens. Most friction injuries can be avoided by using appropriate techniques to move clients so that their skin is never dragged across the linens. Any agent that eliminates contact or decreases the friction between the skin and the linens reduces the potential for injury.*

- Assess factors involved in inadequate dietary intake of protein or kilocalories. Offer nutritional supplements, and support the client during mealtimes. If dietary intake re-mains inadequate, consult with a dietitian about other dietary interventions. *The role nutrition plays in the development of (and to a lesser degree, the healing of) pressure ulcers is not understood, but poor dietary intake of kilocalories, protein, and iron has been associated with the development of pressure ulcers.*

- Maintain the client's current level of activity, mobility, and range of motion. *Frequent turning, repositioning, and movement are essential in reducing the risk of pressure ulcers.*

- For the client on bed rest or who is immobile, provide interventions against the adverse effects of external mechanical forces of pressure, friction, and shear:
  - Reposition all at-risk clients at least every 2 hours, using a written schedule for systematic turning and repositioning.
  - For clients on bed rest, use positioning devices, such as pillows or foam wedges, to protect bony prominences.

- For completely immobile clients, use devices to totally relieve pressure on the heels (the most common method is to raise the heels off the bed). Do not use donut-type devices.

- Avoid placing clients in the side-lying position directly on the trochanter.

- Maintain the head of the bed at the lowest degree of elevation consistent with the client's medical condition and other restrictions. Limit the amount of time the head of the bed is elevated.

- Use assistive devices, such as a trapeze or bed linen, to move clients in bed who cannot assist during transfers and position changes.

- Place any at-risk client on a pressure-reducing device, such as foam, static air, alternating air, gel, or water mattress.

Data indicate that the more spontaneous movements that bedridden, older adult clients make, the lower the incidence of pressure ulcers. Studies reveal that fewer pressure ulcers develop in at-risk clients who are turned every 2 to 3 hours. Proper positioning can reduce pressure on bony prominences. It is difficult to redistribute pressure under heels; suspending the heels is the best method. Donut cushions are more likely to cause than to prevent pressure ulcers. Shearing forces are exerted on the body when the head of the bed is elevated. Lifting (rather than dragging) is less likely to cause injury from friction. Pressure-reducing devices and beds can decrease the incidence of pressure ulcers.

- For chair-bound clients, use pressure-reducing devices. Consider postural alignment, distribution of weight, balance and stability, and pressure relief when positioning these clients. Avoid uninterrupted sitting in a chair or wheelchair. Reposition the client every hour. Teach clients who can do so to shift their weight every 15 minutes. Use a written plan for positioning, movement, and the use of positioning devices. Do not use donut devices. *Prolonged, uninterrupted mechanical pressure results in tissue breakdown. The client's weight should be shifted at least every hour.*

Home Care

Client and family teaching for care of a pressure ulcer also focuses on prevention and includes much of the same information presented in the preceding section. Because many clients with pressure ulcers are older or have other serious illnesses, a caregiver may require teaching on such topics as the following:

- Definition and description of pressure ulcers
- Common locations of pressure ulcers
- Risk factors for the development of pressure ulcers
- Skin care
- Ways to avoid injury
- Diet

Depending on the stage of the pressure ulcer, the nurse teaches the client or caregiver how to care for ulcers that are already present: how to change wet-to-dry dressings, apply skin barriers, and avoid injury and infection. Referrals to a home health agency or community health department can help the family through the lengthy healing process.

THE CLIENT WITH FROSTBITE

Frostbite is an injury of the skin from freezing. If the exposure to freezing temperatures is limited, only the skin and subcutaneous tissues become involved. However, as exposure increases, deeper structures freeze. The skin freezes when the temperature drops to 14° to 24.8°F (210° to 24°C). Frostbite is most common on exposed or peripheral areas of the body, such as the nose, ears, feet, and hands.

As human tissues freeze, ice crystals form and increase intracellular sodium content. Small blood vessels initially vasoconstrict but then vasodilate and become more permeable, causing cellular and tissue swelling. With continued exposure, vasoconstriction and increased viscosity of the blood cause infarction and necrosis of the affected tissue.

Superficial frostbite causes numbness, itching, and prickling. The skin appears cyanotic, reddened, or white. Deeper frostbite causes stiffness and paresthesias. As the skin and tissues thaw, the skin becomes white or yellow and loses its elasticity. The client experiences burning pain. Edema, blisters, necrosis, and gangrene may appear.

Rapid thawing may significantly decrease tissue necrosis. General guidelines for rewarming areas of frostbite follow:

- If you are outdoors, treat superficial frostbite by applying firm pressure with a warm hand or by placing frostbitten hands in the axillae. If the feet are frostbitten, remove wet footwear, dry the feet, and put on dry footwear. Do not rub the areas with snow.
- In the hospital, rapidly rewarm affected areas in circulating warm water, 104° to 105°F (40° to 40.5°C) for 20 to 30 minutes. Do not rub or massage the areas.

Following rewarming, the client is kept on bed rest with the affected parts elevated. Pain medications and anti-inflammatory agents are administered. Blisters are debrided. Whirlpool ther-

apy may be used to clean the skin and debride necrotic tissue. Recovery from frostbite is usually complete if the involved area has not become necrotic. Necrotic tissue may require amputation.

THE CLIENT UNDERGOING CUTANEOUS AND PLASTIC SURGERY

Although many skin disorders are so small and benign that no treatment is necessary, others require some type of surgery of the skin to remove the lesion. Other surgeries and treatments for skin lesions and deformities are used to restore function and change appearance. This section discusses both cutaneous and plastic surgery, as well as other types of treatment modalities used in the care of the client with a skin disorder.

CUTANEOUS SURGERY AND PROCEDURES

The basic types of cutaneous surgery described here are excision, electrosurgery, cryosurgery, curettage, and laser surgery. Two nonsurgical procedures, chemical destruction and sclerotherapy, are also discussed. Most of these procedures are performed in the office or outpatient clinic.

Fusiform Excision

Fusiform excision is the removal of a full thickness of the epidermis and dermis, usually with a thin layer of subcutaneous tissue. It is used to remove tissue for biopsies and for complete removal of benign and malignant lesions of the skin. Most fusiform excisions have a length-to-width ratio of 3 to 1.

Excision of small, superficial lesions is performed under a local anesthetic, and care is taken to place the incision in a way that will provide good cosmetic results. The incision line is usually closed with sutures, and the wound is covered with a dry dressing, an occlusive dressing, or a hydrocolloid dressing.

Electrosurgery

Electrosurgery involves the destruction or removal of tissue with high-frequency alternating current. A variety of surgical procedures may be performed, including *electrodesiccation* (which produces superficial skin destruction), *electrocoagulation* (which produces deeper tissue destruction), and *electrosection* (which can cut through skin and tissue). Electrodesiccation is used to remove benign surface lesions, such as skin tags, keratoses, warts, and angiomas. It is also used to produce hemostasis for capillary bleeding. Electrocoagulation is used to remove telangiectases, warts, and superficial nonmelanoma skin cancers. Electrosection is used to make incisions, excise tissue, and perform biopsies.

Cryosurgery

Cryosurgery is the destruction of tissue by cold or freezing with agents such as fluorocarbon sprays, carbon dioxide snow, nitrous oxide, and liquid nitrogen. Cryosurgery is used to treat many skin lesions (e.g., keratoses, lentigo maligna, venous lakes, nevi, keloids, and Kaposi's sarcoma). The freezing agents are applied topically to the lesion.

The effects of freezing depend on the degree of freeze. Light freezing causes damage to the epidermis with blistering or crusting that heals without scarring. Deeper freezes, used to treat malignant cells, cause edema, necrosis, and tissue slough. The effects of cryosurgery may not be obvious until 24 hours following the treatment. Postoperatively, infection is prevented by applying a topical antibiotic and keeping the treated areas clean. Healing occurs in 2 to 3 weeks.

Curettage

Curettage is the removal of lesions with a curette (a semisharp cutting instrument). The design of the curette allows it to cut through soft or weak tissue, but not through normal tissue. It is used primarily to remove benign and malignant superficial epidermal lesions. Benign lesions removed by curettage include keratoses, nevi, and angiomas. Nonmelanoma skin lesions are removed by curettage if they are small, well-defined, primary tumors. Curettage is also used to remove specimens of tissue for biopsy.

Following curettage, the wound may be treated with electrodesiccation to destroy any remaining malignant cells and to provide hemostasis. These wounds are not closed; rather, they are left open to heal by second intention. Topical antibiotic ointments and dressings may be used in the postoperative period.

Laser Surgery

Laser surgery is used to treat clients with a wide variety of skin disorders, including port-wine stains, telangiectases, and venous lakes. A laser is an intense light that produces a thermal injury on contact with tissue. The injury causes coagulation, vaporization, excision, and ablation (removal of a growth). Argon, pulsed dye, carbon dioxide, and Nd: YAG lasers are used in cutaneous and plastic surgery. A local anesthetic may be used, although pulsed dye laser causes minimal pain and rarely requires anesthesia.

The response differs by type of laser. Following treatment with the argon laser, the lesion appears from white to black in color, a blister forms, and the skin may peel. The area weeps, and an eschar forms; in 10 to 14 days, the eschar separates, revealing an underlying red area. The redness fades over a period of up to 1 year. However, pulsed dye laser does not result in blistering or weeping; only rarely does it result in eschar.

Chemical Destruction

Chemical destruction is the application of a specific chemical to produce destruction of skin lesions. Chemical destruction is used to treat both benign and premalignant lesions. The chemical is applied to the lesion or is used to cause peeling. After application, the treated area forms a thin crust that sloughs off in about a week.

Sclerotherapy

Sclerotherapy is the removal of benign skin lesions with a sclerosing agent that causes inflammation with fibrosis of tissue. Agents that cause therapeutic sclerosis include aethoxysklerol (Sclerodex) and hypertonic sodium chloride. This type of treatment is used for telangiectases and superficial spider veins of the lower extremities. The solution is injected into the affected veins, causing a reaction that closes the lumen of the vein.

PLASTIC SURGERY

Plastic surgery is the alteration, replacement, or restoration of visible portions of the body, performed to correct a structural or cosmetic defect. The word *plastic* comes from the Greek word *plastikos,* which means "able to be molded."

Many skin disorders discussed in this chapter cause changes in appearance. For example, acne may leave deep pitting scars, nevi and keloids are often disfiguring, and skin cancers may require wide excision and skin grafting. These scars, lesions, and wounds often cause embarrassment and alterations in body image. In addition, the removal of lesions may leave unsightly scars or areas of obviously missing tissue.

Cosmetic surgery, also called **aesthetic surgery,** is one of two fields within plastic surgery. Cosmetic surgery enhances the attractiveness of normal features. The other field, **reconstructive surgery,** uses similar techniques; however, its purpose is to improve the function or appearance of parts of the body damaged by trauma, disease, or birth defects. Reconstructive surgeries comprise approximately 60% of all plastic surgeries performed in the United States.

Many of the plastic surgeries permanently alter body image. To provide the client with a preview of what surgery will accomplish, some surgeons integrate computer imaging into preoperative teaching. The computer projects a photograph of the targeted area onto a monitor and uses graphics to demonstrate how the size and or shape of the body part or area will change as a result of the surgery.

Skin Grafts and Flaps

Skin grafts and flaps are used to restore function while also maintaining an acceptable appearance. Both of these procedures involve the movement of skin from one part of the body to another part.

A **skin graft** is a surgical method of detaching skin from a donor site and placing it in a recipient site, where it develops a new blood supply from the base of the wound. Skin grafting is an effective way to cover wounds which have a good blood supply, which are not infected, and in which bleeding can be controlled.

Skin grafts may be either split thickness or full thickness (Figure 14–30 ■). A *split-thickness graft* contains epidermis and only a portion of dermis of the donor site. Split-thickness grafts range in thickness from 0.010 inch to greater than 0.015 inch. A common donor site for a skin graft is the anterior thigh. Skin is removed in sheets from the donor site with a dermatome. Donor sites of split-thickness grafts heal by reepithelialization. A meshed graft is a type of split-thickness graft that is rolled under a special cutting machine to form a mesh pattern with perforations. The perforations allow drainage of serum and blood from under the graft. After healing, however, the skin has a rough appearance. A *full-thickness graft* contains both epidermis and dermis. These layers contain the greatest number of skin elements (sweat glands, sebaceous glands, or

Figure 14–30 ■ Skin depth of split-thickness and full-thickness grafts.

Epidermis
Dermis
Subcutaneous tissue

Thin
Intermediate
Thick

Split-thickness graft
Full-thickness graft

hair follicles) and are best able to withstand trauma. Areas of thin skin are the best donor sites for full-thickness skin grafts. The donor site must be surgically closed and will scar.

Other types of grafts are composite grafts and cultured epithelial grafts. Composite grafts are free grafts and are usually used on the face. They contain skin, subcutaneous tissue, cartilage, or other tissue. Cultured epithelial grafts are made from epithelial cells cultured in vivo, coalesced into sheets, and then used to cover full-thickness wounds. They are used primarily to treat burns.

A **flap** is a piece of tissue whose free end is moved from a donor site to a recipient site while maintaining a continuous blood supply through its connection at the base or pedicle. Flaps carry their own blood supply and are therefore used to cover recipient sites that have a poor blood supply or have sustained a major tissue loss. They are often used for reconstruction or closure of large wounds. Microsurgical techniques, with anastomosis of small blood vessels and nerves, allow reconstruction with free flaps (in which the flap is completely removed from its donor site and moved to the recipient site).

Chemical Peeling

Chemical peeling is the application of a chemical to produce a controlled and predictable injury that alters the anatomy of the epidermis and superficial dermis. The result is skin that appears firmer, smoother, and less wrinkled. This form of cosmetic surgery is more useful in people who have fair, thin skin with fine wrinkling.

Chemical agents used for peeling include phenol, trichloroacetic acid (TCA), and alpha-hydroxy acids (AHA). Phenol, a keratocoagulant, penetrates the epidermis and dermis; regeneration of the epithelium produces the desired results. After treatment, the entire surface of the face except the eyelids is covered with adhesive tape for 1 to 2 days. The adhesive is then removed, and the treated area forms a crust that heals in about a week. TCA has been used for years to obtain the desired effect. A light peel causes mild erythema followed by peeling (as from a mild sunburn) in 3 to 5 days. AHA are organic acids used to produce light to moderate peeling to remove acne, fine lines, seborrheic keratosis, warts, and mild scarring. Both TCA and AHA treatments may be repeated weekly. One complica-

tion of chemical peeling is bleaching of the skin (due to removal of melanocytes).

Liposuction

Liposuction is a method of changing the contours of the body by aspirating fat from the subcutaneous layer of tissue. This treatment is used to remove excess fat from the buttocks, flanks, abdomen, thighs, upper arms, knees, ankles, and chin. It is not a cure for obesity and should not be used as a substitute for weight loss. The procedure is usually done for younger clients because their skin is more elastic. Liposuction may be performed on either an outpatient or inpatient basis.

To aspirate the fat, a small incision is made close to the area, and a suction cannula or curette is inserted and attached to a suction apparatus. The high vacuum pressure caused by the suction machine causes fat cells to emulsify, and they are aspirated out of the body. Following removal of the fat, a pressure dressing is applied to help the skin conform to the new tissue size.

Dermabrasion

Dermabrasion is a method of removing facial scars, severe acne, and pigment from unwanted tattoos. The area is sprayed with a chemical to cause light freezing and is then abraded with sandpaper or a revolving wire brush to remove the epidermis and a portion of the dermis.

Facial Reconstructive Surgery

Many different reconstructive surgeries may be performed to correct deformities or improve cosmetic appearance. Those discussed here are rhinoplasty, blepharoplasty, and rhytidectomy (face-lift).

- A *rhinoplasty* is conducted to improve the appearance of the external nose. The nasal skeleton is reshaped, and the overlying skin and subcutaneous tissue are allowed to redrape over the new framework. A submucous resection of the nasal septum is often done at the same time; this surgery resects a segment of the septal cartilage to improve the nasal airway and also to alter the appearance of the nose. This surgery is done through incisions within the nose, so no visible scars remain after healing.

- A *blepharoplasty* is a cosmetic surgery in which loose skin and protruding periorbital fat is removed from the upper and lower eyelids. With aging, the eyelid skin sags, allowing the periorbital fat to bulge; the skin of the upper eyelid can be so lax that it partially obstructs vision. The procedure is performed under local anesthesia, and excess skin and fat are excised. The incision is made in the normal eyelid lines so that scars are not visible after healing.

- A *rhytidectomy,* or face-lift, is a cosmetic surgery done to improve appearance by removing excess skin (and sometimes fat) from the face and neck. As one ages, the skin of the face and neck tends to become loose and wrinkled. The procedure is usually performed with local anesthesia. To perform the surgery, bilateral incisions are made from the scalp at the temple, in front of the ear in the natural skin line, around the ear lobe, and to the occipital scalp. The skin is then elevated, fat is removed or suctioned, and excess skin is excised. The incision lines are sutured, and a pressure dressing is applied.

NURSING CARE

Nursing care for the client having cutaneous or plastic surgery is highly individualized. It depends on the type of surgery or procedure performed, the type of deficit treated, the reason for the surgery or procedure, the expected results of the treatment, and the response of the client to the lesion or surgery. Although some surgeries, such as skin grafts and flaps, require in-hospital care, many of the surgeries are carried out in the primary care setting, and the client provides self-care at home following or between treatments.

Nursing Diagnoses and Interventions

Although a variety of nursing diagnoses may be appropriate for the client having cutaneous or plastic surgery or procedures, the most common are *Impaired skin integrity, Acute pain,* and *Disturbed body image.*

Impaired Skin Integrity

The client having surgery of the skin has impaired skin integrity. Skin grafts and flaps are performed to repair large wounds, and it is necessary to inflict further wounds to collect the graft or flap from a donor site. Excisions and various cosmetic surgeries cause wounds. Skin is traumatized by freezing, chemicals, abrasion, sclerosing agents, electrical currents, and lasers. Although all of these treatment modalities are conducted to remove lesions, improve function, or improve appearance, they first impair the integrity of the skin. These impairments increase the risk for infection, which would further impair the skin integrity and may negate the benefits of surgery.

Nurses provide preoperative care and teaching, intraoperative assistance, and postoperative care and teaching; in each case, care and teaching are specific to the type of surgical treatment and the individual client. In all cases, the nurse provides appropriate preoperative interventions to prepare the client physically and emotionally for surgery and the postoperative period. The following interventions are appropriate for the client having inpatient skin grafts or flaps.

- Monitor incisions and graft, and flap donor and recipient sites, for manifestations of infection and necrosis:
  - Take and record vital signs every 4 hours.
  - Monitor all wounds for changes in color, consistency, amount, and odor of drainage every 4 to 8 hours.
  - Monitor wounds for increased swelling, redness, and pain every 4 to 8 hours.
  - Monitor and document assessment of graft every 4 hours.
  - Monitor and document temperature, turgor, color, dermal bleeding, and capillary refill of flaps every 4 hours.

When bacterial infection is present, the inflammatory phase of wound healing is prolonged, retarding healing. Increased body temperature and tachycardia are manifestations of infection. The drainage in wounds that become infected is often increased in amount, purulent, thicker, and has a musty or foul odor. Tissue response to infection includes edema, increased erythema, and pain. Grafts and flaps that do not have adequate blood supply will appear black instead of the normal pink-red color.

- Provide care for the donor site:
  - Position the client to minimize pressure on the donor site.
  - Use a bed cradle to keep linens off the area.
  - If the donor site is left open and a heat lamp is to be applied to the area, place the lamp no closer than 2 feet from the wound.
  - Avoid moving the body part containing the donor site, if possible.
  - If the donor site is on the posterior portion of the body, place the client on a special bed (such as a low-pressure or fluidized bed) to decrease pressure and allow air circulation around the donor site.

Minimizing trauma from pressure and movement facilitates healing of the donor site. Leaving the site open to the air and providing heat increase healing. Special beds minimize ischemia and allow donor sites on the posterior side of the body to dry.

- Encourage a diet high in protein, ascorbic acid, vitamins, and minerals. *An adequate protein intake is necessary to supply amino acids for tissue repair. Vitamin C is necessary for collagen formation and wound strength. Vitamins and minerals contribute to the healing process.*
- Change dressings as prescribed, or if the frequency is not indicated, as necessary. Determine which dressings are not to be removed during the healing process and which are to be changed, and whether the wound is to be kept dry or moist.
  - Use aseptic technique and follow standard precautions when changing dressings.
  - Remove old dressings carefully and gently.
  - Choose the appropriate dressing materials.

Donor sites may be covered with an adherent gauze dressing that is allowed to dry and remains adherent through the healing process. Aseptic techniques prevent secondary bacterial infections. Standard precautions protect the nurse from HIV infection. Unless care is taken, the removal of adherent old dressings may damage the wound by traumatizing granulation tissue or wound edges. The use of semipermeable transparent dressings provides an environment that optimizes wound healing by promoting collagen synthesis and the formation of granulation tissue; it also increases cell migration and epithelial resurfacing and prevents the formation of scabs, crusts, and eschar.

Acute Pain

The client having a graft or flap has two wounds; in fact, the donor site may be more painful than the recipient site. Cutaneous surgeries, dermabrasions, and chemical treatments result in blistering, swelling, and loss of epidermal tissue. The client having facial reconstructive surgery has edema.

- Administer pain medications on a regular basis, following guidelines for controlling pain in clients having operative procedures (see Chapter 4). *Established, severe pain is difficult to control and has negative physical and psychological consequences.*
- Use alternative pain relief measures as appropriate and prescribed, such as ice bags or cold compresses. *Cold reduces swelling, acts as a local anesthetic, and decreases pain.*
- Teach the client noninvasive methods of pain relief, such as deep breathing, relaxation, and guided imagery. *Noninvasive methods of pain relief increase the effectiveness of pain medications and also allow the client some control and self-management of pain.*

Disturbed Body Image

Cosmetic surgery is performed for a variety of reasons in adult clients of all ages. Changes in appearance, especially in a society that values youth and beauty, affect one's self-perception. Lesions or scars, especially of the face, may decrease self-esteem and cause a person to avoid social interactions and relationships. With aging, the skin becomes looser and wrinkles appear; this can be a source of anxiety and despair, especially to the woman who has always prided herself on her youthful appearance. Most clients cite one reason for having plastic surgery: to "feel better about myself."

- Provide preoperative teaching:
  - Explain that bruising and swelling will be present and that it will be several weeks before these responses to surgery disappear.
  - Explain that it may take a year for healing to complete and the final results to appear.

Expectations differ; many people expect immediate results. Knowledge of postoperative responses is necessary for the client to adapt to change. The client may need to make arrangements to take time off from work during the initial healing stage.

- Provide time for the client to verbalize feelings and concerns. Be empathetic, and listen nonjudgmentally. *Such nurse-client interaction facilitates acceptance of changes in body image.*
- Refer to a consultant who can provide information on the use of cosmetics and apparel to enhance personal appearance. *Knowledgeable use of cosmetics and clothing can make scars much less noticeable. If the client feels better about appearance, body image is improved.*

Home Care

The nurse teaches the client and family to provide self-care at home after inpatient and outpatient cutaneous and plastic surgery and procedures. The nurse asks about the client's expectations and stresses that final results will not be seen for several months, providing written instructions about the following topics.

- Wound care, including application of topical medications and dressing changes. If the client is to return to the office or clinic for removal of tape or pressure dressings, or for dressing changes in the first weeks after surgery, an appointment is made. For some procedures, the wound is left open to the air.
- Manifestations of wound infection, such as increased temperature, malaise, changes in the appearance of the wound, or changes in drainage. If any of these manifestations occur, the client should notify the health care provider immediately.
- Specific care for the type of surgery or procedure, such as type of oral care, avoiding blowing the nose, or limiting talking.
- Limitations on physical activity, especially lifting or straining.
- When to resume bathing or showering, shampooing the hair, and using cosmetics.
- The need to avoid picking at crusts or scabs. If the healing wound itches, the client should contact the health care provider for a topical medication.
- Use of a 15 (or higher) SPF sunblock when the client is outdoors. This may be prescribed for several months or for the rest of the client's life.

HAIR AND NAIL DISORDERS

THE CLIENT WITH A DISORDER OF THE HAIR

Although hair disorders are not serious threats to health, they may cause embarrassment and a negative body image. Changes in hair growth and pattern occur secondary to other illnesses and treatment for illness and also as a part of the aging process.

The hair grows at various rates. The male beard grows the most rapidly, followed by the hair of the scalp, axillae,

thighs, and eyebrows. Normally, an adult's hair grows at a rate of 10 to 12 mm per month; however, the growth rate is influenced by both the person's state of health and the environment (hair grows faster in hot climates, more slowly in cold climates).

Racial characteristics and gender influence the amount and type of hair. Caucasians have more facial and body hair than do Asians. People of Mongolian or Native American descent have straight hair, those of African descent have wavy to curly hair, and Caucasians have straight to curly hair. In addition, male hair growth characteristics (such as facial hair and hair on the lower extremities) are normal in certain women of some races and families. Women do not normally become bald.

PATHOPHYSIOLOGY

Hair color, growth, and pattern vary from person to person, and they are determined largely by genetic inheritance. However, changes do occur. For example, in some instances, hair loss recurs in successive generations of males in a family; in other cases, hair loss may be the result of chemotherapy. Excessive facial hair may be a response to certain endocrine disorders or to the loss of estrogen after menopause. These changes may seem minor, but they may create psychosocial problems for the person experiencing the changes.

Hirsutism

Hirsutism, also called hypertrichosis, is the appearance of excessive hair in normal and abnormal areas of the body in women. Hirsutism most often occurs in a male distribution (that is, on the upper lip, chin, abdomen, and chest) in women. The excess hair is primarily the result of an increase in androgen levels (especially testosterone) which may be due to any of the following:

- Familial predisposition (considered normal)
- Polycystic ovary syndrome
- Ovarian, adrenal, or pituitary tumors
- Cushing's syndrome
- Central nervous system disorders
- Medications, such as minoxidil, cyclosporine, phenytoin, certain progestins, and anabolic steroids

The manifestations of hirsutism include increased male pattern hair growth, acne, and menstrual irregularities. If the androgen excess is great, defeminization (a decrease in breast size and loss of normal adipose tissue) and virilization (frontal balding, increased muscle mass, deepening of the voice, and enlargement of the clitoris) may occur. Virilization indicates the presence of an androgen-producing tumor (Tierney et al., 2001).

Alopecia

Alopecia is loss of hair, or baldness (Figure 14–31 ■). Alopecia may result from scarring, various systemic diseases, or genetic predisposition. Scarring from trauma, radiation, and severe bacterial, fungal, or viral infections causes permanent and irreversible hair loss over the scarred area. Systemic diseases that may cause alopecia include systemic lupus erythematosus, thyroid disorders, and pituitary insufficiency. The hair loss from these disorders may be reversible. Hair loss from androgenic causes may also occur in the postmenopausal woman. Alopecia may be drug induced and is a side effect of a variety of medications (see Box 14–6).

Types of alopecia follow:

- Male pattern baldness is the most common cause of alopecia in men and is genetically predetermined. The hair loss begins at the temples, with recession of the hairline and baldness of the crown.

Figure 14–31 ■ Alopecia, or baldness, may be the result of scarring, disease, or genetic predisposition.

BOX 14–6	■ Medications Causing Alopecia
■ Thallium	■ Allopurinol
■ Retinoids	■ Propranolol
■ Anticoagulants	■ Indomethacin
■ Antimitotic agents	■ Amphetamines
■ Antithyroid drugs	■ Salicylates
■ Oral contraceptives	■ Levodopa
■ Trimethadione	■ Gentamicin
■ Excessive use of vitamin A	■ Chemotherapy

- Female pattern alopecia begins in women in their 20s and 30s, with progressive thinning and loss of hair over the central part of the scalp. Unlike men, women do not lose hair from the frontal hairline. Many of these women have elevated adrenal androgens.
- Alopecia areata is characterized by round or oval bald patches on the scalp as well as on other hairy parts of the body. The cause is unknown. This type of alopecia is usually self-limiting and reverses without treatment, although it often recurs.
- Alopecia totalis is the loss of all hair on the scalp. This rare condition is irreversible.
- Alopecia universalis is the total loss of hair on all parts of the body.

COLLABORATIVE CARE

Alopecia is diagnosed by assessing the appearance of the hair and hair loss and by assessing the client for other systemic diseases and the use of medications that may cause hair loss. Various treatments are used to restore hair.

The client with hirsutism is examined for hormone levels and indications of other systemic illnesses. Hirsutism is treated by addressing the underlying systemic disorder and stopping medications that may be causing the problem.

Diagnostic Tests

The following diagnostic tests may be ordered for the client with hirsutism.

- Serum testosterone levels are measured; levels above 200 ng/dL indicate the need for further diagnostic work, including a pelvic examination and tests of ovarian function in women.
- Adrenal CT scan may be performed to assess for an adrenal tumor.

Medications

Hirsutism is treated with medications specific to the underlying cause. Oral contraceptives containing estrogen decrease ovarian androgen production and decrease free testosterone levels. Dexamethasone (Decadron) may be prescribed for people with high cortisol levels. Ketoconazole (Nizoral) inhibits androgen production. Antiandrogenic medications cause congenital abnormalities in male infants and are therefore given only to nonpregnant women, who are cautioned to avoid pregnancy while taking the medications.

Male pattern baldness has been successfully treated with topical minoxidil (Loniten) or Rogaine, a commercial product that contains minoxidil. These drugs, which are vasodilators, stimulate vertex hair growth, probably by stimulating the epithelium of the hair follicle. These agents have been most successful in clients who have a recent onset of alopecia or are less than 50 years old. About 40% of clients treated two times a day for a year will have moderate to dense regrowth of hair at the temples (Tierney et al., 2001).

Surgery

Surgical movement of tissue containing hair is used to restore hair or reduce the size of areas of alopecia. These surgical procedures include punch grafting, scalp reduction, and flaps.

- Punch grafting of small hair plugs taken from the back or sides of the scalp is an effective means of replacing hair to areas of alopecia. This procedure is done on an outpatient office or clinic every 1 to 2 months.
- Scalp reduction is done by excising a portion of the affected scalp. In some cases, a tissue expander (such as a silicone balloon) is first implanted under the scalp to enlarge the hair-bearing scalp so that larger areas of alopecia can be removed.
- Flaps from hair-bearing areas of the scalp can be surgically transplanted from adjacent areas into areas of alopecia. This procedure may be done in stages.

NURSING CARE

The client with either hirsutism or alopecia is often self-conscious about appearance and tries a variety of over-the-counter treatments before seeking medical care. Nursing care

for the client with hair disorders focuses on teaching the client self-care and providing support during long-term care. Women with hirsutism are taught to use various means of removing unwanted hair, such as shaving, applying depilatories, waxing, or undergoing electrolysis. Women with mild hirsutism may bleach facial hair to make it less obvious. Clients with alopecia may wear hair pieces or wigs.

THE CLIENT WITH A DISORDER OF THE NAILS

Nail disorders may be due to systemic diseases, trauma, allergies, or irritants. They may also be congenital or genetic. Nails may be discolored, multicolored, malformed, infected, or separated from underlying tissue.

PATHOPHYSIOLOGY

The nail disorders discussed here are separation of the nail, infection, and ingrown toenails.

- **Onycholysis** is the separation of the distal nail plate from the nail bed. It occurs most often in the fingernails. This disorder may result from many different factors, including excessive or prolonged exposure to water, soaps, detergent, alkalies, and industrial keratolytic agents; Candida infections; nail hardeners; and thyroid disorders. Prolonged application of false fingernails may also cause this disorder.
- A **paronychia** is an infection of the cuticle of the fingernails or toenails (Figure 14–32 ■). The disorder often follows a minor trauma and secondary infection with staphylococci, streptococci, or Candida. The acute form begins with a painful inflammation that may progress to an abscess. The chronic form is seen most often in people who have frequent exposure to water. In the chronic form, the skin around the nail is painful, edematous, and infected. The nail plate may become ridged and discolored.
- An **onychomycosis** is a fungal or dermatophyte infection of the nail plate. The nail plate elevates and becomes yellow or white. Psoriasis infections of the nail plate cause the nails to pit.

Figure 14–32 ■ A paronychia is an infection of the cuticle of the fingernails or toenails.

Source: Leonard Morse, Medical Images, Inc.

- An ingrown toenail (*unguis incarnatus*) results when the edge of the nail plate grows into the soft tissue of the toe. Pain and infection may occur. The infection, if untreated, may spread to the bone. This disorder is especially dangerous for the person with diabetes mellitus or peripheral vascular disease.

COLLABORATIVE CARE

The treatment of disorders of the nail vary from pharmacologic treatment to surgical removal. Infections of the nails are treated, depending on the causative agent, with antifungal or antibiotic medications. If the causative agent is a fungus or chronic dermatologic disorder, treatment is difficult and may

not be effective. Persistently painful and/or infected nails are in some cases surgically removed.

NURSING CARE

Nursing care of the client with a disorder of the nail focuses on teaching self-care. Clients with nail disorders that are caused by frequent exposure to water are taught to protect the hands or feet by wearing rubber gloves or boots and to keep the nails as clean and dry as possible. Clients with ingrown toenails are cautioned not to cut into the lateral nail bed, but rather to soak the nail twice a day and insert a piece of cotton or gauze under the softened nail until the nail has grown out enough to trim.

EXPLORE MediaLink

NCLEX review questions, case studies, care plan activities, MediaLink applications, and other interactive resources for this chapter can be found on the Companion Website at www.prenhall.com/lemone.

Click on Chapter 14 to select the activities for this chapter. For animations, video clips, more NCLEX review questions, and an audio glossary, access the Student CD-ROM accompanying this textbook.

TEST YOURSELF

1. Your elderly client has severe xerosis. What topic should be included in your teaching plan?

   a. Take a hot bath every day
   b. Use fabric softeners when laundering clothing
   c. Apply skin lotions after a bath
   d. Maintain a warm environment

2. Which of the following clients is at risk for the development of a candidiasis infection?

   a. An older adult with pruritus
   b. A young woman who is pregnant
   c. An older man with a premalignant skin condition
   d. A young man with multiple nevi

3. What question should be included in a health history of a client with a linear pattern of painful vesicles over the left thorax?

   a. Do you remember being sunburned as a child?
   b. Are you a regular patron of tanning booths?
   c. Have you ever been diagnosed with acne?
   d. Did you have chickenpox when you were young?

4. Of the following, which is most significant to the development of a malignant melanoma?

   a. A change in the color or size of a nevus
   b. Sexual contact with a person who has a herpes virus infection
   c. Inadequate knowledge about infection prevention
   d. A dietary intake of high-calorie foods

5. The rationale for lifting, rather than pulling, a client up in bed is that:

   a. Lifting a client allows a brief period of increased capillary circulation
   b. Lifting a client prevents tissue injury from shearing forces
   c. Pulling a client up in bed decreases tissue ischemia and hypoxia
   d. Pulling a client up in bed promotes capillary blood flow

See Test Yourself answers in Appendix C.

BIBLIOGRAPHY

Agency for Health Care Policy and Research. (1992). *Pressure ulcers in adults: Prediction and prevention.* Rockville, MD: USDHHS.

_____ . (1994). *Treatment of pressure ulcers.* Rockville, MD: USDHHS.

American Cancer Society. (2002). *Cancer facts and figures 2002.* Atlanta: American Cancer Society.

American Melanoma Foundation/National Cancer Institute. (2001). Skin cancer treatment. Available http://cancernet.nci.nih.gov

Appling, S. (1997). Promoting healthy skin. *MEDSURG Nursing, 6*(6), 377–378.

Bielan, B. (1997a). What's your assessment . . . papular urticaria. *Dermatology Nursing, 9*(3), 191, 201.

_____ . (1997b). What's your assessment . . . tinea pedis. *Dermatology Nursing, 9*(2), 105, 117.

Bjorgen, S. (1998). Clinical snapshot: Herpes zoster. *American Journal of Nursing, 98* (2 Continuing Care Extra), 46–47.

Blawat, D., & Banks, P. (1997). Comforting touch: Using topical skin preparations. *Nursing 97, 27*(5), 46–48.

Center for Disease Control. (2001). Cancer prevention and control. Available www.cdc.gov/cancer/nscpep/skin

Boston, M. (1997). Acne: Avoiding permanent damage. *Community Nurse, 3*(4), 15–16.

Davis, P. (1998). Pain from herpes zoster and postherapetic neuralgia. *American Journal of Nursing, 98*(2 Continuing Care Extra), 18, 20.

Hardy, M. (1996). What can you do about your patient's dry skin? *Journal of Gerontological Nursing, 22*(5), 10–18, 52–53.

Johnson, M., & Maas, M. (1997). *Iowa outcome project: Nursing outcomes classification (NOC).* St. Louis: Mosby.

Landow, K. (1998). Hand dermatitis: The perennial scourge. *Postgraduate Medicine, 103*(1), 141–142, 145–148, 151–152.

Lapka, D. (2000). Oncology today. New horizons: Skin cancer. *RN, 63*(7), 32–40.

Lebwohl, M. (1997). Understanding psoriasis. *Women's Health Digest, 3*(3), 159–164.

Leshaw, S. (1998). Itching in active patients: Causes and cures. *Physician & Sportsmedicine, 26*(1), 47–50.

Marghoob, A. (1997). Basal and squamous cell carcinomas. *Postgraduate Medicine, 102*(2), 139–142.

McCloskey, J., & Bulechek, G. (Eds.). (2000). *Iowa intervention project: Nursing interventions classification (NIC)* (3rd ed.). St. Louis: Mosby.

McKay, S. (2000). Why we need to worry about warts. *RN, 63*(9), 68–74.

Metules, T. (2000). Tips for nurses who wash too much. *RN, 63*(3), 34–37.

North American Nursing Diagnosis Association. (2001) *Nursing diagnoses: Definitions & classification 2001–2002.* Philadelphia: NANDA.

Penzer, R., & Finch, M. (2001). Promoting healthy skin in older people. *Nursing Standard, 15*(34), 46–52.

Pieper, B., & Weiland, M. (1997a). Pressure ulcer prevention within 72 hours of admission in a

rehabilitation setting. *Ostomy Wound Management, 43*(8), 14–16, 18, 20.

Pieper, B., Sugrue, M., Weiland, M., Sprague, K., & Heimann, C. (1997b). Presence of ulcer prevention methods used among patients considered at-risk versus those considered not-at-risk. *Journal of WOCN, 24*(4), 191–199.

Porth, C. (2002). *Pathophysiology: Concepts of altered health states* (6th ed.). Philadelphia: Lippincott.

Reifsnider, E. (1997). Common adult infectious skin conditions. *Nursing Practitioner: American Journal of Primary Health Care, 22*(11), 17–18, 20, 23–24.

Rigel, D., & Carucci, J. (2000). Malignant melanoma: Prevention, early detection, and treatment in the 21st century. *CA: A Cancer Journal for Clinicians, 50*(4), 209–213.

Russell, J. (2000). Topical therapy for acne. *American Family Physician, 61*(2), 357–366.

Sarver-Steffensen, J. (1999). When MRSA reaches into long-term care. *RN, 62*(3), 39–41.

Tierney, L., McPhee, S., & Papadakis, M. (Eds.). (2001). *Current medical diagnosis & treatment* (40th ed.). Stamford, CT: Appleton & Lange.

Wilson, B., Shannon, M., & Stang, C. (2001). *Nursing drug guide 2001.* Upper Saddle River, NJ: Prentice Hall.

Yarbo, C., Frogge, M, Goodman, M., & Groenwald, S. (Eds.) (2001). *Cancer nursing: Principles and practice.* (5th ed.). Sudbury, MA: Jones & Bartlett.

Nursing Care of Clients with Burns

LEARNING OUTCOMES

After completing this chapter, you will be able to:

- Apply knowledge of normal integumentary anatomy, physiology, and assessments when providing nursing care for clients with burns (see Chapter 13).

- Discuss types and causative agents of burns.

- Explain burn classification by depth and extent of injury.

- Describe the stages of burn wound healing.

- Explain the pathophysiology, collaborative care, and nursing care for the client with a minor burn.

- Discuss the systemic pathophysiologic effects of a major burn.

- Identify the collaborative care necessary during the emergent/resuscitative stage, the acute stage, and the rehabilitative stage of a major burn.

- Discuss the nursing implications of medications administered to the client with a major burn.

- Discuss the nursing implications for burn wound management.

- Use the nursing process as a framework for providing individualized care to clients with a burn.

www.prenhall.com/lemone
Additional resources for this chapter can be found on the Student CD-ROM accompanying this textbook, and on the Companion Website at www. prenhall.com/lemone. Click on Chapter 15 to select the activities for this chapter.

CD-ROM
- Audio Glossary
- NCLEX Review

Companion Website
- More NCLEX Review
- Case Study
  Full-Thickness Burns
- Care Plan Activity
  Inhalation Injury
- MediaLink Application
  Teaching Plan: Fire Prevention

A **burn** is an injury resulting from exposure to heat, chemicals, radiation, or electric current. A transfer of energy from a source of heat to the human body initiates a sequence of physiologic events that in the most severe cases leads to irreversible tissue destruction. Burns range in severity from a minor loss of small segments of the outermost layer of the skin to a complex injury involving all body systems. Treatments vary from simple application of a topical antiseptic agent in an outpatient clinic to an invasive, multisystem, interdisciplinary health team approach in the aseptic environment of a burn center.

It is estimated that more than 2 million burn injuries occur each year in the United States, and, of those, about 70,000 require hospitalization (Braunwald & Fauci, 2001). The home is the most common site for fire-related burns. Home fires cause 73% of all fire-related deaths, with about 12 people dying in home fires each day. Factors associated with deaths from burns are age (especially children and older adults), careless smoking, alcohol or drug intoxication, and physical and mental disabilities. Occupation is also a factor, with electricians and chemical workers among those at greatest risk (Rutan, 1998).

TYPES OF BURN INJURY

The four types of burn injury are thermal, chemical, electrical, and radiation. Although all four types can lead to generalized tissue damage and multisystem involvement, the causative agents and priority treatment measures are unique to each (Table 15–1).

Thermal Burns

Thermal burns result from exposure to dry heat (flames) or moist heat (steam and hot liquids). They are the most common burn injuries and occur most often in children and older adults. Direct exposure to the source of heat causes cellular destruction that can result in charring of vascular, bony, muscle, and nervous tissue.

Chemical Burns

Chemical burns are caused by direct skin contact with either acid or alkaline agents. More than 25,000 products found in the home or workplace can cause chemical burns. The chemical destroys tissue protein, leading to necrosis. Burns caused by alkalis (such as lye) are more difficult to neutralize than are burns caused by acids. They also tend to have deeper penetration with a correspondingly more severe burn than from acid. Organic compound burns, such as by petroleum distillates, cause cutaneous damage through fat solvent action and may also cause renal and liver failure if absorbed.

Chemical agents are further classified according to the manner by which they structurally alter proteins. Oxidizing agents, such as household bleach, alter protein configuration through the chemical process of reduction. Corrosives, such as lye, cause extensive protein denaturation. Protoplasmic poisons, such as organic compounds, form salts with proteins, inhibiting calcium and other ions needed for cell viability. The severity of the chemical burn is related to the type of agent, the concentration of the agent, the mechanism of action, the duration of contact, and the amount of body surface area exposed. Box 15–1 lists household cleaning agents that may cause burns.

Electrical Burns

The severity of electrical burns depends on the type and duration of current, and amount of voltage. It is particularly difficult to assess the extent of the electrical burn injury, because the destructive processes initiated by the electrical insult are concealed and may persist for weeks beyond the time of the incident. It is difficult to assess the depth and extent of the burn, as electricity follows the path of least resistance, which in the human body tends to lie along muscles, bone, blood vessels, and nerves. Necrosis of the tissue results from impaired blood flow, secondary to blood coagulation at the site of the electrical injury. More than 90% of electrical burn wounds of the extremities that develop gangrene result in amputation.

Alternating current, as is found in conventional households, produces repeated electrical surges that lead to tetanic muscle contractions. Such sustained muscle contractions inhibit respiratory efforts for the duration of contact and result in respiratory arrest. The contractions also cause the person to clamp

TABLE 15–1	Types, Causative Agents, and Priority Treatment Measures for Burns	
Type	**Causative Agent**	**Priority Treatment**
Thermal	Open flame	Extinguish flame (stop, drop, and roll).
	Steam	Flush with cool water.
	Hot liquids (water, grease, tar, metal)	Consult fire department.
Chemical	Acids	Neutralize or dilute chemical.
	Strong alkalis	Remove clothing.
		Consult Poison Control Center.
Electrical	Direct current	Disconnect source of current.
	Alternating current	Initiate CPR if necessary.
	Lightning	Move to area of safety.
		Consult electrical experts.
Radiation	Solar (ultraviolet)	Shield the skin appropriately.
	X-rays	Limit time of exposure.
	Radioactive agents	Move the client away from the radiation source.
		Consult a radiation expert.

BOX 15–1 ■ Household Cleaning Agents That May Cause Burns	
■ Drain cleaners	■ Oven cleaners
■ Lye	■ Toilet bowl cleaners
■ Industrial-strength ammonia	■ Dishwasher detergents
■ Household ammonia	■ Bleach

down on the power source (such as an electrical cord) and thus may increase the duration of contact with the source. Direct current, as in injury from a lightning bolt, exposes the body to very high voltage for an instantaneous period of time. High voltage (lightning) injury usually results in entry and exit wounds. The flash-over effect, a phenomenon unique to lightning injury, actually saves the client from death. It is seen in those instances in which the current travels over the moist surface of the skin rather than through deeper structures.

Radiation Burns

Radiation burns are usually associated with sunburn or radiation treatment for cancer. These kinds of burns tend to be superficial, involving only the outermost layers of the epidermis. All functions of the skin remain intact. Symptoms are limited to mild systemic reactions: headache, chills, local discomfort, nausea, and vomiting. More extensive exposure to radiation or radioactive substances, as in nuclear power accidents, leads to the same degree of tissue damage and multisystem involvement associated with other types of burns.

FACTORS AFFECTING BURN CLASSIFICATION

Tissue damage following a burn is determined primarily by two factors: depth of the burn (the layers of underlying tissue affected) and the extent of the burn (the percentage of body surface area involved).

Depth of the Burn

The depth of burn of injury is determined by the elements of the skin that have been damaged or destroyed. Burn depth results from a combination of the temperature of the burning agent and the length of contact. Burns are classified as either superficial, partial thickness, or full thickness. Characteristics of

burns are described below, summarized in Table 15–2, and illustrated in Figure 15–1 ■.

Superficial Burns

A **superficial burn** (often called a first-degree burn) involves only the epidermal layer of the skin. This type of burn most often results from damage from sunburn, ultraviolet light, minor flash injury (from a sudden ignition or explosion), or mild radiation burn associated with cancer treatment. Because the skin remains intact, this degree of burn is not calculated into the estimates of burn injury. The skin color ranges from pink to bright red, and there may be slight edema over the burned area. Superficial burns involving large body surface areas may be manifested by chills, headache, nausea, and vomiting. The injury usually heals in 3 to 6 days, with dryness and peeling of the outer layer of skin. There is no scar formation. Superficial burns are treated with mild analgesics and the application of water-soluble lotions. Extensive superficial burns, especially in older adults, may require intravenous fluid treatment.

Partial-Thickness Burns

Partial-thickness burns (often called second-degree burns) may be subdivided into superficial partial-thickness and deep dermal partial-thickness burns. The classification depends on the depth of the burn.

A *superficial partial-thickness burn* involves the entire dermis and the papillae of the dermis. Causes may include such injuries as a brief exposure to flash flame or dilute chemical agents, or contact with a hot surface. This burn is often bright red, but has a moist, glistening appearance with blister formation (Figure 15–2 ■). The burned area will blanch on pressure, and touch and pain sensation remain intact. Pain in response to temperature and air is usually severe. These injuries heal within 21 days with minimal or no scarring, but pigment changes are common. Analgesics are administered, and if large blistered areas are disrupted, skin substitutes may be used.

TABLE 15–2 Characteristics of Burns by Depth

Characteristic	Superficial	Split Thickness	Full Thickness
Skin layers lost	Epidermis	Epidermis and dermis	Epidermis, dermis, and underlying tissues
Skin appearance over burn	Red to gray; may have local edema	Fluid-filled blisters; bright pink, may appear waxy white with deep partial-thickness burns	Waxy white; dry, leathery, charred
Skin function	Present	Absent	Absent
Pain sensation	Present	Present	Absent
Manifestations at the burn site	Pain; local edema	Severe pain; edema; weeping of fluid	Little pain; edema
Treatment	Regular cleaning Topical agent of choice	Regular cleaning Topical agent of choice May require skin grafting	Regular cleaning Topical agent of choice Skin substitutes Excision of eschar Skin grafting
Scarring	None	May occur in deep burns	Of grafted area
Time to heal	3 to 6 days	14 to >21 days	Requires skin grafting to heal

Figure 15–1 ■ Burn injury classification according to the depth of the burn.

Full-thickness burn

Partial-thickness burn

Superficial burn

Epidermis

Dermis

Subcutaneous tissue

Muscle

Bone

Normal tissue

Figure 15–2 ■ Partial-thickness burn injury.

Courtesy of Dr. William Dominic, Valley Medical Center.

Figure 15–3 ■ Full-thickness burn injury.

Courtesy of Dr. William Dominic, Valley Medical Center.

A *deep partial-thickness burn* also involves the entire dermis, but extends further into the dermis than a superficial partial-thickness burn. Hair follicles, sebaceous glands, and epidermal sweat glands remain intact (Porth, 2002). Hot liquids or solids, flash flame, direct flame, intense radiant energy, or chemical agents may cause this level of burn wound. The surface of the burn wound appears pale and waxy and may be moist or dry. Large, easily ruptured blisters may be present, or the blisters may look like flat, dry tissue paper. Capillary refill is decreased, and sensation to deep pressure is present. The burn wound is less painful than a superficial partial-thickness burn, but areas of pain and areas of decreased sensation may be present. Deep partial-thickness burn wounds often require more

than 21 days for healing and may convert to a full-thickness injury as necrosis extends the depth of the wound. Contractures are possible, as are hypertrophic scarring and functional impairment. Excision and grafting may be necessary to decrease scarring and loss of function.

Full-Thickness Burns

A **full-thickness burn** (often called a third-degree burn) involves all layers of the skin, including the epidermis, the dermis, and the epidermal appendages (Figure 15–3 ■). The burn wound may extend into the subcutaneous fat, connective tissue, muscle, and bone. Full-thickness burns are caused by prolonged contact with flames, steam, chemicals, or high-voltage electric current.

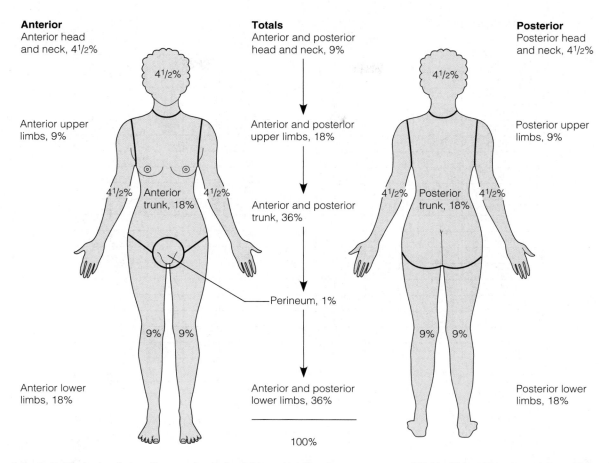

Anterior
Anterior head
and neck, 4¹/₂%

Anterior upper
limbs, 9%

4¹/₂%   Anterior   4¹/₂%
         trunk, 18%

9%   9%

Anterior lower
limbs, 18%

Totals
Anterior and posterior
head and neck, 9%

Anterior and posterior
upper limbs, 18%

Anterior and posterior
trunk, 36%

Perineum, 1%

Anterior and posterior
lower limbs, 36%

100%

Posterior
Posterior head
and neck, 4¹/₂%

Posterior upper
limbs, 9%

4¹/₂%   Posterior   4¹/₂%
         trunk, 18%

9%   9%

Posterior lower
limbs, 18%

Figure 15–4 ■ The "rule of nines" is a method of quickly estimating the percentage of TBSA affected by a burn injury. Although useful in emergency care situations, the rule of nines is not accurate for estimating TBSA for adults who are short, obese, or very thin.

Depending on the cause of injury, the burn wound may appear pale, waxy, yellow, brown, mottled, charred, or nonblanching red. The wound surface is dry, leathery, and firm to the touch. Thrombosed blood vessels may be visible under the surface of the wound. There is no sensation of pain or light touch, as pain and touch receptors have been destroyed. Full-thickness burns require skin grafting to heal.

Extent of the Burn

The extent of the burn injury is expressed as a percentage of the total body surface area (TBSA). There are several methods used for determining the extent of injury. The "rule of nines" is a rapid method of estimation used during the prehospital and emergency care phases. In this method, the body is divided into five surface areas—head, trunk, arms, legs, and perineum—and percentages that equal or total a sum of nines are assigned to each body area (Figure 15–4 ■). For example, a client with burns of the face, anterior right arm, and anterior trunk has burn injury involving 27% of the total body surface area (in this example, face = 4.5%, arm = 4.5%, and trunk = 18% to total 27%). Only partial- and full-thickness burns are included in the estimation.

On the client's admission to the hospital, critical care area, or burn center, more accurate methods for estimating the extent of injury are employed. For example, the Lund and Browder method (Figure 15–5 ■) determines surface area measurements for each body part according to the age of the client.

A recognized system for describing a burn injury, developed by the American Burn Association, uses both the extent and depth of burn to classify burns as minor, moderate, or major (Table 15–3).

BURN WOUND HEALING

Burns heal in the same processes as do other wounds, but the wound healing phases occur more slowly and last longer. The healing process involves four phases: hemostasis, inflammation, proliferation, and remodeling. The following physiologic events occur (Carrougher, 1998):

- *Hemostasis.* Immediately following the injury, platelets coming in contact with the damaged tissue aggregate and degranulate (releasing growth factors). Fibrin is deposited, trapping further platelets, and a thrombus is formed. The thrombus, combined with local vasoconstriction, leads to hemostasis which walls off the wound from the systemic circulation.

- *Inflammation.* Local vasodilation and an increase in capillary permeability follows hemostasis. Neutrophils infiltrate the wound and peak in about 24 hours, and then monocytes predominate. The monocytes are converted into macrophages, which consume pathogens and dead tissue, and also

Area	Age (years)					% 1°	% 2°	% 3°	% Total
	0–1	1–4	5–9	10–15	Adult				
Head	19	17	13	10	7				
Neck	2	2	2	2	2				
Ant. trunk	13	13	13	13	13				
Post. trunk	13	13	13	13	13				
R. buttock	$2\frac{1}{2}$	$2\frac{1}{2}$	$2\frac{1}{2}$	$2\frac{1}{2}$	$2\frac{1}{2}$				
L. buttock	$2\frac{1}{2}$	$2\frac{1}{2}$	$2\frac{1}{2}$	$2\frac{1}{2}$	$2\frac{1}{2}$				
Genitalia	1	1	1	1	1				
R.U. arm	4	4	4	4	4				
L.U. arm	4	4	4	4	4				
R.L. arm	3	3	3	3	3				
L.L. arm	3	3	3	3	3				
R. hand	$2\frac{1}{2}$	$2\frac{1}{2}$	$2\frac{1}{2}$	$2\frac{1}{2}$	$2\frac{1}{2}$				
L. hand	$2\frac{1}{2}$	$2\frac{1}{2}$	$2\frac{1}{2}$	$2\frac{1}{2}$	$2\frac{1}{2}$				
R. thigh	$5\frac{1}{2}$	$6\frac{1}{2}$	$8\frac{1}{2}$	$8\frac{1}{2}$	$9\frac{1}{2}$				
L. thigh	$5\frac{1}{2}$	$6\frac{1}{2}$	$8\frac{1}{2}$	$8\frac{1}{2}$	$9\frac{1}{2}$				
R. leg	5	5	$5\frac{1}{2}$	6	7				
L. leg	5	5	$5\frac{1}{2}$	6	7				
R. foot	$3\frac{1}{2}$	$3\frac{1}{2}$	$3\frac{1}{2}$	$3\frac{1}{2}$	$3\frac{1}{2}$				
L. foot	$3\frac{1}{2}$	$3\frac{1}{2}$	$3\frac{1}{2}$	$3\frac{1}{2}$	$3\frac{1}{2}$				
					Total				

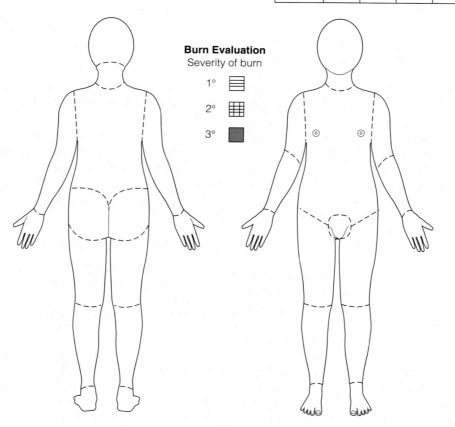

Burn Evaluation
Severity of burn

1° ▤
2° ▦
3° ■

Figure 15–5 ■ The Lund and Browder burn assessment chart. This method of estimating TBSA affected by a burn injury is more accurate than the "rule of nines" because it accounts for changes in body surface area across the life span.

TABLE 15–3 American Burn Association Classification of Burn Injury

Minor Burn Injury	Moderate Burn Injury	Major Burn Injury
Excludes electrical injury, inhalation injury, complicated injuries (such as multiple trauma), and all clients who are considered to be at high risk (such as older adults and those with chronic illnesses)	Excludes electrical injury, inhalation injury, complicated injuries (such as multiple trauma), and all clients who are considered to be at high risk (such as older adults and those with chronic illnesses)	Includes all burns of the hands, face, eyes, ears, feet, and perineum; all electrical injuries, inhalation injuries, multiple trauma injuries, and all clients who are considered to be at high risk
Second-degree burns of less than 15% of the total body surface area in adults	Second-degree burns of 15% to 25% of the total body surface area in adults	Second-degree burns of greater than 25% of the total body surface area in adults
Third-degree burns of less than 2% of the total body surface area not involving special care areas (eyes, ears, face, hands, feet, perineum)	Third-degree burns of less than 10% of the total body surface area not involving special care areas (eyes, ears, face, hands, feet, perineum)	All third-degree burns of 10% or greater of the total body surface area

Note. Burn injuries described in this table (except minor burns) should be treated in a specialized burn center. These criteria have been established by the American Burn Association.

secrete various growth factors. These growth factors stimulate the proliferation of fibroblasts and a deposit of a provisional wound matrix.

- *Proliferation.* Within 3 to 4 days postburn, fibroblasts are the major cell within the wound. Their number peaks at about 14 days after the injury. Granulation tissue begins to form, with complete reepithelialization occurring during this stage. Epithelial cells cover the wound as each cell stretches across the wound surface to join with other epithelial cell sheets or the other side of the wound. The proliferation phase lasts until complete reepithelialization occurs, by epithelial cell migration, surgical intervention, or a combination of the two.

- *Remodeling.* This phase may last for years. Collagen fibers, laid down during the proliferative phase, are reorganized into more compact areas. Scars contract and fade in color. In normal healing following a minor burn injury, the newly formed skin closely resembles its neighboring tissue. However, when a burn injury extends into the dermal layer of skin, two types of excessive scar may develop. A **hypertrophic scar** is an overgrowth of dermal tissue that remains within the boundaries of the wound. A **keloid** is a scar that extends beyond the boundaries of the original wound. People with dark skin are at greater risk for hypertrophic scars and keloids.

THE CLIENT WITH A MINOR BURN

Minor burn injuries consist of superficial burns that are not extensive, superficial split-thickness burns that involve less than 15% of TBSA, and full-thickness burns that involve less than 2% of TBSA, excluding the special care areas (eyes, ears, face, hands, feet, perineum, and joints). Minor burn injuries are not associated with immunosuppression, hypermetabolism, or increased susceptibility to infection.

A minor burn injury is usually treated in an outpatient facility. The goal of therapy is to promote wound healing, eliminate discomfort, maintain mobility, and prevent infection.

PATHOPHYSIOLOGY

Sunburn

Sunburns result from exposure to ultraviolet light. Such injuries, which tend to be superficial, are more commonly seen in clients with lighter skin. Because the skin remains intact, the manifestations in most cases are mild and are limited to pain, nausea, vomiting, skin redness, chills, and headache. Treatment is performed on an outpatient basis and generally consists of applying mild lotions, increasing liquid intake, administering mild analgesics, and maintaining warmth. Older adults should be monitored for evidence of dehydration. Proper use of sunscreen and limiting sun exposure to the less hazardous hours of the day (before 10 A.M. and after 3 P.M.) can prevent sunburn.

Scald Burn

Minor scald burns result from exposure to moist heat and involve superficial and superficial split-thickness burns of less than 15% of TBSA. The goals of therapy are to prevent wound contamination and to promote healing. The nurse teaches the client to apply antibiotic solutions and light dressings and to maintain adequate nutritional intake. Mild analgesics may be ordered to help the client carry out activities of daily living. Tetanus toxoid is administered as appropriate.

COLLABORATIVE CARE

In the outpatient facility, the wound may be washed with mild soap and water. Tar and asphalt can be removed with mineral oil, petroleum ointments, or Medisol (a citrus and petroleum distillate with hydrocarbon structure). Tetanus toxoid booster is recommended for all clients whose immunization histories are in doubt. Although controversy regarding the care of blisters remains, blisters may be managed in one of three ways: left intact, evacuated, or debrided. Follow-up care for the minor burn injury includes twice daily wound cleansing with application of bland ointment, range-of-motion exercises to affected joints, and weekly clinic appointments until the wound heals completely.

NURSING CARE

Although the nurse seldom treats the minor burn in the acute care environment, the burn treatment methods used in the outpatient setting follow the same standard approaches to care. General nursing measures include taking the history, estimating the extent and depth of the injury, cleansing the wound, applying topical agents, dressing the wound, controlling pain, and establishing follow-up care.

Home Care

The nurse should address the following topics to facilitate self-care at home of minor burns.

- How to identify and report manifestations of impaired wound healing:
  - Change in healthy appearance of the wound (altered skin integrity, swelling, blister formation, erythema)
  - Signs of infection (fever, purulent drainage, foul odor)
- Wound care:
  - Daily cleansing with mild soap and water
  - Using sterile technique to change dressings
  - Correct application of ordered topical agents
- Pain management:
  - Use mild analgesics as ordered
  - Use alternative pain management therapies

THE CLIENT WITH A MAJOR BURN

A major burn involves serious injury to the underlying layers of skin and covers a large body surface area. The American Burn Association defines a major burn as one that involves:

- >25% TBSA in adults less than 40 years of age
- >20% TBSA in adults more than 40 years of age

- >10% TBSA full-thickness burn
- Injuries to the face, eyes, ears, hands, feet, or perineum
- High-voltage electrical injuries
- All burn injuries with inhalation injury or major trauma

PATHOPHYSIOLOGY

The pathophysiologic changes that result from major burn injuries involve all body systems. Extensive loss of skin (the body's protective barrier) can result in massive infection, fluid and electrolyte imbalances, and hypothermia. Often the person inhales the products of combustion, thus compromising respiratory function. Cardiac dysrhythmias and circulatory failure are common manifestations of serious burn injuries. A profound catabolic state dramatically increases caloric expenditure and nutritional deficiencies. An alteration in gastrointestinal motility predisposes the client to developing paralytic ileus, and hyperacidity leads to gastric and duodenal ulcerations. Dehydration slows glomerular filtration rates and renal clearance of toxic wastes and may lead to acute tubular necrosis and renal failure. Overall body metabolism may be profoundly altered. Systemic responses to burns are shown in Figure 15–6 ■ and discussed in the following sections.

Integumentary System

Heat transfer to skin is a complex phenomenon. If the microcirculation of the skin remains intact during burning, it cools and protects the deeper portions of the skin and cools the outer surface once the heat source is removed. With extensive burn injury, the integrity of the microcirculation is lost, and the burning process continues even after the heat source is removed.

Burns have a characteristic skin surface appearance that resembles a bull's-eye, with the most severe burn located centrally and the lesser burns located along the peripheral wound edges. Depending on their intensity, burns consist of one, two, or three concentric three-dimensional zones closely corresponding on the skin surface to the depth of the burn.

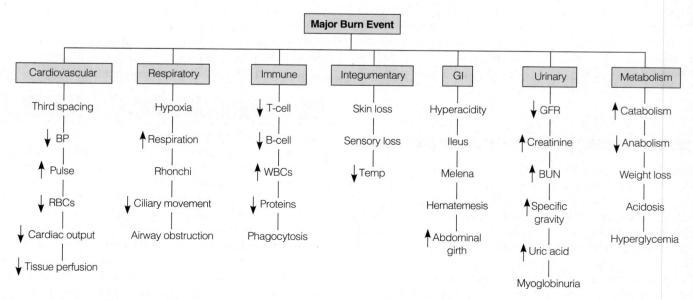

Figure 15–6 ■ Effects of a severe burn on major body systems and metabolism.

- The outer zone of hyperemia blanches on pressure and heals in 2 to 7 days postburn.
- The medial zone of stasis is initially moist, red, and blistered and blanches on pressure. It becomes pale and necrotic on days 3 to 7 postburn.
- The inner zone of coagulation immediately appears leathery and coagulated. It merges with the necrotic zone of stasis in 3 to 7 days postburn.

The overall thickness of the dermis and epidermis varies considerably from one area of the body to another. Similar temperatures produce different depths of injury to different body parts. For example, in the adult, skin covering the medial aspect of the forearm is thinner and more easily damaged than the skin covering the back of the same person. Skin dissipates heat maximally in areas of greatest vascularization. When heat absorption exceeds the rate of dissipation, cellular temperatures rise, and skin tissue is destroyed.

The burn injury results in the formation of necrotic skin and subcutaneous tissue. During the acute stage of the injury, a hard crust (**eschar**) forms, which covers the wound and harbors necrotic tissue. The eschar is characteristically leathery and rigid. Removal of the eschar facilitates healing.

Cardiovascular System

The effects of a major burn are manifested in all components of the vascular system, and include hypovolemic shock (burn shock), cardiac dysrrhythmias (such as ventricular fibrillation), cardiac arrest, and vascular compromise.

Hypovolemic Shock (Burn Shock)

Within minutes of the burn injury, a cascade of cellular events is initiated, and a massive amount of fluid shifts from the intracellular and intravascular compartments into the interstitium. This shift is a type of hypovolemic shock called **burn shock,** and it continues until capillary integrity is restored, usually within 24 to 36 hours of the injury. Although the pathophysiologic mechanisms of postburn vascular changes and fluid volume shifts are not clearly understood, three processes occur early in the postburn phase in clients with ≥ 40% TBSA:

- Increase in microvascular permeability at the burn wound site
- Generalized impairment of cell wall function, resulting in intracellular edema
- Increase in osmotic pressure of the burned tissue, leading to extensive fluid accumulation

During burn shock, the shifting of fluid is the direct result of a loss of cell wall integrity at the site of injury and in the capillary bed. Fluid leaks from the capillaries into interstitial compartments located at the burn wound site and throughout the body, resulting in a decrease in fluid volume within the intravascular space. Plasma proteins and sodium escape into the interstitium, enhancing edema formation. Blood pressure falls as cardiac output diminishes.

Vasoconstriction results as the vascular system attempts to compensate for fluid loss. Abnormal platelet aggregation and white blood cell (WBC) accumulation result in ischemia in the deeper tissue below the burn, leading to eventual thrombosis.

Red blood cells (RBCs) and WBCs remain in the circulation, producing an elevation in erythrocyte and leukocyte counts secondary to hemoconcentration.

The leakage of fluid into the interstitium compromises the lymphatic system, resulting in intravascular hypovolemia and edema at the burn wound site. Edematous body surfaces impair peripheral circulation and result in necrosis of the underlying tissue. During burn shock, potassium ions leave the intracellular compartment, predisposing the client to developing cardiac dysrhythmias. The process of burn shock continues until capillary integrity is restored, usually within 24 hours of the injury.

Burn shock reverses when fluid is reabsorbed from the interstitium into the intravascular compartment. The blood pressure rises as cardiac output increases, and urinary output improves. Diuresis continues from several days to 2 weeks postburn. During this phase, the extra cardiac workload may predispose the older client, or the client with cardiovascular disease, to fluid volume overload.

Cardiac Rhythm Alterations

Burns of more than 40% TBSA cause significant myocardial dysfunction, with a decrease in myocardial contractibility and cardiac output. These changes, which occur prior to a decrease in plasma volume, are believed to be due to the release of substances and oxygen-free radicals from the burn wound and from ischemic myocardial cells. Electrical burns often result in cardiac dysrrhythmias or cardiac arrest caused by heat damage to the myocardium or electrical interference with cardiac electrical activity.

Peripheral Vascular Compromise

Direct heat damage to extremities, especially if circumferential burns are present, results in damage to blood vessels. Circulation to extremities may be further impaired by edema and by peripheral vasoconstriction that occurs during burn shock. In addition, **compartment syndrome** (in which the tissue pressure within a muscle compartment exceeds microvascular pressure, interrupting cellular perfusion) may result from circumferential burns and edema.

Respiratory System

Pulmonary damage may result from either direct inhalation injury or as part of the systemic response to the injury. Inhalation injury is a frequent and often lethal complication of burns. The injury may range from mild respiratory inflammation to massive pulmonary failure. Exposure to heat, asphyxiants, and smoke initiates the pathophysiologic process associated with inhalation injury.

Inflammation occurs at localized sites within the airway and is manifested as hyperemia. As a result, cells are destroyed and the bronchial cilia are rendered inactive. Because the mucociliary transport mechanism no longer functions, the client may develop bronchial congestion and infection.

Interstitial pulmonary edema develops secondary to the escape of fluid from the pulmonary vasculature into the interstitial compartment of the lung tissue. Surfactant is inactivated, resulting in atelectasis and alveolar collapse. Sloughing of the

MediaLink | INHALATION INJURY CARE PLAN

damaged and dead lung tissue occasionally produces debris that may lead to complete airway obstruction.

Upper airway (above the level of the glottis) thermal injury results from the inhalation of heated air or chemicals dissolved in water. Physical findings include the presence of soot, charring, edema, blisters, and ulcerations along the mucosal lining of the oropharynx and larynx. The resulting edema in the airway peaks within the first 24 to 48 hours of injury. Lower airway thermal injury is a rare occurrence. Because the lower airway is protected by laryngeal reflexes, thermal injury below the vocal cords is seldom seen. However, when it does occur, it is typically associated with the inhalation of steam or explosive gases or the aspiration of hot liquids.

Smoke poisoning results when toxic gases and particulate matter, the products of incomplete combustion, deposit directly onto the pulmonary mucosa. The composition of the products of combustion depends on the combustible material, the rate at which the temperature increases, and the amount of ambient oxygen present. Irritant gases and particulate matter have a direct cytotoxic effect. The degree of injury is determined by their solubility in water, duration of exposure, and the size of the particulate or aerosol droplet.

Carbon monoxide, a common asphyxiant, is a colorless, tasteless, odorless gas that has a 200 times greater affinity for hemoglobin than does oxygen. It displaces oxygen to bind with hemoglobin, forming carboxyhemoglobin. As a result, the decrease in arterial oxyhemoglobin produces tissue hypoxia. Carbon monoxide impairs both oxygen delivery and cellular oxygen use. The clinical manifestations of carbon monoxide poisoning range from mild visual impairment to coma and death (Table 15–4).

Gastrointestinal System

Dysfunction of the gastrointestinal system is directly related to the size of the burn wound. Clients with ≥20% TBSA experience decreased peristalsis with resultant gastric distention and increased risk of aspiration. A decrease in or absence of bowel sounds is a manifestation of paralytic ileus (adynamic bowel) secondary to burn trauma. The resulting cessation of intestinal motility leads to gastric distention, nausea, vomiting, and hematemesis.

TABLE 15–4	Manifestations of Carbon Monoxide Poisoning
Level of Carbon Monoxide	**Manifestations**
10% to 20%	Headache, dizziness, nausea, abdominal pain
21% to 40%	Headache, nausea, drowsiness, dizziness, irritability, confusion, stupor, hypotension, bradycardia, skin color ranging from pale to dark red
41% to 60%	Convulsion, coma, hypotension, tachycardia
>60%	Death

Stress ulcers (**Curling's ulcers**) are acute ulcerations of the stomach or duodenum that form following the burn injury. Abdominal pain, acidic gastric pH levels, hematemesis, and melana in the stool may indicate a gastric ulcer.

In addition, ischemia of the intestine from splanchnic vasoconstriction increases the intestinal mucosal permeability. As a result, normal intestinal bacteria move from the lumen of the bowel to extraluminal sites, a process called *bacterial translocation*. This process is believed to be one of the mechanisms causing systemic sepsis and multiple organ dysfunction syndrome.

Urinary System

During the early stages of the burn injury, renal blood flow and glomerular filtration rates are greatly reduced from the decreased intravascular blood volume and the release of antidiuretic hormone (ADH) by the posterior pituitary. Urine output decreases, and serum creatinine and blood urea nitrogen increase.

Dark brown concentrated urine may indicate myoglobinuria, the result of the release of large amounts of dead or damaged erythrocytes after a major burn injury. When large amounts of these pigments are released, the liver cannot keep pace with conjugation and the pigments pass through the glomeruli. The pigments can occlude the renal tubules and cause renal failure, especially when dehydration, acidosis, or shock is also present.

Immune System

The function of the immune system is to protect the human body from invasion by foreign microorganisms. The capillary leak that occurs in the early stages of the burn injury continues throughout the burn shock phase and impairs the active components of both the cell-mediated and humoral immune systems.

The humoral immune system relies on B cells to produce antibodies or immunoglobulins (see Chapter 9). ☾☽ In the burn client, the serum levels of all immunoglobulins are significantly diminished. Serum protein levels remain persistently low throughout the clinical course until wound closure is effected. A marked decrease in T-cell counts results in a reduction of cytotoxic activity and suppression of the cell-mediated immune system.

The compromise in the humoral and cell-mediated immune systems constitutes a state of acquired immunodeficiency, which places the burn client at risk for infection. The period of vulnerability is transient and may last from 1 to 4 weeks following the onset of the burn injury. During this time frame, opportunistic infections can be fatal despite aggressive antimicrobial therapy.

Metabolism

Two distinct phases characterize the body's metabolic response to the burn injury. The ebb phase, occurring during the first 3 days of the injury, is manifested by decreased oxygen consumption, fluid imbalance, shock, and inadequate circulating volume. These responses protect the body from the initial impact of the injury.

A second phase, the flow phase, occurs when adequate burn resuscitation has been accomplished. This phase is characterized by increases in cellular activity and protein catabolism, lipolysis, and gluconeogenesis. The basal metabolic rate (BMR) significantly increases, reaching twice the normal rate. Body weight and heat drop dramatically. Total energy expenditure may exceed 100% of normal BMR. Hypermetabolism persists until after wound closure has been accomplished and may reappear if complications occur.

COLLABORATIVE CARE

The burn team is composed of an interdisciplinary group of health care professionals, who together plan the care and treatment of the burn-injured client during the acute and rehabilitative stages. The burn team consists of the nurse, physician, physical therapist, dietitian, social worker, and burn technician. The team members meet regularly to discuss client progress and to determine collaboratively the most effective regimen of care and psychosocial support.

Stages of Collaborative Care

The clinical course of treatment for the burn client is divided into three stages: the emergent/resuscitative stage, the acute stage, and the rehabilitative stage. Although these stages are useful predictors of the clinical needs of the burn client, it is important to recognize that the process of burn injury is dynamic and that, in many cases, the clinical stage may not be clearly delineated. Assessment and management of the burn-injured client are ongoing processes determined by the clinical picture; they last throughout the course of treatment. Figure 15–7 ■ shows the burn client's progression through the health care system during each clinical stage of burn care.

During each stage, different groups of nurses, physicians, and allied health care specialists collaborate to manage the client's recovery.

The Emergent/Resuscitative Stage

The emergent/resuscitative stage lasts from the onset of injury through successful fluid resuscitation. During this stage, health care workers estimate the extent of burn injury, institute first-aid measures, and implement fluid resuscitation therapies. The client is assessed for shock and evidence of respiratory distress. If indicated, intravenous lines are inserted, and the client may be prophylactically intubated. During this stage, health care workers determine whether the client is to be transported to a burn center for the complex intervention strategies of the professional, interdisciplinary burn team.

Although many burn injuries are treated in local tertiary care facilities, the American Burn Association has developed guidelines for determining whether the client should be transported to a burn center for interdisciplinary approaches to treatment and rehabilitation. Adult clients who should be treated at burn centers include those with:

- Second- or third-degree burns >10% TBSA and older than 50 years of age.
- Second- or third-degree burns >20% TBSA in adults to the age of 50.
- Third-degree burns >5% TBSA in adults of any age.
- Burns involving the hands, feet, face, eyes, ears, or perineum.
- Electrical (including lightning), chemical, and inhalation injuries.
- Circumferential burns of the extremities and/or chest.

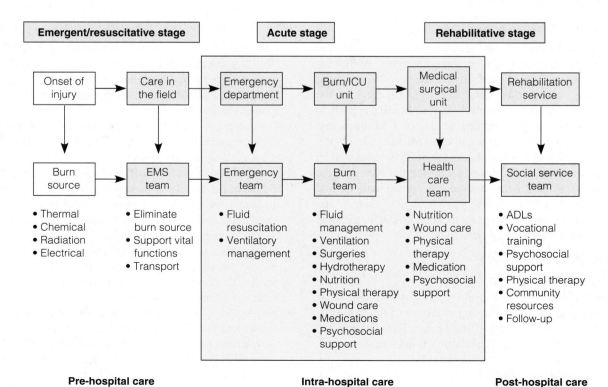

Figure 15–7 ■ The client's progression through the health care system during the emergent, acute, and rehabilitative stages of burn injury.

- Any burn associated with extenuating problems, preexisting illness, fractures, or other trauma.

Acute Stage

The acute stage begins with the start of diuresis and ends with closure of the burn wound (either by natural healing or by using skin grafts). During this stage, wound care management, nutritional therapies, and measures to control infectious processes are initiated. Hydrotherapy and excision and grafting of full-thickness wounds are performed as soon as possible after injury. Enteral and parenteral nutritional interventions are started early in the treatment plan to address caloric needs resulting from extensive energy expenditure. Measures to combat infection are implemented during this stage, including the administration of topical and systemic antimicrobial agents. Pain management constitutes a significant segment of the nursing care plan throughout the clinical course of the burn-injured client. The administration of narcotic pharmaceutical agents must precede all invasive procedures to maximize client comfort and to reduce the anxieties associated with wound debridement and intensive physical therapy.

Rehabilitative Stage

The rehabilitative stage begins with wound closure and ends when the client returns to the highest level of health restoration, which may take years. During this stage, the primary focus is the biopsychosocial adjustment of the client, specifically the prevention of contractures and scars and the client's successful resumption of work, family, and social roles through physical, vocational, occupational, and psychosocial rehabilitation. The client is taught to perform range-of-motion exercises to enhance mobility and to support injured joints.

Prehospital Client Management

Treatment at the injury scene includes measures to limit the severity of the burn and support vital functions. Before attempting to remove the client from the source of burn injury, rescuers must ensure their own safety. Depending on the causative agent, rescuers may need to consult with experts to determine the best way to eliminate the source of the injury. Once the safety of the rescuers has been established, all prehospital interventions are aimed at eliminating the heat source, stabilizing the client's condition, identifying the type of burn, preventing heat loss, reducing wound contamination, and preparing for emergency transport. Restrictive jewelry and clothing is removed at the scene to prevent circumferential constriction of the torso and extremities.

Stop the Burning Process

Emergency measures, by type of injury, include:

THERMAL BURNS. If the thermal injury has been caused by dry heat, smother inflamed clothing or lavage with water. Help the person "stop, drop, and roll" to extinguish the flame and limit the extent of burn. Once the flame has been extinguished, cover the body to prevent hypothermia. If the thermal injury has been caused by moist heat, lavage the area with cool water. Ice is not used for cooling as it causes vasoconstriction and may result in further injury.

CHEMICAL BURNS. For chemical burns, immediately remove the clothing and use a hose or shower to lavage the involved area thoroughly for a minimum of 20 minutes. Many chemicals are in powder form and as much dry chemical needs to be removed as possible before flushing the surface with water. Unusual chemicals may require consultation with the poison control center about appropriate treatment. Protective clothing should be worn during this process to protect the rescuer from chemical exposure.

ELECTRICAL BURNS. Electrical injuries pose serious potential harm to both rescuer and burn victim. Ensure that the source of electrical current has been disconnected, or move the person to safety and away from the energy source using a nonconductive device such as a broomstick. If the person is unresponsive, assess for the presence of cardiac and respiratory function. If indicated, begin cardiopulmonary resuscitation (CPR). A spinal cord injury may be present secondary to the forceful contraction of the muscles of the neck and back during exposure to the current. If possible, place the person in a cervical collar and transport on a spinal board.

RADIATION BURNS. Radiation injuries are usually minor and involve only the epidermal layer of skin. Treatment focuses on helping normal body mechanisms promote wound healing. For severe radiation burns, such as those that result from industrial radiation accidents, trained personnel may need to render the area safe for entry prior to rescue. All interventions are aimed at shielding, establishing distance, and limiting the time of exposure to the radioactive source.

Support Vital Function

The initial assessment of the client's respiratory and hemodynamic status begins with an evaluation of the client's airway, breathing, and circulation (the ABCs of care).

- If the client has no pulse and is not breathing, begin CPR. Establish an airway, and start mouth-to-mouth breathing and chest compressions. Continue CPR until spontaneous cardiopulmonary function returns or until the emergency management team takes over.
- Position the client with the head elevated at greater than 30 degrees, and administer 100% humidified oxygen by face mask. Use nasotracheal suction as necessary to maintain a patent airway. Endotracheal intubation may be necessary if the client has facial edema and inhalation injury. Auscultate the lungs often onsite to monitor respiratory status. Continuous pulse oximetry provides ongoing assessment of the client's oxygen saturation levels.
- Monitor for cardiac dysrrhythmias or arrest. When available, connect the client to a cardiac monitor and observe for dysrhythmias. Elevate burned extremities above the level of the heart to facilitate circulation.
- Initiate fluid replacement therapy for burn wounds that involve more than 20% of the total body surface area. Continuously assess heart and lung sounds and observe level of consciousness, cardiac rate and rhythm, blood pressure, and urine output.
- Cover the client to maintain body temperature and to prevent further wound contamination and tissue damage.

Emergency and Acute Care

Prehospital personnel report to the emergency department staff all findings and medical interventions that occurred at the scene of the injury. The nurse obtains a history of the injury, estimates the depth and extent of the burn, begins fluid resuscitation, and maintains ventilation according to protocol.

Fluid Resuscitation

Fluid resuscitation is the administration of intravenous fluids to restore the circulating blood volume during the acute period of increasing capillary permeability. To counteract the effects of burn shock, fluid resuscitation guidelines are used to replace the extensive fluid and electrolyte losses associated with major burn injuries. Fluid replacement is necessary in all burn wounds that involve ≥20% TBSA.

Crystalloid fluids are administered through two large-bore (14 to 16 gauge) catheters, preferably inserted through unburned skin. Warmed Ringer's lactate solution is the intravenous fluid most widely used during the first 24 hours after burn injury, as it most closely approximates the body's extracellular fluid composition. Several formulas may be used to replace fluid loss. Two commonly used formulas are as follows:

- Parkland formula, in which lactated Ringer's solution is administered 4 mL × kg × % TBSA burn.
- Modified Brooke formula, in which lactated Ringer's solution is administered 2 mL × kg × % TBSA burn.

These formulas specify the volume of fluid to be infused in the first 24 hours after the injury, with 50% of the fluid to be infused during the first 8 hours, followed by the remaining 50% over the next 16 hours (25% per 8 hours). Over the second 24 hours, fluids for clients with larger burns (such as more than 30% TBSA) are changed to a crystalloid solution of 5% dextrose in water titrated to maintain urine output (Bucher & Melander, 1999).

Hourly urine output is often used as the indicator of effective fluid resuscitation, with 30 to 50 cc for an adult considered adequate. (With electrical burns, a urine output of 75 to 100 cc should be maintained). Another valuable indicator is heart rate; if fluid resuscitation is adequate, the rate should be less than 120 beats per minute or in the upper limits of normal for age. A higher rate may indicate a need for additional fluid (Bucher & Melander, 1999).

During the fluid resuscitation stage, the client may require invasive hemodynamic monitoring (see Chapter 29). ⊕⊃ A pulmonary artery catheter can be used to monitor cardiac output, cardiac index, and pulmonary artery wedge pressures. All measurements must be maintained within normal limits to effect adequate fluid resuscitation.

Respiratory Management

Upon the client's admission to the emergency department, several baseline assessments of respiratory status must be obtained: chest X-ray study, ABGs, vital signs, and carboxyhemoglobin levels. Intubation is indicated for all clients with burns of the chest, face, or neck. The primary treatment plan is oriented toward preventing atelectasis and maintaining alveolar oxygen exchange. The following interventions should be initiated.

- Maintain the head of the bed at 30 degrees or greater to maximize the client's ventilatory efforts. Turn the client side to side every 2 hours to prevent hypostatic pneumonia.
- To keep airway passages clear, suction the client frequently, encourage the client to use incentive spirometry hourly, and help the client perform coughing and deep-breathing exercises every 2 hours.
- In the face of impending airway obstruction, the client will require intubation. Nasotracheal tube placement is the preferred route because it seems to be better tolerated and can be more effectively secured. If the client has suffered nasolabial burns, however, the orotracheal route is preferred. Nasotracheal and orotracheal intubation is reserved for short-term ventilatory management. For long-term ventilatory management (i.e., greater than 3 weeks), a tracheostomy is performed.
- Humidification of either room air or oxygen helps prevent the drying of tracheal secretions. Ambient air or oxygen flow is based on ABG results. The client may be placed on a face mask, steam collar, T-piece, mechanical ventilation with PEEP, pressure support ventilation, or high-frequency jet ventilation. The goal of all therapies is to maintain adequate tissue oxygenation with the least amount of inspired oxygen flow necessary.
- Medications to dilate constricted bronchial passages are administered intravenously and as inhalants to control bronchospasms and wheezing. Mucolytic agents liquefy tenacious sputum and aid in expectoration.
- An arterial line is placed in the client with major burn injury for continuous assessment of ABGs. Pulmonary artery pressure catheters may be inserted to measure pulmonary vascular resistance (PVR), pulmonary artery pressure (PAP), pulmonary capillary wedge pressure (PCWP), and mixed venous oxygen saturation (SVO_2). The PVR and PAP rise in the presence of hypoxia. The SVO_2 is the average percentage of hemoglobin bound with oxygen in the venous blood and reflects overall tissue utilization of oxygen. Pulse oximetry monitors arterial oxygen saturation levels.
- Pain medications are administered if the client is not in shock.

After stabilization in the emergency department, the client is transferred to the critical care unit or a specialized burn center (a facility that has a burn physician as director of a specialized nursing unit with dedicated burn beds). In both settings, continuous monitoring of diagnostic tests, administration of medications, pain control, wound management, and nutrition support therapies constitute the initial plan of care.

Diagnostic Tests

The following diagnostic tests are used to evaluate the client's progress and to modify intervention strategies.

- *Urinalysis* indicates the adequacy of renal perfusion and the client's nutritional status. In catabolic states, nitrogen is excreted in large amounts into the urine. Nitrogen loss is measured through 24-hour urine collections for total nitrogen, urea nitrogen, and amino acid nitrogen. *Myoglobinuria,* which manifests as a dark brown, wine-colored urine, signals the development of acute tubular necrosis. Loss of plasma protein and dehydration lead to proteinuria and elevated urine specific gravity. Glycosuria is a transient development following major burn injury; it indicates a need to adjust the nutritional program.

- The *complete blood count* is monitored regularly. Hematocrit is elevated secondary to hemoconcentration and fluid shifts from the intravascular compartment. Hemoglobin is decreased secondary to hemolysis. White blood cells are elevated if infection is present.
- *Serum electrolytes* are monitored regularly. Sodium levels are decreased secondary to massive fluid shifts into the interstitium. Potassium levels initially are elevated during burn shock, as a result of cell lysis and fluid shifts into the extracellular space. Potassium levels decrease after burn shock resolves, as fluid shifts back to intracellular and intravascular compartments.
- *Renal function* test results are closely monitored. Blood urea nitrogen (BUN) is elevated secondary to dehydration. Creatinine is elevated in the presence of renal insufficiency.
- *Total protein, albumin, transferrin, prealbumin, retinol binding protein, alpha 1-acid glycoprotein, and C-reactive protein* indicate protein synthesis and nutritional status. Because of the fluid shifts that occur during the early stages of the burn injury, they are more useful markers during the rehabilitative phase of care.
- *Creatine phosphokinase (CPK)* is elevated following an electrical burn, secondary to extensive muscle damage.
- *Blood glucose* is transiently elevated after major burn injury.
- *Serial ABGs* indicate the presence of hypoxia and acid-base disturbances and indicate client responses to changes in oxygen therapies. The burn-injured client may demonstrate elevated or lowered pH, decreased Pco_2, decreased Po_2, and low-normal bicarbonate levels.
- *Pulse oximetry* allows continuous assessment of oxygen saturation levels. The burn-injured client may have saturation levels below 95%.
- *Serial chest X-ray* studies document changes within the first 24 to 48 hours that may reflect the presence of atelectasis, pulmonary edema, or acute respiratory disease (ARD).
- *Serial electrocardiograms (EKGs)* are necessary to monitor the development of dysrhythmias, especially those associated with hypokalemic and hyperkalemic states.

Medications

Pain Control

Burns often cause excruciating pain. In the early stages of care, intravenously administered narcotics such as morphine, meperidine, or fentanyl are the best means of managing pain. Morphine is the drug of choice. Once the client has been stabilized, it is appropriate to administer narcotics prior to initiating hydrotherapy or intensive exercising routines. The oral, subcutaneous, or intramuscular route of administration should be avoided until hemodynamic stability and unimpaired tissue perfusion returns.

As the client enters the rehabilitative stage of care, alternative therapies for pain control may be added to the plan of care.

Distraction, self-hypnosis, guided imagery, and relaxation techniques are helpful adjuncts in managing pain and coping with loss. Patient-controlled analgesia (PCA) enhances the client's ability to cope with pain. See Chapter 4 for a discussion of strategies for managing pain. ∞

Antimicrobial Agents

Systemic infection is a leading cause of death in major burn patients. Gram-positive organisms such as Staphylococcus and Streptococcus colonize the burn surface during the first week postburn; gram-negative enteric organisms become more common with longer periods of hospitalization. To eliminate infection on the surface of the burn wound, topical antimicrobial therapy is used, depending on protocol. Of the many antimicrobial agents available, the three most widely used are mafenide acetate (Sulfamylon) cream, sulfadiazine (Silvadene) cream, and silver nitrate 0.5% soaks. All three are broad-spectrum antibiotics. The choice of topical antibiotic is based on the extent of the burn wound, the presence of identified bacterial organisms, whether an open (exposing the wound to the air) or closed (using bulky dressings) method of treatment is used, and client response.

The increasing trend is toward prophylactic antibiotic administration in burn clients (Tierney, McPhee, & Papadakis, 2001). Systemic antimicrobial therapy is indicated in the immediate preoperative and postoperative period associated with excision and autografting. Postoperatively, the therapy is discontinued as soon as the client's hemodynamic status returns to normal, usually within the first 24 hours. In the long-term treatment of identified infectious processes, drug administration is limited to the least amount of time required to eradicate the infection. See the box on the following page for nursing implications for topical antimicrobial therapy for the burn client.

Tetanus Prophylaxis

If the client's immunization status is in doubt, tetanus toxoid is administered intramuscularly early in the acute phase of care to prevent *Clostridium tetani* infection.

Preventing Gastric Hyperacidity

Hyperacidity must be controlled to prevent Curling's ulcer. A nasogastric tube is placed during the emergent phase of care, and gastric aspirant is obtained hourly. The gastric pH should be assessed and maintained at levels above 5. To control gastric acid secretion during the acute phase of care, histamine H_2 blockers (e.g., famotidine [Pepcid] and ranitidine [Zantac]) can be administered intravenously, either intermittently or as continuous infusions. As soon as bowel sounds become audible, the client is placed on an antacid regimen.

Treatments

Surgery

Three surgical interventions are commonly employed to manage the burn wound: surgical debridement, escharotomy, and autografting.

ESCHAROTOMY. When the burn eschar forms circumferentially around the torso or extremities, it acts as a tourniquet, impairing circulation. Left unchecked, the affected body part becomes gangrenous.

Medication Administration

Topical Burn Medications

TOPICAL ANTIMICROBIAL AGENTS

Mafenide acetate (Sulfamylon)
Silver nitrate
Silver sulfadiazine (Silvadene)

The use of topical antimicrobial therapy was first investigated more than 60 years ago. Researchers found that the most effective topical agents are those that (1) act against the major pathogens responsible for causing burn wound infection, (2) achieve levels of concentration sufficient to decrease microbial colonization, (3) are rapidly excreted or metabolized, (4) are nontoxic, and (5) are easy to use and inexpensive.

Mafenide Acetate

Mafenide is a synthetic antibiotic closely related chemically, but not pharmacologically, to the sulfonamides. Although the mechanism of action is unclear, the drug appears to interfere with the metabolism of bacterial cells. Mafenide is a bacteriostatic agent effective against many gram-positive and gram-negative organisms.

For topical administration, mafenide is used in an 8.5% cream in a water-miscible base. Following application, the drug is rapidly diffused through the burn eschar and absorbed systemically.

In the general circulation, mafenide metabolizes to a weak carbonic anhydrase inhibitor known as *p*-carboxybenzenesulfonamide, a substance that impairs the renal mechanisms involved in the buffering of blood. Bicarbonate excretion in the urine increases, and ammonia and chloride excretion decreases. To maintain normal acid-base balance, the pulmonary system effects a compensatory hyperventilatory state. If the compensatory hyperventilation is insufficient, the client develops metabolic acidosis.

Nursing Responsibilities

- Use mafenide with caution in clients with renal or pulmonary disease.
- Approximately 3% to 5% of clients develop a hypersensitivity to mafenide, resulting in a maculopapular rash on the unburned areas. Assess the client for the following:

Pruritus	Urticaria
Facial edema	Blisters
Swelling	Eosinophilia

  If hypersensitivity reactions occur, discontinue the drug and administer antihistamines.
- Monitor the client for superinfection within the burn eschar, in the subeschar tissue, or in viable tissue adjacent to the wound.

Client and Family Teaching

- Expect pain or a burning sensation following drug application. Take appropriate measures to control pain before applying the drug.
- Apply the drug to clean, debrided burn wounds once or twice daily. Continue applications until healing is apparent.
- If any signs of allergy develop, discontinue the drug and notify the physician.
- Report any sudden and prolonged increases in respiratory rate.

Silver Nitrate

Silver nitrate is a bacteriostatic agent that inhibits a wide variety of gram-positive and gram-negative organisms. Its antimicrobial effect is due to the actions of silver ions, which markedly alter the microbial cell wall and membrane. Additionally, the drug denatures bacterial protein, thereby inactivating and precipitating the microbes.

Nursing Responsibilities

- Silver nitrate is used as a 0.5% solution in distilled water. Apply the solution to bulky gauze dressings every 2 hours, and provide complete dressing changes twice daily.
- Silver nitrate has limited penetrating ability and is ineffective if used more than 72 hours following a burn injury.
- At the local tissue level, silver nitrate immediately interacts with chloride ions to form a black silver chloride precipitate that discolors both the burn wound and the adjacent tissues. The discoloration significantly hampers visual inspection of the wound.
- High concentrations of the drug result in cellular toxicity of surrounding healthy tissue.
- Because large amounts of water are systemically absorbed from the dressing site, the client may demonstrate a hypotonic state. Hyponatremia and hypochloremic alkalosis are common manifestations in burn-injured clients treated with silver nitrate.

Client and Family Teaching

- Watch for and report any signs and symptoms of hypotonicity: swelling, weight gain, difficulty in breathing.
- This drug causes a black discoloration on all skin surfaces and dressings with which it comes into contact.
- Because discoloration can conceal evidence of infection, watch for systemic manifestations of infection fever, malaise, rapid pulse rate, listlessness.
- Saturate the wound dressings every 2 hours with a 0.5% aqueous solution of the drug. Change the dressings completely twice daily.

Silver Sulfadiazine

Silver sulfadiazine, a sulfonamide, is the most commonly used topical agent. The drug acts on the cell membrane and cell wall of susceptible bacteria and binds to cellular DNA. The drug is bactericidal and effective against a wide variety of gram-negative and gram-positive organisms.

Nursing Responsibilities

- Many clients develop a marked leukopenia in response to this drug, which tends to improve spontaneously over the course of therapy. This finding does not contraindicate use of the drug.
- Hypersensitivity to silver sulfadiazine has been reported in a small number of cases. If the client develops hypersensitivity, administer antihistamine, and change the topical agent.
- If sulfa crystals form in the urine, keep the client well hydrated.
- Treatment with this drug can cause systemic uptake of propylene glycol, which results in an elevated serum osmolality and high urine specific gravity in the client who is not dehydrated. These findings tend to create confusion during the fluid resuscitative stage of care. Whenever the serum osmolality and urine specific gravity fail to correlate with a clinical picture that reflects fluid volume overload (elevated CVP/PCWP, rhonichi/wheezing, edema), suspect systemic propylene glycol uptake.

Client and Family Teaching

- Apply the drug to clean, debrided wounds once or twice daily, completely covering the burn wound at all times.
- Continue applying the drug until healing is apparent.
- If any signs of allergy develop, discontinue the drug and notify the physician.
- Watch for evidence of concentrated urine, and notify the physician.
- If not contraindicated, drink large amounts of fluids to prevent sulfa crystals from forming in the urine.

Figure 15–8 ■ Escharotomy. The surgical procedure consists of removing the eschar formed on the skin and underlying tissue following severe burns. The procedure is particularly helpful in restoring circulation to the extremities of clients when scar tissue forms a tight, constrictive band around the circumference of a limb.

Courtesy of Dr. William Dominic, Valley Medical Center.

To prevent circumferential constriction of the torso or extremity, an **escharotomy** is performed by the physician with a scalpel or by electrocautery (Figure 15–8 ■). A sterile surgical incision is made longitudinally along the extremity or the trunk to release taut skin and allow for expansion caused by edema formation. In the first 24 hours following the procedure, the incision should be gently packed with fine mesh gauze. After 24 hours, the site may be treated with a direct application of a topical antimicrobial agent. See the box below for nursing implications for care of the client undergoing escharotomy.

SURGICAL DEBRIDEMENT. **Surgical debridement** refers to the process of excising the wound to the level of fascia (fascial excision) or sequentially removing thin slices of the burn wound to the level of viable tissue (sequential excision). Because **fascial excision,** or **fasciectomy,** sacrifices potentially viable fat and lymphatic tissue, its use is reserved for clients with extensive or full-thickness burns. The most common technique is electrocautery with cutting and coagulating current capabilities. Sequential excision is performed with the use of a dermatome. Shallow burns and some of moderate depth bleed briskly after one slice. If bleeding does not occur, the procedure is repeated until a viable bed of dermis or subcutaneous fat is reached. Following surgical debridement, the client is returned to the burn unit.

AUTOGRAFTING. A procedure performed in the surgical suite, **autografting** is used to effect permanent skin coverage. Early burn wound excision and skin grafting decreases the hospital stay and enhances rehabilitation. Skin is removed from healthy tissue (donor site) of the burn-injured client and applied to the burn wound (Figures 15–9 ■ and 15–10 ■). (Skin grafts and flaps are discussed in Chapter 14.) After the autograft is applied, the grafted area is immobilized. The site is assessed daily for evidence of adherence. The client resumes range-of-motion exercises 5 days postgraft. As the wound heals, the client may complain of itching, which can be treated with mild lotions.

Cultured epithelial autografting is a technique in which skin cells are removed from unburned sites on the client's body, then minced and placed in a culture medium for growth. Over a 5- to 7-day period, the cells expand 50 to 70 times the size of the initial biopsies. The cells are again separated out and placed in

Nursing Implications for Circumferential Wound Management:

Escharotomy

When a burn wound totally encircles an extremity, the torso, or the neck, the client is at risk for impaired tissue perfusion of the involved area. To prevent arterial occlusion, a circumferential burn wound may need to be excised. An escharotomy is a lengthwise incision made by the physician along the circumferential burn wound to release tension and permit unobstructed arterial blood flow. The nurse continuously assesses the involved area and notifies the physician of the need to perform this emergent procedure, which is done at the bedside. Because only the dead burn wound tissue is excised, the client experiences very little pain.

Nursing Responsibilities
- For circumferential burn wounds of the extremity, assess the extremity for absence of blood flow:
  a. Using a Doppler ultrasound stethoscope, check hourly for the presence of a pulse.
  b. Assess the extremity hourly for warmth, color, sensation, and capillary refill.
  c. Observe for evidence of numbness or tingling.
- For circumferential burn wounds of the torso, assess for evidence of respiratory distress:
  a. Obtain ABGs as needed.

  b. Auscultate lung sounds hourly.
  c. Observe for evidence of cyanosis, tachypnea, anxiety, or restlessness.
- For circumferential burn wounds of the neck, assess for evidence of respiratory distress. Prepare the client for prophylactic intubation.
- Monitor for excessive blood loss, and transfuse the client if indicated.
- Dress the open wound (escharotomy) with topical antimicrobial agents as ordered.

Client Teaching
- Teach the client the importance of reporting any evidence of impaired circulation: numbness, tingling, blue color to the extremity, absence of sensation.
- Assure the client that the procedure will not be painful and will provide immediate relief.
- Teach the client the importance of protecting the open wound (escharotomy) from infection.
- Explain the rationale supporting prophylactic intubation for burn wounds involving the head and neck.
- Provide assurance that all blood loss will be replaced and that bleeding at the site will be controlled.

Figure 15–9 ■ Skin grafting procedure.

Courtesy of Dr. William Dominic, Valley Medical Center.

Figure 15–10 ■ Skin graft for burn injury (autograft).

Courtesy of Dr. William Dominic, Valley Medical Center.

a new culture medium for continued growth. With this technique, enough skin can be grown over a period of 3 to 4 weeks to cover an entire human body. The cells are prepared in sheets and attached to petroleum jelly gauze backing, which is applied to the burn wound site. Problems with infection and lack of attachment have occurred.

Biologic and Biosynthetic Dressings

The terms *biologic dressing* and *biosynthetic dressing* refer to any temporary material that rapidly adheres to the wound bed, promotes healing, and/or prepares the burn wound for permanent autograft coverage. Ideally, these kinds of dressings should be easy to apply and remove, inexpensive, nonantigenic, elastic, able to reduce pain, able to serve as a bacterial barrier, and able to enhance the natural healing process. The dressings are applied to the burn wound as soon as possible. Covering the wound eliminates the loss of water through evaporation, reduces infection, and promotes wound healing. Biologic and biosynthetic dressings that are currently in use include homograft (allograft), heterograft (xenograft), amnionic membranes, and synthetic materials.

Homograft, or **allograft,** is human skin that has been harvested from cadavers. It is stored in skin banks located throughout the nation. The development of methods to achieve prolonged storage of frozen, viable skin has increased the use of this dressing; however, its short supply and expense still pose problems. It is manufactured as strips cut to the pattern of the burn and applied using sterile technique. Under normal circumstances, a homograft is rejected within 14 to 21 days following application.

Heterograft, or **xenograft,** is skin obtained from an animal, usually a pig. Although fresh porcine heterograft is available to some centers, frozen heterograft is much more commonly used. Once applied, heterograft appears to undergo early softening and lysis from enzymatic action from the wound. As a result, frequent changes of the heterograft dressing are necessary. Because of the high infection rates associated with this dressing, silver-nitrate-treated porcine heterograft has been developed to retard microbial growth.

The multiple problems associated with the use of biologic dressings have driven the development of synthetic materials. One such material is Biobrane, a composite material consisting of nylon mesh bonded to silicone that has proved successful in the temporary coverage of second- and third-degree burns. Whereas Biobrane adheres well to moderately clean wounds, it cannot adhere to or lower bacterial counts in grossly contaminated wounds. Biobrane dressing is supplied in various sizes, cut to fit the wound site, and secured with tape or Steri-Strips. It spontaneously separates from the wound when the underlying tissue heals. Hydrocolloid dressings are another type of biosynthetic material. They are occlusive wafers of gumlike materials that provide a water-resistant outer layer for coverage of the donor site. They protect healing tissue from excessive drying, liquefy necrotic tissue, and absorb wound drainage.

If dermal thickness is lost in deep partial-thickness or full-thickness burns, several products can serve as a dermal replacement. Integra is a synthetic dermal substitute and Alloderm is human cadaver allograft dermis that is nonimmunogenic. These products are placed in the wound, and split-thickness autografts are then placed over the dermal replacement. These products are used to provide temporary wound coverage, reduce pain, and facilitate healing.

The most recent temporary skin substitute is TransCyte. This bioengineered substance is derived from human fibroblast cells grown within mesh. As the cells grow, they secrete human dermal collagen, matrix proteins, and growth factors. The product is produced, extensively tested for any infectious agents, and then frozen. It is used for temporary covering for surgically debrided full-thickness and deep partial-thickness burn wounds, and is an alternative to silver sulfadiazine and cadaver skin. TransCyte forms a transparent, protective barrier over the wound surface and is typically applied only once. The best results have been obtained when it was applied within 24 hours of injury.

Wound Management

The outcomes of care for the client with a major burn depends on the prevention and treatment of infection through daily topical wound care, wound monitoring, and wound excision and closure. The goals of wound management are as follows (Bucher & Melander, 1999):

- Remove nonviable tissue.
- Control microbial colonization.
- Promote reepithelialization.
- Achieve wound coverage as early as possible.

DEBRIDING THE WOUND. Burned tissue releases chemical mediators that stimulate phagocytosis in an attempt to digest debris left by decaying necrotic tissue. Necrotic tissue that remains despite phagocytic action retards healing and prolongs inflammation. **Debridement** is the process of removing all loose tissue, wound debris, and eschar (dead tissue) from the wound. Three methods of debridement are employed: mechanical, enzymatic, and surgical (surgical debridement was previously discussed).

A nurse may perform mechanical debridement by applying and removing gauze dressings (wet-to-dry or wet-to-moist), hydrotherapy, irrigation, or scissors and tweezers. During hydrotherapy (in an immersion tank, a shower, or on a spray table) the burn injury may be gently washed with a mild soap or wound cleaner solution to remove dead skin and separate eschar. The solution is then rinsed off with warm saline or tap water. Body hair (except for eyebrows) should be shaved within the burn and to within 2.5 cm of the wound edges. Blistered skin is grasped with a dry gauze and gently removed. The edges of blisters or eschar are trimmed with blunt scissors. The wound is then covered with a topical antimicrobial agent.

Enzymatic debridement involves the use of a topical agent to dissolve and remove necrotic tissue. An enzyme (such as sutilains, collagenase [Santyl], or fibrinolysis-deoxyribonuclease [Elase]) is applied in a thin layer directly to the wound and covered with one layer of fine mesh gauze. A topical antimicrobial agent is then applied and covered with a bulky wet dressing; the wound is immobilized with expandable mesh gauze.

DRESSING THE WOUND. Once the wound has been cleaned and debrided, it may be dressed using one of two methods. In the open method, the burn wound remains open to air, covered only by a topical antimicrobial agent. This method allows the wound to be easily assessed. Topical agents must be frequently reapplied because they tend to rub off onto the bedding.

In the closed method, a topical antimicrobial agent is applied to the wound site, which is covered with gauze or a nonadherent dressing and then gently wrapped with a gauze roll bandage (Figure 15–11 ■). With the closed method, burn wounds are usually dressed twice daily and as needed. Dressings are applied circumferentially in a distal-to-proximal manner. All fingers and toes are wrapped separately.

POSITIONING, SPLINTS, AND EXERCISE. During therapy, the client must be maintained in positions that prevent **contractures** from forming. Because flexion is the natural resting position of joints and extremities, early physical therapy may include maintaining antideformity positions. Splints immobi-

Figure 15–11 ■ Closed method of dressing a burn.

Courtesy of Dr. William Dominic, Valley Medical Center.

lize body parts and prevent contractures of the joints. They are applied and removed according to schedules established by the physical therapist.

Early in the acute phase of care, the physical therapist prescribes active and passive ROM exercises, which are performed every 2 hours at the bedside, most often by physical therapy. Early ambulation is also part of the plan of care once the client's condition becomes stable.

SUPPORT GARMENTS. Applying uniform pressure can prevent or reduce hypertrophic scarring. Tubular support bandages are applied 5 to 7 days postgraft to maintain a tension ranging from 10 to 20 mmHg to control scarring. The client wears custom-made elastic pressure garments for 6 months to a year postgraft.

Nutritional Support

The client with a major burn is in a hypermetabolic and catabolic state. The resting energy expenditure after severe burn injury can increase by as much as 100% above normal levels, depending on the extent of catabolism and the client's physical activity, size, age, and gender. This increase is believed due to heat loss from the burn wound, an increase in beta-adrenergic activity, pain, and infection. As a result, total caloric needs may be as great as 4000 to 6000 kcal per day.

Traditional dietary management based on oral intake seldom meets the kcal requirements necessary to reverse negative nitrogen balance and begin the healing process. Enteral feedings with a nasointestinal feeding tube are therefore instituted within 24 to 48 hours of the burn injury to offset hypermetabolism, improve nitrogen balance, and decrease length of hospital stay. A nasointestinal feeding tube is placed under fluoroscopy, with the tip extending past the pylorus to prevent reflux and aspiration.

Although enteral feeding is the preferred nutritional therapy, it is contraindicated in Curling's ulcer, bowel obstruction, feeding intolerance, pancreatitis, or septic ileus. When the enteral route cannot be used, a central venous catheter is inserted via the subclavian or jugular vein for the administration of total parenteral nutrition (TPN).

TABLE 15–5 Interventions in Various Stages of Burn Injury

Stage of Burn Injury	Onset	End Point	Interventions
Emergent/Resuscitative	Occurrence of burn injury	Successful fluid resuscitation	Remove client from heat source. Initiate first aid. Assess extent of burn injury. Prevent hypothermia. Assess for shock. Determine need for intubation. Determine need for intravenous therapy. Follow protocol for fluid resuscitation. Obtain history. Transport to tertiary care facility.
Acute	Diuresis	Wound closure	Begin hydrotherapy. Determine need for excision of burn wound. Control spread of infection. Institute wound care. Start nutrition support. Graft burn wound. Initiate physical therapy. Manage pain.
Rehabilitative	Wound closure	Return to highest level of health restoration	Prevent scar formation. Continue physical therapy. Address psychosocial, cultural, and spiritual needs. Consider occupational therapy. Consider vocational training. Assess home maintenance management.

NURSING CARE

The client with a major burn has complex, multisystem needs. Table 15–5 lists overall nursing interventions for the emergent, acute, and rehabilitative stages of burn injury.

Health Promotion

Although treatments have improved significantly over the last several decades, there is no cure for burns. Prevention remains the primary goal. With the public's increasing attention to health promotion and disease prevention, the nursing profession currently is well positioned to collaborate with other disciplines to develop initiatives to reduce the number of burn injuries. For example, as client advocates, nurses can alert political leaders to the need to pass legislation aimed at reducing the incidence of burns. Appropriate legislative themes might center on safety in the workplace (e.g., requirements for smoke alarms and sprinkler systems), on the highways (e.g., regulations regarding the transportation of flammable liquids), and in the home (e.g., requirements for safety devices for water heaters and wood-burning stoves, and for self-extinguishing cigarettes). As educators, nurses can develop teaching plans for families and communities to heighten awareness of the problem. As researchers, nurses can investigate conditions leading to burn injury and suggest methods to reduce its prevalence. Working together with health care policymakers and community leaders, nurses can join the effort to lower the number of annual burn cases.

Assessment

Nursing assessment is continuous from the initial contact with the client with a burn injury. This section describes the secondary survey, conducted when the client arrives at the emergency department. Once there, the staff must act quickly to obtain the client's history of the burn injury, including the time of injury, causative agents, early treatment, medical history, and client's age and body weight. In most cases, the client is awake and oriented and able to relate the information during the emergent phase of care. Because changes in sensorium will become evident within the first few hours following a major burn injury, the nurse obtains as much information as is possible immediately on the client's arrival.

- *Time of injury.* In many cases, the client is admitted to the emergency department an hour or more after the injury occurred. The time of the burn injury must be documented as precisely as possible at the scene, because all fluid resuscitation calculations are based on the time of the burn injury, not on the client's time of arrival at the ER.
- *Cause of the injury.* Because the type of burn injury determines which nursing measures take priority, identify the specific causative agent to establish the appropriate plan of care.
- *First-aid treatment.* Prior to the arrival of medical personnel, the client or family may have applied home remedies to treat the burn wound. It is important for the nurse to ascertain and document the nature of all home treatment interventions, including the application of neutralizing agents, liquids, and immobilizing devices used to splint associated injuries.

Meeting Individualized Needs

BURNS IN THE OLDER ADULT

Older adults are at greater risk for burns of all degrees of severity, with burns and fires being a major cause of death. Most burns are accidental, the result of slower reaction times, decreased mobility, visual deficits, a decreased sense of smell, forgetfulness, and impaired sensation. Many older adults are burned by stoves, hot water, hot food, irons, cookware, and heating pads. Older adults with cognitive impairments or dementias may start fires by leaving foods cooking unattended. The most common burns in this age group are the result of catching clothing on fire and scalding from tap water that is too hot.

The care of the older adult with burns often presents unique challenges. They may delay seeking treatment, thus increasing the risk of infection. Their care is often complicated by the presence of other chronic illnesses. They may live alone, and have no one to care for them during rehabilitation. Even small burns have the potential to become lethal in older adults.

Burn prevention topics for older adults are as follows:

- Have a relative or neighbor routinely check for the odor of gas.
- Check the smoke detector battery once a month.
- Wear close-fitting clothing when cooking.
- Use a cooking timer with a loud alarm.
- Never lay anything over a heating device.
- Set the temperature of the hot water heater no higher than 120°F.
- Install antiscald devices in bathroom plumbing.

- *Past medical history.* Clients with histories of respiratory, cardiac, renal, metabolic, neurologic, gastrointestinal, or skin diseases; alcohol abuse; or altered immune states require more intense observation. Known allergies are obtained.
- *Age.* Older adults tend to require more supportive care (see the box above).
- *Medications.* Drugs, either prescribed or recreational, taken by the client prior to the burn injury may further complicate the treatment regimen. Drugs that affect any of the major body systems or cause mood alterations will need to be factored into the treatment plan. As part of the early assessment, obtain and document blood levels of therapeutic pharmaceutical agents and mood-altering substances.
- *Body weight.* During the acute and rehabilitative phases of the burn injury, the client will lose as much as 20% of preburn weight. This fact will have significant implications for all clients, especially for those who are underweight or cachectic at the time of the injury.

Nursing Diagnoses and Interventions

A major burn affects virtually every body system, as well as social, cultural, economic, psychological, and spiritual well-being. Immediate treatment in an intensive care setting is followed by years of rehabilitation and a lifetime of change in what was possible for an individual before the injury. Many nursing diagnoses are appropriate for the client with a major burn injury; those described here are *Altered skin integrity, Deficient fluid volume, Acute pain, Risk for infection, Impaired physical mobility, Imbalanced nutrition: Less than body requirements,* and *Powerlessness.*

Impaired Skin Integrity

The burn injury significantly impairs skin integrity. The severity of wounds varies according to the depth and extent of the burn. General treatment measures are designed to restore normal skin function as quickly as possible. Nursing care focuses on assessing and cleansing the wound and controlling infection.

- Estimate the extent and depth of the burn wound and recalculate extent of unhealed burns weekly. *The severity of the burn injury is the basis for determining which type of interventions are appropriate. Reassessment on a regular basis is necessary to monitor the healing process.*
- Provide daily wound care (including debridement method, dressing method, and medication administration) as prescribed, *to remove dead tissue, control infection, and promote reepithelialization as soon as possible.*
- Provide special skin care to sensitive body areas:
  - Clean burns involving the eyes with normal saline or sterile water, *to prevent corneal and conjunctival drying and adherence.* If contracture of the eyelid develops, apply drops or ointment to the eye, *to prevent corneal abrasion.*
  - Gently wipe burns of the lips with saline-soaked pads. Apply an antibiotic ointment as prescribed. Assess the mouth frequently, and perform mouth care routinely. If an oral endotracheal tube is in place, reposition it often, *to prevent pressure ulcer formation.*
  - Gently debride burns of the nose, and apply mafenide acetate (Sulfamylon) cream. Position nasogastric and nasotracheal tubes, *to prevent excessive pressure.*
  - Apply mafenide acetate (Sulfamylon) cream to burns of the ear. Gently debride and thoroughly clean the wound with a water spray. Do not cover ears with dressings. Do not use pillows; to reduce pressure to the area, use a foam doughnut instead. *Burns of the ears are prone to infection; special positioning devices are necessary to decrease pressure ulcer formation.*

Deficient Fluid Volume

Fluid resuscitation rates are adjusted periodically throughout the emergent stage of care. The nurse should be particularly aware of several situations that may warrant the administration of fluids at rates in excess of the calculations needed to maintain adequate urine output: initial underestimation of the burn size, sequestration of fluid into the lung tissue in inhalation injury, electrical injury (which tends to cause more extensive damage than is immediately visible), full-thickness burns, and inordinately delayed starts of fluid resuscitation.

- Assess blood pressure and heart rate frequently. *Vital signs rapidly deteriorate when fluid resuscitation is inadequate.*

- Monitor hemodynamic status, including CVP and PCWP. *Inadequate fluid resuscitation is manifested by a drop in the central venous pressure and pulmonary capillary wedge pressure.*
- Follow prescribed protocols for intravenous fluid resuscitation. *Therapy for burn shock is aimed at supporting the client through the period of hypovolemic instability.*
- Monitor intake and output hourly. *Report urine outputs of less than 50 mL/h. Intake and output measurements indicate the adequacy of fluid resuscitation, and should range from 30 to 50 mL per hour in an adult.*
- Weigh daily. *Body weight is used to calculate fluid requirements.*
- Test all stools and emesis for the presence of blood. *Occult blood in emesis or stool indicates gastrointestinal bleeding.*
- Maintain a warm environment. *Hypothermia leads to shivering and further loss of body fluid through increased energy expenditure and catabolism.*
- Monitor for fluid volume overload. *Older clients and those with underlying cardiac disease may demonstrate symptoms of congestive heart failure during the fluid resuscitation stage.*

PRACTICE ALERT *Manifestations of fluid overload include weight gain in a short time; an intake that exceeds output; an increase in blood pressure and CVP; jugular vein distention; dyspnea, orthopnea, crackles; and restlessness.* ■

Acute Pain

The client experiences excruciating pain with extensive superficial and all partial-thickness burns. Intense pain is also experienced during wound care and physical therapy. In addition, increased levels of anxiety about treatments and outcomes may further increase the perception of pain.

- Measure the client's level of pain, using a consistent measurement tool. *Pain tolerance is the duration and intensity of pain that the client is able to endure. Pain tolerance differs from one client to the next and may vary in the same client in different situations.*
- Medicate before painful procedures and determine when PCA is appropriate. *The inability to manage pain results in feelings of despair and frustration.*
- Administer intravenous narcotic analgesics as prescribed. *Nurses' fear of precipitating addiction often makes them reluctant to administer narcotics. During the acute stage of burn injury, however, invasive procedures and exposed neurosensory nerve endings dictate the need for narcotic pharmaceutical agents.*

PRACTICE ALERT *Narcotics are never administered orally, subcutaneously, or intramuscularly in the acute stage of a burn.* ■

- Explain all procedures and expected levels of discomfort. *Clients who are prepared for painful procedures and know beforehand the actual sensations they will feel experience less stress.*

- Use methods of nonnarcotic pain control in combination with medications for pain. *Noninvasive pain relief measures (e.g., relaxation, massage, distraction) can enhance the therapeutic effects of pain relief medications.*
- Allow the client to verbalize the pain experience. *Each person experiences and expresses pain in his or her own manner, using various sociocultural adaptation techniques.*

Risk for Infection

From the onset of the burn injury, loss of the body's natural barrier to the external environment increases the risk of infection. Nursing interventions focus on controlling infectious processes. Monitor the results of diagnostic tests, maintain nutritional therapies, and apply antimicrobial agents to monitor and prevent the spread of infection, a major complication of the burn injury.

- Monitor daily for manifestations of wound infection. Remove topical medications and wound exudate and examine the entire wound. *Early manifestations of wound infection include swelling and inflammation in intact skin surrounding the wound; a change in the color, odor, or amount of exudate; increased pain; and loss of previously healed skin grafts.*

PRACTICE ALERT *An increased body temperature, without other manifestations of infection, is not indicative of infection in clients with large burn wounds (in which the hypermetabolic response resets the core temperature to a higher level).* ■

- Monitor for positive blood cultures, *which indicate bacteremia.*
- Monitor for hyperermia, cough, chest pain, wheezing, rhonchi, decreased oxygen saturation, and purulent sputum, *which are manifestations of pneumonia.*
- Monitor for the presence of bacteria in the urine, fever, urgency, frequency, dysuria and superpubic pain, *which are manifestations of urinary tract infections.*

PRACTICE ALERT *If the client has an indwelling catheter, assess the urine for cloudiness and a foul odor, and obtain a urine culture and sensitivity at least weekly.* ■

- Obtain daily WBC counts. *Leukocyte counts are indicators of immune system function, and increase in the presence of infection.*
- Determine tetanus immunization status. *Burn clients are at risk for anaerobic infection caused by* Clostridium tetani.
- Maintain high kcal intake. *Nutritional support provides the nutrients needed to maintain the body's defense mechanisms.*
- Maintain an aseptic environment, using standard precautions (including gloving, gowning, and sterile procedures). *Strict isolation technique deters the development of nosocomial infection.*
- Culture all wounds and body secretions per protocol. *Culture and sensitivity reports identify the presence of infectious microbes and indicate appropriate antimicrobial therapies.*
- Administer prescribed antimicrobial medications, *to decrease invasive wound infections.*

Impaired Physical Mobility

As the burn wound heals and new skin tissue forms, the involved area tends to shrink. Contractures form at the site and significantly limit mobility, especially when a joint is involved. Physical therapy is important, beginning in the early stages of treatment. The nurse institutes ambulation and planned exercise regimens as soon as the client's condition stabilizes.

- Perform active or passive ROM exercises to all joints every 2 hours. Ambulate when stable. *Regular exercise prevents further loss of motion, restores movement, and improves functional status.*
- Apply splints as prescribed. Maintain antideformity positions, and reposition the client hourly. *Splinting and positioning retard the formation of contractures.*

PRACTICE ALERT *Assess all clients, but especially the older adult, for indications of pressure ulcer formation under a splint.* ■

- Maintain limbs in functional alignment, *to preserve joint mobility.*

- Anticipate the need for analgesia. *Administering analgesics promotes the client's comfort during exercising sessions.*

Imbalanced Nutrition: Less Than Body Requirements

The burn injury initiates a complex series of events that have a profound effect on the body's use of nutrients and expenditure of energy. Daily kcal requirements are determined by the nutritionist, and as soon as possible, enteral feedings are initiated. Duodenal tubes are placed to enhance intestinal absorption and retard gastric reflux. Parenteral nutrition is reserved for instances in which enteral feedings are contraindicated. Nursing measures focus on assessing feeding tolerance and use of nutrients.

- Maintain nasogastric/nasointestinal tube placement. *Correct tube placement ensures appropriate absorption of nutrients and prevents aspiration.*
- Maintain enteral/parenteral nutritional support as prescribed. Observe and report any evidence of feeding intolerance: diarrhea, vomiting, excessive gastric residue, abdominal distention, absent bowel sounds, and constipation. *The dietitian, in collaboration with the physician, selects and individualizes the feeding formula according to the client's daily en-*

Nursing Research

Evidence-Based Practice for the Client with a Major Burn

The personal losses resulting from burns include changes in body image and self-concept, altered functional ability, inability to provide self-care, changes in roles and relationships, threats to employment and income, and fear of death. In the initial stage of burn treatment the client gives up most, if not all, control over all aspects of life.

In an investigation of chronic sorrow (Eakes et al., 1998), sorrow is presented as a normal response to an abnormal situation within a model of chronic sorrow. Chronic sorrow is defined as cyclical, with periodic recurrences as long as the disparity created by the loss exists. Characterized as pervasive, permanent, periodic, and potentially progressive in nature, the periodic return of grief is experienced by both individuals and caregivers. Chronic sorrow may be precipitated by a loss without a predictable end such as a chronic health problem or by a circumscribed loss such as the loss of a loved one. Chronic sorrow is most often triggered in individuals with chronic health problems when the individual experiences disparity with accepted social, developmental, or personal norms; and when treatment such as hospitalization brings the ongoing disparity into focus.

Individuals draw on a variety of strategies to cope with the periodic grief associated with chronic sorrow. Positive coping skills include taking part in personal interest and activities, seeking information, living one day at a time, talking with others in the same or similar situation, talking with someone close, and relying on religious or personal beliefs and practices for comfort.

IMPLICATIONS FOR NURSING

It is important that nurses provide interventions for chronic sorrow based on a personal belief that chronic sorrow is normal and

does occur. Being aware of the situations that trigger grief allows the nurse to provide anticipatory guidance drawn from the client's personal coping strategies. Simply asking "what helps?" is often a good way to assess coping strategies. Specific nursing interventions have been identified as being helpful in reducing the emotional pain of grief in clients with chronic health conditions. These interventions are taking time to listen, being empathic, offering support and reassurance, recognizing and focusing on feelings, and appreciating the uniqueness of each client and family. Interventions helpful to caregivers are empathic presence and providing accurate situation-specific information and helpful tips for dealing with the caregiver role.

Critical Thinking in Client Care

1. Support groups are available for clients and care-givers with many different situations of loss. Would you recommend a support group for a young adult with major burns? Why or why not?
2. Why do you think chronic sorrow in a client with severely disfiguring burns differs from that in a client whose child died at the age of 3?
3. Develop a plan for facilitating positive coping strategies for the following clients:
   a. A 22-year-old woman with full-thickness thermal burns over half the face and the skull, with loss of an ear.
   b. A 76-year-old man with deep split-thickness burns of the right hand (he is right-handed) from a hot-water heater explosion.
   c. A 35-year-old single mother of three school-age children, struck by lightning, with burns ranging from superficial to full thickness.

ergy expenditure requirements and feeding tolerance. Failure to maintain rates of infusion predisposes the client to continued catabolism and negative nitrogen balance.

- Weigh the client daily. *Anthropometric measurements indicate the adequacy of nutritional support therapies.*
- Obtain daily laboratory values for protein, iron, CBC, glucose, and albumin. *Decreased serum values indicate inadequate nutritional intake.*

Powerlessness

Usually, the client with a major burn injury endures a lengthy hospital stay involving many treatments and care protocols that are beyond his or her control. During the early stages, much of the care regimen involves excruciating pain. Further, the foreign environment of the burn unit makes it difficult for the client to relate to the immediate surroundings. For example, the need to control infection in the burn unit requires hospital personnel and family members to don sterile clothing prior to coming to the client's bedside. Family members and nursing personnel appear radically different when they are masked and gowned, and their odd appearance can add to the burn-injured client's sense of alienation.

- Allow the client as much control over the surroundings and daily routine as possible. For example, allow the client to choose times of dressing changes. *Powerlessness derives from the belief that one is unable to influence the outcome of a situation.*
- Keep needed items within reach, such as call bell, urinal, water pitcher, and tissues, *to reinforce the client's feelings of control.*
- Allow the client to express feelings. *The nurse can help the client cope by therapeutically listening, displaying a caring presence, clarifying misconceptions, and providing positive feedback* (see the Nursing Research box on previous page).
- Set short-term, realistic goals (e.g., set a goal for the client to ambulate from bedside to chair twice daily). *Small incremental gains are easier to achieve and allow for frequent positive reinforcement.*

Using NANDA, NIC, and NOC

Chart 15–1 shows links between NANDA, NIC, and NOC when caring for the client with a major burn.

CHART 15–1 NANDA, NIC, AND NOC LINKAGES

The Client with a Major Burn

NURSING DIAGNOSES	NURSING INTERVENTIONS	NURSING OUTCOMES
• Impaired Skin Integrity	• Skin Surveillance • Circulatory Precautions • Wound Care • Medication Administration: Skin • Skin Care: Topical Treatments • Positioning • Splinting • Exercise Therapy: Stretching • Exercise Therapy: Joint Mobility • Infection Protection	• Tissue Integrity: Skin • Wound Healing • Risk Control
• Deficient Fluid Volume	• Electrolyte Management Balance • Fluid Management • Fluid Monitoring • Hypovolemia Management • Intravenous Therapy • Shock Management: Volume • Vital Signs Monitoring	• Electrolyte • Fluid Balance
• Anxiety	• Anxiety Reduction • Coping Enhancement	• Anxiety Control • Coping
• Disturbed Body Image	• Body Image Enhancement • Active Listening • Coping Enhancement • Emotional Support • Grief Work Facilitation • Pain Management • Support Group	• Body Image • Grief Resolution

Note. Data from Nursing Outcomes Classification (NOC) by M. Johnson & M. Maas (Eds.), 1997, St. Louis: Mosby; Nursing Diagnoses: Definitions & Classification 2001–2002 by North American Nursing Diagnosis Association, 2001, Philadelphia: NANDA; Nursing Interventions Classification (NIC) by J.C. McCloskey & G. M. Bulechek (Eds.), 2000, St. Louis: Mosby. Reprinted by permission.

Home Care

Client and family teaching is an important component of all phases of burn care. As treatment progresses, the nurse encourages family members to assume more responsibility in providing care. From admission to discharge, the nurse teaches the client and family to assess all findings, implement therapies, and evaluate progress. The following topics should be addressed in preparing the client and family for home care.

- The long-term goals of rehabilitation care: to prevent soft tissue deformity, protect skin grafts, maintain physiologic function, manage scars, and return the client to an optimal level of independence
- Avoiding exposure to people with colds or infections and following aseptic technique meticulously when caring for the wound

- The need for progressive physical activity
- How to apply splints, pressure support garments, and other assistive devices
- Dietary requirements with required kcal
- Alternative pain control therapies, such as guided imagery, relaxation techniques, and diversional activities
- Care of the graft and donor sites
- Referral for occupational therapy, social service, clergy, and/or psychiatric services as appropriate
- Helpful resources:
  - American Burn Association
  - International Society for Burn Injuries
  - American Academy of Facial Plastic and Reconstructive Surgery
  - The Phoenix Society for Burn Survivors, Inc.

Nursing Care Plan
The Client with a Major Burn

Craig Howard, a 39-year-old truck driver, is admitted to the hospital following an accident in which the cab of his truck caught on fire. He was freed from the truck by a passing motorist, who stayed with him until the rescue team arrived and transported him to a local ED. Mr. Howard's wife, Mary, and twin daughters, Jessica and Jane, age 10, have been notified.

ASSESSMENT

On his admission to the ED, Mr. Howard is diagnosed with deep split-thickness and full-thickness burns of the anterior chest, arms, and hands. A quick assessment based on the rule of nines estimates the extent of his burn injury at 36% of TBSA. His vital signs are as follows: T 96.2°F (35.6°C), P 140, R 40, and BP 98/60. In the field, the paramedics had inserted a large-bore central line into Mr. Howard's right subclavian vein and started the rapid infusion of lactated Ringer's solution. Mr. Howard is receiving 40% humidified oxygen via face mask. Initial ABGs are: pH 7.49, P_{O_2} 60 mmHg, P_{CO_2} 32 mmHg, and bicarbonate 22 mEq/L. Lung sounds indicate inspiratory and expiratory wheezing, and a persistent cough reveals sooty sputum production. A Foley catheter is inserted and initially drains a moderate amount of dark, concentrated urine. A nasogastric tube is connected to low-intermittent suction. Mr. Howard is alert and oriented and complains of severe pain associated with the burn injuries. The burn unit is notified, and Mr. Howard is transferred there.

DIAGNOSIS

- *Risk for ineffective airway clearance,* related to increasing lung congestion secondary to smoke inhalation
- *Deficient fluid volume,* related to abnormal fluid loss secondary to burn injury
- *Risk for ineffective tissue perfusion,* related to peripheral constriction secondary to circumferential burn wounds of the arms

EXPECTED OUTCOMES

- Demonstrate a patent airway, as evidenced by clear breath sounds; absence of cyanosis; and vital signs, chest X-ray findings, and ABGs within normal limits.
- Demonstrate adequate fluid volume and electrolyte balance, as evidenced by urine output, vital signs, mental status, and laboratory findings within normal limits.

- Demonstrate adequate tissue perfusion, as evidenced by palpable pulses, warm extremities, normal capillary refill, and absence of paresthesia.

PLANNING AND IMPLEMENTATION

- Prepare for prophylactic nasotracheal intubation to maintain airway patency.
- Initiate fluid resuscitation therapy using the Parkland/Baxter formula to calculate intravenous fluid rate for the first 24 hours postburn.
- Assist the physician to perform escharotomies of both upper extremities.

EVALUATION

The nurse anesthetist inserted a nasotracheal tube and connected Mr. Howard to a T-piece delivering 40% oxygen. Vigorous respiratory toileting has significantly improved his ABGs. Bronchodilators have been parenterally administered and mucolytic agents added to his respiratory treatments. His tracheal secretions have begun to show evidence of clearing. Hourly urine outputs indicate adequate fluid resuscitation. Urine output has been maintained at 50 mL/h, and color and concentration have improved. CVP readings have been maintained at 6 cm H_2O, and blood pressure has increased to 100/64. The pulse rate has decreased to 100.

To improve tissue perfusion of both arms, the physician has performed bilateral escharotomies and the wounds are dressed, using sterile procedure. The extremities have demonstrated improved circulation.

Critical Thinking in the Nursing Process

1. Explain the rationale for the immediate insertion of a Foley catheter and nasogastric tube.
2. An escharotomy was performed on both arms. Why was this procedure necessary in Mr. Howard's case?
3. What is the rationale supporting the intravenous administration of narcotics to control Mr. Howard's pain?
4. Explain the sequence of events that led to a fluid and electrolyte shift during the first 24 to 48 hours after Mr. Howard sustained his injury.

See Evaluating Your Response in Appendix C.

EXPLORE MediaLink

NCLEX review questions, case studies, care plan activities, MediaLink applications, and other interactive resources for this chapter can be found on the Companion Website at www.prenhall.com/lemone.

Click on Chapter 15 to select the activities for this chapter. For animations, video clips, more NCLEX review questions, and an audio glossary, access the Student CD-ROM accompanying this textbook.

TEST YOURSELF

1. A burn caused by exposure to an acidic or basic agent is classified as a/an:
   a. Chemical burn
   b. Thermal burn
   c. Electrical burn
   d. Radiation burn

2. A burn that involves the entire dermis, the dermal papillae, and the hair follicles is classified as what type of burn?
   a. Superficial
   b. Superficial partial thickness
   c. Deep partial thickness
   d. Full thickness

3. Which of the following clients is at greatest risk for burn shock?
   a. One with a 90% superficial burn from a tanning bed
   b. One with 10% TBSA from a gasoline explosion
   c. One with radiation burns following treatment for cancer
   d. One with > 50% TBSA from a high-voltage electrical accident

4. The primary purpose of antimicrobial treatment of the burn wound is to:
   a. Relieve pain
   b. Eliminate infection on the wound surface
   c. Remove eschar
   d. Prevent renal failure

5. Which of the following topics should be included in a presentation on burn prevention at a senior citizen center?
   a. Use a solar-powered nightlight
   b. Do not use the oven for cooking
   c. Set the water heater no higher than 120° F
   d. Check smoke detectors annually

See Test Yourself answers in Appendix C.

BIBLIOGRAPHY

Badger, J. (2001). Burns: The psychological aspects. *American Journal of Nursing, 101*(11), 38–44.

Barnes, A., & Budd, L. (1999). Family-centered burn care. *Canadian Nurse, 95*(6), 24–27.

Braunwald, E., & Fauci, A. (2001). *Harrison's principles of internal medicine* (15th ed.). New York: McGraw-Hill.

Bucher, L., & Melander, S. (1999). *Critical Care Nursing.* Philadelphia: Saunders.

Carrougher, G. (1998). *Burn care and therapy.* St. Louis: Mosby.

Davis, S., & Sheely-Adolphson, P. (1997). Psychosocial interventions: Pharmacologic and psychologic modalities. *Nursing Clinics of North America, 32*(2), 331–342.

DeBoer, S. (2001). Pain control for burn victims: Don't be afraid to administer more morphine than is usual. *American Journal of Nursing, 101*(3), 56.

deRios, M., Novac, A., & Achauer, B. (1997). Sexual dysfunction and the patient with burns. *Journal of Burn Care & Rehabilitation, 18*(1, Pt 1), 37–42.

Docking, P. (1999). Trauma. Electrical burn injuries. *Accident & Emergency Nursing, 7*(2), 70–76.

Eakes, G., Burke, M., & Hainsworth, M. (1998). Middle-range theory of chronic sorrow. *Image: Journal of Nursing Scholarship, 30*(2), 179–184.

Fowler, A. (1998). Nursing management of minor burn injuries. *Emergency Nurse, 6*(6), 31–39.

Greenfield, E., & McManus, A. (1997). Infectious complications. . . prevention and strategies for their control. *Nursing Clinics of North America, 32*(2), 297–309.

Hilton, G. (2001). Emergency: Thermal burns. *American Journal of Nursing, 101*(11), 32–34.

Holm, C., Horbrand, F., von Donnersmarck, G., & Muhlbauer, W. (1999). Acute renal failure in severely burned patients. *Burns, 25*(2), 171–178.

Johnson, M., & Maas, M. (1997). *Nursing outcomes classification (NOC).* St. Louis: Mosby.

Kagan, R., & Smith, S. (2000). Evaluation and treatment of thermal injuries. *Dermatology Nursing, 12*(5), 334–335, 338–344, 347–350.

Kee, J. (2001). *Handbook of laboratory and diagnostic tests* (4th ed.). Upper Saddle River, NJ: Prentice Hall.

Kidd, P., & Wagner, K. (2001). *High-acuity nursing* (3rd ed.). Upper Saddle River, NJ: Prentice Hall.

Lim, J., Rehma, S., & Elmore, P. (1998). Rapid response: Care of burn victims. *AAOHN Journal, 46*(4), 169–180.

Mayes, T., Gottschlich, M., & Warden, G. (1997). Clinical nutrition protocols for continuous quality improvements in the outcomes of patients with burns. *Journal of Burn Care & Rehabilitation, 18*(4), 365–368.

McKirdy, L. (2001). Burn wound cleansing. *Journal of Community Nursing, 15*(5), 24, 26–27, 29.

Menzies, V. (2000). Depression and burn wounds. *Archives of Psychiatric Nursing, 14*(4), 199–206.

McCloskey, J., & Bulechek, G. (Eds.). *Nursing interventions classification (NIC)* (3rd ed.). St. Louis: Mosby.

McKenry, L., & Salerno, E. (1998). *Pharmacology in nursing* (20th ed.). St. Louis: Mosby.

Mertens, D., Jenkins, M., & Warden, G. (1997). Outpatient burn management. *Nursing Clinics of North America, 32*(2), 343–374.

Milner, S., Mottar, R., & Smith, C. (2001). The burn wheel. *American Journal of Nursing, 101*(11), 35–37.

North American Nursing Diagnosis Association. (2001). *Nursing diagnoses: Definitions & classification 2001–2002.* Philadelphia: NANDA.

Porth, C. (2002). *Pathophysiology: Concepts of altered health states* (6th ed.). Philadelphia: Lippincott.

Richard, R. (1999). Assessment and diagnosis of burn wounds. *Advances in Wound Care, 12*(9), 468–471.

Richard, R. (1999). The physiology of burns. *Nursing Times, 95*(34), 25–31.

Rutan, R. (1998). Physiologic response to cutaneous burn injury. In G. Carrougher, *Burn care and therapy* (pp. 1–33). St. Louis: Mosby.

Tierney, L., McPhee, S., & Papadakis, M. (Eds.). (2001). *Current medical diagnosis & treatment* (40th ed.). Stamford, CT: Appleton & Lange.

Wiebelhaus, P., & Hansen, S. (2001). Another choice for burn victims. *RN, 64*(9), 34–37.

Wiebelhaus, P., & Hansen, S. (2001). What you should know about managing burn emergencies. *Nursing, 31*(1), 36–42.

Wiebelhaus, P., Hansen, S., & Hill, H. (2001). Helping patients survive inhalation injuries. *RN, 64*(10), 28–32.

UNIT 4

RESPONSES TO ALTERED ENDOCRINE FUNCTION

Assessing Clients with Endocrine Disorders

www.prenhall.com/lemone

Additional resources for this chapter can be found on the Student CD-ROM accompanying this textbook, and on the Companion Website at www. prenhall.com/lemone. Click on Chapter 16 to select the activities for this chapter.

CD-ROM
- Audio Glossary
- NCLEX Review

Animation
- Endocrine System

Companion Website
- More NCLEX Review
- Functional Health Pattern Assessment
- Case Study
  Endocrine Assessment
- MediaLink Application
  Endocrine Hormones

LEARNING OUTCOMES

After completing this chapter, you will be able to:

- Review the anatomy and physiology of the endocrine glands.

- Explain the functions of the hormones secreted by the endocrine glands.

- Identify specific topics to consider during a health history interview of the client with health problems involving endocrine function.

- Describe techniques for physical assessment of endocrine structure and function.

- Identify abnormal findings that may indicate malfunction of the endocrine system.

The endocrine system is an essential regulator of the body's internal environment. Through hormones secreted by its glands, the endocrine system regulates such varied functions as growth, reproduction, metabolism, fluid and electrolyte balance, and gender differentiation. It also helps the body adapt to constant alterations in the internal and external environment.

REVIEW OF ANATOMY AND PHYSIOLOGY

The major endocrine organs are the pituitary gland, thyroid gland, parathyroid glands, adrenal glands, pancreas, and gonads (reproductive glands). The locations of these glands are illustrated in Figure 16–1 ■. Table 16–1 summarizes the role of the endocrine organs and their hormones. Specific information about the gonads is found in Chapters 46 through 49. ⊂⊃

Pituitary Gland

The pituitary gland (or *hypophysis*) is located in the skull beneath the hypothalamus of the brain. It often is called the "master gland" because its hormones regulate many body functions. The pituitary gland has two parts: the anterior pituitary (or adenohypophysis) and the posterior pituitary (or neurohypophysis). The anterior pituitary is glandular tissue, whereas the posterior pituitary is actually an extension of the hypothalamus.

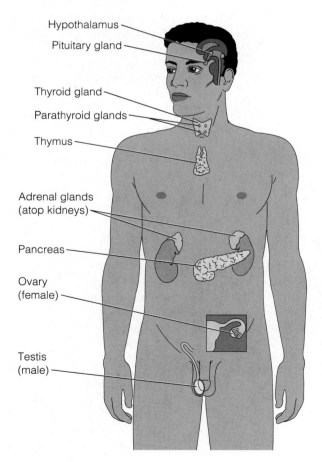

- Hypothalamus
- Pituitary gland
- Thyroid gland
- Parathyroid glands
- Thymus
- Adrenal glands (atop kidneys)
- Pancreas
- Ovary (female)
- Testis (male)

Figure 16–1 ■ Location of the major endocrine glands.

Anterior Pituitary

The *anterior pituitary* has several types of endocrine cells and secretes at least six major hormones (Figure 16–2 ■).

- Somatotropic cells secrete growth hormone (GH) also called *somatotropin*. GH stimulates growth of the body by signaling cells to increase protein production and by stimulating the epiphyseal plates of the long bones.
- Lactotropic cells secrete prolactin (PRL). Prolactin stimulates the production of breast milk.
- Thyrotropic cells secrete thyroid-stimulating hormone (TSH). TSH stimulates the synthesis and release of thyroid hormones from the thyroid gland.
- Corticotropic cells secrete adrenocorticotropic hormone (ACTH). ACTH stimulates release of hormones, especially the *glucocorticoids,* from the adrenal cortex.
- Gonadotropic cells secrete the gonadotropin hormones, follicle-stimulating hormone (FSH), and luteinizing hormone (LH). These hormones stimulate the ovaries and testes (the gonads). In women, FSH stimulates the development of ovarian follicles and induces the secretion of estrogenic female sex hormones. In men, FSH is involved in the development and maturation of sperm. In women, increasing levels of LH work together with FSH to lead to ovulation and the formation of the corpus luteum from an ovarian follicle. In men, LH is called interstitial cell–stimulating hormone (ICSH). This hormone stimulates the interstitial cells of the testes to produce male sex hormones.

Posterior Pituitary

The *posterior pituitary* is made of nervous tissue. Its primary function is to store and release two hormones produced in the hypothalamus:

- Antidiuretic hormone (ADH), also called *vasopressin,* inhibits urine production by causing the renal tubules to reabsorb water from the urine and return it to the circulating blood.
- Oxytocin induces contraction of the smooth muscles in the reproductive organs. In women, oxytocin stimulates the myometrium of the uterus to contract during labor. It also induces milk ejection from the breasts.

Thyroid Gland

The thyroid gland is anterior to the upper part of the trachea and just inferior to the larynx. This butterfly-shaped gland has two lobes connected by a structure called the isthmus.

The glandular tissue consists of follicles filled with a jelly-like colloid substance called thyroglobin, a glycoprotein-iodine complex. Cells within the follicles secrete thyroid hormone (TH), a general name for two similar hormones: *thyroxine* (T_4) and *triiodothyronine* (T_3). The primary role of thyroid hormones is to increase metabolism; they are also responsible for growth and development in children. TH secretion is initiated by the release of TSH by the pituitary gland and is dependent on an adequate supply of iodine.

The thyroid gland also secretes calcitonin, a hormone that decreases excessive levels of calcium in the blood by slowing the calcium-releasing activity of bone cells.

TABLE 16-1 Organs, Hormones, Functions, and Feedback Mechanisms of the Endocrine System

Endocrine Organ	Hormone Secreted	Target Organ and Feedback Mechanism
Thyroid gland	Thyroid hormone (TH): thyroxine (T_4) is the major hormone secreted by the thyroid gland. It is converted to triiodothyronine (T_3) at the target tissues.	Maintains metabolic rate and growth and development of all tissues. T_3 and T_4 are secreted in response to thyroid-stimulating hormone (TSH).
	Calcitonin	Maintains serum calcium levels by decreasing bone resorption and decreasing resorption of calcium in the kidneys whenever levels of plasma calcium are elevated.
Parathyroid gland	Parathyroid hormone (PTH)	Maintains serum calcium levels by stimulating bone resorption and formation and by stimulating kidney resorption of calcium in response to falling levels of plasma calcium.
Adrenal cortex	Mineralocorticoids (e.g., aldosterone)	Promote kidney tubule reabsorption of sodium and water and excretion of potassium in response to elevated levels of potassium and low levels of sodium, thereby increasing blood pressure and blood volume.
	Glucocorticoids (e.g., cortisol)	Help regulate metabolism of carbohydrates, fats, and proteins. Activate anti-inflammatory responses to stressors. Low cortisol levels stimulate hypothalamic secretion of corticotropin-releasing hormone (CRH), which stimulates the anterior pituitary gland to release ACTH, which in turn stimulates the adrenal cortex to secrete cortisol.
	Gonadocorticoids (androgens and small amounts of estrogen and progesterone)	The quantity of sex hormones produced here is small, and the mechanism is not well understood.
Adrenal medulla	Catecholamines (epinephrine and norepinephrine)	Stimulate the heart, constrict blood vessels, inhibit visceral muscles, dilate bronchioles, increase respiration and metabolism, promote hyperglycemia. Secreted in response to physical or psychologic stress.
Anterior pituitary (adenohypophysis)	Growth hormone (GH)	Promotes growth of body tissues by enhancing protein synthesis and promoting use of fat for energy and thus conserving glucose. Release is stimulated by growth hormone releasing hormone (GHRH) in response to low GH levels, hypoglycemia, increased amino acids, low fatty acids, and stress.

Figure 16–2 ■ Actions of the major hormones of the anterior pituitary.

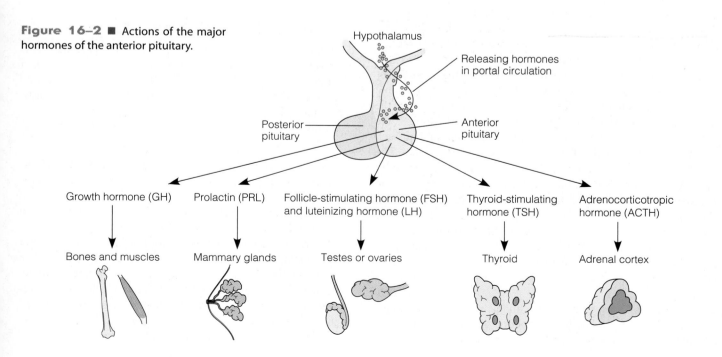

Parathyroid Glands

The parathyroid glands (usually four to six) are embedded on the posterior surface of the lobes of the thyroid gland. They secrete parathyroid hormone (PTH), or *parathormone.* When calcium levels in the plasma fall, PTH secretion increases. PTH also controls phosphate metabolism. It acts primarily by increasing renal excretion of phosphate in the urine, by decreasing the excretion of calcium, and by increasing bone reabsorption to cause the release of calcium from bones. Normal levels of vitamin D are necessary for PTH to exert these effects on bone and kidneys.

Adrenal Glands

The two adrenal glands are pyramid-shaped organs that sit on top of the kidneys. Each gland consists of two parts, which are distinct organs: an inner medulla and an outer cortex.

Adrenal Medulla

The adrenal medulla produces two hormones (also called catecholamines): epinephrine (also called *adrenaline*) and norepinephrine (or *noradrenaline.*) These hormones are similar to substances released by the sympathetic nervous system and thus are not essential to life. Epinephrine increases blood glucose levels and stimulates the release of ACTH from the pituitary; ACTH in turn stimulates the adrenal cortex to release glucocorticoids. Epinephrine also increases the rate and force of cardiac contractions; constricts blood vessels in the skin, mucous membranes, and kidneys; and dilates blood vessels in the skeletal muscles, coronary arteries, and pulmonary arteries.

Norepinephrine increases both heart rate and the force of cardiac contractions. It also vasoconstricts blood vessels throughout the body.

Adrenal Cortex

The adrenal cortex secretes several hormones, all corticosteroids. They are classified into two groups: mineralocorticoids and glucocorticoids. These hormones are essential to life. The release of the mineralocorticoids is controlled primarily by an enzyme called renin. When a decrease in blood pressure or sodium is detected, specialized kidney cells release renin to act on a substance called angiotensinogen, manufactured by the liver. Angiotensinogen is modified by renin and other enzymes to become angiotensin, which stimulates the release of aldosterone from the adrenal cortex. Aldosterone prompts the distal tubules of the kidneys to release increased amounts of water and sodium back into the circulating blood to increase volume and pressure. The glucocorticoids include cortisol and cortisone. These hormones affect carbohydrate metabolism by regulating glucose use in body tissues, mobilizing fatty acids from fatty tissue, and shifting the source of energy for muscle cells from glucose to fatty acids. Glucocorticoids are released in times of stress. An excess of glucocorticoids in the body depresses the inflammatory response and inhibits the effectiveness of the immune system.

Pancreas

The pancreas, located behind the stomach between the spleen and the duodenum, is both an endocrine gland (producing hormones) and an exocrine gland (producing digestive enzymes).

The endocrine cells of the pancreas produce hormones that regulate carbohydrate metabolism. They are clustered in bodies called pancreatic islets (or islets of Langerhans) scattered throughout the gland. Pancreatic islets have at least four different cell types:

- Alpha cells produce glucagon, which decreases glucose oxidation and promotes an increase in the blood glucose level by signaling the liver to release glucose from glycogen stores.
- Beta cells produce insulin, which facilitates the uptake and use of glucose by cells and prevents an excessive breakdown of glycogen in the liver and muscle. In this way, insulin decreases blood glucose levels. Insulin also facilitates lipid formation, inhibits the breakdown and mobilization of stored fat, and helps amino acids move into cells to promote protein synthesis. In general, the actions of glucagon and insulin oppose one another, helping to maintain a stable blood glucose level.
- Delta cells secrete somatostatin, which inhibits the secretion of glucagon and insulin by the alpha and beta cells.
- F cells secrete pancreatic polypeptide, which is believed to inhibit the exocrine activity of the pancreas.

Gonads

The gonads are the testes in men and the ovaries in women. These organs are the primary source of steroid sex hormones in the body. The hormones of the gonads are important in regulating body growth and promoting the onset of puberty.

In men, androgens (primarily testosterone) produced by the testes maintain reproductive functioning and secondary sex characteristics. Androgens also promote the production of sperm. In women, the ovaries secrete estrogens and progesterone to maintain reproductive functioning and secondary sex characteristics. Progesterone also promotes the growth of the lining of the uterus to prepare for implantation of a fertilized ovum.

The structure and functions of the gonads are discussed in Chapter 46. ⊙⊙

AN OVERVIEW OF HORMONES

Hormones are chemical messengers secreted by the endocrine organs and transported throughout the body, where they exert their action on specific cells called target cells. Hormones do not cause reactions directly but rather regulate tissue responses. They may produce either generalized or local effects.

Hormones are transported from endocrine gland cells to target cells in the body in one of four ways:

- Endocrine glands release most hormones, including TH, insulin, and others, into the bloodstream. Some require a protein carrier.
- Neurons release some hormones, such as epinephrine, into the bloodstream. This is called the neuroendocrine route.
- The hypothalamus releases its hormones directly to target cells in the posterior pituitary by nerve cell extension.
- With the paracrine method, released messengers diffuse through the interstitial fluid. This method of transport involves a number of hormonal peptides that are released throughout various organs and cells and act locally. An example is endorphins, which act to relieve pain.

Hormones act by binding to specific receptor sites located on the surfaces of the target cells. These receptors recognize a specific hormone and translate the message into a cellular response. The receptor sites are structured so that they respond only to a specific hormone; in other words, receptors in the thyroid gland are responsive to TSH but not to LH.

Hormone levels are controlled by the pituitary gland and by feedback mechanisms. Although most feedback mechanisms are negative, a few are positive. Negative feedback is controlled much as the thermostat in a house regulates temperature. Sensors in the endocrine system detect changes in hormone levels and adjust hormone secretion to maintain normal body levels. When the sensors detect a decrease in hormone levels, they begin actions to cause an increase in hormone levels; when hormone levels rise above normal, the sensors cause a decrease in hormone production and release. For example, when the hypothalamus or anterior pituitary gland senses increased blood levels of TH, it releases hormones causing a reduction in the secretion of TSH, which in turn prompts a decrease in the output of TH by the thyroid gland.

With positive feedback mechanisms, increasing levels of one hormone cause another gland to release a hormone. For example, the increased production of estradiol (a female ovarian hormone) during the follicular stage of the menstrual cycle in turn stimulates increased FSH production by the anterior pituitary gland. Estradiol levels continue to increase until the ovarian follicle disappears, eliminating the source of the stimulation for FSH, which then decreases. Stimuli for hormone release may also be classified as hormonal, humoral, or neural (Figure 16–3 ■). In hormonal release, hypothalamic hormones stimulate the anterior pituitary to release hormones. Fluctuations in the serum level of these hormones in turn prompt other endocrine glands to release hormones. In humoral release, fluctuations in the serum levels of certain ions and nutrients stimulate specific endocrine glands to release hormones to bring these levels back to normal. In neural release, nerve fibers stimulate the release of hormones.

ASSESSING ENDOCRINE FUNCTION

Function of the endocrine glands is assessed both by a health assessment interview to collect subjective data and a physical assessment to collect objective data. Hormones affect all body tissues and organs, and manifestations of dysfunction are often nonspecific, making assessment of endocrine function often more difficult than assessment of other body systems.

Health Assessment Interview

A health assessment interview to determine problems with the endocrine system may be part of a health screening or total health assessment, or it may focus on a chief complaint (such as increased urination or changes in energy levels). If the client has a problem with endocrine function, the nurse analyzes its onset, characteristics and course, severity, precipitating and relieving factors, and any associated symptoms, noting the timing and circumstances. For example, the nurse may ask the client:

- Describe the swelling you noticed in the front of your neck. When did it begin? Have you noticed any changes in your energy level?
- When did you first notice that your hands and feet were getting larger?
- Have you noticed that your appetite has increased even though you have lost weight?

MediaLink | FUNCTIONAL HEALTH PATTERN ASSESSMENT

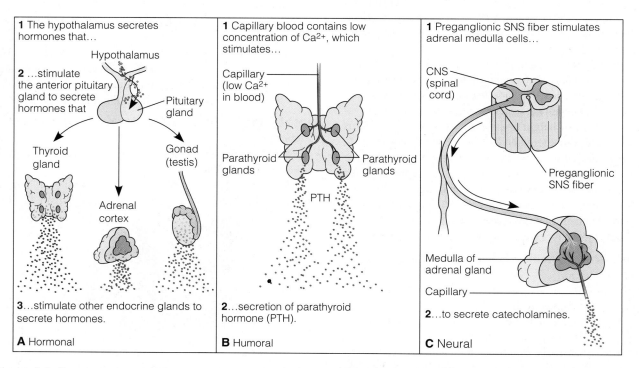

Figure 16–3 ■ Examples of three mechanisms of hormone release: *A,* hormonal; *B,* humoral; *C,* neural.

The health history includes information about the client's medical history, family history, and social and personal history. Ask the client about any changes in normal growth and development as well as in height and weight. Changes in the size of extremities can often be detected by asking whether the client has had to have rings enlarged or to buy increasingly larger gloves and shoes. Enlargement of the neck may be identified by asking whether the client has difficulty finding shirts or blouses with a collar that fits. Also explore changes including difficulty swallowing; increased or decreased thirst, appetite, and/or urination; visual changes; sleep disturbances; altered patterns of hair distribution (such as increased facial hair in women); changes in menstruation; changes in memory or ability to concentrate; and changes in hair and skin texture. Ask the client about any blow to the head, as well as previous hospitalizations, chemotherapy, radiation (especially to the neck), and the use of medications (especially hormones or steroids).

Because many endocrine disorders have a familial tendency, ask the client about a family history of such diseases as diabetes mellitus, diabetes insipidus, thyroid disorders, hypertension, tumors, autoimmune disorders, and obesity. Ask women about problems with pregnancy, menstruation, and/or menopause.

The nurse also asks about the client's occupational and social history. Include questions about the client's satisfaction with occupation, personal relationships, and lifestyle. Other areas of assessment include the client's usual means of coping; use of alcohol, smoking, or drugs; diet; exercise patterns; and sleep patterns. Although the client may not recognize changes in behavior, family members may be able to provide important information.

Physical Assessment

Physical assessment of the endocrine system may be performed as part of a total health assessment, or it may be a focused assessment of clients with known or suspected problems with endocrine function.

The only endocrine organ that can be palpated is the thyroid gland; however, other assessments that provide information about endocrine problems include inspection of the skin, hair and nails, facial appearance, reflexes, and musculoskeletal system. Measurement of height and weight as well as vital signs also provides clues to altered endocrine system function.

The client may sit during the examination. A reflex hammer is used to test deep-tendon reflexes. Prior to the examination, the nurse collects the necessary equipment and explains the techniques to the client to decrease anxiety. Additional techniques for assessing hypocalcemic tetany, a complication of endocrine disorders or surgery, are included in the examination sequence.

Skin Assessments with Abnormal Findings
- Inspect skin color.
  - ✓ Hyperpigmentation may be seen in clients with Addison's disease or Cushing's syndrome.
  - ✓ Hypopigmentation may be seen in diabetes mellitus, hyperthyroidism, or hypothyroidism.
  - ✓ A yellowish cast to the skin might indicate hypothyroidism.
  - ✓ Purple striae over the abdomen and bruising may be present in the client with Cushing's syndrome.

- Palpate the skin, assessing texture, moisture, and the presence of lesions.
  - ✓ Rough, dry skin is often seen in clients with hypothyroidism, whereas smooth and flushed skin can be a sign of hyperthyroidism.
  - ✓ Lesions on the lower extremities might indicate diabetes mellitus.

Nails and Hair Assessment with Abnormal Findings
- Assess texture and condition of nails and hair.
  - ✓ Increased pigmentation of the nails is often seen in clients with Addison's disease.
  - ✓ Dry, thick, brittle nails and hair may be apparent in hypothyroidism; thin, brittle nails and thin, soft hair may be apparent in hyperthyroidism.
  - ✓ Hirsutism (excessive facial, chest, or abdominal hair) may be seen in Cushing's syndrome.

Facial Assessments with Abnormal Findings
- Inspect the symmetry and form of the face.
- Inspect position of eyes.
  - ✓ Variations of form and structure may indicate growth abnormalities such as acromegaly.

Thyroid Gland Assessment with Abnormal Findings
- Palpate the thyroid gland for size and consistency.
  - ✓ Stand behind the client, and place your fingers on either side of the trachea below the thyroid cartilage (Figure 16–4 ■). Ask the client to tilt the head to the right. Now ask the client to swallow. As the client swallows, displace the left lobe while palpating the right lobe. Repeat to palpate the left lobe.
  - ✓ Exophthalmos (protruding eyes) may be seen in hyperthyroidism.
  - ✓ The thyroid may be enlarged in clients with Graves' disease or a goiter.
  - ✓ Multiple nodules may be seen in metabolic disorders, whereas the presence of only one nodule may indicate a cyst or a benign or malignant tumor.
  - ✓ One enlarged nodule suggests malignancy.

Motor Function Assessment with Abnormal Findings
- Assess the deep-tendon reflexes. See Chapter 40 for guidelines on assessment. ∞
  - ✓ Increased reflexes may be seen in hyperthyroidism; decreased reflexes may be seen in hypothyroidism.

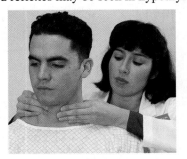

Figure 16–4 ■ Palpating the thyroid gland from behind the client.

Sensory Function Assessment with Abnormal Findings

- Test the client's sensitivity to pain, temperature, vibration, light touch, and stereognosis (the ability to identify an object merely by touch). Compare symmetric areas on both sides of the body, and compare the distal to the proximal regions of the extremities.

  Ask the client to close his or her eyes.
  - To test pain, use the blunt and sharp ends of a new safety pin. Discard the pin after use.
  - To test temperature, use cups or other containers of cold and hot water.
  - To test vibration, use a tuning fork over one of the client's finger or toe joints.
  - To test light touch, use a cotton wisp.
  - To test stereognosis, place in the client's hand a simple, familiar object, such as a rubber band, cotton ball, or button. Ask the client to identify the object.

- ✓ Peripheral neuropathy and paresthesias (altered sensations) may occur in diabetes, hypothyroidism, or acromegaly.

Musculoskeletal Assessment with Abnormal Findings

- Inspect the size and proportions of the client's body structure.
  - ✓ Extremely short stature may indicate dwarfism, which is caused by insufficient growth hormone.
  - ✓ Extremely large bones may indicate acromegaly, which is caused by excessive growth hormone.

Assessing for Hypocalcemic Tetany

- Assess for **Trousseau's sign:** Inflate pressure cuff above antecubital space to occlude blood supply to the arm.
  - ✓ Decreased calcium levels cause the client's hand and fingers to contract (*carpal spasm*).
- Assess for **Chvostek's sign:** Tap your finger in front of the client's ear at the angle of the jaw.
  - ✓ Decreased calcium levels cause the client's lateral facial muscles to contract.

 EXPLORE MediaLink

NCLEX review questions, case studies, care plan activities, MediaLink applications, and other interactive resources for this chapter can be found on the Companion Website at www.prenhall.com/lemone.

Click on Chapter 16 to select the activities for this chapter. For animations, video clips, more NCLEX review questions, and an audio glossary, access the Student CD-ROM accompanying this textbook.

TEST YOURSELF

1. Antidiuretic hormone (ADH) is produced by which endocrine gland?
   a. Pancreas
   b. Adrenals
   c. Thyroid
   d. Pituitary

2. Excessive amounts of glucocorticoids, produced by the adrenal cortex, result in what pathophysiologic health problem?
   a. Inhibited immune response
   b. Increased response to glucagon
   c. Delayed onset of puberty
   d. Decreased metabolic rate

3. When conducting a health history focused on the endocrine system, which of the following questions should be included?
   a. "When did you first notice the pain in your abdomen?"
   b. "Do your children have problems with urination?"
   c. "Are your menstrual periods regular?"
   d. "How did you get this scar on your leg?"

4. What assessments are made when palpating the thyroid gland?
   a. Edema and movement
   b. Size and consistency
   c. Character and texture
   d. Pain and pulse rate

5. Decreased calcium levels can be assessed with Chvostek's sign. To conduct this assessment, the nurse:
   a. Inflates a blood pressure cuff above the antecubital space
   b. Taps the finger in front of the client's ear
   c. Depresses the skin over the shin
   d. Pinches a fold of skin over the sternum

See Test Yourself answers in Appendix C.

BIBLIOGRAPHY

Andresen, G. (1998). Assessing the older patient. *RN, 61*(3), 46–56.

Loriaux, T. (1996). Endocrine assessment: Red flags for those on the front line. *Nursing Clinics of North America, 31*(4), 695–713.

Rusterholtz, A. (1996). Interpretation of diagnostic laboratory tests in selected endocrine disorders.

Nursing Clinics of North America, 31(4), 715–724.

Watson, R. (2001). Assessing endocrine system function in older people. *Nursing Older People, 12*(9), 27–28.

Weber, J., & Kelley, J. (2002). *Health assessment in nursing* (2nd ed.). Philadelphia: Lippincott-Raven.

Wilson, S., & Giddens, J. (2001). *Health assessment for nursing practice.* St. Louis: Mosby.

Winger, J., & Hornick, T. (1996). Age-associated changes in the endocrine system. *Nursing Clinics of North America, 31*(4), 827–844.

Nursing Care of Clients with Endocrine Disorders

MediaLink

www.prenhall.com/lemone
Additional resources for this chapter can be found on the Student CD-ROM accompanying this textbook, and on the Companion Website at www.prenhall.com/lemone. Click on Chapter 17 to select the activities for this chapter.

CD-ROM
- Audio Glossary
- NCLEX Review

Companion Website
- More NCLEX Review
- Case Study
    Hyperthyroidism
- Care Plan Activity
    Cushing's Syndrome
- MediaLink Application
    Exophthalmos

LEARNING OUTCOMES

After completing this chapter, you will be able to:

- Apply knowledge of normal anatomy, physiology, and assessments of the thyroid, parathyroid, adrenal, and pituitary glands when providing nursing care for clients with endocrine disorders (see Chapter 16).

- Identify diagnostic tests used to diagnose disorders of the thyroid, parathyroid, adrenal, and pituitary glands.

- Compare and contrast the manifestations of disorders that result from hyperfunction and hypofunction of the thyroid, parathyroid, adrenal, and pituitary glands.

- Explain the nursing implications for medications prescribed to treat disorders of the thyroid and adrenal glands.

- Provide appropriate nursing care for the client before and after a subtotal thyroidectomy and an adrenalectomy.

- Use the nursing process as a framework for providing individualized care to clients with disorders of the thyroid, parathyroid, adrenal, and pituitary glands.

The thyroid, parathyroid, adrenal, and pituitary glands are part of the endocrine system. Disorders of the structure and function of these glands alter normal hormone levels and the way body tissues use those hormones. When hormone production increases or decreases, people experience alterations in health.

Clients with disorders of the glands discussed in this chapter require nursing care for multiple problems. They often face exhausting diagnostic tests, changes in physical appearance and emotional responses, and permanent alterations in lifestyle. Nursing care is directed toward meeting physiologic needs, providing education, and ensuring psychologic support for the client and family. A holistic approach to the complex needs of clients with these endocrine disorders is an essential component of nursing care.

DISORDERS OF THE THYROID GLAND

Altered thyroid hormone (TH) production or use affects all major organ systems. In the adult, TH changes primarily affect metabolism, cardiovascular function, gastrointestinal function, and neuromuscular function. Thyroid disorders—both hyperthyroidism and hypothyroidism—are among the most common endocrine disorders.

THE CLIENT WITH HYPERTHYROIDISM

Hyperthyroidism (also called **thyrotoxicosis**) is a disorder caused by excessive delivery of TH to the peripheral tissues. Because the primary effect of TH is to increase metabolism and protein synthesis, hyperthyroidism affects all major organ systems of the body. The increase in metabolic rate and the alterations in cardiac output, peripheral blood flow, oxygen consumption, and body temperature are similar to those found in increased sympathetic nervous system activity (Porth, 2002).

The effects of hyperthyroidism are the result of increased circulating levels of TH. This hormonal excess increases the metabolic rate and heightens the sympathetic nervous system's physiologic response to stimulation. The sensitizing effect of abnormally elevated TH levels increases the cardiac rate and stroke volume. As a result, cardiac output and peripheral blood flow increase. Elevated TH levels also increase carbohydrate, protein, and lipid metabolism. Lipids are depleted, and glucose tolerance decreases. Protein degradation increases, resulting in a negative nitrogen balance. Over time, the hypermetabolic effects of excess TH result in caloric and nutritional deficiencies.

PATHOPHYSIOLOGY AND MANIFESTATIONS

Hyperthyroidism results from many different factors, including autoimmune reactions (as in Graves' disease), excess secretion of thyroid-stimulating hormone (TSH) by the pituitary gland, thyroiditis, neoplasms (such as toxic multinodular goiter), and an excessive intake of thyroid medications. The most common etiologies of hyperthyroidism are Graves' disease and toxic multinodular goiter.

The client with hyperthyroidism typically has an increased appetite, yet loses weight and may have hypermotile bowels and diarrhea. Additional manifestations related to hypermetabolism include heat intolerance and increased sweating. The client's hair is fine, and the skin is smooth and warm. Emotional lability is common. The *Multisystem Effects of Hyperthyroidism* are shown on page 446.

Graves' Disease

Graves' disease, the most common cause of hyperthyroidism, is an autoimmune disorder. The serum of more than 90% of clients with Graves' disease contains TSH-R (stim) Ab, an antibody directed against the TSH receptor site in the thyroid follicles (Tierney et al., 2001). When this antibody binds to the TSH receptors, it stimulates hormone synthesis and secretion. The cause is unknown, but there is a hereditary link. Other factors associated with Graves' disease include an immune response against a viral antigen, a defect of the lymphocyte T helper cells, and the presence of other autoimmune disorders (such as myasthenia gravis and pernicious anemia) (Porth, 2002).

Graves' disease is seen 5 times more often in women than in men and occurs most frequently between the ages of 20 and 40. It is seen worldwide, with the incidence often correlated with the amount of iodine in the diet. Increased iodine intake (such as from radiocontrast dyes used in diagnostic tests or from ingestion of kelp tablets) has been associated with an increased frequency of hyperthyroidism.

Clients with Graves' disease have an enlarged thyroid gland (**goiter**) and manifestations of hyperthyroidism (as illustrated in Table 17–1). The hypertrophy of the gland can result from excess TSH stimulation (when the amount of circulating TH is deficient), growth-stimulating immunoglobulins, or substances that inhibit TH synthesis. A goiter may be present in hyperthyroidism or hypothyroidism.

TABLE 17–1 Laboratory Findings in Hyperthyroidism

Test	Normal Values	Findings
Serum TA	Negative to 1:20	Increased
Serum TSH (Sensitive assay)	>1.0 mµ/L	Decreased in primary hyperthyroidism
Serum T_4	5 to 12 mµ/dL	Increased
Serum T_3	80 to 200 ng/dL	Increased
T_3 uptake (T_3RU)	25 to 35 relative percentage	Increased
Thyroid suppression		Increased RAI uptake and T_4 levels

Multisystem Effects of Hyperthyroidism

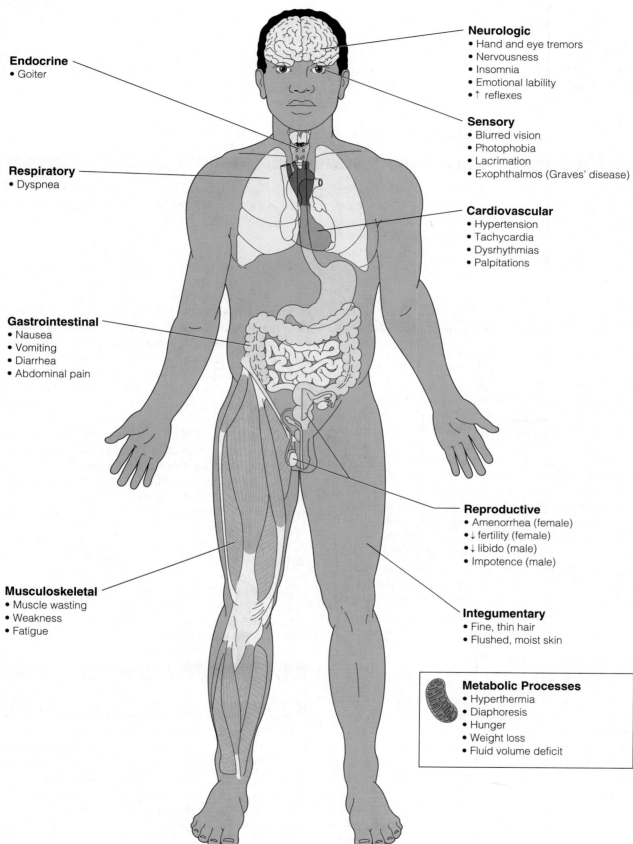

Endocrine
• Goiter

Respiratory
• Dyspnea

Gastrointestinal
• Nausea
• Vomiting
• Diarrhea
• Abdominal pain

Musculoskeletal
• Muscle wasting
• Weakness
• Fatigue

Neurologic
• Hand and eye tremors
• Nervousness
• Insomnia
• Emotional lability
• ↑ reflexes

Sensory
• Blurred vision
• Photophobia
• Lacrimation
• Exophthalmos (Graves' disease)

Cardiovascular
• Hypertension
• Tachycardia
• Dysrhythmias
• Palpitations

Reproductive
• Amenorrhea (female)
• ↓ fertility (female)
• ↓ libido (male)
• Impotence (male)

Integumentary
• Fine, thin hair
• Flushed, moist skin

Metabolic Processes
• Hyperthermia
• Diaphoresis
• Hunger
• Weight loss
• Fluid volume deficit

Figure 17–1 ■ Exophthalmos in a client with Graves' disease. The disease causes edema of fat deposits behind the eyes and inflammation of the extraocular muscles. The accumulating pressure forces the eyes outward from their orbits.

Source: University of Illinois, Custom Medical Stock Photo, Inc.

Proptosis (forward displacement) of the eye occurs in about one-third of cases (Porth, 2002). The forward protrusion of the eyeballs (also called **exophthalmos**) results from an accumulation of fat deposits and inflammation by-products in the retro-orbital tissues. Often the sclera is visible above the iris. The upper lids are often retracted, and the person has a characteristic unblinking stare (Figure 17–1 ■). Proptosis is usually bilateral, but it may involve only one eye. The client may experience blurred vision, diplopia, eye pain, lacrimation, and photophobia. The inability to close the eyelids completely over the protruding eyeballs increases the risk of corneal dryness, irritation, infection, and ulceration. The treatment of Graves' disease does not reverse these changes in the eyes.

Other manifestations include fatigue, difficulty sleeping, hand tremors, and changes in menstruation ranging from decreased flow to amenorrhea. Older clients may present with atrial fibrillation, angina, or congestive heart failure.

Toxic Multinodular Goiter

Toxic multinodular goiter (Figure 17–2 ■) is characterized by small, discrete, independently functioning nodules in the thyroid gland tissue that secrete excessive amounts of TH. It is not known how these nodules grow or become independent, but a genetic mutation of follicle cells is suspected. Elevated TH levels result in manifestations of hyperthyroidism; however, they are slower to develop and differ somewhat from those of Graves' disease. The client with this type of hyperthyroidism is usually a woman in her 60s or 70s who has had a goiter for a number of years.

Excess TSH Stimulation

Overproduction of TSH by the pituitary usually stimulates the thyroid gland to produce excess TH. The elevation in TSH secretion often results from a pituitary adenoma. This secondary form of hyperthyroidism is rare.

Thyroiditis

Thyroiditis (inflammation of the thyroid gland) is most often the result of a viral infection of the thyroid gland. The symp-

Figure 17–2 ■ Toxic multinodular goiter. The formation and growth of numerous nodules in the thyroid gland cause the characteristic massive enlargement of the neck.

Source: Custom Medical Stock Photo, Inc.

toms of thyroiditis are those of acute inflammation and the effects of increased TH. Thyroiditis is an acute disorder that may become chronic, resulting in a hypothyroid state as repeated infections destroy gland tissue. See the discussion of Hashimoto's thyroiditis later in this chapter.

Thyroid Crisis

Thyroid crisis (also called **thyroid storm**) is an extreme state of hyperthyroidism that is rare today because of improved diagnosis and treatment methods (Porth, 2002). When it does occur, those affected are usually people with untreated hyperthyroidism (most often Graves' disease) and people with hyperthyroidism who have experienced a stressor, such as an infection, trauma, untreated diabetic ketoacidosis, or manipulation of the thyroid gland during surgery. Thyroid crisis is a life-threatening condition.

The rapid increase in metabolic rate that results from the excessive TH causes the manifestations of thyroid crisis. The manifestations include hyperthermia, with body temperatures ranging from 102°F (39°C) to 106°F (41°C); tachycardia; systolic hypertension; and gastrointestinal symptoms (abdominal pain, vomiting, diarrhea). Agitation, restlessness, and tremors are common, progressing to confusion, psychosis, delirium, and seizures. The mortality rate is high. Rapid treatment of thyroid crisis is essential to preserve life. Treatment includes relieving respiratory distress, stabilizing cardiovascular function, and reducing TH synthesis and secretion.

COLLABORATIVE CARE

Treatment of hyperthyroidism focuses on reducing the production of TH by the thyroid gland, thus establishing a **euthyroid** (normal thyroid) state, and preventing or treating complications. Depending on the client's age and physical status, either medications, radioactive iodine therapy, or surgery may be used.

Diagnostic Tests

Hyperthyroidism is diagnosed according to the manifestations of the specific disorders causing excessive TH, and by diagnostic test results. Elevated levels of TH (both T_3 and T_4) and increased radioactive iodine (RAI) uptake are diagnostic criteria of hyperthyroidism. Laboratory findings in hyperthyroidism are shown in Table 17–1.

The following diagnostic tests may be ordered:

- *TA test.* Serum thyroid antibodies (TA) are measured to determine whether a thyroid autoimmune disease is causing the client's symptoms. TA is elevated in Graves' disease.
- *TSH test (sensitive assay).* Serum TSH levels are measured and compared with thyroxine (T_4) levels to differentiate pituitary from thyroid dysfunction. The best indicator of primary hyperthyroidism (such as in Graves' disease) is suppression of TSH below 0.1 μg/mL. When the sensitive TSH is not suppressed, the hyperthyroidism is caused by a TSH-secreting pituitary tumor.
- *T_4 test.* Serum thyroxine (T_4) levels are measured to determine TH concentration and to test thyroid gland function. T_4 levels are elevated in hyperthyroidism and in acute thyroiditis.
- *T_3 test.* Serum triiodothyronine (T_3) is measured by radioimmunoassay (T_3RIA), which measures bound and free forms of this hormone. This test is effective for the diagnosis of hyperthyroidism. T_3 levels may also be elevated in thyroiditis.
- *T_3 uptake test.* T_3 uptake (T_3RU) is measured by an in vitro test in which the client's blood is mixed with radioactive T_3; the results are elevated in hyperthyroidism.

- *RAI uptake test.* A radioactive iodine (RAI) uptake test (thyroid scan) measures the absorption of ^{131}I or ^{123}I by the thyroid gland. A calculated dose of radioactive iodine is given orally or intravenously, and the thyroid is then scanned (often after 24 hours). The distribution of radioactivity in the gland is recorded (increased uptake of radioactive iodine is seen in Graves' disease). In addition, the scan reveals the size and shape of the gland.
- *Thyroid suppression test.* RAI and T_4 levels are measured first. The client then takes TH for 7 to 10 days, after which the tests are repeated. Failure of hormone therapy to suppress RAI and T_4 indicates hyperthyroidism.

Medications

Hyperthyroidism is treated by administering antithyroid medications that reduce TH production. Because these drugs do not affect the release or activity of hormone that is already formed, therapeutic effects may not be seen for several weeks. Some commonly prescribed drugs, their actions, and nursing implications are shown in the Medication Administration box below.

Radioactive Iodine Therapy

Because the thyroid gland takes up iodine in any form, radioactive iodine (^{131}I) concentrates in the thyroid gland and damages or destroys thyroid cells so that they produce less TH. Radioactive iodine is given orally. Results typically occur in 6 to 8 weeks. In most instances, the client is not hospitalized during treatment and does not require radiation precautions. This type of therapy is contraindicated in pregnant women

Medication Administration

Hyperthyroidism

IODINE SOURCES

Potassium iodide (SSKI, Thyro-Block)
Potassium iodide (Pima)

Large doses of iodine inhibit TH synthesis and release. Iodine also makes the hyperplastic thyroid less vascular prior to surgery and hastens the ability of other antithyroid drugs to reduce natural hormone output.

Nursing Responsibilities
- Assess for hypersensitivity to iodine before giving medication; for example, ask client about allergies to shellfish.
- Dilute liquid iodine sources in water or orange juice to disguise bitter taste.
- Monitor for increased bleeding tendencies if the client is also taking anticoagulants; iodine increases their effect.

Client and Family Teaching
- The maximum effect of iodine in large doses usually occurs in 1 to 2 weeks.
- Long-term iodine therapy is not effective in controlling hyperthyroidism.

ANTITHYROID DRUGS

Methimazole (Tapazole)
Propylthiouracil (PTU, Propyl-Thracil)

Antithyroid drugs inhibit TH production. They do not affect already formed hormones; thus, several weeks may elapse before the client experiences therapeutic effects.

Nursing Responsibilities
- Monitor for side effects: pruritus, rash, elevated temperature, (for iodides) swelling of the eyelids, anorexia, loss of taste, changes in menstruation.
- Administer drugs at the same time each day to maintain stable blood levels.
- Monitor for symptoms of hypothyroidism: fatigue, weight gain.

Client and Family Teaching
- Watch for unusual bleeding, nausea, loss of taste, or epigastric pain. Report any such symptoms to the physician.
- If you are also taking anticoagulants, report any signs of bleeding.
- If you are taking lithium, be aware of symptoms of hypothyroidism.
- It may take up to 12 weeks before you experience the full effects of the drugs. Take the medication regularly and exactly as prescribed.

because radioactive iodine crosses the placenta and can have negative effects on the developing fetal thyroid gland. Because the amount of gland destroyed is not readily controllable, the client may become hypothyroid and require lifelong TH replacement.

Surgery

Some hyperthyroid clients have such enlarged thyroid glands that pressure on the esophagus or trachea causes breathing or swallowing problems. In these cases, removal of all or part of the gland is indicated. A *subtotal thyroidectomy* is usually performed. This procedure leaves enough of the gland in place to produce an adequate amount of TH. A total **thyroidectomy** is performed to treat cancer of the thyroid; the client then requires lifelong hormone replacement.

Before surgery, the client should be in as nearly a euthyroid state as possible. The client may be given antithyroid drugs to reduce hormone levels and iodine preparations to decrease the vascularity and size of the gland (which also reduces the risk of hemorrhage during and after surgery). Nursing care of the client having a subtotal thyroidectomy is discussed in the box below.

NURSING CARE

Health Promotion

Although hyperthyroidism is not preventable, it is important to teach clients the importance of regular health care provider visits and medication intake.

Assessment

The following data are collected through the health history and physical examination (see Chapter 16). Further focused assessments are described with nursing interventions.

- *Health history:* other diseases, family history of thyroid disease, when symptoms began, severity of symptoms, intake of thyroid medications, menstrual history, changes in weight, bowel elimination
- *Physical assessment:* muscle strength, tremors, vital signs, cardiovascular and peripheral vascular systems, integument, size of thyroid, presence of bruit over thyroid, eyes and vision

NURSING CARE OF THE CLIENT HAVING A SUBTOTAL THYROIDECTOMY

PREOPERATIVE CARE

- Administer ordered antithyroid medications and iodine preparations, and monitor their effects. *Antithyroid drugs are given before surgery to promote a euthyroid state. Iodine preparations are given to the client before surgery to decrease vascularity of the gland, thereby decreasing the risk of hemorrhage.*
- Teach the client to support the neck by placing both hands behind the neck when sitting up in bed, while moving about, and while coughing. *Placing the hands behind the neck provides support for the suture line.*
- Answer questions, and allow time for the client to verbalize concerns. *Because the incision is made at the base of the throat, clients (especially women) are often concerned about their appearance after surgery. Explain that the scar will eventually be only a thin line and that jewelry or scarves may be used to cover the scar.*

POSTOPERATIVE CARE

- Provide comfort measures: Administer analgesic pain medications as ordered, and monitor their effectiveness; place the client in a semi-Fowler's position after recovery from anesthesia; support head and neck with pillows. *Analgesic medications reduce the perception of pain and reduce physical stress during the postoperative period. Positioning the client in a semi-Fowler's position and supporting the head and neck decrease strain on the suture line.*
- Perform focused assessments to monitor for complications:
  a. *Hemorrhage.* Assess dressing (if present) and the area under the client's neck and shoulders for drainage. Monitor blood pressure and pulse for symptoms of hypovolemic shock. Assess tightness of dressing (if present). *The vascularity of the gland increases the risk of hemorrhage. The loca-*

tion of the incision and the position of the client may cause the drainage to run back and under the client. The danger of hemorrhage is greatest in the first 12 to 24 hours after surgery.
  b. *Respiratory distress.* Assess respiratory rate, rhythm, depth, and effort. Maintain humidification as ordered. Assist the client with coughing and deep breathing. Have suction equipment, oxygen, and a tracheostomy set available for immediate use. *Respiratory distress may result from hemorrhage and edema, which may compress the trachea; from tetany and laryngeal spasms resulting from decreased hormones due to removal or damage to the parathyroid glands; and from damage to the laryngeal nerve, causing spasms of the vocal cords. Equipment must be immediately available if the client experiences respiratory distress that requires interventions and treatment.*
  c. *Laryngeal nerve damage.* Assess for the ability to speak aloud, noting quality and tone of voice. *The location of the laryngeal nerve increases the risk of damage during thyroid surgery. Although hoarseness may be due to edema or the endotracheal tube used during surgery and will subside, permanent hoarseness or loss of vocal volume is a potential danger.*
  d. *Tetany.* Assess for signs of calcium deficiency, including tingling of toes, fingers, and lips; muscular twitches; positive Chvostek's and Trousseau's signs; and decreased serum calcium levels. Keep calcium gluconate or calcium chloride available for immediate intravenous use, if necessary. *The parathyroid glands are located in and near the thyroid gland; surgery of the thyroid gland may injure or remove parathyroid glands, resulting in hypocalcemia and tetany. Tetany may occur in 1 to 7 days after thyroidectomy.*

Nursing Diagnoses and Interventions

In planning and implementing nursing care for the client with hyperthyroidism, the nurse considers the client's responses to the systemic effects of the disorder. Although each client may have different needs, nursing diagnoses discussed in this section focus on the most common problems: cardiovascular problems, visual deficits, altered nutrition, and body image disturbance.

Risk for Decreased Cardiac Output

The client with hyperthyroidism is at risk for alterations in cardiac output. Excess TH directly affects the heart, resulting in increased rate and stroke volume. Increases in the metabolic demands and oxygen requirements of peripheral tissues increase the demands on the heart, and systolic hypertension, angina, arrhythmias, or cardiac failure may occur. The client often has palpitations and shortness of breath and is easily fatigued. The risk of complications is greater in clients with pre-existing cardiovascular disorders.

- Monitor blood pressure, pulse rate and rhythm, respiratory rate, and breath sounds. Assess for peripheral edema, jugular vein distention, and increased activity intolerance. *Increased TH increases cardiac rate, stroke volume, and tissue demand for oxygen, causing stress on the heart. This may result in hypertension, arrhythmias, tachycardia, and congestive heart failure.*
- Suggest keeping the environment as cool and free of distraction as possible. Decrease stress by explaining interventions and teaching relaxation procedures. *A physically comfortable and psychologically calm environment can reduce stimuli and stressors. Stress increases circulating catecholamines, which further increase cardiac workload.*
- Encourage the client to balance activity with rest periods. *Rest periods decrease energy expenditure and tissue requirements for oxygen, decreasing demands on the heart by decreasing cardiac workload.*

Disturbed Sensory Perception: Visual

Visual changes that occur in clients with hyperthyroidism include difficulty in focusing, diplopia (double vision), or visual loss. If the client is unable to close the eyelids because of exophthalmos, the risk of corneal dryness with resultant infection or injury increases. Visual deficits may also result from pressure on the optic nerve from retro-orbital edema and the shortening of eye muscles. Although treatment of hyperthyroidism may stop the progression of eye changes, not all symptoms are reversible.

- Monitor visual acuity, photophobia, integrity of the cornea, and lid closure. *The cornea is at risk for dryness, injury, conjunctivitis, and corneal infections. Injury and infection of the cornea can result in further loss of visual acuity.*
- Teach measures for protecting the eye from injury and maintaining visual acuity:
  - Use tinted glasses or shields as protection.
  - Use artificial tears to moisten the eyes.
  - Use cool, moist compresses to relieve irritation.
  - Promptly report any pain or changes in vision.

PRACTICE ALERT *Teach the client to cover or tape the eyelids shut at night if they do not close and to sleep with the head of the bed elevated.* ■

The measures outlined decrease the risk of injury, provide comfort, decrease periorbital edema that can further compromise vision, and ensure immediate care for problems, thereby minimizing the risk of further visual loss.

Imbalanced Nutrition: Less Than Body Requirements

The hypermetabolic state that occurs in hyperthyroidism causes gastrointestinal hypermotility, with nausea, vomiting, diarrhea, and abdominal pain. Although the client may have an increased appetite and eat more than usual, weight loss continues.

- Ask the client to weigh daily (at the same time each day), and keep a record of results. *The inability to meet metabolic demands results in loss of body weight. Regular monitoring detects continued weight loss.*
- In collaboration with a dietitian, teach the client the need for a diet high in carbohydrates and protein and including between-meal snacks. Six small meals a day may be more desirable than three large meals. Caloric intake may need to be increased to 4000 kcal per day if weight loss exceeds 10% to 17% for height and frame. *Increased nutrients as part of a well-balanced diet are necessary to meet metabolic demands. Clients are often better able to increase food intake by eating frequent, small meals. A 1-lb weight gain requires approximately 3500 extra kcal.*
- Monitor nutritional status through results of laboratory data. Serum albumin, transferrin, and total lymphocyte counts are commonly lower than normal in nutritional deficits. *A negative nitrogen balance signifies a catabolic state in which protein is lost and metabolic demands are not being met.*

Disturbed Body Image

Physical changes common in hyperthyroidism include exophthalmos, goiter, tremors, hair loss, increased perspiration, loss of strength, fatigue (see the Nursing Research box on page 451), weight loss, and changes in reproductive and sexual function (amenorrhea in women, impotence in men, and increased libido in both men and women). In addition, the client often has mood changes and insomnia and is constantly nervous and anxious. There may even be periods of psychosis. These changes are frightening not only for the client but also for family members.

- Establish a trusting relationship; encourage the client to verbalize feelings about self and to ask questions about the illness and treatment. Provide reliable information, and clarify misconceptions. *Establishing trust facilitates open sharing of feelings and perceptions.*

Nursing Research

Evidence-Based Practice for Fatigue

This analysis of fatigue (Tiesinga et al., 1996) was conducted to document how it is defined in the literature, and to distinguish dimensions and identify indicators. As defined in this analysis, fatigue is a nonspecific manifestation, often related to different chronic illnesses and their treatments. Fatigue has physical, psychological, and social dimensions.

IMPLICATIONS FOR NURSING

Although nurses both experience fatigue and assess fatigue in clients, little research has been conducted to clearly define and interpret the experience of fatigue. This is important, as the experience of fatigue may well be very different in the client with hyperthyroidism than in the client with fatigue-related radiation treatments. Continued research and the development of accurate

assessment tools will increase the knowledge base necessary to holistic, individualized clinical practice.

Critical Thinking in Client Care

1. What specific pathophysiologic processes in clients with hyperthyroidism or hypothyroidism increase the risk of fatigue?
2. What defining characteristics of the nursing diagnosis *Fatigue* would make implementation of a teaching plan more difficult? How could you adapt your teaching to ensure client and family knowledge?
3. How could fatigue interfere with following a therapeutic regimen that is prescribed? Could fatigue be a major factor when the client is said to be noncompliant? Why or why not?

Home Care

Clients with hyperthyroidism primarily provide self-care at home. Teaching is individualized to meet the client's needs. Address the following topics:

- The client taking oral medications must understand the need for lifelong treatment.
- The client who has a thyroidectomy requires information about postoperative wound care.

- The client having radioactive iodine therapy needs to know the symptoms of hypothyroidism.
- Depending on the age of the client and the support systems available, referral to community health care agencies may be necessary.
- In addition, suggest the following resources:
  - American Thyroid Association
  - Thyroid Foundation of Canada
  - Endocrine Society

MediaLink | ENDOCRINE DISORDER RESOURCES

Nursing Care Plan
A Client with Graves' Disease

Mrs. Juanita Manuel is a 33-year-old mother of four small children. She is a second-year student at the local community college, within one semester of completing the requirements for an associate degree in child care. For the past 3 months, Juanita has been constantly hungry and has eaten more than usual, but she has still lost 15 lb (6.8 kg). She has repeated bouts of diarrhea and often feels nauseated. Her hands shake, she can feel her heart beating rapidly, and she finds herself laughing or crying for no apparent reason.

Mrs. Manuel makes an appointment with her family physician. The nurse at the office completes a health history and physical assessment. When asked how she has been feeling, Mrs. Manuel replies, "Well, I don't know what's wrong with me—but I keep losing weight and I cry at the drop of a hat. I am also just so hot all the time, and I've never had that problem before. I hope I find out what's wrong and it's nothing serious."

ASSESSMENT

The health history indicates that although her appetite has increased, Mrs. Manuel has lost 15 lb (6.8 kg). She states that she has had diarrhea, nausea, palpitations, heat intolerance, and mood changes. Physical assessment findings include the following: T 101°F (38.3°C), P 110, R 24, and BP 162/86. Her skin is moist and warm, her hair thin and fine. She has visible tremors in her hands. Her eyeballs protrude, and she is unable to close her eyelids completely. Her thyroid is enlarged and palpable. Diagnostic tests re-

veal the following abnormal results: T_3, 350 g/dL (normal range: 80 to 200 ng/dL), T_4, 15.1 mg/dL (normal range: 5 to 12 mg/dL). A thyroid scan demonstrates an enlarged thyroid with increased iodine uptake. After the medical diagnosis of Graves' disease is made, Mrs. Manuel is started on the antithyroid medication propylthiouracil, 150 mg orally every 8 hours.

DIAGNOSIS

- *Risk for imbalanced nutrition: Less than body requirements,* related to weight loss of 15 lb (6.8 kg), with present weight 10% less than normal for height
- *Diarrhea,* related to increased peristalsis as evidenced by 8 to 10 liquid stools per day
- *Risk for disturbed sensory perception: Visual,* related to an inability to close the eyelids completely
- *Anxiety,* related to a lack of knowledge about disease process

EXPECTED OUTCOMES

- Gain at least 1 lb (0.45 kg) every 2 weeks.
- Regain normal bowel elimination patterns.
- Maintain normal vision (with no evidence of corneal damage) and verbalize measures to protect her eyes.
- Verbalize medical treatment and self-care needs.
- Verbalize a decrease in anxiety.

(continued on page 452)

Nursing Care Plan
A Client with Graves' Disease (continued)

PLANNING AND IMPLEMENTATION

- Request that she keep a record of daily weight.
- Discuss adopting a high-kcalorie diet. Identify food likes and dislikes, as well as foods that increase diarrhea, before instituting a plan to increase food intake.
- Request that she keep a stool chart, noting the time, type, and precipitating factors for diarrhea stools. Teach comfort measures for irritated anal area (clean washcloth and soap, nonirritating ointment).
- Teach how to apply eye drops (artificial tears).
- Explain the need to elevate the head of the bed to 45 degrees at night, and tape eye shields over eyes before sleep.
- Teach about Graves' disease, the medication's effects and side effects, and the need for continued medical care.

EVALUATION

By her next office visit, Mrs. Manuel has gained 1 lb (0.45 kg) and has discussed her dietary needs with the nurse and her husband.

She is having diarrhea less often. She has safely applied the eye drops and states that she uses the eye shields and elevates the head of her bed at night. The office nurse reviewed the written and verbal information about Graves' disease and the medication prescribed. Mrs. Manuel verbalizes her understanding, stating, "I'll always take my medicine—I never want to feel like that again!" She also says that she feels much less anxious now that she understands what has happened.

Critical Thinking in the Nursing Process

1. What is the pathophysiologic basis for Mrs. Manuel's abnormal vital signs?
2. What is the rationale for having the client with exophthalmos elevate the head of the bed at night?
3. Outline a teaching plan that could be given to clients for home care following a subtotal thyroidectomy.

See Evaluating Your Response in Appendix C.

THE CLIENT WITH HYPOTHYROIDISM

Hypothyroidism is a disorder that results when the thyroid gland produces an insufficient amount of TH. Because a decrease in TH levels decreases metabolic rate and heat production, hypothyroidism affects all body systems (see the *Multisystem Effects of Hypothyroidism* on page 453). Hypothyroidism is more common in women between ages 30 and 60; the incidence rises after age 50. However, the disorder can occur at any stage of life. Careful evaluation of symptoms is important in the older adult because manifestations of hypothyroidism are often thought to be the result of aging instead of a pathologic process.

The hypothyroid state in adults is sometimes called **myxedema.** The term reflects the characteristic accumulation of nonpitting edema in the connective tissues throughout the body. The edema is the result of water retention in mucoprotein (hydrophilic proteoglycans) deposits in the interstitial spaces. The face of a client with myxedema appears puffy, and the tongue is enlarged (Porth, 2002).

PATHOPHYSIOLOGY AND MANIFESTATIONS

Hypothyroidism may be either primary or secondary. Primary hypothyroidism (which is more common) may be caused by congenital defects in the gland, loss of thyroid tissue following treatment for hyperthyroidism with surgery or radiation, antithyroid medications, thyroiditis, or endemic iodine deficiency. The cardiac drug, amiodarone (Cordarone), which contains 75 mg of iodine per 200 mg tablet, is increasingly being implicated in causing thyroid problems (Porth, 2002). Secondary hypothyroidism may result from pituitary TSH deficiency or peripheral resistance to thyroid

hormones. Hypothyroidism has a slow onset, with manifestations occurring over months or even years. With treatment, the mental and physical symptoms rapidly reverse in clients of all ages.

When TH production decreases, the thyroid gland enlarges in a compensatory attempt to produce more hormone. The goiter that results is usually a simple or nontoxic form. People living in certain areas of the world where the soil is deficient in iodine, the substance necessary for TH synthesis and secretion, are more prone to become hypothyroid and develop simple goiter. (Iodine deficiency is discussed below.)

Hypothyroid clients characteristically have the manifestations of goiter, fluid retention and edema, decreased appetite, weight gain, constipation, dry skin, dyspnea, pallor, hoarseness, and muscle stiffness. Many clients have a decreased sense of taste and smell, menstrual disorders, anemias, and cardiac enlargement. The pulse is typically slow. Deficient amounts of TH cause abnormalities in lipid metabolism, with elevated serum cholesterol and triglyceride levels. As a result, the client is at increased risk for atherosclerosis and cardiac disorders. Decreased renal blood flow and glomerular filtration rate reduces the kidney's ability to excrete water, which may cause hyponatremia. Sleep apnea is more common in clients with hypothyroidism. Factors that result in decreased TH (in addition to those described) include iodine deficiency and Hashimoto's thyroiditis. A severe state of hypothyroidism is called *myxedema coma.*

Iodine Deficiency

Iodine is necessary for TH synthesis and secretion. Iodine deficiency may result from certain goitrogenic drugs (which block TH synthesis); lithium carbonate, used to treat bipolar mental disorders; and antithyroid drugs. Goitrogenic compounds in foods such as turnips, rutabagas, and soybeans may

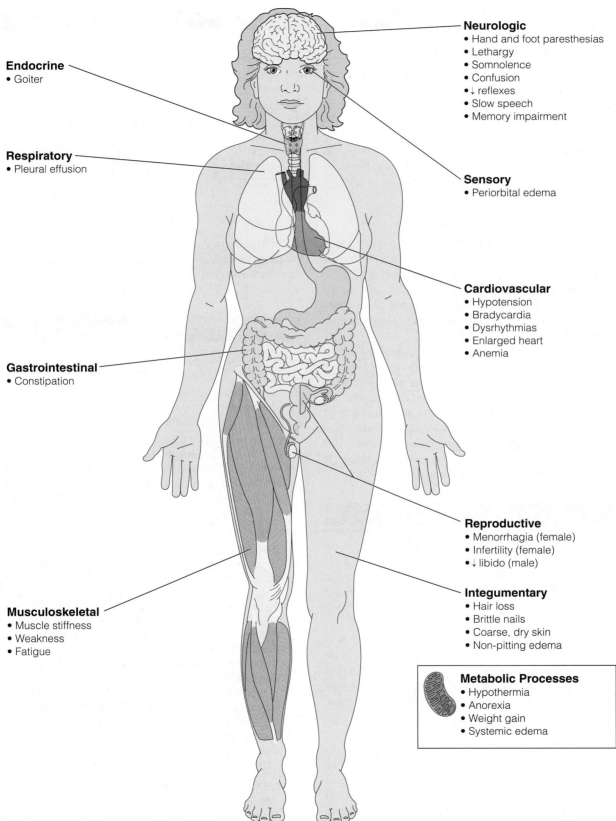

Neurologic
- Hand and foot paresthesias
- Lethargy
- Somnolence
- Confusion
- ↓ reflexes
- Slow speech
- Memory impairment

Endocrine
- Goiter

Respiratory
- Pleural effusion

Sensory
- Periorbital edema

Cardiovascular
- Hypotension
- Bradycardia
- Dysrhythmias
- Enlarged heart
- Anemia

Gastrointestinal
- Constipation

Reproductive
- Menorrhagia (female)
- Infertility (female)
- ↓ libido (male)

Musculoskeletal
- Muscle stiffness
- Weakness
- Fatigue

Integumentary
- Hair loss
- Brittle nails
- Coarse, dry skin
- Non-pitting edema

Metabolic Processes
- Hypothermia
- Anorexia
- Weight gain
- Systemic edema

also block TH synthesis if consumed in sufficient quantities. In areas of the world where the soil is deficient in iodine, dietary intake of iodine may be inadequate. However, the use of iodized salt has reduced this risk in the United States.

Hashimoto's Thyroiditis

Hashimoto's thyroiditis is the most common cause of primary hypothyroidism. In this autoimmune disorder, antibodies develop that destroy thyroid tissue. Functional thyroid tissue is replaced with fibrous tissue, and TH levels decrease. In addition, decreasing levels of TH in the early stages of the disease prompt the gland to enlarge to compensate, causing a goiter. However, as the disease progresses, the thyroid gland becomes smaller. This disorder is more common in women and has a familial link.

Myxedema Coma

Myxedema coma is a life-threatening complication of long-standing, untreated hypothyroidism. It is characterized by severe metabolic disorders (hyponatremia, hypoglycemia, lactic acidosis), hypothermia, cardiovascular collapse, and coma. Myxedema coma, although rare, most commonly occurs during the winter months in older women with long-standing chronic hypothyroidism (Porth, 2002).

Myxedema coma may be precipitated by trauma, infection, failure to take thyroid replacement medications, the use of central nervous system depressants, and exposure to cold temperatures (Porth, 2002). The treatment of myxedema coma addresses the precipitating factors and manifestations and involves maintaining a patent airway; maintaining fluid, electrolyte, and acid-base balance; maintaining cardiovascular status; increasing body temperature; and increasing TH levels. If untreated, the mortality rate is high (Tierney et al., 2001).

COLLABORATIVE CARE

The treatment of the client with hypothyroidism focuses on diagnosis, prevention or treatment of complications, and replacement of the deficient TH. With early and continued treatment, both appearance and mental function return to normal.

Diagnostic Tests

Hypothyroidism is diagnosed by the manifestations and by a decrease in TH, especially T_4. TSH concentration often is increased, because the negative hormonal feedback from TH is lost. The same laboratory and diagnostic tests used to diagnose hyperthyroidism are also used to diagnose hypothyroidism, with opposite results in most cases (see Table 17–2).

Medications

Hypothyroidism is treated with medications that replace TH. Levothyroxine (thyroxine, T_4) is the treatment of choice (Tierney et al., 2001). Medications commonly used to treat hypothyroidism and their nursing implications are shown in the box on this page.

TABLE 17–2 Laboratory Findings in Hypothyroidism

Test	Normal Values	Findings
Serum TA	None to 1:20	Normal
Serum TSH	>1.0 mμ/L	Increased in primary hypothyroidism
Serum T_4	5 to 12 µg/dL	Decreased
Serum T_3	80 to 200 ng/dL	Decreased
T_3 uptake (T_3RU)	25 to 35 relative percentage	Decreased
Thyroid suppression		No change in RAI uptake or T_4 levels

Surgery

If the hypothyroid client has a goiter large enough to cause respiratory difficulties or dysphagia, a subtotal thyroidectomy may be performed (see page 449).

Medication Administration

Hypothyroidism

THYROID PREPARATIONS

Levothyroxine sodium (T_4) (Levoxyl, Levothroid, Synthroid)
Liothyronine sodium (T_3) (Cytomel)
Liotrix ($T_3 - T_4$) (Euthroid, Thyrolar)

Thyroid preparations increase blood levels of TH, thus raising the client's metabolic rate. As a result, cardiac output, oxygen consumption, and body temperature increase. The dosage depends on the drug chosen and the client's degree of thyroid dysfunction, sensitivity to TH, age, body size, and health. The older adult may require lower doses.

Nursing Responsibilities

- Give 1 hour before meals or 2 hours after meals for best absorption.
- Thyroid preparations potentiate the effect of anticoagulant drugs. If the client is also receiving an anticoagulant, monitor for bruising, bleeding gums, and blood in the urine.
- Thyroid medications potentiate the effect of digitalis. If the client is also receiving a digitalis preparation, monitor for signs of digitalis toxicity.
- Monitor for symptoms of coronary insufficiency: chest pain, dyspnea, tachycardia.
- If the client has insulin-dependent diabetes, monitor the effects of insulin. The effect of the insulin may change as thyroid function increases.
- During dose adjustment, take pulse before administering drug. Report pulse >100.

Client and Family Teaching

- Do not substitute brands of drugs or use generic equivalents without the physician's approval.
- The medications must be taken for the rest of one's life.

Medication Administration

Hypothyroidism (continued)

- Report symptoms of excess thyroid hormone to the physician: excess weight loss, palpitations, leg cramps, nervousness, or insomnia.
- If you have diabetes and use insulin, monitor blood glucose levels closely; the thyroid medications may alter the amount of insulin required.
- Thyroid preparations increase the risk of iodine toxicity. Do not use iodized salt or over-the-counter drugs containing iodine.
- If you are also taking an anticoagulant, report any signs of bleeding.
- Report any changes in menstrual periods.
- Take the thyroid preparation each morning to decrease the possibility of insomnia.
- Closely monitor blood pressure and pulse (older clients).
- Avoid excessive intake of foods that are known to inhibit TH utilization such as turnips, cabbage, carrots, spinach, and peaches.

NURSING CARE

Health Promotion

One of the most critical factors in preventing hypothyroidism is education of the public about the necessity of an adequate dietary intake of iodine. The use of iodized salt meets the requirements for hormone production. It is important to teach clients the importance of regular health care provider visits and medication intake.

Assessment

Collect the following data through the health history and physical examination (see Chapter 16). Further focused assessments are described with nursing interventions below. When assessing the older client, be aware of normal changes with aging, outlined in the box below.

- Health history: pituitary diseases, when symptoms began, severity of symptoms, treatment of hyperthyroidism with medications or radioactive iodine, thyroid surgery, treatment of head or neck cancer with radiation, diet, use of iodized salt, bowel elimination, respiratory difficulties

- Physical assessment: muscle strength, deep tendon reflexes, vital signs, cardiovascular and peripheral vascular systems, integument, thyroid gland, weight

Nursing Diagnoses and Interventions

In planning and implementing care for clients with hypothyroidism, the nurse takes into account that the disorder affects all organ systems. Although many nursing diagnoses might be valid, this section focuses on client problems with cardiovascular function, elimination, and skin integrity.

Decreased Cardiac Output

A TH deficit causes a reduction in heart rate and stroke volume, resulting in decreased cardiac output. There may also be an accumulation of fluid in the pericardial sac (from the edema characteristic of hypothyroidism), and coronary artery disease may be present, further compromising cardiac function.

- Monitor blood pressure, rate and rhythm of apical and peripheral pulses, respiratory rate, and breath sounds. *Hypotension indicates decreasing peripheral blood. Fluid in the pericardial sac restricts cardiac function. Monopolysaccharide deposits in the respiratory system decrease vital capacity and cause hypoventilation.*
- Suggest the client avoid chilling; increase room temperature, use additional bed covers, and avoid drafts. *Chilling increases metabolic rate and puts increased stress on the heart.*
- Explain the need to alternate activity with rest periods. Ask the client to report any breathing difficulties, chest pain, heart palpitations, or dizziness. *Activity increases demands on the heart and should be balanced with rest. Symptoms of cardiac stress include dyspnea, chest pain, palpitations, and dizziness.*

Constipation

The hypothyroid client is likely to have a reduced appetite and decreased food intake, a diminished activity level because of muscle aches and weakness, and reduced peristalsis to the point that fecal impactions may occur.

- Encourage a fluid intake of up to 2000 mL per day. Discuss preferred liquids and the best times of day to drink fluids. If kcal intake is restricted, ensure that liquids have no kcal or are low in kcal. *Sufficient fluid intake is necessary to promote proper stool consistency.*

Nursing Care of the Older Adult

VARIATIONS IN ASSESSMENT FINDINGS—HYPOTHYROIDISM

NORMAL CHANGES WITH AGING

- The thyroid gland undergoes some degree of atrophy, fibrosis, and nodularity.
- Hair growth decreases.

- Nails are often thick, brittle, and yellow.
- Facial skin sags, and bones become more prominent.
- Deep tendon reflexes decrease.
- Response to questions may be slower.

- Discuss ways to maintain a high-fiber diet. *Diets high in fiber and fluid produce soft stools. Fiber that is not digested absorbs water, which adds bulk to the stool and assists in the movement of fecal material through the intestines.*

> **PRACTICE ALERT** *High-fiber foods include beans, potatoes, fruits, breads, cereal, crackers, popcorn, and rice.* ■

- Encourage activity as tolerated. *Activity influences bowel elimination by improving muscle tone and stimulating peristalsis.*

Risk for Impaired Skin Integrity

The client with hypothyroidism is at risk for impaired skin integrity related to the accumulation of fluid in the interstitial spaces and to dry, rough skin. Decreased peripheral circulation, decreased activity levels, and slow wound healing further increase the risk. These interventions are outlined for the older client who is hospitalized for surgery or severe hypothyroidism.

- Monitor skin surfaces for redness or lesions, especially if the client's activity is greatly reduced. Use a pressure ulcer risk assessment scale to identify clients at risk. *Hypothyroidism causes dry, rough, edematous skin conditions that increase the risk of skin breakdown.*
- Provide or teach the immobile client measures to promote optimal circulation:
  - Use a turning schedule if the client is on bed rest, or teach the client to change position every 2 hours.

> **PRACTICE ALERT** *Lift the client up in bed to prevent tissue damage from shearing forces.* ■

- Limit the time for sitting in one position; shift weight or lift the body using arm rests every 20 to 30 minutes.
- Use pillows, pads, or sheepskin or foam cushions for bed and/or chair.
- Teach and implement a schedule of range-of-motion exercises.

Prolonged pressure, especially in clients with edema and circulatory impairment, can occlude capillaries and cause hypoxic tissue damage.

- Provide or teach the client measures to maintain skin integrity:
  - Take baths only as necessary; use warm (not hot) water.
  - Use gentle motions when washing and drying skin.
  - Use alcohol-free skin oils and lotions.

Dry skin and edema increase the risk of skin breakdown. Hot water, rough massage, and alcohol-based preparations may increase skin dryness, further impairing the body's ability to maintain skin integrity.

Using NANDA, NIC, and NOC

Chart 17–1 shows links between NANDA, NIC, and NOC when caring for the client with hypothyroidism.

Home Care

Clients with hypothyroidism require lifelong care, primarily at home. Address the following topics.

- The need to take medications for the rest of one's life
- The need for periodic dosage reassessments
- If the client is older or does not have support system, helpful community resources
- Additional resources:
  - American Thyroid Association
  - Thyroid Foundation of Canada
  - Endocrine Society

CHART 17–1   NANDA, NIC, AND NOC LINKAGES

The Client with Hypothyroidism

NURSING DIAGNOSES	NURSING INTERVENTIONS	NURSING OUTCOMES
• Risk for Constipation	• Bowel Management • Constipation Management • Fluid Management	• Bowel Elimination • Hydration
• Excess Fluid Volume	• Fluid Management • Electrolyte Management • Vital Sign Monitoring	• Fluid Balance • Electrolyte Balance
• Activity Intolerance	• Energy Management	• Energy Conservation • Self-Care: Activities of Daily Living
• Altered Thought Processes	• Environmental Management: Safety	• Safety Behavior: Personal

Note. Data from Nursing Outcomes Classification (NOC) *by M. Johnson & M. Maas (Eds.), 1997, St. Louis: Mosby;* Nursing Diagnoses: Definitions & Classification 2001–2002 *by North American Nursing Diagnosis Association, 2001, Philadelphia: NANDA;* Nursing Interventions Classification (NIC) *by J.C. McCloskey & G. M. Bulechek (Eds.), 2000, St. Louis: Mosby. Reprinted by permission.*

Nursing Care Plan
A Client with Hypothyroidism

Jane Lee is a 60-year-old retired nurse living with her husband and daughter on a farm that has been in the family for four generations. Mrs. Lee has gained 10 lb (4.5 kg) in the past few months, even though she is rarely hungry and eats much less than normal. She is always tired and weak—so tired that she has not even been able to help with the chores on the farm or do housework. She is concerned about her appearance and the way she sounds when she talks. Her face is puffy, and her tongue always feels thick. Mr. Lee convinces his wife to make an appointment at a health center in a nearby town.

ASSESSMENT

Brian Henning, RN, completes the health assessment for Mrs. Lee at the health center. He finds that she now weighs 150 lb (68 kg), an increase of 10 lb (4.5 kg) over her weight at her last visit 6 months earlier. Mrs. Lee states that she always feels cold, tired, and weak. She also states that she is constipated, has difficulty remembering things, and looks different. Physical assessment findings include a palpable and bilaterally enlarged thyroid; dry, yellowish skin; nonpitting edema of the face and lower legs; and slow, slurred speech. Diagnostic tests revealed the following abnormal findings: T_3, 56 ng/dL (normal range: 80 to 200 ng/dL); T_4, 3.1 (normal range: 5 to 12 mg/dL); TSH increased. The medical diagnosis of hypothyroidism is made, and Mrs. Lee is started on levothyroxine 0.05 mg daily.

DIAGNOSIS

- *Constipation,* related to decreased peristalsis, as evidenced by hard, formed stools every 4 days
- *Impaired verbal communication,* related to changes in speech patterns and enlarged tongue
- *Low self-esteem,* related to changes in physical appearance and activity intolerance

EXPECTED OUTCOMES

- Regain normal bowel elimination patterns, having a soft, formed stool at least every other day.
- Experience improvement in verbal communication.
- Regain positive self-esteem as medication reduces physical changes and fatigue.

PLANNING AND IMPLEMENTATION

- Teach to increase fluids, bulk, and fiber in the diet to help regain a normal bowel elimination pattern of a soft, formed stool every other day.
- Take medication as prescribed and do not expect immediate reversal of symptoms affecting speech.
- Plan activities around rest periods. Encourage husband and daughter to help with housecleaning and cooking.

EVALUATION

On return to the health center 2 months later, Mrs. Lee reports that she is no longer constipated but that she is continuing to drink six glasses of water and eating oatmeal every day. She no longer feels cold, is regaining her normal energy, and even feels well enough to plant her garden. Her speech is clear and easy to understand. As she leaves the examining room, Mrs. Lee says, "It's hard to believe that I have changed so much—now I look and feel like the 'old' me!"

Critical Thinking in the Nursing Process

1. What physical changes that normally occur with aging are similar to the manifestations of hypothyroidism?
2. Describe the factors that put Mrs. Lee's safety at risk. What alterations in her home environment would you suggest to promote safety until the prescribed medication takes effect?
3. The client taking oral thyroid medications may become hyperthyroid. List the manifestations you would include in a teaching plan to signal this condition.

See Evaluating Your Response in Appendix C.

THE CLIENT WITH CANCER OF THE THYROID

Thyroid cancer is relatively rare, with an estimated rate of 23,000 new cases annually. Thyroid cancer accounts for approximately 1300 cancer deaths a year (American Cancer Society, 2002). The most consistent risk factor is exposure to ionizing radiation to the head and neck during childhood. For example, many adults in their 50s and 60s received X-ray treatments for colds and sinus infections during childhood.

Of the several types of thyroid cancer, the most common types are listed here.

- Papillary thyroid carcinoma is the most common thyroid malignancy. It is usually detected as a single nodule, but may arise from a multinodular goiter. The average age of diagnosis is 42, with 70% of cases occurring in women. Risks for the development of this form are exposure to external X-ray treatments to the head or neck as a child, childhood exposure to radioactive isotopes of iodine in nuclear fallout, and a family history. Papillary thyroid carcinoma is the least aggressive type, but does metastasize to the local and regional lymph nodes and lungs.
- Follicular thyroid cancer is the second most common thyroid malignancy. The average age of diagnosis is 50, with 72% of cases occurring in women. This form is more aggressive, with metastasis commonly found in neck lymph nodes, bone, and lungs.

Thyroid cancer is manifested by a palpable, firm nontender nodule in the thyroid. If undetected, the tumor may grow and impinge on the esophagus or trachea, causing difficulty in swallowing or breathing. Most people with thyroid cancer do not have elevated thyroid hormone levels. The diagnosis is made by measuring thyroid hormones, performing thyroid scans, and by fine-needle biopsy of the nodule. The usual treatment is subtotal or total thyroidectomy. TSH suppression therapy with levothyroxine may be conducted prior to surgery. Radioactive iodine therapy (^{131}I) and chemotherapy are additional therapeutic options. The 5-year survival rate, if the tumor has not metastasized, is 95% (American Cancer Society, 2002). Nursing care for the client with cancer is discussed in Chapter 10.

DISORDERS OF THE PARATHYROID GLANDS

Disorders of the parathyroid glands, hyperparathyroidism and hypoparathyroidism, are not as common as those of the thyroid gland. Hypercalcemia and hypocalcemia (the primary results of alterations in parathyroid function) are discussed in Chapter 5.

THE CLIENT WITH HYPERPARATHYROIDISM

Hyperparathyroidism results from an increase in the secretion of parathyroid hormone (PTH), which regulates normal serum levels of calcium. The increase in PTH affects the kidneys and bones, resulting in the following pathophysiologic changes:

- Increased resorption of calcium and excretion of phosphate by the kidneys, which increases the risk of hypercalcemia and hypophosphatemia
- Increased bicarbonate excretion and decreased acid excretion by the kidneys, which increases the risk of metabolic acidosis and hypokalemia
- Increased release of calcium and phosphorus by bones, with resultant bone decalcification
- Deposits of calcium in soft tissues and the formation of renal calculi

PATHOPHYSIOLOGY AND MANIFESTATIONS

Hyperparathyroidism occurs more often in older adults and is 3 times more common in women. The disorder itself is not common. The three types of hyperparathyroidism are as follows:

- Primary hyperparathyroidism occurs when there is hyperplasia or an adenoma in one of the parathyroid glands. These disorders interrupt the normal regulatory mechanism between serum calcium levels and PTH secretion and increase the absorption of calcium through the gastrointestinal tract.
- Secondary hyperparathyroidism is a compensatory response by the parathyroid glands to chronic hypocalcemia. It is characterized by an increased secretion of PTH.
- Tertiary hyperparathyroidism results from hyperplasia of the parathyroid glands and a loss of response to serum calcium levels. This disorder is most often seen in clients with chronic renal failure.

Many clients with hyperparathyroidism are asymptomatic. When symptoms occur, they are related to hypercalcemia and various musculoskeletal, renal, and gastrointestinal manifestations. Bone reabsorption results in pathologic fractures, while

Manifestations of Hyperparathyroidism

Musculoskeletal System
- Bone pain (back, joints, shins)
- Pathologic fractures (women)
- Muscle weakness
- Muscle atrophy

Renal Effects
- Renal calculi
- Polyuria
- Polydipsia

Gastrointestinal System
- Abdominal pain
- Peptic ulcers
- Pancreatitis
- Nausea
- Constipation

Cardiovascular System
- Arrhythmias
- Hypertension

Central Nervous System
- Paresthesias
- Depression
- Psychosis

Metabolic Effects
- Acidosis
- Weight loss

elevated calcium levels alter neural and muscular activity, leading to muscle weakness and atrophy. Proximal renal tubule function is altered, and metabolic acidosis, renal calculi formation, and polyuria occur.

Manifestations of the effect of hypercalcemia on the gastrointestinal tract include abdominal pain, constipation, anorexia, and peptic ulcer formation. Hypercalcemia also affects the cardiovascular system, causing arrhythmias, hypertension, and increased sensitivity to cardiotonic glycosides (e.g., digitalis preparations). The manifestations of hyperparathyroidism are summarized in the box above.

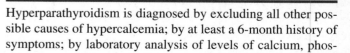

COLLABORATIVE CARE

Hyperparathyroidism is diagnosed by excluding all other possible causes of hypercalcemia; by at least a 6-month history of symptoms; by laboratory analysis of levels of calcium, phosphorus, magnesium, bicarbonate, and chloride; and by bone X-ray studies and scans (Tierney et al., 2002).

Treatment of hyperparathyroidism focuses on decreasing the elevated serum calcium levels. Clients with mild hypercalcemia are urged to drink fluids and keep active. They should avoid immobilization, thiazide diuretics, large doses of vitamins A and D, antacids containing calcium, and calcium supplements. Severe hypercalcemia requires hospitalization and intensive treatment with intravenous saline. Medications to inhibit bone reabsorption and reduce hypercalcemia, such as pamidronate (Aredia) and alendronate (Fosamax), are administered.

Surgical removal of the parathyroid glands affected by hyperplasia or adenoma treats primary hyperparathyroidism. The preoperative and postoperative nursing care of the client having surgery of the parathyroids is essentially the same as that for the client having a thyroidectomy (see page 449).

NURSING CARE

Nursing care of the client with hypercalcemia is discussed in Chapter 5. ∞

THE CLIENT WITH HYPOPARATHYROIDISM

Hypoparathyroidism results from abnormally low PTH levels. The most common cause is damage to or removal of the parathyroid glands during thyroidectomy. The lack of circulating PTH causes hypocalcemia and an elevated blood phosphate level.

PATHOPHYSIOLOGY AND MANIFESTATIONS

Reduced levels of PTH result in impaired renal tubular regulation of calcium and phosphate. In addition, decreased activation of vitamin D results in decreased absorption of calcium by the intestines. The low calcium levels cause changes in neuromuscular activity, affecting peripheral motor and sensory nerves. Hypocalcemia lowers the threshold for nerve and muscle excitability; a slight stimulus anywhere along a nerve or muscle fiber initiates an impulse.

The neuromuscular manifestations that result include numbness and tingling around the mouth and in the fingertips, muscle spasms of the hands and feet, convulsions, and laryngeal spasms. Tetany, a continuous spasm of muscles, is the primary symptom of hypocalcemia. In severe cases of tetany, death may occur. Assessments for **tetany** include Chvostek's sign and

Trousseau's sign (see Chapter 16). The manifestations of hypoparathyroidism are summarized in the box above.

Manifestations of Hypoparathyroidism

Musculoskeletal System
- Muscle spasms
- Facial grimacing
- Carpopedal spasms
- Tetany or convulsions

Integumentary System
- Brittle nails
- Hair loss
- Dry, scaly skin

Gastrointestinal System
- Abdominal cramps
- Malabsorption

Cardiovascular System
- Arrhythmias

Central Nervous System
- Paresthesias (lips, hands, feet)
- Mood disorders (irritability, depression, anxiety)
- Hyperactive reflexes
- Psychosis
- Increased intracranial pressure

COLLABORATIVE CARE

Hypoparathyroidism is diagnosed by low serum calcium levels and high phosphorus levels in the absence of renal failure, an absorption disorder, or a nutritional disorder.

Treatment of hypoparathyroidism focuses on increasing calcium levels. Intravenous calcium gluconate is given immediately to reduce tetany. Long-term therapy includes supplemental calcium, increased dietary calcium, and vitamin D therapy.

NURSING CARE

Nursing care for the client with hypocalcemia is discussed in Chapter 5. ∞

DISORDERS OF THE ADRENAL GLANDS

Disorders of the adrenal cortex or adrenal medulla result in changes in the production of adrenocorticotropic hormone (ACTH). Hormones of the adrenal cortex are essential to life. They maintain homeostasis in response to stressors. Disorders of the adrenal cortex result in complex physical, psychologic, and metabolic alterations that are potentially life threatening. Hormones of the adrenal medulla are not essential to life, because the sympathetic nervous system produces similar body responses. The disorders that occur are hyperfunction and hypofunction of the adrenal cortex and hyperfunction of the adrenal medulla.

THE CLIENT WITH HYPERCORTISOLISM (CUSHING'S SYNDROME)

Cushing's syndrome is a chronic disorder in which hyperfunction of the adrenal cortex produces excessive amounts of circulating cortisol or ACTH. Cushing's syndrome is more common in women, with the average age of onset between 30 and 50 years (Figure 17–3 ■). However, the disorder may occur at any age, especially as the result of pharmacologic therapy. People who take steroids for long periods of time (e.g., for

Figure 17–3 ■ A woman before and after developing Cushing's syndrome. In the photo at right, notice the swollen facial features.

Courtesy of Dr. Charles Wilson, University of California, San Francisco.

the treatment of arthritis, after an organ transplant, or as an adjunct to chemotherapy) are at increased risk for developing the disorder.

PATHOPHYSIOLOGY

Cushing's syndrome may be the result of various causes. The most common etiologies of the disorder are (Porth, 2002):

- The pituitary form, with ACTH hypersecretion by a tumor of the pituitary (called *Cushing's disease*). This is most commonly caused by a small pituitary adenoma, with persistent but disorderly and random overproduction of ACTH.
- The ectopic form, caused by ACTH-secreting tumors (such as small-cell lung cancer). In this form, the ACTH is also random and episodic, but greater than in Cushing's disease.
- The adrenal form, resulting from excessive cortisol secretion by a benign or malignant adrenal tumor. The excess secretion suppresses pituitary ACTH production, resulting in atrophy of the uninvolved adrenal cortex.
- Iatrogenic Cushing's syndrome, resulting from long-term therapy with potent pharmacologic glucocorticoid preparations.

MANIFESTATIONS

The manifestations of Cushing's syndrome result from the ACTH or cortisol excess, and manifest as exaggerated cortisol actions. Obesity and a redistribution of body fat result in fat deposits in the abdominal region (central obesity), fat pads under the clavicle, a "buffalo hump" over the upper back, and a round "moon" face. Changes in protein metabolism cause muscle weakness and wasting, especially in the extremities. Glucocorticoid excess inhibits fibroblasts, resulting in loss of collagen and connective tissue. Thinning of skin, abdominal

striae (reddish purple "stretch marks"), easy bruising, poor wound healing, and frequent skin infections result. Glucose metabolism is altered in the majority of clients, and diabetes mellitus may occur. Electrolyte imbalances also occur with the increased hormone levels. Changes in calcium absorption result in osteoporosis, compression fractures of the vertebrae, fractures of the ribs, and renal calculi. Hypokalemia and hypertension occur as potassium is lost and sodium is retained. Inhibited immune responses increase the risk of infection, and increased gastric acid secretion increases the risk of peptic ulcers. Emotional changes range from depression to psychosis. In women, increasing androgen levels cause hirsutism (excessive facial hair in particular), acne, and menstrual irregularities. The manifestations and effects of Cushing's syndrome are grouped by body system in the box below.

The complications of untreated Cushing's syndrome include electrolyte imbalances (hyperglycemia, hypernatremia, and hypokalemia), hypertension, and emotional disturbances. Increased susceptibility to infections is also a factor. Compression fractures from osteoporosis and aseptic necrosis of the femoral head may result in serious disability. If the client undergoes a bilateral adrenalectomy as a treatment for Cushing's syndrome, an acute deficit of cortisol (addisonian crisis) may result.

COLLABORATIVE CARE

The treatment of Cushing's syndrome includes medications, radiation therapy, or surgery, depending on the etiologic origin of the disorder.

Manifestations of Cushing's Syndrome

Musculoskeletal System
- Weakness
- Muscle wasting
- Osteoporosis

Integumentary System
- Thin, easily bruised skin
- Skin infections
- Poor wound healing
- Eccymosis
- Purple striae (around thighs, breasts, abdomen)
- Hirsutism

Central Nervous System
- Emotional lability
- Psychoses

Gastrointestinal System
- Peptic ulcers

Cardiovascular System
- Hypertension

Renal Effects
- Renal calculi
- Polyuria
- Polydipsia
- Glycosuria

Metabolic Effects
- Hypokalemia
- Hypernatremia
- Truncal obesity

Reproductive System
- Oligomenorrhea or amenorrhea
- Impotence
- Decreased libido

TABLE 17–3 Laboratory Findings in Cushing's Syndrome

	Test	Normal Values	Findings
Serum	Cortisol	8 a.m. to 10 a.m.: 5 to 23 µg/dL 4 p.m. to 6 p.m.: 3 to 13 µg/dL	Increased
	Blood urea nitrogen (BUN)	5 to 25 mg/dL	Normal
	Sodium	135 to 145 mEq/L	Increased
	Potassium	3.5 to 5.0 mEq/L	Increased
	Glucose (serum)	70 to 100 mg/dL	Increased
Urine	17-KS	Male: 5 to 25 mg/24h Female: 5 to 15 mg/24h >65: 4 to 8 mg/24h	Increased

Diagnostic Tests

Cushing's syndrome is diagnosed through a variety of diagnostic tests. Findings are shown in Table 17–3.

- *Plasma cortisol levels* are measured. If Cushing's disease is present, test results show a loss of the normal diurnal variations of higher levels in the morning and lower levels in the afternoon.
- *Plasma ACTH levels* are measured to determine the etiology of the syndrome. Normally, plasma ACTH levels are highest from 7 A.M. to 10 A.M. and lowest from 7 P.M. to 10 P.M. In secondary Cushing's syndrome, ACTH is elevated; in primary Cushing's syndrome, ACTH is decreased.
- *24-hour urine tests* (*17-ketosteroids* and *17-hydroxycorticosteroids*) are conducted to measure free cortisol and androgens; these hormones are increased in Cushing's syndrome.

- *Serum potassium, calcium, and glucose levels* are measured to identify electrolyte imbalances.
- *ACTH suppression test* may be conducted to identify the cause of the disorder. A synthetic cortisol (dexamethasone) is given to suppress the production of ACTH, and plasma cortisol levels are measured. If an extremely high dose of cortisol is necessary to suppress ACTH, the primary disorder is adrenal cortex hyperplasia. If ACTH is not suppressed with the synthetic cortisol, an adrenal tumor is suspected.

Medications

Cushing's syndrome that results from a pituitary tumor is treated by medications as an adjunct to surgery or radiation. Medications are also used for clients with inoperable pituitary or adrenal malignancies. Although the drugs control symptoms, they do not effect a cure. Examples of some commonly prescribed drugs follow:

- Mitotane directly suppresses activity of the adrenal cortex and decreases peripheral metabolism of corticosteroids. It is used to treat metastatic adrenal cancer.
- Metyrapone or ketoconazole (or both) inhibit cortisol synthesis by the adrenal cortex and may be administered to clients with ectopic ACTH-secreting tumors that cannot be surgically removed.
- Somatostatis analog (octreotide) suppresses ACTH secretion in some clients.

Surgery

When Cushing's syndrome is caused by an adrenal cortex tumor, an adrenalectomy may be performed to remove the tumor. Only one adrenal gland is usually involved; however, if an ACTH-producing ectopic tumor is involved, a bilateral adrenalectomy is performed. Lifelong hormone replacement is necessary if both adrenal glands are removed. Nursing care of the client having an adrenalectomy is discussed below.

NURSING CARE OF THE CLIENT HAVING AN ADRENALECTOMY

PREOPERATIVE CARE

- Request a dietary consultation to discuss with the client about a diet high in vitamins and proteins. If hypokalemia exists, include foods high in potassium. *Glucocorticoid excess increases catabolism. Vitamins and proteins are necessary for tissue repair and wound healing following surgery.*
- Use careful medical and surgical asepsis when providing care and treatments. *Cortisol excess increases the risk of infection.*
- Monitor the results of laboratory tests of electrolytes and glucose levels. *Electrolyte and glucose imbalances are corrected before the client has surgery.*
- Teach the client to turn, cough, and perform deep-breathing exercises. *Although they are important for all surgical clients, these activities are even more important for the client who is at risk for infection. Having the client practice and demonstrate the activities increases postoperative compliance.*

POSTOPERATIVE CARE

- Take and record vital signs, measure intake and output, and monitor electrolytes on a frequent schedule, especially during the first 48 hours after surgery. *Removal of an adrenal gland, especially a bilateral adrenalectomy, results in adrenal insufficiency. Addisonian crisis and hypovolemic shock may occur. Cortisol is often given on the day of surgery and in the postoperative period to replace inadequate hormone levels. Intravenous fluids are also administered.*
- Assess body temperature, WBC levels, and wound drainage. Change dressings using sterile technique. *Impaired wound healing increases the risk of infection in clients with adrenal disorders. Use aseptic technique to decrease this risk.*

Surgical removal of the pituitary gland (hypophysectomy) is indicated when Cushing's syndrome is the result of a pituitary disorder. The gland is removed either by a transphenoidal route or by a craniotomy. Nursing care for the client having cranial surgery is discussed in Chapter 42. ↪

NURSING CARE

Health Promotion

Stress the risk of developing Cushing's syndrome for clients taking long-term steroids. The risk of abruptly discontinuing the medications is an essential component of teaching.

Assessment

Collect the following data through the health history and physical examination (see Chapter 16). Further focused assessments are described with nursing interventions below.

- Health history: history of pituitary, adrenal, pancreatic, or pulmonary tumor; frequent infections; gastrointestinal bleeding; stress fractures; pain, changes in weight distribution; change in height; fatigue; weakness; change in appearance; bruising; skin infections; menstrual history; sexual function
- Physical assessment: vital signs, behavior, appearance, fat distribution, face, skin, hair quantity and distribution, muscle size and strength, gait

Nursing Diagnoses and Interventions

The nurse caring for the client with Cushing's syndrome must take a holistic approach to plan and implement interventions for a wide variety of responses, including problems related to fluid and electrolyte balance, injury, infection, and body image. For additional information about clients with alterations in fluid and electrolyte balance, see Chapter 5. ↪

Fluid Volume Excess

The excess cortisol secretion associated with Cushing's syndrome results in sodium and water reabsorption, causing fluid volume excess. The client will have weight gain, edema, and hypertension.

- Ask the client to weigh at the same time each day, and maintain a record of results. *Body weight is an accurate indicator of fluid status. One liter of fluid retention corresponds to about 2 lb (0.9 kg) of body weight.*
- Monitor blood pressure, rate and rhythm of pulse, respiratory rate, and breath sounds. Assess for peripheral edema and jugular vein distention. *Extracellular fluid volume excess resulting from sodium and water retention is manifested by hypertension and a bounding, rapid pulse. There may also be crackles and wheezes, dependent edema, and venous distention.*
- Teach the client and family the reasons for restricting fluid and the importance of limiting fluids if ordered. *Restricting fluid can help decrease the risk of fluid volume excess. Involving the client and family in the plan of care and teaching the rationale for interventions helps achieve goals.*

Risk for Injury

The client with Cushing's syndrome is at risk for injury from several causes. Excess cortisol causes increased absorption of calcium and demineralization of bones, resulting in risk of pathologic fractures. Muscle weakness and fatigue are common, increasing the potential for accidental falls.

- Teach the client and family to maintain a safe environment:
  - Keep unnecessary clutter and equipment out of the way and off the floor.
  - Ensure adequate lighting, especially at night.
  - Encourage the use of assistive devices for ambulation or to ask for help if needed.
  - If the client wears corrective lenses, be sure they are available and clean.
  - Encourage the use of nonskid slippers or shoes.
  - Monitor for signs of fatigue (increased pulse and respirations); plan rest periods.

A well-lighted environment free of clutter decreases the risk of falls and injury. Sensory and motor deficits increase the risk of falls; corrective lenses, assistive devices, and nonslip footwear can decrease this risk. Rest relieves fatigue. To reduce energy expenditure, include alternating periods of rest and activity in daily schedules.

Risk for Infection

Elevated cortisol levels impair the immune response and put the client with Cushing's syndrome at increased risk for infection. Increased cortisol also affects protein synthesis, causing delayed wound healing, and inhibits collagen formation, which results in epidermal atrophy, further inhibiting resistance to infection. In addition, impaired blood flow to edematous tissue results in altered cellular nutrition, which increases the potential for infection. The following interventions are outlined for the client with Cushing's syndrome who is hospitalized.

- Place in a private room, and limit visitors. *The client must avoid exposure to environmental infection.*
- Monitor vital signs and verbalizations of subjective manifestations (e.g., the client's response to, "How do you feel?") every 4 hours. *Increased body temperature and pulse are systemic indicators of infection; however, because Cushing's syndrome impairs the normal inflammatory response, the usual indicators of inflammation may not be present.*

> **PRACTICE ALERT**   *A generalized feeling of malaise may be the primary manifestation of infection.* ■

- Use principles of medical and sterile asepsis when caring for the client, conducting procedures, or providing wound care. *Impaired skin and tissues make aseptic techniques even more necessary to decrease the risk of infection. Intact skin is the first line of defense against infection; if invasive procedures are performed or a wound is present, this defense is lost.*

- If wounds are present, assess the color, odor, and consistency of wound drainage, and look for increased pain in and around the wound. *Cortisol excess delays wound healing and closure.*
- Teach the importance of increasing intake of protein and vitamins C and A. *Protein, vitamin C, and vitamin A are necessary to collagen formation; collagen helps support and repair body tissues.*

Disturbed Body Image

The client with Cushing's syndrome has obvious physical changes in appearance. The abnormal fat distribution, moon face, buffalo hump, striae, acne, and facial hair (in women) all contribute to disruptions in the way clients with this disorder perceive themselves.

- Encourage clients to express feelings and to ask questions about the disorder and its treatment. *The loss of one's normal body image may prompt feelings of hopelessness, powerlessness, anger, and depression. Understanding the disease and adapting to changes from that disease are the first steps in regaining control of one's own body.*
- Discuss strengths and previous coping strategies. Enlist the support of family or significant others in reaffirming the client's worth. *Disturbances in body image are often accompanied by low self-esteem. Self-esteem derives from one's perception of competence and from appraisals of others.*
- Discuss signs of progress in controlling symptoms; for example, decreased facial edema or increased activity tolerance. *Many physical changes from cortisol excess disappear with treatment. Clearly communicate this fact, because the client may believe changes are permanent.*

Using NANDA, NIC and NOC

Chart 17–2 shows links between NANDA, NIC, and NOC when caring for the client with Cushing's syndrome.

Home Care

The client with Cushing's syndrome requires education about self-care at home specific to the type of treatment given. Address the following topics:

- Safety measures to prevent falls if fatigue, weakness, and osteoporosis are present
- Taking medications as prescribed, with information about side effects. Clients often require medications for the rest of their lives, and dosage changes are highly likely.
- Having regular health assessments
- Wearing a medical ID indicating the client has Cushing's syndrome
- Helping the older client with referrals to social services or community health services because of the complexity of the treatment and care required
- Providing helpful resources:
  - American Association of Clinical Endocrinologists
  - Endocrine Society

THE CLIENT WITH CHRONIC ADRENOCORTICAL INSUFFICIENCY (ADDISON'S DISEASE)

Addison's disease is a disorder resulting from destruction or dysfunction of the adrenal cortex. The result is chronic deficiency of cortisol, aldosterone, and adrenal androgens, accompanied by skin pigmentation. It can occur at any age, although it is more common in adults under the age of 60. Like many endocrine disorders, Addison's disease is more common in women.

CHART 17–2 NANDA, NIC, AND NOC LINKAGES

The Client with Cushing's Syndrome

NURSING DIAGNOSES	NURSING INTERVENTIONS	NURSING OUTCOMES
• Risk for Infection	• Infection Protection • Environmental Management • Skin Surveillance • Wound Care	• Risk Control • Risk Detection
• Impaired Skin Integrity	• Infection Control • Skin Surveillance	• Tissue Integrity: Skin
• Risk for Injury	• Fall Prevention • Teaching: Disease Process • Home Maintenance Assistance	• Safety Behavior: Fall Prevention • Safety Behavior: Home Physical Environment
• Disturbed Body Image	• Body Image Enhancement	• Body Image

Note. Data from Nursing Outcomes Classification (NOC) by M. Johnson & M. Maas (Eds.), 1997, St. Louis: Mosby; Nursing Diagnoses: Definitions & Classification 2001–2002 by North American Nursing Diagnosis Association, 2001, Philadelphia: NANDA; Nursing Interventions Classification (NIC) by J.C. McCloskey & G. M. Bulechek (Eds.), 2000, St. Louis: Mosby. Reprinted by permission.

Nursing Care Plan
A Client with Cushing's Syndrome

Sara Domico is a 30-year-old lawyer living in a major metropolitan area. She has never been married, and she shares her life with her cat, Beau, and her parents, who live nearby. Her physician recently diagnosed Ms. Domico as having Cushing's syndrome and admits her to the hospital for surgery for an adrenal cortex tumor (adrenalectomy). She has been having increased muscle weakness, so much so that she has difficulty climbing the one flight of stairs to her apartment. She has also had difficulty sleeping, irregular menstrual periods, and hypertension. Ms. Domico is especially concerned about her protruding abdomen, round face, development of facial hair, and the numerous bruises that have appeared on her skin.

ASSESSMENT
When Ms. Domico arrives at the hospital the morning of surgery, she is admitted by her case manager, Ann Sprengel, RN, CNS. Ann completes a physical assessment that includes abnormal findings of thin lower extremities, an enlarged abdomen, purple striae over the abdomen and buttocks, a round face, and obvious facial hair. Her blood pressure is 160/96. Ms. Domico tells Ann that she is always tired and that sometimes it "just wears me out to walk from the bedroom to the kitchen." Diagnostic tests conducted prior to admission reveal the following abnormal findings (all except cortisol levels are corrected before surgery).

> Glucose: 186 mg/dL (normal range: 70 to 110 mg/dL)
> Sodium: 152 mEq/L (normal range: 135 to 145 mEq/L)
> Potassium: 3.2 mEq/L (normal range: 3.5 to 5.0 mEq/L)
> Calcium: 4.3 mEq/L (normal range: 4.5 to 5.5 mEq/L)
> Cortisol: 35 mg/dL (normal for A.M.: 5 to 23 mg/dL)

DIAGNOSIS
- *Fluid volume excess,* related to sodium retention causing edema and hypertension
- *Risk for injury,* related to generalized fatigue and weakness
- *Risk for infection,* related to impaired immune response and edema
- *Body image disturbance,* related to physical changes secondary to Cushing's syndrome

EXPECTED OUTCOMES
- Regain a normal body fluid balance.

- Remain free of injury.
- Remain free of infection.
- Verbalize understanding of the physical effects of the disease process and realistic expectations of desired changes in appearance.

PLANNING AND IMPLEMENTATION
- Weigh each morning, using the same scale.
- Maintain an accurate record of intake and output.
- Ensure adequate lighting in the room, and wear glasses and shoes when getting out of bed.
- Develop a written schedule of rest and activity periods.
- If agreeable, provide a private room, and restrict visitors to parents at this time.
- Use strict medical and surgical asepsis when providing care.
- Provide time for discussion of the disease and treatment; encourage verbalization of feelings and identify successful coping mechanisms used in the past.
- Encourage turning, coughing, and deep breathing and/or incentive spirometry every 2–4 hours.

EVALUATION
Ms. Domico states that she is "ready to have surgery and start feeling better." She has not fallen or injured herself, and she has remained free of infection. Although edema is still present, she has lost 8 lb (3.6 kg), and her blood pressure is decreased. Ms. Domico has openly discussed her concerns about the way she looks and feels; she understands that symptoms will improve following surgery. She has strong religious beliefs and family support, both of which provide strength and help her cope with the effects of the disorder and the need for any further treatment.

Critical Thinking in the Nursing Process
1. When Ms. Domico was admitted to the hospital, several of her test results were abnormal. Describe the pathophysiologic reason for those results.
2. List the assessments that nurses can make to determine body fluid balance.
3. Develop a plan of care for this client for the nursing diagnosis *Fatigue.*

See Evaluating Your Response in Appendix C.

PATHOPHYSIOLOGY

There are many possible causes of Addison's disease. The etiologies include:

- Autoimmune destruction of the adrenals. This is the most common cause, accounting for about 80% of spontaneous cases (Tierney et al., 2001). It may occur alone, or as part of a polyglandular autoimmune syndrome (PGA). Type 2 PGA is seen in adults, often associated with autoimmune thyroid disease (usually hypothyroidism), type 1 diabetes, primary ovarian or testicular failure, and pernicious anemia.
- Clients who are taking anticoagulants, have major trauma, or are having open heart surgery. Such clients may have bilateral adrenal hemorrhage.

- Adrenoleukodystrophy, an X-linked disorder characterized by an accumulation of very long chain fatty acids in the adrenal cortex, testes, brain, and spinal cord.
- ACTH deficit, resulting from pituitary tumors, pituitary surgery or irradiation, and the use of exogenous steroids.
- Clients who are abruptly withdrawn from long-term, high-dose steroid therapy. Other clients at risk are those with tuberculosis or acquired immune deficiency syndrome (AIDS); the pathogens responsible for either disease can infiltrate and destroy adrenal tissue.

Adrenocortical destruction initially causes a decrease in adrenal glucocorticoid reserve. Basal glucocorticoid secretion is normal, but does not increase in response to stress and surgery. Trauma or infection can precipitate an adrenal crisis. As the destruction of the adrenal cortex continues, even basal secretion of glucocorticoids and mineralocorticoids is deficient. Decreasing plasma cortisol reduces the feedback inhibition of pituitary ACTH and plasma ACTH rises.

Secondary adrenocortical insufficiency occurs when large doses of glucocorticoids are given for their anti-inflammatory and immunosuppressive effects to treat diseases such as arthritis and asthma. Treatment that extends for longer than 4 to 5 weeks suppresses ACTH and cortisol secretion. If the steroid medications are suddenly discontinued, the hypothalamus and pituitary cannot respond normally to the reduced level of circulating glucocorticoids. The client may develop manifestations of chronic adrenocortical insufficiency or, if subjected to stress, adrenal crisis (Tierney et al., 2001).

MANIFESTATIONS

The onset of Addison's disease is slow; the client experiences symptoms after about 90% of the function of the gland is lost. The primary manifestations are the result of elevated ACTH levels and decreased aldosterone and cortisol (see the box below.) Aldosterone deficiency affects the ability of the distal tubules of the nephron to conserve sodium. Sodium is lost, potassium is retained, extracellular fluid is depleted, and the blood volume is decreased. Postural hypotension and syncope are common, and hypovolemic shock may occur. Hyponatremia causes dizziness, confusion, and neuromuscular irritability. Hyperkalemia causes cardiac arrhythmias.

Cortisol insufficiency also causes decreased hepatic glyconeogenesis with hypoglycemia. The client tolerates stress poorly and experiences lethargy, weakness, anorexia, nausea, vomiting, and diarrhea. The increased ACTH levels stimulate hyperpigmentation in about 98% of clients with Addison's disease (Porth, 2002). In Caucasian clients, the skin looks deeply suntanned or bronzed in both exposed and unexposed areas.

Manifestations of Addison's Disease

Integumentary System
- Delayed wound healing
- Hyperpigmentation

Cardiovascular System
- Postural hypotension
- Arrhythmias
- Tachycardia

Central Nervous System
- Lethargy
- Tremors
- Emotional lability
- Confusion

Musculoskeletal System
- Weakness
- Muscle wasting
- Joint pain
- Muscle pain

Gastrointestinal System
- Anorexia
- Nausea and vomiting
- Diarrhea

Reproductive System
- Menstrual changes

Metabolic Effects
- Hyperkalemia
- Hyponatremia
- Hypoglycemia

ADDISONIAN CRISIS

Addisonian crisis is a life-threatening response to acute adrenal insufficiency. This response can occur in any person with Addison's disease; however, it is most commonly precipitated by major stressors, especially if the disease is poorly controlled. Addisonian crisis may also occur in clients who are abruptly withdrawn from glucocorticoid medications or who have hemorrhage into the adrenal glands from either septicemia or anticoagulant therapy.

The client with addisonian crisis may have any of the manifestations of Addison's disease, but the primary symptoms are a high fever, weakness, abdominal pain, severe hypotension, circulatory collapse, shock, and coma. Treatment of the crisis is rapid intravenous replacement of fluids and glucocorticoids. Fluid balance is usually restored in 4 to 6 hours.

COLLABORATIVE CARE

The client with Addison's disease requires early diagnosis and treatment. Medical treatment includes cortisol replacement therapy.

Diagnostic Tests

Addison's disease is diagnosed through findings of decreased levels of cortisol, aldosterone, and urinary 17-ketosteroids. Dehydration may result in increased hematocrit and blood urea nitrogen (BUN). Blood glucose levels are decreased, and potassium is increased. A list of laboratory findings in Addison's disease is shown in Table 17–4. The following diagnostic tests are used:

- *Serum cortisol levels,* which are decreased in adrenal insufficiency
- *Blood glucose levels,* which are decreased in adrenal insufficiency
- *Serum sodium levels,* which are decreased in adrenal insufficiency

TABLE 17–4 Laboratory Findings in Addison's Disease

	Test	Normal Values	Findings
Serum	Cortisol	8 a.m. to 10 a.m.: 5 to 23 µg/dL 4 p.m. to 6 p.m.: 3 to 13 µg/dL	Decreased
	Blood urea nitrogen (BUN)	5 to 25 mg/dL	Increased
	Sodium	135 to 145 mEq/L	Decreased
	Potassium	3.5 to 5.0 mEq/L	Increased
	Glucose (serum)	70 to 100 mg/dL	Decreased
Urine	17-KS	Male: 5 to 25 mg/24h Female: 5 to 15 mg/24h >65: 4 to 8 mg/24h	Low/Absent

- *Serum potassium levels,* which are increased in adrenal insufficiency
- *Blood urea nitrogen (BUN) levels,* which are increased in adrenal insufficiency
- *Urinary 17-hydroxycorticoids* and *17-ketosteroids (17-KS) levels,* which are decreased in adrenal insufficiency
- *Plasma ACTH levels,* which are increased in primary adrenal insufficiency but decreased in secondary adrenal insufficiency
- Possibly *ACTH stimulation test.* (Cortisol levels rise with pituitary deficiency but do not rise in primary adrenal insufficiency.)
- *CT scans* of the head, which identify any intracranial lesion impinging on the pituitary gland

Medications

The primary medical treatment of Addison's disease is replacement of corticosteroids and mineralocorticoids, accompanied by increased sodium in the diet. Hydrocortisone is given orally to replace cortisol; fludrocortisone (Florinef) is given orally to replace mineralocorticoids. Nursing implications in cortisol replacement are given in the box below.

NURSING CARE

Health Promotion

Health promotion interventions for the client with or at risk for Addison's disease focus on careful assessments during anticoagulant therapy, open heart surgery, and trauma treatment. If the disease is present, teaching to prevent or treat an addisonian crisis is essential.

Assessment

Collect the following data through the health history and physical examination (see Chapter 16). Further focused assessments are described with nursing interventions below.

- Health history: weight loss, changes in skin color, nausea and vomiting, anorexia, diarrhea, abdominal pain, weakness, amenorrhea, changes in sexual desire, confusion, intolerance of stress
- Physical assessment: height and weight, vital signs, skin, hair quality and distribution, muscle size and strength

Medication Administration

Addison's Disease

CORTISOL REPLACEMENTS

Cortisone (Cortone, Cortogen)
Hydrocortisone (Cortisol, Hydrocortone, Cortef)
Prednisone (Meticorten, Deltasone, Orasone)
Fludrocortisone acetate (Florinef, F-Cortef)
Dexamethasone (Decadron, Hexadrol, Dexasone)
Prednisolone (Meticortelone)
Methylprednisolone (Medrol, Solu-Medrol)

Adrenocorticosteroids are used for replacement therapy in acute and chronic adrenal insufficiency. These drugs have anti-inflammatory and immunosuppressant effects. They also facilitate coping with stress.

Because corticosteroids are immunosuppressants, their use is contraindicated when an infection is suspected because they mask the signs of infection. Corticosteroids are also contraindicated in many other disorders, including peptic ulcer, Cushing's syndrome, cardiac disease, hyperthyroidism, hypothyroidism, and tuberculosis.

When these drugs are administered in small doses for replacement therapy, side effects are uncommon. Large doses or prolonged therapy may cause a Cushing-like syndrome, with atrophy of the adrenal cortex. Older clients, especially postmenopausal women, are more prone to develop hypertension and osteoporosis when undergoing glucocorticoid therapy. These drugs are used with caution in children and the older adult and are not usually administered to pregnant women.

Nursing Responsibilities
- Establish baseline data, including mental status, neurologic function, vital signs, and weight.
- Identify medications that might interact with corticosteroids: antidiabetic agents, cardiac glycosides, oral contraceptives, anticoagulants.

- Document and report increased blood pressure, edema or weight gain, bleeding or bruising, weakness, or manifestations of Cushing's syndrome.
- Administer oral forms of the drug with food to minimize its ulcerogenic effect.
- Monitor electrolyte levels for increased sodium and decreased potassium.

Client and Family Teaching
- Take medications with food or milk, and report any gastric distress or dark stools.
- Most people need to take the medications for the rest of their lives.
- Consume a diet that is high in potassium, low in sodium, and high in protein.
- Weigh yourself each day at the same time, and report any consistent weight gain, which indicates fluid retention.
- Use safety measures in the home to prevent falls and injuries.
- Corticosteroids may impair the effectiveness of oral contraceptives.
- Take the medication regularly and continuously. *Abruptly discontinuing the medication is dangerous.*
- Obtain a MedicAlert bracelet.
- Monitor for increased stressors (infection, dental work, personal crisis) and increase the dose as indicated by the physician.
- Anticoagulant drugs or insulin may decrease the effectiveness of corticosteroids.
- Report the following to the physician: dizziness on sitting or standing, nausea and vomiting, pain, thirst, feelings of anxiety, malaise, infections.

Nursing Diagnoses and Interventions

The client with Addison's disease requires nursing care for a wide variety of responses to the decrease in cortisol levels. Nursing diagnoses discussed in this section are directed toward problems with fluid and electrolyte balance and compliance with lifelong self-care.

Deficient Fluid Volume

Fluid volume deficit in the client with Addison's disease results from loss of water and sodium, as well as from vomiting and diarrhea. Extracellular fluid volume deficit, decreased cardiac output, hypotension, and hypovolemic shock may occur, especially in crisis situations. Interventions for this diagnosis are outlined for the client who is hospitalized.

- Monitor intake and output, and assess for signs of dehydration: dry mucous membranes; thirst; poor skin turgor; sunken eyeballs; scanty, dark urine; increased urine specific gravity; weight loss; and increased hemoconcentration (increased hematocrit and BUN). *Glucocorticoid and mineralocorticoid depletion causes fluid volume deficit. Fluid volume deficit may reach crisis levels if undetected, causing altered tissue perfusion and hypovolemic shock.*
- Monitor cardiovascular status: Take and record vital signs, assess character of pulses, monitor potassium levels and ECGs. *Fluid volume deficit may lead to hypotension and a rapid, weak, or thready pulse. As aldosterone levels fall, renal excretion of potassium decreases, increasing blood levels of potassium.*

PRACTICE ALERT *Hyperkalemia causes changes in cardiac muscle function, which are reflected in ECG changes.* ■

- Weigh the client daily at the same time and in the same clothing. *Dehydration is manifested by weight loss.*
- Encourage an oral fluid intake of 3000 mL per day and an increased salt intake. *Cortisol deficiency increases fluid loss, leading to extracellular fluid volume depletion. Oral fluid replacement is necessary to balance this loss. An increase in dietary sodium can decrease the hyponatremia characteristic of adrenal insufficiency.*
- Teach to sit and stand slowly, and provide assistance as necessary. *Extracellular fluid volume deficit causes orthostatic hypotension, dizziness, and possible loss of consciousness. These manifestations increase the risk of injury from falls.*

Risk for Ineffective Therapeutic Regimen Management

Clients with Addison's disease must learn to provide lifelong self-care that involves varied components: medications, diet, and recognizing and responding to responses to stress. Changes in lifestyle are difficult to maintain permanently.

- Teach the effects of illness and treatment. Discuss client and family concerns. *Lack of knowledge about the illness, as well as the possibility of complications from disregarding or altering the treatment, can negatively affect compliance.*

- Include the following in the teaching plan:
  - Self-administration of steroids
  - The importance of carrying at all times an emergency kit containing parenteral cortisone and a syringe/needle
  - Wearing a MedicAlert bracelet that says "Adrenal insufficiency—takes hydrocortisone"
  - Increasing oral fluid intake
  - Maintaining a diet high in sodium and low in potassium
  - The necessity of altering the medication dose when experiencing emotional or physical stressors
  - The importance of continuing health care
    One of the most important components of caring for the client with Addison's disease is teaching both the client and family to provide care. The length of treatment and the side effects of medications can discourage compliance.

Home Care

The client with Addison's disease provides self-care at home. One of the most important components of caring for the client with Addison's disease is teaching both the client and family to provide care. Family stability, an awareness of the serious nature of the disease, and the effectiveness of treatment all promote compliance. The length of treatment and the side effects of medications, however, can discourage compliance. In addition to the information in the teaching topics included with nursing diagnoses and interventions, include the following topics:

- The importance of continuing health care
- Referral to social worker, if appropriate
- Referral to community agencies for continued education and support
- Helpful resources:
  - National Institute of Diabetes and Digestive and Kidney Diseases (Addison's disease)
  - Endocrine Society
  - American Association of Clinical Endocrinologists

THE CLIENT WITH PHEOCHROMOCYTOMA

Pheochromocytomas are tumors of chromaffin tissues in the adrenal medulla. These tumors, which are usually benign, produce catecholamines (epinephrine or norepinephrine) that stimulate the sympathetic nervous system. Although many organs are affected, the most dangerous effects are peripheral vasoconstriction and increased cardiac rate and contractility with resultant paroxysmal hypertension. Systolic blood pressure may rise to 200 to 300 mmHg, the diastolic to 150 to 175 mmHg. Attacks are often precipitated by physical, emotional, or environmental stimuli. This condition is life threatening.

A pheochromocytoma is diagnosed by increased catecholamine levels in the blood or urine, by X-ray studies, and by surgical exploration. Surgical removal of the tumor(s) by adrenalectomy is the treatment of choice.

Nursing Care Plan
A Client with Addison's Disease

A 51-year-old unemployed salesman, Mr. Don Sardoff, is brought to the emergency room by his wife, Ellen, at 8 A.M. Mrs. Sardoff tells the emergency room nurse that her husband has not been feeling well for the last week, but that when he got up this morning, he was so weak he couldn't dress himself and didn't know where he was. Mrs. Sardoff also tells the nurse that her husband has been taking a cortisone drug for treatment of his rheumatoid arthritis for the past 2 years, but notes, "We didn't have the money to buy it this month."

ASSESSMENT

On admission to the emergency room, Mr. Sardoff is dehydrated, with dry oral mucous membranes and tongue, poor skin turgor, and sunken eyeballs. His blood pressure is 94/44, and his pulse is rapid and thready. He is weak, dizzy, and disoriented about time and place. Diagnostic tests reveal the following abnormal findings at 8:30 A.M.:

- EKG: widening QRS complex and increased PR interval
- Sodium: 129 mEq/L (normal range: 135 to 145 mEq/L)
- Glucose: 54 mg/dL (normal range: 70 to 110 mg/dL)
- Potassium: 5.3 mEq/L (normal range: 3.5 to 5 mEq/L)
- Cortisol: 2 mg/dL (normal for A.M.: 5 to 23 mg/dL)

The medical orders for Mr. Sardoff include intravenous administration of 5% dextrose in normal saline (D_5NS) at 250 mL/h and hydrocortisone (Solu-Cortef) 200 mg. After the fluids and medication are initiated, Mr. Sardoff is moved to an in-hospital medical bed.

DIAGNOSIS

- *Deficient fluid volume,* related to hypovolemia secondary to adrenal insufficiency
- *Ineffective tissue perfusion: Peripheral,* related to fluid volume deficit
- *Anxiety,* related to lack of knowledge about the effects and treatment of adrenal insufficiency

EXPECTED OUTCOMES

- Regain normal fluid balance.

- Regain normal peripheral perfusion with blood pressure within normal range.
- Verbalize knowledge of the causes and effects of adrenal insufficiency.

PLANNING AND IMPLEMENTATION

- Monitor intake and output closely.
- Take and record weight at the same time daily.
- Monitor blood pressure, pulses, and skin turgor every 2 hours until stable, then 4 times a day.
- Monitor electrolytes, and report abnormal results.
- Discuss a diet that is high in sodium, low in potassium, and has an increased fluid intake (3000 mL per day). Discuss the types of fluids desired and the best times for intake of increased fluids.
- Assist during activity to prevent falls.
- Provide verbal and written instructions, and encourage verbal feedback about the causes and effects of the disease, the effects of medications, the effects of not taking long-term cortisone drugs, the diet, and self-care at home.

EVALUATION

Following treatment for acute adrenal insufficiency, Mr. Sardoff is no longer dehydrated, and his blood pressure has returned to his normal reading of 132/88. He is alert and oriented, and anxious to learn to care for himself at home. After dietary instructions and teaching for self-care that included his wife, Mr. Sardoff verbalizes an understanding of his illness and the need to take his medication carefully and accurately. A referral is made to a social worker for assistance with costs of medications.

Critical Thinking in the Nursing Process

1. Adrenal insufficiency is often diagnosed only when the client becomes seriously ill in response to a stressor. Explain why this statement is or is not true.
2. Describe the physical assessments that are found in the severely dehydrated client.
3. Outline a teaching plan for Mr. Sardoff with foods for a high-sodium, low-potassium diet.

See Evaluating Your Response in Appendix C.

DISORDERS OF THE PITUITARY GLAND

The pituitary gland produces hormones that affect multiple body systems through regulation of endocrine function. Target tissues include the thyroid, adrenal cortex, ovary, uterus, mammary glands, testes, and kidneys. Disorders result from an excess or deficiency of one or more of the pituitary hormones due to a pathologic condition within the gland itself or to hypothalamic dysfunction.

Although disorders of the pituitary cause diverse and serious problems, they are not as common as disorders of other endocrine glands. Hyperpituitarism and hypopituitarism are discussed in this section.

THE CLIENT WITH DISORDERS OF THE ANTERIOR PITUITARY GLAND

Hyperfunction of the anterior pituitary gland, characterized by excess production and secretion of one or more trophic hormones, is usually the result of a pituitary tumor or pituitary hyperplasia. The most common cause of hyperpituitarism is a benign adenoma. The manifestations result from an excess of growth hormone (GH), prolactin (PRL), or ACTH.

Hypofunction of the anterior pituitary gland results in a deficiency of one or more of the gland's hormones. Conditions causing hypopituitarism include pituitary tumors, surgical removal of the pituitary gland, radiation, and pituitary infarction, infection, or trauma.

PATHOPHYSIOLOGY AND MANIFESTATIONS

Growth hormone (also called somatotropin) is produced by cells in the anterior pituitary throughout life. GH is necessary for growth and also contributes to metabolic regulation. GH stimulates all aspects of cartilage growth, and one of its major effects is to stimulate the growth of the epiphyseal cartilage plates of long bones. In addition, other body tissues respond to the metabolic effect of GH with increases in bone width and the growth of visceral and endocrine organs, skeletal and cardiac muscle, skin, and connective tissue. Gigantism and acromegaly (discussed below) result from overstimulation. Growth retardation and short stature result from deficient production of GH.

Hypersecretion of PRL affects reproductive and sexual function. Women may have irregular or absent menses, difficulty in becoming pregnant, and decreased libido. Men may be impotent and have decreased libido. PRL deficiency in postpartal women causes a failure to lactate. An excess secretion of ACTH overstimulates the adrenal cortex, which in turn increases secretion of adrenal hormones. The result is Cushing's syndrome. A deficit of TSH causes hypothyroidism.

Gigantism

Gigantism occurs when GH hypersecretion begins before puberty and the closure of the epiphyseal plates. The person becomes abnormally tall, often exceeding 7 ft (213 cm) in height, but body proportions are relatively normal. Most often the result of a tumor, the condition is rare today as a result of improved diagnosis and treatment.

Acromegaly

Acromegaly, which literally means "enlarged extremities," occurs when sustained GH hypersecretion begins during adulthood, most commonly because of pituitary tumors. As a result of constant stimulation, bone and connective tissue continue to grow. The forehead enlarges, the maxilla lengthens, the tongue enlarges, and the voice deepens (Figure 17–4 ■). Overgrowth of bone and soft tissue in the hands and feet causes clients to buy increasingly larger rings, gloves, and shoes.

Other manifestations include peripheral nerve damage from entrapment of nerves, headache, hypertension, congestive heart failure, seizures, and visual disturbances. Impaired glucose tolerance and diabetes may also occur.

COLLABORATIVE CARE

Acromegaly is treated by surgical removal or irradiation of the pituitary tumor. A transphenoidal or transfrontal surgical procedure is most commonly used (see Chapter 42). ⊖

NURSING CARE

Clients with anterior pituitary disorders require interventions to help in coping with physical and emotional changes, as well as to prevent complications involving other organs and functions of the endocrine system. Nursing care for the client having cranial surgery is discussed in Chapter 42.

Figure 17–4 ■ Manifestations of acromegaly. Progressive alterations in facial appearance include enlargement of the cheekbones and jaw along with thickening of soft-tissue structures such as the nose, lips, cheeks and the flesh above the brows.

THE CLIENT WITH DISORDERS OF THE POSTERIOR PITUITARY GLAND

Disorders of the posterior pituitary are related primarily to excessive or deficient antidiuretic hormone (ADH) secretion. The disorders discussed here are the syndrome of inappropriate ADH secretion and diabetes insipidus.

PATHOPHYSIOLOGY AND MANIFESTATIONS

Antidiuretic hormone is secreted in response to serum osmolality, which is monitored by osmoreceptors in the hypothalamus. When a condition of hyperosmolality occurs, ADH secretion increases, and renal water is reabsorbed. Hypo-osmolality causes the suppression of ADH, and renal water excretion increases.

Syndrome of Inappropriate ADH Secretion

The **syndrome of inappropriate ADH secretion (SIADH)** is characterized by high levels of ADH in the absence of serum hypo-osmolality. This disorder is most often caused by the ectopic production of ADH by malignant tumors (e.g., oat cell carcinoma of the lung, pancreatic carcinoma, leukemia, and Hodgkin's disease). A transient form may follow a head injury, pituitary surgery, or the use of medications such as barbiturates, anesthetics, or diuretics.

Manifestations of SIADH occur as a result of water retention, hyponatremia, and serum hypo-osmolality. Blood volume expands, but the plasma is diluted. Aldosterone is suppressed; as a result, renal excretion of sodium increases. Water moves from the hypotonic plasma and the interstitial spaces into the cells.

Manifestations of SIADH (see Chapter 5 🔗) are usually nonspecific but are related to hyponatremia and water intoxication. Brain cells swell, causing neurologic symptoms: headache, changes in level of consciousness, muscle twitches, and seizures. Usually no edema is present, because water is distributed between the intracellular and extracellular spaces.

Diabetes Insipidus

Diabetes insipidus is the result of ADH insufficiency. The two types are as follows:

- *Neurogenic diabetes insipidus* can either result from a disruption of the hypothalamus and pituitary gland (as from trauma, irradiation, or cranial surgery) or be idiopathic.
- *Nephrogenic diabetes insipidus* is a disorder in which the renal tubules are not sensitive to ADH. This may be familial in origin or the result of renal failure.

Diabetes insipidus may result from brain tumors or infections, pituitary surgery, cerebral vascular accidents, and renal and organ failure. It is also a complication of closed-head trauma with increased intracranial pressure.

A deficit of ADH causes excretion of large amounts of dilute urine (*polyuria*), in some instances as much as 12 L per day. The client has extreme thirst and drinks large volumes of water (*polydipsia*). If unable to replace the water loss, the client becomes dehydrated and hypernatremic. Even though hyperosmolality is present, the urine is dilute and has a low specific gravity.

If this disorder is caused by cerebral injury, symptoms commonly appear 3 to 6 days after the initial injury and last for 7 to 10 days. If the increased intracranial pressure is relieved, symptoms of diabetes insipidus usually disappear. However, diabetes insipidus may also be a chronic illness requiring lifelong treatment and care.

COLLABORATIVE CARE

SIADH is treated by correcting underlying causes, treating the hyponatremia with intravenous hypertonic saline, and restricting oral fluids to less than 800 mL per day.

Diabetes insipidus is also treated by correcting underlying causes, if possible. Other medical interventions include administering intravenous hypotonic fluids, increasing oral fluids, and replacing ADH hormone. Desmopressin acetate, administered intranasally, orally, or parenterally, is the treatment of choice (Tierney et al., 2001).

NURSING CARE

Nursing care for the client with SIADH and diabetes insipidus focuses on client problems with fluid and electrolyte balance, as discussed in Chapter 5.

 EXPLORE MediaLink

NCLEX review questions, case studies, care plan activities, MediaLink applications, and other interactive resources for this chapter can be found on the Companion Website at www.prenhall.com/lemone.

Click on Chapter 17 to select the activities for this chapter. For animations, video clips, more NCLEX review questions, and an audio glossary, access the Student CD-ROM accompanying this textbook.

TEST YOURSELF

1. Graves' disease, the most common cause of hyperthyroidism, is categorized as what type of disorder?

   a. Immune
   b. Infectious
   c. Allergic
   d. Genetic

2. What principle supports the treatment of hyperthyroidism with radioactive iodine?

   a. Radioactive iodine reduces the vascularity of the thyroid gland
   b. Doses of radioactive iodine are too small to be hazardous to other body parts
   c. The thyroid gland takes up iodine in any form
   d. Irradiation of the thyroid gland decreases the risk of hypothyroidism

3. You assess a client with newly diagnosed hypothyroidism as having an enlarged thyroid gland (goiter). What physiologic process causes this enlargement?

   a. An excess of TH stimulates thyroid follicles
   b. An increased dietary iodine intake
   c. A compensatory effort to produce more TH
   d. Tissue hypertrophy in response to increased TH

4. Mrs. Jonah has taken cortisone for her rheumatoid arthritis for several years. What endocrine disorder is she most at risk for developing?

   a. Hyperthyroidism
   b. Hypothyroidism
   c. Acromegaly
   d. Cushing's syndrome

5. Which statement illustrates that the client with Addison's disease understands your teaching?

   a. "I will be sure to stop taking my medications when I have an infection."
   b. "I have purchased an emergency kit and keep it with me all the time."
   c. "I know I should never alter my dose of medications."
   d. "I wonder why I look suntanned all the time."

See Test Yourself answers in Appendix C.

BIBLIOGRAPHY

American Cancer Society. (2002). *Cancer facts & figures.* New York: American Cancer Society.

Burton, M. (1997). Emergency! Pheochromocytoma. *American Journal of Nursing, 97*(11), 57.

Clayton, L., & Dilley, K. (1998). Cushing's syndrome. *American Journal of Nursing, 98*(7), 40–41.

Cooper, D. S. (Ed.). (2001). *Medical management of thyroid disease.* New York: Marcel Dekker, Inc.

Gumowski, J., & Loughran, M. (1996). Disease of the adrenal gland. *Nursing Clinics of North America, 31*(4), 747–768.

Johnson, M., & Maas, M. (Eds.). (1997). *Nursing outcomes classification (NOC).* St. Louis: Mosby.

Kee, J. (2001). *Handbook of laboratory and diagnostic tests with nursing implications* (4th ed.). Upper Saddle River, NJ: Prentice Hall.

McCloskey, J., & Bulechek, G. (Eds.). (2000). *Iowa intervention project: Nursing interventions classification (NIC)* (3rd ed.). St. Louis: Mosby.

McKenry, L., & Salerno, E. (1998). *Pharmacology in nursing* (20th ed.). St. Louis: Mosby.

McPhee, S., Lingappa, V., Ganong, W., & Lange, J. (2000). *Pathophysiology of disease: An introduction to clinical medicine.* New York: Appleton & Lange.

Mead, M. (2000). Thyroid function tests. *Practice Nurse, 19*(6), 283.

New guidelines for detecting thyroid dysfunction. (2000). *Consultant, 40*(9), 1676.

North American Nursing Diagnosis Association. (2001). *Nursing diagnoses: Definitions & classification 2001–2002.* Philadelphia: NANDA.

O'Donnell, M. (1997). Emergency! Addisonian crisis. *American Journal of Nursing, 97*(3), 41.

Porth, C. (2002). *Pathophysiology: Concepts of altered health states* (6th ed.). Philadelphia: Lippincott.

Romeo, J. (1996). Hyperfunction and hypofunction of the anterior pituitary. *Nursing Clinics of North America, 31*(4), 769–778.

Sabol, V. (2001). Addisonian crisis: This life-threatening condition may be triggered by a variety of stressors. *American Journal of Nursing, 101*(7, Advanced Practice Extra), 24AAA, 24CCC–DDD.

Sache, D. (2001). Acromegaly. *American Journal of Nursing, 101*(11), 69, 71, 73–75, 77.

Schilling, J. (1997). Hyperthyroidism: Diagnosis and management of Graves' disease. *Nurse Practitioner, 22*(6), 72, 74–75, 78.

Shannon, M., Wilson, B., & Stang, C. (2002). *Health professional's drug guide 2002.* Upper Saddle River, NJ: Prentice Hall.

Sheppard, M. (2001). Assessing fluid balance. *Nursing Times, 97*(6 Ntplus), XI–XII.

Terpstra, T., & Terpstra, T. L. (2000). Syndrome of inappropriate antidiuretic hormone secretion: Recognition and management. *MEDSURG Nursing, 9*(2), 61–70.

Thyroid disorders and women's health. (2000). *National women's health report, 22*(5), 1–2, 4–6.

Tierney, L., McPhee, S., & Papadakis, M. (Eds.). (2001). *Current medical diagnosis & treatment* (40th ed.). Stamford, CT: Appleton & Lange.

Tiesinga, L., Dassen, T., & Halfens, R. (1996). Fatigue: A summary of the definitions, dimensions, and indicators. *Nursing Diagnosis, 7*(2), 51–62.

Trotto, N. (1999). Hypothyroidism, hyperthyroidism, hyperparathyroidism. *Patient Care, 33*(14), 186–188, 191, 195–200.

Wartofsky, L. (1998). Q & A. . . Thyroid tests and food. *New Choices: Living Even Better After 50, 38*(1), 79.

Yarbro, C., Frogge, M., Goodman, M., & Broenwald, S. (2001). *Cancer nursing: Principles and practice.* Sudbury, MA: Jones and Bartlett.

Nursing Care of Clients with Diabetes Mellitus

MediaLink

www.prenhall.com/lemone
Additional resources for this chapter can be found on the Student CD-ROM accompanying this textbook, and on the Companion Website at www.prenhall.com/lemone. Click on Chapter 18 to select the activities for this chapter.

CD-ROM
- Audio Glossary
- NCLEX Review

Animation
- Glipizide

Companion Website
- More NCLEX Review
- Case Study
  Diabetes Mellitus Type 1
- Care Plan Activity
  Diabetes Mellitus Type 2
- MediaLink Application
  Diabetes Foot Care

LEARNING OUTCOMES

After completing this chapter, you will be able to:

- Apply knowledge of normal endocrine anatomy, physiology, and assessments when providing nursing care for clients with diabetes mellitus (see Chapter 16).

- Describe the prevalence and incidence of diabetes mellitus.

- Explain the pathophysiology, risk factors, manifestations, and complications of type 1 and type 2 diabetes mellitus.

- Compare and contrast the manifestations and collaborative care of hypoglycemia, diabetic ketoacidosis (DKA), and hyperosmolar hyperglycemic state (HHS).

- Identify the diagnostic tests used for screening, diagnosis, and monitoring of diabetes mellitus.

- Discuss the nursing implications for insulin and oral hypoglycemic agents used to treat clients with diabetes mellitus.

- Provide accurate information to clients with diabetes mellitus to facilitate self-management of medications, diet planning, exercise, and self-assessment, including foot care.

- Use the nursing process as a framework for providing individualized care to clients with diabetes mellitus.

Diabetes mellitus (DM) is a common chronic disease of adults. However, depending on the type of diabetes and the age of the client, both client needs and nursing care may vary greatly. Consider the following examples.

- Cheryl Draheim is a 45-year-old schoolteacher. She developed diabetes at age 34 after an automobile accident caused severe pancreatic injuries. Cheryl has always been very careful about taking her insulin, following her diet, and exercising regularly. However, she is beginning to notice that her vision is getting worse and that she is having increasing pain in her legs, especially after standing for long periods of time. Cheryl says that sometimes she believes the disease controls her more than she controls it.

- Tom Chang is 53 years old. Early in his 40s, Tom was diagnosed with type 2 diabetes. Although Tom was taught about the disease and the importance of taking his oral medications, following his diet plan, and getting exercise, he rarely did more than take the medication. Five years ago, he was hospitalized for hyperglycemia and started taking insulin. Last year Tom had a stroke, leaving him unable to walk. He has now been admitted to the hospital for treatment of gangrene of the large toe on his left foot.

- Grace Staples is an independent 82-year-old woman who lives alone and happily takes care of her two cats. She is slightly overweight. Last year, during Grace's annual eye examination, eye changes typical for diabetes were found. She was referred to her family doctor, who diagnosed type 2 diabetes and started her on oral medications. Grace sticks to her diet, walks a mile every day, and plans to live to be 100.

As illustrated in these examples, diabetes mellitus is not a single disorder but a group of chronic disorders of the endocrine pancreas, all categorized under a broad diagnostic label. The condition is characterized by inappropriate hyperglycemia caused by a relative or absolute deficiency of insulin or by a cellular resistance to the action of insulin. Of the several classifications of diabetes, this chapter will focus on the two major types, type 1 and type 2. **Type 1 DM** is the result of pancreatic islet cell destruction and a total deficit of circulating insulin; **type 2 DM** results from insulin resistance with a defect in compensatory insulin secretion.

Diabetes mellitus has been recognized as a disease for centuries. Diabetes derives from a Greek word meaning "to siphon," referring to the increased output of urine. Mellitus derives from a Latin word meaning "sweet." The two words together identify the disease as an outpouring of sweet urine. It was not until 1921 that techniques were developed for extracting insulin from pancreatic tissue and for measuring blood glucose. At the same time, researchers discovered that insulin, when injected, produces a dramatic drop in blood glucose. This meant that diabetes was no longer a terminal illness because hyperglycemia could now be controlled. Since that time, oral hypoglycemic drugs, human insulin products, insulin pumps, home blood glucose monitoring, and transplantation of the pancreas or of pancreatic islet or beta cells have advanced the treatment and care of people with diabetes.

Clients with DM face lifelong changes in lifestyle and health status. Nursing care is provided in many settings for the diagnosis and care of the disease and treatment of complications. A major role of the nurse is that of educator in both hospital and community settings.

INCIDENCE AND PREVALENCE

Approximately 1 million new cases of DM are diagnosed each year in the United States. This chronic illness affects an estimated 17 million people; of that number, 11.1 million have been diagnosed and an estimated 5.9 million are undiagnosed (National Institutes of Health [NIH], 2002, 1999). There is an increased prevalence of diabetes (especially type 2 diabetes) among older adults and in minority populations. See the Focus on Diversity box below.

Diabetes is the sixth leading cause of death by disease in the United States, primarily because of the widespread cardiovascular effects that result in atherosclerosis, coronary artery disease, and stroke. People with diabetes are 2 to 4 times more likely to have heart disease, and 2 to 6 times more likely to have a stroke than people who do not have diabetes. Diabetes is the leading cause of end-stage renal disease (kidney failure), and the major cause of newly diagnosed blindness in people ages 20 to 74. Diabetes also is the most frequent cause of nontraumatic amputations.

Americans with diabetes use a disproportionate share of the nation's health care services. They visit outpatient services and physicians' offices more often than people who do not have the disease, and they require more frequent hospitalizations with longer days of in-hospital treatment. The cost of illness and resulting loss of productivity for people with diabetes exceeds $98 billion per year, according to an estimate by the National Institute for Diabetes and Kidney Disease.

Focus on Diversity

RISK AND INCIDENCE OF DIABETES MELLITUS

- 11.4 million (7.8%) of all non-Hispanic whites have diabetes.
- 2.8 million (13%) of all non-Hispanic African Americans have diabetes, and are 2 times as likely to have diabetes as non-Hispanic whites of similar age. African Americans with type 2 diabetes have higher rates of coronary heart disease, CVA, and end-stage renal disease than do Caucasians with the disease.
- 1.2 million (10.2%) of all Mexican Americans have diabetes, and are 1.9 times as likely to have diabetes as non-Hispanic whites of similar age.
- On average, Hispanic/Latino Americans are about 2 times more likely to have diabetes as non-Hispanic whites of similar age.
- Native Americans are 2.8 times more likely to have diabetes than non-Hispanic whites, and diabetes is especially prevalent in middle-aged and older American Indians. According to the World Health Organization, 50% of the Pima tribe have diabetes, and 90% are diagnosed by age 65 (Burke, 2001).

PATHOPHYSIOLOGY

Overview of Endocrine Pancreatic Hormones and Glucose Homeostasis

Hormones

The endocrine pancreas produces hormones necessary for the metabolism and cellular utilization of carbohydrates, proteins, and fats. The cells that produce these hormones are clustered in groups of cells called the islets of Langerhans. These islets have three different types of cells:

- Alpha cells produce the hormone *glucagon,* which stimulates the breakdown of glycogen in the liver, the formation of carbohydrates in the liver, and the breakdown of lipids in both the liver and adipose tissue. The primary function of glucagon is to decrease glucose oxidation and to increase blood glucose levels. Through *glycogenolysis* (the breakdown of liver glycogen) and *gluconeogenesis* (the formation of glucose from fats and proteins), glucagon prevents blood glucose from decreasing below a certain level when the body is fasting or in between meals. The action of glucagon is initiated in most people when blood glucose falls below about 70 mg/dL.
- Beta cells secrete the hormone *insulin,* which facilitates the movement of glucose across cell membranes into cells, decreasing blood glucose levels. Insulin prevents the excessive breakdown of glycogen in the liver and in muscle, facilitates lipid formation while inhibiting the breakdown of stored fats, and helps move amino acids into cells for protein synthesis. After secretion by the beta cells, insulin enters the portal circulation, travels directly to the liver, and is then released into the general circulation. Circulating insulin is rap-

idly bound to receptor sites on peripheral tissues (especially muscle and fat cells) or is destroyed by the liver or kidneys. Insulin release is regulated by blood glucose; it increases when blood glucose levels increase, and it decreases when blood glucose levels decrease. When a person eats food, insulin levels begin to rise in minutes, peak in 30 to 60 minutes, and return to baseline in 2 to 3 hours.

- Delta cells produce *somatostatin,* which is believed to be a neurotransmitter that inhibits the production of both glucagon and insulin.

Blood Glucose Homeostasis

All body tissues and organs require a constant supply of glucose; however, not all tissues require insulin for glucose uptake. The brain, liver, intestines, and renal tubules do not require insulin to transfer glucose into their cells. Skeletal muscle, cardiac muscle, and adipose tissue do require insulin for glucose movement into the cells.

Normal blood glucose is maintained in healthy people primarily through the actions of insulin and glucagon. Increased blood glucose levels, amino acids, and fatty acids stimulate pancreatic beta cells to produce insulin. As cells of cardiac muscle, skeletal muscle, and adipose tissue take up glucose, plasma levels of nutrients decrease, suppressing the stimulus to produce insulin. If blood glucose falls, glucagon is released to raise glucose levels. Epinephrine, growth hormone, thyroxine, and glucocorticoids (often referred to as glucose counterregulatory hormones) also stimulate an increase in glucose in times of hypoglycemia, stress, growth, or increased metabolic demand. The regulation of blood glucose levels by insulin and glucagon is illustrated in Figure 18–1 ■.

A

B

Figure 18–1 ■ Regulation (homeostasis) of blood glucose levels by insulin and glucagon. *A,* High blood glucose is lowered by insulin release. *B,* Low blood glucose is raised by glucagon release.

Pathophysiology of Diabetes

DM is a group of metabolic diseases characterized by hyperglycemia resulting from defects in the secretion of insulin, the action of insulin, or both. There are four major types of DM. Type I diabetes (5% to 10% of diagnosed cases) was formerly called juvenile-onset diabetes or insulin-dependent diabetes mellitus (IDDM). Type 2 diabetes (90% to 95% of diagnosed cases) was formerly labeled non-insulin-dependent diabetes mellitus (NIDDM) or adult-onset diabetes. The other major types are gestational diabetes (2% to 5% of all pregnancies) and other specific types of diabetes (1% to 2% of diagnosed cases). The classification and characteristics of the four types are described in Table 18–1.

Type 1 Diabetes

Type 1 diabetes most often occurs in childhood and adolescence, but it may occur at any age, even in the 80s and 90s. This disorder is characterized by **hyperglycemia** (elevated blood glucose levels), a breakdown of body fats and proteins, and the development of **ketosis** (an accumulation of ketone bodies produced during the oxidation of fatty acids). Type 1 DM is the result of the destruction of the beta cells of the islets of Langerhans in the pancreas. When beta cells are destroyed, insulin is no longer produced. Although type 1 DM may be classified as either an autoimmune or idiopathic disorder, 90% of the cases are immune mediated. The disorder begins with insulinitis, a chronic inflammatory process that occurs in response to the

TABLE 18–1   Classification and Characteristics of Diabetes

	Classification	Characteristics
I. Type 1 diabetes	A. Immune-mediated	Beta cells are destroyed, usually leading to absolute insulin deficiency. Markers to the immune destruction of the beta cells include islet cell autoantibodies (ICAs) and insulin autoantibodies (IAAs). The rate of beta cell destruction is variable, usually more rapid in infants and children and slower in adults. Destruction of the beta cells has genetic predispositions and is also related to environmental factors as yet undefined.
	B. Idiopathic	Has no known etiologic causes. Most clients are of African or Asian descent. Is strongly inherited. Need for insulin may be intermittent.
II. Type 2 diabetes		May range from predominantly insulin resistance with relative insulin deficiency to a predominantly secretory defect with insulin resistance. There is no immune destruction of beta cells. Initially, and in some cases for the entire life, insulin is not necessary. Most people with this form are obese, or have an increased amount of abdominal fat. Risks for development include increasing age, obesity, and a sedentary lifestyle. Occurs more frequently in women who have had gestational diabetes, and in people with lipid disorders or hypertension. There is a strong genetic predisposition.
III. Other specific types	A. Genetic defects of beta cell	Hyperglycemia occurs at an early age (usually before age 25). This type is referred to as maturity-onset diabetes of the young (MODY).
	B. Genetic defects in insulin action	Are genetically determined. Dysfunctions may range from hyperinsulinemia to severe diabetes.
	C. Diseases of the exocrine pancreas	Acquired processes causing diabetes include pancreatitis, trauma, infection, pancreatectomy, and pancreatic cancer. Severe forms of cystic fibrosis and hemochromatosis may also damage beta cells and impair insulin secretion.
	D. Endocrine disorders	Excess amount of hormones (e.g., growth hormone, cortisol, glucagon, and epinephrine) impair insulin secretion, resulting in diabetes in people with Cushing's syndrome, acromegaly, and pheochromocytoma.
	E. Drug or chemical induced	Many drugs impair insulin secretion, precipitating diabetes in people with predisposing insulin resistance. Examples are nicotinic acid, glucocorticoids, thyroid hormone, thiazides, and dilantin.
	F. Infections	Certain viruses may cause beta cell destruction, including congenital measles, cytomegalovirus, adenovirus, and mumps.
IV. Gestational diabetes mellitus (GDM)		Any degree of glucose intolerance with onset or first recognition during pregnancy.

autoimmune destruction of islet cells. This process slowly destroys beta cell production of insulin, with the onset of hyperglycemia occurring when 80% to 90% of beta cell function is lost. This process usually occurs over a long preclinical period. It is believed that both alpha-cell and beta-cell functions are abnormal, with a lack of insulin and a relative excess of glucagon resulting in hyperglycemia.

RISK FACTORS.   Genetic predisposition plays a role in the development of type 1 DM. Although the risk in the general population ranges from 1 in 400 to 1 in 1000, the child of a person with diabetes has a 1 in 20 to 1 in 50 risk. Genetic markers that determine immune responses—specifically, DR3 and DR4 antigens on chromosome 6 of the human leukocyte antigen (HLA) system—have been found in 95% of people diagnosed with type 1 DM. (HLAs are cell surface proteins, controlled by genes on chromosome 6.) Although the presence of these markers does not guarantee that the person will develop type 1 DM, they do indicate increased susceptibility (Haire-Joshu, 1996).

Environmental factors are believed to trigger the development of type 1 DM. The trigger can be a viral infection (mumps, rubella, or coxsackievirus B4) or a chemical toxin, such as those found in smoked and cured meats. As a result of exposure to the virus or chemical, an abnormal autoimmune response occurs in which antibodies respond to normal islet beta cells as though they were foreign substances, destroying them. The manifestations of type 1 DM appear when approximately 90% of the beta cells are destroyed. However, manifestations may appear at any time during the loss of beta cells if an acute illness or stress increases the demand for insulin beyond the reserves of the damaged cells. The actual cause and exact sequence are not completely understood, but research continues to identify the genetic markers of this disorder and to investigate ways of altering the immune response to prevent or cure type 1 DM.

MANIFESTATIONS.   The manifestations of type 1 DM are the result of a lack of insulin to transport glucose across the cell membrane into the cells (Figure 18–2 ■). Glucose molecules accumulate in the circulating blood, resulting in **hyperglycemia.** Hyperglycemia causes serum hyperosmolality, drawing water from the intracellular spaces into the general circulation. The increased blood volume increases renal blood flow, and the hyperglycemia acts as an osmotic diuretic. The resulting osmotic diuresis increases urine output. This condition is called **polyuria.** When the blood glucose level exceeds the renal threshold for glucose—usually about 180 mg/dL—glucose is excreted in the urine, a condition called **glucosuria.** The decrease in intracellular volume and the increased urinary output cause dehydration. The mouth becomes dry and thirst sensors are activated, causing the person to drink increased amounts of fluid (**polydipsia**).

Because glucose cannot enter the cell without insulin, energy production decreases. This decrease in energy stimulates hunger, and the person eats more food (**polyphagia**). Despite increased food intake, the person loses weight as the body loses water and breaks down proteins and fats in an attempt to restore

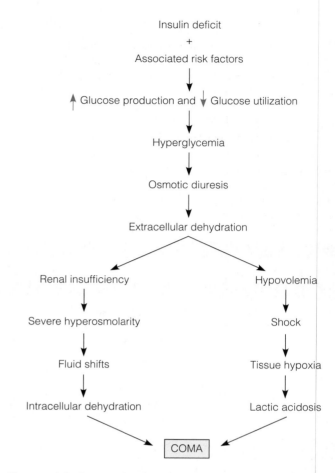

Figure 18–2 ■ Pathophysiologic results of type 1 DM.

energy sources. Malaise and fatigue accompany the decrease in energy. Blurred vision is also common, resulting from osmotic effects that cause swelling of the lenses of the eyes.

Thus, the classic manifestations are polyuria, polydipsia, and polyphagia, accompanied by weight loss, malaise, and fatigue. Depending on the degree of insulin lack, the manifestations vary from slight to severe. People with type 1 DM require an exogenous source of insulin to maintain life.

DIABETIC KETOACIDOSIS.   As the pathophysiology of untreated type 1 DM continues, the insulin deficit causes fat stores to break down, resulting in continued hyperglycemia and mobilization of fatty acids with a subsequent ketosis (see Figure 18–2). **Diabetic ketoacidosis (DKA)** develops when there is an absolute deficiency of insulin and an increase in the insulin counterregulatory hormones. Glucose production by the liver increases, peripheral glucose use decreases, fat mobilization increases, and ketogenesis (ketone formation) is stimulated. Increased glucagon levels activate the gluconeogenic and ketogenic pathways in the liver. In the presence of insulin deficiency, hepatic overproduction of beta-hydroxybutyrate and acetoacetic acids (ketone bodies) causes increased ketone concentrations and an increased release of free fatty acids. As a result of a loss of bicarbonate (which occurs when the ketone is formed), bicarbonate buffering does not occur, and a metabolic acidosis occurs, called DKA. Depression of the central nervous system (CNS) from the accumulation of ketones and the resulting acidosis may cause coma and death if left untreated.

DKA also may occur in a person with diagnosed diabetes when energy requirements increase during physical or emotional stress. Stress states initiate the release of gluconeogenic hormones, resulting in the formation of carbohydrates from protein or fat. The person who is sick, has an infection, or who decreases or omits insulin doses is at a greatly increased risk for developing DKA.

DKA involves four metabolic problems:

- Hyperosmolarity from hyperglycemia and dehydration
- Metabolic acidosis from an accumulation of ketoacids
- Extracellular volume depletion from osmotic diuresis
- Electrolyte imbalances (such as loss of potassium and sodium) from osmotic diuresis

Manifestations of DKA result from severe dehydration and acidosis. These manifestations are summarized in the box below. Laboratory findings include the following:

- Blood glucose levels higher than 250 mg/dL
- Plasma pH less than 7.3
- Plasma bicarbonate less than 15 mEq/L
- Presence of serum ketones
- Presence of urine ketones and glucose
- Abnormal levels of serum sodium, potassium, and chloride

Type 2 Diabetes

Type 2 DM is a condition of fasting hyperglycemia that occurs despite the availability of endogenous insulin (Porth, 2002). Type 2 DM can occur at any age, but it is usually seen in middle-age and older people. Heredity plays a role in its transmission. Although the exact cause of type 2 DM is unknown, several theories have been suggested. These theories include limited beta-cell response to hyperglycemia, peripheral insulin resistance, and insulin-receptor or postreceptor abnormalities. Whatever the cause, there is sufficient insulin production to prevent the breakdown of fats with resultant ketosis; thus, type

2 DM is characterized as a nonketotic form of diabetes. However, the amount of insulin available is not sufficient to lower blood glucose levels through the uptake of glucose by muscle and fat cells.

A major factor in the development of type 2 DM is cellular resistance to the effect of insulin. This resistance is increased by obesity, inactivity, illnesses, medications, and increasing age. In obesity, insulin has a decreased ability to influence glucose metabolism and uptake by the liver, skeletal muscles, and adipose tissue. Although the exact reason for this is not clear, it is known that weight loss may improve the mechanism responsible for insulin receptor-binding or postreceptor activity (McCance & Huether, 2002).

RISK FACTORS. The major risk factors for type 2 DM are:

- History of diabetes in parents or siblings. Although there is no identified HLA linkage, the children of a person with type 2 DM have a 15% chance of developing type 2 DM and a 30% risk of developing a glucose intolerance (the inability to metabolize carbohydrate normally).
- Obesity, defined as being at least 20% over desired body weight or having a body mass index (BMI) of at least 27 kg/m^2. Obesity, especially of the upper body, decreases the number of available insulin receptor sites in cells of skeletal muscles and adipose tissues, a process called *peripheral insulin resistance.* In addition, obesity impairs the ability of the beta cells to release insulin in response to increasing glucose levels.
- Physical inactivity.
- Race/ethnicity (see Box 18–1).
- In women, a history of gestational DM, polycystic ovary syndrome, or delivering a baby weighing more than 9 lb.
- Hypertension ($\geq$130/85 in adults), HDL cholesterol of $\geq$35 mg/dL and/or a triglyceride level of $\geq$250 mg/dL.

MANIFESTATIONS. The person with type 2 DM experiences a slow onset of manifestations and is often unaware of the disease until seeking health care for some other problem. The hyperglycemia in type 2 is usually not as severe as in type 1, but similar symptoms occur, especially polyuria and polydipsia. Polyphagia is not often seen, and weight loss is uncommon. Other manifestations are also the result of hyperglycemia: blurred vision, fatigue, paresthesias, and skin infections. If available insulin decreases, especially in times of physical or emotional stress, the person with type 2 DM may develop DKA, but this occurrence is uncommon.

HYPEROSMOLAR HYPERGLYCEMIC STATE. The metabolic problem called **hyperosmolar hyperglycemic state (HHS)** occurs in people who have type 2 DM. HHS is characterized by a plasma osmolarity of 340 mOsm/L or greater (the normal range is 280 to 300 mOsm/L), greatly elevated blood glucose levels (over 600 mg/dL and often 1000 to 2000 mg/dL), and altered levels of consciousness. HHS is a serious, life-threatening medical emergency and has a higher mortality rate than DKA. Mortality is high not only because the metabolic changes are serious but also because people with diabetes are usually older

---

Manifestations of Diabetic Ketoacidosis (DKA)

Dehydration (from hyperglycemia)

- Thirst
- Warm, dry skin with poor turgor
- Soft eyeballs
- Dry mucous membranes

- Weakness
- Malaise
- Rapid, weak pulse
- Hypotension

Metabolic Acidosis (from ketosis)

- Nausea and vomiting
- Ketone (fruity, alcohol-like) breath odor

- Lethargy
- Coma

Other Manifestations

- Abdominal pain (cause unknown)
- Kussmaul's respirations (increased rate and depth of respirations, with a longer expiration; a compensatory response to prevent a further decrease in pH)

BOX 18–1 ■ Factors Associated with Hyperosmolar Hyper-glycemic State (HHS)

Therapeutic Agents
- Glucocorticoids
- Diuretics
- Beta-adrenergic blocking agents
- Immunosuppressants
- Chlorpromazine
- Diazoxide

Therapeutic Procedures
- Peritoneal dialysis
- Hemodialysis
- Hyperosmolar alimentation (oral or parenteral)
- Surgery

Acute Illness
- Infection
- Gangrene
- Urinary infection
- Burns
- Gastrointestinal bleeding
- Myocardial infarction
- Pancreatitis
- Stroke

Chronic Illness
- Renal disease
- Cardiac disease
- Hypertension
- Previous stroke
- Alcoholism

and have other medical problems that either cause or are caused by HHS. The precipitating factors associated with HHS include infection, therapeutic agents, therapeutic procedures, acute illness, and chronic illness (Box 18–1). The most common precipitating factor is infection. The manifestations of this disorder may be slow to appear, with onset ranging from 24 hours to 2 weeks. The manifestations are initiated by hyperglycemia, which causes increased urine output. With increased output, plasma volume decreases and glomerular filtration rate (GFR) drops. As a result, glucose is retained and water is lost. Glucose and sodium accumulate in the blood and increase serum osmolarity.

Serum hyperosmolarity results in severe dehydration, reducing intracellular water in all tissues, including the brain. The person has dry skin and mucous membranes, extreme thirst, and altered levels of consciousness (progressing from lethargy to coma). Neurologic deficits may include hyperthermia, motor and sensory impairment, positive Babinski's sign, and seizures. Treatment is directed toward correcting fluid and electrolyte imbalances, lowering blood glucose levels with insulin, and treating underlying conditions.

COMPLICATIONS OF DIABETES

The person with DM, regardless of type, is at increased risk for complications involving many different body systems. Alterations in blood glucose levels, alterations in the cardiovascular system, neuropathies, an increased susceptibility to infection, and periodontal disease are common. In addition, the interaction of several complications can cause problems of the feet. The *Multisystem Effects of Diabetes Mellitus* illustration on the next page shows the progression from cardinal signs to acute and late complications for the client with diabetes. A discussion of each of these complications follows; related collaborative care and nursing care are discussed later in the chapter.

Alterations in Blood Glucose Levels

The following discussion provides additional information about hyperglycemia and hypoglycemia. Table 18–2 compares DKA, HHS, and hypoglycemia.

Hyperglycemia

The major problems resulting from hyperglycemia in the person with diabetes are DKA and HHS. Two other problems are the dawn phenomenon and the Somogyi phenomenon.

The **dawn phenomenon** is a rise in blood glucose between 4 A.M. and 8 A.M. that is not a response to hypoglycemia. This condition occurs in people with both type 1 and type 2 DM. The exact cause is unknown but is believed to be related to nocturnal increases in growth hormone, which decreases peripheral uptake of glucose. The **Somogyi phenomena** is a combination of hypoglycemia during the night with a rebound morning rise in blood glucose to hyperglycemic levels. The hyperglycemia stimulates the counterregulatory hormones, which stimulate gluconeogenesis and glycogenolysis and also inhibit peripheral glucose use. This may cause insulin resistance for 12 to 48 hours (McCance & Huether, 2002).

Hypoglycemia

Hypoglycemia (low blood glucose levels) is common in people with type 1 DM and occasionally occurs in people with type 2 DM who are treated with oral hypoglycemic agents. This condition is often called insulin shock, **insulin reaction,** or "the lows" in clients with type 1 DM. Hypoglycemia results primarily from a mismatch between insulin intake (e.g., an error in insulin dose), physical activity, and carbohydrate availability (e.g., omitting a meal). The intake of alcohol and drugs such as chloramphenicol (Chloromycetin), coumadin, monoamine oxidase (MAO) inhibitors, probenecid (Benemid), salicylates, and sulfonamides can also cause hypoglycemia.

The manifestations of hypoglycemia (see below) result from a compensatory autonomic nervous system (ANS) response and from impaired cerebral function due to a decrease in glucose available for use by the brain. The manifestations vary, particularly in older adults. The onset is sudden, and blood

Manifestations of Hypoglycemia

Manifestations Caused by Responses of the Autonomic Nervous System
- Hunger
- Nausea
- Anxiety
- Pale, cool skin
- Sweating
- Shakiness
- Irritability
- Rapid pulse
- Hypotension

Manifestations Caused by Impaired Cerebral Function
- Strange or unusual feelings
- Headache
- Difficulty in thinking
- Inability to concentrate
- Change in emotional behavior
- Slurred speech
- Blurred vision
- Decreasing levels of consciousness
- Seizures
- Coma

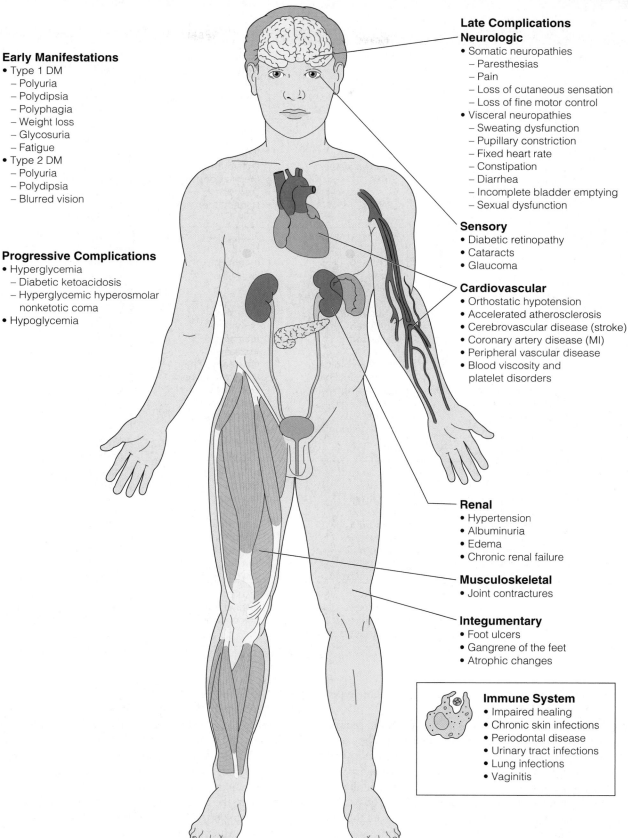

Early Manifestations
- Type 1 DM
  - Polyuria
  - Polydipsia
  - Polyphagia
  - Weight loss
  - Glycosuria
  - Fatigue
- Type 2 DM
  - Polyuria
  - Polydipsia
  - Blurred vision

Progressive Complications
- Hyperglycemia
  - Diabetic ketoacidosis
  - Hyperglycemic hyperosmolar nonketotic coma
- Hypoglycemia

Late Complications
Neurologic
- Somatic neuropathies
  - Paresthesias
  - Pain
  - Loss of cutaneous sensation
  - Loss of fine motor control
- Visceral neuropathies
  - Sweating dysfunction
  - Pupillary constriction
  - Fixed heart rate
  - Constipation
  - Diarrhea
  - Incomplete bladder emptying
  - Sexual dysfunction

Sensory
- Diabetic retinopathy
- Cataracts
- Glaucoma

Cardiovascular
- Orthostatic hypotension
- Accelerated atherosclerosis
- Cerebrovascular disease (stroke)
- Coronary artery disease (MI)
- Peripheral vascular disease
- Blood viscosity and platelet disorders

Renal
- Hypertension
- Albuminuria
- Edema
- Chronic renal failure

Musculoskeletal
- Joint contractures

Integumentary
- Foot ulcers
- Gangrene of the feet
- Atrophic changes

Immune System
- Impaired healing
- Chronic skin infections
- Periodontal disease
- Urinary tract infections
- Lung infections
- Vaginitis

TABLE 18-2 DKA, HHS, and Hypoglycemia Compared

		DKA	HHS	Hypoglycemia
Diabetes Type **Onset** **Cause**		Primary Type 1 Slow ↓ Insulin Infection	Type 2 Slow ↓ Insulin Older age	Both Rapid ↑ Insulin Omitted meal/snack Error in insulin dose
Risk Factors		Surgery Trauma Illness Omitted insulin Stress	Surgery Trauma Illness Dehydration Medications Dialysis Hyperalimentation	Surgery Trauma Illness Exercise Medications Lipodystrophy Renal failure Alcohol intake

Assessments	Skin
	Perspiration
	Thirst
	Breath
	Vital signs
	
	Mental status
	Thirst
	Fluid intake
	Gastrointestinal effects
	
	Level of consciousness
	Energy level
	Other
		Flushed; dry; warm
		None
		Increased
		Fruity
		BP ↓
		P ↑
		R Kussmaul's
		Confused
		Increased
		Increased
		Nausea/vomiting;
		  abdominal pain
		Decreasing
		Weak
		Weight loss
		Blurred vision
			Flushed; dry; warm
			None
			Increased
			Normal
			BP ↓
			P ↑
			R normal
			Lethargic
			Increased
			Increased
			Nausea/vomiting;
			  abdominal pain
			Decreasing
			Weak
			Weight loss
			Malaise
			Extreme thirst
			Seizures
				Pallor; moist; cool
				Profuse
				Normal
				Normal
				BP ↓
				P ↑
				R normal
				Anxious; restless
				Normal
				Normal
				Hunger
				
				Decreasing
				Fatigue
				Headache
				Altered vision
				Mood changes
				Seizures

Laboratory Findings	Blood glucose Plasma ketones Urine glucose Urine ketones Serum potassium Serum sodium Serum chloride Plasma pH Osmolality	>300 mg/dL Increased Increased Increased Abnormal Abnormal Abnormal <7.3 >340 mOsm/L	>600 mg/dL Normal Increased Normal Abnormal Abnormal Abnormal Normal >340 mOsm/L	<50 mg/dL Normal Normal Normal Normal Normal Normal Normal Normal
Treatment		Insulin Treatment Intravenous fluids Electrolytes	Insulin Intravenous fluids Electrolytes	Glucagon Rapid-acting carbohydrate Intravenous solution of 50% glucose

glucose is usually less than 45 to 60 mg/dL. Severe hypoglycemia may cause death.

People who have type 1 DM for 4 or 5 years fail to secrete glucagon in response to a decrease in blood glucose. They then depend on epinephrine to serve as a counterregulatory response to hypoglycemia. However, this compensatory response can become absent or blunted. The person then develops a syndrome called *hypoglycemia unawareness.* The person does not experience symptoms of hypoglycemia, even though it is present. Because treatment is not initiated in the absence of symptoms, the person is likely to have episodes of severe hypoglycemia.

Alterations in the Cardiovascular System

The macrocirculation (large blood vessels) in people with diabetes undergoes changes due to atherosclerosis; abnormalities in platelets, red blood cells, and clotting factors; and changes in arterial walls. It has been established that atherosclerosis has an increased incidence and earlier age of onset in people with diabetes (although the reason is unknown). Other risk factors that contribute to the development of macrovascular disease of diabetes are hypertension, hyperlipidemia, cigarette smoking, and obesity. Alterations in the vascular system increase the risk of the long-term complications of coronary artery disease, cerebral vascular disease, and peripheral vascular disease.

Alterations in the microcirculation in the person with diabetes involve structural defects in the basement membrane of smaller blood vessels and capillaries. (The basement membrane is the structure that supports and serves as the boundary around the space occupied by epithelial cells.) These defects cause the capillary basement membrane to thicken, eventually resulting in decreased tissue perfusion. Changes in basement membranes are believed to be due to one or more of the following: the presence of increased amounts of sorbitol (a substance formed as an intermediate step in the conversion of glucose to fructose), the formation of abnormal glycoproteins, or problems in the release of oxygen from hemoglobin (Porth, 2002). The effects of alterations in the microcirculation affect all body tissues but are seen primarily in the eyes and the kidneys.

Coronary Artery Disease

Coronary artery disease is a major risk factor in the development of myocardial infarction in people with diabetes, especially in the middle to older adult with type 2 DM. Coronary artery disease is the most common cause of death in people with diabetes, accounting for 40% to 60% of all cases of mortality (Haire-Joshu, 1996). People with diabetes who have myocardial infarction are more prone to develop congestive heart failure as a complication of the infarction and are also less likely to survive in the period immediately following the infarction. (Myocardial infarction is fully discussed in Chapter 29.) ⊙⊃

Hypertension

Hypertension (blood pressure ≥140/90 mmHg) is a common complication of DM. It affects 20% to 60% of all people with diabetes, and is a major risk factor for cardiovascular disease and microvascular complications such as retinopathy and nephropathy. Hypertension may be reduced by weight loss, exercise, and decreasing sodium intake and alcohol consumption. If these methods are not effective, treatment with antihypertensive medications is necessary.

Stroke (Cerebrovascular Accident)

People with diabetes, especially older adults with type 2 DM, are 2 to 6 times more likely to have a stroke. Although the exact relationship between diabetes and cerebral vascular disease is unknown, hypertension (a risk factor for stroke) is a common health problem in those who have diabetes. In addition, atherosclerosis of the cerebral vessels develops at an earlier age and is more extensive in people with diabetes (Porth, 1998).

The manifestations of impaired cerebral circulation (see Chapter 41 ⊙⊃) are often similar to those of hypoglycemia or HHS: blurred vision, slurred speech, weakness, and dizziness. People with these manifestations have potentially life-threatening health problems and require constant medical attention.

Peripheral Vascular Disease

Peripheral vascular disease of the lower extremities accompanies both types of DM, but the incidence is greater in people with type 2 DM. Atherosclerosis of vessels in the legs of people with diabetes begins at an earlier age, advances more rap-idly, and is equally common in both men and women. Impaired peripheral vascular circulation leads to peripheral vascular insufficiency with intermittent claudication (pain) in the lower legs and ulcerations of the feet. Occlusion and thrombosis of large vessels and small arteries and arterioles, as well as alterations in neurologic function and infection, result in gangrene (necrosis, or the death of tissue). Gangrene from diabetes is the most common cause of nontraumatic amputations of the lower leg. In people with diabetes, dry gangrene is most common, manifested by cold, dry, shriveled, and black tissues of the toes and feet. The gangrene usually begins in the toes and moves proximally into the foot.

Diabetic Retinopathy

Diabetic retinopathy is the name for the changes in the retina that occur in the person with diabetes. The retinal capillary structure undergoes alterations in blood flow, leading to retinal ischemia and a breakdown in the blood-retinal barrier. Diabetic retinopathy is the leading cause of blindness in people between ages 25 and 74. Retinopathy has three stages:

- *Stage I:* Nonproliferative retinopathy. Dilated veins, microaneurysms, edema of the macula, and the presence of exudates characterize this stage.
- *Stage II:* Preproliferative retinopathy. Retinal ischemia causes infarcts of the nerve fiber layer, with characteristic "cotton wool" patches on the retina. Shunts form between occluded and patent vessels.
- *Stage III:* Proliferative retinopathy. As fibrous tissue and new vessels form in the retina or optic disc, traction on the vitreous humor may cause hemorrhage or retinal detachment.

After 20 years of diabetes, almost all clients with type 1 DM and more than 60% of clients with type 2 DM will have some degree of retinopathy (American Diabetes Association [ADA], 2002). If exudate, edema, hemorrhage, or ischemia occurs near the fovea, the person experiences visual impairment at any stage. In addition, the person with diabetes is at increased risk for developing cataracts (opacity of the lens) as a result of increased glucose levels within the lens itself. Screening for retinopathy is important, as laser photocoagulation surgery has proven beneficial in preventing loss of vision.

Diabetic Nephropathy

Diabetic nephropathy is a disease of the kidneys characterized by the presence of albumin in the urine, hypertension, edema, and progressive renal insufficiency. This disorder is the most common cause of renal failure requiring dialysis or transplantation in the United States. Nephropathy occurs in 20% to 40% of people with diabetes (ADA, 2002).

Despite research, the exact pathologic origin of diabetic nephropathy is unknown; it has been established, however, that thickening of the basement membrane of the glomeruli eventually impairs renal function. It is suggested that an increased intracellular concentration of glucose supports the formation of abnormal glycoproteins in the basement membrane. The accumulation of these large proteins stimulates glomerulosclerosis (fibrosis of the glomerular tissue). Glomerulosclerosis severely impairs the filtering function of the glomerulus, and protein is lost in the urine. *Kimmelstiel-Wilson syndrome* is a type of glomerulosclerosis found only in people with diabetes. In advanced nephropathy, tubular atrophy occurs, and end-stage renal disease results. (Renal failure is discussed in Chapter 27.) ⚭

The first indication of nephropathy is **microalbuminuria,** a low but abnormal level of albumin in the urine. Without specific interventions, people with type 1 DM with sustained microalbuminuria will develop overt nephropathy, accompanied by hypertension, over a period of 10 to 15 years. People with type 2 DM often have microalbuminuria and overt nephropathy shortly after diagnosis, because the diabetes has often been present but undiagnosed for many years. Because the hypertension accelerates the progress of diabetic nephropathy, aggressive antihypertensive management should be instituted. Management includes control of hypertension with ACE inhibitors such as captopril (Capoten), weight loss, reduced salt intake, and exercise.

Alterations in the Peripheral and Autonomic Nervous Systems

Peripheral and visceral neuropathies are disorders of the peripheral nerves and the autonomic nervous system. In people with diabetes, these disorders are often called **diabetic neuropathies.** The etiology of diabetic neuropathies involves (1) a thickening of the walls of the blood vessels that supply nerves, causing a decrease in nutrients; (2) demyelinization of the Schwann cells that surround and insulate nerves, slowing nerve conduction; and (3) the formation and accumulation of sorbitol within the Schwann cells, impairing nerve conduction. The manifestations depend on the locations of the lesions.

Peripheral Neuropathies

The peripheral neuropathies (also called *somatic neuropathies*) include polyneuropathies and mononeuropathies. *Polyneuropathies,* the most common type of neuropathy associated with diabetes, are bilateral sensory disorders. The manifestations appear first in the toes and feet and progress upward. The fingers and hands may also be involved, but usually only in later stages of diabetes. The manifestations of polyneuropathy depend on the nerve fibers involved.

The person with polyneuropathy commonly has distal paresthesias (a subjective feeling of a change in sensation, such as numbness or tingling); pain described as aching, burning, or shooting; and feelings of cold feet. Other manifestations may include impaired sensations of pain, temperature, light touch, two-point discrimination, and vibration. There is no specific treatment for polyneuropathy.

Mononeuropathies are isolated peripheral neuropathies that affect a single nerve. Depending on the nerve involved, manifestations may include the following:

- Palsy of the third cranial (oculomotor) nerve, with headache, eye pain, and an inability to move the eye up, down, or medially
- Radiculopathy, with pain over a dermatome and loss of cutaneous sensation, most often located in the chest

- Diabetic femoral neuropathy, with motor and sensory deficits (pain, weakness, areflexia) in the anterior thigh and medial calf
- Entrapment or compression of the medial nerve at the wrist, resulting in carpal tunnel syndrome with pain and weakness of the hand; the ulnar nerve at the elbow, with weakness and loss of sensation over the palmar surface of the fourth and fifth fingers; and the peroneal nerve at the head of the fibula, with foot drop.

Visceral Neuropathies

The visceral neuropathies (also called *autonomic neuropathies*) cause various manifestations, depending on the area of the ANS involved. These neuropathies may include the following:

- Sweating dysfunction, with an absence of sweating (*anhydrosis*) on the hands and feet and increased sweating on the face or trunk
- Abnormal pupillary function, most commonly seen as constricted pupils that dilate slowly in the dark
- Cardiovascular dysfunction, resulting in such abnormalities as a fixed cardiac rate that does not change with exercise, postural hypotension, and a failure to increase cardiac output or vascular tone with exercise
- Gastrointestinal dysfunction, with changes in upper gastrointestinal motility (*gastroparesis*) resulting in dysphagia, anorexia, heartburn, nausea, and vomiting and altered blood glucose control. Constipation is one of the most common gastrointestinal symptoms associated with diabetes, possibly a result of hypomotility of the bowel. Diabetic diarrhea is not as common, but it does occur and is often associated with fecal incontinence during sleep due to a defect in internal sphincter function.
- Genitourinary dysfunction, resulting in changes in bladder function and sexual function. Bladder function changes include an inability to empty the bladder completely, loss of sensation of bladder fullness, and an increased risk of urinary tract infections. Sexual dysfunctions in men include ejaculatory changes and impotence. Sexual dysfunctions in women include changes in arousal patterns, vaginal lubrication, and orgasm. Alterations in sexual function in people with diabetes are the result of both neurologic and vascular changes.

Increased Susceptibility to Infection

The person with diabetes has an increased risk of developing infections. The exact relationship between infection and diabetes is not clear, but many dysfunctions that result from diabetic complications predispose the person to develop an infection. Vascular and neurologic impairments, hyperglycemia, and altered neutrophil function are believed to be responsible (Porth, 2002).

The person with diabetes may have sensory deficits resulting in inattention to trauma, and vascular deficits that decrease circulation to the injured area; as a result, the normal inflammatory response is diminished and healing is slowed. Nephrosclerosis and inadequate bladder emptying with retention of urine predispose the person with diabetes to pyelonephritis and urinary tract infections. Bacterial and fungal infections of the skin, nails, and mucous membranes are common. Tuberculosis is more prevalent in people with diabetes than in the general population.

Periodontal Disease

Although periodontal disease does not occur more often in people with diabetes, it does progress more rapidly, especially if the diabetes is poorly controlled. It is believed to be caused by microangiopathy, with changes in vascularization of the gums. As a result, gingivitis (inflammation of the gums) and periodontitis (inflammation of the bone underlying the gums) occur.

Complications Involving the Feet

The high incidence of both amputations and problems with the feet in people with diabetes is the result of angiopathy, neuropathy, and infection. People with diabetes are at high risk for amputation of a lower extremity, with increased risk in those who have had DM for more than 10 years, are male, have poor glucose control, or have cardiovascular, retinal, or renal complications.

Vascular changes in the lower extremities of the person with diabetes result in arteriosclerosis. Diabetes-induced arteriosclerosis tends to occur at an earlier age, occurs equally in men and women, is usually bilateral, and progresses more rapidly. The blood vessels most often affected are located below the knee. Blockages form in the large, medium, and small arteries of the lower legs and feet. Multiple occlusions with decreased blood flow result in the manifestations of peripheral vascular disease (see the box below). Peripheral vascular disease is discussed in Chapter 33. ⊝⊃

Diabetic neuropathy of the foot produces multiple problems. Because the sense of touch and perception of pain is absent, the person with diabetes may have some type of foot trauma without being aware of it. The person thus is at increased risk for trauma to tissues of the feet, leading to ulcer development. Infections commonly occur in traumatized or ulcerated tissue (see Figure 18–3 ■).

Despite the many potential sources of foot trauma in the person with diabetes, the most common are cracks and fissures caused by dry skin or infections such as athlete's foot, blisters caused by improperly fitting shoes, pressure from stockings or

Figure 18–3 ■ Ulceration following trauma in the foot of the person with diabetes.

Source: Harry Przekop, Medichrome/The Stock Shop, Inc.

shoes, ingrown toenails, and direct trauma (cuts, bruises, or burns). It is important to remember that the person with diabetic neuropathy who has lost the perception of pain may not be aware that these injuries have occurred. In addition, when a part of the body loses sensation, the person tends to dissociate from or ignore the part, so that an injury may go unattended for days or weeks. The injury may even be forgotten entirely.

Foot lesions usually begin as a superficial skin ulcer. In time, the ulcer extends deeper into muscles and bone, leading to abscess or osteomyelitis. Gangrene can develop on one or more toes; if untreated, the whole foot eventually becomes gangrenous. (Care of the feet, an essential part of client and family education, is discussed later in the chapter.)

DIABETES IN THE OLDER ADULT

Although the older adult may have either type 1 or type 2 DM, most have type 2. The National Institute of Diabetes and Kidney Disease estimates that nearly 11% of the U.S. population between the ages of 65 and 74 have diabetes. The prevalence of diabetes becomes greater with age, increasing from 8.2% with diagnosed diabetes in those age 20 years or older to 18.4% for those equal to or older than age 65 (ADA, 2002). It is predicted that the number of older adults with diabetes will continue to increase, because the incidence of the disease increases with age and because the number of people over 65 is increasing.

Although most older adults with diabetes have type 2 DM, the improved survival rates for people with diabetes have resulted in an increased number of older adults with type 1. The picture is complicated by the fact that blood glucose levels increase with age, beginning in the 50s. For this reason, it is more difficult to diagnose diabetes in the older adult; conversely, the older adult may be mistakenly diagnosed with the disease simply for exhibiting essentially normal age-related changes in glucose. The relationship between normal increases in glucose levels and the presence of diabetes is not yet understood.

Manifestations of Peripheral Vascular Disease

- Loss of hair on lower leg, feet, and toes
- Atrophic skin changes: shininess and thinning
- Cold feet
- Feet and ankles darker than leg
- Dependent rubor, blanching on elevation
- Thick toenails
- Diminished or absent pulses
- Nocturnal pain
- Pain at rest, relieved by standing or walking
- Intermittent claudication
- Patchy areas of gangrene on feet and toes

TABLE 18–3 Implications for Nursing Care of the Older Adult with Diabetes

Health Problem/Complication	Implications for Nursing Care
Urinary incontinence	Polyuria, a classic manifestation of diabetes, often is ignored. This problem also often leads to social isolation.
Decreased thirst	Polydipsia, a classic manifestation of diabetes, often is ignored. This further increases the risk of dehydration and electrolyte imbalances.
Decreased hunger and weight loss	Polyphagia, a classic manifestation of diabetes, often is ignored. The aging process, medications, depression, or lack of socialization may decrease hunger. Weight loss may be gradual and go unnoticed.
Fatigue	Fatigue is a common symptom of diabetes but may be blamed on increased age.
Hypoglycemia	The older adult may have either very mild manifestations or none at all. As a result, hypoglycemia is often ignored until it causes serious effects.
Peripheral neuropathy	Manifestations may be thought to be due to arthritis, and over-the-counter drugs often are used to self-medicate. The risk of falls increases, as does the risk of gangrene and amputation.
Peripheral vascular disease	May go undetected if the person does not get enough exercise to cause claudication. May also impair abilities to climb stairs and walk.
Diabetic retinopathy	May be undetected if the person has cataracts. Diabetic clients also have an increased incidence of cataracts and glaucoma. Deficits in vision threaten independence, mobility, and social interactions.
Hypertension	Treatment with diuretics may further impair glucose tolerance and result in electrolyte imbalances.
Arthritis	Older adults may believe the pain from arthritis to be more important than the diabetes management. Also, depression from chronic pain as well as inactivity and loss of appetite may interfere with diabetes self-care.
Parkinson's disease	The tremors and rigidity of this disease make self-care involving fine and gross motor skills difficult or impossible.
Medications	Older adults commonly take more than one type of medication and are at increased risk for problems relating to drug interactions.

Note. Adapted from "Diabetes Mellitus and the Older Adult" by M. M. Funnell and J. H. Merritt, pp. 755–830, in D. Haire-Joshu (Ed.), Management of Diabetes Mellitus: Perspectives of Care Across the Lifespan (2nd ed.) 1996, St. Louis: Mosby.

The older adult with diabetes has multiple, complex health care problems and needs. The normal physiologic changes of aging may mask manifestations of the onset of diabetes and may also increase the potential for complications. Table 18–3 presents common problems in the older adult that make the diagnosis and management of diabetes more difficult. The older adult with diabetes also has a longer recovery period after surgery or serious illness, often requiring insulin to maintain blood glucose levels.

COLLABORATIVE CARE

The results of a 10-year Diabetes Control and Complications Trial (DCCT), sponsored by the National Institutes of Health (NIH), have significant implications for the management of type 1 DM. People in the study who kept their blood glucose levels close to normal by frequent monitoring, several daily insulin injections, and lifestyle changes that included exercise and a healthier diet reduced by 60% their risk for the development and progression of complications involving the eyes, the kidneys, and the nervous system. Treatment of the client with diabetes focuses on maintaining blood glucose at levels as nearly normal as possible through medications, dietary management, and exercise. Treatment of the acute complications of diabetes (hypoglycemia, DKA, and HHS) is also included in this section.

Diagnostic Tests

Diagnostic tests are conducted for screening purposes to diagnose diabetes, and ongoing laboratory tests are conducted to evaluate the effectiveness of diabetic management. Definitions of normal blood glucose levels vary in clinical practice, depending on the laboratory that performs the assay.

Diagnostic Screening

Three diagnostic tests may be used to diagnose DM, and each must be confirmed, on a subsequent day, with one of the three tests. The diagnostic criteria recommended by the ADA (2002) are:

1. Symptoms of diabetes plus causal plasma glucose (PG) concentration >200 mg/dL (11.1 mmol/L). Causal is defined as any time of day without regard to time since last meal.
2. Fasting plasma glucose (FPG) >126 mg/dL (7.0 mmol/L). Fasting is defined as no caloric intake for 8 hours.
3. Two-hour PG >200 mg/dL (11.1 mmol/L) during an oral glucose tolerance test (OGTT). The test should be performed with a glucose load containing the equivalent of 75 anhydrous glucose dissolved in water (see the Nursing Implications box on the next page).

When using these criteria, the following levels are used for the FPG:

- Normal fasting glucose = 110 mg/dL (6.1 mmol/L)

Nursing Implications for Diagnostic Tests
Oral Glucose Tolerance Test

Preparation of Client
- Have the client eat a diet high in carbohydrates for 3 days before the test.
- If possible, discontinue drugs that may interfere with test results for 3 days before the test:
  a. Corticosteroids
  b. Oral contraceptives
  c. Synthetic estrogens
  d. Phenytoin (Dilantin)
  e. Vitamin C
  f. Aspirin
  g. Thiazide diuretics
  h. Nicotinic acid
- Keep the client NPO except for water for 10 hours before the test.
- The client is given a specified amount of glucose (either 75 g or 100 g) as a lemon-flavor or glucola liquid after fasting blood and urine samples are taken.
- Blood and urine samples are taken after the glucose is ingested at 30 minutes, 1 hour, and 2 hours. In some instances the test may continue for up to 5 hours.
- Observe the client for symptoms of hyperglycemia and hypoglycemia.

Client and Family Teaching
- The procedure for the test.
- Foods that are high in carbohydrates.
- For 10 hours before the test and during the test, the following are not allowed: food, tea, coffee, or alcohol. Smoking is not permitted during the test.
- Nausea, weakness, dizziness, and sweating may be experienced during the test; these symptoms often disappear, but report them to the nurse as soon as they occur.
- Limit activity because increased activity may change the test results. (The client may be requested to remain seated during the test.)

- Impaired fasting glucose = >110 (6.1 mmol/L) and <126 mg/dL (7.0 mmol/L)
- Diagnosis of diabetes = >126 mg/dL (7.0 mmol/L)

When using these criteria, the following levels are used for the OGTT:

- Normal glucose tolerance = 2-hr PG: <140 mg/dL (7.8 mmol/L)
- Impaired glucose tolerance = 2-hr PG: ≥140 (7.8 mmol/L) and <200 mg/dL (11.1 mmol/L)
- Diagnosis of diabetes = 2-hr PG: ≥200 mg/dL (11.1 mmol/L)

Note that although either method may be used to diagnose diabetes, in a clinical setting the FPG is the recommended screening test for nonpregnant adults (ADA, 2002).

Diagnostic Tests to Monitor Diabetes Management
The following diagnostic tests may be used to monitor diabetes management.

- *Fasting blood glucose (FBG).* This test is often ordered, especially if the client is experiencing symptoms of hypoglycemia or hyperglycemia. In most people, the normal range is 70 to 110 mg/dL.
- *Glycosylated hemoglobin (c) (A1C).* This test determines the average blood glucose level over approximately the previous 2 to 3 months. When glucose is elevated or control of glucose is erratic, glucose attaches to the hemoglobin molecule and remains attached for the life of the hemoglobin, which is about 120 days. The normal level depends on the type of assay done, but values above 7% to 9% are considered elevated. The ADA recommends that A1C be performed at the initial assessment, and then at regular intervals, individualized to the medical regimen used.

- *Urine glucose and ketone levels.* These are not as accurate in monitoring changes in blood glucose as blood levels. The presence of glucose in the urine indicates hyperglycemia. Most people have a renal threshold for glucose of 180 mg/dL; that is, when the blood glucose exceeds 180 mg/dL, glucose is not reabsorbed by the kidney and spills over into the urine. This number varies highly, however. **Ketonuria** (the presence of ketones in the urine) occurs with the breakdown of fats and is an indicator of DKA; however, fat breakdown and ketonuria also occur in states of less than normal nutrition.
- *Urine test* for the presence of protein as albumin (*albuminuria*). If albuminuria is present, a 24-hour urine test for creatinine clearance is used to detect the early onset of nephropathy.
- *Serum cholesterol and triglyceride levels.* These are indicators of atherosclerosis and an increased risk of cardiovascular impairments. The ADA (2002) recommends treatment goals to lower LDL cholesterol to <100 mg/dL, raise HDL cholesterol to >45 mg/dL, and lower triglycerides to <150 mg/dL.
- *Serum electrolytes.* Levels are measured in clients who have DKA or HHS to determine imbalances.

Monitoring Blood Glucose
People with diabetes must monitor their condition daily by testing glucose levels. Two types of tests are available. The first type, long used prior to the development of devices to directly measure blood glucose, is urine testing for glucose and ketones. Urine testing is less commonly used today. The second type, direct measurement of blood glucose, is widely used in all types of health care settings and in the home.

Urine Testing for Ketones and Glucose
Urine testing for glucose and ketones was at one time the only available method for evaluating the management of diabetes.

Procedure 18–1 — Testing Urine for Ketones and Glucose

TO TEST THE URINE FOR KETONES

1. Ask the client to void, discard the urine, and drink a full glass of water.
2. Thirty minutes later, collect a urine sample.
3. For Acidtest tablets: Place the tablet on a white paper towel, place 1 drop of urine on the tablet, and wait 30 seconds. If the tablet turns any shade from lavender to deep purple, the test is positive for ketones.

4. For Ketostix: Dip the reagent stick into the urine sample. Wait 15 seconds, and compare the color of the pad at the end of the stick to an accompanying color chart. Purple is indicative of ketones.

TO TEST THE URINE FOR GLUCOSE

1. Follow the same procedure to collect a urine sample.

2. Dip the reagent stick into the urine sample, and wait the time indicated. Compare the color of the pad on the end of the reagent stick with an accompanying color chart. The glucose is expressed as a percentage (for example, 0.5%, 1%, 2%). Remember that normally no glucose is found in the urine, so the presence of glucose is an abnormal manifestation indicating hyperglycemia.

An inexpensive and noninvasive test, it has unpredictable results and cannot be used to detect or measure hypoglycemia. Urine testing is recommended to monitor hyperglycemia and ketoacidosis in people with type 1 DM who have unexplained hyperglycemia during illness or pregnancy. Urine testing may also be used by people who choose not to self-monitor blood glucose by other methods. (See Procedure 18–1.)

Self-Monitoring of Blood Glucose

Self-monitoring of blood glucose (SMBG) allows the person with diabetes to monitor and achieve metabolic control and decrease the danger of hypoglycemia. The ADA recommends that all clients with diabetes must be taught some method of monitoring glycemic control. The timing of SMBG is highly individualized, depending on the person's diagnosis, general disease control, and physical state. SMBG is recommended three or more times a day for clients with type 1 DM. Clients with type 2 DM should be sufficient to help them reach glucose goals. When adding or modifying therapy, clients with both types of DM should test more often than usual. SMBG is also useful when the person is ill or pregnant, or has symptoms of hypoglycemia or hyperglycemia.

The ADA annually publishes a comprehensive list of currently available blood glucose monitoring machines and strips with approximate prices in *Diabetes Forecast*. Most medical insurance policies cover the cost of these machines.

Following is the equipment needed for SMBG.

- Some type of lancet device to perform a finger-stick for obtaining a drop of blood (such as an Autolet, Penlet, or Soft Touch)
- Chemically impregnated test strips that change color when they come into contact with glucose or that can be read by machine (e.g., Glucostix and Chemstrip bG). The strip may also be read by comparing its color with a color chart on the side of the container or on an insert (Figure 18–4 ■).
- A blood glucose monitor (e.g., the Glucometer, the AccuChek, or the One Touch) if the most accurate measurement is desired or recommended. The manufacturer's instructions must be followed carefully. If the timing of the blood on the

Figure 18–4 ■ Determination of blood glucose levels by visual reading. The color of the strip is compared with the color chart on the side of the container.

strip is not exact, the test will not be accurate. In addition, the machine must be cleaned according to the manufacturer's directions to ensure accuracy. Monitors that use no-wipe technology improve the accuracy of glucose measurement. Other monitors are computerized and/or include a memory of previous glucose readings to show a pattern of control.

Factors that may alter blood glucose results when testing with a monitor (Passaniza, 2001) are as follows:

- Increased triglyceride levels, which can interfere with the way light is reflected in light reflectance monitors, such as the AccuChek
- Insufficient amounts of blood on the testing strip, outdated strips, and exposure of the strips to air and humidity
- Both increased and decreased hematocrits, with blood glucose values varying as much as 30% for every 10% change in hematocrit
- High altitudes, which cause a decrease in blood oxygen
- High doses of acetaminophen (Tylenol), ascorbic acid (vitamin C), ibuprofen (Motrin, Advil), salicylates (Aspirin), and tetracycline.

Medications

The pharmacologic treatment for diabetes mellitus depends on the type of diabetes. People with type 1 must have insulin; those with type 2 are usually able to control glucose levels with an oral hypoglycemic medication, but they may require insulin if control is inadequate.

Insulin

The person with type 1 DM requires a lifelong exogenous source of the insulin hormone to maintain life. Insulin is not a cure for diabetes; rather, it is a means of controlling hyperglycemia. Insulin is also necessary in other situations, such as:

- People with diabetes who are unable to control glucose levels with oral antidiabetic drugs and/or diet. Approximately 40% of people with type 2 diabetes require insulin (NIH, 2002).
- People with diabetes who are experiencing physical stress (such as an infection or surgery) or who are taking corticosteroids.
- Women with gestational diabetes who are unable to control glucose with diet.
- People with DKA or HHS.
- People who are receiving high-calorie tube feedings or parenteral nutrition.

SOURCES OF INSULIN. Preparations of insulin are derived from animal (pork pancreas) or synthesized in the laboratory from either an alteration of pork insulin or recombinant DNA technology, using strains of *E. coli* to form a biosynthetic human insulin. Insulin analogs have been developed by modifying the amino acid sequence of the insulin molecule. Although different types are prescribed on an individualized basis, it is standard practice to prescribe human insulin.

INSULIN PREPARATIONS. Insulins are available in rapid-acting, short-acting, intermediate-acting, and long-acting preparations. The trade names and times of onset, peak, and duration of action are listed in Table 18–4.

Insulin lispro (Humalog) is a human insulin analog that is derived from genetically altered *E. coli* that includes the gene for insulin lispro. It is classified as a rapid-acting or ultra-short-acting insulin. Compared to regular insulin, insulin lispro has a more rapid onset (<15 minutes), an earlier peak of glucose lowering (30 to 60 minutes), and a shorter duration of activity (3 to 4 hours). This means that lispro should be administered 15 minutes before a meal, rather than 30 to 60 minutes before as recommended for regular insulin. Clients with type 1 DM usually also require concurrent use of a longer-acting insulin product. Lispro is much less likely than regular insulin to cause tissue changes and may lower the risk of nocturnal hypoglycemia in clients with type 1 DM.

Regular insulin is unmodified crystalline insulin, classified as a short-actin insulin. Regular insulin is clear in appearance and can be given by the intravenous route; the other types are suspensions and could be harmful if given by this route. Regular insulin is also used to treat DKA, to initiate treatment for newly diagnosed type 1 DM, and in combination with intermediate-acting insulins to provide better glucose control.

The onset and peak and duration of action of insulin can be changed by adding zinc, acetate buffers, and protamine. Zinc is added to make lente insulin, and zinc and protamine are added to NPH insulin to prolong their action, and they are classified as intermediate- or long-acting insulins. These preparations appear cloudy when properly mixed prior to injection. Protamine and zinc are foreign substances and may cause hypersensitivity reactions.

Insulin glargine (Lantus) is a 24-hour long-acting rDNA human insulin analog that is given subcutaneously once a day at bedtime to treat clients with both type 1 and type 2 diabetes. It has a relatively constant effect (meaning it does not have a peak time of effect). It may be used in combination with intermediate-acting or long-acting insulins.

CONCENTRATIONS OF INSULIN. Insulin is dispensed as 100 U/mL (U-100) and 500 U/mL (U-500) in the United States. U-100 is the standard insulin concentration used. U-500 insulin

TABLE 18–4	Insulin Preparations			
Preparation	Name	Onset (h)	Peak (h)	Duration (h)
Rapid acting	Lispro	0.25	1–1.5	3–4
Short acting	Regular Regular Humulin (R) Regular Iletin II Velosulin	0.5–1.0	2–3	4–6
Intermediate acting	Lente Humulin (L) Lente Iletin II NPH Humulin (N) NPH Iletin II NPH	2	6–8	12–16
Long acting	Ultralente (U) Lantus	2 (onset and peak not defined)	16–20	24+ 24
Combinations	Humulin 50/50 Humulin 70/30 Novolin 70/30	0.5 0.5 0.5	3 4–8 4–8	22–24 24 24

is only used in rare cases of insulin resistance when clients require very large doses. U-500 and the insulin analog lispro are the only insulins that require a prescription.

INSULIN ADMINISTRATION.   Nursing implications for administering insulin are outlined in the Medication Administration box below and further discussion follows in the chapter. The considerations for administering insulin include routes of administration, syringe and needle selection, preparing the injection, sites of injection, mixing insulins, and insulin regimens.

Routes of Administration.   All insulins are given parenterally, although current research is investigating the development of a nasal spray and an oral preparation of insulin. Only regular insulin is given by both subcutaneous and intravenous routes; all others are given only subcutaneously. If the intravenous route is not available, regular insulin may also be administered intramuscularly in an emergency situation.

Continuous Subcutaneous Insulin Infusion.   Regular insulin is also used in continuous subcutaneous insulin infusion (CSII) devices, often called *insulin pumps* (e.g., Minimed and Disetronic pumps). CSII devices have a small pump that holds a syringe of insulin, connected to a subcutaneous needle by tubing. The pump is about the size of a pager and can be worn on a belt or tucked into a pocket. The needle is placed in the skin, usually in the abdomen. This device delivers a constant amount of programmed insulin throughout each 24-hour period. It also can be used to deliver a bolus of insulin manually (e.g., before meals).

Medication Administration

Insulin

Nursing Responsibilities
- Discard vials of insulin that have been open for several weeks or whose expiration date has passed.
- Refrigerate extra insulin vials not currently in use, but do not freeze them.
- Store insulin in a cool place, and avoid exposure to temperature extremes or sunlight.
- Store compatible mixtures of insulin for no longer than 1 month at room temperature or 3 months at 36° to 46°F (2° to 8°C).
- Discard any vials with discoloration, clumping, granules, or solid deposits on the sides.
- If breakfast is delayed, also delay the administration of rapid-acting insulin.
- Monitor and maintain a record of blood glucose readings 30 minutes before each meal and bedtime (or as prescribed).
- Monitor food intake, and notify the physician if food is not being consumed.
- Monitor electrolytes (especially potassium), blood urea nitrogen (BUN) levels, and creatinine.
- Observe injection sites for manifestations of hypersensitivity, lipodystrophy, and lipoatrophy.
- If symptoms of hypoglycemia occur, confirm by testing blood glucose level, and administer an oral source of a fast-acting carbohydrate, such as juice, milk, or crackers. Hypoglycemic symptoms may vary but commonly include feelings of shakiness, hunger, and/or nervousness accompanied by sweating, tachycardia, or palpitations.
- If symptoms of hyperglycemia occur, confirm by testing blood glucose level, and notify the physician.

Client and Family Teaching
- The manifestations of diabetes mellitus.
- Self-administration of insulin, with a return demonstration.
  a. Wash hands carefully.
  b. Have a vial of insulin, the insulin syringe with needle, and alcohol pads ready to use.
  c. Remove the cover from the needle.
  d. Fill the syringe with an amount of air equal to the number of units of insulin, and insert the needle into the vial.
  e. Push air into the vial, invert the vial, and withdraw the prescribed units of insulin.

  f. Replace the cover over the needle.
  g. Wipe the selected site with alcohol. The injection is less likely to be painful if the alcohol is allowed to dry.
  h. Pinch up a fold of skin, and insert the needle into the tissue at the recommended angle.
  i. Insert the insulin.
  j. Withdraw the needle; if desired, apply firm pressure to the site for a few seconds.
  k. Recap the needle. Many people with diabetes reuse disposable syringes with attached needles without adverse effects. The primary reason for discarding after several uses is that the needle becomes dull and makes the injection painful.
- Follow instructions for mixing insulins (refer to the box on page 490).
- Always keep an extra vial of insulin available.
- Always have a vial of regular insulin available for emergencies.
- Be aware of the signs of hypersensitivity responses, hypoglycemia, and hyperglycemia.
- Keep candy or a sugar source available at all times to treat hypoglycemia, if it occurs.
- Vision may be blurred during the first 6 to 8 weeks of insulin therapy; this is the result of fluid changes in the eye and should clear up in 8 weeks.
- Avoid alcoholic beverages, which may cause hypoglycemia.
- Follow these guidelines for sick days:
  a. Never omit insulin.
  b. Always monitor blood glucose and/or urine ketones at least every 2 to 4 hours.
  c. Always drink plenty of fluids, try to drink at least one glass of water or other calorie-free, caffeine-free liquid each hour.
  d. Get as much rest as possible.
  e. Contact the physician if there is persistent fever, vomiting, shortness of breath, severe pain in the abdomen, dehydration, loss of vision, chest pain, persistent diarrhea, blood glucose levels above 250, or ketones in the urine.
- Establish a plan for rotating injection sites, and observe closely for changes in tissues such as hardness, dimpling, or sunken areas.

Programming the amount of insulin to be delivered is determined by frequent blood glucose monitoring. Several different pumps are available, and each has rechargeable batteries, a syringe, a programmable computer, and a motor and drive mechanism. The rapid-acting insulin analog lispro is an appropriate insulin for insulin pumps, and short-acting regular insulin may also be used. Lispro is not approved for use in pregnancy (Tierney et al., 2001).

Many people with diabetes believe the pump allows more normal regulation of blood glucose and provides greater lifestyle flexibility. Pumps are as safe as multiple-injection therapy when recommended procedures are followed. A potential complication is an undetected interruption in insulin delivery, which may result in a rapid onset of DKA. The needle site must be kept clean and changed on a regular basis (usually every 2 to 3 days) to prevent inflammation and infection. Although the client who chooses an insulin pump has more to learn, many are very satisfied with having more normal glucose control.

Syringe and Needle Selection. Insulin is administered in sterile, single-use, disposable insulin syringes, calibrated in units per milliliter. This means that in U-100 insulin, there are 100 U of insulin in 1 mL. Syringes for administering U-100 insulin can be purchased in either 0.3 mL (30 U), 0.5 mL (50 U), or 1.0 mL (100 U) size. The advantage of the 0.3 mL and 0.5 mL sizes is that the distance between unit markings is greater, making it easier to measure the dose accurately.

Most insulin syringes are manufactured with the needle permanently attached in a 25 to 27 gauge, 0.5 inch size. If this type of syringe is not available, an insulin syringe and a 25 gauge, 0.5 inch, or 0.75 inch needle should be used.

Other special injection products are available for people with physical handicaps. These products include automatic injectors and jet spray injectors. Prefilled syringes are useful for people who are visually impaired or traveling. Prefilled syringes are stable for up to 30 days if stored in the refrigerator.

Preparing the Injection. The vial of insulin in use may be kept at room temperature for up to 4 weeks. Stored vials should be kept in the refrigerator and brought to room temperature prior to administration.

Regular insulin does not require mixing. If the solution is cloudy or discolored, the vial should be discarded. The other types of insulin must be mixed to disperse the particles evenly throughout the solution. Mix the vial by gently rolling it between the hands; vigorous shaking causes bubble formation and frothing, which makes the dose inaccurate. It is critical that no air bubbles remain in the prepared dose, because even a small bubble can displace several units of insulin.

Sites of Injection. Although in theory any area of the body with subcutaneous tissue may be used for injections of insulin, certain sites are recommended (Figure 18–5 ■). The rate of absorption and peak of action of insulin differs according to the site. The site that allows the most rapid absorption is the abdomen, followed by the deltoid muscle, then the thigh, and then the hip. Because of the rapid absorption, the abdomen is the

Figure 18–5 ■ Sites of insulin injection.

recommended site. See Box 18–2 on techniques to minimize painful injections.

When administering insulin, gently pinch a fold of skin and inject the needle at a 90-degree angle. If the person is very thin, a 45-degree angle may be required to avoid injecting into muscle. Routine aspiration to check for blood is not necessary. Do not massage the site after administering the injection, because this may interfere with absorption; pressure, however, may be applied for about 1 minute. Rotation of injection sites is recommended for clients using pork insulin; rotation within sites is recommended for those using human or purified pork insulin. The distance between injections should be about 1 inch (avoiding the area within a 2-inch radius around the umbilicus). Insulin should not be injected into an area to be exercised (such as the thigh before a vigorous walk) or to which heat will be applied; exercise or heat may increase the rate of absorption and cause a more rapid onset and peak of action.

BOX 18–2	■ Techniques to Minimize Painful Injections

■ Inject insulin that is at room temperature.
■ Make sure no air bubbles remain in the syringe before the injection.
■ Wait until alcohol on the skin completely dries before the injection.
■ Relax muscles in the injection area.
■ Penetrate the skin with the needle quickly.
■ Don't change the direction of the needle during insertion or withdrawal.
■ Don't reuse dull needles.

Note: Adapted from "Insulin Administration" by the American Diabetes Association, 1998, Diabetes Care, 21 (Supplement 1), 572–575.

Lipodystrophy. Lipodystrophy (hypertrophy of subcutaneous tissue) or **lipoatrophy** (atrophy of subcutaneous tissue) may result if the same injection sites are used repeatedly, especially with pork and beef insulins. The tissues become hardened and have an orange-peel appearance. The use of refrigerated insulin may trigger the development of tissue atrophy or hypertrophy. These problems rarely occur with the use of human insulins. Lipodystrophy and lipoatrophy alter insulin absorption, delaying its onset or retaining the insulin in the tissue for a period of time instead of allowing it to be absorbed into the body. Lipodystrophy usually resolves if the area is unused for a minimum of 6 months.

Mixing Insulins. When a person with diabetes requires more than one type of insulin, mixing is recommended to avoid administering two injections per dose. Two different concentrations are administered, because a single dose of intermediate-acting or long-acting insulin rarely provides adequate control of blood glucose levels. The procedure for mixing insulins is described in Box 18–3. Following are some general guidelines.

- Commercially mixed insulins are recommended if the insulin ratio is appropriate for the requirements of the client.
- Regular insulin may be mixed with all other types of insulin; it may be injected immediately after mixing or stored for future use.
- NPH insulin and PZI insulin may be mixed only with regular insulin.

- Lente insulin preparations may be mixed with each other; mixing with regular insulin or with PZI and NPH insulin is not recommended.
- Do not mix human and animal insulins.
- Always withdraw regular insulin first to avoid contaminating the regular insulin with intermediate-acting insulin.

Insulin Regimens. The appropriate insulin dosage is individualized by achieving a balance among insulin, diet, and exercise. For most people with diabetes, the timing of insulin action requires two or more injections each day, often a mixture of rapid-acting and intermediate-acting insulins. Timing of the injections depends on blood glucose levels, food consumption, exercise, and types of insulin used. The objective is to avoid daytime hypoglycemia while achieving adequate blood glucose control overnight. Typical insulin regimens are discussed in Table 18–5.

Hypersensitivity Responses. When injected, insulin may cause local and systemic hypersensitivity responses. Manifestations of local reactions are a hardening and reddening of the area that develops over several hours. Local reactions result from a contaminant in the insulin and are more likely to occur when less purified insulin products are used.

Systemic reactions occur rapidly and are characterized by widespread red, intensely pruritic welts. Respiratory difficulty may occur if the respiratory system is involved. Systemic responses are due to an allergy to the insulin itself and are most

---

BOX 18–3 ■ **Mixing Insulins: 10 Units of Regular and 20 Units of NPH**

1. Wash hands.
2. Inspect regular insulin for clarity.
3. Gently rotate NPH insulin to mix well.
4. Wipe off the top of both vials with an alcohol pad.
5. Draw 20 U of air into the syringe, and inject air into the NPH vial (Figure A). Withdraw needle.
6. Draw 10 U of air into the syringe, and inject air into the regular vial (Figure B).
7. Invert the vial, and withdraw 10 U of regular insulin (Figure C). Withdraw the needle.
8. Insert the needle into the NPH vial, and carefully withdraw 20 U of NPH insulin (Figure D).
9. Administer the insulin.
10. Wash hands, and properly dispose of the syringe.

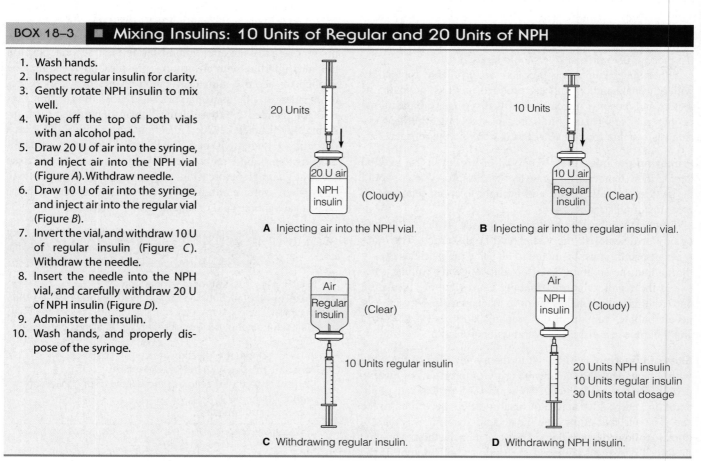

A Injecting air into the NPH vial.

B Injecting air into the regular insulin vial.

C Withdrawing regular insulin.

D Withdrawing NPH insulin.

TABLE 18–5   Insulin Regimens

Regimen	Insulin Type*	General Information
One injection per day	NPH or NPH/R before breakfast	One injection is used to cover all meals (see figure at left). This is a simple regimen, but it is often difficult to control FBG levels, and afternoon hypoglycemia may result from increases in NPH.
Two injections per day	NPH or NPH/R before breakfast and dinner	This regimen is the least complex of those aiming to mimic normal pancreatic function; the person must have a fairly rigid schedule of food intake and exercise.
Three or four injections per day	R before each meal; NPH at dinner or bedtime	This regimen more closely mimics normal pancreatic function; it allows greater choice in mealtimes and exercise (see figure at left). However, each preprandial dose of R must be determined by blood glucose tests.

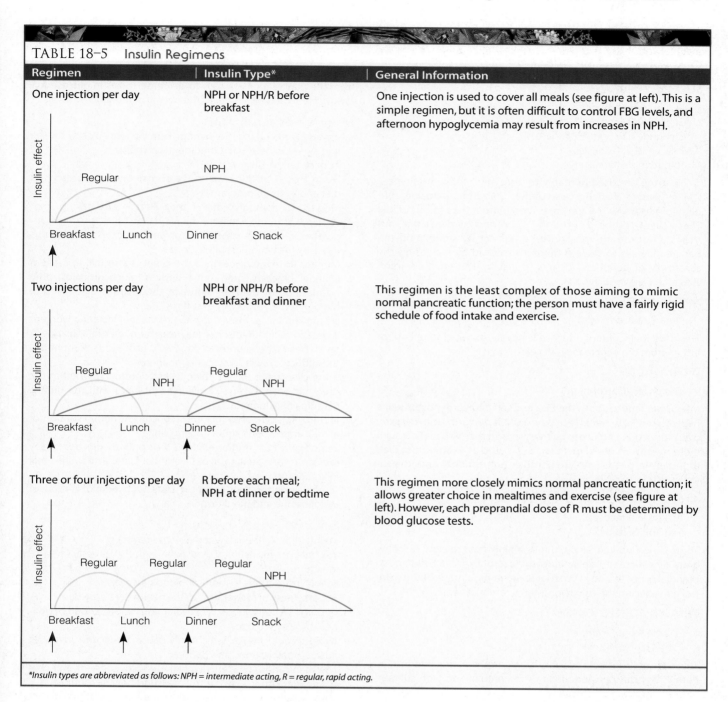

*Insulin types are abbreviated as follows: NPH = intermediate acting, R = regular, rapid acting.

common with beef insulin. The client can be desensitized by administering small doses of purified pork or human insulin, followed by progressively larger doses.

Oral Hypoglycemic Agents

Oral hypoglycemic agents are used to treat people with type 2 DM. Nursing implications for this category of drugs are discussed in the Medication Administration box on page 492.

Aspirin Therapy

People with diabetes are up to 4 times more likely to die from cardiovascular disease. It is recommended that a once daily dose of 75 to 325 mg of enteric-coated aspirin be given to re-duce atherosclerosis in clients with vascular disease or increased cardiovascular risk factors. Aspirin therapy is contraindicated for clients with aspirin allergy, bleeding tendency, recent gastrointestinal bleeding, or active liver disease.

Diet Therapy

The management of diabetes requires a careful balance between the intake of nutrients, the expenditure of energy, and the dose and timing of insulin or oral antidiabetic agents. Although everyone has the same need for basic nutrition, the person with diabetes must eat a more structured diet to prevent hyperglycemia. The goals for dietary management for adults with

Medication Administration

Oral Hypoglycemic Agents

SULFONYLUREAS

Glimepiride (Amaryl)
Glipizide (Glucotrol, Glucotrol XL)
Glyburide (Diaβeta, Micronase)
Tolazamide (Tolinase)
Tolbutamide (Orinase)

These drugs are used primarily to treat mild, nonketotic type 2 DM in people who are not obese. Glyburide, glipizide, and glimepiride are 100 to 200 times more potent than tolbutamide. These clients cannot control the symptoms by diet alone, but they do not require insulin. The drugs act by stimulating the pancreatic cells to secrete more insulin and by increasing the sensitivity of peripheral tissues to insulin. The most common side effect is hypoglycemia.

MEGLITINIDES

Repaglinide (Prandin)

This drug lowers blood glucose levels by stimulating release of insulin from the pancreatic islet cells.

BIGUANIDES

Metformin (Glucophage)

Metformin reduces both the FBG and the degree of postprandial hyperglycemia in clients with type 2 DM. It primarily decreases the overproduction of glucose by the liver, and may also make insulin more effective in peripheral tissues. It is used as an adjunct to diet, especially in clients who are obese or not responding to the sufonylureas.

ALPHA-GLUCOSIDE INHIBITORS

Acarbose (Precose)
Miglitol (Glyset)

These drugs work locally in the small intestine to slow carbohydrate digestion and delay glucose absorption. As a result, postprandial glucose and glycosylated hemoglobin are better controlled, reducing the risk of long-term complications.

THIAZOLIDINEDIONES

Rosiglitazone (Avandia)
Pioglitazone (Actos)

This class of drugs acts by sensitizing peripheral tissue to insulin. Both drugs can be used alone or in combination with sulfonylureas, metformin, and insulin.

D-PHENYLALANINE (AMINO ACID) DERIVATIVE

Netaglinide (Starlix)

This is the first in a new class of oral medications for treatment of type 2 diabetes. It stimulates rapid and short insulin secretion from the pancreatic beta cells to decrease spikes in glucose following meals and also reduces the overall blood glucose level.

Nursing Responsibilities

- Assess clients taking oral hypoglycemic agents closely for the first 7 days to determine therapeutic response.
- Administer the drug with food.
- Teach the client the importance of maintaining a prescribed diet and exercise program.
- Monitor for hypoglycemia if the client is also taking nonsteroidal anti-inflammatory agents (NSAIDs), sulfonamide antibiotics, ranitidine, cimetidine, or beta blockers; these drugs intensify the action of sulfonylureas.
- Monitor for hyperglycemia if the client is also taking calcium channel blockers, oral contraceptives, glucocorticoids, phenothiazines, or thiazide diuretics; these drugs decrease the hypoglycemic responses to sulfonylureas.
- Do not administer these drugs to pregnant or lactating women.
- Assess for side effects: nausea, heartburn, diarrhea, dizziness, fever, headache, jaundice, skin rash, urticaria, photophobia, thrombocytopenia, leukopenia, or anemia.
- If the client is to have a thyroid test, determine whether the drug has been taken; sulfonylureas interfere with the uptake of radioactive iodine.
- Monitor for hypoglycemia with concurrent administration of an oral antidiabetic agent and insulin.
- Temporarily hold metformin for 2 days prior to injection of any radiocontrast agent to avoid potential lactic acidosis if renal failure occurs.
- Closely monitor liver function tests with administration of rosiglitazone and pioglitazone.

Client and Family Teaching

- Maintain prescribed diet and exercise regimen.
- You may need insulin if you have surgery, trauma, fever, or infection.
- Follow instructions to monitor blood glucose.
- Report illness or side effects to the health care provider.
- Undergo periodic laboratory evaluations as prescribed by your health care provider.
- Avoid alcohol intake, which may cause a reaction involving flushing, palpitations, and nausea.
- The medication interferes with the effectiveness of oral contraceptives; other birth control measures may be required.
- Mild symptoms of hyperglycemia may appear if a different agent is begun.
- Take medications as prescribed; for example, once a day at the same time each day. If you are taking acarbose, take the pill with the first bite of food at breakfast, lunch, and dinner.

---

diabetes, based on guidelines established by the ADA (2002), are as follows:

- Maintain as near normal blood glucose levels as possible by balancing food intake with insulin or oral glucose.
- Achieve optimal serum lipid levels.
- Provide adequate calories to maintain or attain reasonable weights, and to recover from catabolic illness.

- Prevent and treat the acute complications of insulin-treated DM, short-term illnesses, and exercise-related problems; or the long-term complications of diabetes.
- Improve overall health through optimal nutrition, using Dietary Guidelines for Americans and the food guide pyramid (see Chapter 2). ∞

Carbohydrates

The ADA recommends that carbohydrates should be individualized to the client's needs, with the combination of carbohydrates and monosaturated fats constituting 60% to 70% of the daily diet. Carbohydrates contain 4 kcal per gram. This group of nutrients consists of plant foods (grains, fruits, vegetables), milk, and some dairy products. Carbohydrates can be divided into simple sugars and complex carbohydrates. Despite a long-held belief, research does not support that sugars are more rapidly digested and therefore aggravate hyperglycemia. Fruits and milk have a lower glycemic response than most starches, and the glycemic response of sucrose is similar to that of bread, rice, and potatoes (ADA, 2002)

The use of sucrose as part of the total carbohydrate content in the diet does not impair blood glucose control in people with diabetes. Sucrose and sucrose-containing foods must be substituted for other carbohydrates gram for gram. Dietary fructose (from fruits and vegetables or from fructose-sweetened foods) produces a smaller rise in plasma glucose than sucrose and most starches, so it may offer an advantage as a sweetening agent. However, large amounts of fructose have potentially adverse effects on serum cholesterol and LDL cholesterol, so amounts used should be controlled.

Protein

The recommended daily protein intake is 15% to 20% of total daily kcal intake. Protein has 4 kcal per gram. Sources of protein should be low in fat, low in saturated fat, and low in cholesterol. Although this amount of protein is much less than that which most people normally consume, it is recommended to help prevent or delay renal complications. To help the client accept the decrease in the amount of protein, the nurse may suggest a less severe restriction at diagnosis with a gradual decrease to take place over a period of years.

Fats

Dietary fats should be low in saturated fat and cholesterol. Saturated fats should be no higher than 10% of the total kcal allowed per day, with dietary cholesterol less than 300 mg per day. Fat has 9 kcal per gram. Sources of the different types of fat include:

- *Saturated fat.* Sources are animal meats (meat and butter fats, lard, bacon), cocoa butter, coconut oil, palm oil, and hydrogenated oils.
- *Polyunsaturated fat.* Sources are oils of corn, safflower, sunflower, soybean, sesame seed, and cottonseed.
- *Monosaturated fat.* Sources are peanut oil, olive oil, and canola oil.

Limiting fat and cholesterol intake may help prevent or delay the onset of atherosclerosis, a common complication of diabetes.

Fiber

Dietary fiber may be helpful in treating or preventing constipation and other gastrointestinal disorders, including colon cancer. It also helps provide a feeling of fullness, and large amounts of soluble fiber may be beneficial to serum lipids. Soluble fiber is found in dried beans, oats, barley, and in some vegetables and fruits (e.g., peas, corn, zucchini, cauliflower, broccoli, prunes, pears, apples, bananas, oranges). Insoluble fiber, which is found in wheat, corn, and in some vegetables and fruits (e.g., carrots, brussels sprouts, eggplant, green beans, pears, apples, strawberries), does facilitate intestinal motility and give a feeling of fullness.

The ideal level of fiber has not been determined, but an intake of 20 to 35 g per day is recommended. An increase in fiber may cause nausea, diarrhea or constipation, and increased flatulence, especially if the person does not also increase fluid intake. Fiber in the diet should therefore be increased gradually.

Sodium

Although the body requires sodium, most people consume much more than is needed each day, especially in processed foods. The recommended daily intake is 1000 mg of sodium per 1000 kcal, not to exceed 3000 mg. The primary concern with sodium is its association with hypertension, a common health problem in people with diabetes. It is suggested that table salt (which is 40% sodium) and processed foods high in sodium be avoided in the diabetes meal plan.

Sweeteners

The diet plan for people with diabetes restricts the amount of refined sugars. As a result, many people use noncaloric sweeteners and foods or drinks made with noncaloric sweeteners. Commercially produced nonnutritive sweeteners are approved for use by the Food and Drug Administration (FDA). Although questions have been raised about the safety of these substances in laboratory animal studies, they are considered safe for use by humans. Included in this category of sweeteners are saccharin (Sweet & Low), aspartame (Nutrasweet, Equal), and acesulfame potassium (Sunnette). The nonnutritive sweeteners have negligent amounts of or no kilocalories and produce very little or no changes in blood glucose levels.

People with diabetes also use nutritive sweeteners, including fructose, sorbitol, and xylitol. The kcal content of these substances is similar to that of table sugar (sucrose), but they cause less elevation in blood glucose. They are often included in foods labeled as "sugar free." Sorbitol may cause flatulence and diarrhea.

Researchers are continuing to study the safety and effectiveness of the sweeteners. In addition, the FDA recommends that the food industry label products with the amount of each ingredient in milligrams per serving and the number of servings per container. When teaching clients about diet, the nurse should include information about the kilocalorie content of sweeteners and the meaning of such words as sugar free and dietetic on labels.

Alcohol

Although drinking alcoholic beverages is not encouraged, neither is it totally prohibited for the client with diabetes. Alcohol consumption may potentiate the hypoglycemic effects of insulin and oral agents. The ADA recommends that men with diabetes consume no more than two drinks and women with diabetes no more than one drink per day. In the following list are guidelines for people who include alcohol in their diet plan.

- The signs of intoxication and hypoglycemia are similar; thus, the person with type 1 DM is at increased risk for an insulin reaction.
- Two oral hypoglycemic agents (chlorpropamide and tolbutamide) may interact with the alcohol, causing headache, flushing, and nausea.
- Liqueurs, sweet wines, wine coolers, and sweet mixes contain large amounts of carbohydrate.
- Light beer is the recommended alcoholic drink.
- Alcohol should be consumed with meals and added to the daily food intake. In most instances, the alcohol is substituted for fat in calculating the diet; a drink with 1.5 oz of alcohol is the equivalent of two fat exchanges (90 kcal). (Food exchanges are discussed below.)

Meal Planning

Several different systems for meal planning are available to the person with diabetes. These systems include a consistent-carbohydrate diabetes meal plan, exchange lists, point systems, food groups, and calorie counting. No matter what system is used, however, it must take into account the person's individualized eating habits, diet history, food values, and special needs. Altering foods and meal patterns are often one of the most difficult parts of diabetes management; careful consideration of individualized preferences enhances compliance with the diet. Although the ADA recommends that a registered dietitian provide the nutrition prescription, nurses must know what is prescribed and be able to reinforce teaching and answer questions.

THE CONSISTENT-CARBOHYDRATE DIABETES MEAL PLAN.
The consistent-carbohydrate diabetes meal plan, which is replacing the traditional exchange list plan, focuses on carbohydrate content. The client eats a similar amount of carbohydrates at each meal or snack each day, based on an individual diet prescription and the food guide pyramid. Carbohydrates in a meal have the most effect on postprandial (after meals) blood glucose levels. They also determine, to a greater extent than do proteins and fats, insulin requirements before meals. Clients should be taught to count carbohydrates so they can administer 1 unit of regular insulin or insulin lispro for each 10 or 15 g of carbohydrate eaten at a meal. This method provides a better connection between food, medications, and exercise.

THE EXCHANGE LISTS.
The exchange list diet is based on the person's ideal (or reasonable) weight, activity level, age, and occupation. These factors determine the total kilocalories that the person may consume each day. After the calories have been determined, the proportions of carbohydrates, proteins, and fats are calculated, using guidelines established by the American Diabetes Association and the American Dietetic Association.

The distribution of foods throughout the day is based on exchange lists. The name and quantity of food that make up one exchange (or serving) are listed; standard household measurements are used. One food portion on the list can be substituted ("exchanged") for another with very little difference in calories or amount of carbohydrates, proteins, and fats. The meal plan prescribes how many exchanges are allowed for each food group per meal and snacks.

DIET PLAN FOR TYPE 1 DIABETES.
Diet and insulin prescription must be integrated for optimal energy metabolism and the prevention of hyperglycemia or hypoglycemia. The goals of the diet plan are to achieve optimal glucose and lipid levels, improve overall health, and maintain reasonable body weight. To meet these goals, the following strategies must be implemented.

- Glucose regulation requires correlating eating patterns with insulin onset and peak of action.
- Meals, snacks, and insulin regimens should be based on the person's lifestyle.
- Meal planning depends on the specific insulin regimen prescribed.
- Snacks are an important consideration in relation to the amount and timing of exercise.
- The diet plan must consider the availability of foods, based on occupational, financial, religious, and ethnic constraints.
- Self-monitoring of blood glucose levels helps the client make adjustments for planned and unplanned changes in routines.

DIET PLAN FOR TYPE 2 DIABETES.
The goals of the diet plan are to improve blood glucose levels, improve overall health, prevent or delay complications, and attain or maintain reasonable body weight. Because the majority of these clients are overweight, weight loss is important and facilitates achieving the other goals.

There are no specific guidelines for the type 2 diet, but in addition to decreasing kilocalories, it is recommended that the client consume three meals of equal size, evenly spaced approximately 4 to 5 hours apart, with one or two snacks. The person with type 2 DM should also decrease fat intake. If the exchange list is difficult to use, calorie counting or designing the diet by grams of fat may be more useful.

Sick-Day Management

When the person with diabetes is sick or has surgery, blood glucose levels increase, even though food intake decreases. The person often mistakenly alters or omits the insulin dose, causing further problems. The guidelines for dietary management during illness focus on preventing dehydration and providing nutrition for promoting recovery. In general, sick-day management includes the following:

- Monitoring blood glucose at least four times a day throughout an illness
- Testing urine for ketones if blood glucose is greater than 240 mg/dL
- Continuing to take the usual insulin dose or oral hypoglycemic agent
- Sipping 8 to 12 oz of fluid each hour
- Substituting easily digested liquids or soft foods if solid foods are not tolerated (The substituted liquids and foods should be carbohydrate equivalents, for example, 1/2 cup sweetened gelatin, 1/2 cup fruit juice, one Popsicle, 1/4 cup sherbet, and 1/2 cup regular soft drink.)
- Calling the health care provider if the client is unable to eat for more than 24 hours or if vomiting and diarrhea last for more than 6 hours.

Diet Plan for the Older Adult

The majority of older adults have type 2 DM and should follow the general guidelines for that diet plan. However, special considerations for the older adult are important if the diet plan is to be followed, including:

- Dietary likes and dislikes
- Who prepares the meals
- Age-related changes in taste perception
- Dental health
- Transportation to buy foods
- Available income

Other factors to consider in planning the diet for the older adult include the age-related decline in kcal requirements, decline in physical activity due to age and/or chronic illnesses, and the onset or progression of other chronic illnesses. The older adult who is overweight should reduce kcal intake to ensure weight loss, but at the same time, careful monitoring for malnutrition is necessary. It is possible for the older adult to revert to normal glucose tolerance if ideal body weight is regained.

Exercise

The third component of diabetes management is a regular exercise program. The benefits of exercise are the same for everyone, with or without diabetes: improved physical fitness, improved emotional state, weight control, and improved work capacity. In people with diabetes, exercise increases the uptake of glucose by muscle cells, potentially reducing the need for insulin. Exercise also decreases cholesterol and triglycerides, reducing the risk of cardiovascular disorders. People with diabetes should consult their primary health care provider before beginning or changing an exercise program. The ability to maintain an exercise program is affected by many different factors, including fatigue and glucose levels. It is as important to assess the person's usual lifestyle before establishing an exercise program as it is before planning a diet. Factors to consider include the client's usual exercise habits, living environment, and community programs. The exercise that the person enjoys most is probably the one that he or she will continue throughout life.

All people with diabetes should follow the recommendations of the ADA when exercising: Use proper footwear, inspect the feet daily and after exercise, avoid exercise in extreme heat or cold, and avoid exercise during periods of poor glucose control. The ADA further recommends that people over age 35 have an exercise-stress electrocardiogram prior to beginning an exercise program.

Type 1 Diabetes

In the person with type 1 DM, glycemic responses to exercise vary according to the type, intensity, and duration of the exercise. Other factors that influence responses include the timing of exercise in relation to meals and insulin injections, and the time of day of the activity. Unless these factors are integrated into the exercise program, the person with type 1 DM has an increased risk of hypoglycemia and hyperglycemia. Following are general guidelines for an exercise program.

- People who have frequent hyperglycemia or hypoglycemia should avoid prolonged exercise until glucose control improves.
- The risk of exercise-induced hypoglycemia is lowest before breakfast, when free-insulin levels tend to be lower than they are before meals later in the day or at bedtime.
- Low-impact aerobic exercises are encouraged.
- Exercise should be moderate and regular; brief, intense exercise tends to cause mild hyperglycemia, and prolonged exercise can lead to hypoglycemia.
- Exercising at a peak insulin action time may lead to hypoglycemia.
- Self-monitoring of blood glucose levels is essential both before and after exercise.
- Food intake may need to be increased to compensate for the activity.
- Fluid intake, especially water, is essential.

Young adults may continue participating in sports with some modifications in diet and insulin dosage. Athletes should begin training slowly, extend activity over a prolonged period, take a carbohydrate source (such as a drink consisting of 5% to 10% carbohydrate) after about 1 hour of exercise, and monitor blood glucose levels for possible adjustments. In addition, a snack should be available after the activity is completed. It may be necessary to omit the usual regular insulin dose prior to an athletic event; even if the athlete is hyperglycemic at the beginning of the event, blood glucose levels will fall to normal after the first 60 to 90 minutes of exercise.

Type 2 Diabetes

An exercise program for the person with type 2 DM is especially important. The benefits of regular exercise include weight loss in those who are overweight, improved glycemic control, increased well-being, socialization with others, and a reduction of cardiovascular risk factors. A combination of diet, exercise, and weight loss often decreases the need for oral hypoglycemic agents. This decrease is due to an increased sensitivity to insulin, increased kcal expenditure, and increased self-esteem. Regular exercise may prevent type 2 DM in high-risk individuals (ADA, 2002).

Following are general guidelines for an exercise program.

- Before beginning the program, have a medical screening for previously undiagnosed hypertension, neuropathy, retinopathy, nephropathy, and cardiac ischemia.
- Begin the program with mild exercises, and gradually increase intensity and duration.
- Self-monitor blood glucose before and after exercise.
- Exercise at least three times a week or every other day, for at least 20 to 30 minutes.
- Include muscle-strengthening and low-impact aerobic exercises in the program.

Treatments

Surgery

Surgical management of diabetes involves replacing or transplanting the pancreas, pancreatic cells, or beta cells. Although it is still in the investigative stage, many researchers believe that transplantation of the tail of the pancreas is the most promising technique for achieving long-term disease control. Islet cell transplantation has had moderate success, and research is continuing. Other research is being conducted in the use of an internally implanted artificial pancreas, or closed-loop artificial beta cell.

Surgery is a stressor that often alters self-management and glycemic control in people with diabetes. In response to stress, levels of catecholamines, cortisol, glucagon, and growth hormones increase, as does insulin resistance. Hyperglycemia occurs, and protein stores are decreased. In addition, diet and activity patterns change, and medication types and dosages vary. As a result, surgical clients who have diabetes are at increased risk for postoperative infection, delayed wound healing, fluid and electrolyte imbalances, hypoglycemia, and DKA.

Preoperatively, all clients should be in the best possible metabolic state. Screening for complications and regular blood glucose monitoring are part of preoperative preparation. Oral hypoglycemic agents may be withheld for 1 or 2 days before surgery, and regular insulin is often administered to the client with type 2 DM during the perioperative period. The client with type 1 DM follows a carefully prescribed insulin regimen individualized to specific needs.

The insulin regimen in the preoperative, intraoperative, and immediate postoperative periods is individualized and may involve any of the following:

- No intermediate- or long-acting insulin is given the day of surgery; regular insulin is given with intravenous glucose.
- Half of the usual intermediate- or long-acting insulin is given before surgery and the remaining half is given in the recovery room.
- The total daily dose of insulin is divided into four equal doses of regular insulin, and one dose is administered subcutaneously every 6 hours. An intravenous solution of 5% dextrose in 0.45% normal saline is administered for fluid replacement, and blood glucose monitoring precedes each insulin dose (Guthrie & Guthrie, 1997).

The surgical procedure should be scheduled for as early as possible in the morning to minimize the length of fasting. If there is no food intake after surgery, intravenous dextrose should be administered, accompanied by subcutaneous regular insulin every 6 hours. The dose can be adjusted to blood glucose levels. Although kcal intake is decreased postoperatively, stress can increase insulin requirements. Glucose control is also affected postoperatively by nausea and vomiting, anorexia, and gastrointestinal suction.

During the postoperative period, the client with type 2 DM may continue to require insulin or may resume oral medications, depending on glucose control. The client with type 1 DM may require reduced insulin as healing progresses and stress diminishes. Regular blood glucose monitoring is essential, as are assessments for hypoglycemia.

Treatment of Hypoglycemia

MILD HYPOGLYCEMIA. When mild hypoglycemia occurs, immediate treatment is necessary. People experiencing hypo-

glycemia should take about 15 g of a rapid-acting sugar. This amount of sugar is found, for example, in three glucose tablets, 1/2 cup of fruit juice or regular soda, 8 oz of skim milk, five Life Savers candies, three large marshmallows, or 3 tsp of sugar or honey. Sugar should not be added to fruit juice. Adding sugar to the fruit sugar already in the juice could cause a rapid rise in blood glucose, with persistent hyperglycemia.

If the manifestations continue, the 15/15 rule should be followed: Wait 15 minutes, monitor blood glucose, and, if it is low, eat another 15 g of carbohydrate. This procedure can be repeated until blood glucose levels return to normal (Haire-Joshu, 1996). People with diabetes should have some source of carbohydrate readily available at all times so that hypoglycemic symptoms can be quickly reversed. If hypoglycemia occurs more than two or three times a week, the diabetes management plan should be adjusted.

SEVERE HYPOGLYCEMIA. People with diabetes who have severe hypoglycemia are often hospitalized. The criteria for hospitalization are one or more of the following:

- Blood glucose is less than 50 mg/dL, and the prompt treatment of hypoglycemia has not resulted in recovery of sensorium.
- The client has coma, seizures, or altered behavior.
- The hypoglycemia has been treated, but a responsible adult cannot be with the client for the following 12 hours.
- The hypoglycemia was caused by a sulfonylurea drug.

If the client is conscious and alert, 10 to 15 g of an oral carbohydrate may be given. If the client has altered levels of consciousness, parenteral glucose or glucagon is administered.

Glucose is administered intravenously as a 25% to 50% solution, usually at a rate of 10 mL over 1 minute by intravenous push, followed by intravenous infusion of 5% dextrose in water (D5W) at 5 to 10 g/h (Haire-Joshu, 1996). This is the most rapid method of increasing blood glucose levels.

Glucagon is an antihypoglycemic agent that raises blood glucose by promoting the conversion of hepatic glycogen to glucose. It is used in severe insulin-induced hypoglycemia and may be given in the recommended dose of 1 mg by the subcutaneous, intramuscular, or intravenous route. Glucagon has a short period of action; an oral (if the client is conscious) or intravenous carbohydrate should be administered following the glucagon to prevent a recurrence of hypoglycemia. If the client has been unconscious, glucagon may cause vomiting when consciousness returns.

Treatment of DKA

DKA requires immediate medical attention. Admission to the hospital is appropriate when the person has a blood glucose of greater than 250 mg/dL, a decreasing pH, and ketones in the urine. If the client is alert and conscious, fluids may be replaced orally. However, alterations in levels of consciousness, vomiting, and acidosis are common, necessitating intravenous fluid replacement. The initial fluid replacement may be accomplished by administering 0.9% saline solution at a rate of 500 to 1000 mL/h. After 2 to 3 hours (or when blood pressure is returning to normal), the administration of 0.45% saline at

Medication Administration

Intravenous Insulin

General Guidelines

- Regular insulin may be given undiluted directly into the vein or through a Y-tube or three-way stopcock.
- Insulin is usually diluted in 0.9% saline or 0.45% saline solution for infusion.
- The glass or plastic infusion container and plastic tubing may reduce insulin potency by at least 20% and possibly by up to 80% before the insulin reaches the venous system.

Nursing Responsibilities

- Monitor blood glucose levels hourly.

- Infuse the insulin solution separately from the hydration solution.
- Flush the intravenous tubing with 50 mL of insulin mixed with normal saline solution to saturate binding sites on the tubing before administering the insulin to the client; this step increases the amount of insulin delivered over the first few hours.
- Do not discontinue the intravenous infusion until subcutaneous administration of insulin is resumed.
- Monitor for manifestations of hypoglycemia.
- Ensure that glucagon is readily available as an antidote for insulin overdose.

200 to 500 mL/h may continue for several more hours. When the blood glucose levels reach 250 mg/dL, dextrose is added to prevent rapid decreases in glucose; hypoglycemia could result in fatal cerebral edema.

Regular insulin is used in the management of DKA and may be given by various routes, depending on the severity of the condition. Mild ketosis may be treated with subcutaneous insulin, whereas severe ketosis requires intravenous insulin infusion. Nursing responsibilities for the client receiving intravenous insulin are described in the Medication Administration box above.

The electrolyte imbalance of primary concern is depletion of body stores of potassium. Initially, serum potassium levels may be normal, but they decrease during treatment. In DKA (and from rehydration), the body loses potassium from increased urinary output, acidosis, catabolic state, and vomiting or diarrhea. Potassium replacement is begun early in the course of treatment, usually by adding potassium to the rehydration fluids. Replacement is essential for preventing cardiac dysrhythmias secondary to hypokalemia. Cardiac rhythms and potassium levels must be monitored every 2 to 4 hours.

Treatment of HHS

HHS is a serious, life-threatening metabolic condition. The client admitted to the intensive care unit for treatment typically manifests blood glucose levels over 700 mg/dL, increased serum osmolarity, and altered levels of consciousness or seizures. Treatment is similar to that of DKA: correcting fluid and electrolyte imbalances and providing insulin to lower hyperglycemia. In general, treatment modalities include the following:

- Establishing and maintaining adequate ventilation
- Correcting shock with adequate intravenous fluids
- Instituting nasogastric suction if comatose to prevent aspiration
- Maintaining fluid volume with intravenous isotonic or colloid solutions
- Administering potassium intravenously to replace losses
- Administering insulin to reduce blood glucose, usually discontinuing administration when blood glucose levels reach 250 mg/dL (Because ketosis is not present, there is no need to continue insulin, as with DKA.)

NURSING CARE

The responses of the person with diabetes to the illness are often complex and individual, involving multiple body systems. Assessments, planning, and implementation differ for the person with newly diagnosed diabetes, the person with long-term diabetes, and the person with acute complications of diabetes. The plan of care and content of teaching also differ according to the type of diabetes, the person's age and culture, and the person's intellectual, psychological, and social resources. However, nursing care often focuses on teaching the client to manage the illness. The Nursing Research box on the following page describes a study of quality of life in people with diabetes.

Health Promotion

Health promotion activities primarily focus on preventing the complications of diabetes. The prevention of the disease has not been determined, although it is recommended that all people should prevent or decrease excess weight, follow a sensible and well-balanced diet, and maintain a regular physical exercise program. Blood glucose screening at 3-year intervals beginning at age 45 is recommended for those in the high-risk groups. These same activities, when combined with medications and self-monitoring, are also beneficial in reducing the onset of complications.

Assessment

The following data are collected through the health history and physical examination (see Chapter 16). ⊖ Further focused assessments are described with nursing interventions below. When assessing the older client, be aware of normal aging changes in all body systems that may alter interpretation of findings.

- Health history: Family history of diabetes; history of hypertension or other cardiovascular problems; history of any change in vision (e.g. blurring) or speech, dizziness, numbness or tingling in hands or feet; pain when walking; frequent voiding; change in weight, appetite, infections, and healing; problems with gastrointestinal function or urination; or altered sexual function

Nursing Research

Evidence-Based Practice for Balancing Quality of Life and Living with Diabetes

Adaptation to and management of a chronic illness such as diabetes are simultaneous and interdependent as the person comes to term with the illness, gains support from caregivers, creates relationships with others, and learns about the illness and its management. This study (Paterson et al., 1998) examined 43 published qualitative reports of the experience of living with diabetes to formulate a comparative analysis of findings. Balance emerged as the predominant metaphor of the experience; to achieve balance the person must learn how to manage the illness, know the body, and foster supportive, collaborative relationships. Although control of blood glucose levels may be a goal established by health care professionals, the research reviewed for this study indicates that a goal of healthy balance more accurately explains peoples' willingness to take part in self-management of diabetes.

IMPLICATIONS FOR NURSING

All teaching plans should be individualized and developed in collaboration with the client. Nurses often focus on diabetes management and control, especially compliance with prescribed regimens. Although clients are sometimes termed "noncompliant," this term conveys judgment about dependence. A focus on balance instead of control may well facilitate new understanding of behavior demonstrated as the client seeks to assert self-control. It is important to also understand that self-control behaviors can change with variations in life and the disease itself, and that each person with diabetes responds uniquely to situations and interventions. Respecting and valuing what a person has learned from living with diabetes is critical to providing effective care.

Critical Thinking in Client Care

1. You are caring for two clients with diabetes who are receiving home care for complications of long-term diabetes. One client follows the medical regimen faithfully, the other adapts it to his own schedule and needs. What differences can you identify in your own reaction to these two different clients? How would these reactions affect your relationship with the clients?
2. Imagine you have just been diagnosed with type 1 diabetes. Make a list of the questions you would have and the areas that would cause you the most difficulty in complying with your medical care.
3. How would you respond if your client tells you, "Sometimes I eat whatever I want to for several days." What do you think this behavior indicates?

TYPE 2 DIABETES CARE PLAN

MediaLink

- Physical assessment: Height/weight ratio, vital signs, visual acuity, cranial nerves, sensory ability (touch, hot/cold, vibration) of extremities, peripheral pulses, skin and mucous membranes (hair loss, appearance, lesions, rash, itching, vaginal discharge)

Nursing Diagnoses and Interventions

Although many different nursing diagnoses are appropriate for the person with diabetes, those discussed in this section address problems with skin integrity, infection, injury, sexuality, coping, and health maintenance. The goals of care are to maintain function, prevent complications, and teach self-management.

Risk for Impaired Skin Integrity

The person with diabetes is at increased risk for altered skin integrity as a result of decreased or absent sensation from neuropathies, decreased tissue perfusion from cardiovascular complications, and infection. In addition, poor vision increases the risk of trauma, and an open lesion is more prone to infection and delayed healing. Impaired skin and tissue integrity, with resultant gangrene, is especially common in the feet and lower extremities.

- Conduct baseline and ongoing assessments of the feet, including:
  - Musculoskeletal assessment that includes foot and ankle joint range of motion, bone abnormalities (bunions, hammertoes, overlapping digits), gait patterns, use of assistive devices for walking, and abnormal wear patterns on shoes.
  - Neurologic assessment that includes sensations of touch and position, pain, and temperature.

- Vascular examination that includes assessment of lower-extremity pulses, capillary refill, color and temperature of skin, lesions, and edema.
- Hydration status, including dryness or excessive perspiration.
- Lesions, fissures between toes, corns, calluses, plantar warts, ingrown or overgrown toenails, redness over pressure points, blisters, cellulitis, or gangrene.

People with diabetes are at significant risk for lower-extremity gangrene. Peripheral neuropathies may result in alterations in the perception of pain, loss of deep tendon reflexes, loss of cutaneous pressure and position sensation, foot drop, changes in the shape of the foot, and changes in bones and joints. Peripheral vascular disease may cause intermittent claudication, absent pulses, delayed venous filling on elevation, dependent rubor, and gangrene. Injuries, lesions, and changes in skin hydration potentiate infections, delayed healing, and tissue loss in the person with diabetes mellitus.

- Teach foot hygiene. Wash the feet daily with lukewarm water and mild hand soap; pat dry, and dry well between the toes. Apply a very thin coat of lubricating cream if dryness is present (but not between the toes). *Proper hygiene decreases the chance of infection. Temperature receptors may be impaired, so the water should always be tested before use.*

PRACTICE ALERT *Teach the person with diabetes to always test the water temperature in the shower or bath before stepping in.* ∎

- Discuss the importance of not smoking if client smokes. *Nicotine in tobacco causes vasoconstriction, further decreasing the blood supply to the feet.*

Meeting Individualized Needs: Foot Care Teaching Session

BUYING AND WEARING SHOES AND STOCKINGS

- Shoes that allow 1/2 to 3/4 inch of toe room are best; there should be room for toes to spread out and wiggle. The lining and inside stitching should be smooth, and the insole soft. The sole should be flexible and cushion the foot. The heel should fit snugly, and the arch support should give good support.
- Do not wear open-toed shoes, sandals, high heels, or thongs; they increase the risk of trauma.
- Buy shoes late in the afternoon, when feet are at their largest; always buy shoes that feel comfortable and do not need to be "broken in."
- Shoes made of natural fibers (leather, canvas) allow perspiration to escape.
- Check the shoes before each wearing for foreign objects, wrinkled insoles, and cracks that might cause lesions.
- Stockings made of wool or cotton allow perspiration to dry.
- Do not wear garters, knee stockings, or panty hose; they may interfere with circulation.
- Wear insulated boots in the winter.

INSPECTING THE FEET

- Check the feet daily for red areas, cuts, blisters, corns, calluses, or cracks in the skin. Check between the toes for cracks or reddened areas.
- Check the skin of the feet for dry or damp areas.
- Use a mirror to check each sole and the back of each heel.
- If you are unable to inspect the feet daily, be sure that someone else does so.

CARE OF TOENAILS

- Cut the toenails after washing, when they are softer and easier to trim.
- Cut the nails straight across with a clipper, and smooth edges and corners with an emery board.
- Do not use razor blades to trim the toenails.
- If you are unable to see well or to reach the feet easily, have someone else trim the nails. If the nails are very thick or ingrown, if the toes overlap, or if circulation is poor, get professional care.

GENERAL INFORMATION

- Never go barefoot. Wear slippers when leaving the bed during the night.
- Do not use commercial corn medicines or pads, chemicals (such as boric acid, iodine, or hydrogen peroxide), or over-the-counter cortisone medications on the feet.
- Do not put heating pads, hot water bottles, or ice packs on the feet. If the feet become cold at night, wear socks or use extra blankets.
- Do not allow the feet to become sunburned.
- Do not put tape on the feet.
- Do not sit with the legs crossed at the knees or ankles.

- Discuss the importance of maintaining blood glucose levels through prescribed diet, medication, and exercise. *Hyperglycemia promotes the growth of microorganisms.*
- Conduct foot care teaching sessions as often as necessary (see the box above). Include information about proper shoe fit and composition, avoiding clothing or activities that decrease circulation to the feet, foot inspections, the care of toenails, and the importance of obtaining medical care for lesions. If the person has visual deficits, is obese, or cannot reach the feet, teach the caregiver how to inspect and care for the feet. Feet should be inspected daily. *Foot care is a priority in diabetes management to prevent serious problems. Many people with diabetes are unaware of lesions or injury until infection and compromised circulation are far advanced. The hows and whys of each component must be included in teaching. A variety of methods may be used, including demonstration, return demonstration, audiovisual aids, and written lists. If the person is wearing shoes and socks, ask him or her to remove them to practice foot care effectively.*

PRACTICE ALERT *Suggest the use of a hand mirror to check the bottom of the feet and the back of the heel.* ■

Risk for Infection

The person with diabetes is at increased risk for infection. The risk of infection is believed to be due to vascular insufficiency that limits the inflammatory response, neurologic abnormalities that limit the awareness of trauma, and a predisposition to bacterial and fungal infections.

- Use and teach meticulous handwashing. *Handwashing is the single most effective method for preventing the spread of infection.*
- Monitor for manifestations of infection: increased temperature, pain, malaise, swelling, redness, discharge, cough. *Early diagnosis and treatment of infections can control their severity and decrease complications.*
- Discuss the importance of skin care. Keep the skin clean and dry, using lukewarm water and mild soap. *People with diabetes are more prone to develop furuncles and carbuncles; the infection often increases the need for insulin. Clean, intact skin and mucous membranes are the first line of defense against infection.*
- Teach dental health measures:
  - Obtain a dental examination every 4 to 6 months.
  - Maintain careful oral hygiene, which includes brushing the teeth with a soft toothbrush and fluoridated toothpaste at least twice a day and flossing as recommended.
  - Be aware of the symptoms requiring dental care: bad breath; unpleasant taste in the mouth; bleeding, red, or sore gums; and tooth pain.
  - If dental surgery is necessary, monitor for need to make adjustments in insulin. *All people with diabetes need to be taught proper oral hygiene, the risk of periodontal disease, and the importance of obtaining dental care for symptoms of oral or dental problems.*
- Teach women with diabetes the symptoms and preventive measures for vaginitis caused by *Candida albicans*. The symptoms are an odorless, white or yellow cheeselike discharge and itching. Sexual transmission is unlikely, but

discomfort may cause the client to avoid sexual activity. *Diabetes is a predisposing factor for* Candida albicans *vaginitis, the most common form of vaginitis. Poor personal hygiene and wearing clothing that keeps the vaginal area warm and moist increase the risk of vaginitis. The infection may spread to the urinary tract, resulting in urinary tract infections; preventing and treating vaginitis decrease this risk.*

PRACTICE ALERT *Teach women with DM to take preventive measures by maintaining good personal hygiene, wiping front to back after voiding, wearing cotton underwear, avoiding tight jeans and nylon pantyhose, and avoiding douching.* ■

Risk for Injury

The person with diabetes is at risk for injury from multiple factors. Neuropathies may alter sensation, gait, and muscle control. Cataracts or retinopathy may cause visual deficits. Hyperglycemia often causes osmotic changes in the lenses of the eye, resulting in blurred vision. In addition, changes in blood glucose alter levels of consciousness and may cause seizures. The impaired mobility, sensory deficits, and neurologic effects of complications of diabetes increase the risk of accidents, burns, falls, and trauma.

- Assess for the presence of contributing or causative factors that increase the risk of injury: blurred vision, cataracts, decreased adaptation to dark, decreased tactile sensitivity, hypoglycemia, hyperglycemia, hypovolemia, joint immobility, unstable gait. *A knowledge base is necessary to develop an individualized plan of care. The risk of injury increases with the number of factors identified.*
- Reduce environmental hazards in the health care facility, and teach the client about safety in the home and in the community.

IN THE HEALTH CARE FACILITY
- Orient the client to new surroundings on admission.
- Keep the bed at the lowest level.
- Keep the floors free of objects.
- Use a night light.
- Check the temperature of the bath or shower water before the client uses it.
- Instruct the client to wear shoes or slippers when out of bed.
- Monitor blood glucose levels regularly.
- Monitor for side effects of prescribed medications, such as dizziness or drowsiness.

IN THE HOME AND COMMUNITY
- Use a night light, preferably one with a soft, nonglare bulb.
- Turn the head away when switching on a bright light.
- Avoid directly looking into headlights when driving at night.
- Test the temperature of the bath or shower water before use.
- Conduct a daily foot inspection.
- Wear shoes and slippers with nonskid soles.
- Do not use throw rugs.
- Install hand grips in the tub and shower and next to the toilet.
- Wear a seat belt when driving or riding in a car.

Strange environments and the presence of hazardous environmental factors increase the risk of falls or other accidents. Glare is often responsible for falls in people with visual deficits. The nurse can reduce factors that increase the risk of injury by implementing care and teaching safe practices during the activities of daily life.

- Monitor for and teach the client and family to recognize and seek care for the manifestations of DKA in the client with type 1 DM: hyperglycemia, thirst, headaches, nausea and vomiting, increased urine output, ketonuria, dehydration, and decreasing level of consciousness. *Blood glucose levels increase if the insulin need is unmet or insufficiently met; the cellular use of fats for fuel results in ketosis. Osmotic diuresis increases urinary output, resulting in thirst and dehydration.*
- Monitor for and teach the client and family to recognize and seek care for the manifestations of HHS in the client with type 2 DM: extreme hyperglycemia, increased urinary output, thirst, dehydration, hypotension, seizures, and decreasing level of consciousness. *HHS is a life-threatening condition requiring recognition and treatment.*

PRACTICE ALERT *Make frequent assessments to monitor for symptoms of HHS in the older adult who has had major surgery.* ■

- Monitor for and teach the client and family to recognize and treat the manifestations of hypoglycemia: low blood glucose, anxiety, headache, uncoordinated movements, sweating, rapid pulse, drowsiness, and visual changes. Teach client and family to carry some form of rapid-acting sugar source at all times. *Severe hypoglycemia causes a decrease in the level of consciousness. The decrease in blood glucose most often results from too much insulin, too little food, or too much exercise.*
- Recommend that the client wear a MedicAlert bracelet or necklace identifying self as a person with diabetes. *In case of sudden, severe illness or accident, a MedicAlert bracelet can allow immediate medical attention for diabetes to be instituted.*

Sexual Dysfunction

Sexuality is a complex and inseparable part of every person. It involves not only physical sexual activities but also a person's self-perception as male or female, roles and relationships, and attractiveness and desirability. Changes in sexual function and in sexuality have been identified in both men and women with diabetes.

Alterations in erectile ability occur in approximately 50% of all men with diabetes. The incidence of impotence increases with the duration of the diabetes and is often associated with peripheral neuropathy. Libido is usually unaffected, even when impotence is present.

Women with diabetes also have alterations in sexual function, although the reason is less clear. The problems reported by women involve decreased desire and decreased vaginal lubrication. Women with diabetes are also at increased risk for vaginitis and may avoid sexual intercourse in order to avoid pain.

- Include a sexual history as a part of the initial and ongoing assessment of the client with diabetes. A specific history form may be used that addresses sexual development, personal and family values, current sexual practices and concerns, and changes desired. Ask a nonthreatening, open-ended question to elicit information, such as, "Tell me about your experience with sexual function since you have been diagnosed with diabetes." *Obtaining accurate information to assess the sexual health of a client is necessary before counseling can begin or referrals can be made.*

> **PRACTICE ALERT** *Sexual function is a private matter, and clients rarely share concerns unless the nurse initiates the discussion.* ■

- Provide information about the actual and potential physical effects of diabetes on sexual function. Include the effect of poor control of blood glucose on sexual function as part of any teaching plan. *Clients benefit from basic information about male and female anatomy and the sexual response cycle, and how diabetes can affect this part of the body. Changes in blood glucose levels not only may cause changes in desire and physical response but also may alter sexual responses as a result of depression, anxiety, and fatigue.*

- Provide counseling or make referrals as appropriate. The nurse is responsible for knowing about sexuality and sexual health throughout the life span and provides information based on knowledge of the effects of illness and treatment on sexual function. For example, men who are impotent may regain the ability to have sexual intercourse through penile implants, suction apparatus, the use of sildenafil citrate (Viagra), or injections of medications (such as yohimbine, an alpha-2 adrenergic blocker) that increase vascular blood flow into the corpus of the penis. Women with decreased vaginal lubrication can decrease painful intercourse by using vaginal lubricants (such as K-Y Jelly) or estrogen creams. *The nurse may make specific suggestions to facilitate positive sexual functioning, referring the client to the appropriate health care provider as necessary for intensive therapy.*

Ineffective Coping

Coping is the process of responding to internal or environmental stressors or potential stressors. When coping responses are ineffective, the stressors exceed the individual's available resources for responding. The person diagnosed with diabetes is faced with lifelong changes in many parts of his or her life. Diet, exercise habits, and medications must be integrated into the person's lifestyle and be carefully controlled. Daily injections may be a reality. Fear of potential complications and of negative effects on the future is common.

If the person is unable to cope successfully with these changes, emotional stress can interfere with glycemic control. In addition, unsuccessful coping often results in noncompliance with prescribed treatment modalities, further impairing glycemic control and increasing the potential for acute and chronic complications.

- Assess the client's psychosocial resources, including emotional resources, support resources, lifestyle, and communication skills. *Chronic illness affects all dimensions of a person's life, as well as the lives of family members and significant others. A comprehensive assessment of strengths and weaknesses is the first step in developing an individualized plan of care to facilitate coping.*

- Explore with the client and family the effects (actual and perceived) of the diagnosis and treatment of diabetes on finances, occupation, energy levels, and relationships. *Common frustrations associated with diabetes are the disease itself, the treatment modalities, and the health care system. Effective coping involves maintaining a healthy self-concept and satisfying relationships, emotional balance, and handling emotional stress.*

- Teach constructive problem-solving techniques. *Problem-focused behaviors include setting attainable and realistic goals, learning about all aspects of the problem, learning new procedures or skills that increase self-esteem, and reaching out to others for support.*

- Provide information about support groups and resources, such as suppliers of products, journals, books, and cookbooks for people with diabetes. *Sharing with others who have similar problems provides opportunities for mutual support and problem solving. Using available resources improves the ability to cope.*

Using NANDA, NIC, and NOC

Chart 18–1 shows links between NANDA, NIC, and NOC when caring for the client with diabetes.

Home Care

Teaching the client and family to self-manage diabetes is a nursing responsibility. Even if a formal teaching plan is developed and implemented by advanced practice nurses, all nurses must be able to reinforce knowledge and answer questions. Teaching is necessary for both the person who is newly diagnosed and for the person who has had diabetes for years. In fact, the latter may need almost as much teaching as the newly diagnosed person (Guthrie & Guthrie, 1997).

The American Diabetes Association recommends that teaching be carried out on three levels. The first level focuses on survival skills, with the person learning basic knowledge and skills to be able to provide diabetes management for the first week or two while he or she adjusts to the idea of having the disease. The second level focuses on home management, emphasizing self-reliance and independence in the daily management of diabetes. The third level aims at improving lifestyle and educating clients to individualize self-management of the illness.

For the hospitalized client with diabetes, teaching should begin on admission. Prior to designing the teaching plan, the nurse makes an initial assessment of the client's and family's knowledge and learning needs, outlining past diabetes management practices and identifying physical, emotional, and sociocultural needs. Educational level, preferred learning methods and style, life experiences, and support systems are also assessed.

It is important that the nurse and client mutually establish goals based on the assessment data. It is equally important that

CHART 18–1 **NANDA, NIC, AND NOC LINKAGES**

The Client with Diabetes

NURSING DIAGNOSES	NURSING INTERVENTIONS	NURSING OUTCOMES
• Ineffective Therapeutic Regimen Management • Imbalanced Nutrition: More than Body Requirements • Fatigue • Risk for Peripheral Neurovascular Dysfunction • Powerlessness • Altered Protection	• Hyperglycemia Management • Nutritional Counseling • Weight Management • Energy Management • Peripheral Sensation • Circulatory Care: Arterial Insufficiency • Self-Esteem Enhancement • Infection Control	• Knowledge: Treatment Regimen • Nutritional Status: Food and Fluid Intake • Knowledge: Diet • Energy Conservation • Circulation Status • Neurological Status • Health Beliefs: Perceived Control • Infection Status

Note. Data from Nursing Outcomes Classification (NOC) by M. Johnson & M. Maas (Eds.), 1997, St. Louis: Mosby; Nursing Diagnoses: Definitions & Classification 2001–2002 by North American Nursing Diagnosis Association, 2001, Philadelphia: NANDA; Nursing Interventions Classification (NIC) by J.C. McCloskey & G. M. Bulechek (Eds.), 2000, St. Louis: Mosby. Reprinted by permission.

family members understand that the responsibility for daily management lies with the client and that the primary role of the family is supportive. The client is the person with the disease, and it is the client who each day must take medications or inject insulin, test blood or urine, calculate and balance foods, exercise, adjust medications, inspect the body for injury, and determine whether and when medical assistance is needed. However, family members require the same knowledge so that they can provide emotional support as well as physical care if necessary.

The following should be included in teaching the client and family about care at home.

- Information about normal metabolism, diabetes mellitus, and how diabetes changes metabolism
- Diet plan: how diet helps keep blood glucose in normal range; number of kcal required and why; amount of carbohydrates, meats, and fats allowed and why; and how to calculate the diet, integrating personal food preferences
- Exercise: how it helps lower blood glucose; the importance of a regular program; types of exercise; integrating personal exercise preferences; how to handle increased activity
- Self-monitoring of blood glucose: how to perform the tests accurately, how to care for equipment, what to do for high or low blood glucose
- Medications:
  - Insulin: type, dosage, mixing instructions (if necessary), times of onset and peak actions, how to get and care for equipment, how to give injections, where to give injections
  - Oral agents: type, dosage, side effects, interaction with other drugs
- Manifestations of acute complications of hypoglycemia and hyperglycemia; what to do when they occur
- Hygiene: skin care, dental care, foot care
- Sick days: what to do about food, fluids, and medications
- Helpful resources:
  - The American Diabetes Association
  - The American Dietetic Association

- National Diabetes Information Clearinghouse
- Department of Veterans Affairs
- Indian Health Service
- National Council of La Raza

Teaching may have to be adapted to the special needs of the older adult. Because 40% of all people with diabetes are over the age of 65, considering the special needs of this population is essential. Uncontrolled diabetes in the older adult increases the potential for functional loss, social disengagement, and increased morbidity and mortality. Education for self-care allows the older adult to be more actively involved in his or her diabetes management and decreases the potential for acute and long-term complications from the disease. Considerations for teaching the older adult with diabetes include the following:

- Changes in diet may be difficult to implement for many reasons. Favorite foods are difficult to give up. Balanced meals at regular intervals may not have been part of the client's lifestyle. Purchasing, storing, and preparing foods may be a problem. Dentures may not fit well. Changes in taste sensation often cause the client to increase the use of salt and sugar.
- Exercise of any type may not have been part of the activities of daily living. Exercise must be individualized for any physical limitations imposed by other chronic illnesses, such as arthritis, Parkinson's disease, chronic respiratory diseases, and/or cardiovascular diseases.
- The diagnosis of a chronic illness threatens independence and self-worth. After years of taking care of self, the older adult with diabetes may now have to depend on others for help in meeting self-care needs. This in turn often leads to withdrawal from social interactions with others.
- Money to purchase medications and supplies often must be taken out of a fixed income.
- Visual deficits make insulin administration difficult or impossible. Visual deficits also interfere with blood glucose monitoring, food preparation, exercises, and foot care.

Nursing Care Plan
A Client with Type 1 Diabetes

Jim Meligrito, age 24, is a third-year nursing student at a large mid-western university. Mr. Meligrito also works 20 hours a week as a campus student security guard. His working hours are 8 P.M. to midnight, five nights a week. He lives with his father, who is also a student. Neither of the two men likes to cook, and they usually eat "whatever is handy." Mr. Meligrito has smoked 8 to 10 cigarettes a day for 5 years. He was diagnosed with type 1 diabetes mellitus at age 12. Although his insulin dosage has varied, he currently takes a total of 32 units of insulin each day, 10 U of NPH and 6 U of regular insulin each morning and evening. He monitors his blood glucose about three times a week. He feels that he is too busy for a regular exercise program and that he gets enough exercise in clinicals and in weekend sports activities. He has not seen a health care provider for over a year.

One day during a 6-hour clinical laboratory in pediatrics, Mr. Meligrito notices that he is urinating frequently, is thirsty, and has blurred vision. He also is very tired but blames all his symptoms on drinking a couple of beers and having had only 4 hours of sleep the night before while studying for an examination, and the stress he has been under lately from school and work. When he remembers that he had forgotten to take his insulin that morning, he realizes he must have hyperglycemia but decides that he will be all right until he gets home in the afternoon. Around noon, he begins having abdominal pain, feels weak, has a rapid pulse, and vomits. When he reports his physical symptoms to his clinical instructor, she sends him immediately to the hospital emergency department, accompanied by another student.

ASSESSMENT
As soon as Mr. Meligrito arrives at the emergency room, his blood glucose level is measured at 300 mg/dL. Urine samples and additional blood samples are sent to the laboratory for analysis. Blood glucose is 330 mg/dL, urine shows the presence of ketones, electrolytes are normal, and pH is 7.1. His vital signs are as follows: T 99°F (37.2°C), P 140, R 28, and BP 102/52. An intravenous infusion of 1000 mL normal (0.9%) saline with 40 mEq of KCl is started at a rate of 400 mL/h. Intravenous regular insulin at 25 mL/h (5 U/h) is begun. Hourly blood glucose monitoring is initiated. Mr. Meligrito is nauseated and lethargic but remains oriented. Three hours later, he has a blood glucose level of 160, and his pulse and blood pressure are normal. He is dismissed from the emergency department after making an appointment for the next morning with the hospital's diabetes nurse educator. When he meets with the diabetes educator, he says that he no longer feels in control of the diabetes or his future goal to become a nurse anesthetist.

DIAGNOSIS
- *Powerlessness* related to a perceived lack of control of diabetes due to present demands on time
- *Deficient knowledge* of self-management of diabetes
- *Risk for ineffective role performance* related to uncertainty about capacity to achieve desired role as registered nurse

EXPECTED OUTCOMES
- Identify those aspects of diabetes that can be controlled and participate in making decisions about self-managing care.

- Demonstrate an understanding of diabetes self-management through planned medication, diet, exercise, and blood glucose self-monitoring activities.
- Explore and clarify Mr. Meligrito's perceptions of his role as a student nurse, verbalizing his ability to meet his expectations.

PLANNING AND IMPLEMENTATION
- Mutually establish specific and individualized short-term and long-term goals for self-management to control blood glucose.
- Provide opportunities to express his feelings about himself and his illness.
- Explore perceptions of his own ability to control his illness and his future, and clarify these perceptions by providing information about resources and support groups.
- Facilitate decision-making abilities in self-managing his prescribed treatment regimen.
- Provide positive reinforcement for increasing involvement in self-care activities.
- Provide relevant learning activities about insulin administration, dietary management, exercise, self-monitoring of blood glucose, and healthy lifestyle.

EVALUATION
After taking an active part in the weekly educational meetings for 2 months, Mr. Meligrito has greatly enhanced his understanding of and compliance with self-management of his diabetes. He states that he finally understands how insulin, food, and exercise affect his body, having previously thought they were "just things I should do when I wanted to." He decides to perform self-management activities one week at a time, rather than think too far into (and thereby feel overwhelmed by) the future. Both son and father have developed a workable meal schedule and weekly grocery list, and they have begun eating breakfast and dinner together. Jim and a friend have arranged to walk 2 to 3 miles three times a week on a community hiking trail. To gain a sense of control over his illness, he has also worked out a schedule that allows time for school, health care, and himself.

Critical Thinking in the Nursing Process
1. What is the pathophysiologic basis for the changes in temperature, pulse, respirations, and blood pressure that occurred on Mr. Meligrito's admission to the hospital emergency department?
2. How can smoking and poor self-management of diabetes increase the risk of long-term complications?
3. Is powerlessness a common response to a chronic illness? Why or why not?
4. Consider that you are teaching Mr. Meligrito and another client, Mr. McDaniel (age 75, newly diagnosed with type 2 DM). What components of your teaching plan would be the same and what components would be different?

See Evaluating Your Response in Appendix C.

EXPLORE MediaLink

NCLEX review questions, case studies, care plan activities, MediaLink applications, and other interactive resources for this chapter can be found on the Companion Website at www.prenhall.com/lemone.

Click on Chapter 18 to select the activities for this chapter. For animations, video clips, more NCLEX review questions, and an audio glossary, access the Student CD-ROM accompanying this textbook.

TEST YOURSELF

1. Increased susceptibility to the development of type 1 diabetes is indicated by which of the following:

   a. Genetic markers that determine immune response
   b. Persistent obesity throughout the adolescent years
   c. Delivery of a baby that weighs less than 6 lb
   d. Excessive amounts of plasma glucagon

2. Diabetic ketoacidosis is the result of which pathologic process?

   a. An excess amount of insulin drives all glucose into the cells
   b. A decreased amount of glucagon causes low protein levels
   c. A deficit of insulin causes fat stores to be used as an energy source
   d. An increase occurs in the breakdown of glucose molecules with hypoglycemia

3. Which of the following clients would be most at risk for the development of type 2 DM?

   a. Young adult who is a professional basketball player
   b. Middle-age man who maintains normal weight

   c. Middle-age woman who is the sole caretaker of her parents
   d. Woman over age 70 who is overweight and sedentary

4. You note that your assigned client has a nursing diagnosis of *Peripheral neurovascular dysfunction* involving both feet. Which of the following assessments would support this diagnosis?

   a. Normal sensation to touch
   b. Loss of normal reflexes
   c. States "I can't feel my feet anymore."
   d. States "I have been having chest pain."

5. Which of the following statements would indicate your client understands teaching about foot care at home?

   a. "I will walk barefooted as long as I am in the house."
   b. "I always buy my shoes as soon as the stores open."
   c. "I will check my feet for cuts and bruises every night."
   d. "If I get a blister, I just put alcohol on it and let it go."

See Test Yourself answers in Appendix C.

BIBLIOGRAPHY

American Diabetes Association. (2002). *Clinical practice recommendations 2002, 25* (Supplement 1).

Batts, M., Gary, T., Huss, K., Hill, M., Bone, L., & Brancatt, F. (2001). Patient priorities and needs for diabetes care among urban African American adults. *Diabetes Educator, 27*(3), 405–412.

Bohannon, N. (1998). Treatment of vulvovaginal candidiasis in patients with diabetes. *Diabetes Care, 21*(3), 451–456.

Bulpitt, C., Palmer, A., Battersby, C., & Fletcher, A. (1998). Association of symptoms of type 2 diabetic patients with severity of disease, obesity, and blood pressure. *Diabetes Care, 21*(1), 111–115.

Burke, D. (2001). Diabetes education for the Native American Population. *Diabetes Educator, 27*(2), 181–189.

Cameron, B. (2002). Making diabetes management routine. *American Journal of Nursing, 102*(2), 26–33.

Carter, J., Gilliland, S., Perez, G., Levin, S., Broussand, B., Valdez, L., Cunningham-Sabo, L., & Davis, S. (1997). Tool chest. Native American

Diabetes Project: Designing culturally relevant education materials. *Diabetes Educator, 23*(2), 133–134.

Fishman, T., Freedline, A., & Town, L. (1997). Helping diabetic patients treat their feet right. *Nursing97, 27*(6), 10–12.

Goldberg, J. M. (2001). Nutrition and exercise. *RN, 64*(7), 34–39.

Guthrie, D., & Guthrie, R. (1997). *Nursing management of diabetes mellitus* (4th ed.). New York: Springer.

Haire-Joshu, D. (Ed.) (1996). *Management of diabetes mellitus: Perspectives of care across the life span* (2nd ed.). St. Louis: Mosby.

Hanna, K., & Guthrie, D. (2001). Health-compromising behavior and diabetes mismanagement among adolescents and young adults. *Diabetes Educator, 27*(2), 223–230.

Hernandez, D. (1998). Microvascular complications of diabetes: Nursing assessment and intervention. *American Journal of Nursing, 98*(6), 26–31.

Johnson, M., & Maas, M. (Eds.). (1997). *Nursing outcomes classification (NOC)*. St. Louis: Mosby.

Kee, J. (1999). *Laboratory & diagnostic tests with nursing implications* (5th ed.). East Norwalk, CT: Appleton & Lange.

Lipton, R., Losy, L., Giachello, A., Mendez, J., & Girotti, M. (1998). Attitudes and issues in treating Latino patients with type 2 diabetes. *Diabetes Educator, 24*(1), 67–71.

Lupo, M. (1997). An overview of foot disease associated with diabetes mellitus. *MEDSURG Nursing, 6*(4), 225–229.

McCance, K., & Huether, S. (2002). *Pathophysiology: The biologic basis for disease in adults and children.* (4th ed.). St. Louis: Mosby.

McCloskey, J. C., & Bulechek, G. M. (Eds.). (2000). *Nursing interventions classification (NIC).* St. Louis: Mosby.

McKenry, L., & Salerno, E. (1998). *Pharmacology in nursing* (20th ed.). St. Louis: Mosby.

National Institutes of Health. (2002). *Diabetes statistics in the United States.* NIH Publication No. 99–3892. Washington, DC: NIH.

North American Nursing Diagnosis Association. (2001). *Nursing diagnoses: Definitions & Classification 2001–2002.* Philadelphia: NANDA.

Passanza, C. (2001). Diabetes update: Monitor options. *RN, 64*(6), 36–43.

Paterson, B., Thorne, S., & Dewis, M. (1998). Adapting to and managing diabetes. *Image: Journal of Nursing Scholarship, 30*(1), 57–62.

Porth, C. (2002). *Pathophysiology: Concepts of altered health states* (6th ed.). Philadelphia: Lippincott.

Robertson, C. (1998). When your patient is on an insulin pump. *RN, 61*(3), 30–33.

Shannon, M., Wilson, B., & Stang, C. (2002). *Health professional's drug guide 2002.* Upper Saddle River, NJ: Prentice Hall.

Stanley, K. (1998). Assessing the nutritional needs of the geriatric patient with diabetes. *Diabetes Educator, 24*(1), 29–30, 35–36, 38.

Strowig, S. (2001). Insulin therapy. *RN, 64*(9), 38–44.

Sullivan, E., & Joseph, D. (1998). Struggling with behavior changes: A special case for clients with diabetes. *Diabetes Educator, 24*(1), 72–77.

Tierney, L., McPhee, S., & Papadakis, M. (Eds.). (2001). *Current medical diagnosis & treatment* (40th ed.). Stamford, CT: Appleton & Lange.

Tkacs, N. (2002). Hypoglycemia unawarenesss. *American Journal of Nursing, 102*(2), 34–41.

Whittemore, R. (2000). Strategies to facilitate lifestyle change associated with diabetes mellitus. *Journal of Nursing Scholarship, 32*(3), 225–232.

UNIT 5

RESPONSES TO ALTERED NUTRITION

Assessing Clients with Nutritional and Gastrointestinal Disorders

MediaLink

www.prenhall.com/lemone
Additional resources for this chapter can be found on the Student CD-ROM accompanying this textbook, and on the Companion Website at www. prenhall.com/lemone. Click on Chapter 19 to select the activities for this chapter.

CD-ROM
• Audio Glossary
• NCLEX Review

Animations
• Digestive System
• Carbohydrates
• Lipids
• Proteins

Companion Website
• More NCLEX Review
• Functional Health Pattern Assessment
• Case Study
  Weight Loss

LEARNING OUTCOMES

After completing this chapter, you will be able to:

■ Review the anatomy and physiology of the gastrointestinal system.

■ Describe the processes of carbohydrate, fat, and protein metabolism.

■ Describe the sources of nutrients and vitamins and their functions in the human body.

■ Identify specific topics to consider during a health history assessment interview of the client with nutritional and gastrointestinal disorders.

■ Describe physical assessment techniques used to evaluate nutritional and gastrointestinal status.

■ Identify abnormal findings that may indicate impairment in gastrointestinal function.

Nutrition is the process by which the body ingests, absorbs, transports, uses, and eliminates food. The digestive organs responsible for these processes are the gastrointestinal tract (also called the alimentary canal) and the accessory digestive organs. The gastrointestinal tract consists of the mouth, pharynx, esophagus, stomach, small intestine, and large intestine. The accessory digestive organs include the liver, gallbladder, and pancreas (Figure 19–1 ■). This chapter discusses the assessment of these organs except the large intestine. Assessment of the large intestine, which is primarily responsible for elimination, is discussed in Chapter 23. ⊗

REVIEW OF ANATOMY AND PHYSIOLOGY

The gastrointestinal (GI) tract is a continuous hollow tube, extending from the mouth to the anus. Once foods are ingested into the mouth, they are subjected to a variety of processes that move them and break them down into end products that can be absorbed from the lumen of the small intestine into the blood or lymph. These digestive processes are as follows:

- Ingestion of food
- Movement of food and wastes
- Secretion of mucus, water, and enzymes
- Mechanical digestion of food
- Chemical digestion of food
- Absorption of digested food

The Mouth

The mouth, also called the oral or buccal cavity, is lined with mucous membranes and is enclosed by the lips, cheeks, palate, and tongue (Figure 19–2 ■).

The lips and cheeks are skeletal muscle covered externally by skin. Their function is to keep food in the mouth during chewing. The palate consists of two regions: the hard palate and the soft palate. The hard palate covers bone and provides a hard surface against which the tongue forces food. The soft palate is primarily muscle; it ends at the back of the mouth as a fold called the uvula. When food is swallowed, the soft palate rises as a reflex to close off the oropharynx.

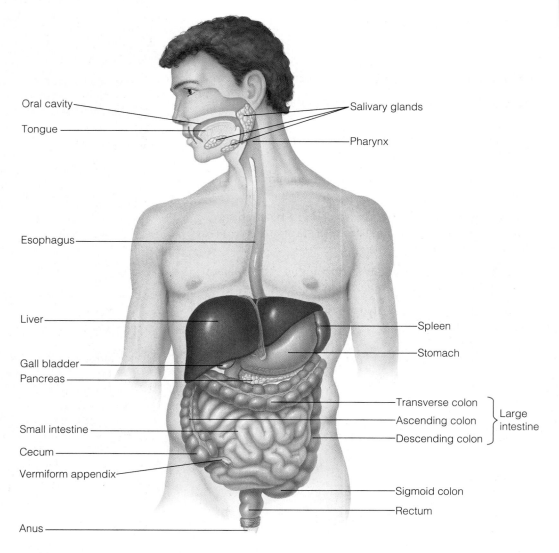

Figure 19–1 ■ Organs of the gastrointestinal tract and accessory digestive organs.

Figure 19–2 ■ Structures of the mouth, the pharynx, and the esophagus.

Hard palate
Oral cavity
Soft palate
Teeth
Gingiva
Tongue
Lingual tonsil
Epiglottis
Trachea

Opening of auditory tube in nasopharynx
Uvula
Palatine tonsil
Oropharynx
Laryngopharynx
Esophagus

The tongue, composed of skeletal muscle and connective tissue, is located in the floor of the mouth. It contains mucous and serous glands, taste buds, and papillae. The tongue mixes food with saliva during chewing, forms the food into a mass (called a bolus), and initiates swallowing. Some papillae provide surface roughness to facilitate licking and moving food; other papillae house the taste buds.

Saliva moistens food so it can be made into a bolus, dissolves food chemicals so they can be tasted, and provides enzymes (such as amylase) that begin the chemical breakdown of starches. Saliva is produced by salivary glands, most of which lie superior or inferior to the mouth and drain into it. The salivary glands include the parotid, the submaxillary, and the sublingual glands.

The teeth chew (masticate) and grind food to break it down into smaller parts. As the food is masticated, it is mixed with saliva. Adults have 32 permanent teeth. The teeth are embedded in the gingiva (gums), with the crown of each tooth visible above the gingiva.

The Pharynx

The pharynx consists of the oropharynx and the laryngopharynx (see Figure 19–2). Both structures provide passageways for food, fluids, and air. The pharynx is skeletal muscles and is lined with mucous membranes. The skeletal muscles move food to the esophagus via the pharynx through **peristalsis** (alternating waves of contraction and relaxation of involuntary muscle). The mucosa of the pharynx contains mucus-producing glands that provide fluid to facilitate the passage of the bolus of food as it is swallowed.

The Esophagus

The esophagus, a muscular tube about 10 inches (25 cm) long, serves as a passageway for food from the pharynx to the stomach (see Figures 19–1 and 19–2). The epiglottis, a flap of cartilage over the top of the larynx, keeps food out of the larynx during swallowing. The esophagus descends through the tho-

rax and diaphragm, entering the stomach at the cardiac orifice. The gastroesophageal sphincter surrounds this opening. This sphincter, along with the diaphragm, keeps the orifice closed when food is not being swallowed.

For most of its length, the esophagus is lined with stratified squamous epithelium; simple columnar epithelium lines the esophagus where it joins the stomach. The mucosa and submucosa of the esophagus lie in longitudinal folds when the esophagus is empty.

The Stomach

The stomach, located high on the left side of the abdominal cavity, is connected to the esophagus at the upper end and to the small intestine at the lower end (Figure 19–3 ■). Normally about 10 inches (25 cm) long, the stomach is a distensible organ that can expand to hold up to 4 L of food and fluid. The

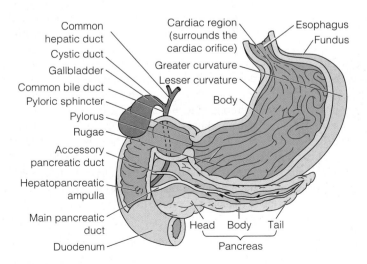

Common hepatic duct
Cystic duct
Gallbladder
Common bile duct
Pyloric sphincter
Pylorus
Rugae
Accessory pancreatic duct
Hepatopancreatic ampulla
Main pancreatic duct
Duodenum

Cardiac region (surrounds the cardiac orifice)
Esophagus
Fundus
Greater curvature
Lesser curvature
Body
Head Body Tail
Pancreas

Figure 19–3 ■ The internal anatomic structures of the stomach, including the pancreatic, cystic, and hepatic ducts; the pancreas; and the gallbladder.

concave surface of the stomach is called the lesser curvature; the convex surface is called the greater curvature. The stomach may be divided into regions extending from the distal end of the esophagus to the opening into the small intestine. These regions are the cardiac region, fundus, body, and pylorus (see Figure 19–3). The pyloric sphincter controls emptying of the stomach into the duodenal portion of the small intestine. The stomach is a storage reservoir for food, continues the mechanical breakdown of food, begins the process of protein digestion, and mixes the food with gastric juices into a thick fluid called **chyme.**

The stomach is lined with columnar epithelial, mucus-producing cells. Millions of openings in the lining lead to gastric glands that can produce 4 to 5 L of gastric juice each day. The gastric glands contain a variety of secretory cells, including the following:

- Mucous cells produce alkaline mucus that clings to the lining of the stomach and protects it from gastric juice.
- Zymogenic cells produce pepsinogen (an inactive form of pepsin, a protein-digesting enzyme).
- Parietal cells secrete hydrochloric acid and intrinsic factor. Hydrochloric acid activates and increases the activity of protein-digesting cells and also is bactericidal. Intrinsic factor is necessary for the absorption of vitamin B_{12} in the small intestine.
- Enteroendocrine cells secrete gastrin, histamine, endorphins, serotonin, and somatostatin. These hormones or hormone-like substances diffuse into the blood. Gastrin is important in regulating secretion and motility of the stomach.

The secretion of gastric juice is under both neural and endocrine control. Stimulation of the parasympathetic vagus nerve increases secretory activity; in contrast, stimulation of sympathetic nerves decreases secretions. The three phases of secretory activity are the cephalic phase, the gastric phase, and the intestinal phase.

- The cephalic phase prepares for digestion and is triggered by the sight, odor, taste, or thought of food. During this initial phase, motor impulses are transmitted via the vagus nerve to the stomach.
- The gastric phase begins when food enters the stomach. Stomach distention (stimulating stretch receptors) and chemical stimuli from partially digested proteins initiate this phase. Gastrin-secreting cells produce gastrin, which in turn stimulates the gastric glands (especially the parietal cells) to produce more gastric juice. Histamine also stimulates hydrochloric acid secretion.
- The intestinal phase is initiated when partially digested food begins to enter the small intestine, stimulating mucous cells of the intestine to release a hormone that promotes continued gastric secretion.

Mechanical digestion in the stomach is accomplished by peristaltic movements that churn and mix the food with the gastric juices to form chyme. Gastric motility is enhanced or retarded by the same factors that affect secretion, namely, distention and the effect of gastrin. After a person eats a normal, well-balanced meal, the stomach empties completely in approximately 4 to 6 hours. Gastric emptying depends on the volume, chemical composition, and osmotic pressure of the gastric contents. The stomach empties large volumes of content more rapidly, while gastric emptying is slowed by solids and fats.

The Small Intestine

The small intestine begins at the pyloric sphincter and ends at the ileocecal junction at the entrance of the large intestine (see Figure 19–1). The small intestine is about 20 ft (6 m) long but only about 1 inch (2.5 cm) in diameter. This long tube hangs in coils in the abdominal cavity, suspended by the mesentery and surrounded by the large intestine. The small intestine has three regions: the duodenum, the jejunum, and the ileum. The duodenum begins at the pyloric sphincter and extends around the head of the pancreas for about 10 inches (25 cm). Both pancreatic enzymes and bile from the liver enter the small intestine at the duodenum. The jejunum, the middle region of the small intestine, extends for about 8 ft (2.4 m). The ileum, the terminal end of the small intestine, is approximately 12 ft (3.6 m) long and meets the large intestine at the ileocecal valve.

Food is chemically digested, and most of it absorbed, as it moves through the small intestine. Circular folds (deep folds of the mucosa and submucosa layers), villi (fingerlike projections of the mucosa cells), and microvilli (tiny projections of the mucosa cells) increase the surface area of the small intestine to enhance absorption of food. Although up to 10 L of food, liquids, and secretions enter the GI tract each day, less than 1 L reaches the large intestine.

Enzymes in the small intestine break down carbohydrates, proteins, lipids, and nucleic acids. Pancreatic amylase acts on starches, converting them to maltose, dextrins, and oligosaccharides; the intestinal enzymes dextrinase, glucoamylase, maltase, sucrase, and lactase further break down these products into monosaccharides. Pancreatic enzymes (trypsin and chymotrypsin) and intestinal enzymes continue to break down proteins into peptides. Pancreatic lipases digest lipids in the small intestine. Triglycerides enter as fat globules and are coated by bile salts and emulsified. Nucleic acids are hydrolyzed by pancreatic enzymes and then broken apart by intestinal enzymes. Both pancreatic enzymes and bile are excreted into the duodenum in response to the secretion of secretin and cholecystokinin, hormones produced by the intestinal mucosa cells when chyme enters the small intestine.

Nutrients are absorbed through the mucosa of the intestinal villi into the blood or lymph by active transport, facilitated transport, and passive diffusion. Almost all food products and water, as well as vitamins and most electrolytes, are absorbed in the small intestine, leaving only indigestible fibers, some water, and bacteria to enter the large intestine.

The Accessory Digestive Organs
The Liver and Gallbladder
The liver is the largest gland in the body, weighing about 3 lb (1.4 kg) in the average-size adult. It is located in the right side of the abdomen, inferior to the diaphragm and anterior to the stomach (see Figure 19–1). The liver has four lobes: right, left,

caudate, and quadrate. A mesenteric ligament separates the right and left lobes and suspends the liver from the diaphragm and anterior abdominal wall. The liver is encased in a fibroelastic capsule.

Liver tissue consists of units called lobules, which are composed of plates of hepatocytes (liver cells). A branch of the hepatic artery, a branch of the hepatic portal vein, and a bile duct communicate with each lobule. Sinusoids, blood-filled spaces within the lobules, are lined with Kupffer cells. These phagocytic cells remove debris from the blood.

The liver performs the following digestive and metabolic functions.

- Secretes bile
- Stores fat-soluble vitamins (A, D, E, and K)
- Metabolizes bilirubin
- Stores blood and releases blood into the general circulation during hemorrhage
- Synthesizes plasma proteins to maintain plasma oncotic pressure
- Synthesizes prothrombin, fibrinogen, and factors I, II, VII, IX, and X, which are necessary for blood clotting
- Synthesizes fats from carbohydrates and proteins to be either used for energy or stored as adipose tissue
- Synthesizes phospholipids and cholesterol necessary for the production of bile salts, steroid hormones, and plasma membranes
- Converts amino acids to carbohydrates through deamination
- Releases glucose during times of hypoglycemia
- Takes up glucose during times of hyperglycemia and stores it as glycogen or converts it to fat
- Alters chemicals, foreign molecules, and hormones to make them less toxic
- Stores iron as ferritin, which is released as needed for the production of red blood cells

Bile production is the liver's primary digestive function. **Bile** is a greenish, watery solution containing bile salts, cholesterol, bilirubin, electrolytes, water, and phospholipids. These substances are necessary to emulsify and promote the absorption of fats. Liver cells make from 700 to 1200 mL of bile daily. When bile is not needed for digestion, the sphincter of Oddi (located at the point at which bile enters the duodenum) is closed, and the bile backs up the cystic duct into the gallbladder for storage.

Bile is concentrated and stored in the gallbladder, a small sac cupped in the inferior surface of the liver. When food containing fats enters the duodenum, hormones stimulate the gallbladder to secrete bile into the cystic duct. The cystic duct joins the hepatic duct to form the common bile duct, from which bile enters into the duodenum (see Figure 19–3).

The Pancreas

The pancreas, a gland located between the stomach and small intestine, is the primary enzyme-producing organ of the digestive system. It is a triangular gland extending across the abdomen, with its tail next to the spleen and its head next to the duodenum (see Figure 19–3). The body and tail of the pancreas

are retroperitoneal, lying behind the greater curvature of the stomach. The pancreas is actually two organs in one, having both exocrine and endocrine structures and functions. The exocrine portion of the pancreas, through secretory units called acini, secretes alkaline pancreatic juice containing many different enzymes. The acini, clusters of secretory cells surrounding ducts, drain into the pancreatic duct. The pancreatic duct joins with the common bile duct just before it enters the duodenum (so that pancreatic juice and bile from the liver enter the small intestine together). The pancreas also has endocrine functions (see Chapter 16). ⊖◉

The pancreas produces from 1 to 1.5 L of pancreatic juice daily. Pancreatic juice is clear and has high bicarbonate content. This alkaline fluid neutralizes the acidic chyme as it enters the duodenum, optimizing the pH for intestinal and pancreatic enzyme activity. The secretion of pancreatic juice is controlled by the vagus nerve and the intestinal hormones secretin and cholecystokinin. Pancreatic juice contains enzymes that aid in the digestion of all categories of foods: lipase promotes fat breakdown and absorption; amylase completes starch digestion; and trypsin, chymotrypsin, and carboxypeptidase are responsible for half of all protein digestion. Nucleases break down nucleic acids.

METABOLISM

After nutrients (carbohydrates, fats, and proteins) are ingested, digested, absorbed, and transported across cell membranes, they must be metabolized to produce and provide energy to maintain life. **Metabolism** is the complex of biochemical reactions occurring in the body's cells. Metabolic processes are either catabolic or anabolic. Catabolism involves the breakdown of complex structures into simpler forms, for example, the breakdown of carbohydrates to produce adenosine triphosphate (ATP), an energy molecule that fuels cellular activity. In the process of anabolism, simpler molecules combine to build more complex structures, for example, amino acids bond to form proteins.

The biochemical reactions of metabolism produce water, carbon dioxide, and ATP (Figure 19–4 ■). The energy value of foods is measured in kilocalories (kcal). A kilocalorie is defined as the amount of heat energy needed to raise the temperature of 1 kilogram (kg) of water 1 degree centigrade.

NUTRIENTS

Nutrients are substances found in food and are used by the body to promote growth, maintenance, and repair. The categories of nutrients are carbohydrates, proteins, fats, vitamins, minerals, and water.

Carbohydrates

The primary sources of carbohydrates (which include sugars and starches) are plant foods. Monosaccharides and disaccharides come from milk, sugar cane, sugar beets, honey, and fruits. Polysaccharide starch is found in grains, legumes, and root vegetables. Following ingestion, digestion, and metabolism, carbohydrates are converted primarily to glucose, the

A Carbohydrates:
composed of simple
sugars (monosaccharides)

Polysaccharide

Monosaccharides

GI digestion
to glucose

Monosaccharides

To
capillary

Cellular
uses

ATP

Excesses
stored
as glycogen
or fat

Glycogen and
fat broken
down for ATP
formation

Broken
down to
glucose
and released
to blood

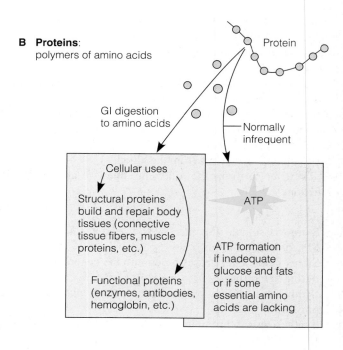

B Proteins:
polymers of amino acids

Protein

GI digestion
to amino acids

Normally
infrequent

Cellular uses

Structural proteins
build and repair body
tissues (connective
tissue fibers, muscle
proteins, etc.)

Functional proteins
(enzymes, antibodies,
hemoglobin, etc.)

ATP

ATP formation
if inadequate
glucose and fats
or if some
essential amino
acids are lacking

C Fats:
made up of
1 glycerol molecule
and 3 fatty acids

Glycerol

Lipid (fat)

Fatty acids

Liver
metabolizes to
ketones, aceto-
acetic acid,
etc.

GI digestion
to fatty acids
and glycerol

Cellular use

Cellular
uses

ATP

Building cell
membranes
and myelin
sheaths

Fat in adipose
tissue insulates
and cushions
body organs;
provides food,
energy stores

Fats are the
primary energy
fuels in many
cells

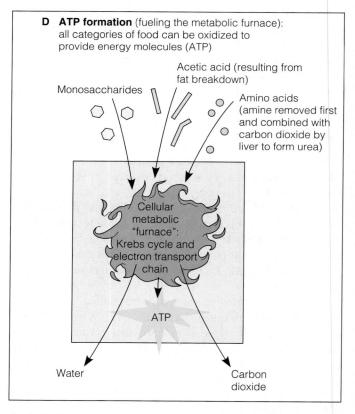

D ATP formation (fueling the metabolic furnace):
all categories of food can be oxidized to
provide energy molecules (ATP)

Acetic acid (resulting from
fat breakdown)

Monosaccharides

Amino acids
(amine removed first
and combined with
carbon dioxide by
liver to form urea)

Cellular
metabolic
"furnace":
Krebs cycle and
electron transport
chain

ATP

Water

Carbon
dioxide

Figure 19–4 ■ A schematic overview of nutrient use by body cells, including *A.* carbohydrates; *B.* proteins; *C,* fats; and *D,* ATP formation.

molecule body cells use to make ATP. Glucose is carefully regulated to maintain cellular functions. Excess glucose in the healthy person is converted to glycogen or fat. Glycogen is stored in the liver and muscles; fat is stored as adipose tissue. Carbohydrate use by the body is shown in Figure 19–4A.

Regardless of source, all carbohydrates supply 4 kcal per gram. The minimum necessary daily carbohydrate intake is unknown, but the recommended daily intake is 125 to 175 g, most of which should be complex carbohydrates (such as milk, potatoes, and whole grains). Excess intake of carbohydrates over time can result in obesity, dental caries, and elevated plasma triglycerides. Over extended periods of time, carbohydrate deficiencies lead to tissue wasting from protein breakdown and metabolic acidosis from an excess of ketones as a by-product of fat breakdown.

Proteins

Proteins are classified as either complete or incomplete. Complete proteins are found in animal products such as eggs, milk, milk products, and meat. They contain the greatest amount of amino acids and meet the body's amino acid requirements for tissue growth and maintenance. Incomplete proteins are found in legumes, nuts, grains, cereals, and vegetables. These sources are low in or lack one or more of the amino acids essential for building complete proteins.

The body uses proteins to build many different structures, including skin keratin, the collagen and elastin in connective tissues, and muscles. They also are used to make enzymes, hemoglobin, plasma proteins, and some hormones. Protein use by the body is shown in Figure 19–4B.

Proteins provide 4 kcal per gram. The recommended daily intake of protein is 56 g for men and 45 g for women. Healthy people with adequate caloric intake have an equal rate of protein synthesis and protein breakdown and loss, reflected as nitrogen balance. If the breakdown and loss of proteins exceeds intake, a negative nitrogen balance results. This may be due to starvation, altered physical states (e.g., from injury or illness), and altered emotional states (such as depression or anxiety). A positive nitrogen balance, which results when protein intake exceeds breakdown, is normal during growth, tissue repair, and pregnancy. Anabolic steroids affect the rate of protein; for example, the adrenal corticosteroids are released in times of stress to increase protein breakdown and conversion of amino acids to glucose. Excessive intake of proteins may lead to obesity, whereas deficits cause weight loss and tissue wasting, edema, and anemia.

Fats (Lipids)

Fats, or lipids, include phospholipids; steroids, such as cholesterol; and neutral fats, more commonly known as triglycerides. Neutral fats are the most abundant fats in the diet. They may be either saturated or unsaturated. Saturated fats are found in animal products (milk and meats) and in some plant products (such as coconut). Unsaturated fats are found in seeds, nuts, and most vegetable oils. Sources of cholesterol include meats, milk products, and egg yolks. Fat use by the body is shown in Figure 19–4C.

Fats are a necessary part of the structure and function of the body. For example:

- Phospholipids are a part of all cell membranes.
- Triglycerides are the major energy source for hepatocytes and skeletal muscle cells.
- Adipose tissue serves as a protection around body organs, as a layer of insulation under the skin, and as a concentrated source of fuel for cellular energy.
- Dietary fats facilitate absorption of fat-soluble vitamins.
- Linoleic acid, an essential fatty acid, helps form prostaglandins, regulatory molecules that assist in smooth muscle contraction, maintenance of blood pressure, and control of inflammatory responses.
- Cholesterol is the essential component of bile salts, steroid hormones, and vitamin D. Fats supply 9 kcal per gram. The recommended intake of fats is 30% or less of the total daily caloric intake. Saturated fats should account for no more than 10% of the total daily caloric intake, and cholesterol intake should not exceed 250 mg per day. When a person consumes more than the body requires, the excess is stored as adipose tissue, increasing the risk of obesity and heart disease. A deficit of fats may cause excessive weight loss and skin lesions.

Vitamins

Vitamins are organic compounds that facilitate the body's use of carbohydrates, proteins, and fats. All of the vitamins except vitamins D and K must be ingested in foods or taken as supplements. Vitamin D is made by ultraviolet irradiation of cholesterol molecules in the skin, and vitamin K is synthesized by bacteria in the intestine. Vitamins are categorized as either fat soluble or water soluble. The fat-soluble vitamins (A, D, E, and K) bind to ingested fats and are absorbed as the fats are absorbed. Water-soluble vitamins (the B complex and C) are absorbed with water in the GI tract (however, vitamin B_{12} must become attached to intrinsic factor to be absorbed). Fat-soluble vitamins are stored in the body, and excesses may cause toxicity; water-soluble vitamins in excess of body requirements are excreted in the urine. The recommended amounts of vitamins, previously labeled recommended daily allowances (RDAs), are now labeled by the National Academy of Sciences as dietary reference intakes (DRIs) per day. DRIs are provided for each vitamin in the following discussion.

Fat-soluble vitamins:
- Vitamin A (retinol) is found in fish liver oils, egg yolk, liver, fortified milk, and margarine. Vitamin A is necessary to vision, skin and mucous membrane integrity, normal reproductive function, and cell membrane structure. The DRI is 1000 µg for men and 800 µg for women.
- Vitamin D is formed by the action of sunlight on cholesterol in the skin. Vitamin D is necessary for blood calcium homeostasis, which in turn is essential to normal blood clotting, bone formation, and neuromuscular function. The DRI is 7.5 µg.
- Vitamin E is found in vegetable oils, margarine, whole grains, and dark green leafy vegetables. Vitamin E is believed to be

an antioxidant; that is, it helps prevent the oxidation of vitamins A and C in the intestine and decreases the oxidation of unsaturated fatty acids to facilitate cell membrane integrity. The DRI is 15 mg.

- Vitamin K is synthesized by coliform bacteria in the large intestine and is found in green leafy vegetables, cabbage, cauliflower, and pork. Vitamin K is essential for the formation of clotting proteins in the liver. The DRI is 2 g.

Water-soluble vitamins:

- Vitamin B_1 (thiamin) is found in lean meats, liver, eggs, green leafy vegetables, legumes, and whole grains. This B vitamin is an essential coenzyme for carbohydrate catabolism and use. It is essential for the healthy functioning of the nerves, muscles, and heart. The DRI is 1.5 mg for men and 1.1 mg for women.
- Vitamin B_2 (riboflavin) is found in liver, egg whites, whole grains, meat, poultry, and fish; a major source is milk. This B vitamin is involved in the catabolism and use of carbohydrates, fats, and proteins, and the use of other B vitamins. It is also important in the production of adrenal hormones. The DRI is 1.7 mg for men and 1.3 mg for women.
- Vitamin B_6 (pyridoxine) is found in meat, poultry, fish, potatoes, tomatoes, sweet potatoes, and spinach. This B vitamin is necessary for amino acid metabolism, formation of antibodies, and formation of hemoglobin. The DRI is 2.2 mg for men and 2 mg for women.
- Vitamin B_{12} (cyanocobalamin) is found in liver, meat, poultry, fish, dairy foods (except butter), and eggs. Vitamin B_{12} is not found in any plant foods, however. It is essential for the production of nucleic acids and of red blood cells in the bone marrow. It also plays an important role in the use of folic acid and carbohydrates and in the healthy functioning of the nervous system. The DRI is 3 µg.
- Vitamin C (ascorbic acid) is found in citrus fruits, fresh potatoes, tomatoes, and green leafy vegetables. Vitamin C acts as an antioxidant and a vasoconstrictor. It also serves in the formation of connective tissue, in the conversion of cholesterol to bile salts, in iron absorption and use, and in the conversion of folic acid to its active form. The DRI is 90 mg for men and 75 mg for women.
- Niacin (nicotinamide) is found in meat, poultry, fish, liver, peanuts, and green leafy vegetables. Niacin plays an important role in the metabolism of carbohydrates and fats and inhibits cholesterol synthesis. It is important for the health of the integumentary, nervous, and digestive systems, and assists in the manufacture of reproductive hormones. The DRI is 19 mg for men and 14 mg for women.
- Biotin is found in liver, egg yolk, nuts, and legumes. Biotin is essential for the catabolism of fatty acids and carbohydrates. It also helps dispose of the waste products of protein catabolism. The DRI is 100 to 200 mg.
- Pantothenic acid is found in meats, whole grains, egg yolk, liver, yeast, and legumes. Pantothenic acid assists in the synthesis of steroids and the heme of hemoglobin. It is essential for the metabolism of carbohydrates and fats and for the manufacture of reproductive hormones. The DRI is 10 mg.

- Folic acid (folacin) is found in liver, dark green vegetables, lean beef, eggs, veal, and whole grains. Folic acid is also synthesized by bacteria in the intestine. Folic acid is the basis of a coenzyme necessary to the manufacture of nucleic acids and is therefore essential for the formation of red blood cells, growth and development, and the health of the nervous system. The RDA is 0.4 mg. (DRI not available.)

Minerals

Minerals work with other nutrients to maintain the structure and function of the body. An adequate supply of calcium, phosphorus, potassium, sulfur, sodium, chloride, and magnesium—as well as other trace elements such as iron, iodine, copper, and zinc—is necessary to health. Most minerals in the body are found in body fluids or are bound to organic compounds. The best sources of minerals are vegetables, legumes, milk, and some meats. Dietary sources for minerals are discussed in Chapter 5. The recommended daily intake for each is as follows:

- Calcium: 1000 mg, although after menopause, women who do not take estrogen supplements should increase their uptake to 1200 mg.
- Phosphorus: 700 mg
- Iron: 15 mg
- Zinc: 12 mg
- Iodine: 150 µg
- Fluoride: 3.1 mg
- Selenium: 55 µg
- Potassium: 2 g

ASSESSING NUTRITIONAL STATUS AND THE GASTROINTESTINAL SYSTEM

The nurse conducts both a health assessment interview (to collect subjective data) and a physical assessment (to collect objective data) to assess the client's nutritional status and gastrointestinal function. Physical assessment of the integumentary system, nervous system, musculoskeletal system, cardiovascular system, and respiratory system may also reflect the client's nutritional status. Table 19–1 summarizes abnormal nutritional assessment findings related to these body systems.

The Health Assessment Interview

This section provides guidelines for collecting subjective data through a health assessment interview specific to nutritional status, the gastrointestinal system, and the accessory digestive organs.

A health assessment interview to determine problems with nutrition and digestion may be conducted during a health screening, may focus on a chief complaint (such as nausea or unexplained weight loss), or may be part of a total health assessment. If the client has a health problem involving nutrition and digestion, analyze its onset, characteristics and course, severity, precipitating and relieving factors, and any associated symptoms, noting the timing and circumstances. For example, ask the client:

- Have you had any episodes of indigestion, nausea, vomiting, diarrhea, or constipation? If so, describe the appearance of what was vomited or the stools and anything that makes

TABLE 19–1 Assessment Findings Due to Malnutrition	
Body System	**Assessment Findings**
Nails	Soft and spoon-shaped in iron deficiency. Splinter hemorrhages in vitamin C deficiency.
Hair	Dry, dull, and scarce in zinc, protein, and linoleic acid deficiencies.
Skin	Flaky and dry in vitamin A, vitamin B, and/or linoleic acid deficiency. Cracks and/or hyperpigmentation in niacin deficiency. Bruising in vitamin C or vitamin K deficiency.
Eyes	Eyes become dry and soft with decrease in vitamin A. Conjunctiva is pale with a decrease in iron, and red with a decrease in riboflavin.
Nervous system	Reflexes are decreased and client may have peripheral neuropathies with thiamine deficiency. Client may be irritable and/or disoriented with thiamine deficiency.
Musculoskeletal system	Muscle wasting is seen with deficits in protein, carbohydrate, and fat metabolism. Calf pain occurs with thiamine deficiency; joint pain may occur with vitamin C deficiency.
Cardiovascular system	Heart size and rate may increase with thiamine deficiency. Diastolic blood pressure may be increased with a high intake of fat. Lowered cardiac output and decreased blood pressure may occur with caloric deficiencies over a long time period.
Respiratory system	Excessive fat can restrict respirations, and excessive fluids can impair gas exchange.
Gastrointestinal system	Cheilosis (sores at corner of mouth) seen in vitamin B-complex deficiencies, especially riboflavin. Stomatitis and spongy, bleeding gums may also be seen in malnutrition.

these problems better or worse. How long have you had these problems?

• What is your usual dietary intake pattern during a 24-hour period?

• Describe what you believe to be a "healthy" diet.

When collecting information about the client's current health status, ask about any changes in weight, appetite, and the ability to taste, chew, or swallow. What is the client's perception of the role of nutrition in maintaining health? Who buys and prepares the food? What medications (prescribed, over-the-counter, or vitamins) is the client currently taking? Does the client take any vitamins, herbal supplements, or other "health-food" items? Does the client consume alcohol (how much and type)? If the client has experienced nausea or vomiting, ask whether the vomitus contains bright red blood, dark (old) blood, bile, or fecal material. If the client is very thin or verbalizes concerns about body size incongruent with the ratio

of height to weight, ask whether the client induces vomiting or uses laxatives to control weight. Ask whether the client has appliances such as braces, bridges, or dentures, and what self-care measures are used for such appliances, as well as oral hygiene practices and frequency of dental visits.

Ask the client to describe any heartburn, indigestion, abdominal discomfort, or pain. Explore the location of the pain, the type of pain, the time it occurs, foods that aggravate or relieve it, and how it is relieved. Abdominal pain is often referred to other sites (see Chapter 4). For example, a client with a liver disorder may experience pain over the right shoulder (Kehr's sign). Epigastric (middle upper abdominal) pain is experienced in cases of acute gastritis, obstruction of the small intestine, and acute pancreatitis. Pain in the right upper quadrant is associated with cholecystitis. Pain in the left upper quadrant may be related to a gastric ulcer.

The health history should include questions about any prior surgeries or trauma of the gastrointestinal tract. Explore the past history of any medical condition that may affect the client's ingestion, digestion, and/or metabolism (for example, Crohn's disease, diabetes mellitus, irritable bowel syndrome, peptic ulcers, or pancreatitis). Other areas significant to assessment of nutritional status and the gastrointestinal system are food allergies (especially to milk, which is evidenced as lactose intolerance with abdominal cramping, excessive flatus, and loose stools) and a family history that may provide clues to increased risk for health problems.

Other questions and leading statements, categorized by functional health patterns, can be found on the Companion Website.

Physical Assessment

Physical assessment of gastrointestinal and nutritional status may be performed as part of a total health assessment, in combination with assessment of the urinary and reproductive systems (problems which may cause clinical manifestations similar to those of the gastrointestinal system), or alone for clients with known or suspected health problems. The techniques of inspection, auscultation, percussion, and palpation are used. Palpation is the last method used in assessing the abdomen, because pressure on the abdominal wall and contents may interfere with bowel sounds and cause pain, ending the examination.

Collect objective data by obtaining **anthropometric measurements** (height, weight, triceps skinfolds, and midarm circumference) and by examining the mouth and abdomen. The equipment necessary for the assessment are a stethoscope, a scale, a tape measure, and skinfold calipers. Prior to the examination, collect all necessary equipment and explain techniques to the client to decrease anxiety. The client may be seated during assessment of the mouth, but is supine during the abdominal assessment.

The quadrants of the abdomen, with related internal structures, are illustrated in Figure 19–5 ■.

Anthropometric Assessment with Abnormal Findings

• Weigh the client and compare the client's actual weight to ideal body weight (IBW) (Table 19–2).

Figure 19–5 ■ The four quadrants of the abdomen, with anatomic location of organs within each quadrant.

RUQ | LUQ

RLQ | LLQ

Midline
Aorta
Bladder
Uterus

◯ = Umbilicus

Right Upper Quadrant
Liver and gallbladder
Pylorus
Duodenum
Head of pancreas
Right adrenal gland
Portion of right kidney
Hepatic flexure of colon
Portions of ascending and
   transverse colon

Left Upper Quadrant
Left lobe of liver
Spleen
Stomach
Body of pancreas
Left adrenal gland
Portion of left kidney
Splenic flexure of colon
Portions of transverse and
   descending colon

Right Lower Quadrant
Lower pole of right kidney
Cecum and appendix
Portion of ascending colon
Bladder (if distended)
Right ovary and salpinx
Right spermatic cord
Right ureter

Left Lower Quadrant
Lower pole of left kidney
Sigmoid colon
Portion of descending colon
Bladder (if distended)
Left ovary and salpinx
Uterus (if enlarged)
Left spermatic cord
Left ureter

TABLE 19–2 Example of a Height and Weight Table

| | Height | | Weight* | | |
	Feet	Inches	Small Frame	Medium Frame	Large Frame
Men **(ages 25–29)**	5	2	128–134	131–134	138–150
	5	3	130–136	133–143	140–153
	5	4	132–138	135–145	142–156
	5	5	134–140	137–148	144–160
	5	6	136–142	139–151	146–164
	5	7	138–145	142–154	149–168
	5	8	140–148	145–157	152–172
	5	9	142–151	148–160	155–176
	5	10	144–154	151–163	158–180
	5	11	146–157	154–166	161–184
	6	0	149–160	157–170	164–188
	6	1	152–164	160–174	168–192
	6	2	155–168	164–178	172–197
	6	3	158–172	167–182	176–202
	6	4	162–176	171–187	181–207
Women **(ages 25–29)**	4	10	102–111	109–121	118–131
	4	11	103–113	111–123	120–134
	5	0	104–115	113–126	122–137
	5	1	106–118	115–129	125–140
	5	2	108–121	118–132	128–143
	5	3	111–124	121–135	131–147
	5	4	114–127	124–138	134–151
	5	5	117–130	127–141	137–155
	5	6	120–133	130–144	140–159
	5	7	123–136	133–147	143–163
	5	8	126–139	136–150	146–167
	5	9	129–142	139–153	149–170
	5	10	132–145	142–156	152–173
	5	11	135–148	145–159	155–176
	6	0	138–151	148–162	158–179

Weight in pounds. Men: allow 5 lb of clothing. Women: allow 3 lb of clothing.
Note. Courtesy of Metropolitan Life Insurance Company, 1983.

TABLE 19–3	Indications of Nutritional Status by Body Weight	
%IBW	%UBW	Nutritional Status
>120	——	Obese
110–120	——	Overweight
80–90	85–95	Mildly undernourished
70–79	75–84	Moderately undernourished
<70	<75	Severely undernourished

TABLE 19–4	Values for Anthropometric Measurements	
		Standard Value
Measurement	Male	Female
Triceps skinfold thickness	12.5 mm	16.5 mm
Midarm circumference	29.3 cm	28.5 cm
Midarm muscle circumference	25.3 cm	23.2 cm

- A weight 10% to 20% less than ideal body weight indicates malnutrition.
- A weight 10% above ideal body weight is considered overweight.
- A weight 20% above ideal body weight is considered obese.
- Calculate the client's percentage of ideal body weight (%IBW).
  - Use the formula in Table 19–3 to determine the presence of obesity and/or malnutrition based on percentage of ideal body weight.
- Calculate the client's percentage of usual body weight (%UBW) to determine weight change, using this formula:

$$\frac{\text{current weight}}{\text{usual weight}} \times 100$$

  - Using %IBW may result in overlooking malnutrition in a very obese client. Refer to Table 19–3 to determine nutritional status based on %UBW.
- Measure triceps skinfold thickness (TSF).
  - Find the midpoint between the client's olecranon and acromion processes.
  - Grasp the skin and fat, and pull it away from the muscle. Apply skinfold calipers for 3 seconds, and record reading (Figure 19–6 ■).
  - Repeat three times, and average the three readings.
  - Compare the client's reading to the standard values shown in Table 19–4.
  - Triceps readings are 10% or more below standards in malnutrition and 10% or more above standards in obesity or overnutrition.
- Measure midarm circumference (MAC).
  - Find the midpoint between the client's olecranon and acromion processes.
  - Wind tape measure around arm (Figure 19–7 ■). Compare the client's reading to the standard values shown in Table 19–4.
- MAC decreases with malnutrition and increases with obesity.
- Calculate midarm muscle circumference (MAMC).
  - Use the client's triceps skinfold measurement and midarm circumference readings to calculate the client's MAMC, using: MAMC = MAC − (0.314 × TSF).
  - Compare the result to the standard values shown in Table 19–4.
- In mild malnutrition, the MAMC is 90% of the standard; in moderate malnutrition, 60% to 90%. In severe malnutrition (muscle wasting), the MAMC is less than 60% of the standard.

Figure 19–6 ■ Measuring triceps skinfold thickness with calipers.

Figure 19–7 ■ Measuring midarm circumference with a tape measure.

Oral Assessment with Abnormal Findings

Note: Wear gloves!

- Inspect and palpate the lips.
  - ✓ *Cheilosis* (painful lesions at corners of mouth) is seen with riboflavin and/or niacin deficiency.
  - ✓ Cold sores or clear vesicles with a red base are seen in herpes simplex I.

- Inspect and palpate the tongue.
  - ✓ Atrophic smooth glossitis is characterized by a bright red tongue. It is seen in B_{12}, folic acid, and iron deficiencies.
  - ✓ Vertical fissures are seen in dehydration.
  - ✓ A black, hairy tongue may be seen following antibiotic therapy.
- Inspect and palpate the buccal mucosa.
  - ✓ *Leukoplakia* (small white patches) may be a sign of a premalignant condition.
  - ✓ A reddened, dry, swollen mucosa may be seen in stomatitis.
  - ✓ *Candidiases* (white cheesy patches that bleed when scraped) may be seen in immune-suppressed clients receiving antibiotics or chemotherapy and in terminally ill clients.
- Inspect and palpate the teeth.
  - ✓ Cavities and excessive plaque are seen with poor nutrition and/or poor oral hygiene.
- Inspect and palpate the gums.
  - ✓ Swollen, red gums that bleed easily (*gingivitis*) are seen in periodontal disease, vitamin C deficiencies, or with hormonal changes.
- Inspect the throat and tonsils.
  - ✓ In acute infections, tonsils are red and swollen and may have white spots.
- Note the client's breath.
  - ✓ Sweet, fruity breath is noted in diabetic ketoacidosis.
  - ✓ Acetone breath may be a sign of uremia.
  - ✓ Foul breath may result from liver disease, respiratory infections, and poor oral hygiene.

Abdominal Assessment with Abnormal Findings

Box 19–1 provides guidelines for abdominal assessment.

- Inspect abdominal contour, skin integrity, venous pattern, and aortic pulsation.
  - ✓ Generalized abdominal distention may be seen in gas retention or obesity.
  - ✓ Lower abdominal distention is seen in bladder distention, pregnancy, or ovarian mass.
  - ✓ General distention and an everted umbilicus is seen with ascites and/or tumors.
  - ✓ A scaphoid (sunken) abdomen is seen in malnutrition or when fat is replaced with muscle.
  - ✓ *Striae* (whitish-silver stretch marks) are seen in obesity and during or after pregnancy.
  - ✓ Spider angiomas may be seen in liver disease.
  - ✓ Dilated veins are prominent in cirrhosis of the liver, ascites, portal hypertension, or venocaval obstruction.
  - ✓ Pulsation is increased in aortic aneurysm.
- Auscultate all four quadrants of the abdomen with the diaphragm of the stethoscope (Figure 19–8 ■). Begin in the lower right quadrant, where bowel sounds are almost always present. Normal bowel sounds (gurgling or clicking) occur every 5 to 15 seconds. Listen for at least 5 minutes in each of the four quadrants to confirm the absence of bowel sounds.
  - ✓ *Borborygmus* (hyperactive high-pitched, tinkling, rushing, or growling bowel sounds) is heard in diarrhea or at the onset of bowel obstruction.
  - ✓ Bowel sounds may be absent later in bowel obstruction, with an inflamed peritoneum, and/or following surgery of the abdomen.
- Auscultate the abdomen for vascular sounds with the bell of the stethoscope (Figure 19–9 ■).
  - ✓ *Bruits* (blowing sound due to restriction of blood flow through vessels) may be heard over constricted arteries. A bruit over the liver may be heard in hepatic carcinoma.

BOX 19–1 ■ Guidelines for Assessing the Abdomen

Ask the client to empty the bladder before beginning the examination. Assist the client to the dorsal recumbent (supine) position, with a small pillow under the head, a pillow under the knees (if desired), and the arms at the sides of the body. Warm the stethoscope before applying it to the client's skin. Ask the client to point to areas that are painful, and explain that those areas will be examined last. Expose the abdomen from below the breasts to the pubic symphysis, and drape the client's thoracic and genital areas. When you document your findings, specify the location by abdominal quadrant.

General guidelines for abdominal assessment are as follows:

1. Inspect the abdomen under a good light source that is shining across the abdomen. Sit at the right side of the client, and note symmetry, distention, masses, visible peristalsis, and respiratory movements. If masses are detected, ask the client to take a deep breath, which decreases the size of the abdominal cavity and makes any abnormality more visible.

2. Auscultate each quadrant of the abdomen, using the diaphragm of the stethoscope. Listen for bowel sounds, arterial bruits, venous hums, and friction rubs.

3. Percuss several areas within each quadrant of the abdomen, using a systematic path. (For example, always begin in the lower left quadrant, then proceed to the lower right quadrant, upper right quadrant, and upper left quadrant, respectively). The predominant percussion tones for the entire abdomen are tympany and dullness. Tympany is present over gas-filled intestines. Dullness is present over the liver, the spleen, an enlarged kidney, or a full stomach. Percuss for fluid, gaseous distention, and masses.

4. Palpate each quadrant of the abdomen for shape, position, mobility, size, consistency, and tenderness of the major abdominal organs. Begin this part of the assessment with light palpation, and increase the depth of palpation to elicit tenderness or better identify organ size and shape. Deep palpation should be conducted only by nurses with considerable experience. Remember to palpate areas of indicated tenderness last and to use gentle pressure. Palpation may be difficult or impossible if the client exhibits muscle guarding from pain or is ticklish. The gallbladder and the spleen are normally not palpable.

✓ A venous hum (continuous medium-pitched sound) may be heard over a cirrhotic liver.

✓ Friction rubs (rough grating sounds) may be heard over an inflamed liver or spleen.

• Percuss the abdomen in all four quadrants (Figure 19–10 ■). Normally, tympany is heard over the stomach and gas-filled bowels.

✓ Dullness is heard when the bowel is displaced with fluid or tumors or filled with a fecal mass.

• Percuss the liver (see Box 19–2 for guidelines for liver percussion and palpation; see Figure 19–11 ■ for landmarks).

✓ In cirrhosis and/or hepatitis, the liver is greater than 6 to 10 cm in the MCL and greater than 4 to 8 cm in the midsternal line (MSL).

• Percuss the spleen for dullness posterior to the midaxilliary line at the level of the 6th to 11th rib (Figure 19–12 ■).

✓ A large area of dullness that extends to the left anterior axillary line on inspiration is associated with an enlarged

Figure 19–8 ■ Auscultating the abdomen with the diaphragm of the stethoscope.

Figure 19–10 ■ Location of sites for systematic percussion of all four quadrants.

Figure 19–9 ■ Location of placement of the stethoscope for auscultation of arteries of the abdomen.

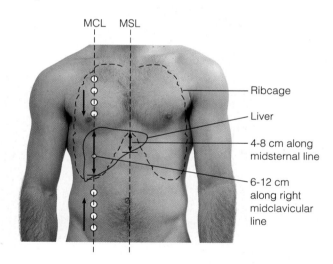

Figure 19–11 ■ Anatomic location of the liver, with the midclavicular line (MCL) and midsternal line (MSL) superimposed. The normal liver span is 6 to 12 cm.

BOX 19–2 ■ Guidelines for Percussing and Palpating the Liver

The size of the liver may be determined by percussion and palpation, as follows:

1. Percuss in the midclavicular line (MCL), beginning below the umbilicus (see Figure 19–11). Begin to percuss over a region of typmpany, and move upward. The first dull percussion tone occurs at the lower border of the liver. Determine the upper liver border by beginning percussion over an area of lung resonance (in the MCL) and percussing downward to the first dull tone, usually at the 5th to 7th interspace. Mark each of these loca-

tions, and measure the distance from one mark to the other to determine liver size. The normal liver size is 6 to 12 cm in the MCL; however, men have larger livers than women.

2. Conduct bimanual palpation of the liver by placing your left hand under the client at the level of the 11th to 12th ribs and applying upward pressure. Place your right hand below the costal margin, ask the client to take a deep breath, and palpate for the liver border. The liver is not normally palpable in a healthy adult, although it may be in very thin people.

spleen and may be related to in trauma, infection, or mononucleosis.

- Percuss for shifting dullness (Figure 19–13 ■).
  - ✓ In a client with ascites, the level of dullness increases when the client turns to the side.
- Palpate the abdomen in all four quadrants.
  - Use a circular motion to move the abdominal wall over underlying structures (Figure 19–14 ■). Feel for masses and note any tenderness or pain the client may have during this part of the exam. Palpate lightly at first (0.5 to 0.75 inch), then deeply (1.5 to 2 inches) with caution.
  - Never use deep palpation in a client who has had a pulsatile abdominal mass, renal transplant polycystic kidneys, or is at risk for hemorrhage.

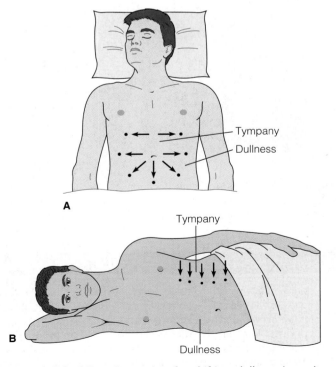

Figure 19–12 ■ Percussing the spleen.

A

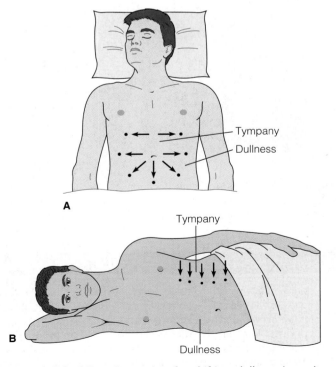

B

Figure 19–13 ■ Percussing for shifting dullness in ascites. *A*, Common percussion tones when the client is lying supine; *B*, changes in percussion tones (shfiting dullness) when the client turns to the side.

- ✓ In cases of peritoneal inflammation, palpation causes abdominal pain and involuntary muscle spasms.
- ✓ Abnormal masses include aortic aneurysms, neoplastic tumors of the colon or uterus, and a distended bladder or distended bowel due to obstruction.
- ✓ A rigid, boardlike abdomen may be palpated when the client has a perforated duodenal ulcer.
- ✓ If a mass is palpated, ask the client to raise head and shoulders. A mass in the abdomen may become more prominent with this maneuver, as will a ventral abdominal wall hernia. If the mass is no longer palpable, it is deeper in the abdomen.
- Palpate for rebound tenderness.
  - ✓ Press the fingers into the abdomen slowly and release the pressure quickly.
    - ✓ In peritoneal inflammation, pain occurs when the fingers are withdrawn.
    - ✓ Right upper quadrant pain occurs with acute cholecystitis.

A

B

Figure 19–14 ■ Light to moderate palpation of the abdomen. *A*, in light palpation, the examiner, keeping the fingers approximated, gently depresses the abdominal wall about 1 cm to assess for large masses, slight tenderness, and muscle guarding. *B*, The examiner performs moderate palpation by using the palm or the side of the hand to depress the abdominal wall to a slightly greater depth than in light palpation. This technique is useful for assessing abdominal organs that move with respiration (such as the liver and the spleen).

✓ Upper middle abdominal pain occurs with acute pancreatitis.

✓ Right lower quadrant pain occurs with acute appendicitis.

✓ Left lower quadrant pain is seen in acute diverticulitis.

- Palpate the liver (Figure 19–15 ■).

✓ An enlarged liver with a smooth, tender edge may indicate hepatitis or venous congestion.

✓ An enlarged, nontender liver may be felt in malignant condition.

✓ Note whether the client guards the abdomen or reports any sharp pain, especially on inspiration.

✓ The client with inflammation of the gallbladder feels sharp pain on inspiration and stops inspiring. This is called Murphy's sign.

Figure 19–15 ■ Palpating the liver with the bimanual method.

EXPLORE MediaLink

NCLEX review questions, case studies, care plan activities, MediaLink applications, and other interactive resources for this chapter can be found on the Companion Website at www.prenhall.com/lemone.

Click on Chapter 19 to select the activities for this chapter. For animations, video clips, more NCLEX review questions, and an audio glossary, access the Student CD-ROM accompanying this textbook.

TEST YOURSELF

1. What is the digestive function of the liver?

   a. To secrete bile
   b. To release glucose
   c. To synthesize plasma proteins
   d. To store iron as ferritin

2. The breakdown of carbohydrates to produce ATP is an example of:

   a. Metabolism
   b. Anabolism
   c. Catabolism
   d. Lipidism

3. During a health history for nutritional problems, it is important to ask the client to describe:

   a. The type, amount, and character of pain experienced
   b. The odor and color of urine

   c. The ability to put joints through full range-of-motion
   d. The usual food and fluid intake for a 24-hour period

4. In which quadrant of the abdomen would you palpate to assess the liver?

   a. Right upper
   b. Right lower
   c. Left upper
   d. Left lower

5. Clients with ascites are assessed for changes in what type of percussion sounds?

   a. Inaudible bowel sounds
   b. Resonance
   c. Alternating amplitude
   d. Shifting dullness

See Test Yourself answers in Appendix C.

BIBLIOGRAPHY

Curl, P., & Warren, J. (1997). Nutritional screening for the elderly: A CNS role. *Clinical Nurse Specialist, 11*(4), 153–158.

Evans-Stoner, N. (1997). Nutrition assessment: A practical approach. *Nursing Clinics of North America, 32*(4), 637–650.

Kirton, C. (1996). Assessing for ascites. *Nursing 96, 26*(4), 53.

Langan, J. (1998). Abdominal assessment in the home: From A to Zzz. *Home Healthcare Nurse, 16*(1), 50–58.

O'Hanlon-Nichols, T. (1998). Basic assessment series: The gastrointestinal system. *American Journal of Nursing, 98*(4), 48–53.

Watson, J., Miller, J., & Tordecilla, L. (2001). Elder oral assessment and care. *MEDSURG Nursing, 10*(1), 37–44.

Watson, R. (2000a). Assessing the gastrointestinal tract in older people: The lower GI tract. *Nursing Older People, 13*(1), 27–28.

_____ . (2000b). Assessing the gastrointestinal tract in older people: The upper GI tract. *Nursing Older People, 12*(10), 27–28.

Weber, J., & Kelley, J. (2002). *Health assessment in nursing* (2nd ed.). Philadelphia: Lippincott-Raven.

Wood, S. (1998). Nutrition assessment. *Nursing Times, 94*(29), insert 2p.

Wright, J. (1997). Seven abdominal assessment signs every emergency nurse should know. *Journal of Emergency Nursing, 23*(5), 446–450.

Nursing Care of Clients with Nutritional Disorders

MediaLink

www.prenhall.com/lemone

Additional resources for this chapter can be found on the Student CD-ROM accompanying this textbook, and on the Companion Website at www.prenhall.com/lemone. Click on Chapter 20 to select the activities for this chapter.

CD-ROM
- Audio Glossary
- NCLEX Review

Companion Website
- More NCLEX Review
- Case Study
  Obesity
- Care Plan Activity
  Malnutrition
- MediaLink Application
  Establishing a Balanced Diet

LEARNING OUTCOMES

After completing this chapter, you will be able to:

- Compare and contrast the pathophysiology and manifestations of nutritional disorders.

- Identify diagnostic tests used to find nutritional disorders.

- Discuss nursing implications for collaborative care for clients with nutritional disorders.

- Provide appropriate nursing care for a client receiving enteral or parenteral nutrition.

- Use appropriate techniques to assess clients with nutritional disorders (see Chapter 19).

- Use the nursing process as a framework for providing individualized nursing care for clients with nutritional disorders.

Obesity and malnutrition, the major nutritional disorders in the world today, affect many systems and organs. They often cause serious health problems, such as hypertension, heart disease, fluid and electrolyte imbalances, disability, and even death.

Clients with nutritional disorders require complex, skilled nursing care. Developmental, sociocultural, psychologic, and physiologic factors may play a role in these disorders: A holistic approach to nursing care is vital. Nursing care focuses on identifying causes, meeting nutritional and physiologic needs, providing client education, and meeting the psychologic needs of clients and families.

THE CLIENT WITH OBESITY

Obesity, an excess of adipose tissue, is one of the most prevalent, preventable health problems in the United States. While obesity is often defined by weight, it is more accurately defined by amount of body fat, or adipose tissue. Adipose tissue is created when energy consumption exceeds energy expenditure. Obesity has serious physiologic and psychologic consequences, and is associated with increased morbidity and mortality. Health-related problems associated with obesity are listed in Box 20–1.

INCIDENCE AND PREVALENCE

Up to one-third of the population in the United States is obese. The incidence of obesity is higher in women, African Americans, and economically disadvantaged people of all races (Braunwald et al., 2001; Tierney et al., 2001). Of particular concern is the increasing incidence of obesity in children and young adults.

OVERVIEW OF NORMAL PHYSIOLOGY

All body activities require energy, including activities of daily living, as well as those necessary to maintain cell and tissue function. Nutrients in food (or enteral or parenteral feedings)

provide this energy and the building blocks for growth and tissue repair. The body stores excess nutrients and energy (measured as kilocalories) to meet the body's needs when required nutrients are unavailable. This ability to store and release energy is important to maintaining body function.

Energy is primarily stored as fat in adipose tissue. Although mature fat cells (adipocytes) do not multiply, the immature cells in adipose tissue can multiply, particularly when exposed to estrogen during puberty, in late adolescence, during breastfeeding, and in middle-aged adults who are overweight. Fat cells store excess energy as **triglycerides,** formed from dietary fats and carbohydrates. The body breaks down the triglycerides in fat cells when needed to provide energy (Porth, 2002).

PATHOPHYSIOLOGY

Obesity occurs when excess calories are stored as fat. It can result from excess energy intake, decreased energy expenditure, or a combination of both.

Appetite, which affects food intake, is regulated by the central nervous system and by emotional factors. The hunger center in the hypothalamus stimulates appetite in response to stimuli such as hypoglycemia. As nutrient levels rise, the satiety center (also in the hypothalamus) sends the message to stop eating. Gastrointestinal filling and hormonal factors also signal *satiety* (a sensation of fullness). Appetite may have little relationship to hunger: People may eat to relieve depression or anxiety.

Several hormones are involved in regulating obesity, including thyroid hormone, insulin, and leptin (a peptide produced by fatty tissue that suppresses appetite and increases energy expenditure). Some studies suggest that leptin resistance is a cause of obesity. Insulin is associated with body fat distribution (Bullock & Henze, 2000). The two major types of body fat distribution are upper body and lower body obesity.

Upper body obesity (also called central obesity) is identified by a waist/hip ratio of greater than 1 in men or 0.8 in women. People with upper body obesity tend to have more intra-abdominal fat and higher levels of circulating free fatty acids (Porth, 2002). As a result, upper body obesity is associated with a greater risk of complications such as hypertension, abnormal blood lipid levels, heart disease, stroke, and elevated insulin levels. Men tend to have more intra-abdominal fat than women, although women develop a central fat distribution pattern after menopause.

Lower body obesity (also known as peripheral obesity), in which the waist/hip ratio is less than 0.8, is more commonly seen in women. The risk for hyperinsulinemia, abnormal lipids, and heart disease is lower in people with lower body obesity than in those with upper body obesity. Lower body obesity may be more difficult to treat, however.

Risk Factors

Many factors contribute to obesity, including genetic, physiologic, psychologic, environmental, and sociocultural factors. There is a strong link between heredity and obesity. A person with one obese parent has a 40% chance of becoming obese;

BOX 20–1 ■ Health-Related Problems in Obesity

- Arthritis
- Atherosclerosis
- Cancers of the breast, uterus, prostate, and colon
- Cholecystitis and cholelithiasis
- Heart failure
- Diabetes mellitus, type 2
- Hiatal hernia
- Postoperative complications
- Hypertension
- Low back pain
- Muscle strains and sprains
- Stress incontinence
- Thrombophlebitis
- Varicosities

MediaLink | OBESITY CASE STUDY

one with two obese parents, an 80% chance. Researchers have reported a strong correlation between the weight of adopted children and their biologic parents.

Physical inactivity is probably the most important factor contributing to obesity. Inactive people may consume fewer calories than active people and continue to gain weight due to lack of energy expenditure.

Environmental influences, such as an abundant and readily accessible food supply, fast-food restaurants, advertising, and vending machines, contribute to increased food intake. Sociocultural influences that contribute to obesity include overeating at family meals, rewarding behavior with food, religious and family gatherings that promote food intake, and sedentary lifestyles.

Psychologic factors, such as low self-esteem, also play a role in obesity. Low self-esteem may precipitate unhealthy eating behaviors, and the resulting weight gain in turn may diminish self-image even further. A person may overeat as a result of anxiety, depression, guilt, or boredom or as a means of getting attention. Some experts characterize overeating as a food addiction and as a coping mechanism for stressful life events.

Complications of Obesity

As obesity increases, adverse consequences of obesity increase. Individuals with **morbid obesity** (those whose weight is more than 100% over ideal body weight) have a risk of dying that is 12 times that of people who are not obese (Braunwald et al., 2001). Obesity increases the risk of insulin resistance and type 2 diabetes. It affects reproductive function in both men and women. Androgen (male sex hormone) levels are reduced in obese men; menstrual irregularities and polycystic ovarian syndrome (PCOS) are more common in obese women. Obesity is a significant risk factor for cardiovascular disease, including hypertension, coronary heart disease, and heart failure. Other health-related problems associated with obesity are listed in Box 20–1.

COLLABORATIVE CARE

Because obesity has many contributing factors, its treatment is far more complex than just reducing the amount of food consumed. Treatment is an ongoing process requiring a number of strategies. Most experts recommend an individualized program of exercise, diet, and behavior modification designed to meet the client's specific needs.

BOX 20–2 ■ Calculating Body Mass Index (BMI)
BMI = weight (kg)/height^2 (m^2)   Normal = BMI 18.5–24.9 kg/m^2 Overweight = BMI 25–29.9 kg/m^2 Obese = BMI > 30 kg/m^2 Morbidly obese = BMI > 40 kg/m^2

Diagnostic Tests

Although body weight may be used to identify obesity, measures of body fat are more accurate. Males at ideal body weight have 10% to 20% body fat, whereas females at ideal body weight have 20% to 30% body fat.

- *Body mass index (BMI)* is used to identify excess adipose tissue. BMI is calculated by dividing the weight (in kilograms) by the height in meters squared (m^2). See Box 20–2.
- *Anthropometry,* skinfold or fatfold measurements, uses calipers to measure skinfold thickness at various sites on the body (see Chapter 19).
- *Underwater weighing (hydrodensitometry)* is considered the most accurate way to determine body fat. This technique involves submerging the whole body and then measuring the amount of displaced water.
- *Bioelectrical impedance* uses a low-energy electrical impulse to determine the percentage of body fat by measuring the electrical resistance of the body.

Other diagnostic tests may be done to help identify a physiologic cause of obesity, as well as complications of obesity.

- A *thyroid profile,* including a T$_3$, T$_4$, and TSH, is done to rule out thyroid disease (see Chapter 16). ⌖
- *Serum glucose* is measured to identify coexisting diabetes mellitus.
- *Serum cholesterol* is measured to assess for elevated levels.
- A *lipid profile* is ordered; high-density lipoprotein (HDL) levels are reduced in obese clients, whereas low-density lipoprotein (LDL) levels are elevated.
- An *electrocardiogram (ECG)* is performed to detect effects of obesity on the heart, such as rate or rhythm disruptions, myocardial infarction, or heart enlargement.

Treatments

Treatment of obesity focuses on changing both eating and exercise habits. A pound of body fat is equivalent to 3500 kcal. To lose 1 pound, therefore, a person must reduce daily caloric intake by 250 kcal for 14 days or increase activity enough to burn the equivalent kcal.

Exercise

Exercise is a critical element in weight loss and maintenance. Physical activity increases energy consumption and promotes weight loss while preserving lean body mass. Physical activity improves physical fitness, decreases appetite, promotes self-esteem, and increases the basal metabolic rate. An exercise or activity program should reflect the client's physical condition, interest, lifestyle, and abilities. Evaluation by a health care practitioner is important before beginning an exercise program. The practitioner instructs the client to increase the duration and intensity of activity and to stop exercising and report symptoms if chest pain or shortness of breath occurs. An aerobic exercise program of 30 minutes of exercise 3 to 5 days a week promotes weight loss while reducing adipose tissue, increasing lean body mass, and promoting long-term weight control.

BOX 20–3 ■ Behavioral Change Strategies for the Obese Client

CONTROLLING THE ENVIRONMENT
- Purchase low-calorie foods.
- Shop from a prepared list and on a full stomach.
- Keep all foods in the kitchen.
- Store all foods in the refrigerator or in the cabinets in opaque containers.
- Prepare exact portions of food to eliminate leftovers.
- Eat all foods in the same place, avoiding the kitchen.
- Avoid eating when watching television or reading.
- Reduce frequency of eating out at restaurants, parties, and picnics.

CONTROLLING PHYSIOLOGIC RESPONSES TO FOOD
- Eat slowly by taking small bites, allowing 20 minutes for a meal.
- Eat a salad or drink a hot beverage before a meal.
- Chew each bite thoroughly and slowly.
- Put eating utensils or food down between bites.
- Concentrate on the eating process, savor the food.
- Stop eating with the first feelings of fullness.

CONTROLLING PSYCHOLOGIC RESPONSES TO FOOD
- Appreciate the aesthetic experience of eating.
- Use attractive dinnerware, and prepare a formal setting for eating.
- Use small plates and cups to make servings of food look larger.
- Concentrate on conversations and socialization during the meal.
- Use nonfood rewards for meeting a goal.
- Acknowledge small successes and improvements in all behavior.
- Substitute other activities for eating (e.g., reading, exercise, hobbies).

Dietary Management

The diet should be low in kilocalories and fat and contain adequate nutrients, minerals, and fiber. The client should eat regular meals with small servings. A gradual, slow weight loss of no more than 1 to 2 pounds per week is recommended. For most people, this means a diet of 1000 to 1500 kcal per day. Fewer than 1200 kcal each day may lead to loss of lean tissue and nutritional deficiencies. The recommended diet generally is low in fat and high in dietary fiber. Excessive calorie restrictions can lead to failure to follow the prescribed diet, feelings of guilt, and overeating. "Yo-yo" dieting (repeated cycles of weight loss and gain) may lead to a metabolic deficiency that makes subsequent weight loss efforts increasingly difficult. Therefore, it is critical that dieters take any weight loss effort seriously and include plans for long-term maintenance. The best approach is to modify dietary intake without severe restrictions, eating a well-balanced, low-fat diet and developing improved eating habits.

Very low calorie diets (VLCD) are generally reserved for clients who are more than 35% overweight. This type of program offers a protein-sparing modified fast (400 to 800 kcal/day or less) under close medical supervision. In a typical program, the client observes a 12-week fast, ingesting only a liquid protein supplement. This initial fast is followed by a 12-week refeeding program with nutrition and behavior modification counseling. The client generally experiences a dramatic and rapid weight loss while maintaining lean body mass. This type of program is indicated for short-term use only and requires very close medical supervision.

Behavior Modification

Behavior modification is a critical component of successful weight management. Strategies such as keeping food records, eliminating cues that precipitate eating, and changing the act of eating are often helpful.

Recording food intake, amount, location of eating, and situations that induce eating often help the dieter gain self-control. These strategies are often most effective when used in combination with other behavior modification approaches.

Researchers have found that most overweight people are stimulated to eat by external cues, such as the proximity to food and the time of day. In contrast, hunger and satiety are the cues that regulate eating in adults of normal weight. Strategies to control food cues include keeping food out of view, eliminating snack foods, and eating only in designated areas. See Box 20–3 for a list of behavior modification strategies.

Other behavior modification approaches focus on helping clients examine factors that affect eating behaviors. Examining lifestyle, personality, and environment helps the client understand eating behaviors and their consequences. The goal is to empower the person who is stimulated to eat to choose activities that are not related to food.

Social support and group programs such as Weight Watchers, Overeaters Anonymous, and Take Off Pounds Sensibly (TOPS) promote weight loss success through peer support. Most organized programs require participants to pay a fee, which may improve compliance.

Medications

Many prescription and over-the-counter drugs have been used to help people lose weight. When used in combination with diet and exercise, drugs can help promote weight loss. Their long-term efficacy, however, is questionable. In addition, tolerance, addiction, and side effects may occur. These products are usually recommended only as an adjunct to therapy and only when traditional therapies have been unsuccessful.

Amphetamines (which have a high potential for abuse) and nonamphetamine appetite suppressants (such as phenteramine) may be used for a short time to promote weight loss. Sibutramine (Meridia) is an appetite suppressant that acts on the CNS. Sibutramine also may increase the metabolic rate, promoting weight loss. It has the additional benefit of lowering

Medication Administration
Drugs to Treat Obesity

APPETITE SUPPRESSANT

- Sibutramine (Meridia)

Sibutramine reduces hunger and increases sensations of satiety by inhibiting the uptake of seroatonin, norepinephrine, and dopamine. It is used to treat obesity in clients with a BMI of >30 kg/m² and obese clients who have risk factors such as diabetes or hypertension.

Nursing Responsibilities

- Assess for contraindications to this drug, such as pregnancy or lactation, use of other appetite suppressants, impaired liver or kidney function, history of coronary heart disease, or alcohol abuse.
- Regularly monitor blood pressure and heart rate during treatment. Increases may indicate need to reduce dose or discontinue treatment.

Client and Family Teaching

- Take as directed; do not exceed recommended dose. Do not take if you may be pregnant or are nursing.
- You may experience difficulty sleeping, nervousness, or palpitations while taking this drug.
- Increase your fluid intake to reduce possible side effects of dry mouth and constipation.

- This drug does not replace diet and exercise for weight loss; continue to follow your prescribed regimen.

LIPASE INHIBITOR

- Orlistat (Xenical)

Orlistat inhibits lipases necessary for the breakdown and absorption of fat, thus decreasing the absorption of dietary fat. Its action is primarily local, within the GI tract, with few systemic effects.

Nursing Responsibilities

- Administer with meals or up to 1 hour following a meal.
- Provide a fat-soluble vitamin supplement (A, D, E, and K) daily. Separate administration time from orlistat by at least 2 hours.

Client and Family Teaching

- Take as directed; do not increase dose. You may skip a dose if you do not consume a meal.
- Use in conjunction with a low-calorie, low-fat diet.
- Common gastrointestinal side effects include oily or fatty stools, flatulence, oily discharge, or frequent stools with difficulty controlling defecation. These side effects may diminish with time or increase if a meal high in fat is consumed.
- Notify your health care provider if you become pregnant while taking this medication.

---

cholesterol and triglyceride levels. Orlistat (Xenical) has a different mechanism of action: It inhibits fat absorption from the GI tract, leading to weight loss. It has the added benefit of lowering blood glucose and cholesterol. See the box above for the nursing implications of these drugs.

Over-the-counter products such as phenylpropanolamine, benzocaine, and bulk-forming agents are commonly used in weight management efforts. Phenylpropanolamine (Acutrim, Dexatrim) is an adrenergic agent that suppresses appetite. This product is contraindicated in clients with hypertension, coronary heart disease, diabetes mellitus, and thyroid disease. Methylcellulose and other bulk-forming products may decrease appetite by producing a sensation of fullness. Clients taking these products may experience flatulence or diarrhea and may need to increase fluid intake.

Surgery

Surgical treatment of obesity generally is limited to morbidly obese clients (BMI of over 40 kg/m² or 100% over ideal body weight). In addition, clients must be able to tolerate surgery and be free of addiction to alcohol or other drugs. A thorough psychologic evaluation is done before surgery.

The most common surgical procedures used in the United States to treat obesity are the vertical banded gastroplasty and Roux-en-Y gastric bypass (Figure 20–1 ■). These procedures reduce stomach capacity. Although the risk for postoperative complications is high, the mortality rate for these procedures is low. Possible postoperative complications include anasto-

Gastroplasty   Vertical banding   Gastric bypass

Figure 20–1 ■ Surgical procedures to treat obesity.

mosis leak with peritonitis, abdominal wall hernia, wound infections, deep vein thrombosis, nutritional deficiencies, and gastrointestinal symptoms (Tierney et al., 2001). Clients may lose as much as half their initial body weight following surgery.

Maintaining Weight Loss

Losing weight and maintaining that loss are two separate but related issues. Most experts agree that the majority of dieters regain lost weight within a 2-year period. The potential risks associated with regaining weight make maintenance a critical issue. Clients are encouraged to continue exercise, self-monitoring, and treatment support. Long-term weight loss and maintenance mean a lifelong commitment to significant lifestyle changes, including food and eating habits, activity and exercise routines, and behavior modification.

NURSING CARE

Health Promotion

Maintaining a healthy weight throughout the life span begins in childhood. Obese children and teenagers become obese adults. Promote healthy eating, including a diet rich in whole grains, fruits, and vegetables and low in fat. Encourage all children and adults to maintain an active lifestyle, engaging in at least 30 minutes of aerobic activity daily. Encourage parents to limit time children spend watching television, using the computer, and playing video games. Discuss the effect of smoking and excess alcohol use on nutrition and activity.

Adults commonly gain about 20 pounds between early and middle adulthood. Encourage clients to reduce the amount of calories consumed as energy needs change.

Assessment

Collect the following data through the health history and physical examination (see Chapter 19).

- Health history: risk factors; current and usual weight; recent weight gains or losses; perception of weight and effect on health; usual diet and food intake; exercise/activity patterns; prior weight-loss efforts; current medications; coexisting disorders such as cardiovascular disease and diabetes
- Physical examination: vital signs; weight and height; skinfold measurements; waist/hip ratio; BMI

Nursing Diagnoses and Interventions

Nursing care for overweight and obese clients is community based and holistic, focusing on both physiologic and psychologic responses to weight and appearance.

Imbalanced Nutrition: More Than Body Requirements

Although many factors contribute to obesity, it always involves an imbalance of kcal consumption to energy expenditure.

- Encourage the client to identify the factors that contribute to excess food intake. *Identification of cues to eating helps the client eliminate or reduce these cues.*
- Establish realistic weight-loss goals and exercise/activity objectives. *Small, reasonable goals, such as loss of 1 to 2 pounds per week, increase the likelihood of success.*
- Assess the client's knowledge and discuss well-balanced diet plans. Provide necessary teaching about diet. *Knowledge empowers the client to participate and make appropriate diet choices.*
- Discuss behavior modification strategies, such as self-monitoring and environmental management. *Behavior modification, diet, and exercise are critical to promoting successful, long-term weight loss.*

Activity Intolerance

Obese clients may experience excess fatigue, tachycardia, and shortness of breath with activity due to the physiologic effects of excess weight as well as a sedentary lifestyle. A medical evaluation may be needed before beginning an exercise program.

- Assess current activity level and tolerance of that activity. Assess vital signs. *This provides baseline information to plan an activity program and assess response to that activity.*
- After medical clearance, plan with the client a program of regular, gradually increasing exercise. Consider a consultation with an exercise physiologist. *An individualized exercise program promotes activities within the client's physical capabilities.*

Ineffective Therapeutic Regimen Management

Most overweight or obese clients experience some difficulty integrating all the components of a weight-loss program into a daily routine. For a weight loss and maintenance program to be successful, the overweight client must modify dietary intake in a world of daily temptations. There may be many obstacles to exercise, including a busy schedule, activity intolerance, impaired physical mobility, lack of equipment, and the embarrassment of being fat.

- Discuss ability and willingness to incorporate changes into daily patterns of diet, exercise, and lifestyle. *This provides data from which to set realistic goals with the client.*
- Help the client identify behavior modification strategies and support systems for weight loss and maintenance. *Weight loss and maintenance are most successful if the client establishes lifestyle patterns that promote interest and motivation and thus exercise and diet management. Family and social support is critical to successful adherence to the therapeutic regime.*
- Have the client establish strategies for dealing with "stress" eating or interruptions in the therapeutic regime. *A sense of failure associated with overeating or lack of exercise can lead to further overeating. Identifying positive strategies to deal with these situations promotes self-acceptance and limits self-punishment through overeating.*

Chronic Low Self-Esteem

Although many obese clients may have accepted their weight and body appearance on some level, most overweight and obese individuals verbalize the experience of "fat prejudice" in their family, workplace, or community. Obese clients may experience ridicule, prejudice, and health problems attributed to being "fat." These experiences, coupled with day-to-day problems such as finding attractive clothing or a chair large enough to sit on can affect self-esteem. Many clients report that "fat" jokes or comments contribute to a sense of negative self-worth.

- Encourage the client to verbalize the experience of being overweight, and validate the client's experience. *This provides baseline data to use in developing individualized interventions to addresses self-esteem issues.*
- Set small goals with the client and offer positive feedback and encouragement. *Small goals provide more opportunities for success. Positive feedback and encouragement provide a comfortable environment in which to develop self-esteem.*
- Refer for counseling as appropriate. *Many clients benefit from counseling for issues related to self-esteem.*

CHART 20-1   NANDA, NIC, AND NOC LINKAGES

The Obese Client

NURSING DIAGNOSES	NURSING INTERVENTIONS	NURSING OUTCOMES
• Imbalanced Nutrition: More than Body Requirements	• Nutrition Management • Weight Reduction Assistance • Behavior Modification	• Nutritional Status • Nutrient Intake • Weight Control
• Disturbed Body Image	• Body Image Enhancement	• Body Image
• Chronic Low Self-Esteem	• Self-Esteem Enhancement	• Self-Esteem

Note. Data from Nursing Outcomes Classification (NOC) by M. Johnson & M. Maas (Eds.), 1997, St. Louis: Mosby; Nursing Diagnoses: Definitions & Classification 2001–2002 by North American Nursing Diagnosis Association, 2001, Philadelphia: NANDA; Nursing Interventions Classification (NIC) by J.C. McCloskey & G. M. Bulechek (Eds.), 2000, St. Louis: Mosby. Reprinted by permission.

Using NANDA, NIC, and NOC

Chart 20–1 shows links between NANDA nursing diagnoses, NIC, and NOC for obese clients.

Home Care

Weight reduction usually occurs in community-based settings. Weight loss and maintenance requires a long-term commitment

Nursing Care Plan
A Client with Obesity

Sam Elliott, age 57, has gained 30 pounds since his retirement 2 years ago. The most active thing he does each day is "puttering around" and "walking to the end of the driveway to get the mail." His diet includes juice, oatmeal, muffin, and coffee with cream for breakfast; donuts and coffee with friends midmorning; a bologna-and-cheese sandwich with chips and a root beer for lunch; and cheese, crackers, and wine before a dinner of meat, potatoes, vegetables, and dessert. He tells the nurse, "I have never had to diet. I just don't know how to get this weight off."

ASSESSMENT
Mr. Elliott is 5' 8" (173 cm) tall and weighs 201 lb (91.2 kg). His BMI is 30.1 kg/m². His cholesterol is 240 mg/dL (normal 150 to 200 mg/dL) with an HDL of 37 mg/dL (normal male value > 45 mg/dL) and an LDL of 180 mg/dL (normal <130 mg/dL). His BP is 138/90. His fasting blood glucose is normal at 103 mg/dL. His ECG shows normal sinus rhythm. He reports fatigue and shortness of breath with activity. His health care provider has advised a weight loss of 30 pounds and a regular exercise program.

DIAGNOSES
- *Imbalanced nutrition: More than body requirements* related to food intake in excess of energy expenditure
- *Risk for ineffective therapeutic regimen management* related to knowledge deficit
- *Activity intolerance* related to sedentary lifestyle

EXPECTED OUTCOMES
- Lose 1 pound each week.
- Walk 30 minutes 5 days each week.
- Verbalize an understanding of the relationship between weight loss, weight control, and exercise.
- Identify behavior modification strategies to avoid overeating.
- Identify support systems for behavior modification.

PLANNING AND IMPLEMENTATION
- Assess weight and blood pressure once or twice each week.
- Discuss current eating habits and strategies to reduce fat and calorie intake.
- Discuss cues that promote eating. Identify strategies to eliminate or reduce eating cues.
- Teach to keep a food diary to examine and change eating habits.
- Discuss the role of regular exercise in weight loss and weight control. Instruct to maintain an exercise record to track the intensity and duration of activity.
- Discuss lifestyle and behavior modification strategies to promote successful weight loss and control.

EVALUATION
Two weeks after changing his diet and beginning to exercise, Mr. Elliott has lost 2 pounds. He has maintained a food diary. He has identified boredom as a cue to eating. In light of that fact, he has started volunteering at the local hospital, where he is working with children. He is walking for 30 minutes 5 days a week. He plans to increase his activity periods to 45 minutes. He verbalizes commitment to a lifelong plan of exercising and eating a low-fat diet. His BP has ranged from 132/76 to 136/84. He plans to have the employee health nurse at the hospital check his weight and BP each week and to join Weight Watchers for ongoing support.

Critical Thinking in the Nursing Process
1. What are some possible pathophysiologic bases for Mr. Elliott's abnormal cholesterol, HDL, and LDL levels?
2. Develop a teaching plan for a group of overweight men and women.
3. Identify potential barriers to losing weight and strategies to reduce or eliminate these barriers.

See Evaluating Your Response in Appendix C.

by the client, family, and support systems. Address the following topics with the client and family.

- Lifestyle changes are more effective than diets. Fad diets promote rapid weight loss but often are not nutritionally sound or may be difficult to maintain for a lifetime.
- All household members should consume a diet that is nutritionally sound, low in fat, and high in fiber.
- Establish realistic weight loss goals and a system of nonfood rewards for achieving each goal.
- Identify an "exercise buddy" or support system to promote continued physical activity.
- Expect occasional failures. Resume prescribed diet and exercise routine as soon as possible; the goal is long-term weight management.
- Community resources such as Weight Watchers, TOPS, or health care–based programs provide information, strategies, and support for successful weight management.

THE CLIENT WITH MALNUTRITION

Malnutrition results from inadequate intake of nutrients. There may be a lack of major nutrients (calories, carbohydrates, proteins, and fats) or micronutrients such as vitamins and minerals. Malnutrition may be caused by inadequate nutrient intake, impaired absorption and use of nutrients, or increased metabolic needs.

INCIDENCE AND PREVALENCE

Malnutrition is a widespread cause of disease and mortality throughout the world. It is endemic in regions affected by famine. Groups at risk for malnutrition in the United States include the young, poor, elderly, homeless, low-income women, and ethnic minorities. Even when food is plentiful, clients may be undernourished because of poor food choices.

More than half of all hospitalized clients are malnourished (Braunwald et al., 2001). Malnutrition may be present on admission or develop as a result of surgery or serious illness. See Box 20–4 for conditions commonly associated with malnutrition.

PATHOPHYSIOLOGY

Carbohydrates and fats in the diet are the body's primary energy source. Approximately 15% to 25% of the body is fat, the

BOX 20–4	■ Conditions Associated with Malnutrition

■ Acute respiratory failure	■ Gastrointestinal disorders
■ Aging	■ Neurologic disorders
■ AIDS	■ Renal disease
■ Alcoholism	■ Short bowel syndrome
■ Burns	■ Surgery
■ COPD	■ Trauma
■ Eating disorders	

body's energy reservoir. The remainder (muscles, bones, other body tissues and organs) is lean body mass, metabolically active tissue. Proteins in the diet primarily are used to maintain this tissue. Glycogen and proteins in this lean body mass also act as energy stores.

When dietary intake does not meet the body's energy needs, the body uses glycogen, body proteins, and lipids (fats) to support metabolism. In **starvation** (inadequate dietary intake), glycogen initially is used to provide energy. After the first 24 hours of starvation, gluconeogenesis (formation of glucose from proteins) is the major source of energy. As starvation continues, the body breaks down fats into free fatty acids and ketones, which provide energy for the brain. The size of all body compartments is reduced as body fats and muscle proteins are used to meet energy needs. As lean body mass is reduced, metabolically active tissue is lost, and energy expenditure decreases.

The stress of acute illness or trauma produces a different response. The acute stress response produces a state of hypermetabolism and **catabolism** (cell and tissue breakdown). This hypermetabolic state increases energy expenditure and nutrient needs. Lean body mass is broken down to meet these needs. If untreated, up to half of the body's protein stores can be used within 3 weeks.

Many hospitalized clients are malnourished (starved) on admission. Surgery or illness promote a stress response, resulting in **protein-calorie malnutrition (PCM)**. In PCM, both protein and calories are deficient. Chronic protein deficiency with adequate calories to meet energy needs is called **kwashiorkor.** When both proteins and calories are insufficient to meet the body's needs, PCM is known as **marasmus.**

Risk Factors

Risk factors for malnutrition include the following:

- Age—older adults are at greater risk for malnutrition due to a variety of factors (see the Meeting Individualized Needs box on page 530)
- Poverty, homelessness, inadequate food storage and preparation facilities
- Functional health problems that limit mobility or vision
- Oral or gastrointestinal problems that affect food intake, digestion, and absorption
- Chronic pain or chronic diseases such as pulmonary, cardiovascular, renal, or endocrine disorders
- Medications or treatments that affect appetite
- Acute problems such as infection, surgery, or trauma

Manifestations and Complications

The manifestations of malnutrition may vary among clients. Weight loss is the most apparent manifestation of malnutrition. The malnourished client may have a body weight of less than 90% of ideal. Body mass also is reduced (see Box 20–2), as is skinfold thickness. Other manifestations include a wasted appearance, dry and brittle hair, and pale mucous membranes. Peripheral or abdominal edema may be present. Manifestations of specific nutritional deficiencies may be present (Table 20–1). See page 531 for the *Multisystem Effects of Malnutrition.*

Meeting Individualized Needs

NUTRITION FOR THE OLDER ADULT

Older adults are at greater risk for malnutrition. Age-related changes that contribute to this problem include changes in taste and smell, a higher incidence of gastrointestinal disease, poor oral health, loss of teeth or ill-fitting dentures, anorexia caused by medications, and functional limitations that impair the ability to shop and cook. Psychosocial issues also contribute to the problem. Older adults living on fixed incomes, many at the poverty level, may not be able to afford well-balanced meals. Loss of appetite is a problem commonly seen with depression. Social isolation and loneliness contribute to the problem. Eating is a social event, and older adults who eat alone may not eat as well as those who share meals with companions, and may consume too few, or too many, calories.

Conduct a thorough assessment to determine nutritional status. Assess psychological factors that influence eating habits, such as loneliness, isolation, and depression. Note the client's general appearance and obtain a diet history, including information about foods and nutrients the client consumes, and recent weight loss or gain. Review laboratory values, including complete blood count, total protein, and albumin.

Teaching for Home Care

To maintain nutritional status, the older client should be advised to:

- Eat a well-balanced diet.
- Eat fresh fruits and vegetables.
- Shop wisely to get the most value for the money.
- Avoid processed foods.
- Avoid foods high in fat.
- Drink adequate fluids.
- Exercise regularly.
- Contact local agencies for the availability of congregate meals (e.g., at local senior centers) or home-delivered meals (e.g., Meals-on-Wheels).

Subcutaneous fat and muscle proteins are broken down in PCM, impairing mobility and increasing the risk for skin and tissue breakdown (pressure ulcers). Protein synthesis is inhibited and wound healing delayed. Serum albumin levels fall, leading to abdominal edema, diarrhea, and impaired nutrient absorption. Immune function is impaired, increasing the risk of infection. Cardiac output falls, and the risk for postural hypotension increases.

TABLE 20–1	Manifestations of Specific Nutrient Deficiencies
Deficiency	**Assessment Data**
Calorie	Weight Loss Weakness, listlessness Loss of subcutaneous fat Muscle wasting
Protein	Thin or sparse hair Flaking skin Hepatomegaly
Vitamin A	Night blindness Altered taste and smell Dry, scaling, rough skin
Thiamine	Confusion, apathy Cardiomegaly, dyspnea Muscle cramping and wasting Paresthesia, neuropathy Ataxia
Riboflavin	Cheilosis, stomatitis Neuropathy, glossitis
Vitamin C	Swollen, bleeding gums Delayed wound healing Weakness, depression Easy bruising
Iron	Smooth tongue Listlessness, fatigue Dyspnea

COLLABORATIVE CARE

The goal of treatment for the malnourished client is to restore ideal body weight while replacing and restoring depleted nutrients and minerals. The client's age, severity of malnutrition, and coexisting health problems help determine interventions. Treatment may include oral supplementation, tube feedings, or total parenteral nutrition (TPN).

Diagnostic Tests

As with obesity, the standard measurements to assess for malnutrition include height, weight, calculation of BMI, and skinfold measurements. A BMI of less than 18 to 20 kg/m^2 may indicate malnutrition. The following laboratory studies also may be ordered.

- *Serum albumin* is reduced in PCM, and may be below 3.0 mg/dL.
- The *total lymphocyte count* is evaluated by multiplying the WBC by the percentage of lymphocytes. The total lymphocyte count is reduced in PCM.
- *Serum electrolytes* are measured. Potassium levels are low in severe malnutrition.

The following specialized procedures to evaluate the extent of malnutrition may be ordered.

- *Bioelectric impedance analysis* measures body fat and total body water. Differences in the conductivity of a weak current (measured between the hands and feet) allow calculation of body fat and water (current flows more slowly through fat tissue than through water).
- *Total daily energy expenditure* (which includes resting energy expenditure, energy needed for digestion, plus physical activity needs) may be measured to help determine the client's calorie intake needs.

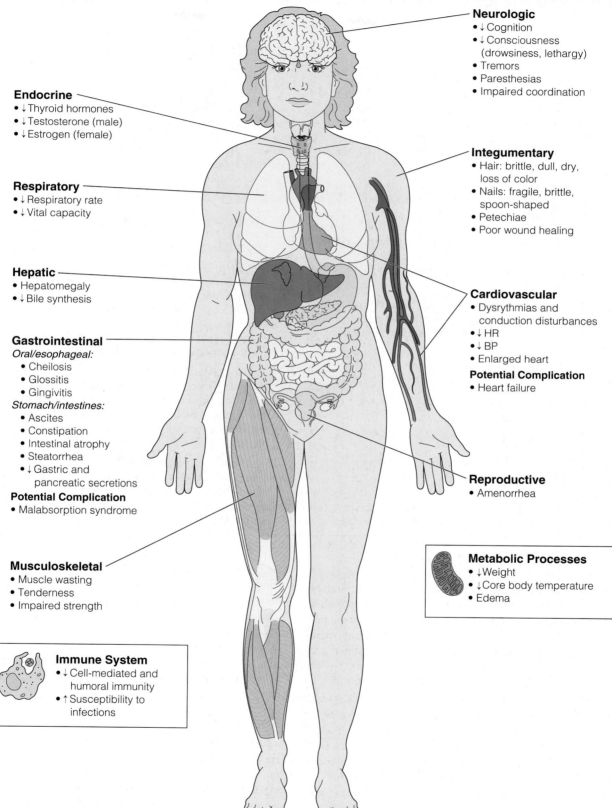

Neurologic
- ↓ Cognition
- ↓ Consciousness (drowsiness, lethargy)
- Tremors
- Paresthesias
- Impaired coordination

Endocrine
- ↓ Thyroid hormones
- ↓ Testosterone (male)
- ↓ Estrogen (female)

Respiratory
- ↓ Respiratory rate
- ↓ Vital capacity

Integumentary
- Hair: brittle, dull, dry, loss of color
- Nails: fragile, brittle, spoon-shaped
- Petechiae
- Poor wound healing

Hepatic
- Hepatomegaly
- ↓ Bile synthesis

Cardiovascular
- Dysrythmias and conduction disturbances
- ↓ HR
- ↓ BP
- Enlarged heart

Potential Complication
- Heart failure

Gastrointestinal
Oral/esophageal:
- Cheilosis
- Glossitis
- Gingivitis

Stomach/intestines:
- Ascites
- Constipation
- Intestinal atrophy
- Steatorrhea
- ↓ Gastric and pancreatic secretions

Potential Complication
- Malabsorption syndrome

Reproductive
- Amenorrhea

Musculoskeletal
- Muscle wasting
- Tenderness
- Impaired strength

Metabolic Processes
- ↓ Weight
- ↓ Core body temperature
- Edema

Immune System
- ↓ Cell-mediated and humoral immunity
- ↑ Susceptibility to infections

Medication Administration
Vitamin & Mineral Supplements

FAT-SOLUBLE VITAMINS

Vitamin A
Vitamin D
Vitamin E
Vitamin K

The fat-soluble vitamins are absorbed in the gastrointestinal tract. Vitamins A and D are stored in the liver.

All fat-soluble vitamins may become toxic if taken in excess amounts.

Nursing Responsibilities
- Monitor for manifestations of vitamin excess as well as for adverse effects from vitamin administration.
- Monitor carefully for hypersensitivity reactions during the parenteral administration. Have emergency equipment available.
- Administer vitamin A with food.
- Do not administer vitamin K intravenously.

Client and Family Teaching
- Teach the importance of eating a well-balanced diet. If indicated, provide lists of foods high in specific vitamins.
- Caution that excessive intake of these vitamins may lead to vitamin toxicity.

WATER-SOLUBLE VITAMINS

Vitamin C (ascorbic acid)
Vitamin B complex:
  Thiamine (B_1)
  Riboflavin (B_2)
  Niacin (Nicotinic acid)
  Pyridoxine hydrochloride (B_6)
  Pantothenic acid
  Biotin

These vitamins are used to prevent or treat deficiency problems. If the diet is deficient in one vitamin, it is usually deficient in other vitamins as well; therefore, multivitamin preparations are often administered. Most of these vitamins are well absorbed from the gastrointestinal tract.

Nursing Responsibilities
- Monitor for responses to replacement therapy.
- Monitor for hypersensitivity reactions from parenteral administration. Have emergency equipment available.

Client and Family Teaching
- Do not exceed the recommended daily allowances for the specific vitamin.

MINERALS

Sodium	Copper	Manganese
Potassium	Fluoride	Chromium
Magnesium	Iodine	Selenium
Calcium	Zinc	

Minerals are inorganic chemicals that are vital to a variety of physiologic functions. Also called trace elements, these minerals are part of a balanced diet. Recommended daily allowances have not been established for all mineral substances. The dosage of prescribed minerals depends on the specific deficiency, route of administration, and the client's general health.

Nursing Responsibilities
- Monitor for manifestations of mineral imbalance.
- Prior to administration dilute oral mineral preparations.
- Prior to the administration of iodine, assess for history of hypersensitivity to iodine or seafood; if hypersensitive notify the physician.

Client and Family Teaching
- Encourage the client to avoid exceeding the known recommended daily allowances of the mineral.
- Instruct the client to take minerals other than fluoride and zinc with or after meals.

Medications

Malnourished clients generally require supplemental vitamins and minerals to restore these essential micronutrients. A multivitamin and mineral supplement may be given, or therapy may be tailored to correct specific deficiencies. See the box above for nursing implications of vitamin and mineral supplements.

Fluid and Dietary Management

Fluids and nutrients are carefully reintroduced in severely malnourished clients. First, fluid and electrolyte imbalances are corrected, with particular attention paid to restoring normal potassium, magnesium, and calcium levels, as well as acid-base balance. Once fluid and electrolyte imbalances are corrected, protein and calories are gradually reintroduced into the diet. Vitamin and mineral supplements are provided along with refeeding. Fat and lactose are reintroduced into the diet last.

Gradual refeeding is necessary to prevent electrolyte imbalances from developing as potassium, magnesium, phosphorus, and glucose move into the cells. Heart failure may occur due to depressed cardiac function. Abnormalities in gastrointestinal function can lead to malabsorption and diarrhea with refeeding (Tierney et al., 2001). Commercially available nutritional supplements (such as Carnation Instant Breakfast, Ensure, and Sustacal) may supplement protein and calorie intake. Administering 2 ounces of nutritional supplement with each medication given (unless the medication must be given on an empty stomach) may be an effective way to increase clients' calorie and protein intake (Bender et al., 2000).

Enteral Nutrition

Enteral nutrition, or tube feeding, may be used to meet calorie and protein requirements in clients unable to consume adequate food. Indications for tube feedings include difficulty swallowing, unresponsiveness, oral or neck surgery or trauma, anorexia, or serious illness. Tube feedings may provide part or all of a client's nutritional needs.

Tube feedings are usually administered through a soft, small-caliber nasogastric or nasoduodenal tube with a weighted

Nursing Research

Evidence-Based Practice for Determining Feeding Tube Placement

The auscultatory method of determining the location for feeding tubes on initial placement and prior to initiating feeding is commonly recommended in nursing textbooks and is frequently used. The premise is that injecting a small amount of air into the tube will produce a distinctive sound if the tube is correctly located, presumably in the stomach. Sounds produced by tubes located in the esophagus, intestines, and respiratory tract are presumed to be different enough to alert the nurse to the improper location. However, based on a series of studies (Metheny et al., 1998), the auscultory method for determining placement is not reliable. This is especially true for small-bore feeding tubes. Testing the pH level of aspirates from newly inserted feeding tubes and of tubes from clients receiving intermittent feedings can help distinguish gastric from respiratory and intestinal placement. Based on the pH of a large number of samples of aspirates from feeding tubes, a pH between 0 and 4 suggests gastric placement and a pH of 7 or greater indicates respiratory placement. As the tube advances through the stomach into the intestine, pH levels increase and the color of the aspirate changes. If placement in the small intestine is required, a confirmatory X-ray should be taken. These researchers recommend that the pH method be used rather than the auscultory method and that protocols be updated to reflect current information.

IMPLICATIONS FOR NURSING

With the advent of small-bore nasogastric and nasointestinal feeding tubes and the increasing use of gastrostomy and jejunostomy feeding tubes, more and more clients are receiving enteral feedings. Nurses need to use alternative methods to auscultation to determine correct initial and continued placement of these tubes. Aspiration of contents and pH testing is more effective for determining tube placement.

Critical Thinking in Client Care

1. This study investigated differences in auscultatory sounds through small-lumen feeding tubes. Would the sound be more noticeably different with the larger bore tubes used for gastric lavage and drainage?
2. What other methods for determining tube placement are recommended in fundamentals and skills texts?
3. Compare the normal pH of aspirates obtained from the respiratory tract, esophagus, stomach, duodenum, and jejunum.
4. Develop a teaching plan for the client being discharged with a gastrostomy or jejunostomy feeding tube.

---

mercury tip. They also can be administered through a gastrostomy or jejunostomy tube. Small-bore feeding tubes are easily displaced; appropriate tube placement should be periodically checked by aspirating the tube and checking the pH of aspirated contents. A pH of <4 indicates placement in the stomach; pH >6 indicates the tube is in the jejunum. See the Nursing Research box above.

Most tube feeding formulas provide 1 kcal/mL with approximately 14% of the calories from protein, 60% from carbohydrates, and 25% to 30% from fat. Administering 1500 mL per day provides the recommended daily intake of all vitamins and minerals. Formulas that provide more calories per mL, more grams of protein, added fiber, or lower fat also are available. Commercial products provide instructions for initiating therapy. Some formulas are initially diluted to half strength for the first day of therapy. If tolerated, the formula is given at three-fourths strength on the second day and at full strength thereafter. Some formulas are started with smaller volumes of full-strength formula with a gradual increase in volume. Formulas may be administered as a bolus feeding or as a continuous- drip feeding regulated by a feeding pump.

Aspiration and diarrhea are the most common complications of enteral feedings. Continuous infusion of the formula reduces the risk of aspiration. The risk also is reduced by placing the feeding tube in the jejunum rather than the stomach. To avoid aspiration, the nurse elevates head of the bed at least 30 degrees during feeding and for at least 1 hour after feeding. Formulas that contain fiber can reduce the incidence of diarrhea. Fluid and electrolyte status is monitored carefully, and additional water is administered as needed.

Parenteral Nutrition

Total parenteral nutrition (TPN), also known as *hyperalimentation,* is the intravenous administration of carbohydrates (high concentrations of dextrose), protein (amino acids), electrolytes, vitamins, minerals, and fat emulsions. These solutions usually are administered through a central vein, such as the subclavian vein (Figure 20–2 ■).

TPN is initiated when a client's nutritional requirements cannot be met through diet, enteral feedings, or peripheral vein infusions. Clients who have undergone major surgery or trauma or are seriously undernourished are often candidates for TPN. TPN is used for both short- and long-term management of nutritional deficiencies, and many clients are discharged to home with TPN and monitored by home health nurses.

To begin therapy, the physician inserts the central venous catheter under aseptic conditions. The location of the catheter tip is confirmed by X-ray. A triple-lumen catheter is most commonly used. This type of catheter permits administration of medications, intralipids, or blood through other lumens. Parenteral nutrition solutions are mixed using sterile technique under a laminar-flow-air hood. A commonly used solution includes 500 mL of 50% dextrose, 500 mL of an 8.5% amino acid solution, electrolytes, minerals, and vitamins. The sterility of the solution is maintained, and no medication, other than intralipids, is added to the solution or to the lumen through which the TPN is being administered. Most hospitals have specific policies and procedures for changing the tubing and the dressing at the insertion site as well as for hanging new containers. TPN solutions are always administered with an infusion pump to ensure the correct rate of infusion.

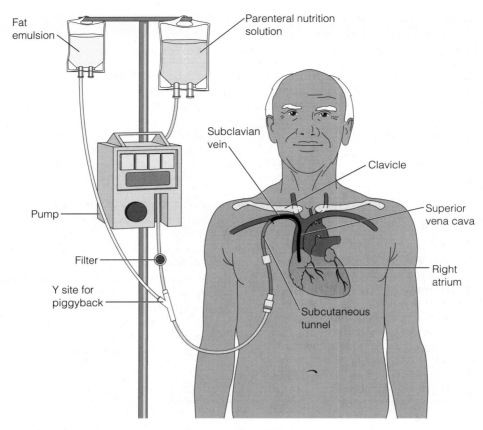

Figure 20–2 ■ Total parenteral nutrition through a catheter in the right subclavian vein.

The client receiving parenteral nutrition is at risk for mechanical, metabolic, and infectious complications. Pneumothorax, hemothorax, brachial plexus injury, and improper position are possible complications of central venous catheter insertion. Once in place, the catheter may dislodge, leak, or break and become an embolus. Clots also may form within or around the catheter.

Fluid overload is a risk with parenteral nutrition, particularly in older adults. The high-glucose formulas can lead to osmotic diuresis or shifts of electrolytes, potassium and phosphorus in particular, into the cells. Blood glucose and serum electrolyte levels are carefully monitored during treatment. Long-term use of parenteral nutrition can lead to gallstone formation and liver disease.

Disruption of the skin barrier and administration of a solution high in glucose presents a risk for infection in clients receiving TPN. The temperature and other manifestations of infection are carefully monitored. Meticulous sterile technique is used for site and catheter care and bag and tubing changes.

NURSING CARE

Health Promotion

Aggressive nursing assessment and interventions can help prevent malnutrition associated with hospitalization or long-term care. In hospitalized clients, carefully monitor food intake.

When the client is placed on NPO status for surgery or tests, ask the care provider to restore diet orders as soon as possible. If allowed, encourage family members to provide favorite foods to promote intake. In long-term care settings, promote socialization during meals. Assess food likes and dislikes for clients, and provide foods they are likely to eat.

Assessment

Collect nutritional assessment data on admission and periodically (once or twice a week) during long-term institutionalization.

- Health history: usual daily dietary pattern (type and amount of foods consumed); usual weight and recent changes; appetite and food tolerance; specific food likes and dislikes; difficulty swallowing; problems such as anorexia, nausea, diarrhea, or constipation; history of surgery and/or chronic diseases (e.g., chronic lung disease) and medications
- Physical examination: height, weight, skinfold thickness, BMI; vital signs; general appearance, muscle wasting, mobility; skin and mucous membranes; bowel sounds; laboratory studies

Nursing Diagnoses and Interventions

The complex effects of malnutrition on multiple body systems place the client at high risk for a number of other problems. This section addresses problems with nutrition, infections, fluid volume, and skin integrity.

Imbalanced Nutrition: Less Than Body Requirements

The nurse plays a critical role in the ongoing assessment of the malnourished client, while collaborating with the multidisciplinary team to provide nutritional therapies.

- If the client is able to eat, provide an environment and nursing measures that encourage eating. Eliminate foul odors, provide oral hygiene before and after meals, make meals appetizing, and offer frequent, small meals including preferred foods. Consult with the nutrition support team to provide adequate protein, calories, minerals, and vitamins. *Oral hygiene and a pleasant environment make food more appetizing. Small, frequent meals are generally more appealing and less overwhelming to a client with anorexia. Many clients require complicated nutritional therapy such as enteral or parenteral therapy to meet nutritional needs.*
- Provide a rest period before and after meals. *Eating requires energy, and the malnourished client may have decreased physical strength and energy.*
- Assess knowledge and provide appropriate teaching. *Lack of knowledge often contributes to undernutrition. Education empowers the client to make healthy choices.*

Risk for Infection

Malnourished clients have a much higher risk for infection than well-nourished people. Malnutrition affects many components of the immune system, including the skin, mucous membranes, and lymph tissue and cells.

- Monitor temperature and assess for manifestations of infection every 4 hours. *Although the baseline temperature may be subnormal in malnourished clients, any elevation from baseline may indicate infection. Manifestations of infection may include chills, malaise, erythema, and leukocytosis. Early detection of infection may prevent complications.*
- Maintain medical asepsis when providing care and surgical asepsis when carrying out procedures. *Handwashing is the best strategy to prevent the spread of pathogens. Sterile technique is required for procedures such as inserting central lines and changing dressings.*

- Teach the signs and symptoms of infection, good handwashing technique, and factors that increase the risk for infection. *Knowledge empowers the client to participate in self-care, thus reducing exposure to infectious pathogens.*

Risk for Deficient Fluid Volume

The client with malnutrition may also have a fluid volume deficit. Difficulty swallowing food and fluids or administration of hyperosmolar nutritional solutions may lead to dehydration or electrolyte disturbances.

- Monitor oral mucous membranes, urine specific gravity, level of consciousness, and laboratory findings every 4 to 8 hours. *Dry mucous membranes, increased urine specific gravity, decreased level of consciousness, and electrolyte imbalances may indicate dehydration.*
- Weigh daily and monitor intake and output. *Daily weights and intake and output measurements help monitor fluid balance.*
- If allowed, offer fluids frequently in small amounts, considering the client's preferences. *Frequent, small amounts of fluids are better tolerated and promote adequate intake.*

Risk for Impaired Skin Integrity

Skin integrity depends on adequate nutrition. Loss of subcutaneous tissue and muscle increase the risk of pressure ulcers. In addition, healing is impaired in malnourished clients.

- Assess skin every 4 hours. *Baseline and ongoing assessments allow prompt identification of early manifestations of skin breakdown.*
- Turn and position at least every 2 hours. Encourage passive and active range-of-motion exercises. *These measures reduce pressure and promote oxygenation of cells.*
- Keep skin dry and clean, and minimize shearing forces. Keep linens smooth, clean, and dry. Provide therapeutic beds, mattresses, or pads. *These nursing measures promote comfort and reduce the risk of skin breakdown.*

Using NANDA, NIC, and NOC

Chart 20–2 shows links between NANDA nursing diagnoses, NIC, and NOC for the client with malnutrition.

CHART 20–2 NANDA, NIC, AND NOC

The Malnourished Client

NURSING DIAGNOSES	NURSING INTERVENTIONS	NURSING OUTCOMES
• Imbalanced Nutrition: Less than Body Requirements • Adult Failure to Thrive • Ineffective Protection • Ineffective Therapeutic Regimen Management	• Fluid Monitoring • Weight Gain Assistance • Nutrition Therapy • Infection Protection • Teaching: Procedure/Treatment	• Nutritional Status: Nutrient Intake • Nutritional Status • Immune Status • Knowledge: Treatment Regimen

Note. Data from Nursing Outcomes Classification (NOC) by M. Johnson & M. Maas (Eds.), 1997, St. Louis: Mosby; Nursing Diagnoses: Definitions & Classification 2001–2002 by North American Nursing Diagnosis Association, 2001, Philadelphia: NANDA; Nursing Interventions Classification (NIC) by J.C. McCloskey & G. M. Bulechek (Eds.), 2000, St. Louis: Mosby. Reprinted by permission.

Nursing Care Plan
A Client with Malnutrition

Rose Chow is an 88-year-old widow who lives alone. She typically rises early and has a cup of tea before spending her morning puttering in her garden. She consumes her main meal of the day at lunch, which usually includes rice and some vegetables. For dinner, she generally eats a bowl of rice with "whatever seems to be in the refrigerator." She admits to little interest in cooking or eating since her husband died 10 years ago and her group of friends has been "dying off, too."

ASSESSMENT

Mrs. Chow weighs 95 lb (43.1 kg) and is 5'3" (160 cm) tall, for a BMI of 16.8. She reports weighing 118 lb (53.5 kg) 5 years ago. Her triceps skinfold thickness measurement is 11 mm (normal values for a female: >13 mm). Her skin is pale, and she appears thin and wasted. Her temperature is 97°F (36.1°C). Diagnostic test results include serum albumin 2.9 g/dL (normal 3.4 to 4.8 g/dL) and serum cholesterol 130 mg/dL (normal 150 to 200 mg/dL). A diagnosis of protein-calorie malnutrition is made, and a 1500-calorie per day diet is recommended.

DIAGNOSES

- *Imbalanced nutrition: Less than body requirements* related to lack of knowledge and inadequate food intake
- *Risk for infection* related to protein-calorie malnutrition
- *Impaired social interaction* related to widowhood and reduced social support group

EXPECTED OUTCOMES

- Gain at least 1 pound per week.
- Verbalize understanding of nutritional requirements and identify strategies to incorporate requirements into daily diet after discharge.
- Remain infection free, evidenced by normal vital signs.

- Identify strategies to increase social interaction, such as participating in senior citizens' lunches at local senior center.

PLANNING AND IMPLEMENTATION

- Weigh weekly at a consistent time of day.
- Refer to dietitian for evaluation of nutritional needs.
- Teach about nutritional requirements, and plan an eating program that includes high-calorie, high-protein foods and supplements and reflects her food preferences. Encourage small, frequent meals.
- Encourage to keep a food intake diary.
- Teach strategies to reduce risks for infection.
- Provide information about communal meals available to seniors in the community, and help Mrs. Chow develop a plan to participate.

EVALUATION

One month later, Mrs. Chow has gained 3 pounds and reports feeling "more energetic." A friend is helping her shop to ensure that she purchases foods to maintain her protein, calorie, and nutrient intake. She has begun attending senior lunches twice a week, and is enjoying "being around people again." Although she still doesn't enjoy cooking like she used to, she is using prepared foods and supplements to maintain her nutrient intake.

Critical Thinking in the Nursing Process

1. What is the physiologic basis for Mrs. Chow's low albumin and cholesterol levels?
2. Mrs. Chow asks, "Can I get better by just taking more vitamins?" How will you respond?
3. Design a teaching plan for a Hispanic client with protein-calorie malnutrition.

See Evaluating Your Response in Appendix C.

Home Care

Clients with malnutrition may be cared for at home or in the hospital with diet, enteral, or parenteral therapy. Each year, it is more common to see clients managing tube feeding or TPN at home. Teaching for the client and family includes the following topics.

- Diet recommendations and use of nutritional supplements
- Where to obtain recommended foods and nutritional supplements
- If continuing enteral or parenteral nutrition, how to (1) prepare and/or handle solutions, (2) add them to either the feeding tube or central line, (3) manage infusion pumps, (4) care for the feeding tube or central catheter, (5) recognize and manage problems and complications, and (6) how and when to notify the health care provider of problems.

THE CLIENT WITH AN EATING DISORDER

Eating disorders are characterized by severely disturbed eating behavior and weight management. Eating disorders are more common in affluent societies where food is plentiful. Women are much more commonly affected than men. **Anorexia nervosa** is characterized by a body weight less than 85% of expected for age and height, and an intense fear of gaining weight. Anorexia nervosa affects about 0.5% to 1% of women in the United States. **Bulimia nervosa,** which affects 1% to 3% of women in the United States, is characterized by recurring episodes of binge eating followed by purge behaviors such as self-induced vomiting, use of laxatives or diuretics, fasting, or excessive exercise.

ANOREXIA NERVOSA

Anorexia nervosa typically begins during adolescence. Clients with anorexia nervosa have a distorted body image and irrational fear of gaining weight. They maintain weight loss by restricted calorie intake, often accompanied by excessive exercise. Some clients may exhibit binge–purge behavior. A number of risk factors, both biologic and psychosocial, have been identified for anorexia nervosa. Abnormal levels of neurotransmitters and other hormones may play a role. Women who develop anorexia nervosa tend to be obsessive

TABLE 20–2   Manifestations and Complications of Anorexia Nervosa and Bulemia Nervosa

Disorder	Manifestations	Complications
Anorexia nervosa	• Weight < 85% of normal, muscle wasting • Fear of weight gain, refusal to eat • Disturbed body image, excessive exercise • Amenorrhea • Skin and hair changes • Hypotension, bradycardia • Hypothermia • Constipation • Insomnia	• Electrolyte and acid-base disturbances • Reduced cardiac muscle mass, low cardiac output, dysrhythmias • Anemia • Hypoglycemia, elevated serum uric acid levels • Osteoporosis • Enlarged salivary glands • Delayed gastric emptying • Abnormal liver function
Bulimia nervosa	• Weight often normal; may be slightly overweight • Binge–purge behavior • Oligomenorrhea or amenorrhea • Lacerations of palate; callous on fingers or dorsum of hand	• Enlarged salivary glands • Stomatitis, loss of dental enamel • Fluid, electrolyte, and acid-base imbalances • Dysrhythmias • Esophageal tears, stomach rupture

and perfectionistic. Family, social, or occupational (e.g., a career in modeling or ballet) pressures to maintain low body weight also contribute.

The manifestations and complications of anorexia nervosa are listed in Table 20–2. Clients who engage in binge–purge behavior have a higher risk for complications.

BULIMIA NERVOSA

Bulimia nervosa develops in late adolescence or early adulthood, often following a diet. The client with bulimia typically reports binge eating followed by purging 5 to 10 times per week (Braunwald et al., 2001). Foods consumed during a binge often are high calorie, high fat, and sweet. After binge eating, the client induces vomiting (usually by stimulating the gag reflex), or may take excessive quantities of laxatives or diuretics. In contrast to anorexia, the client's weight often is normal. Fluid and electrolyte balance, in contrast, may be severely disrupted by loss of fluid and gastrointestinal secretions. The complications of bulimia nervosa (Table 20–2) primarily result from the purging behavior.

COLLABORATIVE CARE

Eating disorders, anorexia nervosa in particular, are difficult to effectively treat. Because of the intense fear of weight gain and the distorted body image of clients with anorexia, they strongly resist increasing food intake. A combination of nutritional, behavioral, and psychologic treatment is necessary.

Clients with anorexia nervosa may require hospitalization, particularly if their weight is less than 75% of normal. Refeeding is gradually introduced to avoid complications such as heart failure. Meals must be supervised and a firm but empathetic attitude conveyed about the importance of adequate food intake. Psychologic treatment focuses on providing emotional support during weight gain and helping the client base their

self-esteem on factors other than weight (e.g., personal relationships, satisfaction with achieving occupational goals) (Braunwald et al., 2001).

An antidepressant drug such as fluoxetine (Prozac) may benefit the client with bulimia nervosa. Cognitive behavioral therapy also is used to treat bulimia, focusing on excessive concerns about weight, persistent dieting, and binge–purge behaviors.

NURSING CARE

Nurses can be instrumental in identifying clients with anorexia nervosa or bulimia nervosa and referring them for treatment. It is particularly important to identify these disorders early to prevent adverse effects on growth and increase the success of treatment.

The nurse is an integral part of the eating disorders treatment team. Although *Imbalanced nutrition: Less than body requirements* is a primary nursing diagnosis for clients with anorexia or bulimia, the following nursing diagnoses also should be considered.

- *Ineffective sexuality patterns*
- *Chronic low self-esteem*
- *Disturbed body image*
- *Ineffective family therapeutic regimen management*

When planning and implementing care, consider the following nursing activities.

- Regularly monitor weight, using standard conditions. *Weight gain or loss provides information about the effectiveness of care, as well as the client's risk for complications.*
- Monitor food intake during meals, recording percentage of meal and snack consumed. Maintain close observation for at least one hour following meals; do not allow client alone in bathroom. *Observing the client during and after meals helps*

prevent disposal of food and purging behavior after eating. Recording actual food intake allows accurate calculation of calorie intake.

- Serve balanced meals, including all nutrient groups. Increase serving size gradually. *The client may find "normal" food servings overwheming, reducing the desire to eat. Calorie intake is initially limited to prevent complications associated with refeeding, then gradually increased.*
- Serve frequent, small feedings of cold or room temperature foods. *Cool foods reduce sensations of early satiety, promoting greater food intake at a meal or snack.*
- Administer a multivitamin and mineral supplement to replace losses.

Clients with anorexia nervosa or bulimia nervosa require extended treatment of the disorder. Involvement of the family and social support persons is vital to success. Encourage family members to participate in teaching and diet counseling sessions. Discuss the value of family therapy to address issues that have contributed to the disorder. Emphasize the need to provide consistent messages of support for healthy eating habits. Discuss using rewards for food and calorie intake rather than weight gain. Provide referrals to a dietitian, nutritional support team, counseling, and support groups for people with eating disorders.

 EXPLORE MediaLink

NCLEX review questions, case studies, care plan activities, MediaLink applications, and other interactive resources for this chapter can be found on the Companion Website at www.prenhall.com/lemone.

Click on Chapter 20 to select the activities for this chapter. For animations, video clips, more NCLEX review questions, and an audio glossary, access the Student CD-ROM accompanying this textbook.

TEST YOURSELF

1. Of the following noted in a client's history, which does the nurse identify as the greatest risk factor for obesity?

   a. Adopted at 2 months of age
   b. Usual diet includes "fast food" lunches twice a week
   c. Does not engage in regular activity
   d. Allergic to chocolate and strawberries

2. A client on a reduced calorie diet asks the nurse what she can do to lose weight faster, because most weeks she loses no more than 0.5 lb. "At this rate, it will take me years to get to my goal!" The most appropriate response by the nurse would be:

   a. "Let's reevaluate your long-term goal. Perhaps it was set too low for you."
   b. "A pound of body fat equals 3500 calories. Let's reevaluate your diet and exercise plan for calorie intake and expenditure."
   c. "Perhaps we should look into a diet supplement since you are unable to stick with your prescribed diet plan."
   d. "You sound frustrated. Would you like to take some time off from your diet and exercise plan?"

3. An expected finding in a client admitted with a diagnosis of protein-calorie malnutrition would be:

   a. Recent 5 lb weight loss
   b. Increased skinfold thickness measurements
   c. Hyperactive bowel sounds
   d. Anxiety and agitation

4. Before administering an intermittent enteral feeding, the nurse confirms placement of the small bore feeding tube in the stomach by:

   a. Instilling water and listening for the gastric gurgle
   b. Withdrawing the tube slightly, then reinserting it
   c. Aspirating gastric contents and check for a pH of <4
   d. Obtaining a flat-plate X-ray of the stomach

5. The nurse identifies which of the following as a realistic goal for a client with anorexia nervosa?

   a. Will consume 100% of a 2500 calorie diet
   b. Will gain 2 pounds per week
   c. Will rest alone in room following meals
   d. Will participate in family counseling

See Test Yourself answers in Appendix C.

BIBLIOGRAPHY

Ackley, B. J., & Ladwig, G. B. (2002). *Nursing diagnosis handbook: A guide to planning care* (5th ed.). St. Louis: Mosby.

Ainley, H. (2001). Analysis. . . managing obesity. *Practice Nurse, 22*(3), 14–15.

Bender, S., Pusateri, M., Cook, A., Ferguson, M., & Hall, J. C. (2000). Malnutrition: Role of the TwoCal® HN med pass program. *MEDSURG Nursing, 9*(6), 284–295.

Braunwald, E., Fauci, A. S., Kasper, D. L., Hauser, S. L., Longo, D. L., & Jameson, J. L. (2001). *Harrison's principles of internal medicine* (15th ed.). New York: McGraw-Hill.

Bullock, B. A., & Henze, R. L. (2000). *Focus on pathophysiology.* Philadelphia: Lippincott.

Cammons, A. R., & Hackshaw, H.S. (2000). Are we starving our patients? *American Journal of Nursing, 100*(5), 43–46.

Crogan, N. L., Shultz, J. A., & Massey, L. K. (2001). Nutrition knowledge of nurses in long-term care facilities. *Journal of Continuing Education in Nursing, 32*(4), 171–176.

Deglin, J. H., & Vallerand, A. H. (2001). *Davis's drug guide for nurses* (7th ed.). Philadelphia: F.A. Davis.

Devlin, M. (2000). The nutritional needs of the older person. *Professional Nurse, 16*(3), 951–955.

Dudek, S. G. (2000). Malnutrition in hospitals: Who's assessing what patients eat? *American Journal of Nursing, 100*(4), 36–42.

Ferguson, M., Cook, A, Bender, S., Rimmasch, H., & Voss, A. (2001). Diagnosing and treating involuntary weight loss. *MEDSURG Nursing, 10*(4), 165–175.

Gallo, J. J., Busby-Whitehead, J., Rabins, P. V., Silliman, R. A., & Murphy, J. B. (Eds.). (1999). *Reichel's care of the elderly: Clinical aspects of aging* (5th ed.). Philadelphia: Lippincott Williams & Wilkins.

Green, S., & O'Kane, M. (2001). Obesity. *Practice Nurse, 22*(3), 20, 22, 24.

Jeffrey, S. (2001). The role of the nurse in obesity management. *Journal of Community Nursing, 15*(3), 20, 22, 26.

Johnson, M., Bulechek, G., Dochterman, J. M., Maas, M., & Moorhead, S. (2001). *Nursing diagnoses, outcomes, & interventions.* St. Louis: Mosby.

Ledsham, J., & Gough, A. (2000). Screening and monitoring patients for malnutrition. *Professional Nurse, 15*(11), 695–698.

Lehne, R. A. (2001). *Pharmacology for nursing care* (4th ed.). Philadelphia: Saunders.

Malarkey, L.M., & McMorrow, M.E. (2000). *Nurse's manual of laboratory tests and diagnostic procedures* (2nd ed.). Philadelphia: Saunders.

Meeker, M. H., & Rothrock, J. C. (1999). *Alexander's care of the patient in surgery* (11th ed.). St. Louis: Mosby.

Metheny, N. A., & Titler, M. G. (2001). Assessing placement of feeding tubes. *American Journal of Nursing, 101*(5), 36–45.

Metheny, N., Wehrle, M., Wiersema, L., & Clark, J. (1998). pH, color, and feeding tubes. *RN, 61*(1), 25–27.

North American Nursing Diagnosis Association. (2001). *NANDA nursing diagnoses: Definitions & classification 2001–2002.* Philadelphia: NANDA.

Nutrition. Clinical guidelines to manage malnutrition in nursing homes. (2001). *Geriatric Nursing, 22*(1), 46.

Orbanic, S. (2001). Understanding bulimia. *American Journal of Nursing, 101*(3), 35–41.

Porth, C. M. (2002). *Pathophysiology: Concepts of altered health states* (5th ed.). Philadelphia: Lippincott.

Robinson, F. (2001). Analysis . . . management of excess weight in primary care. *Practice Nurse, 21*(5), 16, 19.

Saunders, C. S. (2001). Diet and nutrition in your practice. Intervening in the obesity epidemic. *Patient Care for the Nurse Practitioner, 4*(3), 12–14, 16, 18+.

Tierney, L. M., McPhee, S. J., & Papadakis, M. A. (2001). *Current medical diagnosis & treatment* (40th ed.). New York: Lange Medical Books/McGraw-Hill.

Vender, S., Pusateri, M., Cook, A., Ferguson, M., & Hall, J.C. (2000). Malnutrition: Role of the TwoCal® med pass program. *MEDSURG Nursing, 9*(6), 284–295.

Nursing Care of Clients with Upper Gastrointestinal Disorders

MediaLink

www.prenhall.com/lemone

Additional resources for this chapter can be found on the Student CD-ROM accompanying this textbook, and on the Companion Website at www.prenhall.com/lemone. Click on Chapter 21 to select the activities for this chapter.

CD-ROM
- Audio Glossary
- NCLEX Review

Animations
- Mouth and Throat
- Ranitidine

Companion Website
- More NCLEX Review
- Case Study
  Peptic Ulcer Disease
- Care Plan Activity
  Peptic Ulcer Disease and Pain
- MediaLink Application
  Oral Cancer

LEARNING OUTCOMES

After completing this chapter, you will be able to:

- Describe the pathophysiology of common disorders of the mouth, esophagus, and stomach.

- Relate the manifestations of upper gastrointestinal disorders to the pathophysiologic processes.

- List diagnostic tests used to identify disorders of the upper gastrointestinal tract.

- Discuss the nursing implications for collaborative care measures used to treat clients with upper gastrointestinal disorders.

- Use knowledge of normal anatomy and physiology and assessments to provide nursing care for clients with upper gastrointestinal disorders (see Chapter 19).

- Use the nursing process to assess needs, plan, and implement individualized care for the client with an upper gastrointestinal disorder.

The upper gastrointestinal tract includes the mouth, esophagus, stomach, and proximal small intestine. Food and fluids, ingested through the mouth, move through the esophagus to the stomach. The stomach and upper intestinal tract (duodenum and jejunum) are responsible for the majority of food digestion. When an acute or chronic disease process interferes with the function of this portion of the gastrointestinal (GI) tract, nutritional status can be affected and the client may experience symptoms that interfere with lifestyle.

Nurses provide both acute care for the hospitalized client and teaching about the skills and knowledge needed to manage these conditions at home.

DISORDERS OF THE MOUTH

Inflammations, infections, and neoplastic lesions of the mouth affect food ingestion and nutrition. Oral lesions may have a variety of causes, including infection, mechanical trauma, irritants such as alcohol, and hypersensitivity. Appropriate treatment of the disorder, any underlying factors, and associated symptoms is essential.

THE CLIENT WITH STOMATITIS

Stomatitis, inflammation of the oral mucosa, is a common disorder of the mouth. It may be caused by viral (herpes simplex) or fungal (Candida albicans) infections, mechanical trauma (e.g., cheek biting), and irritants such as tobacco or chemotherapeutic agents.

PATHOPHYSIOLOGY

The oral mucosa, which lines the oral cavity, is a relatively thin, fragile layer of stratified squamous epithelial cells. The blood supply to the oral mucosa is rich. Frequent exposure to the environment, a rich blood supply, and the oral mucosa's delicate nature increase the risk of infection or inflammation, reaction to toxins, and trauma.

The clinical manifestations of stomatitis vary according to its cause. Table 21–1 outlines common causes of stomatitis with their manifestations and treatment. Chemotherapy or chemical irritation may result in generalized redness, swelling, and ulcerations.

COLLABORATIVE CARE

Stomatitis is diagnosed by direct physical examination and, if indicated, cultures, smears, and evaluation for systemic illness. Treatment addresses both the underlying cause and any coexisting illnesses. An undiagnosed oral lesion present for more than 1 week and that does not respond to therapy must be evaluated for malignancy.

Direct smears and cultures of lesions may be obtained to identify causative organisms. If systemic illness is suspected, a variety of diagnostic tests may be ordered to identify the underlying cause.

General treatment measures include using a topical anesthetic, such as 2% viscous lidocaine, as an oral rinse. This

TABLE 21–1 Manifestations and Treatment of Common Stomatitis Conditions

Type	Cause	Manifestations	Complications
Cold sore, fever blister	Herpes simplex virus	• Initial burning at site • Clustered vesicular lesions on lip or oral mucosa	• Self-limiting • Acyclovir to shorten course
Aphthous ulcer (canker sore, ulcerative stomatitis)	Unknown, may be type of herpes virus	• Well-circumscribed, shallow erosions with white or yellow center encircled by red ring • Less than 1 cm in diameter • Painful	• Topical steroid ointment • Amlexanox oral paste (Aphthasol) • Oral prednisone
Candidiasis (thrush)	*Candida albicans*	• Creamy white, curdlike patches • Red, erythematous mucosa	• Fluconazole (Diflucan) • Ketoconazole (Nizoral) • Clotrimazole troches • Nystatin vaginal troches (dissolved orally) or mouth rinse
Necrotizing ulcerative gingivitis (trench mouth, Vincent's infection)	Infection with spirochetes and bacilli or systemic infection	• Acute gingival inflammation and necrosis • Bleeding, halitosis • Fever • Cervical lymphadenopathy	• Correct any underlying disorders • Warm, half-strength peroxide mouthwashes • Oral penicillin

solution is not swallowed to avoid impairment of the swallowing mechanism. Orabase, a protective paste, may be applied to oral ulcers to promote comfort. Triamcinolone acetonide may be mixed in Orabase to reduce inflammation and promote healing. Sodium bicarbonate mouthwashes may provide relief and promote cleansing, whereas alcohol-based mouthwashes may cause pain and burning.

Fungal infections often are treated with a nystatin oral suspension; clients "swish and swallow" the solution. Clotrimazole lozenges also treat oral fungal infections. If the infection does not resolve, oral antifungal medications such as fluconazole or ketoconazole may be used. Antifungals are usually continued for at least 3 days after symptoms disappear.

Herpetic lesions may be treated with topical or oral acyclovir. Acyclovir ointment provides comfort and lubrication while limiting the spread of the virus. Acyclovir capsules reduce the severity of symptoms and the duration of the lesions.

Bacterial infections are treated with antibiotics based on cultures and smears. Oral penicillin is the treatment of choice if the client is not allergic and the cultured bacteria is sensitive. Nursing implications for selected drugs used to treat stomatitis are outlined below.

NURSING CARE

Nursing care for the client with stomatitis focuses not only on the oral inflammation, but also on any underlying systemic diseases and the effects of the condition on the client's comfort and nutrition.

Nursing Diagnoses and Interventions
Impaired Oral Mucous Membrane
Stomatitis disrupts the integrity of the oral mucous membrane. Regardless of cause, the pain and symptoms of stomatitis must be relieved to promote comfort as well as food and fluid intake.

- Assess and document oral mucous membranes and the character of any lesions every 4 to 8 hours. *Baseline and ongoing assessment data provide the basis for evaluation.*
- Assist with thorough mouth care after meals, at bedtime, and every 2 to 4 hours while awake. If unable to tolerate a toothbrush, offer sponge or gauze toothettes. Avoid using alcohol-based mouthwashes. *Mouth care promotes hygiene, comfort, and healing. Alcohol-based mouthwashes may be irritating to mucous membranes, causing pain and further tissue damage.*
- Assess knowledge and teach about condition, mouth care, and treatments. Instruct to avoid alcohol, tobacco, and spicy or irritating foods. *Knowledge promotes client participation in the plan of care and compliance. Alcohol, tobacco, and hot, spicy rough foods may injure the inflamed mucous membranes.*

Imbalanced Nutrition: Less Than Body Requirements
Oral lesions and pain may limit oral intake, which may in turn lead to nutritional deficits. Anorexia and general malaise may also contribute to decreased intake.

- Assess food intake as well as the client's ability to chew and swallow. Weigh daily. Provide appropriate assistive de-

Medication Administration
Drugs Used to Treat Stomatitis

TOPICAL ORAL ANESTHETICS

Orajel	Anbesol
Viscous lidocaine	Triamcinolone acetonide

These drugs reduce the pain associated with mucous membrane lesions or stomatitis. They provide temporary relief of pain. Any oral lesion that persists longer than 1 week should be evaluated by an oral surgeon.

Nursing Responsibilities
- Instruct the client to seek medical attention for any oral lesion that does not heal within 1 week.
- Monitor for local hypersensitivity reactions, and discontinue use if they occur.

Client and Family Teaching
- Apply every 1 to 2 hours as needed.
- Perform oral hygiene after meals and at bedtime.

TOPICAL ANTIFUNGAL AGENTS

Clotrimazole	Nystatin

These products help in the topical treatment of candidiasis. Their effects are primarily local rather than systemic.

Nursing Responsibilities
- Instruct the client to dissolve lozenges in the mouth.

- Instruct the client to rinse mouth with oral suspension for at least 2 minutes and expectorate or swallow as directed.
- These drugs are contraindicated in pregnancy.

Client and Family Teaching
- Take medication as prescribed.
- Do not eat or drink 30 minutes after medication.
- Contact physician if symptoms worsen.
- Perform good oral hygiene after meals and at bedtime; remove dentures at bedtime.

ANTIVIRAL AGENT

Acyclovir (Zovirax)

Acyclovir is useful in the treatment of oral herpes simplex virus. It helps reduce the severity and frequency of infections. It interferes with the DNA synthesis of herpes simplex virus.

Nursing Responsibilities
- Start therapy with acyclovir as soon as herpetic lesions are noted.
- Administer with food or on an empty stomach.

Client and Family Teaching
- The virus remains latent and can recur during stressful events, fever, trauma, sunlight exposure, and treatment with immunosuppressive drugs.
- Take the medication as ordered, and contact the physician if symptoms worsen.

vices such as straws or feeding syringes. *Adequate nutrition is essential for healing. Daily weights allow monitoring of the adequacy of food intake. Assistive devices may allow food intake while avoiding irritation of ulcerations or lesions.*

- Encourage a high-calorie, high-protein diet considerate of food preferences. Offer soft, lukewarm, or cool foods or liquids such as eggnogs, milk shakes, nutritional supplements, popsicles, and puddings frequently in small amounts. Obtain nutritional consultation. *Oral intake may be limited, and enriched foods and liquids enhance nutrition. A nutritional consultation can help ensure an adequate diet and assist in meeting nutritional needs.*

Home Care

Clients with stomatitis generally provide self-care. Include the following topics in teaching for home care.

- Managing any underlying health conditions and ongoing treatments such as chemotherapy
- The recommended diet and oral hygiene regime
- Nutritional supplements to help meet nutritional requirements
- Prescribed medication, its route, side effects, frequency of administration, and signs and symptoms to report
- The importance of completing the full course of antibiotic, antiviral, or antifungal treatment
- Manifestations to report and the importance of follow-up care

THE CLIENT WITH ORAL CANCER

Oral cancer, malignancy of the oral mucosa, may develop on the lips, tongue, floor of the mouth, or other oral tissues. It is uncommon, accounting for only 5% of all cancers. It has, however, a high rate of morbidity and mortality. The incidence of this type of head and neck cancer is twice as high in men as in women, and it is seen more often in men over 40. The stage of an oral cancer determines the prognosis, treatment, and degree of disability. The primary risk factors for oral cancer are smoking, drinking alcohol, and chewing tobacco. Marijuana use, occupational exposures to chemicals, and viruses such as human papilloma virus (HPV) also may contribute to the risk for oral cancer.

PATHOPHYSIOLOGY AND MANIFESTATIONS

Oral cancer is usually a squamous cell carcinoma. Most early cancers of the mouth, lips, tongue, or pharynx present as inflamed areas with irregular, ill-defined borders. More advanced cancers appear as deep ulcers that are fixed to deeper tissues. Early lesions involve the mucosa or submucosa, whereas more advanced tumors may involve the tongue, oropharynx, mandible, or maxilla.

The earliest symptom of oral cancer is a painless oral ulceration or lesion (Figure 21–1 ■). Later symptoms vary and may include difficulty speaking, swallowing, or chewing; swollen lymph nodes; and blood-tinged sputum. See the box above for

Figure 21–1 ■ Oral cancer.

Source: Biophoto Associates/Photo Researchers, Inc.

Manifestations of Oral Cancer

- White patches (leukoplakia)
- Red patches (erythroplakia)
- Ulcers
- Masses
- Pigmented areas (brownish or black)
- Fissures
- Asymmetry of the head, face, jaws, or neck

other manifestations of oral cancer. Any oral lesion that does not heal or respond to treatment within 1 to 2 weeks should be evaluated for malignancy.

COLLABORATIVE CARE

The first component of treatment is eliminating any causative factors such as chewing tobacco, smoking, or drinking alcohol. Tumor staging then determines therapy. A biopsy of the oral lesion allows direct visualization of cells to determine the presence or absence of cancerous cells. Staging may require additional diagnostic studies such as CT scans or an MRI.

Radiation and chemotherapy may be considered based on age, tumor stage, general condition, and preferences. Radiation therapy may be used preoperatively to "shrink" the tumor or postoperatively to limit the risks of metastasis. Chemotherapy may be indicated depending on the stage of the tumor. See Chapter 10 for more information about radiation and chemotherapy to treat cancer.

Following the biopsy and staging of the tumor, surgery is generally indicated, although an advanced or extensive tumor may be considered unresectable. If the tumor involves surrounding tissues, the cosmetic effects of surgery are important considerations. The goal of surgery is removal of the lesion and potentially cancerous surrounding tissue or lymph nodes. Advanced carcinomas may require extensive excision or a *radical neck dissection,* a potentially disfiguring procedure in which the lymph nodes and muscles of the neck are removed. A tracheostomy is performed at the time of surgery. The tracheostomy may be temporary, but often is permanent. See Chapter 35 ⊖⊖ for more information about caring for a client following radical neck dissection and a tracheostomy

NURSING CARE

Health Promotion

Reducing or eliminating tobacco use (smoking and smokeless tobacco) and excess alcohol consumption can significantly reduce the incidence of oral cancer. Teach children and adolescents about the dangers of using tobacco and alcohol. Emphasize the relationship between smokeless tobacco and oral cancer. Discuss strategies to deal with peer pressure to use tobacco and alcohol.

Assessment

Early precancerous oral lesions are very treatable. Unfortunately, these lesions usually are painless, so diagnosis and treatment often is delayed. Assess the oral cavity of all clients, particularly those with risk factors for oral cancer.

- Health history: complaints of oral lesions that fail to heal; use (current or past) of tobacco products or excess alcohol
- Physical examination: Inspect and palpate lips and oral mucosa (including tongue and floor of mouth under the tongue) for tumors or lesions. Lesions may appear as velvety red or white patches that do not scrape off, or as ulcers or areas of necrosis.

Nursing Diagnoses and Interventions

The mouth allows food ingestion, and the lips are integral to verbal and nonverbal expression. The head, mouth, and lips are important to self-perception and body image. Nursing diagnoses discussed in this section consider such problems as airway clearance, nutrition, communication, and body image.

Risk for Ineffective Airway Clearance

The location and the extent of an oral cancer and its excision may compromise the airway. Swelling of adjacent tissues, increased oral secretions, or difficulty swallowing may contribute to respiratory distress. If extensive surgery is performed, a tracheostomy usually is performed to maintain airway patency.

PRACTICE ALERT | *In the initial postoperative period, assess airway patency and respiratory status at least hourly. A patent airway is vital to maintain respirations and oxygenation of tissues. Frequent assessment allows early identification of possible airway compromise.* ■

- Unless contraindicated, place in Fowler's position, supporting arms. Assist the client to turn, cough, and deep

breathe at least every 2 to 4 hours. *Fowler's position promotes lung expansion. Turning, coughing, and deep breathing help maintain a patent airway by preventing pooling of secretions.*
- Maintain adequate hydration (2000 to 3000 mL per day unless contraindicated) and humidity of inspired air. *Adequate hydration helps thin and loosen secretions.*

Imbalanced Nutrition: Less Than Body Requirements

Surgery affects oral food and fluid intake. Enteral feedings or total parenteral nutrition may be required. A gastrostomy tube usually is inserted during surgery to maintain nutrition. If an oral diet is permitted, anorexia or pain may affect intake.

- Weigh daily. Assess oral intake for adequacy of protein, calories, and nutrients. *Daily weights and nutritional assessments provide information about the adequacy of diet.*
- Offer soft, bland foods with supplements as indicated. Provide small, frequent feedings, making mealtimes pleasant. *Soft, bland foods may be better tolerated following oral surgery. Large meals may be overwhelming; small, frequent meals promote food and nutrient intake.*
- Provide enteral feedings per gastrostomy tube as ordered. Elevate the head of the bed 30 to 40 degrees. *Enteral feedings maintain nutritional status in the client who is unable to consume foods orally. Elevating the head of the bed reduces the risk of regurgitation and aspiration of gastric contents.*
- Assess for gastric residual volume per facility protocol for the type of feeding (intermittent or continuous). See the Nursing Research box page 545. Notify the physician of volumes greater than 200 mL or 50% of previous feeding if feeding is intermittent. *Excess residual volume may increase the risk for aspiration.*
- Consider a nutritional consultation to assess diet and plan appropriate supplements. *A registered dietitian can calculate energy requirements and develop an individualized diet plan to meet nutritional requirements.*

Impaired Verbal Communication

Oral surgery can interfere with communication. Effective communication is vital to postoperative recovery and prevention of complications.

- Before surgery, establish and practice a communication plan such as using a magic slate or flash cards. *Practicing communication techniques reduces fear and anxiety while promoting communication.*
- Provide ample time for communication efforts and do not answer for the client. Be alert for nonverbal communications. Use yes/no questions and simple phrases. *Providing adequate time allows the client opportunity to express ideas and thoughts. Nonverbal communication provides cues regarding comfort or other needs. Simple yes/no questions are easily answered nonverbally.*
- If indicated, refer to or consult with a speech therapist. *A speech therapist can help promote or restore effective communication.*

Nursing Research

Evidence-Based Practice for Clients with Enteral Feeding Tubes

Practices and protocols for assessing gastric residual volume in clients with nasogastric or gastrostomy feeding tubes are inconsistent. Researchers have come to varying conclusions about the amount of gastric residual volume that is safe and does not increase gastric distention and the risk for aspiration. In one study, while more than 30% of the clients had residual volumes greater than 150 mL, only 4% had evidence of formula in their airways. In an extensive review of the literature regarding measurement of gastric residual volume, Edwards and Metheny (2000) also found that nursing practice often was inconsistent with hospital protocols.

IMPLICATIONS FOR NURSING

Gastric motility slows following surgery or trauma, in diabetes, sepsis, or electrolyte imbalance, and with medications such as narcotic analgesics. Excessive gastric distention appears to increase the risk for aspiration of gastric contents. However, when enteral feedings are withheld unnecessarily, the nutritional status of the client is at risk. Impaired nutrition affects healing and recovery.

The authors suggest a protocol for enteral infusions that includes: (1) checking residual volume every 4 hours; (2) assessing the client and contacting the physician if the residual volume is greater than 200 mL or 50% of the previous bolus feeding; and (3) withholding the feeding only when directed to do so by the physician (Edwards & Metheny, 2000).

Critical Thinking in Client Care

1. What factors might influence the accuracy of residual volume measurements? What measures can be taken to obtain accurate measurements?
2. What would be the effect of withholding one bolus feeding of 240 mL of a standard enteral formula? If this is repeated daily for a week, what is the cumulative effect?
3. One reason frequently cited for avoiding checking residual volume is the risk of plugging the feeding tube. Identify measures to prevent this potential problem.

PRACTICE ALERT *Provide an emergency call system and respond promptly. Make all staff aware that the client cannot respond over an intercom system by posting an alert on the intercom. Nonverbal clients rely on an emergency call system to summon help. Answering promptly reduces fear and anxiety and maintains safety.* ∎

Disturbed Body Image

Radical surgery of the head or neck seriously affects body image. An altered speech pattern and any disfigurement affect the ability to feel attractive or effective in work or social roles. Clients may defer lifesaving surgery to postpone disfiguring interventions or therapies.

- Assess coping style, self-perception, and responses to altered appearance or function. *This information can be used to identify appropriate interventions and care.*
- Encourage verbalization of feelings regarding perceived and actual changes. *Nonjudgmental acceptance of feelings and fears helps establish trust.*
- Provide emotional support, encourage self-care, and provide decision-making opportunities. *Self-care promotes self-acceptance and independence. Giving choices empowers the client to participate in care.*

Using NANDA, NIC, and NOC

Chart 21–1 shows links between NANDA nursing diagnoses, NIC, and NOC when caring for the client with oral cancer.

CHART 21–1 NANDA, NIC, AND NOC LINKAGES

The Client with Oral Cancer

NURSING DIAGNOSES	NURSING INTERVENTIONS	NURSING OUTCOMES
• Impaired Oral Mucous Membrane	• Oral Health Restoration	• Oral Health • Self-Care: Oral Hygiene
• Acute Pain	• Pain Management • Patient-Controlled Analgesia (PCA) Assistance	• Comfort Level • Pain Control
• Risk for Imbalanced Nutrition: Less Than Body Requirements	• Nutrition Management • Fluid Monitoring • Swallowing, Therapy	• Nutritional Status • Nutritional Status: Food and Fluid Intake

Note. Data from Nursing Outcomes Classification (NOC) by M. Johnson & M. Maas (Eds.), 1997, St. Louis: Mosby; Nursing Diagnoses: Definitions & Classification 2001–2002 by North American Nursing Diagnosis Association, 2001, Philadelphia: NANDA; Nursing Interventions Classification (NIC) by J.C. McCloskey & G. M. Bulechek (Eds.), 2000, St. Louis: Mosby. Reprinted by permission.

Home Care

Discharge planning for the client with oral cancer depends on the type of treatment planned and surgery performed. Depending on the client's age, condition, and availability of support systems, referral to community health care agencies may be an essential component of care. Visits from home care nurses can assist in meeting health care needs.

Discuss the following topics with the client and family members or care providers:

- Diagnosis and prescribed care
- Monitoring for new lesions or recurrences
- Diet, nutrition, and activity
- Pain management
- Airway management, care of incision, and signs and symptoms to report

Nursing Care Plan
A Client with Oral Cancer

Juan Chavez, a married 44-year-old farmer, has two adult children. He and his wife raise and sell fruits and vegetables. Two months ago, Mr. Chavez developed a sore on his tongue that would not heal. Mr. Chavez tells his admission nurse, Sara Bucklin, "The doctor says he will have to remove part of my tongue," and anxiously asks, "Will I ever look the same? How will I be able to talk?"

ASSESSMENT

Mr. Chavez's admission history reveals that he has been healthy, but has smoked two packs of cigarettes a day for over 20 years, and usually drinks two to four beers per day. He admits to being anxious and fearful of surgery and its outcomes. He says he quit smoking and drinking 2 weeks ago. The biopsy report is positive for squamous cell carcinoma of the tongue. Mr. Chavez has no enlarged cervical nodes and says he has no bloody sputum or saliva, difficulty swallowing, chewing, or talking. His weight is in the normal range for his height. A wide excision of the oral lesion is planned.

DIAGNOSES

- *Risk for ineffective airway clearance* related to oral surgery
- *Risk for imbalanced nutrition: Less than body requirements* related to oral surgery
- *Impaired verbal communication* related to excision of a portion of the tongue
- *Disturbed body image* related to surgical excision of the tongue

EXPECTED OUTCOMES

- Maintain a patent airway and remain free of respiratory distress.
- Maintain a stable weight and level of hydration.
- Effectively communicate with staff and family using a magic slate and flash cards.
- Communicate an increased ability to accept changes in body image.

PLANNING AND IMPLEMENTATION

- Assess airway patency and respiratory status every hour until stable.

- Maintain semi-Fowler's position, supporting arms. Encourage to turn, cough, and deep breathe every 2 to 4 hours.
- Teach the importance of activity, turning, coughing, and deep breathing.
- Monitor daily weights.
- Consult with dietitian to assess calorie needs and plan appropriate enteral feeding. Assess response to enteral feedings.
- Demonstrate and allow to practice using magic slate and flash cards prior to surgery.
- Allow adequate time for communication efforts.
- Keep emergency call system in reach at all times and answer light promptly. Alert all staff of inability to respond verbally.
- Encourage expression of feelings regarding perceived and actual changes.
- Provide emotional support, encourage self-care and participation in decision making.

EVALUATION

At the time of discharge, Mr. Chavez has maintained his weight and has started on oral liquids, including supplements and enriched liquids. His airway has remained clear, and he is effectively coughing and deep breathing. He has used the magic slate to communicate throughout his hospital stay. He is regaining use of his tongue, and can speak a few words. Although initially distressed, he is communicating an increased ability to cope with loss of part of his tongue. He and his wife say they understand his discharge instructions, including diet, activity, follow-up care, and signs and symptoms to report.

Critical Thinking in the Nursing Process

1. What measures can you, as a nurse, implement to reduce the incidence of oral cancer?
2. Plan a health education program for young athletes who chew tobacco.
3. Mr. Chavez's wife calls you 2 weeks after discharge. She tells you that he refuses to try to talk and is relying on his magic slate to communicate. How will you respond?

See Evaluating Your Response in Appendix C.

DISORDERS OF THE ESOPHAGUS

The esophagus plays an essential role in the ingestion of food and liquids. Disorders of the esophagus can be inflammatory, mechanical, or cancerous. Because of its location and neighboring organs, the symptoms of esophageal disorders may mimic those of a variety of other illnesses.

THE CLIENT WITH GASTROESOPHAGEAL REFLUX DISEASE

Gastroesophageal reflux is the backward flowing of gastric contents into the esophagus. When this occurs, the client experiences heartburn. Many people with gastroesophageal reflux have few symptoms, while others develop inflammatory esophagitis as a result of exposure to gastric juices.

Gastroesophageal reflux disease (GERD) is a common gastrointestinal disorder that affects 15% to 20% of adults. As many as 10% of people experience daily symptoms such as heartburn and indigestion (Braunwald et al., 2001; Mattonen, 2001; Tierney et al., 2001).

PATHOPHYSIOLOGY

Normally, the lower esophageal sphincter remains closed except during swallowing. Reflux (backflow) of gastric contents into the esophagus is prevented by pressure differences between the stomach and the lower esophagus. The diaphragm, the lower esophageal sphincter, and the location of the gastroesophageal junction below the diaphragm help maintain this pressure difference (Figure 21–2 ■).

Gastroesophageal reflux may result from transient relaxation of the lower esophageal sphincter, an incompetent lower esophageal sphincter, and/or increased pressure within the stomach (Figure 21–3 ■). Factors contributing to gastroesophageal reflux include increased gastric volume (e.g., after meals), positioning that allows gastric contents to remain close to the gastroesophageal junction (e.g., bending over, lying down), and increased gastric pressure (e.g., obesity or wearing tight clothing). A hiatal hernia may contribute to GERD.

Gastric juices contain acid, pepsin, and bile, which are corrosive substances. Esophageal peristalsis and bicarbonate in salivary secretions normally clear and neutralize gastric juices in the esophagus. During sleep, however, and in clients with impaired esophageal peristalsis or salivation, the esophageal mucosa is damaged by gastric juices, causing an inflammatory response. With prolonged exposure, esophagitis develops. Superficial ulcers develop, and the mucosa becomes red, friable (easily torn), and may bleed. If untreated, scarring and esophageal stricture may develop.

MANIFESTATIONS AND COMPLICATIONS

GERD causes heartburn, usually after meals, with bending over, or when reclining. Regurgitation of sour material into the mouth, or difficulty and pain with swallowing may develop. Other manifestations may include atypical chest pain, sore throat, and hoarseness. See the Manifestations box on page 548. Aspiration of gastric contents can cause hoarseness or respiratory symptoms.

Complications include esophageal strictures and Barrett's esophagus. Strictures can lead to dysphagia. Barrett's esophagus

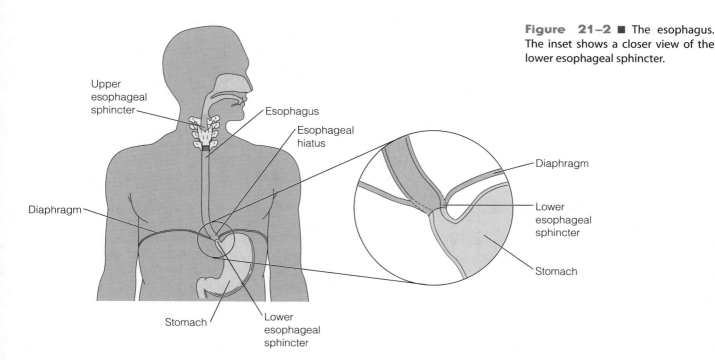

Figure 21–2 ■ The esophagus. The inset shows a closer view of the lower esophageal sphincter.

Transient lower esophageal
sphincter relaxation

Incompetent lower esophageal
sphincter

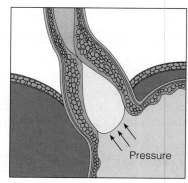

Increased intragastric pressure

Figure 21–3 ■ Mechanisms of gastroesophageal reflux.

Manifestations of GERD

- Heartburn
- Regurgitation
- Pain after eating
- Dysphagia
- Chest pain
- Belching

is characterized by changes in the cells lining the esophagus and an increased risk of developing esophageal cancer (Porth, 2002).

COLLABORATIVE CARE

Often the diagnosis of GERD is made by the history of symptoms and predisposing factors. Collaborative care focuses on lifestyle changes, diet modification, and for more severe cases, drug therapy. Surgery is reserved for clients who develop serious complications.

Diagnostic Tests

Diagnostic tests that may be ordered for clients with manifestations of GERD include:

- *Barium swallow* to evaluate the esophagus, stomach, and upper small intestine.
- *Upper endoscopy* to permit direct visualization of the esophagus. Tissue may be obtained for biopsy to establish the diagnosis and rule out malignancy. See the accompanying box for nursing care of the client undergoing an upper endoscopy.
- *24-hour ambulatory pH monitoring* may be performed to establish the diagnosis of GERD. For this test, a small tube with a pH electrode is inserted through the nose into the esophagus. The electrode is attached to a small box worn on the belt which records the data. The data are later analyzed by computer.
- *Esophageal manometry* measures pressures of the esophageal sphincters and esophageal peristalsis.

Medications

Antacids, such as Mylanta or Maalox, relieve mild or moderate symptoms by neutralizing stomach acid. Gaviscon, which forms a floating barrier between the gastric contents and the esophageal mucosa when the client is upright, may also be used.

Nursing Implications for Diagnostic Tests: Upper Endoscopy

Client Preparation

- Schedule at least 2 days after barium swallow or upper gastrointestinal series.
- Ensure the informed consent is signed prior to premedication.
- Encourage questions, and provide answers and support.
- Withhold food and fluids for 6 to 8 hours before the procedure.
- Remove dentures and eyewear. Provide mouth care.

Client and Family Teaching

- Do not eat or drink anything for 6 to 8 hours before the procedure.
- The procedure is somewhat uncomfortable but requires only 20 to 30 minutes to complete.
- A local anesthetic will be used in your throat and you will be given a sedative during the procedure.
- After the procedure, you will be allowed to eat and drink as soon as your gag reflex returns and you are able to swallow.
- You may experience mild bloating, belching, or flatulence following the procedure.
- Contact your physician immediately if you develop any of the following: difficulty swallowing; epigastric, substernal or shoulder pain; vomiting blood or black tarry stools; or fever.

Histamine$_2$-receptor (H$_2$-receptor) blockers reduce gastric acid production and are effective in treating GERD symptoms. When treating GERD, H$_2$-receptor blockers are usually given twice a day or more frequently for a prolonged period of time. Cimetidine, ranitidine, famotidine, and nizatidine are all approved by the FDA for the treatment of GERD and are available over the counter.

Omeprazole (Prilosec), lansoprazole (Prevacid), pantoprazole (Protonix), and rabeprazole (Aciphex) are proton-pump inhibitors (PPIs) that reduce gastric secretions. PPIs promote healing of erosive esophagitis as well as relieve symptoms. An 8-week course of treatment is initially prescribed, although some clients may require 3 to 6 months of therapy.

A promotility agent, such as metoclopramide (Reglan), may be ordered to enhance esophageal clearance and gastric emptying. Metoclopramide is used to treat clients with regurgitation, symptoms of indigestion, and nighttime symptoms. However, it is not recommended for long-time use. See the Medication Administration box below for the nursing implications of drugs used to treat GERD.

Dietary and Lifestyle Management

GERD is a chronic condition. Dietary and lifestyle changes are important to reduce symptoms and long-term effects of the disorder. Acidic foods such as tomato products, citrus fruits, spicy foods, and coffee are eliminated from the diet. Fatty foods, chocolate, peppermint, and alcohol relax the lower esophageal

---

Medication Administration

Drugs Used to Treat GERD, Gastritis, and Peptic Ulcer Disease

ANTACIDS

Maalox	Gaviscon	Gelusil	Tums
Mylanta	Aludrox	Riopan	Amphojel

Antacids buffer or neutralize gastric acid, usually acting locally. Antacids are used in GERD, gastritis, and peptic ulcer disease to relieve pain and prevent further damage to esophageal and gastric mucosa.

Nursing Responsibilities

- Antacids interfere with the absorption of many drugs given orally; separate administration times by at least 2 hours.
- Monitor for constipation or diarrhea resulting from antacid therapy. Notify the physician should either develop; a different antacid may be ordered.
- Although most antacids have little systemic effect, electrolyte imbalances can develop. Monitor serum electrolytes, particularly sodium, calcium, and magnesium levels.

Client and Family Teaching

- Take your antacid frequently as prescribed, 1 to 3 hours after meals and at bedtime. To be effective, the antacid must be in your stomach.
- Avoid taking an antacid for approximately 2 hours before and 1 hour after taking another medication.
- Shake suspensions well prior to administration.
- Chew tablets thoroughly, and follow with 4 to 6 ounces of water.
- Report worsening symptoms, diarrhea, or constipation to your primary care provider.
- Continue taking the antacid for the duration prescribed. While pain and discomfort often are relieved soon after treatment begins, healing takes 6 to 8 weeks.

H$_2$-RECEPTOR BLOCKERS

Cimetidine (Tagamet)	Ranitidine (Zantac)
Famotidine (Pepcid)	Nizatidine (Axid)

H$_2$-receptor blockers reduce acidity of gastric juices by blocking the ability of histamine to stimulate acid secretion by the gastric parietal cells. As a result, both the volume and concentration of hydrochloric acid in gastric juice is reduced. H$_2$-receptor blockers are given orally or intravenously. Both prescription and over-the-counter preparations are available.

Nursing Responsibilities

- To ensure absorption, do not give an antacid within 1 hour before or after giving an H$_2$-receptor blocker.
- When administered intravenously, do not mix with other drugs. Administer in 20 to 100 mL of solution over 15 to 30

minutes. Rapid intravenous injection as a bolus may cause dysrhythmias and hypotension.
- Monitor for interaction with such drugs as oral anticoagulants, beta blockers, benzodiazepines, tricyclic antidepressants, and others. H$_2$-receptor blockers may inhibit the metabolism of other drugs, increasing the risk of toxicity.

Client and Family Teaching

- Take the drug as directed, even if pain and gastric discomfort are relieved early in the course of therapy.
- Take at bedtime if once-a-day dosing is ordered. If spaced through the day, take before meals. Avoid taking antacids for 1 hour before and 1 hour after taking this drug.
- To promote healing, avoid cigarette smoking (which increases gastric acid secretion) and gastric mucosal irritants such as alcohol, aspirin, and NSAIDs.
- Long-term use of these drugs can lead to gynecomastia (breast enlargement) and impotence in men and breast tenderness in women. Discontinuing the drug will reverse these effects.
- Report possible adverse effects such as diarrhea, confusion, rash, fatigue, malaise, or bruising to your care provider.

PROTON-PUMP INHIBITORS

Lansoprazole (Prevacid)
Omeprazole (Prilosec)
Pantoprazole (Protonix)
Rabeprazole (Aciphex)

Proton-pump inhibitors (PPIs) are the drugs of choice for severe GERD. PPIs inhibit the hydrogen-potassium-ATP pump, reducing gastric acid secretion. Initially, the PPI may be given twice a day, with the dose reduced to once daily (at bedtime) after 8 weeks.

Nursing Responsibilities

- Administer before breakfast and at bedtime if ordered twice a day; at bedtime if once a day.
- Do not crush tablets.
- Monitor liver function tests for possible abnormal values, including increased AST, ALT, alkaline phosphatase, and bilirubin levels.

Client and Family Teaching

- Take the drug as ordered for the full course of therapy, even if symptoms are relieved.
- Do not crush, break, or chew tablets.
- Avoid cigarette smoking, alcohol, aspirin, and NSAIDs while taking this drug as these substances may interfere with healing.
- Report black tarry stools, diarrhea, or abdominal pain to your primary care provider.

(continued on page 550)

MediaLink | RANITIDINE ANIMATION

Medication Administration

Drugs Used to Treat GERD, Gastritis, and Peptic Ulcer Disease (continued)

ANTI-ULCER AGENT

Sucralfate (Carafate)

Sucralfate reacts with gastric acid to form a thick paste which adheres to damaged gastric mucosal tissue. It protects gastric mucosa and promotes healing through this local action.

Nursing Responsibilities

- Administer on an empty stomach, 1 hour before meals and at bedtime.
- Do not crush tablets.
- Separate administration time from antacids by at least 30 minutes.

Client and Family Teaching

- Take as directed, even after symptoms have been relieved.
- Do not crush or chew tablets; shake suspension well.
- Increase your intake of fluids and dietary fiber to prevent constipation.

PROMOTILITY AGENT

Metoclopramide (Reglan)

By acting on the central nervous system, metoclopramide stimulates upper gastrointestinal motility and gastric emptying. As a result, nausea, vomiting, and symptoms of GERD are reduced.

Nursing Implications

- Do not administer this drug to clients with possible gastrointestinal obstruction or bleeding, or a history of seizure disorders, pheochromocytoma, or Parkinson's disease.
- Monitor for extrapyramidal side effects (e.g., difficulty speaking or swallowing, loss of balance, gait disruptions, twitching or twisting movements, weakness of arms or legs) or manifestations of tardive dyskinesia (uncontrolled rhythmic facial movement, lip-smacking, tongue rolling). Report immediately.
- Give oral doses 30 minutes before meals and at bedtime.
- May be given by direct intravenous push over 1 to 2 minutes, or diluted by slow infusion over 15 to 30 minutes.

Client and Family Teaching

- Take this drug as directed. If you miss a dose, take as soon as you remember unless it is close to time for the next dose.
- Do not drive or engage in other activities that require alertness if this drug makes you drowsy.
- Avoid using alcohol or other CNS depressants while you are taking this drug.
- Immediately contact your health care provider if you develop involuntary movements of your eyes, face, or limbs.

---

sphincter or delay gastric emptying, so should be avoided. The client is advised to maintain ideal body weight, eat smaller meals, refrain from eating for 3 hours before bedtime, and stay upright for 2 hours after meals. Elevating the head of the bed on 6- to 8-inch blocks often is beneficial. Stopping smoking is a necessary lifestyle change. Avoiding tight clothing and avoiding bending may help to relieve symptoms.

Surgery

Surgery may be used for clients who do not respond to pharmacologic and lifestyle management. Antireflux surgeries increase pressure in the lower esophagus, inhibiting gastric content reflux. Laparoscopic procedures for GERD include tightening the lower esophageal sphincter with an endoscopic suturing system or burning spots on the muscle surrounding the lower esophageal sphincter to create scar tissue (Mattonen, 2001). An open surgical procedure known as Nissen fundoplication also may be done (Figure 21–4 ■).

NURSING CARE

Assessment

Assessment data related to GERD include the following:

- Health history: manifestations such as frequent heartburn; intolerance of foods that are acidic, spicy, or fatty; regurgitation of acidic gastric juice; increased symptoms when bending over, lying down, or wearing tight clothing; difficulty swallowing
- Physical assessment: Epigastric tenderness

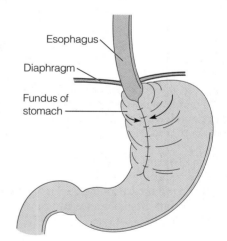

Esophagus

Diaphragm

Fundus of stomach

Figure 21–4 ■ Nissen fundoplication. The fundus of the stomach is wrapped around the lower esophagus and the edges are sutured together.

Nursing Diagnoses and Interventions

Pain

The epigastric pain associated with GERD can be severe, interfering with rest and causing anxiety.

- Provide small, frequent meals. Restrict intake of fat, acidic foods, coffee, and alcohol. *Limiting the size of meals reduces pressure in the stomach, reducing esophageal reflux. Fatty, acidic foods, coffee, and alcohol increase gastric acidity and interfere with gastric emptying, increasing the incidence of gastroesophageal reflux.*

CHART 21–2 NANDA, NIC, AND NOC LINKAGES

The Client with GERD

NURSING DIAGNOSES	NURSING INTERVENTIONS	NURSING OUTCOMES
• Pain: Heartburn	• Behavior Modification	• Pain: Disruptive Effects
• Imbalanced Nutrition: Less Than Body Requirements	• Nutrition Management • Nutrition Monitoring	• Nutritional Status: Food and Fluid Intake
• Ineffective Health Maintenance	• Teaching: Individual	• Knowledge: Treatment Regimen

Note. Data from Nursing Outcomes Classification (NOC) by M. Johnson & M. Maas (Eds.), 1997, St. Louis: Mosby; Nursing Diagnoses: Definitions & Classification 2001–2002 by North American Nursing Diagnosis Association, 2001, Philadelphia: NANDA; Nursing Interventions Classification (NIC) by J.C. McCloskey & G. M. Bulechek (Eds.), 2000, St. Louis: Mosby. Reprinted by permission.

- Instruct to stop smoking. Refer to a smoking cessation clinic or program as needed. *Cigarette smoking increases gastric acidity and interferes with healing of damaged mucosa.*
- Administer antacids, H_2-receptor blockers, and proton-pump inhibitors as ordered. Instruct client to continue therapy as prescribed, even after symptoms have been relieved. *These drugs neutralize or reduce gastric acid secretion, relieving symptoms and promoting healing.*
- Discuss the long-term nature of GERD and its management. *Lifestyle changes need to be continued after healing and symptom relief to manage the long-term effects of GERD.*

Using NANDA, NIC, and NOC

Chart 21–2 shows links between NANDA nursing diagnoses, NIC, and NOC for clients with GERD.

Home Care

GERD is a lifelong condition best managed by the client. Teach the client and family about continuing management strategies, including dietary changes, remaining upright after meals, and avoiding eating for at least 3 hours before bedtime. Suggest elevating the head of the bed on 6- to 8-inch wooden blocks placed under the legs. Discuss the need for continued gastric acid reduction using antacids, H_2-receptor blockers, or proton-pump inhibitors. All are effective to reduce the acidity of gastric juices. Antacids, the most cost-effective measure, require frequent doses to neutralize gastric acid. H_2-receptor blockers, also available over the counter, are a cost-effective management strategy that require only twice-a-day dosing.

THE CLIENT WITH HIATAL HERNIA

A **hiatal hernia** occurs when part of the stomach protrudes through the esophageal hiatus of the diaphragm into the thoracic cavity. While hiatal hernia is thought to be a common problem, most affected individuals are asymptomatic. The incidence of hiatal hernia increases with age.

In a *sliding hiatal hernia,* the gastroesophageal junction and the fundus of the stomach slide upward through the esophageal hiatus (Figure 21–5A). Several factors may contribute to a sliding hiatal hernia, including weakened gastroesophageal-diaphragmatic anchors, shortening of the esophagus, or increased intra-abdominal pressure. Small sliding hiatal hernias produce few symptoms.

In a *paraesophageal hiatal hernia,* the junction between the esophagus and stomach remains in its normal position below the diaphragm while a part of the stomach herniates through the esophageal hiatus (Figure 21–5B). A paraesophageal hernia can become incarcerated (constricted) and strangulate, impairing blood flow to the herniated tissue. Clients with

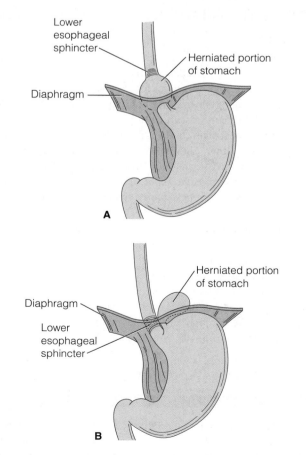

Figure 21–5 ■ Hiatal hernias. *A,* Sliding hiatal hernia. *B,* Paraesophageal hiatal hernia.

Manifestations of Hiatal Hernia

- Reflux, heartburn
- Substernal chest pain
- Occult bleeding
- Feeling of fullness
- Dysphagia
- Belching, indigestion

paraesophageal hernia may develop gastritis, or chronic or acute gastrointestinal bleeding. The manifestations of hiatal hernias are listed in the box above.

A barium swallow or an upper endoscopy may be done to diagnose hiatal hernia. Many clients with hiatal hernia require no treatment. If symptoms are present, treatment measures such as those for clients with GERD may be ordered. If medical management is ineffective or the hernia becomes incarcerated, surgery may be required. The most common surgical procedure is the Nissen fundoplication (see Figure 21–4). This surgery prevents the gastroesophageal junction from slipping into the thoracic cavity.

Nursing care for the client with a hiatal hernia is similar to that for the client with GERD. If surgery is performed, nursing care is similar to that for clients undergoing gastric or thoracic surgery (see Chapter 7). ⟲⟳

THE CLIENT WITH IMPAIRED ESOPHAGEAL MOTILITY

Disorders of esophageal motility can cause dysphagia or chest pain. **Achalasia,** a disorder of unknown etiology, is characterized by impaired peristalsis of the smooth muscle of the esophagus and impaired relaxation of the lower esophageal sphincter. The client experiences gradually increasing dysphagia with both solid foods and liquids. Fullness in the chest during meals, chest pain, and nighttime cough are additional manifestations. Other clients may experience **diffuse esophageal spasm** that causes nonperistaltic contraction of esophageal smooth muscle. This disorder causes chest pain and/or dysphagia. The chest pain can be severe, and usually occurs at rest.

Treatment of achalasia may include endoscopically guided injection of botulinum toxin into the lower esophageal sphincter or balloon dilation of the LES. Botulinum toxin injection lowers LES pressure, but may need to be repeated every 6 to 9 months. Balloon dilation tears muscle fibers in the LES, reducing its pressure (Figure 21–6 ■). A laparoscopic myotomy (incision into the circular muscle layer of the LES) also reduces pressure and relieves symptoms.

THE CLIENT WITH ESOPHAGEAL CANCER

Cancer of the esophagus is a relatively uncommon malignancy in the United States. It does, however, have a high mortality rate, primarily because symptoms often are not recognized until late in the course of the disease.

Lower esophageal sphincter

Figure 21–6 ■ Balloon dilation of the lower esophageal sphincter.

PATHOPHYSIOLOGY AND MANIFESTATIONS

Squamous cell carcinoma is the most common type of esophageal cancer. It usually affects the middle or distal portion of the esophagus. Squamous cell cancer is much more common in blacks than in whites. Cigarette smoking and chronic alcohol use are strong risk factors for squamous cell esophageal tumors.

Adenocarcinoma, nearly as common as squamous cell, is more common in whites. It usually develops in the distal portion of the esophagus. Adenocarcinoma is commonly associated with Barrett's esophagus, a possible complication of chronic GERD and achalasia.

The most common symptom of esophageal carcinoma is progressive dysphagia. Other manifestations are listed in the box below. The cancer often is advanced and incurable by the time the disease is diagnosed.

Manifestations of Esophageal Cancer

- Dysphagia
- Weight loss
- Regurgitation
- Chest pain
- Anemia
- GERD-like symptoms
- Anorexia
- Persistent cough

COLLABORATIVE CARE

Controlling dysphagia and maintaining nutritional status is an essential goal of therapy for clients with esophageal cancer, regardless of the stage of the disease. Treatment may involve surgery, radiation therapy, and/or chemotherapy.

Diagnostic Tests

Diagnostic and staging procedures for esophageal cancer may include esophagography, bronchoscopy, and scans to detect metastasis. The following diagnostic tests may be done.

- *Barium swallow* to identify irregular mucosal patterns or narrowing of the lumen, which suggest esophageal cancer.
- *Esophagoscopy* to allow direct visualization of the tumor and obtain tissue for biopsy.
- *Chest X-ray, CT scans,* or *MRI* to identify possible tumor metastases to other organs or tissues.
- *Complete blood count (CBC)* may indicate anemia due to chronic blood loss. *Serum albumin levels* may be low due to malnutrition, and *liver function tests (ALT, alkaline phosphatase, AST,* and *bilirubin)* are elevated if liver metastases are present.

Treatments

The treatment of esophageal cancer depends on the stage of the disease, as well as factors such as the client's condition and preference.

Clients with early, "curable" esophageal cancer may be treated with surgery alone. Surgery involves resection of the affected portion of the esophagus, and possible anastamosis of the stomach to the remaining esophagus. Mediastinal lymph nodes may be resected at the time of surgery. Other approaches to early esophageal cancer include combined radiation and chemotherapy, or a combination of radiation therapy and chemotherapy prior to surgical resection of the tumor. Complications associated with radiation therapy to the esophagus include perforation, hemorrhage, and strictures. When the tumor has spread locally or to distant sites, palliative therapy relieves dysphagia and pain (Tierney et al., 2001). Palliative therapy may include surgical resection, radiation therapy, or local treatments such as wire stents or laser therapy to keep the esophagus patent.

NURSING CARE

Health Promotion

Health promotion measures to reduce the risk for and incidence of esophageal cancer include educating people (especially young people) about the dangers of cigarette smoking and excess alcohol use. Refer to smoking cessation and alcohol treatment programs as indicated.

Assessment

Early diagnosis and treatment of esophageal cancer can make a difference in the client's prognosis. Collect the following assessment data related to esophageal cancer.

- Health history: current symptoms such as chest pain, dysphagia, odynophagia (pain with swallowing), coughing or hoarseness; duration of symptoms; recent weight loss; smoking history; current and past patterns of alcohol consumption
- Physical examination: weight; general health status; skin color; supraclavicular and cervical lymph nodes for lymphadenopathy

Nursing Diagnoses and Interventions

Imbalanced Nutrition: Less Than Body Requirements

The client diagnosed with esophageal cancer may already suffer from some degree of malnutrition because of difficulty and pain with swallowing. Enteral nutrition via nasogastric feeding tube or gastrostomy tube or parenteral nutrition maintain nutritional status after surgery or if the tumor is inoperable and obstruction occurs. See Chapter 20 for nursing interventions related to enteral and parenteral feedings.

Risk for Ineffective Airway Clearance

After surgery for esophageal cancer, the client is at high risk for aspiration and difficulty maintaining a patent airway due to disruption of the esophagus and incision into the thoracic cavity.

- Assess mental and respiratory status (including rate, depth, breath sounds, and oxygen saturation levels) every hour during the initial postoperative period. *Altered mental status increases the risk for aspiration. An increased respiratory rate, dyspnea, diminished breath sounds, or decreased oxygen saturation levels may indicate impaired airway clearance or possible aspiration pneumonia.*
- Encourage coughing and deep breathing every 2 to 4 hours and as needed. *These activities help mobilize respiratory secretions.*
- Verify enteral tube feeding placement by checking the pH of gastric aspirate (see Chapter 20). Stop enteral feedings if feelings of fullness or nausea occur. Suction gastrointestinal contents as needed, positioning the client on the side. *Overdistention of the stomach or delayed gastric emptying may result in regurgitation of stomach contents. Nausea or a feeling of fullness may indicate stomach overdistention. Suctioning and positioning limit the risk of aspiration.*

Anticipatory Grieving

Upon a diagnosis of cancer, the client and family may experience a grief reaction. The pessimistic prognosis associated with esophageal cancer and the disruptions in relationships may result in an intense sense of loss. Chapter 11 discusses care of client experiencing grief and loss.

Using NANDA, NIC, and NOC

Chart 21–3 shows links between NANDA nursing diagnoses, NIC, and NOC for clients with esophageal cancer.

CHART 21-3 NANDA, NIC, AND NOC LINKAGES

The Client with Esophageal Cancer

NURSING DIAGNOSES	NURSING INTERVENTIONS	NURSING OUTCOMES
• Impaired Swallowing	• Aspiration Precautions • Positioning	• Aspiration Control • Swallowing Status
• Imbalanced Nutrition: Less Than Body Requirements	• Fluid Monitoring • Nutrition Management	• Nutritional Status: Food and Fluid Intake
• Fear	• Anxiety Reduction	• Anxiety Control

Note. Data from Nursing Outcomes Classification (NOC) by M. Johnson & M. Maas (Eds.), 1997, St. Louis: Mosby; Nursing Diagnoses: Definitions & Classification 2001–2002 by North American Nursing Diagnosis Association, 2001, Philadelphia: NANDA; Nursing Interventions Classification (NIC) by J.C. McCloskey & G. M. Bulechek (Eds.), 2000, St. Louis: Mosby. Reprinted by permission.

Home Care

Most care for clients with esophageal cancer is provided in community-based and home settings. Include the following topics in client and family teaching for home care:

• Planned treatment options including the risks, benefits, and potential adverse effects of each

• Wound and follow-up care following surgery
• How to prepare, implement, and care for tube feedings or home parenteral nutrition

Based on the client's needs and prognosis, referral to a home health agency and/or hospice may be appropriate.

DISORDERS OF THE STOMACH AND DUODENUM

The stomach and upper small intestine (duodenum and jejunum) are responsible for the majority of food digestion. The major disorders that affect digestion are gastritis, peptic ulcer disease, and cancer of the stomach. Nursing roles in managing these disorders include both acute care for the hospitalized client and teaching to give the client the skills and knowledge to manage these conditions at home.

OVERVIEW OF NORMAL PHYSIOLOGY

Normally, the stomach is protected from the digestive substances it secretes—namely hydrochloric acid and pepsin—by the **gastric mucosal barrier** (Figure 21-7 ■). The gastric mucosal barrier includes:

• An impermeable hydrophobic lipid layer that covers gastric epithelial cells. This lipid layer prevents diffusion of water-soluble molecules, but substances such as aspirin and alcohol can diffuse through it.
• Bicarbonate ions secreted in response to hydrochloric acid secretion by the parietal cells of the stomach. When bicarbonate (HCO_3^-) secretion is equal to hydrogen ion (H^+) secretion, the gastric mucosa remains intact. Prostaglandins, chemical messengers involved in the inflammatory response, support bicarbonate production and blood flow to the gastric mucosa.
• Mucus gel that protects the surface of the stomach lining from the damaging effects of pepsin and traps bicarbonate to neutralize hydrochloric acid. This gel also acts as a lubricant, preventing mechanical damage to the stomach lining from its contents.

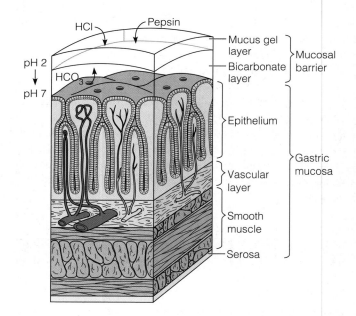

Figure 21-7 ■ The gastric mucosa and mucosal barrier. The mucus gel and bicarbonate of the mucosal barrier protect the gastric mucosa (the epithelial, vascular, and smooth muscle layers) from damage by digestive substances such as hydrochloric acid and pepsin.

When an acute or chronic irritant disrupts the mucosal barrier, or when disease alters the processes that maintain the barrier, the gastric mucosa becomes irritated and inflamed. Lipid-soluble substances such as aspirin and alcohol penetrate the gastric mucosal barrier, leading to irritation and possible inflammation. Bile acids also break down the lipids in the mucosal barrier, increasing the potential for irritation (Porth, 2002). In addition, aspirin and other nonsteroidal anti-inflammatory drugs (NSAIDs) inhibit prostaglandins. Aspirin and NSAIDs also alter the nature of gastric mucus, affecting its protective function.

THE CLIENT WITH GASTRITIS

Gastritis, inflammation of the stomach lining, results from irritation of the gastric mucosa. Gastritis is common, and may be caused by a variety of factors. The most common form of gastritis, **acute gastritis,** is generally a benign, self-limiting disorder associated with the ingestion of gastric irritants such as aspirin, alcohol, caffeine, or foods contaminated with certain bacteria. Manifestations of acute gastritis may range from asymptomatic to mild heartburn to severe gastric distress, vomiting, and bleeding with **hematemesis** (vomiting blood).

Chronic gastritis is a separate group of disorders characterized by progressive and irreversible changes in the gastric mucosa (Porth, 2002). Chronic gastritis is more common in the elderly, chronic alcoholics, and cigarette smokers. When symptoms of chronic gastritis occur, they are often vague, ranging from a feeling of heaviness in the epigastric region after meals to gnawing, burning, ulcerlike epigastric pain unrelieved by antacids.

PATHOPHYSIOLOGY

Acute Gastritis

Acute gastritis is characterized by disruption of the mucosal barrier by a local irritant. This disruption allows hydrochloric acid and pepsin to come into contact with the gastric tissue, resulting in irritation, inflammation, and superficial erosions. The gastric mucosa rapidly regenerates, generally making acute gastritis a self-limiting disorder, with resolution and healing occurring within several days.

The ingestion of aspirin or other NSAIDS, corticosteroids, alcohol, and caffeine is commonly associated with the development of acute gastritis. Accidental or purposeful ingestion of a corrosive alkali (such as ammonia, lye, Lysol, and other cleaning agents) or acid leads to severe inflammation and possible necrosis of the stomach. Gastric perforation, hemorrhage, and peritonitis are possible results. Iatrogenic causes of acute gastritis include radiation therapy and administration of certain chemotherapeutic agents.

Erosive Gastritis

A severe form of acute gastritis, **erosive** or **stress-induced gastritis,** occurs as a complication of other life-threatening conditions such as shock, severe trauma, major surgery, sepsis, burns, or head injury. When these erosions follow a major burn, they are called **Curling's ulcers,** after Thomas Curling, a British physician, who first described them in 1842. When stress ulcers occur following head injury or central nervous system surgery, they are referred to as **Cushing's ulcers,** after Harvey Cushing, a U.S. surgeon.

The primary mechanisms leading to erosive gastritis appear to be ischemia of the gastric mucosa resulting from sympathetic vasoconstriction, and tissue injury due to gastric acid. As a result, multiple superficial erosions of the gastric mucosa develop. Maintaining the gastric pH at greater than 3.5 and inhibiting gastric acid secretion with medications help prevent erosive gastritis.

Manifestations

The client with acute gastritis may have mild symptoms such as **anorexia** (loss of appetite), or mild epigastric discomfort relieved by belching or defecating. More severe manifestations include abdominal pain, nausea, and vomiting. Gastric bleeding may occur, with hematemesis or **melena** (black, tarry stool that contains blood). Erosive gastritis is not typically associated with pain. The initial symptom often is painless gastric bleeding occurring 2 or more days after the initial stressor. Bleeding typically is minimal, but can be massive. Corrosive gastritis can cause severe bleeding, signs of shock, and an *acute abdomen* (severely painful, rigid, boardlike abdomen) if perforation occurs. See the Manifestations box below.

Chronic Gastritis

Unrelated to acute gastritis, chronic gastritis is a progressive disorder that begins with superficial inflammation and gradually leads to atrophy of gastric tissues. The initial stage is characterized by superficial changes in the gastric mucosa and a decrease in mucus. As the disease evolves, glands of the gastric mucosa are disrupted and destroyed. The inflammatory process involves deep portions of the mucosa, which thins and atrophies. There appear to be at least two different forms of chronic gastritis, classified as type A and type B.

Type A gastritis, the less common form of chronic gastritis, usually affects people of Northern European heritage. This

Manifestations of Acute and Chronic Gastritis

ACUTE GASTRITIS

Gastrointestinal	**Systemic**
• Anorexia	• Possible shock
• Nausea and vomiting	
• Hematemesis	
• Melena	
• Abdominal pain	

CHRONIC GASTRITIS

Gastrointestinal	**Systemic**
• Vague discomfort after eating; may be asymptomatic	• Anemia
	• Fatigue

type of gastritis is thought to have an autoimmune component. In type A or autoimmune gastritis, the body produces antibodies to parietal cells and to intrinsic factor. These antibodies destroy gastric mucosal cells, resulting in tissue atrophy and the loss of hydrochloric acid and pepsin secretion. Because intrinsic factor is required for the absorption of vitamin B_{12}, this immune response also results in pernicious anemia. For further discussion of pernicious anemia, see Chapter 32. ∞

Type B gastritis is the more common form of chronic gastritis. Its incidence increases with age, reaching nearly 100% in people over the age of 70. Type B gastritis is caused by chronic infection of the gastric mucosa by *Helicobacter pylori* (*H. pylori*), a gram-negative spiral bacterium. *H. pylori* infection causes inflammation of the gastric mucosa, with infiltration by neutrophils and lymphocytes. The outermost layer of gastric mucosa thins and atrophies, providing a less effective barrier against the autodigestive properties of hydrochloric acid and pepsin.

Infection with *H. pylori* also is associated with an increased risk for peptic ulcer disease. *H. pylori* infection significantly increases the risk of developing gastric cancer. See the sections that follow for more information about these disorders.

Manifestations

Chronic gastritis is often asymptomatic until atrophy is sufficiently advanced to interfere with digestion and gastric emptying. The client may complain of vague gastric distress, epigastric heaviness after meals, or ulcerlike symptoms. These symptoms typically are not relieved by antacids. In addition, the client may experience fatigue and other symptoms of anemia. If intrinsic factor is lacking, paresthesias and other neurologic manifestations of vitamin B_{12} deficiency may be present. See the Manifestations box on previous page.

COLLABORATIVE CARE

Acute gastritis is usually diagnosed by the history and clinical presentation. In contrast, the vague symptoms of chronic gastritis may require more extensive diagnostic testing.

Clients with acute and chronic gastritis are generally managed in community settings. The client requires acute care only when nausea and vomiting are severe enough to interfere with normal fluid and electrolyte balance and nutritional status. If hemorrhage results, surgical intervention may be required.

Diagnostic Tests

Diagnostic tests that may be ordered for the client with gastritis include the following:

- *Gastric analysis* to assess hydrochloric acid secretion. A nasogastric tube is passed into the stomach, and pentagastrin is injected subcutaneously to stimulate gastric secretion of hydrochloric acid. Secretion may be decreased in clients with chronic gastritis.

- *Hemoglobin, hematocrit,* and *red blood cell indices* are evaluated for evidence of anemia. The client with gastritis may develop pernicious anemia because of parietal cell destruction, or iron-deficiency anemia because of chronic blood loss.
- *Serum vitamin B_{12} levels* are measured to evaluate for possible pernicious anemia. Normal values for vitamin B_{12} are 200 to 1000 pg/mL, with lower levels seen in older adults.
- *Upper endoscopy* may be done to inspect the gastric mucosa for changes, identify areas of bleeding, and obtain tissue for biopsy. Bleeding sites may be treated with electro- or laser coagulation or injected with a sclerosing agent during the procedure. See the Nursing Implications box on page 548 for client preparation and teaching related to an upper endoscopy.

Medications

Drugs such as a proton-pump inhibitor (PPI), histamine$_2$ (H$_2$)-receptor blocker, or sucralfate may be ordered to prevent or treat acute stress gastritis. PPIs and H$_2$-receptor blockers reduce the amount or effects of hydrochloric acid on the gastric mucosa. Lansoprazole (Prevacid) and omeprazole (Prilosec) are examples of PPIs. H$_2$-receptor blockers include cimetidine (Tagamet), ranitidine (Zantac), famotidine (Pepcid), and nizatidine (Axid). These drugs also are available in nonprescription strength. Sucralfate (Carafate) works locally to prevent the damaging effects of acid and pepsin on gastric tissue. It does not neutralize or reduce acid secretion. Nursing implications for drugs commonly used in managing gastritis are included in the Medication Administration box on pages 549–550.

The client with type B chronic gastritis may be treated to eradicate the *H. pylori* infection. This generally involves combination therapy consisting of two antibiotics (such as metronidazole and clarithromycin or tetracycline) and a PPI. In some cases, eradication of the infection is not warranted, and the client is treated symptomatically.

Treatments

In acute gastritis, gastrointestinal tract rest is provided by 6 to 12 hours of NPO status, then slow reintroduction of clear liquids (broth, tea, gelatin, carbonated beverages), followed by ingestion of heavier liquids (cream soups, puddings, milk) and finally a gradual reintroduction of solid food.

If nausea and vomiting threaten fluid and electrolyte balance, intravenous fluids and electrolytes are ordered.

Gastric Lavage

Acute gastritis resulting from ingestion of a poisonous or corrosive substance (acid or strong alkali), is treated with immediate dilution and removal of the substance. Vomiting is not induced because it might further damage the esophagus and possibly the trachea; instead, **gastric lavage,** washing out of the stomach contents, is performed. See Procedure 21–1.

Procedure 21–1

Gastric Lavage

When it is important to remove or dilute gastric contents rapidly, gastric lavage, irrigation or washing out of the stomach, may be indicated. In acute poisoning or ingestion of a caustic substance, a large-bore 30- to 36- French nasogastric tube is inserted, and lavage performed. When gastric hemorrhage occurs, lavage may be used to remove blood from the GI tract. Because the GI tract is not sterile, clean technique is appropriate for use, although the solution used will generally be sterile.

- Obtain baseline assessment, including vital signs, abdominal inspection, girth, and bowel sounds. *It is important to have assessment data documented prior to instituting the procedure for comparison.*
- Explain the procedure, answering questions and clarifying perceptions. Instruct to report any pain, difficulty breathing, or other problems during the procedure. *A client who is able to understand and cooperate with the procedure will tolerate lavage better. The client may be aware of symptoms of complications such as perforation or tube displacement before they are evident to the nurse.*
- Place in semi-Fowler's or Fowler's position. If unable to tolerate elevation of the head of the bed because of hypotension, place in left side-lying position. *Elevating of the head of the bed or side-lying position will minimize the risk of aspiration.*
- Insert a nasogastric tube if one is not already in place. Verify tube placement by aspirating gastric contents and test pH of aspirate. *Proper placement is vital to prevent aspiration or overdistention of the small bowel with irrigating solution.*

CLOSED SYSTEM IRRIGATION

- Wearing clean gloves, connect bag or bottle of normal saline irrigating solution to nasogastric tube using a Y connector. Attach drainage or suction tube to other arm of connector (Figure 21–8 ■). Empty the stomach, clamp drain tube or turn off suction, and allow 50 to 200 mL of solution

to run into stomach by gravity. Stop solution and allow to drain or suction out. Repeat until ordered amount has been used or desired results are obtained, for example, no further clots and solution returns clear or light pink. Measure the amount of drainage, subtracting the amount of irrigant instilled, to obtain gastric output. *The closed system minimizes the risk of contact with body fluids for the nurse. Measuring gastric output is important in monitoring fluid balance.*

INTERMITTENT OPEN SYSTEM

- Wearing clean gloves and other personal protective equipment as necessary (gown and face protection), empty the stomach using suction or a 50-mL catheter-tip syringe. Measure and discard the aspirate. Using the syringe, draw up approximately 50 mL of irrigation solution, and instill it using gentle pressure. Aspirate the nasogastric tube, and discard the solution into a measuring container. Continue this procedure until the desired amount of irrigant or desired results have been

obtained. *Manual irrigation with a catheter-tip syringe may be more effective in removing clots from the stomach and nasogastric tube.*
- Continue to monitor vital signs (including temperature), tolerance of the procedure, and other assessment data. *The client may be unstable and require continuous reevaluation Gastric lavage may cause hypothermia; therefore, monitor temperature and indications of hypothermia, such as lethargy and changes in cardiac rate and rhythm.*
- If the aspirate has not cleared to light pink or pink-tinged after 20 to 30 minutes of lavage or if the client is unable to tolerate the procedure, notify the physician. *Medical or surgical intervention may be necessary to stop hemorrhage in some instances.*
- On completion of lavage, provide mouth and nares care. Continue to monitor vital signs, abdominal status, and other assessment data.
- Document the procedure, including the amount and type of irrigant used, gastric output character and amount, and the client's condition and tolerance of the procedure.

Figure 21–8 ■ The client with a closed system gastric lavage.

NURSING CARE

Health Promotion

Teach all clients and community members about measures to prevent acute gastritis. Food contaminated with bacteria is a significant cause of acute gastritis. Discuss food safety measures such as fully cooking meats and egg products, and promptly refrigerating foods after cooking to avoid bacterial growth. Stress that food contaminated with potential pathogens often looks, smells, and tastes good, making it difficult to identify. Teach clients to abstain from eating or drinking anything during an acute episode of vomiting, then reintroduce clear liquids gradually once vomiting has stopped (2 to 4 hours after the last episode of vomiting). Suggest using liquids such as Pedialyte or sport drinks to replace lost electrolytes and fluid. Instruct clients to avoid milk and milk products until they easily tolerate clear liquids and solid foods such as dry toast or saltine crackers.

Assessment

Assessment data to collect for clients with acute or chronic gastritis include the following:

- Health history: current symptoms and their duration; relieving and aggravating factors; history of ingestion of toxins, contaminated food, alcohol, aspirin, or NSAIDs; other medications
- Physical examination: vital signs including orthostatic vitals if indicated; peripheral pulses; general appearance; abdominal assessment including appearance, bowel sounds, and tenderness

Nursing Diagnoses and Interventions

In planning and implementing nursing care for the client with acute or chronic gastritis, consider both the direct effects of the disorder on the gastrointestinal system and nutritional status as well as its effects on lifestyle and psychosocial integrity. This section focuses on problems of fluid balance and nutrition.

Deficient Fluid Volume

Nausea, vomiting, and abdominal distress are the primary manifestations of acute gastritis. The risk for fluid and electrolyte imbalance is high because of inadequate intake of food and fluids, and abnormal losses of fluids and electrolytes with vomiting.

PRACTICE ALERT *Tachycardia, tachypnea, and hypotension, especially orthostatic hypotension, may indicate fluid volume deficit. Electrolyte or acid-base imbalances resulting from vomiting may cause cardiac dysrhythmias or changes in respirations.* ■

- Monitor and record vital signs at least every 2 hours until stable, then every 4 hours. Check for orthostatic hypotension.
- Weigh daily. Monitor and record intake and output; record urine output every 1 to 4 hours as indicated. *Daily weights are an accurate indicator of fluid volume. Urine output of less than 30 mL per hour indicates decreased cardiac output and a need for prompt fluid replacement.*

- Monitor skin turgor, color, and condition and status of oral mucous membranes frequently. Provide skin and mouth care frequently. *Skin turgor and mucous membrane assessments indicate hydration status. Good skin and mouth care are necessary to maintain skin and mucous membrane integrity.*
- Monitor laboratory values for electrolytes and acid-base balance. Report significant changes or deviations from normal. *Electrolytes are lost through vomiting, increasing the risk of electrolyte and acid-base imbalances. These imbalances, in turn, affect multiple body systems.*
- Administer oral or parenteral fluids as ordered. *Oral fluids may be withheld until vomiting has ceased, then gradually reintroduced. Intravenous fluids restore or maintain hydration until adequate oral intake is resumed.*
- Administer antiemetic and other drugs as ordered to relieve vomiting and facilitate oral feeding. Encourage fluids as soon as feasible. *The oral route is preferred for fluid and nutrient intake; medications may be used to allow earlier resumption of feeding.*

PRACTICE ALERT *Ensure safety: Place call light within reach, put up the side rails, instruct to avoid getting up without assistance. Orthostatic hypotension may lead to syncope and to falls if the client attempts to get up without assistance.* ■

Imbalanced Nutrition: Less Than Body Requirements

Manifestations of chronic gastritis may lead to reduced food intake and malnutrition. The client often associates these unpleasant sensations with eating, and may gradually reduce food intake. Associated anorexia also contributes to poor food intake.

- Monitor and record food and fluid intake and any abnormal losses (such as vomiting). *Careful monitoring can help in developing a dietary plan to meet the caloric needs of the client.*
- Monitor weight and laboratory studies such as serum albumin, hemoglobin, and red blood cell indices. *Weights and laboratory values provide data regarding nutritional status and the effectiveness of interventions.*
- Arrange for dietary consultation to determine caloric and nutrient needs and develop a dietary plan. Consider food preferences and tolerances in menu planning. *A diet high in protein, vitamins, and minerals may be prescribed to meet nutritional needs of the client with chronic gastritis. In addition, specific food intolerances may need to be considered. Planning to include preferred foods in the diet helps ensure consumption of the prescribed diet.*
- Provide nutritional supplements between meals or frequent small feedings as needed. *Many clients with chronic gastritis tolerate small, frequent feedings better than three large meals per day.*
- Maintain tube feedings or parenteral nutrition as ordered. Refer to Chapter 20 for further information on enteral and parenteral feedings.

CHART 21–4 NANDA, NIC, AND NOC LINKAGES		
The Client with Gastritis or Peptic Ulcer Disease		
NURSING DIAGNOSES	**NURSING INTERVENTIONS**	**NURSING OUTCOMES**
• Pain • Nausea • Risk for Deficient Fluid Volume • Ineffective Health Maintenance • Fatigue	• Medication Management • Nausea Management • Fluid/Electrolyte Management • Teaching: Disease Process • Energy Management	• Comfort Level • Nutritional Status: Food and Fluid Intake • Hydration • Knowledge: Treatment Regimen • Nutritional Status: Energy

Note. Data from Nursing Outcomes Classification (NOC) by M. Johnson & M. Maas (Eds.), 1997, St. Louis: Mosby; Nursing Diagnoses: Definitions & Classification 2001–2002 by North American Nursing Diagnosis Association, 2001, Philadelphia: NANDA; Nursing Interventions Classification (NIC) by J.C. McCloskey & G. M. Bulechek (Eds.), 2000, St. Louis: Mosby. Reprinted by permission.

Using NANDA, NIC, and NOC

Chart 21–4 shows links between NANDA nursing diagnoses, NIC, and NOC when caring for a client with gastritis.

Home Care

Because acute or chronic gastritis is usually managed in community-based settings, teaching is vital. For the client with acute gastritis, teaching focuses on managing acute symptoms, reintroducing fluids and solid foods, indicators of possible complications (e.g., continued vomiting, signs of fluid and electrolyte imbalance), and preventing future episodes.

Provide the following information for clients with chronic gastritis.

• Maintaining optimal nutrition
• Helpful dietary modifications
• Using prescribed medications
• Avoiding known gastric irritants, such as aspirin, alcohol, and cigarette smoking

Referral to smoking-cessation classes or programs to treat alcohol abuse may be necessary.

THE CLIENT WITH PEPTIC ULCER DISEASE

Peptic ulcer disease (PUD), a break in the mucous lining of the gastrointestinal tract where it comes in contact with gastric juice, is a chronic health problem. PUD affects approximately 10% of the population or 4 million people in the United States every year (Braunwald et al., 2001; Tierney et al., 2001).

Peptic ulcers occur in any area of the gastrointestinal tract exposed to acid-pepsin secretions, including the esophagus, stomach, or duodenum. **Duodenal ulcers** are the most common. They usually develop between the ages of 30 and 55, and are more common in men than women. **Gastric ulcers** more often affect older clients, between the ages of 55 and 70. Ulcers are more common in people who smoke and who are chronic users of NSAIDs. Alcohol and dietary intake do not seem to cause PUD, and the role of stress is uncertain. Although the incidence of PUD has dramatically decreased, the incidence of

BOX 21–1 ■ Risk Factors for Peptic Ulcer Disease

■ *H. pylori* infection
  ■ Low socioeconomic status
  ■ Crowded, unsanitary living conditions
  ■ Unclean food or water
■ Use of NSAIDs
  ■ Advanced age
  ■ History of ulcer
  ■ Concurrent use of other drugs such as glucocorticoids or other NSAIDs
■ Cigarette smoking
■ Family history of PUD
■ Possible risk factors: psychological stress; alcohol and/or caffeine consumption

gastric ulcers is increasing, believed due to the widespread use of NSAIDs (Tierney et al., 2001).

Risk Factors

Chronic *H. pylori* infection and use of aspirin and NSAIDs are the major risk factors for PUD. Contributing risk factors are listed in Box 21–1. Overall, an estimated one in six clients infected with *H. pylori* develop PUD. Of the NSAIDs, aspirin is the most ulcerogenic. A strong familial pattern suggests a genetic factor in the development of PUD. Cigarette smoking is a significant risk factor, doubling the risk of PUD. Cigarette smoking inhibits the secretion of bicarbonate by the pancreas and possibly causes more rapid transit of gastric acid into the duodenum.

PATHOPHYSIOLOGY

The innermost layer of the stomach wall, the gastric mucosa, consists of columnar epithelial cells, supported by a middle layer of blood vessels and glands, and a thin outer layer of smooth muscle. The mucosal barrier of the stomach, a thin coating of mucous gel and bicarbonate, protects the gastric mucosa. The mucosal barrier is maintained by bicarbonate secreted by the epithelial cells, by mucus gel production stimulated by prostaglandins, and by an adequate blood supply to the mucosa (see the overview of normal physiology on page 554).

An **ulcer,** or break in the gastrointestinal mucosa, develops when the mucosal barrier is unable to protect the mucosa from damage by hydrochloric acid and pepsin, the gastric digestive juices.

H. pylori infection, found in about 70% of people who have PUD, is unique in colonizing the stomach. It is spread person to person (oral–oral or fecal–oral), and contributes to ulcer formation in several ways. The bacteria produce enzymes that reduce the efficacy of mucus gel in protecting the gastric mucosa. In addition, the host's inflammatory response to *H. pylori* contributes to gastric epithelial cell damage without producing immunity to the infection. Although the gastric mucosa is the usual site for *H. pylori* infection, this infection also contributes to duodenal ulcers. This is possibly related to increased gastric acid production associated with *H. pylori* infection.

NSAIDs contribute to PUD through both systemic and topical mechanisms. Prostaglandins are necessary for maintaining the gastric mucosal barrier. NSAIDs interrupt prostaglandin synthesis by disrupting the action of the enzyme cyclooxygenase (COX). The two forms of this enzyme are COX-1 and COX-2. The COX-1 enzyme is necessary to maintain the integrity of the gastric mucosa, but the anti-inflammatory effects of NSAIDs are due to their ability to inhibit the COX-2 enzyme. The COX-2 selective NSAIDs are less damaging to the gastric mucosa because they have less effect on the COX-1 enzyme. In addition to their systemic effect, aspirin and many NSAIDs cross the lipid membranes of gastric epithelial cells, damaging the cells themselves.

The ulcers of PUD may affect the esophagus, stomach, or duodenum. They may be superficial or deep, affecting all layers of the mucosa (Figure 21–9 ■). Duodenal ulcers, the most common, usually develop in the proximal portion of the duodenum,

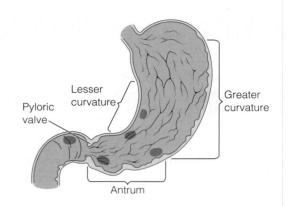

Figure 21–10 ■ Common sites affected by peptic ulcer disease.

close to the pyloris (Figure 21–10 ■). They are sharply demarcated and usually less than 1 cm in diameter (Figure 21–11 ■). Gastric ulcers often are found on the lesser curvature and the area immediately proximal to the pylorus. Gastric ulcers are associated with an increased incidence of gastric cancer.

Peptic ulcer disease may be chronic, with spontaneous remissions and exacerbations. Exacerbations of the disease may be associated with trauma, infection, or other physical or psychologic stressors.

MANIFESTATIONS

Pain is the classic symptom of peptic ulcer disease. The pain is typically described as gnawing, burning, aching, or hungerlike and is experienced in the epigastric region, sometimes radiating to the back. The pain occurs when the stomach is empty (2 to 3 hours after meals and in the middle of the night) and is relieved by eating with a classic "pain-food-relief" pattern. The client may complain of heartburn or regurgitation and may vomit.

The presentation of peptic ulcer disease in the older adult is often less clear, with vague and poorly localized discomfort, perhaps chest pain or dysphagia, weight loss, or anemia. In the older adult, a complication of PUD such as upper GI hemorrhage or perforation of the stomach or duodenum may be the presenting symptom.

Figure 21–9 ■ Erosion and ulcerations of the upper gastrointestinal tract.

Figure 21–11 ■ A superficial peptic ulcer.

Source: SPL/Photo Researchers, Inc.

Manifestations of PUD Complications

HEMORRHAGE

- Occult or obvious blood in the stool
- Hematemesis
- Fatigue
- Weakness, dizziness
- Orthostatic hypotension
- Hypovolemic shock

OBSTRUCTION

- Sensations of epigastric fullness
- Nausea and vomiting
- Electrolyte imbalances
- Metabolic alkalosis

PERFORATION

- Severe upper abdominal pain, radiating to the shoulder
- Rigid, boardlike abdomen
- Absence of bowel sounds
- Diaphoresis
- Tachycardia
- Rapid, shallow respirations
- Fever

Complications

The complications associated with peptic ulcers include hemorrhage, obstruction, and perforation. See the box above for the manifestations of these complications.

Among people with PUD, 10% to 20% experience **hemorrhage** as a result of ulceration and erosion into the blood vessels of the gastric mucosa. In the older adult, bleeding is the most frequent complication. When small blood vessels erode, blood loss may be slow and insidious, with occult blood in the stool the only initial sign. If bleeding continues, the client becomes anemic and experiences symptoms of weakness, fatigue, dizziness, and orthostatic hypotension. Erosion into a larger vessel can lead to sudden and severe bleeding with hematemesis, melena, or **hematochezia** (blood in the stool), and signs of hypovolemic shock.

Gastric outlet obstruction may result from edema surrounding the ulcer, smooth muscle spasm, or scar tissue. Generally, obstruction is a gradual rather than an acute process. Symptoms include a feeling of epigastric fullness, accentuated ulcer symptoms, and nausea. If the obstruction becomes complete, vomiting occurs. Hydrochloric acid, sodium, and potassium are lost in vomitus, potentially leading to fluid and electrolyte imbalance and metabolic alkalosis.

The most lethal complication of PUD is **perforation** of the ulcer through the mucosal wall. When perforation occurs, gastric or duodenal contents enter the peritoneum, causing an inflammatory process and peritonitis. Chemical peritonitis from the hydrochloric acid, pepsin, bile, and pancreatic fluid is immediate; bacterial peritonitis follows within 6 to 12 hours from gastric contaminants entering the normally sterile peritoneal cavity. When an ulcer perforates, the client has immediate, severe upper abdominal pain, radiating throughout the abdomen and possibly to the shoulder. The abdomen becomes rigid and boardlike, with absent bowel sounds. Signs of shock may be present, including diaphoresis, tachycardia, and rapid, shallow respirations. Classic symptoms of perforation may not be present in an older adult. The older adult may instead present with mental confusion and other nonspecific symptoms. This atypical presentation can lead to delays in diagnosis and treatment, increasing the associated mortality rate.

Zollinger-Ellison Syndrome

Zollinger-Ellison syndrome is peptic ulcer disease caused by a gastrinoma, or gastrin-secreting tumor of the pancreas, stomach, or intestines. Gastrinomas may be benign, although 50% to 70% are malignant tumors. Gastrin is a hormone that stimulates the secretion of pepsin and hydrochloric acid. The increased gastrin levels associated with these tumors result in hypersecretion of gastric acid, which in turn causes mucosal ulceration.

The peptic ulcers of Zollinger-Ellison syndrome may affect any portion of the stomach or duodenum, as well as the esophagus or jejunum. Characteristic ulcerlike pain is common. The high levels of hydrochloric acid entering the duodenum may also cause diarrhea and **steatorrhea** (excess fat in the feces), from impaired fat digestion and absorption. Complications of bleeding and perforation are often seen with Zollinger-Ellison syndrome. Fluid and electrolyte imbalances may also result from persistent diarrhea with resultant losses of potassium and sodium in particular.

COLLABORATIVE CARE

Treatment for PUD focuses on eradicating *H. pylori* infection and treating or preventing ulcers related to use of NSAIDs.

Diagnostic Tests

- *Upper GI series* using barium as a contrast medium can detect 80% to 90% of peptic ulcers. It commonly is the diagnostic procedure chosen first; it is less costly and less invasive than gastroscopy. Small or very superficial ulcers may be missed, however.
- *Gastroscopy* allows visualization of the esophageal, gastric, and duodenal mucosa and direct inspection of ulcers. Tissue also can be obtained for biopsy. Nursing care of the client undergoing a gastroscopy is outlined in the box on page 548.
- Biopsy specimens obtained during a gastroscopy can be tested for the presence of *H. pylori* using several different methods. In the *biopsy urease test*, the specimen is put into a gel containing urea. If *H. pylori* is present, the urease that it produces changes the color of the gel, often within minutes. Biopsy specimen cells also can be microscopically examined or cultured for evidence of *H. pylori*.
- Noninvasive methods of detecting *H. pylori* infection include *serologic testing* (to detect IgG antibodies through ELISA) and the *urea breath test*. In this test, radiolabeled urea is given orally. The urease produced by *H. pylori* bacteria converts the urea to ammonia and radiolabeled carbon dioxide, which can then be measured as the client exhales. This test also can be used to evaluate the effectiveness of treatment to eradicate *H. pylori*.

- If Zollinger-Ellison syndrome is suspected, *gastric analysis* may be performed to evaluate gastric acid secretion. Stomach contents are aspirated through a nasogastric tube and analyzed. In Zollinger-Ellison syndrome, gastric acid levels are very high.

Medications

The medications used to treat PUD include agents to eradicate *H. pylori*, drugs to decrease gastric acid content, and agents that protect the mucosa. Nursing responsibilities related to selected drugs to treat GERD, gastritis, and PUD are found in the Medication Administration box on pages 549–550.

Eradication of *H. pylori* is often difficult. Combination therapies that use two antibiotics with either bismuth or proton-pump inhibitors (e.g., a combination of omeprazole, metronidazole, and clarithromycin or bismuth subsalicylate, tetracycline, and metronidazole) are necessary. With complete eradication of *H. pylori*, reinfection rates are less than 0.5% per year.

In clients who have NSAID-induced ulcers, the NSAID in use should be discontinued if at all possible. If this is not possible, twice-daily PPIs enable ulcer healing.

Medications that decrease gastric acid content include proton-pump inhibitors and the H_2-receptor antagonists.

- Proton pump inhibitors bind the acid-secreting enzyme (H^+, K^+ ATPase) that functions as the proton pump, disabling it for up to 24 hours. These drugs are very effective, resulting in over 90% ulcer healing after 4 weeks. Compared to the H_2-receptor blockers, the proton-pump inhibitors provide faster pain relief and more rapid ulcer healing.
- Histamine$_2$-receptor blockers inhibit histamine binding to the receptors on the gastric parietal cells to reduce acid secretion. These drugs are very well tolerated and have few serious side effects; however, drug interactions can occur. These drugs must be continued for 8 weeks or longer for ulcer healing.

Agents that protect the mucosa include sucralfate, bismuth, antacids, and prostaglandin analogs.

- Sucralfate binds to proteins in the ulcer base, forming a protective barrier against acid, bile, and pepsin. Sucralfate also stimulates the secretion of mucus, bicarbonate, and prostaglandin.
- Bismuth compounds (Pepto-Bismol) stimulate mucosal bicarbonate and prostaglandin production to promote ulcer healing. In addition, bismuth has an antibacterial action against *H. pylori*. There are very few side effects, other than a harmless darkening of stools.
- Prostaglandin analogs (misoprostol) promote ulcer healing by stimulating mucus and bicarbonate secretions and by inhibiting acid secretion. Although not as effective as the other drugs discussed, misoprostol is used to prevent NSAID-induced ulcers.
- Antacids stimulate gastric mucosal defenses, thereby aiding in ulcer healing. They provide rapid relief of ulcer symptoms, and are often used as needed to supplement other antiulcer medications. Antacids are inexpensive, but clients often have difficulty with a regular regimen because the drugs must be taken frequently and may cause either constipation (from the

aluminum-type antacids) or diarrhea (from the magnesium-based antacids). Antacids also interfere with the absorption of iron, digoxin, some antibiotics, and other drugs.

Treatments

Dietary Management

In addition to pharmacologic treatment, clients are encouraged to maintain good nutrition, consuming balanced meals at regular intervals. It is important to teach clients that bland or restrictive diets are no longer necessary. Mild alcohol intake is not harmful. Smoking should be discouraged, as it slows the rate of healing and increases the frequency of relapses.

Surgery

The identification of *H. pylori* as a cause of PUD and the availability of drugs to treat the infection and heal peptic ulcers has all but eliminated surgery as a treatment option for peptic ulcer disease. Older clients, however, may have undergone gastric resection surgery for PUD, and may have long-term complications related to the surgery. See the section on gastric cancer for more information about gastric surgery and its potential complications.

Treatment of Complications

The client hospitalized with a complication of PUD such as bleeding, gastrointestinal obstruction, or perforation and peritonitis requires additional interventions to restore homeostasis.

In hemorrhage associated with PUD, initial interventions focus on restoring and maintaining circulation. Normal saline, lactated Ringer's, or other balanced electrolyte solutions are administered intravenously to restore intravascular volume if signs of shock (tachycardia, hypotension, pallor, low urine output, and anxiety) are present. Whole blood or packed red blood cells may be administered to restore hemoglobin and hematocrit levels.

Gastroscopy with direct injection of a clotting or sclerosing agent into the bleeding vessel may be performed. Laser photocoagulation, using light energy, or electrocoagulation, which uses electric current to generate heat, can also be done via gastroscopy to seal bleeding vessels.

The client is kept NPO until bleeding is controlled. Antacids are administered hourly via the nasogastric tube to protect the bleeding ulcer from gastric acid and to prevent acid reflux. H_2-receptor blockers such as cimetidine, ranitidine, and famotidine are administered intravenously until the client can resume oral intake. Surgery may be necessary if medical measures are ineffective in controlling bleeding. Older adults who experience bleeding as a complication of PUD are more likely to rebleed or require surgery to control the hemorrhage. See page 568 for nursing care of the client having gastric surgery.

Repeated inflammation, healing, scarring, edema, and muscle spasm can lead to gastric outlet (pyloric) obstruction. Initial treatment includes gastric decompression with nasogastric suction and administration of intravenous normal saline and potassium chloride to correct fluid and electrolyte imbalance. H_2-receptor blockers are given intravenously as well. Balloon dilation of the gastric outlet may be done via upper endoscopy. If these measures are unsuccessful in relieving obstruction, surgery may be required.

Gastric or duodenal perforation resulting in contamination of the peritoneum with gastrointestinal contents often requires immediate intervention to restore homeostasis and minimize peritonitis. Intravenous fluids maintain fluid and electrolyte balance. Nasogastric suction removes gastric contents and minimizes peritoneal contamination. Placing the client in Fowler's or semi-Fowler's position allows peritoneal contaminants to pool in the pelvis. Intravenous antibiotics aggressively treat bacterial infection from intestinal flora. Laparoscopic surgery or an open laparotomy may close the perforation.

NURSING CARE

Health Promotion

Although it is difficult to predict which clients will develop peptic ulcer disease, promote health by advising clients to avoid risk factors such as excessive aspirin or NSAID use and cigarette smoking. In addition, encourage clients to seek treatment for manifestations of gastroesophageal reflux disease (GERD) or chronic gastritis, both of which also are associated with *H. pylori* infection.

Assessment

Collect the following subjective and objective data when assessing the client with peptic ulcer disease.

- Health history: complaints of epigastric or left upper quadrant pain, heartburn, or discomfort; its character, severity, timing and relationship to eating, measures used for relief; nausea or vomiting, presence of bright blood or "coffee-ground" appearing material in vomitus; current medications including use of aspirin or other NSAIDs; cigarette smoking and use of alcohol or other drugs
- Physical examination: general appearance including height and weight relationship; vital signs including orthostatic measurements; abdominal examination including shape and contour, bowel sounds, and tenderness to palpation; presence of obvious or occult blood in vomitus and stool

Nursing Diagnoses and Interventions

Pain

The pain of peptic ulcer disease is often predictable and preventable. Pain is typically experienced 2 to 4 hours after eating, as high levels of gastric acid and pepsin irritate the exposed mucosa. Measures to neutralize the acid, minimize its production, or protect the mucosa often relieve this pain, minimizing the need for analgesics.

- Assess pain, including location, type, severity, frequency, and duration, and its relationship to food intake or other contributing factors.

PRACTICE ALERT *Avoid making assumptions about pain. Acute pain may indicate a complication, such as perforation (often heralded by sudden, severe epigastric pain and a rigid, boardlike abdomen) or it may be totally unrelated to PUD (e.g., angina, gallbladder disease, or pancreatitis).* ∎

- Administer proton-pump inhibitors, H$_2$-receptor antagonists, antacids, or mucosal protective agents as ordered. Monitor for effectiveness and side effects or adverse reactions. *The pain associated with PUD is generally caused by the effect of gastric juices on exposed mucosal tissue. These medications reduce pain and promote healing by reducing acid production, neutralizing acid, or providing a barrier for the damaged mucosa.*
- Teach relaxation, stress-reduction, and lifestyle management techniques. Refer for stress management counseling or classes as indicated. *Although there is no clear relationship between stress and PUD, measures to relieve stress and promote physical and emotional rest help reduce the perception of pain and may reduce ulcer genesis.*

Sleep Pattern Disturbance

Nighttime ulcer pain, which typically occurs between 1:00 and 3:00 A.M., may disrupt the sleep cycle and result in inadequate rest. Anticipation of pain may lead to insomnia or other sleep disruptions.

- Stress the importance of taking medications as prescribed. *The bedtime dose of proton-pump inhibitor or H$_2$-receptor blocker minimizes hydrochloric acid production during the night, reducing nighttime pain.*
- Instruct to limit food intake after the evening meal, eliminating any bedtime snack. *Eating before bed can stimulate the production of gastric acid and pepsin, increasing the likelihood of nighttime pain.*
- Encourage use of relaxation techniques and comfort measures such as soft music as needed to promote sleep. *Once the pain associated with PUD has been controlled, these measures help reduce anxiety and reestablish a normal sleep pattern.*

Imbalanced Nutrition: Less Than Body Requirements

In an attempt to avoid discomfort, the client with peptic ulcer disease may gradually reduce food intake, sometimes jeopardizing nutritional status. Anorexia and early satiety are additional problems associated with PUD.

- Assess current diet, including pattern of food intake, eating schedule, and foods that precipitate pain or are being avoided in anticipation of pain. *The client may not realize the extent of self-imposed dietary limitations, especially if symptoms have persisted for an extended time. Assessment increases awareness and also helps identify the adequacy of nutrient intake.*
- Refer to a dietitian for meal planning to minimize PUD symptoms and meet nutritional needs. Consider normal eating patterns and preferences in meal planning. *Although no specific diet is recommended for PUD, clients should avoid foods that increase pain. Six small meals per day often help increase food tolerance and decrease postprandial discomfort.*
- Monitor for complaints of anorexia, fullness, nausea, and vomiting. Adjust dietary intake or medication schedule as indicated. *PUD and resultant scarring can lead to impaired gastric emptying, necessitating a treatment change.*

PRACTICE ALERT *Advise the client to report increasing or persistent symptoms of anorexia, nausea and vomiting, or fullness to the care provider. ■*

- Monitor laboratory values for indications of anemia or other nutritional deficits. Monitor for therapeutic and side effects of treatment measures such as oral iron replacement. Instruct the client taking oral iron replacement to avoid using an antacid within 1 to 2 hours of taking the iron preparation. *Anemia can result from poor nutrient absorption or chronic blood loss in clients with PUD. Oral iron supplements may cause GI distress, nausea, and vomiting; if these side effects are intolerable, notify the physician for a possible change of therapy. Antacids bind with oral iron preparations, blocking absorption.*

Deficient Fluid Volume

Erosion of a blood vessel with resultant hemorrhage is a significant risk for the client with peptic ulcer disease. Acute bleeding can lead to hypovolemia and fluid volume deficit, which can lead to a decrease in cardiac output and impaired tissue perfusion.

PRACTICE ALERT *Monitor and record blood pressure and apical pulse every 15 to 30 minutes until stable; monitor central venous pressure or pulmonary artery pressure as indicated. Insert a Foley catheter and monitor urinary output hourly. Weigh daily. Continuous monitoring of cardiac output parameters is essential in clients with an acute hemorrhage to identify possible shock and intervene at an early stage. ■*

- Monitor stools and gastric drainage for overt and occult blood. Assess gastric drainage (vomitus or from a nasogastric tube) to estimate the amount and rapidity of hemorrhage. *Drainage is bright red with possible clots in acute hemorrhage; dark red or the color of coffee grounds when blood has been in the stomach for a period of time. Hematochezia (stool containing red blood and clots) is present in acute hemorrhage; melena (black, tarry stool) is an indicator of less acute bleeding. When small vessels are disrupted, bleeding may be slow and not overtly evident. With chronic or slow gastrointestinal bleeding, the risk of a fluid volume deficit is minimal; anemia and activity intolerance are more likely.*
- Maintain intravenous therapy with fluid volume and electrolyte replacement solutions; administer whole blood or packed cells as ordered. *Both fluids and electrolytes are lost through vomiting, nasogastric drainage, and diarrhea in an episode of acute bleeding. To prevent shock, it is essential to maintain a blood volume and cardiac output sufficient to perfuse body tissues. Whole blood and packed cells replace both blood volume and red blood cells, providing additional oxygen-carrying capacity to meet cell needs.*
- Insert a nasogastric tube and maintain its position and patency; if ordered, irrigate with sterile normal saline until returns are clear. Initially, measure and record gastric output every hour (be sure to subtract the volume of irrigant), then every 4 to 8 hours. *Nasogastric suction removes blood from*

the gastrointestinal tract, preventing vomiting and possible aspiration. Irrigation with sterile saline solution at room temperature has a vasoconstrictive effect, slowing active bleeding. Water is not used as an irrigant to avoid water intoxication. Sterile solution is used because of the possibility of perforation. Gastric output is replaced milliliter for milliliter with a balanced electrolyte solution to maintain homeostasis.

- Monitor hemoglobin and hematocrit, serum electrolytes, BUN, and creatinine values. Report abnormal findings. *Hemoglobin and hematocrit are lower than normal with acute or chronic GI bleeding. In acute hemorrhage, initial results may be within normal range because both cells and plasma are lost. Loss of fluids and electrolytes with gastric drainage and diarrhea will alter normal levels. Digestion and absorption of blood in the GI tract may result in elevated BUN and creatinine levels.*
- Assess abdomen, including bowel sounds, distention, girth, and tenderness every 4 hours and record findings. *Borborygmi or hyperactive bowel sounds with abdominal tenderness are common with acute GI bleeding. Increased distention, increasing abdominal girth, absent bowel sounds, or extreme tenderness with a rigid, boardlike abdomen may indicate perforation.*
- Maintain bed rest with the head of the bed elevated. Ensure safety. *Loss of blood volume may cause orthostatic hypotension with resultant syncope or dizziness upon standing.*

Using NANDA, NIC, and NOC

Chart 21–4 shows links between NANDA nursing diagnoses, NIC, and NOC when caring for a client with peptic ulcer disease (see page 559).

Home Care

Peptic ulcer disease is managed in home and community-based settings; only its complications typically require treatment in an acute care setting. Provide the following information when preparing the client for home care.

- Prescribed medication regimen, including desired and potential adverse effects
- Importance of continuing therapy even when symptoms are relieved
- Relationship between peptic ulcers and factors such as NSAID use and smoking. If indicated, refer to a smoking-cessation clinic or program.
- Importance of avoiding aspirin and other NSAIDs; stress the necessity of reading the labels of over-the-counter medications for possible aspirin content
- Manifestations of complications that should be reported to the care provider, including increased abdominal pain or distention, vomiting, black or tarry stools, lightheadedness, or fainting
- Stress and lifestyle management techniques that may help prevent exacerbation. Refer to resources for stress management, such as classes, counseling, and formal or informal groups.

Nursing Care Plan
A Client with Peptic Ulcer Disease

Sean O'Donnell is a 47-year-old police officer who lives and works in a metropolitan area. Mr. O'Donnell has had "heartburn" and abdominal discomfort for years, but thought it went along with his job. Last year, after becoming weak, lightheaded, and short of breath, he was found to be anemic and was diagnosed as having a duodenal ulcer. He took omeprazole (Prilosec) and ferrous sulfate for 3 months before stopping both, saying he had "never felt better in his life." Mr. O'Donnell has now been admitted to the hospital with active upper GI bleeding.

ASSESSMENT

Rachel Clark is Mr. O'Donnell's admitting nurse and case manager. On initial assessment, Mr. O'Donnell is alert and oriented, though very apprehensive about his condition. Skin pale and cool; BP 136/78, P 98; abdomen distended and tender with hyperactive bowel sounds; 200 mL bright red blood obtained on nasogastric tube insertion. Hemoglobin 8.2 g/dL and hematocrit 23% on admission. Mr. O'Donnell is taken to the endoscopy lab where his bleeding is controlled using laser photocoagulation. On his return to the nursing unit, he receives two units of packed red blood cells and intravenous fluids to restore blood volume. A 5-day course of high-dose oral omeprazole (40 mg bid) is ordered to prevent rebleeding, and Mr. O'Donnell is allowed to begin a clear liquid diet 24 hours after his endoscopy. Tissue biopsy obtained during endoscopy confirms the presence of H. pylori infection.

DIAGNOSES

- *Deficient fluid volume* related to acute bleeding duodenal ulcer
- *Risk for injury* related to acute blood loss
- *Fear* related to threat to well-being
- *Ineffective therapeutic regimen management* related to lack of knowledge regarding PUD and its treatment

EXPECTED OUTCOMES

- Maintains normal blood pressure, pulse, and urine output (>30 mL/hr).
- Remains free of injury.
- Seeks information to reduce fear.
- Identifies and uses coping strategies to manage fear.
- Describes prescribed therapeutic regimen.
- Verbalizes ability to manage prescribed regimen.

PLANNING AND IMPLEMENTATION

- Place call light within reach and encourage to ask for help when getting up or ambulating. Remind to rise slowly from lying to sitting and sitting to standing.
- Discuss situation and provide information about all procedures and treatments.
- Reassure about the effectiveness of treatment in reducing the risk for further bleeding.
- Discuss current and planned treatment measures; stress the importance of completing the prescribed treatment to reduce the risk of further ulcer development.
- Encourage to avoid using aspirin or NSAIDs in the future; suggest alternative medications such as acetaminophen.
- Discuss stress reduction techniques and refer for stress reduction counseling or workshops as indicated.

EVALUATION

Mr. O'Donnell is discharged 48 hours after admission. He has had no further evidence of bleeding, and has resumed a regular diet. His hemoglobin and hematocrit remain low, and he has a prescription for ferrous sulfate. He will complete the prescribed high-dose omeprazole regimen at home, then begin treatment with omeprazole, amoxicillin, and clarithromycin (Biaxin) to eradicate the H. pylori infection detected during endoscopy. After 2 weeks of this regimen, he will continue taking omeprazole at bedtime for 4 to 8 weeks. He verbalizes a good understanding of his treatment and the importance of completing the entire regimen. Mr. O'Donnell expresses concern about his ability to "keep his cool on the inside" when under stress. Ms. Clark, his case manager, gives him the names of several resources to help with stress management in case he wants help.

Critical Thinking in the Nursing Process

1. How does H. pylori infection contribute to the development of peptic ulcers?
2. Describe the physiologic responses to fear and anxiety. Why is it important to alleviate fear and its physical consequences in clients with PUD?
3. What suggestions can you make to help Mr. O'Donnell manage his complex treatment regimen over the next 3 months?
4. Develop a teaching plan that includes stress reduction techniques Mr. O'Donnell can use while performing his duties as a police officer.

See Evaluating Your Response in Appendix C.

THE CLIENT WITH CANCER OF THE STOMACH

Worldwide, cancer of the stomach is the most common cancer (other than skin cancer); but it is less common in the United States, with an estimated 21,500 new cases annually. The incidence of gastric cancer is highest in Hispanics, African Americans, and Asian Americans, with men affected twice as often as women. Older adults are more likely to develop gastric cancer: The mean age at time of diagnosis is 63. People in lower socioeconomic groups are more often affected by gastric cancer.

Risk Factors

H. pylori infection is a major risk factor for cancer of the distal portion of the stomach; from 35% to 89% of cases can be attributed to this infection. Other risk factors are a genetic predisposition, chronic gastritis, pernicious anemia, gastric polyps, and carcinogenic factors in the diet (such as smoked foods and nitrates). Achlorhydria, a lack of hydrochloric acid in the stomach, is a known risk factor. The risk for gastric cancer also is increased in people who have had a partial gastric resection.

PATHOPHYSIOLOGY

Adenocarcinoma, which involves the mucus-producing cells of the stomach, is the most common form of gastric cancer. These carcinomas may arise anywhere on the mucosal surface of the stomach but are most frequently found in the distal portion. Half of all gastric cancers occur in the antrum or pyloric region (Porth, 2002). Gastric cancer begins as a localized lesion (in situ), then progresses to involve the mucosa or submucosa (early gastric carcinoma). Lesions may spread by direct extension to tissues surrounding the stomach, the liver in particular. The lesion may ulcerate or appear as a polypoid (polyplike) mass (Figure 21–12 ■). Lymph node involvement and metastasis occur early due to the rich blood and lymphatic supply to the stomach. Metastatic lesions are often found in the liver, lungs, ovaries, and peritoneum.

MANIFESTATIONS

Few symptoms are associated with gastric cancer. Unfortunately, the disease is often quite advanced and metastases are usually present at the time of diagnosis. Early symptoms are vague, including feelings of early satiety, anorexia, indigestion, and possibly vomiting. The client may experience ulcerlike pain unrelieved by antacids, typically occurring after meals. As the disease progresses, weight loss occurs, and the client may be **cachectic** (in very poor health and malnourished) at the time of diagnosis. An abdominal mass may be palpable, and occult blood may be present in the stool, indicating gastrointestinal bleeding.

COLLABORATIVE CARE

Diagnostic Tests

Anemia detected by a CBC often is the first indication of gastric cancer. An upper GI X-ray with barium swallow is useful to identify lesions, and ultrasound or other radiologic techniques may identify a mass. Upper endoscopy with visualization and biopsy of the lesion provides the definitive diagnosis.

Surgery

When gastric cancer is identified prior to the development of metastasis, surgical removal of part or all of the stomach and regional lymph nodes is the treatment of choice. **Partial gastrectomy** involves removal of a portion of the stomach, usually the distal half to two-thirds. In partial gastrectomy, the surgeon constructs an anastamosis from the remainder of the stomach directly to the duodenum or to the proximal jejunum. The **gastroduodenostomy,** or **Billroth I,** and the **gastrojejunostomy,** or **Billroth II,** are commonly used partial gastrectomy procedures (Figure 21–13 ■ A and B).

Early Gastric Cancer

- Mucosa
- Muscularis mucosa
- Submucosa
- Muscularis
- Lymph node
- Serosa

Polypoid Carcinoma

- Lymph node metastasis

Ulcerating Carcinoma

Figure 21–12 ■ The spread and forms (polypoid and ulcerating) of gastric cancer.

A **total gastrectomy,** removal of the entire stomach, may be done for diffuse cancer that is spread throughout the gastric mucosa but limited to the stomach. In a total gastrectomy, the surgeon constructs an anastamosis from the esophagus to the duodenum or jejunum. Total gastrectomy with **esophago-jejunostomy** is illustrated in Figure 21–13C.

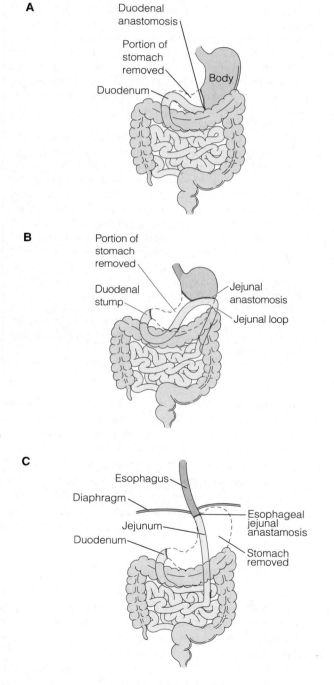

Figure 21-13 ■ Partial and total gastrectomy procedures. *A,* Partial gastrectomy with anastomosis to the duodenum. *B,* Partial gastrectomy with anastomosis to the jejunum. *C,* Total gastrectomy with anastomosis of the esophagus to the jejunum.

Nursing care of the client who has undergone gastric surgery is outlined in the box on page 568.

Complications

Several long-term complications may develop following gastrectomy procedures. **Dumping syndrome** is the most common problem. It may follow a partial gastrectomy with duodenal or jejunal anastamosis. When the pylorus has been resected or bypassed, a hypertonic, undigested food bolus may rapidly enter the duodenum or jejunum. Water is pulled into the lumen of the intestine by the hyperosmolar character of the chyme, resulting in decreased blood volume and intestinal dilation. Peristalsis is stimulated, and intestinal motility is increased.

Early symptoms of dumping syndrome occur within 5 to 30 minutes after eating. These symptoms result from intestinal dilation, peristaltic stimulation, and hypovolemia caused by undigested food in the proximal small intestine. Manifestations include nausea with possible vomiting, epigastric pain with cramping and borborygmi (loud, hyperactive bowel sounds), and diarrhea. Systemic symptoms from the hypovolemia and reflex sympathetic stimulation include tachycardia, orthostatic hypotension, dizziness, flushing, and diaphoresis.

The entry of hyperosmolar chyme into the jejunum also causes a rapid rise in the blood glucose. This stimulates the release of an excessive amount of insulin, leading to hypoglycemic symptoms 2 to 3 hours after the meal. The pathogenesis and clinical manifestations of dumping syndrome are represented in Figure 21–14 ■. Dumping syndrome is typically self-limiting,

Figure 21–14 ■ The pathogenesis and manifestations of dumping syndrome.

NURSING CARE OF THE CLIENT HAVING GASTRIC SURGERY

PREOPERATIVE NURSING CARE

- See Chapter 7 for routine preoperative care and teaching.
- Insert a nasogastric tube if ordered preoperatively. *Although it is often inserted in the surgical suite just prior to surgery, the nasogastric tube may be placed preoperatively to remove secretions and empty stomach contents.*

POSTOPERATIVE NURSING CARE

- Provide routine care for the surgical client as outlined in Chapter 7.
- Assess position and patency of nasogastric tube, connecting it to low suction. Gently irrigate with sterile normal saline if tube becomes clogged. *The nasogastric tube will be placed in surgery to avoid disruption of the gastric suture lines and should be well secured. If repositioning or tube replacement is needed, notify the surgeon. Patency must be maintained to keep the stomach decompressed, reducing pressure on sutures.*
- Assess color, amount, and odor of gastric drainage, noting any changes in these parameters or the presence of clots or bright bleeding. *Initial drainage is bright red. It becomes dark, then clear or greenish-yellow over the first 2 to 3 days. A change in the color, amount, or odor may indicate a complication such as hemorrhage, intestinal obstruction, or infection.*
- Maintain intravenous fluids while nasogastric suction is in place. *The client on nasogastric suction is not only unable to take oral food and fluids but also is losing electrolyte-rich fluid through the nasogastric tube. If replacement fluid and electrolytes are not maintained, the client is at risk for dehydration imbalances of sodium, potassium, and chloride; and metabolic alkalosis.*

- Provide antiulcer and antibiotic therapy as ordered. *These medications may be ordered for the postoperative client, depending on the procedure performed. Antibiotic therapy is a common preventive measure for infection that may result from contamination of the abdominal cavity with gastric contents.*
- Monitor bowel sounds and abdominal distention. *Bowel sounds indicate resumption of peristalsis. Increasing distention may indicate third-spacing, obstruction or infection.*
- Resume oral food and fluids as ordered. Initial feedings are clear liquids, progressing to full liquids and then frequent small feedings of regular foods. Monitor bowel sounds and for abdominal distention frequently during this period. *Oral feedings are reintroduced slowly to minimize trauma to the suture lines by possible gastric distension.*
- Encourage ambulation. *Ambulation stimulates peristalsis.*
- Begin discharge planning and teaching. Consult with a dietitian for diet instructions and menu planning; reinforce teaching. Teach the client about potential postoperative complications, such as abdominal abscess, dumping syndrome, postprandial hypoglycemia, or pernicious anemia. Also, teach the client to recognize signs and symptoms and preventive measures. *The client's gastric capacity is reduced after partial gastrectomy, necessitating a corresponding reduction in meal size. Changes in gastric emptying and reduction in gastric secretions may change the client's tolerance for many foods, requiring slow reintroduction of these foods. Dumping syndrome, postprandial hypoglycemia, and pernicious anemia are possible long-term complications of partial gastrectomy. For most clients, dietary modifications can control both dumping syndrome and postprandial hypoglycemia.*

---

lasting 6 to 12 months after surgery; however, a small percentage of people continue to experience long-term symptoms.

Dumping syndrome is managed primarily by a dietary pattern that delays gastric emptying and allows smaller boluses of undigested food to enter the intestine. Meals should be small and more frequent. Liquids and solids are taken at separate times instead of together during a meal. The amount of proteins and fats in the diet is increased, because they exit the stomach more slowly than carbohydrates. Carbohydrates, especially simple sugars, are reduced. The client is instructed to rest in a recumbent or semirecumbent position for 30 to 60 minutes after meals. Anticholinergics, sedatives, and antispasmodics may be prescribed.

Anemia may be a chronic problem after a major gastric resection. Iron is absorbed primarily in the duodenum and proximal jejunum; rapid gastric emptying or a gastrojejunostomy may interfere with adequate absorption.

The cells of the stomach produce intrinsic factor, required for the absorption of vitamin B_{12}. Vitamin B_{12} deficiency leads to pernicious anemia. Because of hepatic stores of vitamin B_{12}, symptoms of anemia may not be seen for 1 to 2 years after surgery. Vitamin B_{12} levels are routinely monitored following extensive gastric resections.

Other nutritional problems seen following surgery include folic acid deficiency and decreased absorption of calcium and vitamin D. Poor absorption of nutrients, combined with the inability to eat large meals, puts the client at risk for weight loss in addition to the more specific nutrient deficiencies. Nearly 50% of clients who have gastric surgery experience significant weight loss, primarily because of insufficient calorie intake. Factors contributing to insufficient intake of calories include early satiety (feeling of fullness), decreased stomach size, and altered emptying patterns.

Other Therapies

Radiation or chemotherapy may be used to eliminate any lymphatic or metastatic spread. For the client with more advanced disease, treatment is palliative and may include surgery and chemotherapy. These clients may require a gastrostomy or jejunostomy feeding tube (Figure 21–15 ■).

See the box on page 569 for nursing care of the client with a gastrostomy or jejunostomy tube.

Because gastric cancer is generally advanced by the time of diagnosis, the prognosis is poor. The 5-year survival rate of all clients treated for gastric carcinoma is 10%.

NURSING CARE OF THE CLIENT WITH A GASTROSTOMY OR JEJUNOSTOMY TUBE

Clients who have had extensive gastric surgery or who require long-term enteral feedings to maintain nutrition may have a gastrostomy or jejunostomy tube inserted.

PROCEDURE

Gastrostomy tubes are surgically placed in the stomach, with the stoma in the epigastric region of the abdomen (see Figure 21–15). Jejunostomy tubes are placed in the proximal jejunum. Immediately following the procedure, the tube may be connected to low suction or plugged. If the client has been receiving tube feedings, these may be reinitiated shortly after tube placement.

NURSING CARE

- Assess tube placement by aspirating stomach contents and checking the pH of aspirate to determine gastric or intestinal placement. A pH of 5 or less indicates gastric placement; the pH is generally 7 or higher with intestinal placement. *Recent studies show auscultation to be ineffective in determining feeding tube placement. Measuring the pH of aspirate from the tube is more reliable as a means of determining tube placement.*
- Inspect the skin surrounding the insertion site for healing, redness, swelling, and the presence of any drainage. If drainage is present, note the color, amount, consistency, and odor. *Changes in the insertion site, drainage, or lack of healing may indicate an infection.*
- Assess the abdomen for distention, bowel sounds, and tenderness *to evaluate functioning of the gastrointestinal tract.*
- Until the stoma is well healed, use sterile technique for dressing changes and site care. Clean technique is appropriate for use once healing is complete. *Sterile technique reduces the risk of wound contamination by pathogens that can lead to infec-*

tion. *Once healing has occurred, clean technique is acceptable because the gastrointestinal tract is not a sterile body cavity.*
- Wearing clean gloves, remove old dressing. Cleanse the site with saline or soap and water, and rinse as appropriate. A well-healed stoma may be cleansed in the shower with the tube clamped or plugged. Pat dry with 4X4 gauze pads, and allow to air dry. Apply Stomadhesive, karaya, or other protective agents around tube as needed to protect the skin. *Gastric acid and other wound drainage is irritating to the skin. Meticulous care is important to maintain the integrity of the skin surrounding the stoma.*
- Redress the wound using a stoma dressing or folded 4X4 gauze pads. *Do not cut gauze pads, because threads may enter the wound, causing irritation and increasing the risk of inflammation.*
- Irrigate the tube with 30 to 50 mL of water, and clean the tube inside and out as indicated or ordered. Soft gastric tubes may require cleaning of the inner lumen with a special brush to maintain patency. *Tube feeding formulas may coat the inside of the gastrostomy tube and eventually cause it to become occluded. Regular irrigation with water and brushing as indicated maintain tube patency.*
- Provide mouth care or remind the client to do so. *When feedings are not being taken orally, the usual stimulus to do mouth care is lost. In addition, salivary fluids may not be as abundant, and oral mucous membranes may become dry and cracked.*
- If indicated, teach the client and family how to care for the tube and feedings. Refer to a home health agency or visiting nurse for support and reinforcement of learning. *Gastrostomy tubes are often in place long term. When the client and family are able to assume care, independence and self-image are enhanced.*

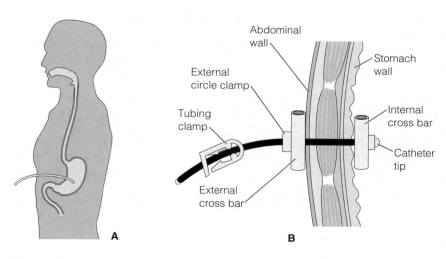

Figure 21–15 ■ Gastrostomy. *A,* Gastrostomy tube placement. *B,* The tube is fixed against both the abdomen and stomach walls by cross bars.

NURSING CARE

Health Promotion

Although the exact causes of gastric cancer are unknown, contributing factors such as *H. pylori* infection and consumption of foods preserved with nitrates have been identified. To reduce their risk of developing gastric cancer, encourage clients with known *H. pylori* infection to complete the prescribed course of treatment and verify that it has eradicated the infection. With all clients, discuss the relationship between gastric cancer and consumption of foods preserved with nitrates (such as bacon and other processed meats), and encourage limited consumption of these products.

Assessment

Assessment data related to gastric cancer include the following:

- Health history: manifestations such as anorexia, early satiety, indigestion, or vomiting; epigastric pain after meals; recent unintentional weight loss
- Physical assessment: general appearance, weight for height; abdominal distention or a palpable upper abdominal mass; occult blood in stool or vomitus

Nursing Diagnoses and Interventions

Imbalanced Nutrition: Less Than Body Requirements

The client with gastric cancer may be malnourished because of anorexia, early satiety, and increased metabolic needs related to the tumor. Extensive gastric resection also makes it difficult to consume an adequate diet. Malnourishment, in turn, impairs healing and the client's ability to tolerate cancer treatment.

- Consult with dietitian for a complete nutrition assessment and diet planning. *The client is at risk for protein-calorie malnutrition, which impairs the ability to heal and recover from extensive surgery.*
- Weigh daily. Monitor laboratory values such as hemoglobin, hematocrit, and serum albumin levels. *Daily weights are a valuable measurement of both fluid and nutritional status. Laboratory values provide further evidence of nutritional status.*
- Provide preferred foods; have family prepare meals when possible. Provide supplemental feedings between meals. *Small, frequent feedings and preferred foods encourage intake of nutrients.*

PRACTICE ALERT *Assess ability to consume adequate nutrients. Nausea and feelings of early satiety may impair nutrient consumption, indicating a need to institute enteral or parenteral feedings.* ∎

- Arrange for visitors to be present during meals. *Eating is a social function as well as a physiologic one. Companionship often improves food intake.*
- Administer pain and antiemetic medications as needed before meals. *Pain and nausea suppress the appetite; relief promotes food intake.*

Anticipatory Grieving

- Encourage family members to spend as much time as possible with the client. *The family may feel helpless and ineffectual. Supporting family members' presence can encourage this vital interaction.*
- Do not negate denial if present. *Denial is a coping mechanism that protects the client from hopelessness.*
- Allow clients to talk openly if desired about their condition and the prognosis. *Acceptance of the client's fears helps reduce anxiety and promote coping behaviors.*
- Actively listen to the client's and family's expressions of grieving. Avoid interrupting or offering meaningless words of consolation. *Being present and active listening are often the most effective interventions for the grieving client.*

Home Care

Although the client with gastric cancer may be hospitalized for surgery, most care is provided in the home and community-based settings such as hospice care. When preparing the client and family for home care, discuss the following topics.

- Care of incision and feeding tube (if present) or central venous line
- Maintaining nutrition and preventing complications of surgery such as dumping syndrome
- Pain management

Provide referrals to home care agencies, hospice, and cancer support groups as appropriate. Provide information about services available through the local chapter of the American Cancer Society.

Nursing Care Plan
A Client with Gastric Cancer

George Harvey is a 61-year-old estate attorney who lives with his wife, Harriet. For the last 3 months, Mr. Harvey has had increasing anorexia and difficulty eating. He has lost 10 pounds. His physician has diagnosed gastric cancer, and Mr. Harvey is admitted for a partial gastrectomy and gastrojejunostomy. The oncologist has recommended postoperative chemotherapy and radiation. Mr. Harvey reports that the doctor told him "that will give me the best chance for cure."

ASSESSMENT

On admission before surgery, Mr. Harvey tells his nurse, Lauren Walsh, that he has eaten very little in the past few weeks. He asks, "What will happen to my wife if something happens to me? I'm afraid this cancer will get me." Mr. Harvey weighs 147 lb (67 kg) and is 72 inches (183 cm) tall. He is pale and thin; his vital signs are BP 148/86, P 92, R 18, and T 97.8° F PO. A firm mass is palpable in the left epigastric region. The rest of his physical assessment data are within normal limits. Mr. Harvey's hemoglobin is 12.8 g/dL, hematocrit is 39%, and serum albumin level is 3.2 g/dL, indicating that he is mildly malnourished. All other preoperative laboratory and diagnostic studies are within normal limits.

DIAGNOSES

- *Imbalanced nutrition: Less than body requirements* related to anorexia and difficulty eating
- *Acute pain* related to surgical incision and manipulation of abdominal organs
- *Risk for ineffective airway clearance* related to upper abdominal surgery
- *Anticipatory grieving* related to recent diagnosis of cancer

EXPECTED OUTCOMES

- Maintain present weight during hospitalization.
- Resume a high-calorie, high-protein diet by time of discharge.
- Verbalize effective pain management, maintaining a reported pain level of 3 or less on a scale of 1 to 10.
- Maintain a patent airway and clear breath sounds.
- Verbalize feelings regarding diagnosis and participate in decision making.

PLANNING AND IMPLEMENTATION

- Weigh daily.
- Maintain nasogastric tube placement, patency, and suction as ordered.
- Maintain intravenous fluids and total parenteral nutrition as ordered until oral food intake is resumed.
- Arrange for diet teaching, including strategies to prevent dumping syndrome, before discharge.
- Maintain patient-controlled analgesia (PCA) until able to take oral analgesics.
- Assess respiratory status including rate, depth, and breath sounds every hour initially, then every 4 hours.
- Assist to cough, deep breathe, and use inspirometer every 2 to 4 hours and as needed. Splint abdomen during coughing.
- Encourage verbalization of feelings about diagnosis and perceived losses.
- Encourage participation in decision making.

EVALUATION

Mr. Harvey's weight remained stable through his hospitalization. On discharge he is taking a high-protein, high-calorie diet in six small feedings per day. He and his wife have reviewed his diet with the dietitian and are planning on using some dietary supplements at home to meet protein needs. He verbalizes an understanding of measures to prevent dumping syndrome, including separating his intake of solid foods and liquids. Mr. Harvey is using oral analgesics in the morning and at bedtime to control his pain. He and his wife have begun to discuss the meaning of his diagnosis. Mrs. Harvey tells the discharge nurse, "We are going to a support group called 'Coping with Cancer' when George is stronger."

Critical Thinking in the Nursing Process

1. What is the rationale for maintaining nasogastric suction after gastrojejunostomy?
2. Develop a preoperative teaching plan for a client undergoing an partial gastrectomy.
3. Mr. Harvey calls you just before the initial dose of chemotherapy and says, "Everyone tells me that chemotherapy will cause vomiting, and I don't think I can take being sick again." How would you respond?
4. Design interventions to ensure adequate nutrition for people with advanced gastric cancer.

See Evaluating Your Response in Appendix C.

EXPLORE MediaLink

NCLEX review questions, case studies, care plan activities, MediaLink applications, and other interactive resources for this chapter can be found on the Companion Website at www.prenhall.com/lemone.

Click on Chapter 21 to select the activities for this chapter. For animations, video clips, more NCLEX review questions, and an audio glossary, access the Student CD-ROM accompanying this textbook.

TEST YOURSELF

1. The nurse assessing for oral cancer risk factors in a client with a persistent sore on his tongue asks about:

   a. Consumption of highly spiced foods
   b. Thumb sucking or pacifier use as a child
   c. Regular use of dental floss
   d. Tobacco use in any form

2. The nurse teaching a client with gastroesophageal reflux disease includes which of the following instructions?

   a. This is a benign disease requiring no treatment
   b. Elevate the head of the bed on 6- to 8-inch blocks
   c. Take antacids or H_2-receptor blockers only when symptoms are severe
   d. Surgery frequently is required to relieve manifestations of the disease

3. The nurse evaluates his teaching of a client with acute stress gastritis as effective when the client states that she will:

   a. Avoid using aspirin or NSAIDs for routine pain relief
   b. Consume only bland foods
   c. Return for yearly upper endoscopy exams
   d. Fully cook all meats, poultry, and egg products

4. The nurse identifies which of the following nursing diagnoses as highest priority for the client admitted with peptic ulcer disease and possible perforation:

   a. *Acute pain*
   b. *Ineffective health maintenance*
   c. *Nausea*
   d. *Impaired tissue integrity: Gastrointestinal*

5. Following a partial gastrectomy for gastric cancer, a client complains of nausea, abdominal pain and cramping, and diarrhea after eating. Recognizing manifestations of dumping syndrome, the nurse recommends:

   a. Fasting for a period of 6 to 12 hours before meals
   b. Decreasing the protein content of meals
   c. Frequent small meals that contain solid foods or liquids, but not both
   d. A diet rich in carbohydrates to maintain blood glucose levels

See Test Yourself answers in Appendix C.

BIBLIOGRAPHY

Ackley, B.J., & Ladwig, G. B. (2002). *Nursing diagnosis handbook: A guide to planning care* (5th ed.). St. Louis: Mosby.

Ahya, S. N., Flood, K., & Paranjothi, S. (Eds.). (2001). *The Washington manual of medical therapeutics* (30th ed.). Philadelphia: Lippincott Williams & Wilkins.

Braunwald, E., Fauci, A. S., Kasper, D. L., Hauser, S. L., Longo, D. L., & Jameson, J. L. (2001). *Harrison's principles of internal medicine* (15th ed.). New York: McGraw-Hill.

Brooks-Brunn, J. A. (2000). Esophageal cancer: An overview. *MEDSURG Nursing, 9*(5), 248–254.

Bullock, B. A., & Henze, R. L. (2000). *Focus on pathophysiology*. Philadelphia: Lippincott.

Chait, M. M. (2000). The many complications of gastroesophageal reflux disease. *Home Health Care Consultant, 7*(1), 25–27.

Edwards, S. J., & Metheny, N. A. (2000). Measurement of gastric residual volume: State of the science. *MEDSURG Nursing, 9*(3), 125–128.

Gallo, J. J., Busby-Whitehead, J., Rabins, P. V., Silliman, R. A., & Murphy, J. B. (Eds.). (1999). *Reichel's care of the elderly: Clinical aspects of aging* (5th ed.). Philadelphia: Lippincott Williams & Wilkins.

Galvin, T. J. (2001). Dysphagia: Going down and staying down. *American Journal of Nursing, 101*(1), 37–42.

Johnson, M., Bulechek, G., Dochterman, J. M., Maas, M., & Moorhead, S. (2001). *Nursing diagnoses, outcomes, & interventions*. St. Louis: Mosby.

Malarkey, L. M., & McMorrow, M. E. (2000). *Nurse's manual of laboratory tests and diagnostic procedures* (2nd ed.). Philadelphia: Saunders.

Mattonen, M. C. (2001). Managing heartburn in adults. *MEDSURG Nursing, 10*(5), 269–276.

McManus, T. J. (2000). *Helicobacter pylori*. An emerging infectious disease. *Nurse Practitioner, 25*(8), 40, 43–44, 47–48+.

Meeker, M. H., & Rothrock, J. C. (1999). *Alexander's care of the patient in surgery* (11th ed.). St. Louis: Mosby.

Metheny, N. A., & Titler, M. G. (2001). Assessing placement of feeding tubes. *American Journal of Nursing, 101*(5), 36–45.

North American Nursing Diagnosis Association. (2001). *NANDA Nursing diagnoses: Definitions & classification 2001–2002*. Philadelphia: NANDA.

Porth, C. M. (2002). *Pathophysiology: Concepts of altered health states* (6th ed.). Philadelphia: Lippincott.

Resto, M. A. (2000). Hospital extra. Gastroesophageal reflux disease. *American Journal of Nursing, 100*(9), 24D, 24F, 24H.

Terrado, M., Russell, C., & Bowman, J. B. (2001). Dysphagia: An overview. *MEDSURG Nursing, 10*(5), 233–248.

Tierney, L. M., McPhee, S. J., & Papadakis, M. A. (2001). *Current medical diagnosis & treatment* (40th ed.). New York: Lange Medical Books/McGraw-Hill.

Walton, J. C., Miller, J., & Tordecilla, L. (2001). Elder oral assessment and care. *MEDSURG Nursing, 10*(1), 37–44.

Wilkinson, J. M. (2000). *Nursing diagnosis handbook with NIC interventions and NOC outcomes* (7th ed.). Upper Saddle River, NJ: Prentice Hall Health.

Nursing Care of Clients with Gallbladder, Liver, and Pancreatic Disorders

www.prenhall.com/lemone

Additional resources for this chapter can be found on the Student CD-ROM accompanying this textbook, and on the Companion Website at www.prenhall.com/lemone. Click on Chapter 22 to select the activities for this chapter.

CD-ROM
- Audio Glossary
- NCLEX Review

Animation
- Cirrhosis

Companion Website
- More NCLEX Review
- Case Study
  Hepatitis B
- Care Plan Activity
  Hepatitis A
- MediaLink Application
  Treatment of Liver Cancer

LEARNING OUTCOMES

After completing this chapter, you will be able to:

- Describe the pathophysiology of commonly occurring disorders of the gallbladder, liver, and exocrine pancreas.

- Relate knowledge of normal anatomy and physiology to the manifestations and effects of biliary, hepatic, and pancreatic disorders.

- Discuss diagnostic tests, including client preparation, used to identify biliary, hepatic, and pancreatic disorders.

- Discuss nursing implications for dietary and pharmacologic interventions used for clients with these disorders.

- Provide appropriate nursing care for the client who has surgery of the gallbladder, liver, or pancreas.

- Relate changes in normal assessment data to the pathophysiology and manifestations of gallbladder, liver, and exocrine pancreatic disorders.

- Use the nursing process to plan and provide individualized care for clients with disorders of the gallbladder, liver, or exocrine pancreas.

Gallbladder, liver, and exocrine pancreatic disorders may occur as primary disorders, or develop secondarily to other disease processes. One organ's functioning frequently affects that of another. Duct inflammation or obstruction, and changes in the multiple functions of these organs, can cause significant health effects.

Clients with a gallbladder, liver, or pancreatic disorder may experience pain, multiple metabolic and nutritional disturbances, and altered body image. Nursing care addresses physiologic and psychosocial needs of the client and family.

GALLBLADDER DISORDERS

Altered bile flow through the hepatic, cystic, or common bile duct is a common problem. It often leads to inflammation and other complications. Gallstones are the most common cause of obstructed flow. Tumors and abscesses also can obstruct bile flow.

THE CLIENT WITH CHOLELITHIASIS AND CHOLECYSTITIS

Cholelithiasis is the formation of stones (*calculi*) within the gallbladder or biliary duct system. Cholelithiasis is a common problem in the United States, affecting more than 10% of men and 20% of women by age 65 (Tierney et al., 2001).

PHYSIOLOGY REVIEW

Normally, bile is formed by the liver and stored in the gallbladder. Bile contains bile salts, bilirubin, water, electrolytes, cholesterol, fatty acids, and lecithin. In the gallbladder, some of the water and electrolytes are absorbed, further concentrating the bile. Food entering the intestine stimulates the gallbladder to contract and release bile through the common bile duct and sphincter of Oddi into the intestine. The bile salts in bile increase the solubility and absorption of dietary fats.

PATHOPHYSIOLOGY AND MANIFESTATIONS
Cholelithiasis

Gallstones form when several factors interact: abnormal bile composition, biliary stasis, and inflammation of the gallbladder. Most gallstones (80%) consist primarily of cholesterol; the rest contain a mixture of bile components. Excess cholesterol in bile is associated with obesity, a high-calorie, high-cholesterol diet, and drugs that lower serum cholesterol levels. When bile is supersaturated with cholesterol, it can precipitate out to form stones. Biliary stasis, or slowed emptying of the gallbladder, contributes to cholelithiasis. Stones do not form when the gallbladder empties completely in response to hormonal stimulation. Slowed or incomplete emptying allows cholesterol to concentrate and increases the risk of stone formation. Finally, inflammation of the gallbladder allows excess water and bile salt reabsoprtion, increasing the risk for lithiasis. Box 22–1 lists the risk factors for cholelithiasis.

PRACTICE ALERT *Certain very low-calorie diets are associated with a high risk of cholelithiasis. Increased cholesterol concentration in the bile and decreased gallbladder contractions associated with fasting increase the risk of gallstone formation.* ■

BOX 22–1	■ Risk Factors for Cholelithiasis

- Age
- Family history of gallstones
- Race or ethnicity: Native American (either Northern or Southern hemisphere); Northern European heritage
- Obesity, hyperlipidemia
- Rapid weight loss
- Female gender; use of oral contraceptives
- Biliary stasis: pregnancy, fasting, prolonged parenteral nutrition
- Diseases or conditions: cirrhosis; ileal disease or resection; sickle cell anemia; glucose intolerance

Most gallstones are formed in the gallbladder. They then may migrate into the ducts (Figure 22–1 ■), leading to *cholangitis* (duct inflammation). Although some people with cholelithiasis are asymptomatic, many develop manifestations. Early manifestations of gallstones may be vague: epigastric fullness or mild gastric distress after eating a large or fatty meal. Stones that obstruct the cystic duct or common bile duct lead to distention and increased pressure behind the stone. This causes **biliary colic,** a severe, steady pain in the epigastric region or right upper quadrant of the abdomen.

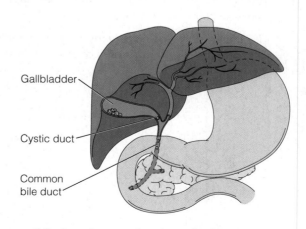

Gallbladder
Cystic duct
Common bile duct

Figure 22–1 ■ Common locations of gallstones.

The pain may radiate to the back, right scapula, or shoulder. The pain often begins suddenly following a meal, and may last as long as 5 hours. It often is accompanied by nausea and vomiting.

Obstruction of the common bile duct may cause bile reflux into the liver, leading to jaundice, pain, and possible liver damage. If the common duct is obstructed, pancreatitis (discussed later in this chapter) is a potential complication.

Cholecystitis

Cholecystitis is inflammation of the gallbladder. *Acute cholecystitis* usually follows obstruction of the cystic duct by a stone. The obstruction increases pressure within the gallbladder, leading to ischemia of the gallbladder wall and mucosa. Chemical and bacterial inflammation often follow. The ischemia can lead to necrosis and perforation of the gallbladder wall.

Acute cholecystitis usually begins with an attack of biliary colic. The pain involves the entire right upper quadrant (RUQ), and may radiate to the back, right scapula, or shoulder. Movement or deep breathing may aggravate the pain. The pain usually lasts longer than biliary colic, continuing for 12 to 18 hours. Anorexia, nausea, and vomiting are common. Fever often is present, and may be accompanied by chills. The RUQ is tender to palpation.

Chronic cholecystitis may result from repeated bouts of acute cholecystitis or from persistent irritation of the gallbladder wall by stones. Bacteria may be present in the bile as well. Chronic cholecystitis often is asymptomatic.

Complications of cholecystitis include *empyema,* a collection of infected fluid within the gallbladder; gangrene and perforation with resulting peritonitis or abscess formation; formation of a fistula into an adjacent organ (such as the duodenum, colon, or stomach); or obstruction of the small intestine by a large gallstone (*gallstone ilius*). Table 22–1 compares the manifestations and complications of acute cholelithiasis with those of cholecystitis.

COLLABORATIVE CARE

Treatment of the client with cholelithiasis or cholecystitis depends of the acuity of the condition and the client's overall health status. When gallstones are present but asymptomatic and the client has a low risk for complications, conservative treatment is indicated. However, when the client experiences frequent symptoms, has acute cholecystitis, or has very large stones, the gallbladder and stones are usually surgically removed.

Diagnostic Tests

Diagnostic tests are ordered to identify the presence and location of stones, identify possible complications, and help differentiate gallbladder disease from other disorders.

- *Serum bilirubin* is measured. Elevated direct (conjugated) bilirubin may indicate obstructed bile flow in the biliary duct system (see Box 22–2).
- *Complete blood count (CBC)* may indicate infection and inflammation if the WBC is elevated.
- *Serum amylase* and *lipase* are measured to identify possible pancreatitis related to common duct obstruction.
- *Abdominal X-ray* (flat plate of the abdomen) may show gallstones with a high calcium content.
- *Ultrasonography of the gallbladder* is a noninvasive exam that can accurately diagnose cholelithiasis. It also can be used to assess emptying of the gallbladder.
- *Oral cholecystogram* is performed using a dye administered orally to assess the gallbladder's ability to concentrate and excrete bile.
- *Gallbladder scans* use an intravenous radioactive solution that is rapidly extracted from the blood and excreted into the biliary tree to diagnose cystic duct obstruction and acute or chronic cholecystitis.

Medications

Clients who refuse surgery or for whom surgery is inappropriate may be treated with a drug to dissolve the gallstones.

TABLE 22–1	Manifestations and Complications of Cholelithiasis and Cholecystitis	
Manifestations	Cholelithiasis	Cholecystitis
Pain	• Abrupt onset • Severe, steady • Localized to epigastrium and RUQ of abdomen • May radiate to back, right scapula, and shoulder • Lasts 30 minutes to 5 hours	• Abrupt onset • Severe, steady • Generalized in RUQ of abdomen • May radiate to back, right scapula, and shoulder • Lasts 12 to 18 hours • Aggravated by movement, breathing
Associated symptoms	• Nausea, vomiting	• Anorexia, nausea, vomiting • RUQ tenderness and guarding • Chills and fever
Complications	• Cholecystitis • Common bile duct obstruction with possible jaundice and liver damage • Common duct obstruction with pancreatitis	• Gangrene and perforation with peritonitis • Chronic cholecystitis • Empyema • Fistula formation • Gallstone ilius

BOX 22–2 ■ Sorting Out Total, Direct, and Indirect Bilirubin Levels

When serum bilirubin levels are drawn, the results usually are reported as the total bilirubin, direct bilirubin, and indirect bilirubin levels. Most bilirubin is formed from hemoglobin, as aging or abnormal RBCs are removed from circulation and destroyed. It is then bound to protein and transported to the liver. This protein-bound bilirubin is called *indirect* or *unconjugated* bilirubin. Once in the liver, bilirubin is separated from the protein and converted to a soluble form, *direct* or *conjugated* bilirubin. Conjugated bilirubin is then excreted in the bile.

- **Total** (serum) **bilirubin,** the total bilirubin in the blood, includes both indirect and direct forms. In adults, the normal total bilirubin is 0.3 to 1.2 mg/dL or SI 5 to 21 μmol/L. Total bilirubin levels increase when more is being produced (e.g., RBC hemolysis), or when its metabolism or excretion are impaired (e.g., liver disease or biliary obstruction).
- **Direct** (conjugated) **bilirubin** levels, normally 0 to 0.2 mg/dL or SI <3.4 μmol/L in adults, rise when its excretion is impaired by obstruction within the liver (e.g., in cirrhosis, hepatitis, exposure to hepatotoxins) or in the biliary system.
- **Indirect** (unconjugated) **bilirubin** levels, normally <1.1 mg/dL or SI <19 μmol/L in adults, rise in RBC hemolysis (e.g., sickle cell disease or transfusion reaction).

Ursodiol (Actigall) and chenodiol (Chenix) reduce the cholesterol content of gallstones, leading to their gradual dissolution. These drugs are most effective in treating stones with high cholesterol content. They are less effective in treating radiopaque stones with high calcium salt content. Ursodiol is generally well tolerated with few side effects, while chenodiol has a high incidence of diarrhea at therapeutic doses. It also is hepatotoxic, so periodic liver function studies are required during therapy.

The primary disadvantages of pharmacologic treatment for gallstones include its cost, long duration (2 years or more), and the high incidence of recurrent stone formation when treatment is discontinued. If infection is suspected, antibiotics may be ordered to cure the infection and reduce associated inflammation and edema. Clients with pruritus (itching) due to severe obstructive jaundice and an accumulation of bile salts on the skin may be given cholestyramine (Questran). This drug binds with bile salts to promote their excretion in the feces. A narcotic analgesic such as morphine may be required for pain relief during an acute attack of cholecystitis.

Treatments

Surgery

Laparoscopic cholecystectomy (removal of the gallbladder) is the treatment of choice for symptomatic cholelithiasis or cholecystitis. This minimally invasive procedure has a low risk of complications and generally requires a hospital stay of less than 24 hours. Not all clients are candidates for laparoscopic cholecystectomy, and there is a risk that a laparoscopic cholecystectomy may be converted to a *laparotomy* (surgical opening into the abdomen) during the procedure. See the box below for nursing care for a client having laparoscopic cholecystectomy.

When stones are lodged within the ducts, a **cholecystectomy** with common bile duct exploration may be done. A T-tube (Figure 22–2 ■) is inserted to maintain patency of the duct and promote bile passage while the edema decreases. Excess bile is collected in a drainage bag secured below the surgical site. If it is suspected that a stone has been retained following surgery, a postoperative cholangiogram via the T-tube or direct visualization of the duct with an endoscope may be performed. See the box on page 577 for nursing care for a client with a T-tube.

Some clients who are poor surgical risks and for whom laparoscopic cholecystectomy is inappropriate may have either a *cholecystostomy* to drain the gallbladder, or a *choledochostomy* to remove stones and position a T-tube in the common bile duct.

Dietary Management

Food intake may be eliminated during an acute attack of cholecystitis, and a nasogastric tube inserted to relieve nausea and vomiting. Dietary fat intake may be limited, especially if the

NURSING CARE OF THE CLIENT WITH LAPAROSCOPIC CHOLECYSTECTOMY

BEFORE SURGERY

- Provide routine preoperative care as ordered (see Chapter 7).
- Reinforce teaching about the procedure and postoperative expectations, including pain management, deep breathing, and mobilization. *Preoperative teaching reduces anxiety and promotes rapid postoperative recovery.*

AFTER SURGERY

- Provide routine postoperative recovery care as outlined in Chapter 7.
- Assist to chair at bedside as allowed. *Early mobilization promotes lung ventilation and circulation, reducing the potential for postoperative complications.*

- Advance oral intake from ice chips to regular diet as tolerated. *Oral intake can be rapidly resumed due to minimal disruption of the gastrointestinal tract during surgery.*
- Provide and reinforce teaching: pain management, incision care, activity level, postoperative follow-up appointments. *With early discharge, the client and family assume responsibility for the majority of postoperative care. A clear understanding of this care and expected needs reduces anxiety and the risk of postoperative complications.*
- Initiate follow-up contact 24 to 48 hours after discharge to evaluate adequacy of pain control, incision management, and discharge understanding. *Contact following discharge provides an opportunity to evaluate care and reinforce teaching.*

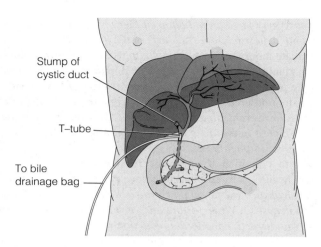

Figure 22–2 ■ T-tube placement in the common bile duct. Bile fluid flows with gravity into a drainage collection device below the level of the common bile duct.

client is obese. If bile flow is obstructed, fat-soluble vitamins (A, D, E, and K) and bile salts may need to be administered.

Other Therapies

In some cases, shock wave lithotripsy may be used with drug therapy to dissolve large gallstones. In *extracorporeal shock wave lithotripsy (ESWL),* ultrasound is used to align the stones with the source of shock waves and the computerized lithotripter. Positioning is of prime importance throughout the procedure, which usually takes an hour. Mild sedation may be given during the procedure. Postprocedure nursing care includes monitoring for biliary colic that may result from the gallbladder contracting to remove stone fragments, nausea, and transient hematuria. *Percutaneous cholecystostomy,* ultrasound-guided drainage of the gallbladder, may be done in high-risk clients to postpone or even eliminate the need for surgery.

Complementary Therapies

The herb goldenseal has been used in treating cholecystitis. One of the active ingredients in goldenseal, berberine, stimu-

lates secretion of bile and bilirubin. It also inhibits the growth of many common pathogens, including those known to infect the gallbladder. A study of the effectiveness of berberine in clients with cholecystitis demonstrated relief of all symptoms. Goldenseal can stimulate the uterus, so it is contraindicated for use during pregnancy. It also should not be used by nursing mothers.

NURSING CARE

Health Promotion

While most risk factors for cholelithiasis cannot be controlled or modified, several can. Modifiable risk factors include obesity, hyperlipidemia, extreme low-calorie diets, and diets high in cholesterol. Encourage clients who are obese to increase their activity level and follow a low-carbohydrate, low-fat, low-cholesterol diet to promote weight loss and reduce their risk for developing gallstones. Discuss the dangers of "yo-yo" dieting, with cycles of weight loss followed by weight gain, and of extremely low calorie diets. Encourage clients with high serum cholesterol levels to discuss using cholesterol-lowering drugs with their primary care provider.

Assessment

Assessment data related to cholelithiasis and cholecystitis include the following:

- Health history: current manifestations, including RUQ pain, its character and relationship to meals, duration, and radiation, nausea and vomiting or other symptoms; duration of symptoms; risk factors or previous history of symptoms; chronic diseases such as diabetes, cirrhosis, or inflammatory bowel disease; current diet; use of oral contraceptives or possibility of pregnancy
- Physical assessment: current weight; color of skin and sclera; abdominal assessment including light palpation for tenderness; color of urine and stool

NURSING CARE OF THE CLIENT WITH A T-TUBE

- Ensure that the T-tube is properly connected to a sterile container; keep the tube below the level of the surgical wound. *This position promotes the flow of bile and prevents backflow or seepage of caustic bile onto the skin. The tube itself decreases biliary tree pressure.*
- Monitor drainage from the T-tube for color and consistency; record as output. Normally, the tube may drain up to 500 mL in the first 24 hours after surgery; drainage decreases to less than 200 mL in 2 to 3 days, and is minimal thereafter. Drainage may be blood tinged initially, changing to green-brown. Report excessive drainage immediately (after 48 hours, drainage greater than 500 mL is considered excessive). *Stones or edema and inflammation can obstruct ducts below the tube, requiring treatment.*

- Place in Fowler's position. *This promotes gravity drainage of bile.*
- Assess skin for bile leakage during dressing changes. *Bile irritates the skin; it may be necessary to apply skin protection with karaya or another barrier product.*
- Teach client how to manage the tube when turning, ambulating, and performing activities of daily living. *Direct pulling or traction on the tube must be avoided.*
- If indicated, teach care of the T-tube, how to clamp it, and signs of infection. *Clients may be discharged home with the tube in place. Reporting early signs of infection facilitates prompt treatment.*

Nursing Diagnoses and Interventions

Priority nursing diagnoses for the client with cholelithiasis or cholecystitis often include pain related to biliary colic or surgery, imbalanced nutrition related to the effects of altered bile flow and to nausea and anorexia, and risk for infection related to potential rupture of an acutely inflamed gallbladder. Nursing interventions for the client who has undergone a laparoscopic or open cholecystectomy are similar to those for other clients having abdominal surgery. See Chapter 7. ⊖⊃

Pain

The pain associated with cholelithiasis can be severe. Sometimes a combination of interventions is indicated.

- Discuss the relationship between fat intake and the pain. Teach ways to reduce fat intake (see Box 22–3). *Fat entering the duodenum initiates gallbladder contractions, causing pain when gallstones are present in the ducts.*
- Withhold oral food and fluids during episodes of acute pain. Insert nasogastric tube and connect to low suction if ordered. *Emptying the stomach reduces the amount of chyme entering the duodenum and the stimulus for gallbladder contractions, thus reducing pain.*
- For severe pain, administer meperidine or other narcotic analgesia as ordered. *Recent research indicates that morphine is no more likely to cause spasms of the sphincter of Oddi than meperidine.*
- Place in Fowler's position. *Fowler's position decreases pressure on the inflamed gallbladder.*
- Monitor vital signs, including temperature, at least every 4 hours. *Bacterial infection often is present in acute cholecystitis, and may cause an elevated temperature and respiratory rate.*

Imbalanced Nutrition:
Less Than Body Requirements

The client with severe gallbladder disease may develop nutritional imbalances related to anorexia, pain and nausea following meals, and impaired bile flow that alters absorption of fat and fat-soluble vitamins (A, D, E, K) from the gut.

- Assess nutritional status, including diet history, height and weight, and skinfold measurements (see Chapters 19 and 20). ⊖⊃ *Even though often obese, clients with gallbladder*

BOX 22–3	■ Examples of High-Fat Foods

- ■ Whole-milk products (e.g., cream, ice cream, cheese)
- ■ Doughnuts, deep-fried
- ■ Avocados
- ■ Sausage, bacon, hot dogs
- ■ Gravies with fat, cream
- ■ Most nuts (e.g., pecans, cashews)
- ■ Corn chips and potato chips
- ■ Butter and cooking oils
- ■ Fried foods (e.g., cheeseburgers, hamburgers, french fries)
- ■ Peanut butter
- ■ Chocolate candies

---

disease may have an imbalanced diet or may have specific vitamin deficiencies, particularly of the fat-soluble vitamins.

- Evaluate laboratory results, including serum bilirubin, albumin, glucose, and cholesterol levels. Report abnormal results to the primary care provider. *Elevated serum bilirubin may indicate impaired bilirubin excretion due to obstructed bile flow. A low serum albumin may indicate poor nutritional status. Glucose intolerance and hypercholesterolemia are risk factors for cholelithiasis.*
- Refer to a dietitian or nutritionist for diet counseling to promote healthy weight loss and reduce pain episodes. *A low-carbohydrate, low-fat, higher-protein diet reduces symptoms of cholecystitis. While fasting and very-low-calorie diets are contraindicated, a moderate reduction in calorie intake and increased activity levels promote weight loss.*
- Administer vitamin supplements as ordered. *Clients who do not absorb fat well due to obstructed bile flow may require supplements of the fat-soluble vitamins.*

Risk for Infection

An acutely inflamed gallbladder may become necrotic and rupture, releasing its contents into the abdominal cavity. While the resulting infection often remains localized, peritonitis can result from chemical irritation and bacterial contamination of the peritoneal cavity.

PRACTICE ALERT *Rupture of an acutely inflamed gallbladder may be heralded by abrupt but transient pain relief as contents are released from the distended gallbladder into the abdomen. Promptly report this change to the physician.* ■

Following open cholecystectomy (*laparotomy*), the risk for pulmonary infection is significant due to the high abdominal incision.

- Monitor vital signs including temperature every 4 hours. Promptly report vital sign changes or temperature elevation. *Tachycardia, increased respiratory rate, or an elevated temperature may indicate an infectious process.*
- Assess abdomen every 4 hours and as indicated (e.g., when pain level changes abruptly). *Increasing abdominal tenderness or a rigid, boardlike abdomen may indicate rupture of the gallbladder with peritonitis.*
- Assist to cough and deep breathe or use incentive spirometer every 1 to 2 hours while awake. Splint abdominal incision with a blanket or pillow during coughing. *The high abdominal incision of an open cholecystectomy interferes with effective coughing and deep breathing, increasing the risk of atelectasis and respiratory infections such as pneumonia.*
- Place in Fowler's position and encourage ambulation as allowed. *Fowler's position and ambulating promote lung expansion and airway clearance, reducing the risk of respiratory infections.*
- Administer antibiotics as ordered. *Antibiotics may be given preoperatively to reduce the risk of infection from infected gallbladder contents, and may be continued postoperatively to prevent infection.*

CHART 22–1 LINKAGES BETWEEN NANDA, NIC, AND NOC

The Client with Gallbladder Disease

NURSING DIAGNOSES	NURSING INTERVENTIONS	NURSING OUTCOMES
• Pain	• Pain Management • Patient-Controlled Analgesia Assistance	• Pain Control
• Imbalanced Nutrition: Less Than Body Requirements • Ineffective Health Maintenance	• Fluid Monitoring • Nutrition Management • Nutrition Monitoring • Teaching: Procedure /Treatment • Decision-Making Support	• Nutritional Status: Food and Fluid Intake • Knowledge: Treatment Regimen • Participation: Health Care Decisions

Data from Nursing Outcomes Classification (NOC) *by M. Johnson & M. Maas (Eds.), 1997, St. Louis: Mosby;* Nursing Diagnoses: Definitions & Classification 2001–2002 *by North American Nursing Diagnosis Association, 2001, Philadelphia: NANDA;* Nursing Interventions Classification (NIC) *by J.C. McCloskey & G. M. Bulechek (Eds.), 2000, St. Louis: Mosby. Reprinted by permission.*

Using NANDA, NIC, and NOC

Chart 22–1 shows links between NANDA nursing diagnoses, NIC, and NOC when caring for a client with cholelithiasis or cholecystitis.

Home Care

Teaching varies, depending on the choice of treatment options for cholelithiasis and cholecystitis. If surgery is not an option, teach about medications that dissolve stones, their use and adverse effects (diarrhea is a common side effect), and maintaining a low-fat, low-carbohydate diet if indicated. Include an explanation about the role of bile and the function of the gallbladder in terms that the client and family can understand.

Provide appropriate preoperative teaching for the planned procedure. Discuss the possibility of open cholecystectomy even when a laparoscopic procedure is planned. Teach postoperative self-care measures to manage pain and prevent complications. If the client will be discharged with a T-tube, provide instructions about its care (see the Nursing Care box on page 577). Discuss manifestations of complications to report to the physician. Stress the importance of follow-up appointments.

Following cholecystectomy, a low-fat diet may be initially recommended. Refer the client and food preparer to a dietitian to review low-fat foods. Higher fat foods may be gradually added to the diet as tolerated.

Nursing Care Plan
A Client with Cholelithiasis

Joyce Red Wing is a 44-year-old married mother of three children. A member of the Chickasaw tribe, she is active in tribal activities and works part time as a cook at a community kitchen. Recently Mrs. Red Wing has noticed a dull pain in her upper abdomen that gets worse after eating fatty foods; nausea and sometimes vomiting accompany the pain. She had a similar pain after the birth of her last child. She is diagnosed with cholelithiasis, and is admitted for a laparoscopic cholecystecomy.

ASSESSMENT

David Corbin, RN, takes Mrs. Red Wing's admission history. It includes intolerance to fatty foods and intermittent "stabbing" abdominal pain that radiates to her back. Her usual diet includes tacos or fried bread and biscuits with gravy for breakfast. She reports "not wanting to eat much of anything lately." She states she has never had surgery before and hopes "everything goes well." Physical assessment includes T 100° F (37.7° C), P 88, R 20, and BP 130/84. She has had a recent 5 lb weight loss, currently weighing 130 lb (59 kg). She is 63 inches (160 cm) tall. Abdominal examination elicits tenderness in the right upper abdominal quadrant.

She has no jaundice, chills, or evidence of complications.

DIAGNOSES

- *Imbalanced nutrition: Less than body requirements* related to anorexia and recent weight loss
- *Pain* related to inflamed gallbladder and surgical incisions
- *Risk for infection* related to potential bacterial contamination of abdominal cavity
- *Anxiety* related to lack of information about perioperative experience

EXPECTED OUTCOMES

- Maintain present weight within 5 lb (2.3 kg) over the next 3 weeks.
- Resume regular diet, decreasing intake of foods high in fat.
- Verbalize adequate pain control after surgery and with activity resumption.
- Remain free of infection.
- Verbalize a decrease in anxiety before surgery.

(continued on page 580)

Nursing Care Plan
A Client with Cholelithiasis (continued)

PLANNING AND IMPLEMENTATION

- Teach about the gallbladder and the function of bile.
- Discuss pre- and postoperative care, including self-care following discharge.
- Promote mobility as soon as allowed after surgery.
- Teach home care of stab wounds and recognition of signs of infection.
- Review specific high-fat foods to avoid and ways to maintain her weight.
- Provide analgesia as needed postoperatively. Teach appropriate analgesic use after discharge.

EVALUATION

Mrs. Red Wing is discharged the morning after her surgery. She is afebrile, has no signs of infection, and is able to appropriately care for her stab wounds. She identifies signs of infection and talks about ways to reduce her fat intake while keeping her weight stable. She verbalizes understanding of initial activity restrictions and resumption of normal activities. Mrs. Red Wing states, "It wasn't as bad as I thought it would be at first." She has an appointment to see her surgeon in 1 week.

Critical Thinking in the Nursing Process

1. What is the rationale for a low-fat diet with cholelithiasis? Discuss nutritional practices as they relate to the medical problem and Mrs. Red Wing's culture.
2. How would your discharge teaching for Mrs. Red Wing differ if she had had an open cholecystectomy instead of a laparoscopic cholecystectomy?
3. Design a nursing care plan for Mrs. Red Wing for the nursing diagnosis: *Fatigue*.

See Evaluating Your Response in Appendix C.

THE CLIENT WITH CANCER OF THE GALLBLADDER

Gallbladder cancer is rare, primarily affecting people over age 65. Women are more likely to develop the disorder. Manifestations of gallbladder cancer include intense pain and a palpable mass in the RUQ of the abdomen. Jaundice and weight loss are common. Gallbladder cancers spread by direct extension to the liver, and metastasize via the blood and lymph system.

At the time of diagnosis, the cancer usually is too advanced to treat surgically. Ninety-five percent of clients with primary cancer of the gallbladder die within 1 year. Radical and extensive surgical interventions may be performed, but the prognosis is poor regardless of treatment (Tierney et al., 2001). Nursing care is palliative, focusing on maintaining comfort and independence to the extent possible.

LIVER DISORDERS

The liver is a complex organ with multiple metabolic and regulatory functions. Optimal liver function is essential to health. Because of the significant amount of blood in the liver at all times, it is exposed to the effects of pathogens, drugs, toxins, and possibly malignant cells. As a result, liver cells may become inflamed or damaged, or cancerous tumors may develop.

THE CLIENT WITH HEPATITIS

Hepatitis is inflammation of the liver. It is usually caused by a virus, although it may result from exposure to alcohol, drugs and toxins, or other pathogens. Hepatitis may be acute or chronic in nature. Cirrhosis, discussed in the next section, is a potential consequence of severe hepatocellular damage.

PATHOPHYSIOLOGY AND MANIFESTATIONS

The essential functions of the liver are multiple. One of its primary functions is the metabolism and elimination of bilirubin. Bilirubin is a breakdown product of hemoglobin, released when RBCs are broken down and destroyed. This insoluble form of bilirubin (unconjugated bilirubin) is metabolized by the liver into a soluble form (conjugated bilirubin), which is then eliminated in bile. The liver also metabolizes carbohydrates, proteins, and fats. Most drugs are metabolized in the liver, and substances such as alcohol and many toxins are detoxified. These metabolic functions and bile elimination are disrupted by the inflammation of hepatitis. See Chapter 19 for more information about the liver. ∞

Viral Hepatitis

At least five viruses are known to cause hepatitis: hepatitis A virus (HAV), hepatitis B virus (HBV), hepatitis C virus (HCV), the hepatitis B-associated delta virus (HDV), and hepatitis E virus (HEV). These viruses differ from one another in mode of transmission, incubation period, the severity and type of liver damage they cause, and their ability to become chronic or develop a carrier (asymptomatic) state. Table 22–2 identifies unique features of the primary hepatitis viruses. Two additional

TABLE 22–2	Comparison of Types of Viral Hepatitis				
Virus	**Hepatitis A (HAV)**	**Hepatitis B (HBV)**	**Hepatitis C (HCV)**	**Hepatitis D (HDV)**	**Hepatitis E (HEV)**
Mode of transmission	Fecal–oral	Blood & body fluids; perinatal	Blood & body fluids	Blood & body fluids; perinatal	Fecal–oral
Incubation (in weeks)	2–6	6–24	5–12	3–13	3–6
Onset	Abrupt	Slow	Slow	Abrupt	Abrupt
Carrier state	No	Yes	Yes	Yes	Yes
Possible complications	Rare	Chronic hepatitis Cirrhosis Liver cancer	Chronic hepatitis Cirrhosis Liver cancer	Chronic hepatitis Cirrhosis Fulminant hepatitis	May be severe in pregnant women
Laboratory findings	Anti-HAV antibodies present	Positive HBsAg (HBV surface antigen); anti-HBV antibodies present	Anti-HCV antibodies present	Positive HDVAg (delta antigen) early; anti-HDV antibodies later	Anti-HEV antibodies present

viruses, hepatitis F and hepatitis G, have recently been identified. Their characteristics are yet to be defined.

Hepatitis viruses replicate in the liver, damaging liver cells (hepatocytes). The viruses provoke an immune response that causes inflammation and necrosis of hepatocytes as well. Although the extent of damage and the immune response vary among the different hepatitis viruses, the disease itself usually follows a predictable pattern.

No manifestations are present during the incubation period after exposure to the virus. The *prodromal* or *preicteric* (before jaundice) *phase* may begin abruptly or insidiously, with general malaise, anorexia, fatigue, and muscle and body aches. These manifestations often are mistaken for the flu. Nausea, vomiting, diarrhea, or constipation may develop, as well as mild RUQ abdominal pain. Chills and fever may be present.

The *icteric* (jaundiced) *phase* usually begins 5 to 10 days after the onset of symptoms. It is heralded by jaundice of the sclera, skin, and mucous membranes. Inflammation of the liver and bile ducts prevents bilirubin from being excreted into the small intestine. As a result, the serum bilirubin levels are elevated, causing yellowing of the skin and mucous membranes. Pruritus may develop due to deposition of bile salts on the skin. The stools are light brown or clay colored because bile pigment is not excreted through the normal fecal pathway. Instead, the pigment is excreted by the kidneys, causing the urine to turn brown.

During the icteric phase, the initial prodromal manifestations usually diminish even though the serum bilirubin increases. The appetite increases, and the temperature returns to normal. When uncomplicated, spontaneous recovery usually begins within 2 weeks of the onset of jaundice.

The *convalescent phase* follows jaundice and lasts several weeks. During this time, manifestations gradually improve: Serum enzymes decrease, liver pain decreases, and gastrointestinal symptoms and weakness subside. See the box on this page for the manifestations of each phase of hepatitis.

Hepatitis A

Hepatitis A, or *infectious hepatitis,* often occurs in either sporadic attacks or mild epidemics. It is transmitted by the fecal–oral route via contaminated food, water, shellfish, and direct contact with an infected person. The virus is in the stool of infected persons up to 2 weeks before symptoms develop. Although hepatitis A usually has an abrupt onset, it is typically a benign and self-limited disease with few long-term consequences. Symptoms last up to 2 months.

Hepatitis B

Hepatitis B can cause acute hepatitis, chronic hepatitis, fulminant hepatitis, or a carrier state. This virus is spread through contact with infected blood and body fluids. Health care workers are at risk through exposure to blood and needle-stick injuries. Other high-risk groups for hepatitis B include injection drug users, people with multiple sex partners, men who have sex with other men, and people frequently exposed to blood products (such as people on hemodialysis). Hepatitis B is a major risk factor for primary liver cancer.

Manifestations of Acute Hepatitis

PREICTERIC PHASE
- "Flulike" symptoms: malaise, fatigue, fever
- Gastrointestinal: anorexia, nausea, vomiting, diarrhea, constipation
- Muscle aches, polyarthritis
- Mild right upper abdominal pain and tenderness

ICTERIC PHASE
- Jaundice
- Pruritus
- Clay-colored stools
- Brown urine
- Decrease in preicteric phase symptoms (e.g., appetite improves; no fever)

POSTICTERIC/CONVALESCENT PHASE
- Serum bilirubin and enzymes return to normal levels
- Energy level increases
- Pain subsides
- Gastrointestinal: minimal to absent

MediaLink | HEPATITIS B CASE STUDY

In hepatitis B, liver cells are damaged by the immune response to this antigen. Damage may affect only portions or the majority of the liver. The liver shows evidence of injury and scarring, regeneration, and proliferation of inflammatory cells (Bullock & Henze, 2000).

Hepatitis C

Hepatitis C, formerly known as non-A, non-B hepatitis, is the primary worldwide cause of chronic hepatitis, cirrhosis, and liver cancer (Porth, 2002). It is transmitted through infected blood and body fluids. Injection drug use is the primary risk factor for HCV infection. The initial manifestations of this type of hepatitis often are mild and nonspecific. The disease often is recognized long after exposure occurred, when secondary effects of the disease (such as chronic hepatitis or cirrhosis) develop.

Hepatitis Delta

Hepatitis delta (HDV) only causes infection in people who also are infected with hepatitis B. It can cause acute or chronic infection, and can increase the severity of HBV infection (Porth, 2002). It is transmitted in the same manner as HBV.

Hepatitis E

Hepatitis E is rare in the United States. It is transmitted by fecal contamination of water supplies in developing areas such as southeast Asia, parts of Africa, and Central America. It primarily affects young adults. It can cause fulminant, fatal hepatitis in pregnant women.

Chronic Hepatitis

Chronic hepatitis is chronic infection of the liver. While it may cause few symptoms, it is the primary cause of liver damage leading to cirrhosis, liver cancer, and liver transplantation. Three of the known hepatitis viruses cause chronic hepatitis: HBV, HCV, and HDV. Manifestations of chronic hepatitis include malaise, fatigue, and hepatomegaly. Occasional icteric (jaundiced) periods may occur. Liver enzymes, particularly serum aminotransferase levels, typically are elevated.

Fulminant Hepatitis

Fulminant hepatitis is a rapidly progressive disease, with liver failure developing within 2 to 3 weeks after the onset of symptoms. Although uncommon, it is usually related to HBV with concurrent HDV infection.

Toxic Hepatitis

Many substances, including alcohol, certain drugs, and other toxins, can directly damage liver cells. Alcoholic hepatitis can result from chronic alcohol abuse or from an acute toxic reaction to alcohol. Alcoholic hepatitis causes necrosis of hepatocytes and inflammation of the liver parenchyma (functional tissue). Unless alcohol intake is avoided, progression to cirrhosis is common.

Other potential hepatotoxins include acetaminophen, benzene, carbon tetrachloride, halothane, chloroform, and poisonous mushrooms. These substances directly damage liver cells, leading to necrosis. The degree of damage often depends on age and the extent of exposure (dose) to the hepatoxin. Acetaminophen is a common cause of hepatocellular damage.

Hepatobiliary Hepatitis

Hepatobiliary hepatitis is due to cholestasis, the interruption of the normal flow of bile. Cholestasis may result from obstruction of the hepatic duct with stones or inflammation secondary to cholelithiasis. Other agents, such as oral contraceptives and allopurinol (a drug used to lower uric acid levels), also can cause cholestasis. When bile flow is disrupted, the liver parenchyma may become inflamed. Reestablishing bile flow by removing the stone or other causative agent is the treatment for hepatobiliary hepatitis.

COLLABORATIVE CARE

Management of hepatitis focuses on determining its cause, providing appropriate treatment and support, and teaching strategies to prevent further liver damage. Effective management begins with thorough assessment of diagnostic and laboratory data.

Diagnostic Tests

Liver function tests, such as blood levels of bilirubin and enzymes commonly released when liver cells are damaged, are obtained. These include the following:

- *Alanine aminotransferase (ALT)* is an enzyme contained within each liver cell. When liver cells are damaged, it is released into the blood. Levels may exceed 1000 IU/L or more in acute hepatitis.
- *Aspartate aminotransferase (AST)* is an enzyme found predominantly in heart and liver cells. AST levels rise when liver cells are damaged; with severe damage, blood levels may be 20 to 100 times normal values (Malarkey & McMorrow, 2000).
- *Alkaline phosphatase (ALP)* is an enzyme present in liver cells and bone. Serum ALP levels often are elevated in hepatitis.
- *Gamma-glutamyltransferase (GGT)* is an enzyme present in cell membranes. Its blood levels rise in hepatitis and obstructive biliary disease, and remain elevated until function is restored.
- *Lactic dehydrogenase (LDH),* an enzyme present in many body tissues, is a nonspecific indicator of tissue damage. Its isoenzyme, LDH5, is a specific indicator of liver damage.
- *Serum bilirubin* levels, including *conjugated* and *unconjugated,* are elevated in viral hepatitis due to impaired bilirubin metabolism and obstruction of the hepatobiliary ducts by inflammation and edema. The bilirubin level decreases as inflammation and edema subside.
- Laboratory tests for viral antigens and their specific antibodies may be done to identify the infecting virus and its state of activity. These tests are summarized in Table 22–2.
- A *liver biopsy* may be done to detect and evaluate chronic hepatitis. (Nursing implications for this test are outlined in the box on page 590.)

Medications

Prevention

Hepatitis A and hepatitis B are preventable diseases. Vaccines are available, as are preparations to prevent the disease following known or suspected exposure.

VACCINES. Hepatitis A vaccine provides long-term protection against HAV infection. It is an inactivated whole virus vaccine available in pediatric and adult formulations. Although more than 95% of adults achieve immunity after one dose of the vaccine, two doses are recommended for full protection. See Table 22–3.

Three doses of hepatitis B vaccine provide immunity to HBV infection in 90% of healthy adults. Hepatitis B vaccine is a recombinant vaccine. Vaccines produced by different manufacturers may be used interchangeably, although their dosages differ. Older adults are less likely to achieve immunity than younger adults. Clients on hemodialysis and people who are immunocompromised may need larger or more doses of the vaccine to achieve adequate protection. Serologic testing for immunity is recommended on completion of the series for people in these high-risk groups.

POSTEXPOSURE PROPHYLAXIS. Postexposure prophylaxis may be recommended for household or sexual contacts of people with HAV or HBV and other people who are known to have been exposed to these viruses. It is not necessary if the exposed person has been vaccinated and is known to be immune.

Hepatitis A prophylaxis is provided by a single dose of immune globulin (IG) given within 2 weeks after exposure. IG is recommended for all people with household or sexual contact with a person known to be infected with hepatitis A. See Table 22–3 for further recommendations.

Hepatitis B postexposure prophylaxis is indicated for people exposed to the hepatitis B virus. Hepatitis B immune globulin (HBIG) is given to provide for short-term immunity. HBV vaccine may be given concurrently. Candidates for postexposure prophylaxis include those with known or suspected percutaneous or permucosal contact with infected blood, sexual partners of clients with acute HBV or who are HBV carriers, and household contacts of clients with acute HBV infection (Atkinson, et al, 2000).

Treatment

In most cases of acute viral hepatitis, pharmacologic treatment of the infection is not indicated. Acute hepatitis C may be treated with interferon alpha, an antiviral agent, to reduce the risk of chronic hepatitis C.

Interferon alpha is used to treat both chronic hepatitis B and chronic hepatitis C. Interferon alpha interferes with viral replication, reducing the viral load. It is given by intramuscular or

TABLE 22–3   CDC Recommendations for Hepatitis Prevention in Adults

Disease/Strategy	Immunization	Adverse Reactions	Population Recommendations
Hepatitis A Prevention	Hepatitis A vaccine (Havrix; VAQTA), 2 doses (initial dose with booster in 6–12 months) IM into deltoid muscle	Pain at injection site	• Children >2 yr • International travelers • Homosexual men • Drug users • Persons with clotting-factor disorders, chronic liver disease, hepatitis C • Persons with occupational risk
Postexposure prophylaxis	Standard immune globulin IM into large muscle mass within 2 weeks of exposure	Rare; risk of anaphylaxis in people with IgA deficiency	• Close contacts of people with known hepatitis A • People potentially exposed to hepatitis A at child care center or restaurant with infected food handler
Hepatitis B Prevention	Recombinant hepatitis B vaccine (Recombivax HB; Engerix-B), 3 doses (initial dose followed by doses at 4 weeks and 5 months later) given IM into deltoid muscle	Pain at injection site; fatigue, headache	• Infants and adolescents • Adults with increased risk of HBV • Homosexual males; heterosexuals with multiple sexual partners • Injection drug users • Long-term male prisoners • People on hemodialysis • Health care workers
Postexposure prophylaxis	Hepatitis B immune globulin (HBIG) given IM into large muscle mass within 24 hr to 7 days of exposure, second dose 28 to 30 days after exposure; concurrent initiation of hepatitis B vaccine series	Infrequent; muscle stiffness, pain	• Infants born to women with HBV infection • Percutaneous or permucosal exposure to HBV when unvaccinated or antibody response is negative or unknown

Note. From *Epidemiology and Prevention of Vaccine-Preventable Diseases* (6th ed.) by Centers for Disease Control and Prevention (CDC), January 2000, Atlanta: Department of Health and Human Services.

subcutaneous injection. Virtually all clients treated with interferon alpha develop a flulike syndrome with fever, fatigue, muscle aches, headache, and chills. Acetaminophen helps alleviate some of these adverse effects. Depression also is a common adverse effect of this drug.

An alternate drug for treating chronic hepatitis B is lamivudine (Epivir HBV), an antiviral drug that can reduce liver inflammation and fibrosis. Although it has minimal side effects, clients may become resistant to the beneficial effects of lamivudine.

The treatment of choice for chronic hepatitis C is combination therapy of interferon alpha with ribavirin (Rebetol), an oral antiviral drug. This combination therapy improves the response rate over either drug used alone. Ribavirin has two major adverse effects: hemolytic anemia and birth defects. Blood counts are obtained before and during treatment to detect early signs of hemolytic anemia. Because of the risk for birth defects, this drug is contraindicated for use during pregnancy, and two reliable methods of birth control must be used by women taking the drug and female sexual partners of men taking the drug.

Treatments

Treatment of acute hepatitis also includes as-needed bed rest, adequate nutrition as tolerated, and avoidance of strenuous activity, alcohol, and agents that are toxic to the liver. In most cases, clinical recovery takes 3 to 16 weeks.

Complementary Therapies

Milk thistle, with its active ingredient silymarin, has been used by herbalists to treat liver disease for over 2000 years. Clinical studies have demonstrated that treatment with silymarin promotes recovery and reduces complications in clients with viral hepatitis. It also is beneficial for clients who have liver damage due to toxins, cirrhosis, and alcoholic liver disease. Silymarin's beneficial effects are attributed to its ability to promote liver cell growth, block toxins from entering and damaging liver cells, and reduce liver inflammation. It also is a powerful antioxidant.

Herbalists also may use licorice root to treat hepatitis. It has both antiviral and anti-inflammatory effects. Long-term use of licorice root, however, can lead to hypertension and affect fluid and electrolyte balance.

Herbal preparations also may be used to relieve the adverse effects of interferon alpha. Ginger can help relieve nausea, and St. John's wort is used for the depression associated with interferon alpha.

NURSING CARE

Health Promotion

Nurses play an instrumental role in preventing the spread of hepatitis. Stress the importance of hygiene measures such as handwashing after toileting and before all food handling. Discuss the dangers of injection drug use, and, with drug users, of sharing needles or other equipment. Encourage all sexually active clients to use safer sexual practices such as abstinence, mutual monogamy, and barrier protection (such as male or female condoms).

Discuss recommendations for hepatitis A and hepatitis B vaccine with people in high or moderate risk groups for these infections. Encourage all people with known or probable exposure to HAV or HBV to obtain postexposure prophylaxis.

Assessment

Collect assessment data related to hepatitis, such as the following:

- Health history: current manifestations, including anorexia, nausea, vomiting, abdominal discomfort, changes in bowel elimination or color of stools; muscle or joint pain, fatigue; changes in color of skin or sclera; duration of symptoms; known exposure to hepatitis; high-risk behaviors such as injection drug use or multiple sexual partners; previous history of liver disorders; current medications, prescription and over the counter
- Physical assessment: vital signs including temperature; color of sclera and mucous membranes; skin color and condition; abdominal contour and tenderness; color of stool and urine

Nursing Diagnoses and Interventions

Clients with acute or chronic hepatitis usually are treated in community settings; rarely is hospitalization required. Nursing care focuses on preventing spread of the infection to others and promoting the client's comfort and ability to provide self-care.

Risk for Infection (Transmission)

An important goal when caring for clients with acute viral hepatitis is preventing spread of the infection.

- Use standard precautions. Practice meticulous handwashing. *The hepatitis viruses are spread by direct contact with feces or blood and body fluids. Standard precautions and good handwashing protect both health care workers and other clients from exposure to the virus.*
- For clients with HAV or HEV, use standard precautions and contact isolation if fecal incontinence is present. *The fecal–oral route is the primary mode of transmission of these viruses. Other hepatitis viruses are transmitted through blood and other body fluids.*
- Encourage prophylactic treatment of all members of household and intimate sexual contacts. *Prophylactic treatment of people in close contact with the client decreases their risk of contacting the disease, or if already infected, the severity of the disease.*

PRACTICE ALERT *If the client diagnosed with hepatitis A is employed as a food handler or child care worker, contact the local health department to report possible exposure of patrons. Maintain confidentiality. Prophylactic treatment of people who have possibly been exposed to the virus can prevent a local epidemic of the disease.* ■

Fatigue

Fatigue, and possible weakness, is common in acute hepatitis. Although bed rest is rarely indicated, adequate rest periods and limitation of activities may be necessary. Many clients with acute hepatitis may be unable to resume normal activity levels for 4 or more weeks.

- Encourage planned rest periods throughout the day. *Adequate rest is necessary for optimal immune function.*
- Assist to identify essential activities and those that can be deferred or delegated to others. *Identifying essential and nonessential activities promotes the client's sense of control.*
- Suggest using level of fatigue to determine activity level, with gradual resumption of activities as fatigue and sense of well-being improves. *Fatigue associated with activity is an indicator of appropriate and inappropriate activity levels. As recovery progresses, increasing activity levels are tolerated with less fatigue.*

Imbalanced Nutrition:
Less Than Body Requirements

Adequate nutrition is important for immune function and healing in clients with acute or chronic hepatitis.

- Help plan a diet of appealing foods that provides a high kilocaloric intake of approximately 16 carbohydrate kilocalories per kilogram of ideal body weight. *Sufficient energy is required for healing; adequate carbohydrate intake can spare protein.*
- Encourage planning food intake according to symptoms of the disease. Discuss eating smaller meals and using between-meal snacks to maintain nutrient and calorie intake. *Clients with acute hepatitis often are more anorexic and nauseated in the afternoon and evening; planning the majority of calorie intake in the morning helps maintain adequate intake. Limiting fat intake and the size of meals may reduce the incidence of nausea.*
- Instruct to avoid alcohol intake and diet drinks. *Alcohol avoidance is vital to prevent further liver damage and pro-mote healing. Diet drinks (e.g. diet sodas or juice drinks) provide few calories when an increased calorie intake is needed for healing.*
- Encourage use of nutritional supplements such as Ensure or Instant Breakfast drinks to maintain calorie and nutrient intake. *Nutritional supplement drinks are an additional source of concentrated calories and nutrients.*

Disturbed Body Image

Jaundice and associated rashes and itching can affect the client's body image. Nursing measures to prevent skin breakdown and address body image are discussed in the following section on cirrhosis.

Using NANDA, NIC, and NOC

Chart 22–2 shows links between NANDA nursing diagnoses, NIC, and NOC when caring for a client with hepatitis.

Home Care

Provide discharge teaching to clients and their families for home care. Include the following topics.

- Recommended prophylactic treatment
- Infection control measures such as frequent handwashing, not sharing eating utensils, avoiding food handling or preparation activities by the client with hepatitis A; abstaining from sexual relations during acute infection and using barrier protection if a carrier or for chronic infection
- Managing fatigue and limited activity
- Promoting nutrient intake
- Avoiding hepatic toxins such as alcohol, acetaminophen, and selected other drugs; encourage to alert all care providers to presence of infection
- Recommended follow-up

If chronic hepatitis B or C is being treated with medications, teach how to administer the drug, its dosing schedule, precautions, and management of adverse effects. Stress the importance of keeping follow-up appointments, including recommended laboratory testing.

Medialink | HEPATITIS A CARE PLAN

CHART 22–2 LINKAGES BETWEEN NANDA, NIC, AND NOC

The Client with Hepatitis

NURSING DIAGNOSES	NURSING INTERVENTIONS	NURSING OUTCOMES
• Fatigue	• Energy Management	• Energy Conservation
• Imbalanced Nutrition: Less Than Body Requirements	• Nutrition Management	• Nutritional Status: Nutrient Intake
• Ineffective Health Maintenance	• Self-Responsibility Facilitation	• Self-Direction of Care
	• Teaching: Disease Process	• Treatment Behavior: Illness or Injury
• Social Isolation	• Family Involvement Promotion	• Social Support
	• Social System Enhancement	

Data from Nursing Outcomes Classification (NOC) by M. Johnson & M. Maas (Eds.), 1997, St. Louis: Mosby; Nursing Diagnoses: Definitions & Classification 2001–2002 by North American Nursing Diagnosis Association, 2001, Philadelphia: NANDA; Nursing Interventions Classification (NIC) by J.C. McCloskey & G. M. Bulechek (Eds.), 2000, St. Louis: Mosby. Reprinted by permission.

THE CLIENT WITH CIRRHOSIS

Cirrhosis is the end stage of chronic liver disease. It is a progressive, irreversible disorder, eventually leading to liver failure. Cirrhosis is the tenth leading cause of death in the United States (Tierney et al, 2001). **Alcoholic** or **Laënnec's cirrhosis** is the most common type of cirrhosis in North America and many parts of Europe and South America (Braunwald et al., 2001). Cirrhosis also may result from chronic hepatitis B or C; prolonged obstruction of the biliary (bile drainage) system; long-term, severe right heart failure; and other uncommon liver disorders.

PHYSIOLOGY REVIEW

The portal venous system is the primary source of blood flow to the liver. This venous system drains blood from the abdominal organs.

The essential functions of the liver include the metabolism of proteins, carbohydrates, and fats. It also is responsible for the metabolism of steroid hormones and most drugs. It synthesizes blood proteins, albumin and clotting factors in particular. The liver detoxifies alcohol and other toxic substances. Ammonia, a toxic by-product of protein metabolism, is converted to urea in the liver for elimination by the kidneys. The liver produces bile, an essential substance for absorbing fats and eliminating bilirubin from the body. Minerals and fat-soluble vitamins are stored in the liver, as is glycogen (stored carbohydrate for energy reserves). The Kupffer cells that line the sinusoids phagocytize foreign cells and damaged blood cells. See Chapter 19 for more information about the liver.

PATHOPHYSIOLOGY

In cirrhosis, functional liver tissue is gradually destroyed and replaced by fibrous scar tissue. As hepatocytes and liver lobules are destroyed, the metabolic functions of the liver are lost. Structurally abnormal nodules encircled by connective tissue form. This fibrous connective tissue forms constrictive bands that disrupt blood and bile flow within liver lobules. Blood no longer flows freely through the liver to the inferior vena cava. This restricted blood flow leads to portal hypertension, increased pressure in the portal venous system.

Alcoholic Cirrhosis

Alcoholic or Laënnec's cirrhosis is the end result of alcoholic liver disease. Alcohol causes metabolic changes in the liver: triglyceride and fatty acid synthesis increases, and the formation and release of lipoproteins decrease, leading to fatty infiltration of hepatocytes (fatty liver). At this stage, abstinence from alcohol can allow the liver to heal. With continued alcohol abuse, the disease progresses. Inflammatory cells infiltrate the liver (alcoholic hepatitis), causing necrosis, fibrosis, and destruction of functional liver tissue. In the final stage of alcoholic cirrhosis, regenerative nodules form, and the liver shrinks and develops a nodular appearance (Bullock & Henze, 2000). Malnutrition commonly accompanies alcoholic cirrhosis.

Biliary Cirrhosis

When bile flow is obstructed within the liver or in the biliary system, retained bile damages and destroys liver cells close to the interlobular bile ducts. This leads to inflammation, fibrosis, and formation of regenerative nodules.

Posthepatic Cirrhosis

Advanced progressive liver disease resulting from chronic hepatitis B or C or from an unknown cause is known as posthepatic or postnecrotic cirrhosis. Chronic viral hepatitis appears to be the leading cause of posthepatic cirrhosis in the United States (Braunwald et al., 2001). The liver is shrunken and nodular, with extensive liver cell loss and fibrosis.

MANIFESTATIONS AND COMPLICATIONS

Early in the course of cirrhosis, few manifestations may be present. The liver usually is enlarged and may be tender. A dull, aching pain in the RUQ may be present. Other early signs include weight loss, weakness, and anorexia. Bowel function is disrupted with diarrhea or constipation (Porth, 2002).

As the disease progresses, manifestations related to liver cell failure and portal hypertension develop. Impaired metabolism causes such manifestations as bleeding, ascites, gynecomastia (breast enlargement) in men and infertility in women, jaundice, and neurologic changes. Portal hypertension accounts from such manifestations as ascites, peripheral edema, anemia, and low WBC and platelet counts. See *Multisystem Effects of Cirrhosis* on page 587.

Portal Hypertension

Portal hypertension, elevated pressure in the portal venous system, causes blood to be rerouted to adjoining lower pressure vessels. This *shunting* of blood involves collateral vessels. Affected veins, which become engorged and congested, are located in the esophagus, rectum, and abdomen. Portal hypertension increases the hydrostatic pressure in vessels of the portal system. Increased hydrostatic pressure in the capillaries pushes fluid out, contributing to ascites formation.

Splenomegaly

The spleen enlarges (**splenomegaly**) as portal hypertension causes blood to be shunted into the splenic vein. Splenomegaly increases the rate at which red and white blood cells and platelets are removed from circulation and destroyed. This increased blood cell destruction leads to anemia, leukopenia, and thrombocytopenia (Porth, 2002).

Ascites

Ascites is the accumulation of plasma-rich fluid in the abdominal cavity. Although portal hypertension is the primary cause of ascites, decreased serum proteins and increased aldosterone also contribute to the fluid accumulation. *Hypoalbuminemia,* low serum albumin, decreases the colloidal osmotic pressure of plasma. This pressure normally holds fluid in the intravascular compartment; when plasma colloidal osmotic pressure decreases, fluid escapes into extravascular compartments.

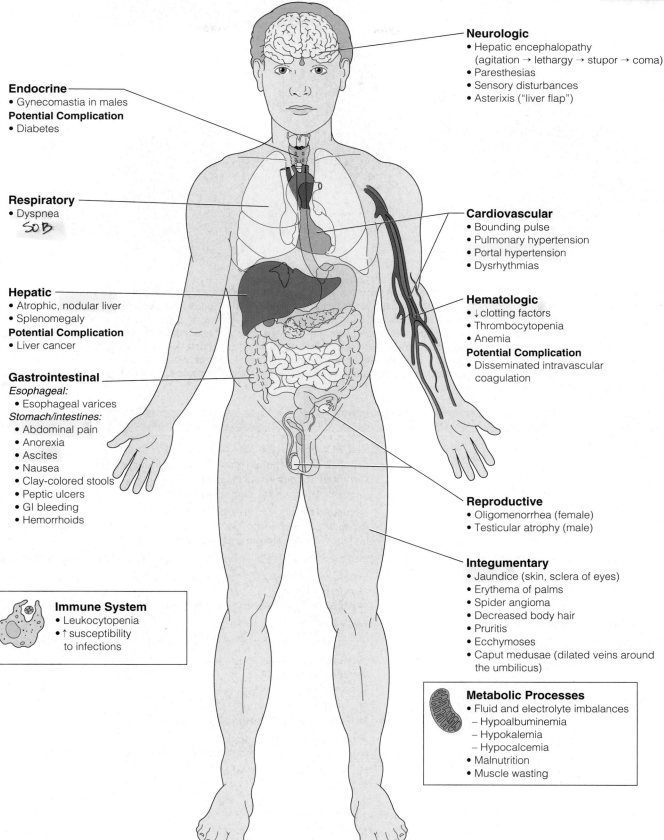

Neurologic
- Hepatic encephalopathy
  (agitation → lethargy → stupor → coma)
- Paresthesias
- Sensory disturbances
- Asterixis ("liver flap")

Endocrine
- Gynecomastia in males

Potential Complication
- Diabetes

Respiratory
- Dyspnea
  SOB

Cardiovascular
- Bounding pulse
- Pulmonary hypertension
- Portal hypertension
- Dysrhythmias

Hepatic
- Atrophic, nodular liver
- Splenomegaly

Potential Complication
- Liver cancer

Hematologic
- ↓ clotting factors
- Thrombocytopenia
- Anemia

Potential Complication
- Disseminated intravascular
  coagulation

Gastrointestinal
Esophageal:
- Esophageal varices

Stomach/intestines:
- Abdominal pain
- Anorexia
- Ascites
- Nausea
- Clay-colored stools
- Peptic ulcers
- GI bleeding
- Hemorrhoids

Reproductive
- Oligomenorrhea (female)
- Testicular atrophy (male)

Integumentary
- Jaundice (skin, sclera of eyes)
- Erythema of palms
- Spider angioma
- Decreased body hair
- Pruritis
- Ecchymoses
- Caput medusae (dilated veins around
  the umbilicus)

Immune System
- Leukocytopenia
- ↑ susceptibility
  to infections

Metabolic Processes
- Fluid and electrolyte imbalances
  – Hypoalbuminemia
  – Hypokalemia
  – Hypocalcemia
- Malnutrition
- Muscle wasting

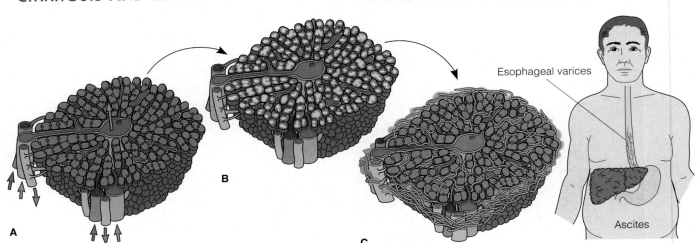

A. The portal vein (draining the capillary beds of the gut) provides 75% of the liver's blood supply; the hepatic artery provides the remainder. Venous and arterial blood mixes as it flows through the sinusoids and into the central hepatic vein, and from there into the inferior vena cava. *B.* Long-standing liver cell necrosis (from chronic infection, toxins such as alcohol, or obstructed bile flow) eventually overwhelms the liver's regenerative capacity, leading to fibrosis and scarring. Isolated hepatocytes continue to regenerate, forming nodules amongst the fibrous scar tissue. *C.* These nodules and scar tissue restrict blood flow through the liver, increasing pressure and congestion in the portal venous system. Blood is diverted into lower pressure collateral vessels, which become engorged, forming visible surface veins, hemorrhoids, and esophageal varices. Esophageal varices push the mucosa into its lumen, increasing the risk for trauma and bleeding due to food roughage or gastric reflux.

Manifestations of Cirrhosis with Underlying Cause

MANIFESTATION	UNDERLYING PATHOPHYSIOLOGY
Edema, ascites	• Impaired plasma protein synthesis (hypoalbuminemia) • Disrupted hormone balance and fluid retention • Increased pressure in portal venous system
Bleeding, bruising	• Decreased clotting factor synthesis • Increased platelet destruction by enlarged spleen • Impaired vitamin K absorption and storage
Esophageal varices, hemorrhoids	• Increased pressure in portal venous system with collateral vessel development
Gastritis, anorexia, diarrhea	• Engorged veins in gastrointestinal system • Alcohol ingestion • Impaired bile synthesis and fat absorption
Abdominal wall vein distention (caput medusae)	• Portal hypertension
Jaundice	• Impaired bilirubin metabolism and excretion
Malnutrition, muscle wasting	• Impaired nutrient metabolism • Impaired fat absorption • Impaired hormone metabolism
Anemia, leukopenia, increased risk for infection	• Bleeding • Increased blood cell destruction by spleen
Asterixis, encephalopathy	• Accumulated metabolic toxins • Impaired ammonia metabolism and excretion
Gynecomastia, infertility, impotence	• Altered sex hormone metabolism

Hyperaldosteronism, an increase in aldosterone, causes sodium and water retention, contributing to ascites and generalized edema. See the box above for selected manifestations of cirrhosis and their underlying pathophysiology.

Esophageal Varices

Esophageal varices are enlarged, thin-walled veins that form in the submucosa of the esophagus. See the *Pathophysiology Illustration* feature above. These collateral vessels form when blood

BOX 22–4 ■	Factors Precipitating Hepatic Encephalopathy

- High serum ammonia level
- Constipation
- Blood transfusions
- Gastrointestinal bleeding
- Medications: sedatives, tranquilizers, narcotic analgesics, anesthetics
- Hypoxia
- High-protein diet
- Severe infection
- Surgery

is shunted from the portal system due to portal hypertension. The thin-walled varices may rupture, causing massive hemorrhage; even eating high-roughage foods can precipitate bleeding. Thrombocytopenia, platelet deficiency, and impaired production of clotting factors by the liver contribute to the risk for hemorrhage.

Hepatic Encephalopathy

Hepatic encephalopathy results from accumulation of neurotoxins in the blood. Ammonia, a by-product of protein metabolism, contributes to hepatic encephalopathy. Ammonium ion is produced as proteins and amino acids are broken down by bacteria in the intestinal tract. Normally, the ammonia produced is then converted by the liver to urea before entering the general circulation. As functional liver tissue is destroyed, ammonia can no longer be converted to urea, and it accumulates in the blood. Other nervous system depressants, such as narcotics and tranquilizers, can contribute to hepatic encephalopathy. Box 22–4 lists selected precipitating factors for hepatic encephalopathy. *Asterixis* (liver flap), a flapping tremor of the hands when the arms are extended, is an early sign. Changes in personality and mentation develop; agitation, restlessness, impaired judgment, and slurred speech also are early manifestations of hepatic encephalopathy. As it progresses, confusion, disorientation, and incoherence develop. Deep coma is the final stage of hepatic encephalopathy.

Hepatorenal Syndrome

Although the cause is unclear, renal failure with azotemia (excess nitrogenous waste products in the blood), sodium retention, oliguria, and hypotension may develop in clients with advanced cirrhosis and ascites. The syndrome may be precipitated by gastrointestinal bleeding, aggressive diuretic therapy, or by an unknown cause (Braunwald et al., 2001).

COLLABORATIVE CARE

Care for the client with cirrhosis is holistic, addressing physiologic, psychosocial, and spiritual needs. The importance of including the family in the plan of care cannot be overemphasized, particularly if alcohol abuse is identified as the cause. Treatment includes medications to help regulate protein metabolism, maintenance of fluid and electrolyte balance, and supportive therapies, including treatment of underlying problems, such as malnutrition, anemia, bleeding, encephalopathy, renal failure, and infections.

Diagnostic Tests

Studies to confirm the diagnosis of cirrhosis and identify its cause and effects are performed. Diagnostic tests may include the following:

- *Liver function studies* include *ALT, AST, alkaline phosphatase,* and *gamma-glutamyl transferase (GGT)*. All may be elevated in cirrhosis, but usually not as severely as in acute hepatitis. Elevations in these enzymes may not correlate well with the extent of liver damage in cirrhosis.
- *CBC with platelets* is done. A low RBC count, hemoglobin, and hematocrit demonstrate anemia related to bone marrow suppression, increased RBC destruction, bleeding, and deficiencies of folic acid and vitamin B_{12}. Platelets are low, related to increased destruction by the spleen. Leukopenia (low WBC count) also relates to splenomegaly.
- *Coagulation studies* show a prolonged prothrombin time due to impaired production of coagulation proteins and lack of vitamin K.
- *Serum electrolytes* are measured. Hyponatremia is common, due to hemodilution. Hypokalemia, hypophosphatemia, and hypomagnesemia also are frequently seen, related to malnutrition and altered renal excretion of these electrolytes.
- *Bilirubin* levels are usually elevated in severe cirrhosis, including both direct (conjugated) and indirect (unconjugated) bilirubin.
- *Serum albumin* levels show hypoalbuminemia due to impaired liver production.
- *Serum ammonia* levels are elevated, as the liver fails to effectively convert ammonia to urea for renal excretion.
- *Serum glucose* and *cholesterol* levels frequently are abnormal in clients with cirrhosis.
- *Abdominal ultrasound* is performed to evaluate liver size, detect ascites, and identify liver nodules. Ultrasound may be used in conjunction with *doppler studies* to evaluate blood flow through the liver and spleen (Tierney et al., 2001).
- *Esophagascopy* (upper endoscopy) may be done to determine the presence of esophageal varices.
- *Liver biopsy* is not always necessary to diagnose cirrhosis, but may be done to distinguish cirrhosis from other forms of liver disease. See the box on page 590 for nursing implications for a client having a liver biopsy. Figure 22–3 ■ shows the site and position for liver biopsy. Biopsy may be deferred if the bleeding time is prolonged (such as a prothrombin time [PT] greater than 3 seconds over the control).

Medications

Medications are used to treat the complications and effects of cirrhosis; they do not reverse or slow the process of cirrhosis itself. Known hepatotoxic drugs and alcohol are avoided, as are drugs metabolized by the liver (e.g., barbiturates, sedatives, hypnotics, and acetaminophen). Several groups of drugs are commonly prescribed. See the Medication Administration box on page 591 for nursing responsibilities and client teaching for commonly used drugs in clients with cirrhosis.

- Diuretics reduce fluid retention and ascites. Spironolactone (Aldactone) is frequently the drug of first choice because it

Liver
Diaphragm
Lung
6th rib

A

B   C   D

Figure 22–3 ■ Liver biopsy. *A,* The client exhales completely, then holds his or her breath. This brings the liver and diaphragm to their highest position. *B,* The biopsy needle is inserted into the liver. *C,* Approximately 1 mL of saline is injected to clear the needle of blood and tissue. *D,* The needle is advanced, and a tissue sample is aspirated. Pressure is applied to the site immediately after the needle is withdrawn. The specimen is sent to the laboratory for analysis.

addresses one of the causes of ascites—increased aldosterone levels. If additional diuresis is necessary, a loop diuretic such as furosemide (Lasix) may be added to the regimen.

- Medications to reduce the nitrogenous load and lower serum ammonia levels are added when manifestations of hepatic encephalopathy develop. Two commonly administered medications are lactulose and neomycin. Both exert their effects locally, in the bowel. Lactulose reduces the number of ammonia-forming organisms in the bowel and increases the acidity of colon contents, converting ammonia into ammonium ion. Ammonium ion is not absorbable, and is excreted in the feces. Neomycin sulfate is a locally acting antibiotic that also reduces the number of ammonia-forming bacteria in the bowel.
- The beta-blocker nadolol (Corgard) may be given together with isosorbide mononitrate (Ismo, Imdur, Monoket) to prevent rebleeding of esophageal varices. This drug combination also lowers hepatic venous pressure.
- Ferrous sulfate and folic acid are given as indicated to treat anemia. Vitamin K may be ordered to reduce the risk of bleeding. When bleeding is acute, packed red blood cells, fresh frozen plasma, or platelets may be administered to restore blood components and promote hemostasis.
- Antacids are prescribed as indicated. A drug regimen to treat *H. pylori* infection may also be effective (see Chapter 21). ⊘
- Oxazepam (Serax), a benzodiazepine antianxiety/sedative drug, is not metabolized by the liver, and may be used to treat acute agitation.

Nursing Implications for Diagnostic Tests

Liver Biopsy

Preparation of Client
- Review chart for signed consent form.
- Withhold food and fluids per policy, usually 4 to 6 hours preprocedure.
- Assess and record baseline vital signs.
- Review prothrombin time (PT) and platelet count; administer vitamin K as ordered.
- Instruct to empty bladder immediately before the biopsy.
- Place in supine position on far right side of bed; turn head to left and extend right arm above head to improve access to the biopsy site.

Client and Family Teaching
- Discuss preparation for the biopsy and expected sensations during the procedure.
- Hold your breath following expiration during needle insertion to keep diaphragm and liver high and stabilized in the abdominal cavity.
- Obtaining the tissue sample usually requires only 10 to 15 seconds; there may be some pain or discomfort during this time.
- Direct pressure is applied to the site immediately after the needle is removed; you will be placed on your right side to maintain site pressure.
- You may develop pain in the right shoulder as the anesthetic loses effect.
- You will be monitored for bleeding after the procedure.
- Food and fluids are withheld for 2 hours after the biopsy; you then can resume your usual diet.
- Avoid coughing, lifting, or straining for 1 to 2 weeks.

Treatments

Treatment of cirrhosis is supportive, directed at slowing the progression to liver failure and reducing complications.

Dietary and Fluid Management
Dietary support is an essential part of care for the client with cirrhosis. Dietary needs change as hepatic function fluctuates.

- Sodium intake is restricted to under 2 g/day, and fluids are restricted as necessary to reduce ascites and generalized edema. Fluids are often limited to 1500 mL/day. Fluid needs are calculated based on response to diuretic therapy, urine output, and serum electrolyte values.
- Unless serum ammonia levels are high, a palatable diet with adequate calories and 75 to 100 g of protein per day is recommended. If hepatic encephalopathy is present, protein is restricted to 60 to 80 g/day (Tierney et al., 2001). When encephalopathy resolves and serum ammonia levels stabilize, protein intake is allowed as tolerated. The diet is high is calories and includes moderate fat intake to promote healing. Parenteral nutrition is used as needed to maintain nutritional status when food intake is limited.
- Vitamin and mineral supplements are ordered based on laboratory values. Deficiencies in the B-complex vitamins, particularly thiamin, folate, and B_{12}, and the fat-soluble vita-

Medication Administration

The Client with Cirrhosis

DIURETICS

Spironolactone (Aldactone)   Furosemide (Lasix)

Spironolactone is a potassium-sparing diuretic that competes with aldosterone. It reduces ascites by increasing renal excretion of fluid and decreasing aldosterone levels. Furosemide is a loop diuretic that promotes the excretion of potassium. Drugs may be given in combination if serum potassium level permits.

Nursing Responsibilities

- Monitor ECG, serum potassium, BUN, creatinine levels, and hydration status.
- Weigh daily.
- Carefully monitor intake and output.
- Monitor for signs of hyperkalemia if taking spironolactone alone: bradycardia; widening QRS, spiking T waves, or ST segment depression on ECG, diarrhea; and muscle twitching.
- Assess for hyponatremia: confusion, lethargy, apprehension.

Client and Family Teaching

- Maintain diet and fluid restrictions as prescribed.
- Report increases in weight or edema.
- Immediately report signs of hyponatremia, hyperkalemia, or hypokalemia (see Chapter 5).
- Expect increased urinary output; take medications in morning hours to avoid nocturia.

LAXATIVES

Lactulose (Cephulac, Chronulac)

Lactulose is a disaccharide laxative that is not absorbed by the gastrointestinal tract. It reduces the number of ammonia producing bacteria and lowers the pH in the colon. The lower pH (increased acidity) converts ammonia to ammonium ion, a nonabsorbable form that is excreted in the feces. Lactulose also pulls water into the bowel lumen, increasing the number of daily stools.

Nursing Responsibilities

- Assess bowel sounds and abdominal girth.
- Maintain accurate stool chart.
- Adjust dose to achieve two to three soft stools per day.
- Monitor electrolytes and hydration.

Client and Family Teaching

- Drink adequate fluids.
- Report diarrhea; if present, decrease dose.
- This drug may cause nausea. Continue taking the drug; taking it with crackers or a soft drink may reduce nausea.

ANTI-INFECTIVE AGENTS

Neomycin sulfate (Neo Tabs)

Neomycin sulfate is a nonsystemic aminoglycoside antibiotic that reduces intestinal bacteria and decreases ammonia production in the bowel lumen. The drug may be administered as an oral or rectal preparation.

Nursing Responsibilities

- Monitor hearing, renal, and neurologic functions. Drug is ototoxic, nephrotoxic, and neurotoxic.
- Prior to administration, check for previous hypersensitivity reaction.
- Monitor intake and output.
- Monitor BUN and creatinine levels.
- If the client is taking digitalis, monitor levels; oral neomycin interferes with its absorption.

Client and Family Teaching

- Report dizziness, tinnitus (ringing in ears), hearing loss, headaches, tremors, or vision changes immediately.
- Keep follow-up appointments.
- Maintain fluids, avoid dehydration. (Teach signs of dehydration.)

---

mins A, D, and E are common. These vitamins may need to be administered in a water-soluble form. Clients with alcohol-induced cirrhosis are at high risk for magnesium deficiency, which needs to be replaced.

Complication Management

Paracentesis, aspiration of fluid from the peritoneal cavity, may be a diagnostic or a therapeutic procedure. It may be done therapeutically to relieve severe ascites that does not respond to diuretic therapy. The goal of paracentesis is to relieve respiratory distress caused by excess fluid in the abdomen. Ascites fluid may be withdrawn in moderate amounts of 500 mL to 1 L daily to reduce the risk of fluid and electrolyte imbalances. Large-volume paracentesis, withdrawal of 4 to 6 L of fluid at one time, may be used. Albumin is often administered intravenously during large volume paracentesis to maintain intravascular volume as the pressure of the ascites fluid in the abdomen is relieved. Nursing implications for the client undergoing paracentesis are listed in the box on page 592. Figure 22–4 ■ shows insertion sites and client positioning during paracentesis.

Figure 22–4 ■ Sites and position for paracentesis. *A,* Potential sites of needle or trocar insertion to avoid abdominal organ damage. *B,* The client sits comfortably; in this position, the intestines float back and away from the insertion site.

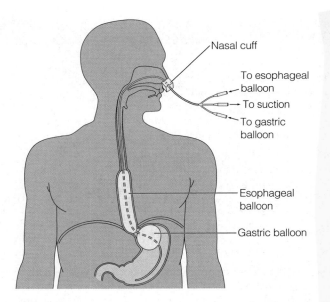

Figure 22–5 ■ Triple-lumen nasogastric tube (Sengstaken-Blakemore) used to control bleeding esophageal varices.

Labels on figure: Nasal cuff; To esophageal balloon; To suction; To gastric balloon; Esophageal balloon; Gastric balloon

Bleeding esophageal varices are life threatening and require intensive care management. Restoration of hemodynamic stability is the first priority. A central line is inserted and central venous and pulmonary artery pressures are monitored (see Chapter 30). ⬤ Blood is given to restore blood volume, and fresh frozen plasma may be administered to restore clotting factors. Somatostatin or octreotide, drugs that constrict blood vessels in the gut, are given intravenously to reduce blood flow in the portal venous system. Vasopressin, a drug that produces generalized vasoconstriction, also may be used.

When the blood pressure and cardiac output have stabilized, upper endoscopy is performed to evaluate and treat the varices. A large nasogastric tube is inserted prior to endoscopy, and **gastric lavage** (irrigation of the stomach with large quantities of normal saline) is performed to improve visualization. During endoscopy, the varices may be banded or sclerosed to reduce the risk of recurrent bleeding. In *banding (variceal ligation)*, small rubber bands are placed on varices to occlude blood flow. *Endoscopic sclerosis* involves injecting a sclerosing agent directly into the varices to induce inflammation and clotting. See Chapter 21 ⬤ for the nursing implications of endoscopy.

Balloon tamponade of bleeding varices may be used if bleeding cannot be controlled through vasoconstriction or if endoscopy is unavailable. A multiple-lumen nasogastric tube (such as a Sengstaken-Blakemore tube or a Minnesota tube) is inserted, and the gastric and esophageal balloons are inflated to apply direct pressure on the bleeding varices (Figure 22–5 ■). Tension is applied to the tube to further compress the varices. Balloon tamponade carries a number of risks, including aspiration, airway obstruction, and tissue ischemia and necrosis. An endotracheal tube is inserted prior to nasogastric intubation to support the airway and reduce the risk of aspiration. This short-term measure is used only until more definitive treatment can be done.

Transjugular intrahepatic portosystemic shunt (TIPS) is used to relieve portal hypertension and its complications of esophageal varices and ascites. A channel is created through the liver tissue using a needle inserted transcutaneously (Figure 22–6 ■). An expandable metal stent is inserted into this channel, to allow blood to flow directly from the portal vein into the hepatic vein, bypassing the cirrhotic liver. The shunt relieves pressure in esophageal varices and allows better control of fluid retention with diuretic therapy. Stenosis and occlusion of the shunt are frequent complications. TIPS also increases the risk of developing hepatic encephalopathy (due to decreased perfusion of the liver and impaired ammonia metabolism) and may reduce long-term survival. It generally is used as a short-term measure until liver transplant is performed.

Surgery

Liver transplantation is indicated for some clients with irreversible, progressive cirrhosis. A decline in functional status, increasing bilirubin levels, falling albumin levels, and increasing problems with complications that respond poorly to treatment are indications for liver transplantation. Malignancy, active alcohol or drug abuse, and poor surgical risk are contraindications for the surgery. See the box on the next page for nursing care of the client having a liver transplant.

NURSING CARE

Health Promotion

For most clients, high-risk behaviors are the risk factors for cirrhosis. With all clients (including children and young adults), stress the relationship between alcohol and drug abuse and liver disorders. While many clients tolerate alcohol use in

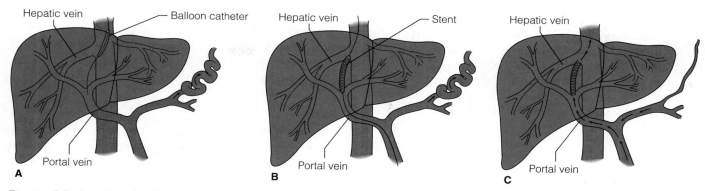

Figure 22–6 ■ Transjugular intrahepatic portosystemic shunt (TIPS). *A,* Guided by angiography, a balloon catheter inserted via the jugular vein is advanced to the hepatic veins and through the substance of the liver to create a portacaval (portal vein-to-vena cava) channel. *B,* A metal stent is positioned into the channel, and expanded by inflating the balloon. *C,* The stent remains in place after the catheter is removed, creating a shunt for blood to flow directly from the portal vein into the hepatic vein.

NURSING CARE OF THE CLIENT UNDERGOING LIVER TRANSPLANTATION

PREOPERATIVE CARE

- Obtain a complete nursing history and physical examination. *A complete preoperative nursing assessment provides baseline data for comparison after surgery.*
- Provide routine preoperative care as ordered (see Chapter 7). *Preoperative care is similar to that provided for other clients undergoing major surgery.*
- Discuss preoperative and postoperative expectations with the client and family. Introduce to the intensive care unit, and discuss anticipated drainage tubes and supportive measures in the immediate postoperative period. Provide information about visiting policies and family accommodations (if available). *Preoperative teaching helps relieve anxiety in the client and family members. Clients return from surgery to an intensive care or specialized care unit. Restrictions on the number of visitors and the time they may spend with the client are common.*
- Once a donor liver is located, check for evidence of infection; if no infection is present, begin preoperative antibiotics as ordered. *An acute or chronic infection may contraindicate liver transplantation as drugs given postoperatively to suppress rejection of the transplanted organ also impair the ability to fight infection.*

POSTOPERATIVE CARE

- Provide routine postoperative care as outlined in Chapter 7.
- Maintain airway and ventilatory support until awake and alert. *Until the new liver clears the anesthesia, the client requires measures to support respirations and ventilation.*
- Monitor temperature and implement rewarming measures (such as warming blankets, heating lamps, and head covers) as indicated. *The client often is hypothermic after liver transplant, necessitating careful rewarming while maintaining hemodynamic stability.*
- Frequently monitor hemodynamic pressures, including arterial blood pressure, central venous pressure, and pulmonary artery pressures. *Postoperative fluid volume status may be difficult to determine without careful pressure measurements. The rate and type of fluids administered are determined by hemodynamic status.*

- Monitor urine output hourly; maintain careful intake and output records. Weigh daily. *Urine output and weight provide additional information about fluid volume status. In addition, renal function may be altered after liver transplant; acute renal failure is a significant risk. See Chapter 27 for more information about acute renal failure and its management.*
- Monitor for signs of active bleeding, including excess drainage, increasing abdominal girth, bloody nasogastric drainage, black tarry stools, tachypnea, tachycardia, diminished peripheral pulses, or pallor. Report immediately. *Altered coagulation in the early postoperative period increases the risk for bleeding. Blood products to replace volume and clotting factors may be necessary.*
- Monitor serum electrolytes and laboratory values related to blood coagulation, liver function, and renal function. Report abnormal results or significant changes immediately. *Electrolyte imbalances are common postoperatively. Altered liver or renal function tests may indicate rejection of the transplanted liver or acute renal failure. Other early signs of transplant rejection include fever, a drop in bile output, or a change in bile color and viscosity (Urden, Stacy, & Lough, 2002).*
- Monitor neurologic status. *With good function of the transplanted organ, mental status should clear within days of the transplant.*
- Provide discharge teaching:
  a. Teach how to reduce risk of infection, and signs of infection to report.
  b. Instruct to recognize and report signs of organ rejection.
  c. Discuss all medications, including their purpose, schedule, adverse effects, and potential long-term effects. Stress the importance of complying with all prescribed medications and postoperative precautions for the remainder of the client's life.
  d. Discuss possible changes in body image and psychologic responses to receiving a transplanted organ. Refer to a counselor or support group as indicated.
  e. Refer for home health services for continued assessment and teaching.
  f. Stress importance of continued follow-up with transplant team and primary care provider.

moderation with no adverse effects on the liver, excess alcohol use is the leading cause of cirrhosis. Injection drug use also is a significant risk factor, increasing the risk for contracting blood-borne hepatitis (B, C, or D). These types of viral hepatitis can lead to chronic hepatitis and, ultimately, to cirrhosis. Discuss abstinence or safer sex practices as another measure to prevent viral hepatitis and potential liver damage.

Assessment

Assessment data related to cirrhosis includes the following:

- Health history: current manifestations, including abdominal pain or discomfort, recent weight loss, weakness, and anorexia; altered bowel elimination; excess bleeding or bruising; abdominal distension; jaundice, pruritus; altered libido or impotence; duration of symptoms; history of liver or gallbladder disease; pattern and extent of alcohol or injection drug use; use of other prescription and nonprescription drugs.
- Physical assessment: vital signs; mental status; color and condition of skin and mucous membranes; peripheral pulses and presence of peripheral edema; abdominal assessment including appearance, shape and contour, bowel sounds, abdominal girth, percussion for liver borders, and palpation for tenderness and liver size.

Nursing Diagnoses and Interventions

Nursing care of the client with cirrhosis presents many challenges because liver function affects all body systems. The nurse is responsible for coordinating care among care providers. Many nursing diagnoses may apply. The diagnoses discussed in this section focus on problems with fluid and electrolyte balance, altered thought processes, risk for bleeding, skin integrity, and nutrition.

Excess Fluid Volume

Cirrhosis affects water and salt regulation due to portal hypertension, hypoalbuminemia, and hyperaldosteronism. Signs of fluid volume overload and portal hypertension may develop: ascites, peripheral edema, internal hemorrhoids and varices, and prominent abdominal wall veins. Careful monitoring is necessary, as treatment measures can lead to further fluid and electrolyte imbalances.

- Weigh daily. Assess for jugular vein distention, measure abdominal girth daily, and check for peripheral edema. Monitor intake and output. *Careful assessment is important to detect fluid shifts.*
- Assess urine specific gravity. *Specific gravity measures the concentration of urine, an indicator of hydration.*

PRACTICE ALERT *Monitor the client with cirrhosis for signs of impaired renal function, such as oliguria, a fixed specific gravity of about 1.012, central edema (around the eyes and of the face), and increasing serum creatinine and BUN levels. Such signs may indicate hepatorenal syndrome or acute renal failure from another cause.* ∎

- Provide a low-sodium diet (500 to 2000 mg/day) and restrict fluids as ordered. *Excess sodium leads to water retention, and can increase fluid volume, ascites, and portal hypertension.*

Disturbed Thought Processes

Accumulated nitrogenous waste products and other metabolites affect mental status and thought processes. Effects of hepatic encephalopathy can range from mild confusion to agitation to coma.

- Assess neurologic status, including level of consciousness and mental status. Observe for signs of early encephalopathy: changes in handwriting, speech, and asterixis. *Early identification of evidence of encephalopathy allows prompt intervention—subtle changes in neurologic functioning are important!*

PRACTICE ALERT *Closely monitor clients who have experienced gastrointestinal bleeding for signs of hepatic encephalopathy. Blood in the intestinal tract is digested as a protein, increasing serum ammonia levels and the risk for hepatic encephalopathy.* ∎

- Avoid factors that may precipitate hepatic encephalopathy. Avoid hepatotoxic medications and CNS depressant drugs. *Cautious use of medications and close monitoring can eliminate iatrogenic causes of encephalopathy.*
- If possible, plan for consistent nursing care assignments. *Consistent care providers facilitate early identification of subtle neurologic changes indicative of hepatic encephalopathy.*
- Provide low-protein diet as prescribed; teach the family the importance of maintaining diet restrictions. *Nitrogenous by-products from dietary protein increase serum ammonia levels.*
- Administer medications or enemas as ordered to reduce nitrogenous products. Monitor bowel function and provide measures to promote regular elimination and prevent constipation. *Oral or rectally administered (per enema) medications are ordered to reduce intestinal bacteria and the ammonia they produce. Regular bowel elimination promotes protein and ammonia elimination in the feces.*
- Orient to surroundings, person, and place; provide simple explanations and reassurance. *Modification of verbal interactions to level of understanding and mental status may reduce anxiety and agitation.*

Ineffective Protection

Impaired coagulation, esophageal varices, and possible acute gastritis place the client with cirrhosis at significant risk for hemorrhage. Clotting is altered by vitamin K deficiency, impaired manufacture of coagulation factors II, VII, IX, and X, and increased platelet destruction due to splenomegaly.

- Monitor vital signs; report tachycardia or hypotension. *Increased pulse and decreasing blood pressure may indicate hypovolemia due to hemorrhage.*
- Institute bleeding precautions (see Box 22–5). *Preventive measures can decrease the risk for active bleeding.*
- Monitor coagulation studies and platelet count. Report abnormal results. *Coagulation studies help determine the risk for bleeding and the need for treatment.*
- Carefully monitor the client who has had bleeding esophageal varices for evidence of rebleeding: hematemasis,

BOX 22–5 ■ Bleeding Precautions

■ Prevent constipation.
■ Avoid rectal temperatures or enemas.
■ Avoid injections; if needed, use small-gauge needle and apply gentle pressure.
■ Monitor platelet count, PT, and PTT.
■ Assess for ecchymotic areas and areas of purpura.
■ Apply pressure to bleeding sites. After venipuncture, apply direct pressure for at least 5 minutes.
■ Use only a soft toothbrush.
■ Avoid blowing nose.
■ Assess oral cavity for bleeding gums.

hematochezia (bright blood in the stool) or tarry stools, signs of hypovolemia or shock. *Rebleeding is common following variceal hemorrhage, especially within the first week.*

PRACTICE ALERT *Carefully monitor the respiratory status of the client with a Sengstaken-Blakemore or Minnesota tube. Displacement of the tube can obstruct the airway unless an endotracheal tube is in place. The esophageal balloon prevents the client from swallowing oral secretions, increasing the risk for aspiration. Keep the head of the bed elevated to 45 degrees to reduce the risk of aspiration and promote gas exchange.* ■

Impaired Skin Integrity

Severe jaundice with bile salt deposits on the skin may cause pruritus. Scratching related to the pruritus damages the skin and impairs its integrity. Malnutrition, particularly protein deficiency, and edema also increase the risk for tissue breakdown and impaired skin integrity.

- Use warm water rather than hot water when bathing. *Hot water increases pruritus.*
- Use measures to prevent dry skin: Apply an emollient or lubricant as needed to keep skin moist, avoid soap or preparations with alcohol, and do not rub the skin. *Dry skin contributes to pruritus.*

- If indicated, apply mittens to the hands to prevent scratching. *Clients with encephalopathy may not understand the need to refrain from scratching.*
- Institute measures to prevent skin and tissue breakdown: Turn at least every 2 hours, use an alternating pressure mattress, and frequently assess skin condition. *Frequent position changes relieve pressure and promote circulation and tissue oxygenation.*
- Administer prescribed antihistamine (to relieve pruritus) cautiously. *Decreased liver function increases the risk for altered drug responses.*

Imbalanced Nutrition: Less than Body Requirements

The client with cirrhosis is at risk for malnutrition for a number of reasons: possible chronic alcohol use, anorexia, impaired vitamin and mineral absorption, and impaired protein metabolism. In addition, salt and protein restrictions may make the diet less palatable and appealing to the client.

- Weigh daily. Instruct to weigh at least weekly at home. *Weight is a good indicator of both nutritional status and fluid balance. Short-term weight fluctuations tend to reflect fluid balance, while longer-term changes in weight are more reflective of nutritional status.*
- Provide small meals with between meal snacks. *A small meal is more appealing for an anorexic client. Between-meal snacks help maintain adequate calorie and nutrient intake.*
- Unless protein is restricted due to impending hepatic encephalopathy, promote protein and nutrient intake by providing nutritional supplements such as Ensure or Instant Breakfast. *The sodium and protein content of all meals and snacks must be calculated when maintaining restrictions of these nutrients.*
- Arrange for consultation with a dietitian for diet planning while hospitalized and at home. *The dietitian can provide detailed instructions, sample menus, and suggestions for improving the palatability of the diet and promoting intake.*

Using NANDA, NIC, and NOC

Chart 22–3 shows links between NANDA nursing diagnoses, NIC, and NOC for the client with cirrhosis.

CHART 22–3 LINKAGES BETWEEN NANDA, NIC, AND NOC

The Client with Cirrhosis

NURSING DIAGNOSES	NURSING INTERVENTIONS	NURSING OUTCOMES
• Disturbed Thought Processes	• Reality Orientation • Environmental Management: Safety	• Cognitive Orientation • Neurological Status: Consciousness
• Fatigue	• Energy Management	• Energy Conservation
• Ineffective Health Maintenance	• Self-Responsibility Facilitation	• Health-Promoting Behavior
• Ineffective Protection	• Bleeding Precautions	• Coagulation Status
• Risk for Impaired Skin Integrity	• Skin Surveillance	• Tissue Integrity: Skin and Mucous Membranes

Data from Nursing Outcomes Classification (NOC) by M. Johnson & M. Maas (Eds.), 1997, St. Louis: Mosby; Nursing Diagnoses: Definitions & Classification 2001–2002 by North American Nursing Diagnosis Association, 2001, Philadelphia: NANDA; Nursing Interventions Classification (NIC) by J.C. McCloskey & G. M. Bulechek (Eds.), 2000, St. Louis: Mosby. Reprinted by permission.

Nursing Care Plan
A Client with Alcoholic Cirrhosis

Richard Wright is a 48-year-old divorced father of two teenagers. Mr. Wright has been admitted to the community hospital with ascites and malnutrition. He has had three previous hospital stays for cirrhosis, the most recent 6 months ago.

ASSESSMENT

Mr. Wright is lethargic but responds appropriately to verbal stimuli. He complains of "spitting up blood the past week or so" and says, "I'm just not hungry." He has lost 20 lb (9 kg) since his previous admission. He is jaundiced and has petechiae and ecchymoses on his arms and legs. Liz Mowdi, Mr. Wright's nurse, notes pitting pretibial edema. Abdominal assessment reveals a tight, protuberant abdomen with caput medusae. The liver margin is not palpable; the spleen is enlarged. Vital signs are T 100°F (37.7°C), P 110, R 24, and BP 110/70.

Abnormal laboratory results include WBC 3700/mm³ (normal 4300 to 10,800/mm³); RBC 4.0 million/mm³ (normal 4.6 to 5.9 million/mm³); platelets 75,000/mm³ (normal 150,000 to 350,000/mm³); serum ammonia 105 μm/dL (normal 35 to 65 μm/dL); total bilirubin 4.9 μg/dL (normal 0.1 to 1.0 μg/dL); and serum sodium 150 mEq/L (normal 135 to 145 mEq/L). Potassium, hemoglobin, hematocrit, total protein, and albumin levels are markedly decreased. Hepatic enzymes are elevated. Blood urea nitrogen and creatinine levels are marginally elevated. Oxygen saturation (O_2 sat) is 88% (normal range: 96% to 100%) per pulse oximetry.

Endoscopy shows bleeding from gastric ulcer, and the diagnosis of alcoholic cirrhosis with gastritis is made. Mr. Wright is started on Aldactone, 25 mg PO q8h; Riopan, 30 mL 2 hr p.c. and hs; lactulose, 30 mL q h until onset of diarrhea, then 15 mL t.i.d.; and low-protein, 800 mg sodium diet; fluid restriction of 1500 mL/day.

DIAGNOSES

- *Impaired gas exchange* related to pressure of ascites fluid on the diaphragm as manifested by tachypnea and decreased oxygen saturation
- *Excess fluid volume* related to electrolyte imbalance and hypoalbuminemia as manifested by ascites and peripheral edema
- *Imbalanced nutrition: less than body requirements* related to anorexia and possible alcohol abuse manifested by weight loss and low serum protein levels
- *Disturbed thought processes* related to effects of high ammonia levels as manifested by lethargy
- *Ineffective protection* related to impaired platelet formation and malnutrition

EXPECTED OUTCOMES

- Respiratory rate and O_2 sats will be within normal limits.
- Abdominal girth will decrease by 1 to 2 cm per day; peripheral edema will decrease.
- Will gain 1 lb (0.45 kg) per week without evidence of increased fluid retention. Serum albumin levels will return to normal range.
- Will be alert and oriented; serum ammonia levels are within normal range.
- Will demonstrate no further evidence of active bleeding.
- Will verbalize willingness to join a community support group.

PLANNING AND IMPLEMENTATION

- Weigh daily.
- Provide high-calorie, low-salt, low-protein diet with between-meal snacks.
- Maintain stool chart.
- Assign same nurses to care as much as possible to facilitate evaluation of mental status. Promptly report changes in status or laboratory values.
- Measure abdominal girth every 8 hr, marking level of measurement.
- Institute bleeding precautions.
- Elevate head of bed; assist to chair with legs elevated t.i.d. as tolerated.
- Include significant others in care and teaching; refer to community agencies for discharge follow-up.

EVALUATION

A week after admission, Mr. Wright's ascites has decreased and no further active bleeding is noted. His serum protein levels have increased, and his laboratory values are improving. No further bruising is noted during hospitalization. Although he shows a 5 lb weight loss as excess water is eliminated, he is consuming 100% of his diet. His serum ammonia levels have returned to normal. On discharge, O_2 sat is 96%; respirations are 18. Lactulose will be continued on discharge.

Ms. Mowdi provides both written and verbal information about the medication and cirrhosis, including measures to prevent complications. Mr. Wright and his children express interest in Alcoholics Anonymous and Al Anon and are referred to those agencies. Prior to discharge, follow-up appointments are made with a psychiatric social worker and a primary caregiver.

Critical Thinking in the Nursing Process

1. Describe the relationship between portal hypertension, liver dysfunction, and ascites.
2. Outline a 1-day menu for a low-protein, low-sodium high-calorie diet.
3. What is the pathophysiologic basis for hepatic encephalopathy? What are the nursing responsibilities related to lactulose and neomycin?
4. Design a nursing care plan for Mr. Wright for the diagnosis *Ineffective coping*.

See Evaluating Your Response in Appendix C.

Home Care

Cirrhosis is a chronic, progressive disease. As such, the client and family assume major roles in managing the disease and its manifestations and in preventing complications. Teaching topics for home care include:

- The absolute necessity of avoiding alcohol and other hepatotoxic drugs. Suggest in-patient or community-based alcohol treatment programs and Alcoholics Anonymous as indicated.
- Diet and fluid intake restrictions and recommendations. Include suggestions to promote nutritional intake and increase the flavor of food when sodium is restricted.
- Prescribed medications; their timing, intended and adverse effects, and manifestations to report to the primary care provider.
- Bleeding precautions (see Box 22–5).
- Manifestations of potential complications to be reported to the primary care provider. Stress the importance of promptly reporting evidence of gastrointestinal bleeding for prompt intervention for potential hemorrhage.
- Skin care techniques to reduce pruritus and the risk of damage.
- Ways to manage fatigue and conserve energy.

Provide referrals for home health services, dietary consultation, social services, and counseling as needed by the client and family. Suggest local support groups where available. If appropriate, suggest hospice services for the client with end-stage liver disease.

THE CLIENT WITH CANCER OF THE LIVER

Primary liver cancer is uncommon in the United States, accounting for only 0.5% to 2% of all cancers (Porth, 2002). It is, however, a common malignancy worldwide. Hepatocellular carcinoma is common in parts of Asia and Africa, where the incidence is as high as 500 cases per 100,000 people. This higher incidence is linked to chronic hepatitis B or C infection. The incidence of primary liver cancer is higher in men than it is in women. It typically develops in the fifth or sixth decade of life (Braunwald et al., 2001). The prognosis for primary liver cancer is poor, in part because the disease often is advanced at the time of diagnosis. Metastasis to the liver from primary tumors of the lung, breast, and gastrointestinal tract are relatively common.

PATHOPHYSIOLOGY

About 80% to 90% of primary hepatic cancers arise from the liver's parenchymal cells (hepatocellular carcinoma); the remainder form in the bile ducts (cholangiocarcinoma). Regardless of the origin, the progress of the disease is similar. Several etiologic factors have been identified (Box 22–6). Most primary liver cancer in the United States is related to alcoholic cirrhosis, HBV, or HCV.

The underlying pathophysiology of primary liver cancer is damage to hepatocellular DNA. This damage may be caused by integration of HBV or HCV into the DNA or by repeated cycles of cell necrosis and regeneration that facilitate DNA mutations. HBV and aflatoxins damage a specific tumor sup-

---

BOX 22–6 ■ Suspected Causes of Primary Liver Cancer

- Chronic hepatitis C infection
- Chronic hepatitis B infection
- Cirrhosis, regardless of type
- Chronic aflatoxin (a toxin produced by *Aspergillus* molds) exposure
- Arsenic-contaminated water
- Carcinogens in food
- Possible hormonal factors (e.g., long-term use of androgens)

---

pressor gene, p53. Tumors may be limited to one specific area, may occur as nodules throughout the liver, or may develop as surface infiltrates. The tumor interferes with normal hepatic function, leading to biliary obstruction and jaundice, portal hypertension, and metabolic disruptions (hypoalbuminemia, hypoglycemia, and bleeding disorders). It also may secrete bile products and produce hormones (paraneoplastic syndrome) that may lead to polycythemia, hypoglycemia, and hypercalcemia (Bullock & Henze, 2000). Tumors usually grow rapidly and metastasize early.

MANIFESTATIONS

Initial manifestations of liver cancer develop insidiously and often are masked by the presence of cirrhosis or chronic hepatitis. Weakness, anorexia, weight loss, fatigue, and malaise are common early manifestations. Abdominal pain and a palpable mass in the right upper quadrant are common presenting symptoms. See the box below for manifestations of primary liver cancer. Ascites and jaundice may be present at diagnosis. Signs of liver failure with portal hypertension, splenomegaly, and altered metabolism develop as the tumor progresses. Most clients die within 6 months of the diagnosis (Porth, 2002).

COLLABORATIVE CARE

Liver tumors are identified by CT scans and MRI. A liver biopsy may be done to confirm the diagnosis and identify the tumor type or origin. See the box on page 590 for the nursing implications of liver biopsy. Serum αfetoprotein (AFP) levels, normally low in nonpregnant adults, rise in most clients with hepatocellular cancer.

Manifestations of Primary Liver Cancer

- Malaise
- Anorexia
- Lethargy
- Weight loss
- Fever of unknown origin
- Feeling of abdominal fullness
- Painful right upper quadrant mass
- Manifestations of liver failure

Small, localized tumors may be surgically resected, offering the only viable chance for cure. Most tumors, however, have spread extensively or have distant metastasis at the time of diagnosis, so this is frequently not an option. Liver transplantation may be done; however, the tumor may recur in the transplanted organ.

Radiation therapy is used to shrink the tumor, decreasing pressure on surrounding organs and reducing pain. Chemotherapy may be used as primary treatment or adjunctive therapy. Direct continuous hepatic arterial infusion with an implanted pump has shown promise in prolonging survival rates. See Chapter 10 for nursing care for clients receiving radiation therapy or chemotherapy. 🔗

NURSING CARE

Encourage clients with risk factors for primary liver cancer to avoid alcohol and other substances that may further damage the liver. Urge them to discuss regular screening for liver tumors (such as serum AFP levels) with their primary care physician.

Both the client and the family need extensive nursing support. Controlling pain is a priority. Because of the poor prognosis, early referral for hospice services may be appropriate.

Nursing diagnoses, interventions, and teaching for the client with liver cancer are similar to those for clients with cirrhosis.

THE CLIENT WITH LIVER TRAUMA

Blunt or penetrating trauma to the abdomen can damage the liver. Liver trauma is frequently seen in combination with injuries to other abdominal organs. Motor vehicle crashes, stab or gunshot wounds, and iatrogenic sources such as liver biopsy are among the causes of these injuries.

PATHOPHYSIOLOGY

Liver trauma generally causes bleeding due to the vascularity of the organ. Liver injury may cause a surface hematoma, hematoma within the liver parenchyma, laceration of liver tissue, or disruption of vessels leading to or from the liver. Severe bleeding can rapidly disrupt hemodynamic stability and lead to shock.

PRACTICE ALERT
Bleeding due to liver trauma may not be immediately apparent. Instruct the client with apparent or potential liver trauma to immediately report light-headedness, rapid heart rate, shortness of breath, thirst, or increasing abdominal pain. ■

COLLABORATIVE CARE

Diagnostic peritoneal lavage is often used along with CT scan to diagnose liver trauma. The procedure is performed by making a small abdominal incision into the peritoneum (after the bladder has been emptied), and inserting a small catheter into the peritoneal cavity. If blood is immediately detected, the client is taken directly to surgery for abdominal exploration. If frank bleeding is not apparent, a liter of isotonic fluid is instilled into the abdomen, then drained and sent for laboratory analysis.

Intravenous fluids, fresh frozen plasma, platelets, and other clotting factors are administered to restore blood volume and promote hemostasis. Hemodynamic status is closely monitored; continued instability may indicate a need for surgical intervention to control hemorrhage. Postoperative nursing care focuses on preventing pulmonary complications, such as atelectasis, and detecting and preventing infection.

NURSING CARE

Nursing care of the client with liver trauma focuses on fluid management and other supportive care related to shock. Keeping family members informed is an important aspect of care, especially during the period of client instability. Diagnoses include the following:

- *Deficient fluid volume* related to hemorrhage
- *Risk for infection* related to wound or abdominal contamination
- *Ineffective protection* related to impaired coagulation

THE CLIENT WITH LIVER ABSCESS

Liver abscesses usually are bacterial or amebic (protozoal) in origin. Bacterial abscesses may follow trauma or surgical procedures, including biopsy. Multiple or single abscesses occur most commonly in the right lobe. Amebic abscesses most frequently occur following infestation of the liver by *Entamoeba histolytica*. Amebic infestation is associated with poor hygiene, unsafe sexual practices, or travel in areas where drinking water is contaminated.

PATHOPHYSIOLOGY

Following bacterial or amebic invasion of the liver, healthy tissue is destroyed, leaving an area of necrosis, inflammatory exudate, and blood. This damaged region becomes walled off from the healthy liver tissue. Pyogenic (bacterial) liver abscess may be caused by cholangitis, or distant or intra-abdominal infections, such as peritonitis or diverticulitis. *Escherichia coli* is the most frequently identified causative organism. The onset of pyogenic abscess is usually sudden, causing acute symptoms such as fever, malaise, vomiting, hyperbilirubinemia, and pain in the right upper abdomen.

The infection pathway for amebic hepatic abscesses usually is the portal venous circulation from the right colon. Generally, the onset of amebic abscess is insidious.

COLLABORATIVE CARE

Hepatic abscess is diagnosed through biopsy, hepatic aspirate, blood and fecal cultures, and CT scan and ultrasound studies. Therapy is based on identifying the causative organism through laboratory cultures. Pyogenic abscesses are treated with antibiotics to which the causitive organism is sensitive.

Pharmacologic agents used for amebic hepatic abscess are the same as those used for intestinal amebic infestation (see Chapter 24); combination therapy is commonly used. Two commonly used drugs for treating amebic liver abscesses are metronidazole (Flagyl) and iodoquinol (Diquinol). Both medications can cause gastrointestinal symptoms. Bone marrow suppression is a risk with metronidazole.

If the abscess does not respond to antibiotic therapy, percutaneous aspiration or surgical drainage may be done. In these procedures, a *percutaneous closed-catheter drain* is placed in the abscess to promote drainage of purulent material.

NURSING CARE

A major aspect of nursing care is prevention; teaching clients to avoid contaminated water and foods is especially important. Nursing interventions include teaching hikers to treat water and food handlers to wash hands thoroughly.

Clients who have a liver abscess require supportive care to prevent dehydration from the accompanying fever, nausea, vomiting, and anorexia. Careful monitoring of fluid and electrolyte status is indicated, as are comfort measures for abdominal pain. Possible nursing diagnoses include the following:

- *Risk for deficient fluid volume,* related to effects of prolonged fever and vomiting
- *Deficient knowledge* about transmission of amebic abscess
- *Activity intolerance,* related to pain and weakness

EXOCRINE PANCREAS DISORDERS

The pancreas is both an exocrine and an endocrine gland. It is made up of two basic cell types, each having different functions. The exocrine cells produce enzymes that empty through ducts into the small intestine, whereas the endocrine cells produce hormones that enter the bloodstream directly. Disorders of the exocrine pancreas affect the secretion and glandular control of digestive enzymes, whereas disorders of the endocrine pancreas affect the production of hormones necessary for normal carbohydrate, protein, and fat metabolism. Disorders of the exocrine pancreas are discussed in this section of the chapter; diabetes mellitus, a disorder of the endocrine pancreas, is discussed in Chapter 18. ⊖⊃

THE CLIENT WITH PANCREATITIS

Pancreatitis, or inflammation of the pancreas, is characterized by release of pancreatic enzymes into the tissue of the pancreas itself, leading to hemorrhage and necrosis. Pancreatitis may be either acute or chronic. About 5000 new cases of acute pancreatitis are diagnosed every year in the United States. It is a serious disease, with a mortality rate of approximately 10% (Braunwald et al., 2001). Alcoholism and gallstones are the primary risk factors for acute pancreatitis.

The incidence of chronic pancreatitis is less clear, because many people with chronic pancreatitis do not have classic manifestations of the disease. Clients with pancreatitis may have long-term effects of the disease, with chronic changes in enzyme and hormone production.

PHYSIOLOGY REVIEW

Knowledge of the normal structure and functions of the exocrine pancreas is important to understand how inflammation affects it and the client. The exocrine pancreas consists of lobules of acinar cells. The acinar cells secrete digestive enzymes and fluids (pancreatic juices) into ducts that empty into the main pancreatic duct (the duct of Wirsung). The pancreatic duct joins the common bile duct and empties into the duodenum through the ampulla of Vater (in some people the main pancreatic duct empties directly into the duodenum). The epithelial lining of the pancreatic ducts secretes water and bicarbonate to modify the composition of the pancreatic secretions. Pancreatic enzymes are secreted primarily in an inactive form and are activated in the intestine, a modification that prevents digestion of pancreatic tissue by its own enzymes (Porth, 2002). The pancreatic enzymes, with related functions, are as follows:

- Proteolytic enzymes, including trypsin, chymotrypsin, carboxypolypeptidase, ribonuclease, and deoxyribonuclease, which break down dietary proteins
- Pancreatic amylase, which breaks down starch
- Lipase, which breaks down fats into glycerol and fatty acids

PATHOPHYSIOLOGY

Acute Pancreatitis

Acute pancreatitis is an inflammatory disorder that involves self-destruction of the pancreas by its own enzymes through autodigestion. The milder form of acute pancreatitis, *interstitial edematous pancreatitis,* leads to inflammation and edema of pancreatic tissue. It often is self-limiting. The more severe form, *necrotizing pancreatitis,* is characterized by inflammation, hemorrhage, and ultimately necrosis of pancreatic tissue. Acute pancreatitis is more common in middle adults; its incidence is higher in men than in women. Acute pancreatitis is usually associated with gallstones in women and with alcoholism in men. Some clients recover completely, others experience recurring attacks, and still others develop chronic pancreatitis. The mortality and symptoms depend on the severity and type of pancreatitis: With mild pancreatic edema, mortality is low (6%); with severe necrotic pancreatitis, the mortality rate is high (23%) (Porth, 2002).

Although the exact cause of pancreatitis is not known, the following factors may activate pancreatic enzymes within the pancreas, leading to autodigestion, inflammation, edema, and/or necrosis.

- Gallstones may obstruct the pancreatic duct or cause bile reflux, activating pancreatic enzymes in the pancreatic duct system.
- Alcohol causes duodenal edema, and may increase pressure and spasm in the sphincter of Oddi, obstructing pancreatic outflow. It also stimulates pancreatic enzyme production, thus raising pressure within the pancreas.

Other factors associated with acute pancreatitis include tissue ischemia or anoxia, trauma or surgery, pancreatic tumors, third-trimester pregnancy, infectious agents (viral, bacterial, or parasitic), elevated calcium levels, and hyperlipidemia. Some medications have been linked with this disorder, including thiazide diuretics, estrogen, steroids, salicylates, and nonsteroidal anti-inflammatory drugs (NSAIDs). Regardless of the precipitating factor, the pathophysiologic process begins with the release of activated pancreatic enzymes into pancreatic tissue. Activated proteolytic enzymes, trypsin in particular, digest pancreatic tissue and activate other enzymes such as phospholipase A, which digests cell membrane phospholipids, and elastase, which digests the elastic tissue of blood vessel walls. This leads to proteolysis, edema, vascular damage and hemorrhage, and necrosis of parenchymal cells. Cellular damage and necrosis releases activated enzymes and vasoactive substances that produce vasodilation, increase vascular permeability, and cause edema. A large volume of fluid may shift from circulating blood into the retroperitoneal space, the peripancreatic spaces, and the abdominal cavity.

Manifestations

Acute pancreatitis develops suddenly, with an abrupt onset of continuous severe epigastric and abdominal pain. This pain commonly radiates to the back and is relieved somewhat by sitting up and leaning forward. The pain often is initiated by a fatty meal or excessive alcohol intake.

Other manifestations include nausea and vomiting; abdominal distention and rigidity; decreased bowel sounds; tachycardia; hypotension; elevated temperature; and cold, clammy skin. Within 24 hours, mild jaundice may appear. Retroperitoneal bleeding may occur 3 to 6 days after the onset of acute pancreatitis; signs of bleeding include bruising in the flanks (Turner's sign) or around the umbilicus (Cullen's sign). See the Manifestations box on this page.

Complications

Systemic complications of acute pancreatitis include intravascular volume depletion with acute tubular necrosis and renal failure (see Chapter 27 ⚭ for more information about acute renal failure), and acute respiratory distress syndrome (ARDS). Acute renal failure usually develops within 24 hours after the

---

Manifestations of Acute and Chronic Pancreatitis

ACUTE PANCREATITIS
- Abrupt onset of severe epigastric and LUQ pain, may radiate to back
- Nausea, vomiting; fever
- Decreased bowel sounds; abdominal distention and rigidity
- Tachycardia, hypotension; cold, clammy skin
- Possible jaundice
- Positive Turner's sign (flank ecchymosis) or Cullen's sign (peri-umbilical ecchymosis)

CHRONIC PANCREATITIS
- Recurrent epigastric and LUQ pain, radiates to back
- Anorexia, nausea and vomiting, weight loss
- Flatulence, constipation
- Steatorrhea

---

onset of acute pancreatitis. Manifestations of ARDS may be seen 3 to 7 days after its onset, particularly in clients who have experienced severe volume depletion. See Chapter 36 for more information about ARDS.

Localized complications include pancreatic necrosis, abscess, pseudocysts, and pancreatic ascites. Pancreatic necrosis causes an inflammatory mass which may be infected. It may lead to shock and multiple organ failure. A pancreatic abscess may form late in the course of the disease (6 or more weeks after its onset), causing an epigastric mass and tenderness (Tierney et al., 2001). Pancreatic pseudocysts, encapsulated collections of fluid, may develop both within the pancreas itself and in the abdominal cavity. They may impinge on other structures, or may rupture, causing generalized peritonitis. Rupture of a pseudocyst or of the pancreatic duct can lead to pancreatic ascites. Pancreatic ascites is recognized by gradually increasing abdominal girth and persistent elevation of the serum amylase level without abdominal pain.

Chronic Pancreatitis

Chronic pancreatitis is characterized by gradual destruction of functional pancreatic tissue. In contrast to acute pancreatitis, which may completely resolve with no long-term effects, chronic pancreatitis is an irreversible process that eventually leads to pancreatic insufficiency. Alcoholism is the primary risk factor for chronic pancreatitis in the United States. Malnutrition is a major worldwide risk factor. About 10% to 20% of chronic pancreatitis is idiopathic, with no identified cause. A genetic mutation on a gene associated with cystic fibrosis may play a role in these cases. Children or young adults with cystic fibrosis may develop chronic pancreatitis as well.

In chronic pancreatitis related to alcoholism, pancreatic secretions have an increased concentration of insoluble proteins. These proteins calcify, forming plugs that block pancreatic ducts and the flow of pancreatic juices. This blockage leads to inflammation and fibrosis of pancreatic tissue. In other cases, a stricture or stone may block pancreatic outflow, causing chronic obstructive pancreatitis. In chronic pancreatitis, recurrent episodes of inflammation eventually lead to fibrotic changes in the parenchyma of the pancreas, with loss of exocrine function. This leads to malabsorption from pancreatic insufficiency. If endocrine function is disrupted as well, clinical diabetes mellitus may develop.

Manifestations and Complications

Chronic pancreatitis typically causes recurrent episodes of epigastric and left upper abdominal pain that radiates to the back. This pain may last for days to weeks. As the disease progresses, the interval between episodes of pain becomes shorter. Other manifestations include anorexia, nausea and vomiting, weight loss, flatulence, constipation, and **steatorrhea** (fatty, frothy, foul-smelling stools caused by a decrease in pancreatic enzyme secretion). See page 600.

Complications of chronic pancreatitis include malabsorption, malnutrition, and possible peptic ulcer disease. Pancreatic pseudocyst or abscess may form, or stricture of the common bile duct may develop. Diabetes mellitus may develop, and there is an increased risk for pancreatic cancer. Narcotic addiction related to frequent, severe pain episodes is common.

COLLABORATIVE CARE

Acute pancreatitis often is a mild, self-limiting disease. Treatment focuses on reducing pancreatic secretions and providing supportive care. Treatment to eliminate the causative factor is begun after the acute inflammatory process resolves. Severe necrotizing pancreatitis may require intensive care management. Treatment for chronic pancreatitis often focuses on managing pain and treating malabsorption and malnutrition.

Diagnostic Tests

The laboratory tests that may be ordered when pancreatitis is suspected are summarized in Table 22–4. Diagnostic studies include the following:

- *Ultrasonography* can identify gallstones, a pancreatic mass, or pseudocyst.
- *Computed tomography (CT) scan* may be ordered to identify pancreatic enlargement, fluid collections in or around the pancreas, and perfusion deficits in areas of necrosis.
- *Endoscopic retrograde cholangiopancreatography (ERCP)* may be performed to diagnose chronic pancreatitis and to differentiate inflammation and fibrosis from carcinoma.
- *Endoscopic ultrasonography* can detect changes indicative of chronic pancreatitis in the pancreatic duct and parenchyma.
- *Percutaneous fine-needle aspiration biopsy* may be performed to differentiate chronic pancreatitis from cancer of the pancreas; the cells that are aspirated are examined for malignancy.

Medications

The treatment of acute pancreatitis is largely supportive. Narcotic analgesics such as morphine sulfate are used to control pain. Antibiotics often are prescribed to prevent or treat infection.

Clients with chronic pancreatitis also require analgesics, but are closely monitored to prevent drug dependence. Narcotics are avoided when possible. Pancreatic enzyme supplements are given to reduce steatorrhea (see the Medication Administration box on page 602). H_2 blockers such as cimetidine (Tagamet) and ranitidine (Zantac), and proton-pump inhibitors such as omeprazole (Prilosec) may be given to neutralize or decrease gastric secretions. Octreotide (Sandostatin), a synthetic hormone, suppresses pancreatic enzyme secretion and may be used to relieve pain in chronic pancreatitis.

Fluid and Dietary Management

Oral food and fluids are withheld during acute episodes of pancreatitis to reduce pancreatic secretions and promote rest of the organ. A nasogastric tube may be inserted and connected to suction. Intravenous fluids are administered to maintain vascular volume, and total parenteral nutrition (TPN) is initiated. Oral food and fluids are begun once the serum amylase levels

TABLE 22–4	Laboratory Tests in Exocrine Pancreatic Disorders	
Test	**Normal Value**	**Significance**
Serum amylase	25 to 125 U/L	Rises within 2 to 12 hours of onset of acute pancreatitis to 2 to 3 times normal. Returns to normal in 3 to 4 days.
Serum lipase	<200 U/L	Levels rise in acute pancreatitis; remains elevated for 7 to 14 days.
Serum trypsinogen	<80 µg/L	Elevated in acute pancreatitis; may be decreased in chronic pancreatitis.
Urine amylase	4 to 37 U/L/2h	Urine amylase levels rise in acute pancreatitis.
Serum glucose	70 to 110 mg/dL	May be transient elevation in acute pancreatitis.
Serum bilirubin	0.1 to 1.0 mg/dL	Compression of the common duct may increase bilirubin levels in acute pancreatitis.
Serum alkaline phosphatase	30 to 95 U/L	Compression of the common duct may increase levels in acute pancreatitis.
Serum calcium	8.9 to 10.3 mg/dL or 4.5 to 5.5 mEq/L	Hypocalcemia develops in up to 25% of clients with acute pancreatitis.
White blood cells	4500/mm^3 to 10,000/mm^3	Leukocytosis indicates inflammation and is usually present in acute pancreatitis.

Medication Administration

The Client with Chronic Pancreatitis

PANCREATIC ENZYME REPLACEMENT

Pancrelipase (Lipancreatin)

Pancrelipase enhances the digestion of starches and fats in the gastrointestinal tract by supplying an exogenous source of the enzymes protease, amylase, and lipase. The drug promotes nutrition and decreases the number of bowel movements.

Nursing Responsibilities

- Assess for allergy to pork protein.
- Monitor frequency and consistency of stools.
- Weigh every other day. Record weights.

- Give with meals; if not enteric coated, H_2 antagonists or antacids may be given concurrently to prevent destruction of the enzymes by hydrochloric acid.
- Monitor for side effects: rash, hives, respiratory difficulty, hematuria, hyperuricemia, or joint pain.

Client and Family Teaching

- Take with meals or snacks.
- If medicine is enteric coated, do not crush, chew, or mix with alkaline foods (e.g., milk, ice cream)
- Be sure to follow prescribed diet.

---

have returned to normal, bowel sounds are present, and pain disappears. A low-fat diet is ordered, and alcohol intake is strictly prohibited.

Surgery

If the pancreatitis is the result of a gallstone lodged in the sphincter of Oddi, an *endoscopic transduodenal sphincterotomy* may be performed to remove the stone. When cholelithiasis is identified as a causative factor, a cholecystectomy is performed once the acute pancreatitis has resolved. Surgical procedures to promote drainage of pancreatic enzymes into the duodenum or resection of all or part of the pancreas may be done to provide pain relief in clients with chronic pancreatitis. Large pancreatic pseudocysts may be drained endoscopically or surgically.

Complementary Therapies

Several complementary therapies may be used in conjunction with traditional treatments for clients with acute or chronic pancreatitis. Fasting or use of low-salt, low-fat vegetarian diets may reduce episodes of recurrent pain. Qigong, a system of gentle exercise, meditation, and controlled breathing, is believed to balance the flow of qi (a vital life force) through the body. Qigong lowers the metabolic rate, and may reduce the stimulation of pancreatic enzyme secretion. Magnetic field therapy also may be employed for clients with pancreatitis. All complementary therapies should be prescribed by a trained and competent practitioner.

NURSING CARE

Health Promotion

Teach clients who abuse alcohol about the risk for developing pancreatitis. Advise abstinence to reduce this risk, and refer to an alcohol treatment program or Alcoholics Anonymous.

Assessment

Assessment data related to acute or chronic pancreatitis include the following:

- Health history: current manifestations; abdominal pain (location, nature, onset and duration, identified precipitating

factors); anorexia, nausea or vomiting; flatulence, diarrhea, constipation, or stool changes; recent weight loss; history of previous episodes or gallstones; alcohol use (extent and duration); current medications
- Physical assessment: vital signs including orthostatic vitals and peripheral pulses; temperature; skin temperature and color, presence of any flank or periumbilical ecchymoses; abdominal assessment including bowel sounds, presence of distention, tenderness, or guarding

Nursing Diagnoses and Interventions

Nursing care for the client with acute pancreatitis focuses on managing pain, nutrition, and maintaining fluid balance.

Pain

Obstruction of pancreatic ducts and inflammation, edema, and swelling of the pancreas caused by pancreatic autodigestion cause severe epigastric, left upper abdominal, or midscapular back pain. The pain often is accompanied by nausea and vomiting, abdominal tenderness, and muscle guarding.

- Using a standard pain scale (see Chapter 4 ⊕), assess pain, including location, radiation, duration, and character. Note nonverbal cues of pain: restlessness or remaining rigidly still; tense facial features; clenched fists; rapid, shallow respirations; tachycardia; and diaphoresis. Administer analgesics on a regular schedule. *Pain assessment before and after analgesic administration measures its effectiveness. Administering analgesics on a regular schedule prevents pain from becoming established, severe, and difficult to control. Unrelieved pain has negative consequences; for example, pain, anxiety, and restlessness may increase pancreatic enzyme secretion.*

PRACTICE ALERT
Regularly assess respiratory status (at least every 4 to 8 hours), including respiratory rate, depth, and pattern; breath sounds; oxygen saturation and arterial blood gas results. Report tachypnea, adventitious or absent breath sounds, oxygen saturation levels below 92%, PaO_2 <70 mmHg or $PaCO_2$ >45 mmHg. Severe abdominal pain causes shallow respirations and hypoventilation, and suppresses cough effectiveness, which can lead to pooling of secretions, atelectasis, and pneumonia. ∎

- Maintain nothing by mouth (NPO) status and nasogastric tube patency as ordered. *Gastric secretions stimulate hormones that stimulate pancreatic secretion, aggravating pain. Eliminating oral intake and maintaining gastric suction reduces gastric secretions. Nasogastric suction also decreases nausea, vomiting, and intestinal distention.*
- Maintain bed rest in a calm, quiet environment. Encourage use of nonpharmacologic pain management techniques such as meditation and guided imagery. *Decreasing physical movement and mental stimulation decreases metabolic rate, gastrointestinal secretion, pancreatic secretions, and resulting pain. Adjunctive pain relief measures enhance the effectiveness of analgesics (see Chapter 4).*
- Assist to a comfortable position, such as a side-lying position with knees flexed and head elevated 45 degrees. *Sitting up, leaning forward, or lying in a fetal position tend to decrease pain caused by stretching of the peritoneum by edema and swelling.*
- Remind family and visitors to avoid bringing food into the client's room. *The sight or smell of food may stimulate secretory activity of the pancreas through the cephalic phase of digestion.*

Imbalanced Nutrition:
Less Than Body Requirements

The effects of pancreatitis and its treatment may result in malnutrition. Inflammation increases metabolic demand and frequently causes nausea, vomiting, and diarrhea. At a time of increased metabolic demand, NPO status and gastric suction further decrease available nutrients. In the client with chronic pancreatitis, loss of digestive enzymes affects the digestion and use of nutrients.

- Monitor laboratory values: serum albumin, serum transferrin, hemoglobin, and hematocrit. *Serum albumin, serum transferrin (which transports iron in the blood), hemoglobin, and hematocrit levels are decreased in malnutrition. Decreased pancreatic enzymes affect protein catabolism and absorption; decreased transferrin affects iron absorption and transport, thereby decreasing hematocrit and hemoglobin levels.*
- Weigh daily or every other day. *Short-term weight changes (over hours to days) accurately reflect fluid balance, whereas weight changes over days to weeks reflect nutritional status.*
- Maintain stool chart; note frequency, color, odor, and consistency of stools. *Protein and fat metabolism are impaired in pancreatitis; undigested fats are excreted in the stool. Steatorrhea indicates impaired digestion and, possibly, an increase in the severity of pancreatitis.*
- Monitor bowel sounds. *The return of bowel sounds indicates return of peristalsis; nasogastric suction usually is discontinued within 24 to 48 hours thereafter.*
- Administer prescribed intravenous fluids and/or TPN. *Intravenous fluids are given to maintain hydration. TPN is used to provide fluids, electrolytes, and kilocalories when fasting is prolonged (more than 2 to 3 days).*
- Provide oral and nasal care every 1 to 2 hours. *Fasting and nasogastric suction increase the risk for mucous membrane irritation and breakdown.*

- When oral intake resumes, offer small, frequent feedings. Provide oral hygiene before and after meals. *Oral hygiene decreases oral microorganisms that can cause foul odor and taste, decreasing appetite. Small, frequent feedings reduce pancreatic enzyme secretion and are more easily digested and absorbed.*

Risk for Deficient Fluid Volume

Acute pancreatitis can lead to a fluid shift from the intravascular space into the abdominal cavity (third spacing). Third spacing of fluid may cause hypovolemic shock, affecting cardiovascular function, respiratory function, renal function, and mental status.

- Assess cardiovascular status every 4 hours or as indicated, including vital signs, cardiac rhythm, hemodynamic parameters (central venous and pulmonary artery pressures); peripheral pulses and capillary refill; skin color, temperature, moisture, and turgor. *These measurements are indicative of fluid volume status and are used to monitor response to treatment. Stable values are as follows: heart rate less than 100; blood pressure within 10 mmHg of baseline; central venous pressure 0 to 8 mmHg; pulmonary wedge pressure 8 to 12 mmHg; cardiac output approximately 5 L/min; and skin warm, dry, with good turgor and color. (See Chapter 6 for a full discussion of hypovolemic shock.)*
- Monitor renal function. Obtain hourly urine output; report if less than 30 mL per hour. Weigh daily. *Urine output of less than 30 mL per hour indicates decreased renal perfusion or acute renal failure, a major complication of acute pancreatitis. Weight changes are an effective indicator of fluid volume status.*
- Monitor neurologic function, including mental status, level of consciousness, and behavior. *Hypotension and hypoxemia may decrease cerebral perfusion, causing changes in mental status, decreased level of consciousness, and changes in behavior. In addition, alcohol withdrawal is a risk in the client with acute pancreatitis.*

Using NANDA, NIC, and NOC

Chart 22–4 shows links between NANDA nursing diagnoses, NIC, and NOC for the client with acute or chronic pancreatitis.

Home Care

The client with pancreatitis is often acutely ill and, along with family members, needs information about both hospital procedures and self-care at home following discharge. During the acute stage, keep explanations brief and simple.

Prior to discharge, teach the client and family about the disease and how to prevent further attacks of inflammation. Include the following topics as appropriate.

- Alcohol can cause stones to form, blocking pancreatic ducts and the outflow of pancreatic juice. Continued alcohol intake is likely to cause further inflammation and destruction of the pancreas. Avoid alcohol entirely.
- Smoking and stress stimulate the pancreas and should be avoided.

CHART 22-4 LINKAGES BETWEEN NANDA, NIC, AND NOC

The Client with Pancreatitis

NURSING DIAGNOSES	NURSING INTERVENTIONS	NURSING OUTCOMES
• Pain	• Pain Management	• Pain Control
• Deficient Fluid Volume	• Fluid Management	• Fluid Balance
	• Hypovolemia Management	
• Imbalanced Nutrition: Less than Body Requirements	• Nutrition Management	• Nutritional Status: Food and Fluid Intake
• Ineffective Breathing Pattern	• Respiratory Monitoring	• Respiratory Status: Ventilation

Data from Nursing Outcomes Classification (NOC) *by M. Johnson & M. Maas (Eds.), 1997, St. Louis: Mosby;* Nursing Diagnoses: Definitions & Classification 2001–2002 *by North American Nursing Diagnosis Association, 2001, Philadelphia: NANDA;* Nursing Interventions Classification (NIC) *by J.C. McCloskey & G. M. Bulechek (Eds.), 2000, St. Louis: Mosby. Reprinted by permission.*

• If pancreatic function has been severely impaired, discuss appropriate use of pancreatic enzymes, including timing, dose, potential side effects, and monitoring of effectiveness.

• A low-fat diet is recommended. Provide a list of high-fat foods to avoid. Crash dieting and binge eating also should be avoided as they may sometimes precipitate attacks. Spicy foods, coffee, tea, or colas, and gas-forming foods, stimulate gastric and pancreatic secretions and may precipitate pain. Avoid them if this occurs.

• Report symptoms of infection (fever of 102°F (38.8°C) or more, pain, rapid pulse, malaise) as a pancreatic abscess may develop after initial recovery.

Refer to a dietitian or nutritionist for diet teaching as needed. If appropriate, refer to community agencies, such as Alcoholics Anonymous, or to an alcohol treatment program. Provide referrals to community or home health agencies as needed for continued monitoring and teaching at home.

Nursing Care Plan
A Client with Acute Pancreatitis

Rose Schliefer is a 59-year-old wife, mother of three, and grandmother of four. She has been hospitalized for the past 6 weeks for acute hemorrhagic pancreatitis and pseudocyst. The pancreatitis was caused by gallstones. Mrs. Schliefer spent 3 weeks in intensive care, and then underwent surgery to remove the gallstones and to insert drains into the pseudocyst. Prior to discharge, she had progressed to a soft, high-carbohydrate, low-fat diet; had all drains removed; and was able to walk in the hall. Mrs. Schliefer was referred to a community health agency in her home town for continued follow-up.

ASSESSMENT

Lee Quinn, the community health nurse, assesses Mrs. Schliefer at home after discharge. Mrs. Schliefer is thin and appears anxious and tired. She states that she lost 30 lb (13.6 kg) in the hospital and now weighs only 102 lb (46 kg). She is 66 inches (168 cm) tall. Her vital signs are within normal limits. Mrs. Schliefer has a well-healed upper abdominal scar and two round wounds (from drains) on each side of her abdomen. The wounds are closed but still have scabs. Her skin is cool and dry, and turgor is poor. She is alert and oriented and responds appropriately to questions. Blood glucose levels are normal. Mrs. Schliefer states that her main problems are lack of energy and lack of appetite for the low-fat diet that has been ordered. Mrs. Schliefer's husband and daughters express concern about their ability to provide care. Although they have been taught all about the disease

and how to provide care, they still are not sure they know exactly what should be done now that Mrs. Schliefer is at home.

DIAGNOSES

• *Fatigue* related to decreased metabolic energy production
• *Imbalanced nutrition: Less than body requirements* related to prolonged hospitalization, dietary restrictions, and impaired digestion
• *Bathing/hygiene self-care deficit* (Level II: requires help of another person, supervision, and teaching) related to decreased strength and endurance
• *Risk for caregiver role strain* related to inexperience with caregiving tasks

EXPECTED OUTCOMES

• Set priorities for daily and weekly activities, and incorporate a rest period into daily activity.
• Gain 3 to 4 lb.
• Bathe and maintain personal hygiene without assistance.
• Family members will verbalize comfort with providing necessary care.

PLANNING AND IMPLEMENTATION

• Explain causes of fatigue. Review effects of pancreatitis, surgery, and acute illness on energy levels.
• Develop activity goals, incorporating small, incremental steps toward achieving goal. Mrs. Schliefer indicates that she wants to cook a meal for the whole family. To reach this goal, she will:

Nursing Care Plan

A Client with Acute Pancreatitis (continued)

a. Schedule the meal when her energy level is highest.
b. List actions necessary to prepare the meal and delegate difficult tasks to family members.
c. Ask daughters to reorganize the kitchen to avoid unnecessary steps.
d. Plan the meal no sooner than the third week after being home.
- Instruct to:
  a. Rest in bed each day from 1:00 P.M. to 3:00 P.M.
  b. Eat six small meals a day with family members or friends.
  c. Sit and rest quietly for 15 minutes before eating.
- Discuss dietary restrictions and how to adapt them to usual diet.
- Advice to use shower chair and develop self-care goals for bathing and hygiene in small steps. Add self-care tasks gradually as tolerated.
- Discuss division of responsibilities for physical care, home maintenance, and medical care with family members.
- Encourage family discussion of concerns about future; acknowledge family strengths.

EVALUATION

One month after discharge, Mrs. Schliefer and her family have established new routines based on her energy levels. Mrs. Schliefer now fixes lunch because she feels best during midday. She and her husband share this time together without interruption. Mrs. Schliefer still rests during the day but can now provide self-care. She has gained only 2 lb, but states that she is getting used to the new diet and that "things are even starting to taste good without butter." She also says that sitting quietly before meals is helpful and that she prefers eating six small meals a day. Mr. and Mrs. Schliefer and their daughters agree that their initial worries about Mrs. Schliefer's care have been resolved; now they all know what they must do, and the future looks much brighter.

Critical Thinking in the Nursing Process

1. Your client with acute pancreatitis is also an alcoholic. Describe assessments that indicate the beginnings of withdrawal.
2. Discuss the pathophysiologic basis of hypovolemic shock in acute necrotic pancreatitis.
3. Outline a teaching plan that includes specific foods to omit and to include in a high-carbohydrate, low-protein, low-fat diet.
4. Develop a plan of care for the nursing diagnosis, *Impaired home maintenance management*.

See Evaluating Your Response in Appendix C.

THE CLIENT WITH PANCREATIC CANCER

Cancer of the pancreas accounts for approximately 2% of all cancers. It is, however, one of the most lethal cancers: More than 98% of people with pancreatic cancer die. An estimated 30,300 new cases occurred in the United States in 2002, with approximately 29,700 deaths from cancer of the pancreas (American Cancer Society, 2002). The incidence of pancreatic cancer increases after age 50. The incidence is slightly higher in women than men, and is higher in blacks than in whites. Most cancers of the pancreas occur in the exocrine pancreas, are adenocarcinomas, and cause death within 1 to 3 years after diagnosis.

The major risk factor for cancer of the pancreas is smoking; the incidence is twice as high in smokers as in nonsmokers. Other risk factors are exposure to industrial chemicals or environmental toxins, high-fat diet, chronic pancreatitis, and diabetes mellitus.

Cancer of the pancreas has a slow onset, with manifestations of anorexia, nausea, weight loss, flatulence, and dull epigastric pain. The pain increases in severity as the tumor grows. Other manifestations depend on the location of the tumor. Cancer of the head of the pancreas, which is the most common site, often obstructs bile flow through the common bile duct and the ampulla of Vater, resulting in jaundice, clay-colored stools, dark urine, and pruritus. Cancer of the body of the pancreas presses on the celiac ganglion, causing pain that increases when the person eats or lies supine. Cancer of the tail of the pancreas often causes no symptoms until it has metastasized. Other late manifestations include a palpable abdominal mass and ascites. Because the manifestations are nonspecific, up to 85% of clients with cancer of the pancreas do not seek health care until the cancer becomes too far advanced for a cure.

Early cancers of the head of the pancreas may be resectable. A pancreatoduodenectomy (commonly called Whipple's procedure) is performed to remove the head of the pancreas, the entire duodenum, the distal third of the stomach, a portion of the jejunum, and the lower half of the common bile duct. The common bile duct is then sutured to the end of the jejunum, and the remaining pancreas and stomach are sutured to the side of the jejunum (Figure 22–7 ■). Radiation and chemotherapy are often used in addition to surgery.

Postoperative nursing care of the client undergoing Whipple's procedure is outlined on page 606. Immediate postoperative care is often provided in the intensive care unit.

The client with pancreatic cancer has multiple problems requiring nursing care. Chapter 10 ⬡ provides a discussion of care of the client with cancer; the nursing diagnoses and interventions discussed for the client with pancreatitis are also appropriate for the client with pancreatic cancer.

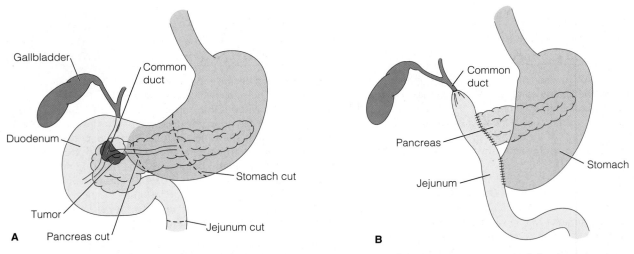

Figure 22–7 ■ Pancreatoduodenectomy (Whipple's procedure): *A,* areas of resection; *B,* appearance following resection.

NURSING CARE OF THE CLIENT UNDERGOING WHIPPLE'S PROCEDURE

PREOPERATIVE CARE

- Provide routine preoperative nursing care as outlined in Chapter 7. ⊙⊙
- Clarify teaching and learning as needed. Provide psychologic support for client and family. *The client and family faced with a diagnosis of pancreatic cancer may require reinforcement of teaching as anxiety, fear, and possible denial can interfere with learning.*

POSTOPERATIVE CARE

- Provide postoperative care as outlined in Chapter 7.
- Maintain in semi-Fowler's position. *Semi-Fowler's position facilitates lung expansion and reduces stress on the anastomosis and suture line.*
- Maintain low gastrointestinal suction. If drainage is not adequate, obtain an order to irrigate, using minimal pressure. Do not reposition nasogastric tube. *Pressure within the operative area from retained secretions increases intraluminal pressure and places stress on the suture line. Forceful irrigations and repositioning of the nasogastric tube may disrupt the suture line.*
- Maintain pain control using analgesics as prescribed (PCA, infusion, or given on a regular basis). Assess effectiveness of pain management. *Doses higher than normal may be required if narcotic analgesics have been used prior to surgery to manage pain.*

Increased pain may indicate complications such as disruption of suture line, leakage from anastomosis, or peritonitis. Adequate pain management increases resistance to stress, facilitates healing and increases the ability to cough, deep breathe, and change position.

- Assist with coughing, deep breathing, and changing position every 1 to 2 hours. Splint incision during coughing and deep breathing. *The location of the incision makes coughing and deep breathing more painful. The prolonged surgical procedure, anesthesia, location of incision, and immobility increase the risk of retained secretions, atelectasis, and pneumonia. Changing position facilitates drainage of secretions; effective coughing and deep breathing remove secretions and open distal alveoli.*
- Monitor for complications:
  a. Take vital signs every 2 to 4 hours or as indicated; immediately report changes (such as elevated temperature; hypotension; weak, thready pulse; increased or difficult respirations).
  b. Assess skin color, temperature, moisture, and turgor.
  c. Measure urinary output, gastrointestinal output, and drainage from any other tubes; monitor amount and type of would drainage.
  d. Assess level of consciousness.
  e. Monitor results of laboratory tests, especially arterial blood gases, hemoglobin, and hematocrit.

The major complications following Whipple's procedure are hemorrhage, hypovolemic shock, and hepatorenal failure. The assessments listed provide information about the client's status and alert the nurse to abnormal findings that signal the onset of these complications.

EXPLORE MediaLink

NCLEX review questions, case studies, care plan activities, MediaLink applications, and other interactive resources for this chapter can be found on the Companion Website at www.prenhall.com/lemone.

Click on Chapter 22 to select the activities for this chapter. For animations, video clips, more NCLEX review questions, and an audio glossary, access the Student CD-ROM accompanying this textbook.

TEST YOURSELF

1. When assessing the client admitted for a laparoscopic chole-cystectomy, the nurse would expect to find:
   a. History of intermittent episodes of right upper quadrant pain
   b. Significant jaundice of the sclera and skin
   c. Complaints of recurrent heartburn and acid reflux
   d. Ascites and peripheral edema

2. During an outbreak of hepatitis A traced to a food handler at a local restaurant, the nurse teaches staff at the restaurant that the most cost-effective means of protecting customers from further outbreaks is to:
   a. Insist that all food handlers be immunized against hepatitis A
   b. Test all new employees for hepatitis A antigen
   c. Wash hands thoroughly before handling food and after using the bathroom
   d. Use gloves for handling food if any cuts or scrapes are on hands

3. The nurse would evaluate teaching as effective when a client with chronic hepatitis C states which of the following?
   a. "I will reduce my alcohol intake and use only acetaminophen for pain relief."
   b. "I understand that I must return to the doctor every year for a follow-up liver biopsy."

   c. "Even though no treatment is available for this disease, I plan to live a long life."
   d. "I will avoid donating blood and will use barrier protection during sex."

4. A client hospitalized with cirrhosis, ascites, and mild hepatic encephalopathy suddenly vomits 200 mL of bright red blood. Which of the following should the nurse do first?
   a. Insert a nasogastric tube
   b. Place in Fowler's position
   c. Contact the physician
   d. Check stool for occult blood

5. A 54-year-old woman admitted with acute pancreatitis says, "I don't understand how I got this disease. I thought alcoholics got pancreatitis—I never drink." Which of the following is the most appropriate response by the nurse?
   a. "Was there a time in your life that you did drink heavily?"
   b. "It also is prevalent in smokers; do you smoke cigarettes?"
   c. "Gallstones also are a risk factor. We'll evaluate for them."
   d. "Intravenous drug use is a risk factor. Do you use drugs by injection?"

See Test Yourself answers in Appendix C.

BIBLIOGRAPHY

Ackley, B.J., & Ladwig, G. B. (2002). *Nursing diagnosis handbook: A guide to planning care* (5th ed.). St. Louis: Mosby.

American Cancer Society. (2002). *Cancer facts and figures 2002*. Atlanta: Author.

Atkinson, W., Wolfe, C., Humiston, S., & Nelson, R. (Eds.). (2000). *Epidemiology and prevention of vaccine-preventable diseases* (6th ed.). Atlanta: Centers for Disease Control.

Bockhold, K. M. (2000). Who's afraid of hepatitis C? *American Journal of Nursing, 100*(5), 26–31.

Braunwald, E., Fauci, A. S., Kasper, D. L., Hauser, S. L., Longo, D. L., & Jameson, J. L. (2001). *Harrison's principles of internal medicine* (15th ed.). New York: McGraw-Hill.

Bullock, B. A., & Henze, R. L. (2000). *Focus on pathophysiology*. Philadelphia: Lippincott.

Cole, L. (2001). Acute pancreatitis. *Nursing, 31*(12), 58–63.

Deglin, J. H., & Vallerand, A. H. (2001). *Davis's drug guide for nurses* (7th ed.). Philadelphia: F.A. Davis.

Dill, B., Dill, J. E., Berkhouse, L., & Palmer, S. T. (1999). Endoscopic ultrasound for chronic abdominal pain and gallbladder disease. *Gastroenterology Nursing, 22*(5), 209–212.

Dougherty, A. S., & Dreher, H. M. (2001). Hepatitis C: Current treatment strategies for an emerging epidemic. *MEDSURG Nursing, 10*(1), 9–13.

Farrar, J. A. (2001). Emergency! Acute cholecystitis. *American Journal of Nursing, 101*(1), 35–36.

Fontaine, K. L. (2000). *Healing practices: Alternative therapies for nursing*. Upper Saddle River, NJ: Prentice Hall Health.

Hession, M. C. (1998). Factors influencing successful discharge after outpatient laparoscopic sholecystectomy. *Journal of Perianesthesia Nursing, 13*(1), 11–15.

Johnson, M., Bulechek, G., Dochterman, J. M., Maas, M., & Moorhead, S. (2001). *Nursing diagnoses, outcomes, & interventions*. St. Louis: Mosby.

Johnson, M., Maas, M., & Moorhead, S. (Eds.). (2000). *Nursing outcomes classification (NOC)* (2nd ed.). St. Louis: Mosby.

Klainberg, M. (1999). Primary biliary cirrhosis. *American Journal of Nursing, 99*(12), 38–39.

Kuhn, M. A. (1999). *Complementary therapies for health care providers.* Philadelphia: Lippincott.

Lehne, R. A. (2001). *Pharmacology for nursing care* (4th ed.). Philadelphia: Saunders.

Malarkey, L.M., & McMorrow, M.E. (2000). *Nurse's manual of laboratory tests and diagnostic procedures* (2nd ed.). Philadelphia: Saunders.

Marx, J. F. (1998). Understanding the varieties of viral hepatitis. *Nursing, 28*(7), 43–49.

McCloskey, J. C., & Bulechek, G. M. (Eds.). (2000). *Nursing interventions classification (NIC)* (3rd ed.). St. Louis: Mosby.

Meeker, M. H., & Rothrock, J. C. (1999). *Alexander's care of the patient in surgery* (11th ed.). St. Louis: Mosby.

North American Nursing Diagnosis Association. (2001). *NANDA nursing diagnoses: Definitions & classification 2001–2002.* Philadelphia: NANDA.

Porth, C. M. (2002). *Pathophysiology: Concepts of altered health states* (6th ed.). Philadelphia: Lippincott.

Savage, R. B., Hussey, M. J., & Hurie, M. B. (2000). A successful approach to immunizing men who have sex with men against hepatitis B. *Public Health Nursing, 17*(3), 202–206.

Shovein, J. T., Damazo, R. J., & Hyams, I. (2000). Hepatitis A: How benign is it? *American Journal of Nursing, 100*(3), 43–47.

Springhouse. (1999). *Nurse's handbook of alternative & complementary therapies.* Springhouse, PA: Author.

Thorn, K. (1999). Hepatitis C: The lurking dragon. *Case Manager, 10*(4), 55–62.

Tierney, L. M., McPhee, S. J., & Papadakis, M. A. (2001). *Current medical diagnosis & treatment* (40th ed.). New York: Lange Medical Books/McGraw-Hill.

Urden, L. D., Stacy, K. M., & Lough, M. E. (2002). *Thelan's critical care nursing: Diagnosis and management* (4th ed.). St. Louis: Mosby

Wilkinson, J. M. (2000). *Nursing diagnosis handbook with NIC interventions and NOC outcomes* (7th ed.). Upper Saddle River, NJ: Prentice Hall Health.

Williamson, L. (1998). Self-destruction in the pancreas. *Nursing Times, 94*(29), 57–59.

Wrobleski, D. M., Barth, M. M., & Oyen, L. J. (1999). Necrotizing pancreatitis: Pathophysiology, diagnosis, and acute care management. *AACN Clinical Issues, 10*(4), 464–477.

ELIMINATION PATTERNS

Unit 6
Responses to Altered Bowel Elimination

Unit 7
Responses to Altered Urinary Elimination

Functional Health Patterns with Related Nursing Diagnoses

HEALTH PERCEPTION HEALTH MANAGEMENT
- Perceived health status
- Perceived health management
- Health care behaviors: health promotion and illness prevention activities, medical treatments, follow-up care

VALUE-BELIEF
- Values, goals, or beliefs (including spirituality) that guide choices or decisions
- Perceived conflicts in values, beliefs, or expectations that are health related

COPING-STRESS-TOLERANCE
- Capacity to resist challenges to self-integrity
- Methods of handling stress
- Support systems
- Perceived ability to control and manage situations

NUTRITIONAL-METABOLIC
- Daily consumption of food and fluids
- Favorite foods
- Use of dietary supplements
- Skin lesions and ability to heal
- Condition of the integument
- Weight, height, temperature

Part 3 Elimination Patterns NANDA Nursing Diagnoses
- Bowel Incontinence
- Constipation
- Perceived Constipation
- Risk for Constipation
- Diarrhea
- Impaired Urinary Elimination
- Functional Urinary Incontinence
- Reflex Urinary Incontinence
- Stress Urinary Incontinence
- Total Urinary Incontinence
- Urge Urinary Incontinence
- Risk for Urge Urinary Incontinence
- Urinary Retention
- Self-Care Deficit: Toileting

SEXUALITY-REPRODUCTIVE
- Satisfaction with sexuality or sexual relationships
- Reproductive pattern
- Female menstrual and perimeno-pausal history

ELIMINATION
- Patterns of bowel and urinary excretion
- Perceived regularity or irregularity of elimination
- Use of laxatives or routines
- Changes in time, modes, quality or quantity of excretions
- Use of devices for control

ROLE-RELATIONSHIP
- Perception of major roles, relationships, and responsibilities in current life situation
- Satisfaction with or disturbances in roles and relationships

ACTIVITY-EXERCISE
- Patterns of personally relevant exercise, activity, leisure, and recreation
- ADLs which require energy expenditure
- Factors that interfere with the desired pattern (e.g., illness or injury)

SELF-PERCEPTION–SELF-CONCEPT
- Attitudes about self
- Perceived abilities, worth, self-image, emotions
- Body posture and movement, eye contact, voice and speech patterns

SLEEP-REST
- Patterns of sleep and rest/relaxation in a 24-hr period
- Perceptions of quality and quantity of sleep and rest
- Use of sleep aids and routines

COGNITIVE-PERCEPTUAL
- Adequacy of vision, hearing, taste, touch, smell
- Pain perception and management
- Language, judgment, memory, decisions

RESPONSES TO ALTERED BOWEL ELIMINATION

Assessing Clients with Bowel Elimination Disorders

MediaLink

www.prenhall.com/lemone

Additional resources for this chapter can be found on the Student CD-ROM accompanying this textbook, and on the Companion Website at www.prenhall.com/lemone. Click on Chapter 23 to select the activities for this chapter.

CD-ROM
- Audio Glossary
- NCLEX Review

Companion Website
- More NCLEX Review
- Functional Health Pattern Assessment
- Case Study
    Irritable Bowel Syndrome

LEARNING OUTCOMES

After completing this chapter, you will be able to:

- Review the anatomy and physiology of the small and large intestines.

- Explain the physiologic processes involved in bowel elimination.

- Identify specific topics for consideration during a health history interview of the client with problems of bowel elimination.

- Describe physical assessment techniques of bowel function.

- Identify manifestations of impairment of bowel function.

After foods are eaten and broken down into usable elements, nutrients are absorbed and indigestible materials are eliminated. Bowel elimination is the end process in digestion. This chapter describes the structure and function of the large intestine, including the rectosigmoid region and the anus, as well as the assessment of bowel function. The anatomy and physiology of the small intestine are discussed more fully in Chapter 19; ⌘ the information in this chapter is provided as a base for understanding health problems from altered bowel function. In addition, this chapter discusses the function of the small intestine in the absorption of digested end products. Malabsorption (impaired absorption of nutrients) is discussed fully in Chapter 24. ⌘

REVIEW OF ANATOMY AND PHYSIOLOGY
The Small Intestine

The small intestine begins at the pyloric sphincter and ends at the ileocecal junction at the entrance of the large intestine. The small intestine is about 20 feet (6 m) long, but only about 1 inch (2.5 cm) in diameter. This long tube hangs in coils in the abdominal cavity, suspended by the mesentery and surrounded by the large intestine.

The small intestine has three regions: the duodenum, the jejunum, and the ileum. The duodenum begins at the pyloric sphincter and extends around the head of the pancreas for about 10 inches (25 cm). Both pancreatic enzymes and bile from the liver enter the small intestine at the duodenum. The jejunum is the middle region of the small intestine. It extends for about 8 feet (2.4 m). The ileum, the terminal end of the small intestine, is approximately 12 feet (3.6 m) long and meets the large intestine at the ileocecal valve.

Food is chemically digested and mostly absorbed as it moves through the small intestine. Circular folds (deep folds of the mucosa and submucosa layers), villi (fingerlike projections of the mucosa cells), and microvilli (tiny projections of the mucosa cells) all increase the surface area of the small intestine to enhance absorption of food. Although up to 10 L of food, liquids, and secretions enter the gastrointestinal tract each day, most is digested and absorbed in the small intestine; less than 1 L reaches the large intestine.

Enzymes in the small intestine break down carbohydrates, proteins, lipids, and nucleic acids.

- Pancreatic amylase acts on starches, converting them to maltose, dextrins, and oligosaccharides; the intestinal enzymes dextrinase, glucoamylase, maltase, sucrase, and lactase further break down these products into monosaccharides.
- Proteins are broken down into peptides by the pancreatic enzymes trypsin and chymotrypsin and by intestinal enzymes. Pancreatic enzymes (trypsin and chymotrypsin) and intestinal enzymes continue to break down proteins into peptides
- Pancreatic lipases break down lipids in the small intestine.
- Triglycerides enter as fat globules, and are then coated by bile salts and emulsified.
- Nucleic acids are hydrolyzed by pancreatic enzymes, then broken apart by intestinal enzymes.

Both pancreatic enzymes and bile are excreted into the duodenum in response to the secretion of secretin and cholecystokinin, hormones produced by the intestinal mucosa cells when chyme enters the small intestine.

Nutrients are absorbed through the mucosa of the intestinal villi into the blood or lymph by active transport, facilitated transport, and passive diffusion. Almost all food products and water, as well as vitamins and most electrolytes, are absorbed in the small intestine, leaving only indigestible fibers, some water, and bacteria to enter the large intestine.

The Large Intestine

The large intestine, or colon, begins at the ileocecal valve and terminates at the anus (Figure 23–1 ■). It is about 5 feet (1.5 m) long. The large intestine frames the small intestine on three sides and includes the cecum, the appendix, the colon, the rectum, and the anal canal.

The first section of the large intestine is the cecum. The appendix is attached to its surface as an extension. The appendix, a twisted structure in which bacteria can accumulate, may become inflamed.

The colon is divided into ascending, transverse, and descending segments. The ascending colon extends along the right side of the abdomen to the hepatic flexure, where it makes a right-angle turn. The next segment, called the transverse colon, crosses the abdomen to the splenic flexure. At this juncture, the descending colon descends down the left side of the abdomen and ends at the S-shaped sigmoid colon. The sigmoid colon terminates at the rectum.

The rectum is a mucosa-lined tube approximately 12 cm in length (Figure 23–2 ■). The rectum has three transverse folds (*valves of Houston*) that retain feces yet allow flatus to be passed through the anus. The rectum ends at the anal canal, which terminates at the anus.

The anus, a hairless, dark-skinned area, is the end of the digestive tract. It has both an internal involuntary sphincter and an external voluntary sphincter. The sphincters are usually open only during defecation. The anorectal junction separates the rectum from the anal canal and may be the site of internal hemorrhoids (clusters of dilated veins in swollen anal tissue).

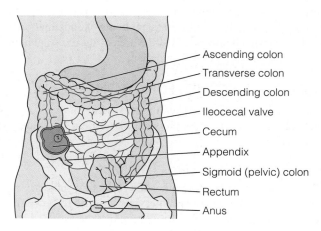

Ascending colon
Transverse colon
Descending colon
Ileocecal valve
Cecum
Appendix
Sigmoid (pelvic) colon
Rectum
Anus

Figure 23–1 ■ Anatomy of the large intestine.

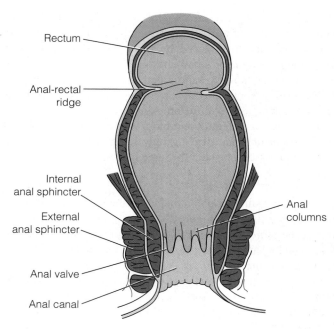

Figure 23–2 ■ Structure of the rectum and anus.

The major function of the large intestine is to eliminate indigestible food residue from the body. The large intestine absorbs water, salts, and vitamins formed by the food residue and bacteria. The semiliquid chyme that passes through the ileocecal valve is formed into feces as it moves through the large intestine. Feces are moved along the intestine by peristalsis, waves of alternating contraction and relaxation. Goblet cells lining the large intestine secrete mucus that facilitates the lubrication and passage of feces.

The defecation reflex is initiated when feces enter the rectum and stretch the rectal wall. This spinal cord reflex causes the walls of the sigmoid colon to contract and the anal sphincters to relax. This reflex can be suppressed by voluntary control of the external sphincter. Closing the glottis and contracting the diaphragm and abdominal muscles to increase intra-abdominal pressure facilitates expulsion of feces; this movement is called *Valsalva's maneuver.* Prolonged suppression of defecation can result in a weakened reflex that may in turn lead to *constipation* (infrequent and often uncomfortable passage of hard, dry stool). Frequent bouts of constipation may lead to external hemorrhoids at the area of the external hemorrhoidal plexus.

ASSESSING BOWEL FUNCTION

The nurse conducts both a health assessment interview (to collect subjective data) and a physical assessment (to collect objective data).

Health Assessment Interview

This section provides guidelines for collecting subjective data through a health assessment interview specific to bowel function. Problems with bowel elimination may be assessed as part of a health screening, may focus on a chief complaint (such as abdominal pain or change in bowel patterns), or may be part of a total health assessment. The assessment of bowel sounds is a common part of routine assessments.

Clients may feel embarrassed and hesitant to provide information about bowel elimination patterns. To promote effective rapport, remain nonjudgmental and ask for less personal information first.

If the client has a health problem involving bowel function, analyze its onset, characteristics and course, severity, precipitating and relieving factors, and any associated symptoms, noting the timing and circumstances. For example, ask the client:

- Can you describe the type of cramping and abdominal pain you are experiencing?
- Have you ever had bleeding from your rectum?
- Have you noticed increased constipation since your surgery?

Begin the interview by inquiring about any medical conditions that may influence the client's bowel elimination pattern, such as a stroke or spinal cord impairment, inflammatory gastrointestinal diseases, endocrine disorders, and allergies. Note any recent travel to other countries. Information about the client's psychosocial history is also important. Assess the client's lifestyle for any patterns of psychologic stress and/or depression, which may alter bowel elimination patterns. Depression may be associated with constipation, whereas *diarrhea* (frequent passage of loose, watery stools) may occur in situations of high stress and anxiety. Explore the client's activities of daily living, including exercise, sleep-rest patterns, and dietary and fluid intake. Changes in activities of daily living can influence bowel elimination patterns.

Determine whether the client has had any lower abdominal pain or rectal pain, which may be associated with a distended colon filled with gas or fluid. Crampy, colicky pains occur with diarrhea and/or constipation. Sudden onset of lower abdominal cramping occurs in obstruction of the colon. Left lower abdominal pain is associated with diverticulitis. Rectal pain may occur with stool retention and/or hemorrhoids.

Ask the client to describe the frequency and character of the stools. Ask about any history of diarrhea, constipation, or bleeding from the rectum, and collect information about the use of laxatives, suppositories, or enemas. Anticholinergic drugs, antihistamines, tranquilizers, or narcotics may cause constipation.

If the client has an **ostomy** (surgical opening into the bowel), ask about skin care problems, consistency of stool, foods that cause problems, the number of times that the client empties the appliance bag each day, and irrigation habits. Finally, explore the client's feelings about the appliance.

To obtain information about the client's nutritional status, ask about changes in weight, appetite, food preferences, food intolerances, special diets, and any cultural or ethnic influences on dietary intake. Ask whether the client is experiencing nausea and vomiting; if so, determine any relation to food intake, and ask the client to describe character of the emesis. In addition, ask about indigestion, the use of antacids or other over-the-counter medications, herbal preparations, and episodes of diarrhea and its character.

Explore any family history of colon cancer, colitis, gallbladder disease, or malabsorption syndromes, such as lactose intolerance and celiac sprue. Assess the client's risk factors for cancer, including age greater than 50; family member with colon cancer; history of endometrial, ovarian, or breast cancer; and previous diagnoses of colon inflammation, polyps, or cancer.

Other questions and leading statements, categorized by functional health patterns, can be found on the Companion Website.

Physical Assessment

The function of the bowels is assessed through a rectal examination, an anal examination, and examination of the client's stool. A complete assessment also includes inspection of the abdomen and auscultation of bowel sounds. Guidelines for abdominal assessment and assessment of bowel sounds are outlined in Chapter 19. ∞

Physical assessment of the abdomen may be performed as part of a total health assessment, in combination with assessment of the urinary and reproductive systems (problems which may cause clinical manifestations similar to those of the gastrointestinal system), or alone for clients with known or suspected health problems. The techniques of inspection, auscultation, percussion, and palpation are used. Palpation is the last method used in assessing the abdomen, because pressure on the abdominal wall and contents may interfere with bowel sounds and cause pain, ending the examination.

Necessary equipment includes water-soluble lubricant, material for testing the stool, and disposable gloves for the examiner. Ask the client to empty the bladder before the examination and lie in the supine position. Have the client turn to the left lateral (Sims') position for the rectal examination. The older client or the client with limited mobility may need assistance in assuming this position.

Explain what will happen during the examination, and encourage the client to take deep, regular breaths to increase relaxation. Explain that during the examination, it may feel as though the client is about to have a bowel movement and that sometimes flatus (gas) is passed. Assure the client that this is normal. Ensure that the examination area is private and the client is draped properly to prevent unnecessary exposure.

Abdominal Assessment with Abnormal Findings (✓)

- Inspect the abdomen.
  - ✓ Retention of flatus (gas) or stool may cause generalized abdominal distention.
  - ✓ Malnutrition causes a scaphoid (concave) abdomen.
- Auscultate the four quadrants of the abdomen with the diaphragm of the stethoscope. Begin in the lower right quadrant, where bowel sounds are almost always present. Normal bowel sounds (gurgling or clicking) occur every 5 to 15 seconds. Listen for at least 5 minutes in each of the four quadrants to confirm the absence of bowel sounds.
  - ✓ High-pitched, tinkling, rushing, or growling bowel sounds may be heard in the client who has diarrhea or who is experiencing the onset of a bowel obstruction.

  - ✓ Bowel sounds may be absent in later stages of a bowel obstruction or after surgery of the abdominal organs.

Perianal Assessment with Abnormal Findings (✓)

- Inspect the perianal area. Wearing gloves, spread the client's buttocks apart. Observe the area, and ask client to bear down as if they were trying to have a bowel movement.
  - ✓ Swollen, painful, longitudinal breaks in the anal area may appear in clients with anal fissures. (These are caused by the passing of large, hard stools, or by diarrhea.)
  - ✓ Dilated anal veins appear with hemorrhoids.
  - ✓ A red mass may appear with prolapsed internal hemorrhoids.
  - ✓ Doughnut-shaped red tissue at the anal area may appear with a prolapsed rectum.
- Palpate the anus and rectum. Lubricate the gloved index finger and ask the client to bear down. Touch the tip of your finger to the client's anal opening. Flex the index finger, and slowly insert it into the anus, pointing the finger towards the umbilicus (Figure 23–3 ■). Rotate the finger in both directions to palpate any lesions or masses. (The prostate or cervix may also be examined at this time. See Chapter 46.) ∞
  - ✓ Movable, soft masses may be polyps.
  - ✓ Hard, firm, irregular embedded masses may indicate carcinoma.

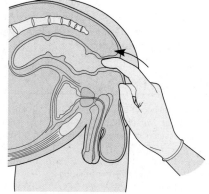

Figure 23–3 ■ Digital examination of the anus and rectum.

BOX 23–1 ■ Assessing Stool Characteristics

Inspect feces for color, odor, and consistency after the rectal exam or after defecation. Both hands are gloved.

COLOR

■ Blood *on* the stool results from bleeding from the sigmoid colon, anus, or rectum. Blood *within* the stool indicates bleeding from the colon due to ulcerative colitis, diverticulosis, or tumors. Black, tarry stools, called **melena,** occur with upper gastrointestinal bleeding. Oral iron may turn stools black and mask melena.

■ Grayish or whitish stools can result from biliary tract obstruction due to lack of bile in stool.

■ Greasy, frothy, yellow stools, called **steatorrhea,** may appear with fat malabsorption.

ODOR

■ Distinct, foul odors may be noted with stools containing blood or extra fat or in cases of colon cancer.

CONSISTENCY

■ Hard stools or long, flat stools may result from a spastic colon or bowel obstruction due to a tumor or hemorrhoids. Hard stools may also result from ingestion of oral iron.

■ Mucousy, slimy feces may indicate inflammation and occur in irritable bowel syndrome.

■ Watery, diarrhea stools appear with malabsorption problems, irritable bowel syndrome, emotional or psychologic stress, ingestion of spoiled foods, or lactose intolerance.

Fecal Assessment with Abnormal Findings (✓)

• Inspect the client's feces. After palpating the rectum, withdraw your finger gently. Inspect any feces on the glove. Note color and/or presence of blood. Also use gloved fingers to note consistency.

   ✓ See Box 23–1 for information about stool characteristics.

• Test the feces for occult blood. Use a commercial testing kit.

   ✓ A positive occult blood test requires further testing for colon cancer or gastrointestinal bleeding due to peptic ulcers, ulcerative colitis, or diverticulosis.

• Note the odor of the feces.

   ✓ Distinctly foul odors may be noted with stools containing blood or extra fat or in cases of colon cancer.

EXPLORE MediaLink

NCLEX review questions, case studies, care plan activities, MediaLink applications, and other interactive resources for this chapter can be found on the Companion Website at www.prenhall.com/lemone.

Click on Chapter 23 to select the activities for this chapter. For animations, video clips, more NCLEX review questions, and an audio glossary, access the Student CD-ROM accompanying this textbook.

TEST YOURSELF

1. What is the major function of the large intestine?
   a. To produce hormones necessary to digest food
   b. To break down lipids, proteins, and carbohydrates
   c. To secrete bile into the small intestine
   d. To eliminate undigested food residue

2. The appendix is attached to the surface of what segment of the large intestine?
   a. Cecum
   b. Ascending colon
   c. Transverse colon
   d. Rectum

3. Which of the following questions or statements would be appropriate for the client with an ostomy?

   a. "Have you had any bleeding from your hemorrhoids?"
   b. "Has your appetite changed lately?"
   c. "Tell me about your family."
   d. "Describe the consistency of your stools."

4. What assessment technique is used to assess bowel sounds?
   a. Inspection
   b. Palpation
   c. Percussion
   d. Auscultation

5. What term is used to describe black, tarry stools?
   a. Occult blood
   b. Hematemesis
   c. Melena
   d. Steatorrhea

See Test Yourself answers in Appendix C.

BIBLIOGRAPHY

Dammel, T. (1997). Fecal occult-blood testing: Looking for hidden danger. *Nursing97, 27*(7), 44–45.

Goff, K. (1997). Assessment of the gastrointestinal tract. *Support Line, 19*(2), 3–7.

Hall, G., Karstens, M., Rakel, B., Swanson, E., & Davidson, A. (1995). Managing constipation using a research-based protocol. *MEDSURG Nursing, 4*(1), 11–18.

Kirton, C. (1997). Assessing bowel sounds. *Nursing97, 27*(3), 64.

Langan, J. (1998). Abdominal assessment in the home: From A to Zzz. *Home Healthcare Nurse, 16*(1), 50–58.

Lyneham, J. (2001). Physical examination (abdomen, thorax and lungs): A review. *Australian Journal of Advanced Nursing, 18*(3), 31.

Watson, R. (2001). Assessing the gastrointestinal tract in older people. 2: The lower GI tract. *Nursing Older People, 13*(1), 27–28.

Weber, J., & Kelley, J. (2002). *Health assessment in nursing* (2nd ed.). Philadelphia: Lippincott.

Wilson, S., & Giddens, J. (2001). *Health assessment for nursing practice* (2nd ed.). St. Louis: Mosby.

Wright, J. (1997). Seven abdominal assessment signs every emergency nurse should know. *Journal of Emergency Nursing, 23*(5), 446–450.

Nursing Care of Clients with Bowel Disorders

MediaLink

www.prenhall.com/lemone
Additional resources for this chapter can be found on the Student CD-ROM accompanying this textbook, and on the Companion Website at www.prenhall.com/lemone. Click on Chapter 24 to select the activities for this chapter.

CD-ROM
- Audio Glossary
- NCLEX Review

Companion Website
- More NCLEX Review
- Case Study
  Irritable Bowel Syndrome
- Care Plan Activity
  Irritable Bowel Syndrome
- MediaLink Application
  Crohn's Disease

After completing this chapter, you will be able to:

- Relate the effects and manifestations of bowel disorders to normal physiology and assessment findings (Chapter 23).

- Discuss the pathophysiology, manifestations, and management of bowel absorption and elimination disorders.

- List diagnostic tests used to identify disorders of the small and large bowel.

- Discuss the nursing implications of medications used in managing bowel absorption and elimination disorders.

- Discuss care of clients with a colostomy or ileostomy.

- Provide appropriate nursing care for the client before and after intestinal surgery.

- Provide appropriate teaching for clients with bowel absorption and elimination disorders and their families.

- Use the nursing process as a framework for providing individualized care to clients with disorders of bowel absorption and elimination.

Disorders of intestinal absorption and bowel elimination can affect health, comfort, and well-being. Bowel function can be affected by inflammations, infections, tumors, obstructions, or changes in structure.

Clients with intestinal disorders often face extensive diagnostic testing, surgery, and permanent changes in physical appearance and lifestyle. Nursing care is directed toward meeting the client's physiologic needs, providing emotional support, and educating the client to adapt to changes in lifestyle.

DISORDERS OF INTESTINAL MOTILITY

Few body functions respond as readily to internal and external influences as the process of defecation. Factors affecting the gastrointestinal (GI) tract directly, such as food intake and bacterial population, affect the number and consistency of stools. Indirect factors, such as psychologic stress or voluntary postponement of defecation, also affect elimination.

In modern society, "normal" bowel elimination patterns vary widely. For some clients, two to three stools per day is the usual pattern. Others may normally have as few as three stools per week. It is important to evaluate each client's elimination pattern against his or her own normal pattern.

THE CLIENT WITH DIARRHEA

Diarrhea is an increase in the frequency, volume, and fluid content of the stool. In diarrhea, the water content of feces is increased, usually due to either malabsorption or water secretion in the bowel. It is a symptom rather than a primary disorder.

Diarrhea may be acute or chronic. Acute diarrhea, which usually lasts less than a week, is usually due to an infectious agent. Chronic diarrhea (diarrhea that persists longer than 3 to 4 weeks) may be caused by inflammatory bowel disorders, malabsorption, or even endocrine disorders.

PATHOPHYSIOLOGY

About 1500 mL of digested material enters the large intestine daily. Most of the water and some of the solutes are reabsorbed in the bowel, leaving only about 200 mL of feces to be eliminated.

Large volume diarrhea, characterized by both increased numbers and volume of stools, is caused by increased water content of the stool. This increased water content may result from either osmotic or secretory processes. Water may be pulled into the bowel lumen by osmosis when the feces contains osmotically active molecules. Some stool softeners and laxatives work on this principle. When the lactose in milk is not broken down and absorbed, the lactose molecules exert an osmotic draw, causing diarrhea. The diarrhea associated with cholera and *Escherichia coli* infection is caused by increased water secretion in the small and large intestines. Unabsorbed dietary fat, some cathartics and other drugs, and other factors can cause secretory diarrhea.

Small volume diarrhea, characterized by frequent small stools, is usually caused by inflammation or disease of the colon. Diseases that affect the intestinal mucosa, such as inflammatory bowel disease, cause an exudative diarrhea. The mucosal inflammation causes plasma, serum proteins, blood, and mucus to accumulate in the bowel, increasing fecal bulk and fluidity. An increased rate of propulsion within the bowel can also decrease the amount of water normally absorbed from the chyme, leading to diarrhea. For this reason, laxatives that increase bowel motility and bowel resection or bypass can lead to diarrhea.

MANIFESTATIONS AND COMPLICATIONS

The manifestations of diarrhea depend on its cause, duration, and severity, as well as the area of bowel affected and the client's general health. Diarrhea can present as several large, watery stools daily, or very frequent small stools that contain blood, mucus, or exudate.

Diarrhea can have devastating effects. Water and electrolytes are lost in diarrheal stool. This can lead to dehydration, particularly in the very young, the older adult, or the debilitated client unable to respond to thirst. With severe diarrhea, vascular collapse and hypovolemic shock may occur. Potassium and magnesium are lost, potentially leading to hypokalemia and hypomagnesemia. The loss of bicarbonate in the stool can lead to metabolic acidosis. See Chapter 5 ⟨⟩ for further discussion of the effects of these imbalances.

COLLABORATIVE CARE

Management of diarrhea focuses on identifying and treating the underlying cause. In addition, the diarrhea itself may need to be treated to promote comfort and to prevent complications. The history (including the onset and associated circumstances of the diarrhea) and physical examination often provide enough information to identify its cause.

Diagnostic Tests

The following laboratory and diagnostic tests may be ordered to help identify the cause of diarrhea.

- *Stool specimen* is obtained for gross and microscopic examination. Gross examination includes volume and water content, and the presence of any blood, pus, mucus, or excess fat. Microscopic examination evaluates the presence of WBCs, unabsorbed fat, and parasites. WBCs in the stool may indicate a bacterial infection or mucosal ulceration. Because parasites, ova, or larvae may not be continuously present in stool, a series of three specimens, spaced 2 to 3 days apart, is obtained when parasitic infection is suspected.

- *Stool culture* is ordered when an enteric pathogen is suspected (e.g., for persistent or bloody diarrhea accompanied by fever and/or recent travel out of the country).
- *Serum electrolytes, serum osmolality,* and *arterial blood gases* may be ordered to assess for adverse effects of diarrhea. Increased serum osmolality indicates water loss and dehydration. Other potential imbalances include hypokalemia, hypomagnesemia, and metabolic acidosis as a result of diarrhea. The serum sodium may be increased or decreased, depending on the type of diarrhea.
- *Sigmoidoscopy* allows direct examination of the bowel mucosa. Stool may also be obtained during sigmoidoscopy for microscopic examination. The preparation and teaching for a client undergoing sigmoidoscopy is in the box below.
- *Tissue biopsy* may be performed to identify chronic inflammatory processes, infection, and other causes of diarrhea. For biopsy, a small section of tissue (which may include the mucosal and muscle layers) is removed and examined for gross microscopic and histologic (cell character) changes.

Nursing Implications for Diagnostic Tests

Sigmoidoscopy

Client Preparation

- Ensure the presence of a signed informed consent form.
- Generally, clear liquid or a light diet is ordered for the evening before the procedure.
- Instruct to take a laxative.
- Administer an enema or rectal suppository before the procedure as ordered.

Client and Family Teaching

Before Procedure

- The procedure takes approximately 15 minutes.
- A mild sedative or tranquilizer may be given during the procedure.
- You may be positioned on your left side or in the knee-chest position.
- The scope will be inserted through the anus into the sigmoid colon.
- Feces may be suctioned.
- A biopsy may be taken. Polyps may be removed.
- Taking deep breaths when you feel discomfort may help you relax.

After Procedure

- Sit up slowly to avoid dizziness or lightheadedness.
- You may pass large amounts of flatus if air was instilled into the bowel.
- Report any abdominal pain, fever, chills, or rectal bleeding.
- If a polyp is removed, avoid heavy lifting for 7 days, and avoid high-fiber foods for 1 to 2 days.

Medications

Antidiarrheal medications are used sparingly or not at all until the cause of diarrhea has been identified. In diarrhea associated with botulism or bacillary dysentery, giving an antidiarrheal agent can worsen or prolong the disease by slowing elimination of the toxin from the bowel. Once the underlying cause for diarrhea has been established, specific medications may be ordered to treat the underlying cause. Antibiotics are used with caution because they alter the normal bacterial population of the bowel and may actually worsen diarrhea. A balanced electrolyte solution may be required to replace fluid losses. Intravenous or oral potassium preparations may also be prescribed.

Opium and some of its derivatives, anticholinergics, absorbants, and demulcents are commonly used as antidiarrheal preparations. Specific preparations, their method of action, and the nursing implications for these medications are outlined in the box below and on the following page.

Medication Administration

Antidiarrheal Preparations

ABSORBANTS AND PROTECTANTS

Kaolin and pectin (Kaopectate, Donnagel-MB), Charcoal
Bismuth subsalicylate (Pepto-Bismol)

Absorbant preparations act locally in the intestines to bind substances that can cause diarrhea. Absorbants are safe and are generally available over the counter. Their efficacy has not been proved, although bismuth subsalicylate has been shown to be somewhat effective in preventing and managing traveler's diarrhea, usually related to contaminated water supplies. Bismuth salts also have a protective and antimicrobial effect.

Nursing Responsibilities

- Assess for contraindications to antidiarrheal therapy, such as some infections or chronic inflammatory bowel disease, including ulcerative colitis.
- If fever is present, check with physician before giving the medication.
- Administer these medications at least 1 hour before or 2 hours after other oral medications; they may interfere with the absorption of other drugs.
- Observe the client's response to the medication. Constipation is a potential problem.

Client and Family Teaching

- Take the recommended dosage at the onset of diarrhea and after each loose stool.
- Do not take any of these preparations for more than 48 hours. If diarrhea persists, notify the physician.
- Do not give antidiarrheal medications to debilitated older clients without physician supervision.
- Chew bismuth subsalicylate tablets, rather than swallowing them whole, for maximal effectiveness. This medication may cause harmless darkening of the tongue and stool.
- If you are allergic to aspirin, use bismuth subsalicylate with caution; as a general rule, avoid taking aspirin while taking bismuth subsalicylate.

(continued on page 620)

Medication Administration

Antidiarrheal Preparations (continued)

OPIUM AND OPIUM DERIVATIVES

Camphorated tincture of opium (Paregoric)
Tincture of opium (laudanum, opium tincture)
Difenoxin (Motofen)
Diphenoxylate (Lomotil, Lotrol, others)
Loperamide hydrochloride (Imodium)

Opium and its derivatives act on the central nervous system (CNS) to decrease the motility of the ileum and colon, slowing transit time and promoting more water absorption. They also decrease the sensation of a full rectum and increase anal sphincter tone. Paregoric and tincture of opium have a greater potential for abuse and are prescription drugs subject to controls under the federal Controlled Substance Act of 1970. Difenoxin, diphenoxylate, and loperamide are derivatives of opium with few analgesic, euphoric, or abuse-promoting effects and are in more common use today.

Nursing Responsibilities

- Assess for contraindications to antidiarrheal or narcotic medications prior to giving these drugs.
- Administer paregoric undiluted with water.
- Do not administer difenoxin and diphenoxylate to clients receiving monoamine oxidase inhibitors (MAOI); hypertensive crises may occur.
- Observe closely for increased effects of other CNS depressants, such as alcohol, narcotic analgesics, or barbiturate sedatives.
- Observe for abdominal distention; toxic megacolon may occur if these drugs are given to the client with ulcerative colitis.

Client and Family Teaching

- Take the medication as recommended at the onset of diarrhea and after each loose stool.

- These drugs may be habit forming, use for no more than 48 hours.
- Avoid using alcohol and over-the-counter cold preparations while taking these drugs.
- These preparations may cause drowsiness, avoid driving or operating machinery while taking them.

ANTICHOLINERGICS

Atropine
Belladonna alkaloids (Donnagel, Donnatal)

Anticholinergic medications reduce bowel spasticity and acid secretion in the stomach. They are used to treat diarrhea that is associated with peptic ulcer disease and irritable bowel syndrome. These are nonspecific drugs; their systemic effects are their major drawback.

Nursing Responsibilities

- Assess for contraindications to atropine and other anticholinergic medications: glaucoma, prostatic hypertrophy, and gastrointestinal or genitourinary obstruction.
- Observe for side effects, such as eye pain, impaired urination, or constipation.

Client and Family Teaching

- Take only as directed, stop the drug and notify the physician if you develop eye pain, impaired urination, constipation.
- Do not operate machinery while taking this medication; drowsiness may occur.
- Hard candies help relieve oral dryness associated with these preparations.

Dietary Management

Fluid replacement is of primary importance in managing the client with diarrhea. If the client is able to tolerate oral fluids (i.e., if the client is not experiencing nausea and vomiting), an oral glucose/balanced electrolyte solution provides the best fluid replacement. Commercial preparations such as Gatorade and other sports drinks are available, as are pediatric solutions (e.g., Pedialyte), which can be used for adults as well as children. A solution of 5 mL (1 teaspoon) each of table salt and baking soda and 4 teaspoons (20 mL) of granulated sugar added with desired flavoring (such as lemon extract or juice) to 1 quart (1 L) of water can be made at home to replace water and electrolytes.

Solid food is withheld in the first 24 hours of acute diarrhea to rest the bowel. After that time, frequent, small, soft feedings can be added. Milk and milk products are added last, because the lactose they contain frequently aggravates the diarrhea. Raw fruits and vegetables, fried foods, bran, whole-grain cereals, condiments, spices, coffee, and alcoholic beverages are avoided during the recovery period.

Clients with chronic diarrhea may benefit by eliminating specific foods from the diet (see the Meeting Individual Needs box on page 621). Foods and nonfood substances that may aggravate diarrhea are outlined in Table 24–1. The diet should be high in calories and nutritional value. Vitamin supplements

TABLE 24–1 Foods That May Aggravate Chronic Diarrhea

Foods	Reason
Milk, ice cream, yogurt, soft cheeses, cottage cheese	Contain lactose; not tolerated by clients with lactase deficiency who cannot digest lactose.
Apple juice, pear juice, grapes, honey, dates, nuts, figs, fruit-flavored soft drinks	Contain fructose; when consumed in large quantities, fructose may not be totally absorbed, causing an osmotic draw of fluid into the bowel.
Table sugar	Contains sucrose; not tolerated by clients with sucrase deficiency.
Apple juice, pear juice, sugarless gums and mints	May contain sorbitol or mannitol, sugars that are not absorbed and can cause osmotic draw.
Antacids	Magnesium-containing antacids decrease bowel transit time and contain poorly absorbed salts that can exert an osmotic draw.
Coffee, tea, cola drinks, over-the-counter analgesics	Contain caffeine, which can decrease bowel transit time.

Meeting Individualized Needs

LACTOSE INTOLERANCE

The enzyme lactase is necessary to digest and absorb lactose, or "milk sugar," a disaccharide found in milk. Lactase deficiency is common in adults; only about 30% of people worldwide are able to efficiently digest and absorb lactose throughout their lives. Lactose intolerance is common in Native North Americans and Southeast Asians. Scandinavians and other northern Europeans have the lowest incidence of lactose intolerance (Whitney & Rolfes, 2002).

may be necessary, particularly the fat-soluble vitamins (A, D, E, and K). Clients with severe chronic diarrhea may require parenteral nutrition (see Chapter 20 ⊙).

Complementary Therapies

Herbal or homeopathic therapies may be used to help relieve diarrhea. Herbal treatments may include a strong tea of black pepper, chamomile, coriander, rosemary, sandalwood, or thyme. Homeopathic practitioners may use podophyllum tablets to treat diarrhea (Fontaine, 2000). Refer the client to a qualified practitioner for more information about using complementary therapies to treat diarrhea.

NURSING CARE

Health Promotion

Teach all clients about the importance of handwashing as a measure to prevent the spread of infectious diseases, including those that cause diarrhea. Teach safe food handling techniques to prevent bacterial contamination, and discuss measures to ensure safe drinking water. For clients planning to travel outside the United States or to wilderness areas, teach measures to purify water for drinking and cooking.

Assessment

The nursing assessment can help identify the cause of the client's diarrhea, as well as early signs of complications. Collect the following assessment data.

- Health history: duration and extent of diarrhea; associated symptoms; dietary intake; recent travel out of the country or to wilderness areas; previous history of diarrhea; chronic diseases; prescription and nonprescription medications
- Physical examination: vital signs (including orthostatic vitals); peripheral pulses; skin temperature, moisture, turgor; color and moisture of mucous membranes; abdominal contour and girth; bowel sounds; stool for obvious or occult blood, pus, mucus, or steatorrhea (bulky, foul-smelling stool)

Nursing Diagnoses and Interventions

Nursing care of the client with diarrhea focuses on identifying the cause, relieving the symptoms, preventing complications, and preventing the potential spread of infection to others.

Diarrhea

Nursing interventions for diarrhea focus helping the client recover a normal elimination pattern without adverse consequences.

- Monitor and record the frequency and characteristics of bowel movements *to provide a measure of the effectiveness of treatment.*
- Measure abdominal girth and auscultate bowel sounds every 8 hours as indicated. *Loud, rushing bowel sounds (borborygmi) indicates increased peristalsis, and may be heard in clients with acute diarrhea. Diminished or absent bowel sounds may indicate a complication of treatment, such as constipation or toxic megacolon.*
- Use standard precautions, including gloves and handwashing. *Standard precautions help prevent the spread of infection to others.*
- Provide ready access to bathroom, commode, or bedpan. *The client may have little warning of the need to defecate. Easily accessed toileting facilities reduce the risk for soiling or injury.*
- Administer antidiarrheal medications as prescribed, *to promote comfort and prevent excess fluid loss.*
- Limit food intake if the diarrhea is acute, reintroducing solid foods slowly, in small amounts, *to allow the bowel to rest and mucosa to heal in acute diarrhea states.*

Risk for Deficient Fluid Volume

The increased water content of diarrheal stool places the client at risk for fluid deficit.

- Record intake and output; weigh daily; assess skin turgor, mucous membranes, and urine specific gravity every 8 hours. *These assessments help monitor fluid volume status.*

PRACTICE ALERT *Assess skin turgor over the sternum in the older adult. Loss of subcutaneous fat associated with aging makes skin turgor assessment on the arms less reliable.* ■

- Monitor vital signs, including orthostatic blood pressures. *Orthostatic hypotension is identified by a drop in BP of more than 10 mmHg and pulse increase of 10 BPM when changing from a lying to a sitting position or from a sitting to a standing position. It is an indicator of fluid volume deficit.*

PRACTICE ALERT *Institute safety precautions such as providing assistance when ambulating for the client with orthostatic hypotension. The fall in blood pressure with position changes can cause lightheadedness and syncope.* ■

- Provide fluid and electrolyte replacement solutions as indicated. Ensure ready access to fluids; assist the debilitated client with fluid intake. Notify the care provider if the client is unable to tolerate oral fluids. *Oral fluids are encouraged as tolerated to prevent dehydration. Intravenous fluids are necessary if oral fluids are not tolerated. An intake of 3000 mL per day or more is often needed to replace fluid losses.*

Risk for Impaired Skin Integrity

Decreased extracellular fluid volume and the irritating effects of diarrheal stool increase the risk for skin breakdown.

- Assist with cleaning the perianal area as needed. Use warm water, a gentle cleanser, and soft cloths. *Cleansing removes irritating substances in the stool. Gentle cleansing helps maintain integrity of dehydrated skin.*
- Apply protective ointment to the perianal area. *Moisture-barrier ointments or creams protect the skin from excoriation and help prevent tissue breakdown.*

Using NANDA, NIC, and NOC

Chart 24–1 shows links between NANDA nursing diagnoses, NIC, and NOC for the client with diarrhea.

Home Care

Acute and chronic diarrhea generally are managed by the client in the home. Teach the client and family members about the following subjects.

- Causes of diarrhea (as directed by the diagnosis)
- Importance of handwashing and hygiene measures
- Importance of maintaining adequate fluid intake to replace lost water and electrolytes
- Use of a balanced electrolyte solution such as Gatorade or a similar product (purchased or home prepared) for fluid replacement
- Recommendations to limit food intake during acute diarrhea, and resume gradually with small feedings of foods that have a constipating effect: applesauce, bananas, crackers, rice, potatoes
- To avoid foods high in fiber, milk products, and caffeine
- Ways to maintain nutrition if chronic diarrhea is a problem: frequent small meals, nutritional supplements, vitamin supplements
- Precautions and limitations of antidiarrheal preparations
- Importance of seeking medical intervention if diarrhea continues or recurs

THE CLIENT WITH CONSTIPATION

Constipation is defined as the infrequent (two or fewer bowel movements weekly) or difficult passage of stools. Constipation affects older adults more frequently than younger people. Recent studies indicate that approximately 20% to 35% of people over age 65 report recurrent constipation and laxative use. Although fecal transit in the large intestine slows with aging, the increased incidence of constipation is thought to relate more to impaired general health status, increased medication use, and decreased physical activity in the older adult.

PATHOPHYSIOLOGY AND MANIFESTATIONS

Constipation may be a primary problem or a symptom of another disease or condition. Acute constipation, a definite change in the bowel elimination pattern, often is caused by an organic process. A change in bowel patterns that persists or becomes more frequent or severe may be due to a tumor or other partial bowel obstruction. With chronic constipation, functional causes that impair storage, transport, and evacuation mechanisms impede the normal passage of stools. Common causes of constipation are listed in Table 24–2.

Psychogenic factors are the most frequent causes of chronic constipation. These factors include postponing defecation when the urge is felt, and the perception of satisfaction with defecation. Clients often abuse the use of laxatives and enemas to stimulate a bowel movement when constipation is perceived. Overuse of these measures can lead to real intestinal problems that worsen the condition. For example, *cathartic colon,* impaired colonic motility and changes in bowel structure, mimics ulcerative colitis in that the normal pouchlike or saccular appearance of the colon is lost. *Melanosis coli* is a brownish-black discoloration of the colon mucosa. Both conditions may be caused by long-term laxative use.

With significant constipation or long-term dependence on laxatives or enemas, **fecal impaction** may develop. Impaction

---

CHART 24–1 LINKS BETWEEN NANDA, NIC, AND NOC

The Client with Altered Bowel Motility

NURSING DIAGNOSES	NURSING INTERVENTIONS	NURSING OUTCOMES
• Diarrhea	• Diarrhea Management • Fluid / Electrolyte Management	• Bowel Elimination • Electrolyte and Acid-Base Balance • Fluid Balance
• Constipation	• Bowel Management • Constipation / Impaction Management	• Bowel Elimination • Symptom Control
• Bowel Incontinence	• Bowel Incontinence Care • Bowel Training • Perineal Care	• Bowel Continence • Tissue Integrity: Skin and Mucous Membranes

Note. Data from Nursing Outcomes Classification (NOC) by M. Johnson & M. Maas (Eds.), 1997, St. Louis: Mosby; Nursing Diagnoses: Definitions & Classification 2001–2002 by North American Nursing Diagnosis Association, 2001, Philadelphia: NANDA; Nursing Interventions Classification (NIC) by J.C. McCloskey & G. M. Bulechek (Eds.), 2000, St. Louis: Mosby. Reprinted by permission.

TABLE 24–2	Selected Causes of Constipation
Factor	**Related Cause**
Activity	Lack of exercise; bed rest
Dietary	Highly refined, low-fiber foods; inadequate fluid intake
Drugs	Antacids containing aluminum or calcium salts; narcotic analgesics; anticholinergics; many antidepressants, tranquilizers, and sedatives; antihypertensives, such as ganglionic blockers, calcium-channel blockers, beta-adrenergic blockers, and diuretics; iron salts
Large bowel	Diverticular disease, inflammatory disease, tumor, obstruction; changes in rectal or anal structure or function
Psychogenic	Voluntary suppression of urge; perceived need to defecate on schedule; depression
Systemic	Advanced age; pregnancy; neurologic conditions (trauma, multiple sclerosis, tumors, cerebrovascular accident, Parkinsonism); endocrine and metabolic disorders (hypothyroidism, hypercalcemia, uremia, porphyria)
Other	Chronic laxative or enema use

Nursing Implications for Diagnostic Tests

Barium Enema

Client Preparation

Ensure presence of a signed informed consent for the procedure.

- Provide or instruct to follow a clear liquid diet for 24 hours prior to the test. All food and fluids may be withheld for 8 hours prior to the test.
- Administer or instruct to use laxatives, enemas, or suppositories as ordered the evening prior to the procedure. Additional bowel preparation may be ordered for the morning just prior to the procedure.

Client and Family Teaching

Before Procedure
- The procedure takes approximately 1 hour.
- The barium will be instilled through a lubricated tube inserted into your rectum. You will experience a sensation of fullness, and may feel the need to defecate.
- You will be positioned on the left side, on your back, and prone during this procedure.
- A fluoroscope will be used to follow the progress of the barium, and X-rays will be taken.
- You will expel the barium in the bathroom.

After Procedure
- Following the procedure, a laxative will be given.
- The stools may be white for the next 1 to 2 days.

may also occur following barium administration for radiologic exam. The impaction is felt as a rock-hard or puttylike mass of feces in the rectum. Abdominal cramping and a full sensation in the rectal area may be manifestations of impaction. Watery mucus or liquid stool may be passed around the impaction, causing the client to complain of diarrhea.

COLLABORATIVE CARE

Initial evaluation of constipation is based on the history and physical examination. The abdomen may appear somewhat distended, and bowel sounds may be reduced. If an impaction is present, digital examination of the rectum reveals a palpable hard or puttylike fecal mass.

Simple or chronic constipation is treated with education (a daily bowel movement is not necessary for health), and modification of diet and exercise routines. If the problem is acute or does not resolve, further diagnostic examination may be ordered.

Diagnostic Tests

- *Serum electrolytes* and *thyroid function tests* may be done to identify metabolic and endocrine problems that may contribute to constipation.
- *Barium enema* may be ordered to evaluate bowel structure and to identify tumors or diverticular disease. Barium is instilled into the large intestine and X-rays are taken. Nursing care for the client undergoing a barium enema is described in the following box.

- *Sigmoidoscopy* or *colonoscopy* may also be used to evaluate constipation, particularly when the problem is acute and a tumor or obstruction is suspected. A flexible endoscope is used to inspect bowel mucosa and structure. Suspicious lesions may be biopsied at the time of the scope. See the box on page 624 for nursing care for the client having a colonoscopy.

Medications

Laxative and cathartic preparations to promote stool evacuation were among the earliest drugs. Milder preparations are generally known as laxatives; cathartics have a stronger effect. Most laxatives are appropriate only for short-term use. Cathartics and enemas interfere with normal bowel reflexes and should not be used for simple constipation. Laxatives should never be given if a bowel obstruction or impaction is suspected, nor to people with abdominal pain of undetermined origin (Tierney et al., 2001). When the bowel is obstructed, laxatives or cathartics may cause serious mechanical damage and perforate the bowel.

The only laxatives that are appropriate and safe for long-term use are bulking agents, such as psyllium seed, calcium polycarbophil, and methylcellulose. These agents act by increasing the bulk of the feces and drawing water into the bowel to soften it. Commonly prescribed laxatives and cathartics are discussed in the Medication Administration box on page 624.

Nursing Implications for Diagnostic Tests

Colonoscopy

Client Preparation
- Ensure presence of a signed informed consent for the procedure.
- A liquid diet may be prescribed for 2 days prior to the procedure, and the client is usually NPO for 8 hours just before the procedure.
- Administer or instruct the client in bowel preparation procedures such as taking citrate of magnesia or polyethylene glycol the evening before.
- Sedation is usually given during the procedure.

Client and Family Teaching

Before Procedure
- Explain dietary restrictions and their purpose.

- The procedure takes 30 minutes to 1 hour.
- The scope is inserted through the anus and advanced to the cecum.
- A biopsy may be taken, and polyps may be removed.
- Discomfort is minimal.
- Arrange for transportation as you may not be allowed to drive for 24 hours after the procedure.

After Procedure
- You may have increased flatus as air is instilled into the bowel during the procedure.
- Report any abdominal pain, chills, fever, rectal bleeding, or mucopurulent discharge.
- If a polyp has been removed, avoid heavy lifting for 7 days, and avoid high-fiber food for 1 to 2 days.

Medication Administration

Laxatives and Cathartics

BULK-FORMING AGENTS
> Bran
> Calcium polycarbophil (Fibercon)
> Methylcellulose (Citrucel)
> Psyllium hydrophilic mucilloid (Metamucil, Effer-Syllium)

Bulk-forming agents are the only safe laxatives for long-term use. They contain vegetable fiber, which is not digested or absorbed in the gut. This natural fiber creates bulk and draws water into the intestine, softening the stool mass.

Nursing Responsibilities
- Mix the agent with a full glass of cool liquid just prior to administering.
- Do not administer to clients with possible stool impaction or bowel obstruction.

Client and Family Teaching
- Drink at least 6 to 8 full glasses of nonalcoholic fluid per day. Adequate hydration is necessary to produce the drugs laxative effect.
- These agents may be mixed with water, milk, or fruit juice.
- Take the drug in the morning or with meals. To reduce the risk of impaction, do not take at bedtime.
- Because of the increased risk of impaction, check with the physician before increasing dietary fiber while you are taking these agents.

WETTING AGENTS
> Docusate (Colace, Surfak, Doxidan, others)

Wetting agents reduce stool surface tension and form an emulsion of fat and water, softening the stool. They are used primarily to prevent straining and reduce the discomfort of expelling hard stools.

Nursing Responsibilities
- Administer with ample fluids to promote softening effect.
- Wetting agents may alter the absorption of other drugs. Do not administer within 1 hour of other oral medications.

- Do not attempt to crush or open caplets; a liquid form is available for clients who cannot swallow pills or capsules.

Client and Family Teaching
- Do not use for more than 1 week or less unless specifically recommended by the physician.
- Take the medication in the morning or evening, but avoid taking it with other medications.
- Adequate fluid is necessary to obtain the beneficial effect of the drug. Drink 6 to 8 glasses of nonalcoholic fluid per day.

OSMOTIC AND SALINE LAXATIVES/CATHARTICS
> Lactulose (Rhodialose)
> Sorbitol
> Magnesium hydroxide (Milk of Magnesia)
> Magnesium citrate
> Polyethylene glycol (Klean-Prep)

Laxatives in this group contain poorly absorbed salts or carbohydrates that remain in the bowel, increasing osmotic pressure and drawing water into the intestine. Stool volume increases, consistency decreases, and peristalsis is stimulated. Many of these agents also have an irritant effect on the bowel, further stimulating peristalsis. They are used to stimulate rapid or complete bowel evacuation to relieve constipation and to prepare the bowel for diagnostic and surgical procedures. They should be limited to acute, short-term use; chronic use may suppress normal bowel reflexes.

Nursing Responsibilities
- Assess for possible contraindications to osmotic or saline laxatives, including bowel ulceration or obstruction, dehydration, electrolyte imbalances, heart failure (which may be aggravated by the sodium content), or renal failure.
- Administer with a full glass of liquid, preferably in the morning to avoid sleep disturbance.
- Monitor fluid and electrolyte status: skin turgor, mucous membranes, intake and output; daily weight, and laboratory studies, such as hemoglobin and hematocrit levels, serum osmolality and electrolytes, and urine specific gravity.

Medication Administration

Laxatives and Cathartics (continued)

Client and Family Teaching

- Do not use these agents on a routine basis to treat or prevent constipation.
- Chill the solution to increase its palatability.
- Expect some abdominal cramping.
- Use only as directed. Increase fluid intake to at least 6 to 8 glasses of nonalcoholic fluid.
- Notify the physician if adverse effects occur, including abdominal pain, bloody stool, excessive skin or mucous membrane dryness, rapid weight loss, dizziness, or other unusual symptoms.
- These agents work in 3 to 6 hours; take them in the morning or early evening to avoid sleep disturbance.

IRRITANT OR STIMULANT LAXATIVES

Bisacodyl (Dulcolax, Bisco-Lax, Carter's Liver Pills, Codylax, others)
Phenolphthalein (Evac-U-Gen, Evac-U-Lax, Feen-A-Mint, Phenolax, others)
Cascara sagrada
Senna (Senna laxative, Fletcher's Castoria)
Castor oil

Stimulant laxatives work by stimulating the motility and secretion of intestinal mucosa. Their use results in watery stool, often accompanied by abdominal cramping and pain. They are used to relieve constipation, although they should not be used as the initial treatment. Stimulant laxatives are also used for preparing the bowel for diagnostic testing.

Nursing Responsibilities

- Assess for potential contraindications to these laxatives, including abdominal pain and cramping, nausea and vomiting, anal or rectal fissures.
- Administer on an empty stomach to minimize the effects of food on its dissolution and absorption.
- Do not crush enteric-coated bisacodyl tablets or administer with alkaline products. This may hasten their dissolution in the stomach, leading to gastric distress.

Client and Family Teaching

- Discourage the use of this type of laxative, even in over-the-counter preparations, for the initial or continuing relief of constipation.
- Do not use the laxative for more than 1 week; chronic use can be habit forming and may suppress normal bowel reflexes.

- These laxatives are excreted in breast milk and should not be used by lactating women.
- Phenolphthalein-containing products may discolor the urine pink or red. Report possible hypersensitivity manifestations, such as difficulty breathing, dizziness or lightheadedness, or skin rashes, to the primary care provider, and stop taking the medication.

LUBRICANTS

Mineral oil

Mineral oil is the only lubricant laxative available. It acts by forming an oily coat on the fecal mass, preventing the reabsorption of water, and resulting in softer stool. Problems associated with the use of mineral oil as a laxative include reduced absorption of the fat-soluble vitamins A, D, E, and K; possible damage to the liver and spleen due to systemic absorption, and potential pneumonitis from aspiration of oil droplets into the lungs.

Nursing Responsibilities

- Assess for possible contraindications to use of mineral oil, including advanced age, preexisting lung disease, and hemorrhoids or other rectal lesions.
- Do not give mineral oil concurrently with wetting agents or stool softeners, because these increase the potential for systemic absorption and increase the effects of the mineral oil.
- Administer mineral oil in the evening before bedtime to reduce the effect on the absorption of fat-soluble vitamins and minimize the risk of aspiration.
- Assess for manifestations of vitamin deficiency. Monitor the client taking oral anticoagulants for evidence of increased bleeding, such as bleeding gums, easy bruising, or melena.

Client and Family Teaching

- Long-term use of mineral oil is not recommended because of its risks and adverse effects.
- Do not use mineral oil if hemorrhoids or rectal lesions are present, leakage of the oil through the anal sphincter may cause itching and interfere with healing.
- Suck on a lemon or orange slice after taking oral mineral oil to reduce the oily aftertaste.

Dietary Management

Foods that have a high fiber content are recommended. Vegetable fiber is largely indigestible and unabsorbable, so it increases stool bulk. Fiber also helps draw water into the fecal mass, softening the stool and making defecation easier. Raw fruits and vegetables are good sources of dietary fiber, as is cereal bran. Use 2 to 3 teaspoons of unprocessed bran with meals (sprinkled on fruit or cereal) or up to 1/4 cup daily to supply adequate fiber.

Fluids are also important to maintain bowel motility and soft stools. The client should drink 6 to 8 glasses of fluid per day.

In older adults, constipation may be due to inadaquate food intake. Carefully evaluate diet history and usual daily intake.

Enemas

Significant or chronic constipation or a fecal impaction may require the administration of an enema. As a general rule, enemas should be used only in acute situations and only on a short-term basis. They may also be ordered to prepare the bowel for diagnostic testing or examination. The following types of enemas may be prescribed.

- A saline enema using 500 to 2000 mL of warmed physiologic saline solution is the least irritating to the bowel.

- Tap-water enemas use 500 to 1000 mL of water to soften feces and irritate the bowel mucosa, stimulating peristalsis and evacuation.
- Soap-suds enemas consist of a tap-water solution to which soap is added as a further irritant.
- Phosphate enemas (e.g., Fleet) use a hypertonic saline solution to draw fluid into the bowel and irritate the mucosa, leading to evacuation.
- Oil retention enemas instill mineral or vegetable oil into the bowel to soften the fecal mass. The instilled oil is retained overnight or for several hours before evacuation.

The repeated use of enemas can lead not only to impaired bowel function, but also to fluid and electrolyte imbalances. Tap-water and phosphate enemas are particularly likely to cause these problems. In acute conditions with risk of bowel obstruction, perforation, ulceration, or other problem, enemas should not be administered until their safe use can be established.

NURSING CARE

Health Promotion

Education can prevent constipation. Teach clients the importance of maintaining a diet high in natural fiber. Foods such as fresh fruits, vegetables, whole-grain products, and bran provide natural fiber. Encourage reducing consumption of meats and refined foods, which are low in fiber and can be constipating. Emphasize the need to maintain a high fluid intake every day, particularly during hot weather and exercise. Discuss the relationship between exercise and bowel regularity. Encourage clients to engage in some form of exercise, such as walking daily.

Discuss normal bowel habits, and explain that a daily bowel movement is not the norm for all people. Encourage clients to respond to the urge to defecate when it occurs. Suggest setting aside a time, usually following a meal, for elimination.

Assessment

To assess the client with real or perceived constipation, collect the following data.

- Health history: usual and current pattern of defecation, including time of day, amount, and stool consistency; usual diet, fluid intake, and activity pattern; possible contributing factors such as narcotic analgesics, activity limitations, painful hemorrhoids, perianal surgery; chronic diseases such as endocrine or neurologic disorders; prescribed and nonprescription medications
- Physical examination: abdominal girth and shape, bowel sounds, tenderness, and percussion tone; digital exam of the rectum if impaction is suspected.

For discussion of constipation in the older adult see the box on this page.

Nursing Diagnoses and Interventions

Nursing interventions for the client with constipation focus chiefly on education.

Meeting Individualized Needs

THE OLDER ADULT

Constipation and perceived constipation are common problems in older adults. While constipation is not a normal consequence of aging, factors such as slowed peristalsis, lowered activity levels, reduced food and fluid intake, and decreased sensory perception contribute to the higher incidence of constipation seen in the elderly. Chronic diseases such as diabetes, mobility problems, and medications also increase the risk of constipation in older adults.

Cultural influences and advertising lead many older adults to believe that a daily bowel movement is important for health. This belief contributes to an increased incidence of perceived constipation in the elderly. Because of this perception, the older adult may come to rely on laxatives, suppositories, or enemas to facilitate regular bowel movements. These external aids to defecation can further impair the ability to maintain "normal" bowel habits: a movement of soft stool every 2 to 3 days.

Constipation

Whether real or perceived, constipation is disruptive to the client's activities of daily living (ADLs) and life satisfaction.

- Monitor pattern of defecation and stool consistency. *This information helps establish the client's usual pattern of defecation and differentiate between actual and perceived constipation.*
- Provide additional fluids to maintain an intake of at least 2500 mL per day. *A generous fluid intake helps maintain soft stool consistency and promote intestinal motility.*
- Encourage drinking a glass of warm water before breakfast. Provide time and privacy following breakfast for bowel elimination. *This helps develop a pattern of natural elimination; the warm water provides mild stimulation of bowel peristalsis.*
- Consult with the dietitian to provide a diet high in natural fiber unless contraindicated. Provide foods such as natural bran, prunes, or prune juice. *Natural fiber adds bulk to the stool and has a mild stimulant effect.*
- Encourage activities such as ambulation or chair exercises (range of motion, stretching, wheelchair lifts, etc.) as tolerated. *Activity stimulates peristalsis and strengthens abdominal muscles, facilitating elimination.*
- If indicated, consult with primary care provider about the use of bulk laxatives, stool softeners, or other laxatives as needed. *Laxatives may be necessary to relieve acute constipation. Clients with long-term activity or diet restrictions or impaired abdominal muscle strength may need a bulk-forming laxative to maintain normal elimination patterns and prevent constipation.*

Using NANDA, NIC, and NOC

See Chart 24–1 on page 622 for links between NANDA nursing diagnoses, NIC, and NOC for the client with constipation.

Home Care

Include the following topics when teaching for home care measures to prevent and treat constipation.

- Increasing dietary fiber intake by including fresh fruits and vegetables, whole grains, high-fiber breakfast cereals, and unprocessed bran in the diet (Bran can be sprinkled on cereals, mixed into bread or muffin recipes, or mixed with fruit juice to increase its palatability.)
- Maintaining fluid intake of 6 to 8 glasses of water per day (unless contraindicated)
- Suggestions for remaining physically active to promote bowel function and maintain muscle tone
- Responding to the urge to defecate when perceived
- Appropriate use of laxatives:
  - Do not use laxatives, suppositories, or enemas on a regular basis.
  - Bulk-forming agents provide insoluble fiber, and are safe for long-term use; it is important to drink at least 6 to 8 glasses of water daily when using these (or any) laxatives.
  - Other laxatives such as milk of magnesia, docusate (Colase, DSS, others), bisacodyl (Dulcolax, others), cascara, or castor oil should be used only occasionally to relieve constipation.
- The need to report any change in bowel habits such as new or persistent constipation or diarrhea, abdominal pain, black or bloody stools, nausea or anorexia, weakness, or unexplained weight loss to the primary care provider.

THE CLIENT WITH IRRITABLE BOWEL SYNDROME

Irritable bowel syndrome (IBS), also known as spastic bowel or functional colitis, is a motility disorder of the gastrointestinal tract. It is a functional disorder with no identifiable organic cause. IBS is often characterized by abdominal pain with constipation, diarrhea, or both.

Irritable bowel syndrome is common, affecting up to 20% of people in Western civilization. It usually affects young people, although may also be prevalent in older adults. Women are affected 2 to 3 times more frequently than men (Braunwald et al., 2001).

PATHOPHYSIOLOGY

In IBS, it appears that central nervous system (CNS) regulation of the motor and sensory functions of the bowel are altered. Clients with IBS often experience increased motor reactivity of the small bowel and colon in response to stimuli such as food intake, hormonal influences, and physiologic or psychologic stress. Sensory responses from the gut also are exaggerated in response to the movement of chime through the bowel (Braunwald et al., 2001). Hypersecretion of colonic mucus is a common feature of the syndrome.

Manifestations of Irritable Bowel Syndrome

- Abdominal pain
  - May be relieved by defecation
  - May be intermittent and colicky or dull and continuous
- Altered bowel elimination
  - Constipation
  - Diarrhea
  - Mucous stools
- Abdominal bloating and flatulence
- Abdominal tenderness, especially over sigmoid colon
- Possible nausea, vomiting

A lower visceral pain threshold is often found in clients with IBS. Clients may complain of pain, bloating, and distention when intestinal gas levels are normal.

Psychologic factors such as depression or anxiety have been linked to IBS; however, they have not been identified as causes of the disorder. Clients with underlying psychologic factors may be more likely to seek medical attention for symptoms, but normal psychologic profiles are noted in clients with the disorder who do not seek medical attention (Tierney et al., 2001). Recent research does indicate a correlation between emotional, physical, and sexual abuse and IBS. Again, however, causation could not be established.

MANIFESTATIONS

Irritable bowel syndrome is characterized by abdominal pain that often is relieved by defecation and a change in bowel habits (see the box above). The pain may be either colicky, occurring in spasms, or dull and continuous. Altered patterns of defecation may include:

- A change in frequency
- Abnormal stool form (hard or lumpy, loose or watery)
- Altered stool passage (straining, urgency, or a sensation of incomplete evacuation)
- Passage of mucus

The client may also complain of abdominal bloating and excess gas. Other manifestations include nausea, vomiting, and anorexia; fatigue, headache, depression, or anxiety. The abdomen is often tender to palpation, particularly over the sigmoid colon.

COLLABORATIVE CARE

Irritable bowel syndrome is diagnosed based on the presence of abdominal pain or discomfort that has two of the following three characteristics: (1) relieved by defecation; (2) associated with a change in frequency of elimination; (3) associated with a change in stool form (Tierney et al., 2001). Management is directed toward relieving manifestations and reducing or eliminating precipitating factors. Stress reduction measures, exercises, or counseling may benefit the client.

Diagnostic Tests

The primary purpose of diagnostic testing is to rule out other causes of abdominal pain and altered fecal elimination.

- *Stool* may be examined for *occult blood, ova and parasites,* and *culture.* A stool smear for WBCs may also be done; an elevated WBC count may indicate an inflammatory or infectious process.
- *Complete blood count (CBC) with differential* and *erythrocyte sedimentation rate (ESR)* are evaluated. Anemia may indicate blood loss and a possible tumor, polyps, or other organic problem. An elevated WBC may indicate bacterial infection, and an elevated ESR is seen with many inflammatory processes.
- *Sigmoidoscopy* or *colonoscopy* may be ordered to visually examine bowel mucosa, measure intraluminal pressures, and biopsy suspicious lesions. In IBS, the bowel appears normal, with increased mucus, marked spasm, and possible hyperemia (increased redness), but no suspicious lesions. Intraluminal pressures are often increased. The procedure itself may stimulate manifestations of the syndrome. Nursing care related to these procedures is found in the Nursing Implications boxes on pages 619 and 624.
- *Small bowel series (upper GI series with small bowel follow-through)* and *barium enema* may be ordered. For the small bowel series, an oral barium preparation is administered, and the small intestine is examined under fluoroscopy. With IBS, the entire GI tract may show increased motility. The box below outlines nursing care of the client undergoing a small bowel series. Nursing care of the client having a barium enema is described in the Nursing Implications box on page 623.

Medications

Although not curative, medications may be prescribed to manage the symptoms of IBS. Bulk-forming laxatives (such as bran, methylcellulose, or psyllium) may help reduce bowel spasm and normalize the number and form of bowel movements. An anticholinergic drug such as dicyclomine (Antispas, Bentyl, others) or hyoscyamine (Anaspaz, others) may be ordered to inhibit bowel motility by interfering with parasympathetic stimulation of the gastrointestinal tract. It relieves postprandial abdominal pain when given 30 to 60 minutes before meals. In clients with diarrhea, loperamide (Imodium) or diphenoxylate (Lomotil) may be used prophylactically to prevent diarrhea in selected situations.

New drugs that affect GI motility by altering serotonin receptors in the GI tract are being researched. The initial approved drug, alosetron, was later withdrawn from the market due to severe complications associated with its use.

Antidepressant drugs, including tricyclics and selective serotonin reuptake inhibitors (SSRIs), may help relieve abdominal pain associated with IBS. While the anticholinergic side effects of the tricyclics (such as desipramine [Norpramin] and imipramine [Tofranil]) may help decrease diarrhea, they have more adverse effects than SSRIs such as sertraline (Zoloft) and fluoxetine (Prozac).

Dietary Management

Many clients with IBS benefit from additional dietary fiber. Adding bran to meals provides added bulk and water content to the stool, reducing the incidence of both loose diarrheal stools and hard, constipated stools. Other dietary changes are specific to individual triggers for IBS symptoms. Some clients may benefit from limiting lactose, fructose, or sorbitol intake (see Table 24–1). When excess gas and flatulence is a problem, reducing the intake of gas-forming foods, such as beans, cabbage, apple and grape juices, nuts, and raisins, may be helpful. Caffeinated drinks, such as coffee, tea, and soft drinks, act as gastrointestinal stimulants; limiting intake of these fluids may also prove beneficial.

Complementary Therapies

Herbal preparations may provide some benefit for clients with IBS. Herbs with an antispasmotic effect, such as anise, chamomile, peppermint, and sage, may be used to reduce the manifestations of IBS. Refer the client to a certified herbologist or naturopathic physician for treatment.

Nursing Implications for Diagnostic Tests

Small Bowel Series

Client Preparation

- Ensure the presence of a signed informed consent for the procedure.
- A low-residue diet may be ordered for 48 hours preceding the examination, and a tap-water enema or cathartic may be given the evening before.
- Instruct to withhold all food for 8 hours and water for 4 hours before the examination.
- Withhold medications affecting bowel motility for 24 hours prior to examination if possible (unless prescribed as part of the preparation procedure).

Client and Family Teaching

- Although the test is not uncomfortable, it requires several hours to complete. Bring reading material, paperwork, or crafts along to occupy time.
- For a small bowel exam, the barium may be administered orally, or instilled through a weighted tube inserted into the small bowel, or endoscopically.
- Increase intake of fluids for at least 24 hours after the procedure to facilitate evacuation of the barium. A laxative or cathartic may be prescribed.
- Stool will be chalky white for up to 72 hours after the exam. Normal stool color will return on complete evacuation of barium.

NURSING CARE

Clients with irritable bowel syndrome rarely require acute care for IBS as a primary problem. However, nurses frequently interact with these clients in clinics and other outpatient settings.

Assessment

Careful assessment is important to help identify the effects of IBS on the client. Collect the following assessment data.

- Health history: current symptoms, their onset and duration; current treatment measures; effect of symptoms on lifestyle; careful exploration of history of emotional, physical, or sexual abuse
- Physical examination: apparent general state of health; abdominal shape and contour, bowel sounds, tenderness

Nursing Diagnoses and Interventions

The primary nursing responsibility is education; providing referrals and counseling are additional nursing responsibilities to clients who have irritable bowel syndrome.

The following nursing diagnoses may be appropriate for clients with IBS.

- *Constipation* related to altered gastrointestinal motility
- *Diarrhea* related to altered gastrointestinal motility and excess mucous secretion
- *Anxiety* related to situational stress
- *Ineffective coping* related to effects of disorder on lifestyle

Refer to the previous sections on diarrhea and constipation for selected nursing interventions.

Home Care

Include the following topics in teaching for the client with irritable bowel syndrome.

- The nature of the disorder and the reality of the client's symptoms
- The relationship between irritable bowel syndrome and stress, anxiety, and depression
- Stress- and anxiety-reduction techniques, such as meditation, visualization, exercise, "time out," and progressive relaxation
- Dietary influences that may contribute to IBS and suggested dietary changes, such as additional fiber and water intake
- The use and role of prescribed medications, their adverse effects, and when to contact the physician
- The importance of routine follow-up appointments and of notifying the primary care provider if manifestations change (such as blood in the stool, significant constipation or diarrhea, increasing abdominal pain, or weight loss)

Refer the client to a counselor or other mental health professional for assistance in dealing with psychologic factors.

THE CLIENT WITH FECAL INCONTINENCE

Fecal incontinence, the loss of voluntary control of defecation, occurs less frequently than urinary incontinence but is no less distressing to the client. Multiple factors contribute to fecal in-

BOX 24–1 ■ Selected Causes of Fecal Incontinence

Neurologic Causes
- Spinal cord injury or disease
- Head injury, stroke, or brain tumor
- Degenerative neurologic disease, such as multiple sclerosis, amyotrophic lateral sclerosis (ALS), dementia
- Diabetic neuropathy

Local Trauma
- Obstetric tears
- Anorectal injury
- Anorectal surgery with sphincter damage

Inflammatory Processes
- Infection
- Radiation

Other Physiologic Causes
- Diarrhea
- Stool impaction
- Pelvic floor relaxation or loss of sphincter tone
- Tumors

Psychologic Causes
- Depression
- Confusion and disorientation

continence, including both physiologic and psychologic conditions (Box 24-1). Bowel incontinence is usually considered a manifestation of a disorder rather than a disorder unto itself. Clients often do not reveal fecal incontinence in discussing health concerns. Little information is available about its incidence and prevalence. Because many of the etiologic factors are more prevalent in the older adult, older clients are more often affected.

PHYSIOLOGY REVIEW

To understand the pathophysiology of fecal incontinence, it is necessary to understand the normal mechanisms of defecation. The rectum is normally empty. When it is distended by feces entering from the sigmoid colon, the defecation reflex is stimulated. This reflex causes involuntary relaxation of the internal sphincter and stimulates the urge to defecate. When the external sphincter, which is under both voluntary and autonomic (involuntary) control, relaxes, defecation occurs. Adults normally can override the defecation reflex by voluntary contraction of the external sphincter and pelvic floor muscles. The wall of the rectum gradually relaxes, and the urge to defecate subsides.

PATHOPHYSIOLOGY

The most common causes of fecal incontinence are those that interfere with either sensory or motor control of the rectum and anal sphincters. If the external sphincter is paralyzed as a result of spinal cord injury or disease, defecation occurs automatically when the internal sphincter relaxes with the defecation reflex. If sphincter muscles have been damaged or excessive pelvic floor relaxation has occurred, it may not be possible to override the defecation reflex with voluntary control.

Age-related changes in anal sphincter tone and response to rectal distention increase the risk for fecal incontinence in older adults. Resting and maximal anal sphincter pressures are decreased, particularly in older women. In addition, less rectal distention is needed to produce sustained relaxation of the anal sphincter in older females.

COLLABORATIVE CARE

The diagnosis of fecal incontinence is based on the client's history. Physical examination of the pelvic floor and anus is performed to evaluate muscle tone and rule out a fecal impaction. Impaired sphincter muscle may be palpable on digital exam. *Anorectal manometry* or a rectal motility test may be used to evaluate the functional ability of the sphincter muscles. A small, flexible balloon catheter is introduced into the rectum, and pressures are measured in the rectum and internal and external sphincters. Normally, rectal dilation causes the internal sphincter to relax and the external sphincter to contract. *Sigmoidoscopy* also may be used to examine the rectum and anal canal.

Management of fecal incontinence is directed toward the identified cause. Medications to relieve diarrhea or constipation may be prescribed. A high-fiber diet, ample fluids, and regular exercise are helpful for many clients. Exercises to improve sphincter and pelvic floor muscle tone (Kegel exercises) may be of long-term benefit. See Chapter 26 ⊂⊃ for more information about Kegel exercises.

A bowel training program to establish a regular pattern of elimination often is effective. The client is taught to establish a regular time of day for elimination, usually 15 to 30 minutes after breakfast. A stimulant, such as a cup of coffee, a rectal suppository, or even a phosphate enema, may be given to prompt defecation. Clients with neurologic incontinence may learn to stimulate the anal canal digitally to initiate defecation.

Dietary changes may be useful in managing fecal incontinence. If incontinence occurs only when stools are loose or liquid, increasing dietary fiber or using a bulking agent to increase stool bulk and solidity may be effective (Bliss et al., 2001). When incontinence of solid stool occurs, a low-residue diet of foods that are easily digested and absorbed may be prescribed to reduce the frequency of defecation. Clients also may benefit from using loperimide before meals and prophylactically before running errands or leaving the house. (Tierney et al., 2001). Biofeedback therapy may be used for mentally alert clients with intact sphincter muscles but low muscle tone. With motivation and reinforcement, clients achieve improved sphincter control in response to a stimulus.

When damage to the sphincter or rectal prolapse (protrusion of rectal mucous membrane through the anus) is the cause of fecal incontinence, surgical repair is the treatment of choice. Surgery may also be indicated when conservative measures have not been effective. Permanent colostomy, the creation of an opening from the large bowel on the abdominal wall, is a last-choice option for some clients, but it can control fecal output when other measures fail.

NURSING CARE

Assessment

- Health history: extent, onset, and duration of incontinence; identified contributing factors; history of spinal cord or anorectal injury or surgery; chronic diseases such as diabetes, multiple sclerosis, or other neurologic disorders
- Physical examination: mental status; general health; examination of perineal tissues, digital rectal examination

Nursing Diagnoses and Interventions

Bowel Incontinence

Nurses are often responsible for instituting bowel training programs and other measures to manage fecal incontinence.

- Teach caregivers to place the client on a toilet or commode and provide for privacy at a certain time of day. *Placing the client in a normal position to defecate at a consistent time of day stimulates the defecation reflex and helps reestablish a pattern of stool evacuation.*
- If necessary, insert a glycerine or bisacodyl (Dulcolax) suppository 15 to 20 minutes before positioning on the toilet or commode. *This helps to stimulate evacuation. Once a regular elimination pattern is established, it may be possible to discontinue suppository use.*
- Maintain a caring, nonjudgmental manner in providing care. *This promotes a feeling of acceptance when the client may feel unacceptable.*

PRACTICE ALERT
Provide room odor control with deodorizer tablets, sprays, or other devices. Controlling odor is important to preserve the client's self-esteem. ■

Risk for Impaired Skin Integrity

Good skin care is vital for the client with fecal incontinence. Stool contains enzymes and other irritating substances that promote skin breakdown when they are not promptly removed. This can lead to pressure ulcers, particularly when a neurologic disorder (such as spinal cord injury, dementia, or stroke) impairs mobility.

- Clean the skin thoroughly with mild soap and water after each bowel movement. *Toilet tissue may be more irritating to the skin and less effective in removing fecal material.*
- Apply a skin barrier cream or ointment after each bowel movement. *These help protect the skin from irritating substances in the feces.*
- If incontinence pads or briefs are used, check frequently for soiling and change when feces is noted. *Although these help protect bedding and clothing from soilage, they can contribute to skin breakdown if they are not checked and changed frequently.*

Using NANDA, NIC, and NOC

Chart 24–1 on page 622 shows links between NANDA nursing diagnoses, NIC, and NOC for the client with fecal incontinence.

Nursing Research

Evidence-Based Practice for Fecal Incontinence

Fecal incontinence is a distressing problem, particularly for clients residing in a community setting. In a prospective study, researchers at the University of Minnesota, Minneapolis, evaluated the effects of fiber supplementation on a group of community-living adults who were incontinent of loose or liquid stools.

Study participants recorded their dietary intake and stool characteristics and collected their stool for 8 days before addition of a fiber supplement. Participants were then randomly assigned to take psyllium, gum arabic, or placebo while continuing their usual diet. They again collected their stool and recorded dietary intake and stool characteristics for the final 8 days of the supplementation period.

On conclusion of the study period, the proportion of incontinent stools in subjects in both the psyllium and gum arabic groups was less than half that of the control group. Stool consistency also improved in the two groups taking fiber supplements.

IMPLICATIONS FOR NURSING

Fiber supplements are readily available in pharmacies and grocery stores as bulk-forming laxatives. These supplements have few contraindications and few adverse effects (other than a potential increase in flatus) when taken as directed with ample fluid. Nurses should feel comfortable recommending them for clients who have fecal incontinence associated with loose or liquid stool consistency.

Critical Thinking in Client Care

1. Why is fecal incontinence more frequently associated with loose or liquid stools than with soft, formed stools?
2. How do bulk-forming laxatives work to prevent constipation and reduce the frequency of liquid or loose stools?
3. What teaching will you provide for the client taking a bulk-forming laxative?

Note. From "Supplementation with dietary fiber improves fecal incontinence" by D. Bliss, H. Jung, K. Savik, A. Lowry, M. LeMoine, L. Jensen, C. Werner, & K. Schaffer (2001), Nursing Research, 50(4), 203–213.

Home Care

Managing fecal incontinence is a challenging problem for the client and family caregivers. For the client with intact cognition, it can be psychologically devastating. The client may become socially isolated from fear of odor or clothing soilage. Self-esteem may suffer from a sense of lost control over body functions and the inability to provide self-care. It is important to stress that incontinence is never normal (i.e., aging alone is not a cause of incontinence) and often is treatable. Encourage the client to seek medical evaluation of the problem.

Topics of instruction for the client and family include:

- Recommended dietary measures such as consuming a high-fiber diet and ample fluids to maintain soft, formed stool, or a low-residue diet to reduce the number of stools
- Suggestions for regular exercise to stimulate bowel peristalsis and regular evacuation
- Use of bulk-forming laxatives, such as psyllium seed (Metamucil) to provide stool bulk and reduce the number of small, liquid stools. See the box above for research supporting the use of psyllium or gum arabic to reduce incontinent episodes.
- Prescribed medications (such as loperamide to reduce the number of stools), their appropriate use, and management of adverse effects (such as constipation)
- Bowel training program instructions, including techniques for digital anal stimulation, inserting suppositories, or administering enemas as recommended
  - For digital anal simulation, teach to insert a lubricated gloved finger through the anal sphincter into the rectum 1.5 to 2 inches while seated on the toilet or commode, then use a circular side-to-side movement to gently stretch the rectal wall until the internal sphincter relaxes.
- The importance of good skin care, particularly if neurologic impairment is present
- The potential benefits and associated risks of biofeedback and surgical treatment, if recommended

Provide referrals for home care or community health services as indicated.

ACUTE INFLAMMATORY AND INFECTIOUS DISORDERS

The GI tract is particularly vulnerable to inflammation and infection because of its continual exposure to the external environment. Although most pathogens affecting the GI tract are ingested in food or water, infection also may be spread by direct contact, possibly by the respiratory route. Pathogens may also be transmitted sexually through anal intercourse.

Acute disease of the GI tract may be caused by the pathogen itself or by a bacterial or other toxin. Acute inflammatory disorders such as appendicitis and peritonitis result from contamination of damaged or normally sterile tissue by the client's own endogenous or resident bacteria.

THE CLIENT WITH APPENDICITIS

Appendicitis, inflammation of the vermiform appendix, is a common cause of acute abdominal pain. It is the most common reason for emergency abdominal surgery in the United States

(Tierney et al., 2001). Appendicitis can occur at any age, but is more common in adolescents and young adults and slightly more common in males than females.

PATHOPHYSIOLOGY

The appendix is a tubelike pouch attached to the cecum just below the ileocecal valve. It is usually located in the right iliac region, at an area designated as McBurney's point (Figure 24–1 ■). The function of the appendix is not fully understood, although it regularly fills with and empties digested food.

Obstruction of the proximal lumen of the appendix is apparent in most acutely inflamed appendices. The obstruction is often caused by a **fecalith**, or hard mass of feces. Other obstructive causes include a calculus or stone, a foreign body, inflammation, a tumor, parasites (e.g., pinworms), or edema of lymphoid tissue. Following obstruction, the appendix becomes distended with fluid secreted by its mucosa. Pressure within the lumen of the appendix increases, impairing its blood supply and leading to inflammation, edema, ulceration, and infection. Purulent exudate forms, further distending the appendix. Within 24 to 36 hours, tissue necrosis and gangrene result, leading to perforation if treatment is not initiated. Perforation results in bacterial peritonitis, which may remain localized.

Appendicitis can be classified as simple, gangrenous, or perforated, depending on the stage of the process. In *simple appendicitis,* the appendix is inflamed but intact. When areas of tissue necrosis and microscopic perforations are present in the appendix, the disorder is called *gangrenous appendicitis.* A *perforated appendix* shows evidence of gross perforation and contamination of the peritoneal cavity.

MANIFESTATIONS AND COMPLICATIONS

Continuous mild generalized or upper abdominal pain is the initial characteristic symptom of acute appendicitis. Over the next 4 hours, the pain intensifies and localizes in the right lower quadrant of the abdomen. It is aggravated by moving, walking, or coughing. On palpation, localized and rebound tenderness are noted at McBurney's point. **Rebound tenderness** is demonstrated by relief of pain with direct palpation of McBurney's point followed by pain on release of pressure. Extension or internal rotation of the right hip increases the pain. In addition to pain, a low-grade temperature, anorexia, nausea, and vomiting are often present.

Pain and local tenderness may be less acute in older adults, delaying the diagnosis (Tierney et al., 2001). This can present a significant problem; the course of acute appendicitis in older adults is more virulent and complications develop sooner. Pregnant women may develop right lower quadrant, periumbilical, or right subcostal (under the rib cage) pain due to displacement of the appendix by the distended uterus (Tierney et al., 2001).

Perforation, peritonitis, and abscess are possible complications of acute appendicitis. Perforation is manifested by increased pain and a high fever. It can lead to a small, localized abscess, local peritonitis, or significant generalized peritonitis. (Peritonitis is discussed in the next section of this chapter.)

A less common disorder is chronic appendicitis, characterized by chronic abdominal pain and recurrent acute attacks at intervals of several months or more. Other conditions, such as inflammatory bowel disease and renal disorders, often cause symptoms attributed to chronic appendicitis.

COLLABORATIVE CARE

Because the acutely inflamed appendix can perforate within 24 hours, rapid diagnosis and treatment are important. Because of this urgency and the low incidence of surgical complications, diagnostic testing and preoperative treatment are limited. The client is admitted to the hospital, and intravenous fluids are initiated. Oral food and fluids are withheld until a diagnosis is confirmed. Once the diagnosis is established, an appendectomy is performed.

Diagnostic Tests

Laboratory tests are used to help confirm the diagnosis and rule out other possible causes for the symptoms. The following tests may be ordered.

- *WBC count with differential* is obtained. With appendicitis, the total white count is elevated ($10,000/mm^3$ to $20,000/mm^3$), with an increased number of immature WBCs.
- *Urinalysis* is performed to rule out a urinary tract infection or other urologic cause of the client's symptoms.
- *Abdominal X-rays* are taken with the client in the flat and upright positions. A fecalith or calculus may be noted in the right lower quadrant, or a localized ileus may be noted.
- *Abdominal ultrasound* is the most effective test for diagnosing acute appendicitis. In this noninvasive test, high-frequency sound waves are reflected back to a Doppler device to create a computer-generated image. The test requires fewer than 30 minutes to complete. Ultrasound examination has reduced the incidence of exploratory surgery and is particularly useful with clients with atypical symptoms, such as older adults.

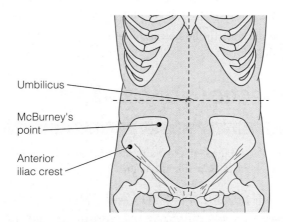

Umbilicus

McBurney's point

Anterior iliac crest

Figure 24–1 ■ McBurney's point, located midway between the umbilicus and the anterior iliac crest in the right lower quadrant. It is the usual site for localized pain and rebound tenderness due to appendicitis.

- *Pelvic examination* is generally performed on female clients of childbearing age to rule out a gynecologic disorder, tubal pregnancy, or pelvic inflammatory disease (PID).
- *Intravenous pyelogram (IVP)* may be used to differentiate appendicitis from possible urinary tract disease.

Medications

Prior to surgery, intravenous fluids are given to restore or maintain vascular volume and prevent electrolyte imbalance. Antibiotic therapy with a third-generation cephalosporin effective against many gram-negative bacteria, such as cefoperazone (Cefobid), cefotaxime (Claforan), ceftazidime (Fortaz), or ceftriaxone (Rocephin), is initiated prior to surgery. The antibiotic is repeated during surgery and continued for at least 48 hours postoperatively. The nursing implications for cephalosporin antibiotics are discussed in Chapter 8. ⊖⊙ Note that antibiotic therapy alone is not generally used to treat acute appendicitis.

Surgery

The treatment of choice for acute appendicitis is an **appendectomy,** surgical removal of the appendix. Either a laparoscopic approach (insertion of an endoscope to view abdominal contents) or laparotomy (surgical opening of the abdomen) may be used for appendectomy. Laparoscopic appendectomy requires a very small incision through which the laparoscope is inserted. This procedure has several advantages: (1) direct visualization of the appendix allows definitive diagnosis without laparotomy; (2) postoperative hospitalization is short; (3) postoperative complications are infrequent; and (4) recovery and resumption of normal activities is rapid.

An open appendectomy is performed by laparotomy. A small transverse incision is made at McBurney's point; the appendix is isolated and ligated (tied off) to prevent contamination of the site with bowel contents, and then removed (Figure 24–2 ■). Laparotomy generally is used when the ap-

Figure 24–2 ■ Appendectomy. The appendix and cecum are brought through the incision to the surface of the abdomen. The base of the appendix is clamped and ligated; the appendix is then removed.

pendix has ruptured. It allows removal of contaminants from the peritoneal cavity by irrigation with sterile normal saline. Occasionally the wound may be left unsutured for periodic irrigation. Recovery is generally uneventful. Refer to Chapter 7 ⊖⊙ for further discussion of preoperative and postoperative nursing care.

NURSING CARE

Assessment

Because appendicitis can rapidly progress from inflammation to perforation, prompt assessment is vital. Obtain the following assessment data.

- Health history: current manifestations, including onset, duration, progression, and aggravating or relieving factors; most recent food or fluid intake; known medication or other allergies; current medications; history of chronic diseases
- Physical examination: vital signs including temperature; apparent general health; abdominal shape and contour, bowel sounds, tenderness to light palpation

Nursing Diagnoses and Interventions

Preoperative nursing care is directed toward preparing the client physically and psychologically for emergency surgery. Limited time is available for preoperative teaching.

> **PRACTICE ALERT** *Keep the client with suspected appendicitis NPO, and do not administer laxatives or enemas, which may cause perforation of the appendix. No heat should be applied to the abdomen; this may increase circulation to the appendix and also cause perforation.* ■

Risk for Infection

Preventing complications during the preoperative and postoperative periods is a primary nursing care goal. Perforation and peritonitis are the most likely preoperative complications; postoperative complications include wound infection, abscess, and possible peritonitis.

> **PRACTICE ALERT** *Assess abdominal status frequently, including distention, bowel sounds, and tenderness. Increasing generalized pain, a rigid, boardlike abdomen, and abdominal distention may indicate developing peritonitis.* ■

- Monitor vital signs, including temperature. *Tachycardia and rapid shallow respirations may indicate perforation of the appendix with resulting peritonitis. Fever may develop as well, and the blood pressure may fall if sepsis is present.*
- Maintain intravenous infusion until oral intake is adequate. *Intravenous fluids are given to maintain vascular volume and to provide a route for antibiotic administration.*
- Assess wound, abdominal girth, and postoperative pain. *Swelling of the wound, increased abdominal girth, or an increase in pain may indicate infection or peritonitis.*

Pain

The client with appendicitis experiences pain before and after surgery. Analgesia is limited until the diagnosis is established. Postoperative pain is controlled by narcotic or nonnarcotic analgesics.

- Assess pain, including its character, location, severity, and duration. Report any unexpected changes in the nature of pain. *Both preoperatively and postoperatively, the client's pain provides important clues about the diagnosis and possible complications such as rupture of the appendix or peritonitis.*

> **PRACTICE ALERT** *Sudden relief of preoperative pain may signal rupture of the distended and edematous appendix.* ■

- Administer analgesics as ordered. *Preoperatively, pain medication can be given after a diagnosis is established. Postoperatively, provide analgesics to maintain comfort and enhance mobility.*
- Assess effectiveness of medication 30 minutes after administration. Report unrelieved pain. *Pain unrelieved by prescribed analgesic may indicate a complication or the need for further assessment. For example, continued abdominal discomfort and distention may indicate excess intestinal gas which may be better relieved by ambulation.*

Using NANDA, NIC, and NOC

Chart 24–2 shows links between NANDA nursing diagnoses, NIC, and NOC for the client with appendicitis or peritonitis.

Home Care

Preoperative teaching may be limited by pain and the emergent nature of surgery. Explain why food and fluids are not permitted during this time. If time allows, teach postoperative turning, coughing, deep breathing, and pain management.

With uncomplicated appendectomy, the client often is discharged either the day of surgery or the day following surgery. Postoperative teaching includes:

- Wound or incision care, including handwashing and dressing change procedures as indicated.
- Instructions to report fever, increased abdominal pain, swelling, redness, drainage, bleeding, or warmth of the operative site to the physician.
- Activity limitations (e.g., lifting, driving), if any.
- Returning to work.

Provide a referral for community health or home health care nursing services as indicated, for example, if the client has preexisting illness or difficulty performing activities of daily living and self-care.

THE CLIENT WITH PERITONITIS

Peritonitis, inflammation of the peritoneum, is a serious complication of many acute abdominal disorders. It is usually caused by enteric bacteria entering the peritoneal cavity through a perforated ulcer, ruptured appendix, perforated diverticulum (discussed later in this chapter), necrotic bowel, or during abdominal surgery. Pelvic inflammatory disease, gallbladder rupture, or abdominal trauma also can lead to peritonitis.

PHYSIOLOGY REVIEW

The peritoneum is a double-layered serous membrane lining the walls (parietal peritoneum) and organs (visceral peritoneum) of the abdominal cavity. There is a potential space

---

CHART 24–2 LINKS BETWEEN NANDA, NIC, AND NOC

The Client with Appendicitis or Peritonitis

NURSING DIAGNOSES	NURSING INTERVENTIONS	NURSING OUTCOMES
• Acute Pain	• Analgesic Administration • Patient-Controlled Analgesia (PCA) Assistance	• Comfort Level • Pain Control
• Deficient Fluid Volume	• Fluid Management • Hypovolemia Management	• Electrolyte and Acid-Base Balance • Fluid Balance
• Imbalanced Nutrition: Less Than Body Requirements	• Nutrition Monitoring	• Nutritional Status
• Ineffective Breathing Pattern	• Positioning • Respiratory Monitoring	• Respiratory Status: Ventilation
• Risk for Infection	• Incision Site Care • Wound Care	• Wound Healing: Primary Intention • Wound Healing: Secondary Intention

Note: Data from Nursing Outcomes Classification (NOC) by M. Johnson & M. Maas (Eds.), 1997, St. Louis: Mosby; Nursing Diagnoses: Definitions & Classification 2001–2002 by North American Nursing Diagnosis Association, 2001, Philadelphia: NANDA; Nursing Interventions Classification (NIC) by J.C. McCloskey & G. M. Bulechek (Eds.), 2000, St. Louis: Mosby. Reprinted by permission.

Nursing Care Plan
A Client with Acute Appendicitis

Jamie Lynn is a 19-year-old college student majoring in physical therapy. Ms. Lynn arrives at the emergency department at 1:00 A.M. complaining of general lower abdominal pain that had started the previous evening. By midnight, the pain was more localized over the right lower quadrant. She also reports nausea and vomiting.

ASSESSMENT

Sue Grady, RN, completes the admission assessment in the emergency department. Ms. Lynn is complaining of nausea and severe abdominal pain, stating, "Walking makes my stomach hurt worse." Physical assessment findings include: T 100.2°F (37.8°C), P 84, R 16, and BP 110/70; skin warm to touch; abdomen flat and guarded, with marked tenderness in right lower quadrant. Ms. Lynn's complete blood count shows WBC 14,000/mm³; neutrophils 81.1%; lymphocytes 12.5%. The diagnosis of acute appendicitis is made, and Ms. Lynn is transferred to surgery for a laparoscopic appendectomy.

DIAGNOSIS

- *Impaired skin integrity* related to surgical incisions
- *Pain* related to surgical intervention
- *Anxiety* related to situational crisis

EXPECTED OUTCOMES

- Incisions will heal without infection or complications.
- Will verbalize adequate pain relief.
- Will verbalize decreased anxiety.
- Returns to preoperative activities.

PLANNING AND IMPLEMENTATION

- Assess pain using a pain scale; provide analgesics as needed.
- Teach pain management following discharge.
- Teach abdominal splinting during coughing, turning, or ambulating as needed.
- Teach home care of incisions.
- Discuss activity limitations as ordered.
- Instruct to report fever or warmth, redness, or drainage from the incisions.

EVALUATION

On discharge the following evening, Ms. Lynn is fully ambulatory. Her appetite has returned, and she is tolerating food and fluids well. Her temperature is normal. The nurse provides Ms. Lynn with written and verbal information on postoperative care following an appendectomy.

Critical Thinking in the Nursing Process

1. What is the pathophysiologic basis for Ms. Lynn's elevated WBC?
2. How would Ms. Lynn's postoperative care and teaching differ if she had undergone a laparotomy instead of a laparoscopic appendectomy?
3. Outline a teaching plan to give to clients for home care following an appendectomy.
4. Develop a care plan for Ms. Lynn for the nursing diagnosis, *Anxiety* related to a situational crisis.

See Evaluating Your Response in Appendix C.

---

between the parietal and visceral layers of the peritoneum that contains a small amount of serous fluid. This space, the peritoneal cavity, normally is sterile.

PATHOPHYSIOLOGY

Peritonitis results from contamination of the normally sterile peritoneal cavity by infection or a chemical irritant. Chemical peritonitis often precedes bacterial peritonitis. Perforation of a peptic ulcer or rupture of the gallbladder releases gastric juices (hydrochloric acid and pepsin) or bile into the peritoneal cavity, causing an acute inflammatory response.

Bacterial peritonitis usually is caused by infection by *Escherichia coli, Klebsiella, Proteus,* or *Pseudomonas* bacteria, which normally inhabit the bowel. Inflammatory and immune defense mechanisms are activated when bacteria enter the peritoneal space. These defenses can effectively eliminate small numbers of bacteria, but may be overwhelmed by massive or continued contamination. When this occurs, mast cells release histamine and other vasoactive substances, causing local vasodilation and increased capillary permeability. Polymorphonuclear leukocytes (PMNs, a type of WBC) infiltrate the peritoneum to phagocytize bacteria and foreign matter. Fibrinogen-rich plasma exudate promotes bacterial destruc-

tion and forms fibrin clots to seal off and segregate the bacteria. This process helps limit and localize the infection, allowing host defenses to eradicate it. Continued contamination, however, leads to generalized inflammation of the peritoneal cavity. The inflammatory process causes fluid to shift into the peritoneal space (third spacing). Circulating blood volume is depleted, leading to hypovolemia. *Septicemia,* systemic disease caused by pathogens or their toxins in the blood, may follow.

MANIFESTATIONS

Manifestations of peritonitis depend on the severity and extent of the infection, as well as the age and general health of the client. Both local and systemic manifestations are present (see the box on page 636). The client often presents with evidence of an *acute abdomen,* an abrupt onset of diffuse, severe abdominal pain. The pain may localize and intensify near the area of infection. Movement may intensify the pain. The entire abdomen is tender, with guarding or rigidity of abdominal muscles. The acute abdomen is often described as boardlike. Rebound tenderness may be present over the area of inflammation. Peritoneal inflammation inhibits peristalsis, resulting in a paralytic ileus. (Paralytic ileus is discussed in a

Manifestations of Peritonitis

Abdominal Manifestations
- Diffuse or localized pain
- Tenderness with rebound
- Boardlike rigidity
- Diminished or absent bowel sounds
- Distention
- Anorexia, nausea, and vomiting

Systemic Manifestations
- Fever
- Malaise
- Tachycardia
- Tachypnea
- Restlessness
- Confusion or disorientation
- Oliguria

later section of this chapter.) Bowel sounds are markedly diminished or absent, and progressive abdominal distention is noted. Pooling of GI secretions may cause nausea and vomiting. Systemic manifestations of peritonitis include fever, malaise, tachycardia and tachypnea, restlessness, and possible disorientation. The client may be oliguric and show signs of dehydration and shock.

The older, chronically debilitated, or immunosuppressed client may present with few of the classic signs of peritonitis. Increased confusion and restlessness, decreased urinary output, and vague abdominal complaints may be the only manifestations present. These clients are at increased risk for delayed diagnosis, contributing to a higher mortality rate.

Complications

Complications of peritonitis may be life threatening. Abscess formation is common. The very defense mechanisms designed to isolate and localize the infection can protect it from immune responses and systemic antibiotics. Fibrous adhesions in the abdominal cavity are a late complication and may lead to subsequent obstruction.

Without prompt and effective treatment, septicemia and septic shock can develop. Fluid loss into the abdominal cavity may also lead to hypovolemic shock. These potentially lethal complications require immediate, aggressive intervention to prevent multiple organ failure and death. Shock and its management are discussed in Chapter 6. ⊙⊘

The overall mortality rate associated with peritonitis is about 40%. Clients with other medical conditions, older clients, and those with greater bacterial contamination have a higher risk of dying. Young people with perforated ulcers or appendicitis, those with less extensive bacterial contamination, and those who receive early surgical intervention have mortality rates of less than 10%.

COLLABORATIVE CARE

Care of the client with peritonitis focuses on establishing the diagnosis and identifying and treating its cause as well as the peritonitis. Preventing complications is an important aspect of care.

Diagnostic Tests

Diagnostic testing is done to establish the diagnosis of peritonitis, rule out other disorders, and help identify the cause. The following tests may be ordered.

- *WBC count* is elevated to approximately 20,000/mm^3 in peritonitis. Increased numbers of immature blood cells are present as the bone marrow releases them in response to the infection.
- *Blood cultures* are ordered to identify the possible presence of bacteria in the blood (*bacteremia*). Bacteremia often precedes *septicemia,* a potential complication of peritonitis.
- *Liver* and *renal function studies* and *serum electrolytes* may be ordered to evaluate the systemic effects of peritonitis and help guide treatment.
- *Abdominal X-rays* (supine and standing) are obtained to detect intestinal distention, air-fluid levels (indicative of ileus or bowel obstruction), and free air under the diaphragm (indicative of GI perforation).
- *Paracentesis* is performed to obtain peritoneal fluid for analysis (see Chapter 22). ⊙⊘ In peritonitis, the fluid contains increased protein and WBCs. Bacteria may be present. Amylase in the fluid may indicate acute pancreatitis. Peritoneal fluid analysis helps establish the diagnosis and underlying cause of acute peritonitis.

Medications

Until the infecting organism has been identified, a broad-spectrum antibiotic effective against organisms commonly implicated in peritonitis is prescribed. Once culture results have been obtained, antibiotic therapy is modified to the specific organism(s) responsible. Cephalosporin antibiotics are often prescribed if gram-negative enteric bacteria are suspected. Other antibiotics that may be ordered include ampicillin (Omnipen, Polycillin, others), metronidazole (Flagyl, others), clindamycin (Cleocin), or an aminoglycoside antibiotic such as gentamycin (Garamycin) or amikacin (Amikin). Nursing implications for antibiotic therapy are discussed in Chapter 8. ⊙⊘

In addition to antibiotic therapy, analgesics are usually ordered to promote comfort.

Surgery

If the cause of peritonitis is a perforation, gangrenous bowel, or inflamed appendix, a laparotomy is done to close the perforation or remove the damaged and inflamed tissue. If an abscess is present, it also may be surgically drained or removed.

Peritoneal lavage, washing of the peritoneal cavity with copious amounts of warm isotonic fluid, may be done during surgery. This procedure dilutes residual bacteria and removes gross contaminants, blood, and fibrin clots. In rare instances, peritoneal lavage may be continued for several days following surgery. The solution is infused into the upper portion of the peritoneal cavity and removed via drains in the pelvic cul-de-sac. Careful attention to fluid and electrolyte status and strict aseptic technique are necessary.

Clients who have had laparotomy for peritonitis often return from surgery with either Penrose or closed drain systems such as a Jackson-Pratt drain. In some cases, the incision may be left unsutured. With severe and long-standing peritonitis, the abdomen may be closed temporarily with polypropylene mesh containing a nylon zipper or Velcro to allow repeated exploration of the abdomen and drainage of infectious sites.

Treatments

Intravenous fluids and electrolyte replacements are administered to maintain vascular volume and fluid and electrolyte balance. Parenteral nutrition is given until adequate oral intake resumes. The client is placed on bed rest in Fowler's position to help localize the infection and promote lung ventilation. Oxygen is often ordered to facilitate cellular metabolism and healing.

Intestinal Decompression

The inflammatory process of peritonitis often draws large amounts of fluid into the abdominal cavity and the bowel. In addition, peristaltic activity of the bowel is slowed or halted by the inflammation, causing **paralytic ileus** (or *ileus*), impaired propulsion or forward movement of bowel contents. Intestinal decompression is used to relieve abdominal distention, facilitate closure, and minimize postoperative respiratory problems. A nasogastric or long intestinal tube is inserted and connected to continuous drainage (Figure 24–3 ■). If prolonged intestinal decompression is anticipated, a jejunostomy may be performed for comfort. Suction is maintained until peristalsis resumes, bowel sounds are present, and the client is passing flatus. Food and fluids are withheld until intestinal motility has returned and suction is discontinued.

Weighted Balloon

Figure 24–3 ■ The weighted tip or inflated balloon at the end of an intestinal tube is drawn into the intestine by gravity and peristalsis.

NURSING CARE

As noted earlier, peritonitis is a serious illness. Early recognition and treatment are important to minimize the risk of complications.

Assessment

- Health history: complaints of pain, its onset, character, severity, location, aggravating and relieving factors; associated symptoms such as anorexia, nausea, vomiting; current and previous history of peptic ulcer disease, gallbladder disease, other related conditions; chronic diseases; current medications
- Physical examination: vital signs including temperature; level of consciousness; skin color, temperature, warmth, capillary refill and turgor; abdominal shape, contour, bowel sounds, tenderness, and guarding

Nursing Diagnoses and Interventions

Clients with peritonitis require intensive nursing and medical care to prevent complications and recover fully. Nursing care priorities include pain; altered fluid balance; altered protection due to infection, drains, and possibly repeated surgeries; and anxiety.

Pain

Abdominal distention and acute inflammation contribute to the pain associated with peritonitis. Surgery further disrupts abdominal muscles and other tissues, causing pain. Effective pain management promotes immune function, healing, mobility, and recovery.

- Assess pain, including its location, severity (using a standard pain scale), and type. Monitor analgesic effectiveness. Report changes to the primary care provider.

> **PRACTICE ALERT** *Unrelieved pain or a change in the location, severity, or type of pain may indicate spread of infection, abscess formation, or other complications of peritonitis.* ■

- Place in Fowler's or semi-Fowler's position with the knees and feet elevated. *This position reduces stress on abdominal structures and facilitates respirations, promoting comfort.*
- Administer analgesics as ordered on a routine basis or using patient-controlled analgesia (PCA). *Routine analgesic administration maintains a therapeutic blood level and helps maintain comfort, facilitating healing and movement.*
- Teach and assist with adjunctive pain management techniques such as meditation, visualization, massage, and progressive relaxation. *Adjunctive measures augment analgesics and help promote a sense of control over pain.*

Deficient Fluid Volume

In peritonitis, significant amounts of fluid are drawn into the abdominal cavity and bowel, reducing vascular volume and cardiac output. This fluid also may be lost from the body by intestinal suction or through drains placed in the abdomen during surgery. An unsutured incision causes additional significant fluid loss.

- Maintain accurate intake and output records. Measure urine output every 1 to 2 hours; report output of less than 30 mL/hr. Measure gastrointestinal output at least every 4 hours. *Intake and output records provide valuable information about fluid volume status.*

> **PRACTICE ALERT** *Urine output of less than 30 mL/hr may indicate hypovolemia, decreased cardiac output, and impaired tissue perfusion.* ∎

- Monitor vital signs and hemodynamic parameters such as central venous pressure, cardiac output, and pulmonary artery pressures every hour or as indicated. *These measurements provide important information about fluid and vascular volumes as well as cardiovascular status.*
- Weigh daily. *Weight is an accurate indicator of fluid status. Rapid weight gains or losses reflect changes in fluid volume.*
- Assess skin turgor, color, temperature, and mucous membranes at least every 8 hours. *Warm, dry skin with poor turgor and dry, shiny mucous membranes indicates dehydration.*
- Measure or estimate fluid losses through abdominal drains and on dressings. *Significant amounts of exudative fluid may be lost.*
- Monitor laboratory values, including hemoglobin and hematocrit, urine specific gravity, serum osmolality and electrolytes, and ABGs. Report changes to the physician. *Laboratory results provide information about fluid and electrolyte status and acid-base balance.*
- Administer intravenous fluids and electrolytes as ordered. Gastrointestinal drainage may be replaced milliliter for milliliter with a balanced electrolyte solution. *Intravenous fluids are necessary to meet daily fluid intake needs, as well as replace continuing losses of water and electrolytes.*
- Provide good skin care and frequent oral hygiene. *Fluid deficit increases the risk of skin breakdown and ulceration of mucous membranes.*

Ineffective Protection
Repeated surgeries, an unsutured incision, and the presence of drains interrupt skin integrity and the body's first line of defense against microorganisms. In addition, immune defenses are stressed by the infection and potential malnutrition. As a result, the risk for impaired healing and further infection is increased.

- Monitor temperature, pulse rate, and for localized signs of infection such as redness and swelling around incisions and drain sites, increased or purulent drainage, and cloudy or malodorous urine. *Impaired defenses increase the risk for extension of the infection or unrelated infections.*
- Obtain cultures of purulent drainage from any site. *Early identification of any additional infection allows timely intervention.*
- Monitor WBC and differential, serum protein, and albumin. *An increased WBC with a higher percentage of immature cells present in the blood is an indicator of infection and normal immune response. Serum albumin and protein levels are indicators of nutritional status as well as immune function.*
- Practice meticulous handwashing and use standard precautions at all times. *Handwashing reduces transient bacteria on the skin and remains the most important method of controlling infection. Standard precautions reduce the risk of spreading infection to or from the client.*
- Use strict aseptic technique for dressing changes, wound care, and irrigations. *Disruption of the protective barrier of the skin increases the risk of contamination and further infection.*
- Maintain fluid balance and nutritional status through enteral or parenteral feedings, as indicated. *Adequate nutrition and fluid balance are necessary for optimal immune system function.*

> **PRACTICE ALERT** *An acute infection such as peritonitis causes a stress response with excess energy expenditure and loss of body proteins and cell mass. Glycogen stores are rapidly depleted, and body proteins are used to meet energy needs. Withholding food further complicates this process, leading to rapid development of protein-calorie malnutrition (PCM). PCM impairs the immune response and slows healing.* ∎

Anxiety
The severity and potential threat to life associated with peritonitis present a situational crisis for the client and family. Anxiety is a common response.

- Assess the client's and family's anxiety level and present coping skills. *Interventions need to be tailored to the needs and strengths of the client and family.*
- Present a calm, reassuring manner. Encourage expression of concerns; listen carefully, and acknowledge their validity. *This helps establish trust.*
- Maintain consistent caregiver assignments. *Consistency of nursing care and care providers helps reduce anxiety. Complex wound care and irrigation procedures are best performed by people who are very familiar with prescribed techniques.*
- Explain all treatments, procedures, tests, and examinations. *An increased understanding of what is being done can reduce anxiety.*
- Reinforce and clarify information as needed. *This improves understanding and promotes acceptance.*
- Teach and assist with relaxation techniques such as meditation, visualization, and progressive relaxation. *These measures promote positive coping skills and reduce physical manifestations of anxiety.*

Using NANDA, NIC, and NOC
Linkages between NANDA nursing diagnoses, NIC, and NOC for the client with peritonitis are illustrated in Chart 24–2.

Home Care

Teaching for the client with peritonitis is vital during hospitalization and prior to discharge. Provide brief but complete explanations of procedures, examinations, and expected sensations throughout hospitalization to reduce anxiety and improve cooperation.

Teaching for home care includes the following topics:

- Wound care procedures, including dressing changes or irrigations. Provide verbal and written instructions, and allow opportunities to practice and demonstrate the procedure prior to discharge.
- Where to obtain necessary supplies.
- Prescribed medications, including name and purpose of the drug, potential adverse effects, and their management.
- Manifestations of further infection (redness, heat, swelling, purulent drainage, chills, and fever) and potential complications to be reported to the care provider.
- Prescribed activity restrictions.
- Instructions for a high-calorie, high-protein diet for healing and optimal immune function.

Provide a referral to home health services for assessment, wound care, and further teaching, as needed.

THE CLIENT WITH GASTROENTERITIS

Gastroenteritis, or enteritis, is an inflammation of the stomach and small intestine. Enteritis may be caused by bacteria, viruses, parasites, or toxins. Upper GI symptoms such as anorexia, nausea, and vomiting are common. Diarrhea of varying intensity and abdominal discomfort are nearly universal features of gastroenteritis.

The infectious organism usually enters the body in contaminated water or food. For this reason, gastroenteritis often is called "food poisoning." Viruses commonly cause acute diarrheal illness. Diarrhea due to rotaviruses or the Norwalk virus occurs year-round in both adults and children. These illnesses are generally mild and self-limited, but can have severe consequences in the very young, the very old, or in people with impaired immune function.

PATHOPHYSIOLOGY

Bacterial or viral infection of the GI tract produces inflammation, tissue damage, and manifestations by two primary mechanisms.

- *The production of exotoxins.* A number of bacteria produce and excrete an exotoxin that enters the surrounding environment (intestinal lumen), causing damage and inflammation. Exotoxins in the GI tract are often referred to as *enterotoxins.* They impair intestinal absorption and can cause secretion of significant amounts of electrolytes and water into the bowel, resulting in diarrhea and fluid loss. Common bacterial enterotoxins include those produced by *Staphylococcus, Clostridium perfringens, Clostridium botulinum,* some strains of *Escherichia coli,* and *Vibrio cholerae.*
- *Invasion and ulceration of the mucosa.* Other bacteria, including some *Shigella, Salmonella,* and *Escherichia coli* species, damage tissue more directly. They invade the intestinal mucosa of the small bowel or colon, producing microscopic ulceration, bleeding, fluid exudate, and water and electrolyte secretion.

In some cases, the mechanism of injury is unclear. It may be a combination of direct and toxic damage. The Norwalk virus damages the mucosa of the jejunum, with fluid and electrolyte secretion.

MANIFESTATIONS AND COMPLICATIONS

Although the manifestations of bacterial and viral enteritis vary according to the organism involved, several features are common (see the box below). Anorexia, nausea, and vomiting are caused by distension of the upper GI tract by unabsorbed chyme and excess water. Bowel distention, along with irritation of the bowel mucosa and gas production due to fermentation of undigested food, also lead to abdominal pain and cramping. *Borborygmi,* excessively loud and hyperactive bowel sounds, are another result. The abdomen is often distended and tender.

Diarrhea is usually predominant with enteritis. Fluid is secreted into the bowel lumen, and the unabsorbed chyme and electrolytes create an osmotic draw of fluid into the bowel. Motility is stimulated, and stools become watery and frequent. Loss of fluids and electrolytes through diarrhea can lead to the most serious manifestations of enteritis. Fluid volume can be rapidly depleted, leading to dehydration and hypovolemia. Orthostatic hypotension may be noted initially, along with an elevated temperature. If fluid loss continues, hypovolemic shock may develop.

Electrolyte and acid-base imbalances may result from gastroenteritis. Extensive vomiting can lead to metabolic alkalosis due to the loss of hydrochloric acid from the stomach. When diarrhea predominates, metabolic acidosis is more likely. Potassium is lost in either case, leading to hypokalemia. Hyponatremia may develop if fluids are replaced with pure water. Headache, cardiac irregularities, changes in respiratory rate

Manifestations of Gastroenteritis

Gastrointestinal Effects
- Anorexia, nausea, and vomiting
- Abdominal pain and cramping
- Borborygmi
- Diarrhea

General Effects
- Malaise, weakness, and muscle aches
- Headache
- Dry skin and mucous membranes
- Poor skin turgor
- Orthostatic hypotension, tachycardia
- Fever

and pattern, malaise and weakness, muscle aching, and signs of neuromuscular irritability are the possible manifestations of these disturbances in homeostasis.

Several gastrointestinal infections produce specific effects that are discussed below and summarized in Table 24–3.

Traveler's Diarrhea

People traveling to another country frequently develop diarrhea within 2 to 10 days, particularly when there is a significant difference in climate, sanitation standards, or food and drink. Strains of enterotoxin-producing *E. coli,* shigella species, and *Camylobacter* are the most frequent causes of traveler's diarrhea (Tierney et al., 2001). Other bacteria and viruses also may cause traveler's diarrhea.

Up to 10 or more loose stools per day and abdominal cramping are common manifestations. Nausea and vomiting are less frequent; fever is rare. Symptoms usually resolve within 2 to 5 days. Complications are rare.

TABLE 24–3 Selected Bacterial Infections of the Bowel

Disease and Organism	Incubation	Pathogenesis	Manifestations	Management
Traveler's diarrhea: *Escherichia coli*	24 to 72 hours	Enterotoxin causes hypersecretion of the small intestine.	Abrupt onset of diarrhea; vomiting rare	Prophylactic bismuth subsalicylate; anti-diarrheals such as loperamide or diphenoxylate; 3- to 5-day course of norfloxacin, ciprofloxacin, or trimethoprim-sulfamethoxazole
Staphylococcal food poisoning	2 to 8 hours	Enterotoxin impairs intestinal absorption and affects vomiting centers in the brain.	Severe nausea and vomiting; abdominal cramping and diarrhea; headache and fever	Fluid and electrolyte replacement as needed
Botulism: *Clostridium botulinum*	1.5 to 8 days	Absorbed enterotoxin produces neuro-muscular blockade and progressive paralysis.	Diplopia, pupils fixed and dilated; dry mouth, dysphagia; progressive cephalocaudal weakness and paralysis; GI symptoms minimal; respiratory failure possible complication	Gastric lavage to remove toxin from gut; administration of botulinus antitoxin; respiratory, fluid, and nutritional support
Cholera: *Vibrio cholerae*	1 to 3 days	Enterotoxin affects entire small intestine, causing secretion of water and electrolytes into bowel lumen.	Severe diarrhea with "rice water stool," grey, cloudy, odorless, with no blood or pus; vomiting; thirst, oliguria, muscle cramps, weakness; dehydration and vascular collapse	Oral or intravenous rehydration; possible antimicrobial therapy with ampicillin, tetracycline, trimethoprim-sulfamethoxazole, others
Hemorrhagic colitis: *E. coli*	1 to 3 days	Enterotoxin causes direct mucosal damage in large intestine; also toxic to vascular endothelial cells.	Severe abdominal cramping, watery diarrhea that becomes grossly bloody; fever; possible complications: hemolytic uremic syndrome and thrombotic thrombocytopenic purpura	Supportive care with fluid replacement and bland diet; may require dialysis or plasmapheresis for complications
Salmonellosis: *Salmonella*	8 to 48 hours	Superficial infection of the GI tract without invasion or production of toxins.	Diarrhea with abdominal cramping, nausea, and vomiting; low-grade fever, chills, weakness	Treatment of symptoms; trimethoprim-sulfamethoxazole, ampicillin, or ciprofloxacin for severe illness
Shigellosis (bacillary dysentery): *Shigella*	1 to 4 days	Local tissue invasion, primarily involving large intestine and distal ileum; endotoxin causes fluid and electrolyte secretion into bowel lumen.	Watery diarrhea with severe abdominal cramping and tenesmus; lethargy	Fluid and electrolyte replacement; correction of acidosis; antibiotic therapy with trimethoprim-sulfamethoxazole, ciprofloxacin, or ampicillin

Staphylococcal Food Poisoning

Certain foods provide an excellent medium for staphylococcal growth when contaminated and left at room temperature. Examples include meats and fish, dairy products (e.g., custards), and bakery products (e.g., cream-filled pastries). The organism itself does not affect the bowel; the toxin it produces, however, impairs intestinal absorption and acts on receptors in the gut, stimulating the medullary center to produce vomiting.

The onset of staphylococcal food poisoning is abrupt, occurring within 2 to 8 hours after consuming the contaminated food. Nausea and vomiting are severe. Manifestations typically last 3 to 6 hours, and include abdominal cramping, diarrhea, headache, and fever. Complications such as fluid and electrolyte imbalances are rare, but may develop in older adults and people with underlying chronic disease processes.

Botulism

Botulism is a severe, life-threatening form of food poisoning caused by *Clostridium botulinum.* These spore-forming anaerobic bacteria grow in improperly preserved foods, such as home-canned vegetables, smoked meats, and vacuum-packed fish. The spores are highly resistant to heat; a temperature of 248°F for 30 minutes is required to kill the bacteria. The bacterial toxin, however, is easily destroyed by temperatures as low as 176°F.

The bacterial toxin is absorbed into the bloodstream from the intestines. It blocks release of acetylcholine, a neurotransmitter, from nerve endings, causing bilateral and symmetric neurologic symptoms. Cranial nerves are often affected first, followed by descending weakness or paralysis. Diplopia (double vision) and loss of accommodation are common initial symptoms, often accompanied by dry mouth and dysphagia. Nausea, vomiting, and abdominal cramps may occur. Diarrhea is rare with botulism. As neuromuscular paralysis progresses, respiratory muscles become progressively weaker. Respiratory muscle paralysis may lead to death unless ventilatory support is provided. Sensation is not impaired, and the client remains mentally alert.

Cholera

Cholera is an acute diarrheal illness caused by strains of *Vibrio cholerae.* It is endemic in parts of Asia, the Middle East, and Africa. Epidemics occur periodically. Cholera is spread by the fecal–oral route through contaminated water or food. The organism produces an enterotoxin, enzymes, and other substances that affect the entire small intestine. Water and electrolytes are secreted into the bowel lumen in response to the toxin. The enzymes and other substances produced by the bacteria may affect mucous protection of bowel endothelium.

Cholera ranges in severity from very mild, with few or no symptoms, to acute and fulminant. Its onset is typically abrupt, with severe, frequent, watery diarrhea. Up to 1 L of stool may be passed in an hour, rapidly producing depleting fluid volume. Stool is often described as "rice water stool" and characteristically gray and cloudy, with no fecal odor, blood, or pus. Vomiting may accompany the diarrhea. Other manifestations relate to the loss of fluid and electrolytes: thirst, oliguria, muscle cramps, weakness, and significant signs of dehydration. Metabolic acidosis and hypokalemia develop. If untreated, circulatory collapse and acute renal failure may occur.

Recovery from cholera usually occurs spontaneously within 3 to 6 days. With prompt and adequate fluid replacement, mortality is less than 1%.

Escherichia coli Hemorrhagic Colitis

Most pathologic forms of *E. coli* bacteria cause little more than common traveler's diarrhea. Some strains, such as serotype 0157:H7, produce a potent enterotoxin in the large intestine after being ingested. This toxin damages bowel mucosa and the endothelial cells of blood vessels in the GI tract. If absorbed, the toxin can damage other blood vessels as well, such as those of the kidney.

Cattle provide the reservoir for *E. coli* 0157:H7. It is usually spread through undercooked beef (hamburger in particular) and unpasteurized milk or apple juice. It may also be spread by direct contact via the fecal–oral route. The onset of hemorrhagic colitis is abrupt, with severe abdominal cramping and watery diarrhea that becomes grossly bloody within 24 hours. Fever may be present.

Hemolytic uremic syndrome and thrombotic thrombocytopenic purpura are significant complications of *E. coli* hemorrhagic colitis, affecting about 5% of people with the disease. Children and older adults have the highest risk for developing complications.

Salmonellosis

Salmonellosis is food poisoning caused by ingesting raw or improperly cooked meat, poultry, eggs, and dairy products contaminated with *Salmonella* bacteria. These bacteria cause superficial infection of the GI tract, rarely invading further. They do not produce a toxin.

Symptoms develop 8 to 48 hours after ingesting the bacteria. Diarrhea may be violent with abdominal cramping, nausea, and vomiting. A low-grade fever, chills, and weakness may accompany GI manifestations. The disease usually is self-limited, resolving within 3 to 5 days, although bacteremia may develop.

Shigellosis (Bacillary Dysentery)

Shigellosis (or bacillary dysentery) occurs worldwide, accounting for up to 5% to 10% of diarrheal illness in some regions. It may be endemic or occur in epidemics. Humans are the reservoir for *Shigella* organisms, which are spread directly via the fecal–oral route or indirectly through contaminated food, fomites (such as inanimate objects), and vectors (such as fleas). The incubation period for shigellosis is 1 to 4 days.

Shigella organisms infect the lower intestine, and sometimes the distal ilium. They invade the tissue, causing inflammation, and they produce an enterotoxin. The result is watery diarrhea containing blood, mucus, and inflammatory exudate. The onset of diarrhea is abrupt, with severe abdominal cramping, and *tenesmus,* a sensation of urgent and continuing need to defecate. Lethargy is common; rarely, neurologic symptoms occur.

In adults, shigellosis is usually mild and self-limiting. Older adults and debilitated clients are at risk for volume depletion and electrolyte imbalances. Secondary infection is another potential complication, as is acute blood loss from mucosal ulcerations.

COLLABORATIVE CARE

The goals of care for gastroenteritis are to manage the symptoms, prevent complications, identify the cause of the infection, and prevent its spread. The history and manifestations provide valuable cues about the cause. Diagnostic testing is used to identify the pathogen and evaluate its effects. In most cases, treatment is supportive, directed toward relieving symptoms, restoring fluid and electrolyte balance, and maintaining function.

Diagnostic Tests

If symptoms are severe or do not resolve within about 48 hours, laboratory testing is used to identify the causative organism and to assess fluid, electrolyte, and acid-base balance.

- *Stool specimen for culture, ova and parasites, and fecal leukocytes.* Stool culture usually reveals the infective organism, but may require up to 6 weeks for some bacteria, making it impractical. In infections such as botulism, the toxin itself may be isolated in the stool. Contamination of the stool by urine or treatment with antibiotics, bismuth subsalicylate (Pepto-Bismol), or mineral oil may interfere with pathogen growth, altering stool culture results. Use a clean bedpan or collection device to obtain the stool specimen, and instruct the client to avoid mixing the stool with urine or toilet tissue.

- *Gram stain of vomitus* may reveal staphylococci in staphylococcal food poisoning.
- *Serum toxin levels* may be ordered, particularly if botulism is suspected.
- *Serum osmolality and electrolytes,* and *arterial blood gases* assess fluid, electrolyte, and acid-base balance. Common imbalances associated with enteritis and diarrhea are outlined in Table 24–4.

A *sigmoidoscopy* may be done to differentiate inflammatory bowel disease from infectious processes. It does not replace stool cultures, because the lesions associated with some infectious processes are indistinguishable from those of ulcerative colitis. Nursing care of the client undergoing a sigmoidoscopy is included in the Nursing Implications box on page 619.

Medications

Acute enteritis usually resolves spontaneously, and no drug treatment is required. If the client is severely ill and symptoms are prolonged, medications may be prescribed.

Antibiotic therapy may used to treat cholera, salmonellosis, or shigellosis. Trimethoprim-sulfamethoxazole (Septra, Bactrim), ciprofloxacin (Cipro), ampicillin (Ampicin, Omnipen, Polycillin-N, others), or another antibiotic may be prescribed. Stool culture is obtained prior to starting antibiotics, but treatment may begin before culture results are available. A presumptive diagnosis based on history and presenting symptoms guides the choice of antibiotic.

An antidiarrheal drug may be prescribed to promote comfort and reduce fluid loss. Nursing measures related to antidiarrheal medications are outlined in the Nursing Implications box on page 619. It is vital to remember that antidiarrheal

TABLE 24–4	Laboratory Values Associated with Enteritis and Diarrhea	
Test	**Normal Value**	**Change with Significant Diarrhea**
Serum osmolality	275 to 295 mOsm/kg	Increased; levels above 320 mOsm/kg indicate significant dehydration
Serum potassium	3.5 to 5.0 mEq/L	Decreased due to loss through stool and vomitus; levels below 2.5 mEq/L are critical
Serum sodium	136 to 148 mEq/L	Decreased due to loss through stool and vomitus; may be significant when fluid losses are replaced with pure water; levels below 120 mEq/L may be critical
Serum chloride	96 to 106 mEq/L	Increased when sodium loss is greater than chloride loss; decreased with severe diarrhea and with vomiting; possible critical values are below 80 mEq/L or above 115 mEq/L
Blood gases		
• pH	Arterial: 7.35 to 7.45	Decreased in metabolic acidosis, a possible result of severe diarrhea; increased in metabolic alkalosis, a possible result of severe vomiting and chloride loss; values below 7.25 or above 7.55 are critical
• P_{CO_2}	Arterial: 35 to 45 mmHg	Typically decreased in metabolic acidosis as the body attempts to eliminate excess acid by "blowing off" CO_2; increased with metabolic alkalosis as the body retains CO_2 in an attempt to normalize pH
• Bicarbonate	22 to 26 mEq/L	Decreased in metabolic acidosis; increased in metabolic alkalosis
Hematocrit	Males: 40% to 50% Females: 37% to 47%	Increased with dehydration and hypovolemia as a result of concentration of blood cells
Urine specific gravity	1.010 to 1.025	Increased with dehydration and hypovolemia as kidneys attempt to conserve fluid

agents are not used to treat botulism. In fact, cathartics may be ordered to promote removal of the toxin from the bowel.

Botulism antitoxin is administered as soon as possible if botulism is suspected. The antitoxin may be given prophylactically, when ingestion of the bacteria or toxin is suspected. If the antitoxin is given more than 72 hours after symptom onset it may not be effective. The antitoxin neutralizes circulating toxin. It does not displace toxin bound to nerve endings, so existing paralysis continues when it is given. Botulism antitoxin is made from horse serum, so it can provoke an anaphylactic response and serum sickness (see Chapter 9). ᴳᴰ Sensitivity testing and progressive desensitization is recommended prior to administering the antitoxin. This may not always be possible because of symptom progression. Keep epinephrine at the bedside to treat potential anaphylaxis.

Treatments

Replacing lost fluids and electrolytes is vital when vomiting and/or diarrhea are severe or prolonged. In many cases of enteritis, fluid and electrolyte replacement are all that is required until the infection resolves.

Oral rehydration is preferred for replacing physiologic fluids. An oral glucose-electrolyte solution is often well tolerated in sips, even when vomiting is present. Commercial preparations such as Gatorade, All-Sport, and Pedialyte are available. A solution of 5 mL (1 teaspoon) table salt, 5 mL baking soda, 20 mL (4 teaspoons) granulated sugar, and flavoring (such as lemon extract or juice) to 1 L (1 quart) of water also is effective.

Intravenous rehydration may be necessary with severe diarrhea and fluid loss. In some cases, a combination of oral and intravenous fluids may be used to replace lost fluids and maintain vascular volume. Balanced electrolyte solutions, such as glucose in normal saline, Ringer's solution, and others, are used. Lactated Ringer's solution or another alkalinizing solution may be ordered if metabolic acidosis is present.

Gastric lavage and catharsis—in effect, "washing out" the stomach and intestines—may be done to remove unabsorbed toxin from the GI tract if botulism is suspected. The client with botulism is closely observed for signs of respiratory distress. Respiratory support with endotracheal intubation or tracheostomy and mechanical ventilation may be required (see Chapter 36).

Plasmapheresis (plasma exchange therapy) may be performed to remove circulating toxins for botulism or hemorrhagic colitis caused by *E. coli*. In plasmapheresis, harmful components in plasma are removed by withdrawing blood, separating the plasma from the blood cells, and returning the cells with an equal amount of albumin or human plasma to the client. This procedure is usually done in a series, rather than as a single treatment. Informed consent is required for plasmapheresis. Potential complications include those associated with intravenous catheters, shifts in fluid balance, and altered blood clotting.

Acute tubular necrosis and renal failure associated with hemorrhagic colitis may necessitate dialysis to remove wastes and prevent severe fluid and electrolyte imbalances and meta-

bolic acidosis. Although acute renal failure often resolves spontaneously and renal function resumes, dialysis can be lifesaving. Either hemodialysis or peritoneal dialysis may be used, generally as a temporary measure. Nursing care related to acute renal failure and dialysis is discussed in Chapter 27. ᴳᴰ

NURSING CARE

Few clients with acute enteritis require hospitalization. Most are treated in outpatient and community settings. Assessment, education, and support of self-care measures are major nursing responsibilities.

Health Promotion

Nurses play a significant role in preventing enteritis as educators, community health providers, and advocates for environmental safety.

Teach the importance of proper food handling and maintaining appropriate temperatures. Adequate cooking of meat products is vital to prevent disorders such as staphylococcal food poisoning, *E. coli* hemorrhagic colitis, and salmonellosis. Emphasize the importance of not consuming raw meat products, and cooking hamburger in particular to the point that no redness is noted in the meat. The highly pathogenic *E. coli* serotype 0157:H7 is present in the gut of infected animals. Meats from the animal may be contaminated with bowel contents. The organism is readily destroyed by heat, so cuts of meat such as steaks or roasts are less likely to cause infection, since the organism is on the outside of the meat. However, the process of grinding hamburger allows *E. coli* to be mixed throughout the meat. Thorough cooking destroys the organism. This pathogen (and others) may also be spread through unpasteurized milk. Discuss the dangers of consuming milk that has not been pasteurized and encourage clients to avoid it.

Dairy products, eggs, and egg products left at room temperature provide a good growth medium for bacteria. Discuss the importance of prompt refrigeration of meats and these products to minimize this risk.

Nonacidic canned foods, such as vegetables, mushrooms, meats, and fish, are potential sources of botulism toxin. The high temperatures required to destroy the bacteria and its spores are achieved only by pressure canning with appropriate pressures and duration. Emphasize the importance of following directions precisely when home-canning foods. Advise boiling home-canned foods for 10 to 15 minutes to destroy any potential toxin. Any food that is discolored or comes from a can or jar that has been damaged or does not have a tight seal should be destroyed without tasting or touching. Food contaminated with botulism may have no unusual odor or color. If the seal is questionable, discard the food.

Many gastrointestinal infections are spread through contaminated water. Encourage travelers to consume only bottled water unless local water supplies are clearly safe. Water purification tablets are available for hikers and campers, and may also be used when traveling abroad.

Assessment

- Health history: onset, duration, and severity of symptoms; recent activities such as attending a picnic or potluck, international travel, or camping; other affected members of the household; measures taken to relieve symptoms or replace fluids
- Physical examination: vital signs including temperature and orthostatic vitals; skin color, temperature, moisture, and turgor; peripheral pulses and capillary refill; abdominal shape, contour, bowel sounds, tenderness

Nursing Diagnoses and Interventions

Diarrhea and fluid volume deficit are priority nursing diagnoses. See the earlier section of this chapter on diarrhea for specific nursing interventions related to these diagnoses.

Other nursing diagnoses that may be appropriate for the client with acute enteritis are as follows:

- *Risk for aspiration* related to impaired swallow reflex (botulism)
- *Nausea* related to effects of infection or toxins on GI tract and vomiting center of the brain
- *Impaired home maintenance* related to lack of knowledge about safe food preparation and storage practices
- *Impaired spontaneous ventilation* related to respiratory muscle paralysis (botulism)
- *Impaired urinary elimination* related to effects of enterotoxin on renal function (*E. coli* hemorrhagic colitis)

Home Care

Discuss the following topics when preparing the client for home care.

- The importance of good handwashing, particularly before handling food and after each bowel movement
- The need to wash clothing and linens contaminated with feces separately in hot water and detergent
- Oral solutions to replace lost fluids and electrolytes
- Appropriate use of antidiarrheal medications if recommended
- Symptoms of complications to report to the health care-provider

THE CLIENT WITH A PROTOZOAL BOWEL INFECTION

Parasites live within, upon, or at the expense of other organisms. Parasitic intestinal infections are common in developing countries. They include both protozoal and helminthic infections (discussed in the next section of this chapter). Parasites that infect the bowel usually enter the GI tract through the mouth by the fecal–oral route; some are spread by direct contact or through sexual activity.

Of the protozoal bowel infections, only giardiasis is common in the United States. Amebiasis is found chiefly in the tropics and where sanitation is poor. Cryptosporidiosis, a form of coccidiosis, is an important worldwide cause of sporadic mild diarrhea, traveler's diarrhea, and severe diarrhea in people who are immunocompromised.

PATHOPHYSIOLOGY AND MANIFESTATIONS

The most common protozoal infections of the bowel are discussed below and summarized in Table 24–5.

Giardiasis

Giardiasis is a protozoal infection of the upper small intestine caused by *Giardia lamblia*. It is the most common intestinal protozoal pathogen in the United States, affecting children more often than adults. Humans are the reservoir for *Giardia*. It is spread by the fecal–oral route, usually in contaminated food or water. It is also spread by direct contact.

When the cyst form of the organism is ingested, trophozoites emerge in the duodenum and jejunum, attaching themselves to the intestinal mucosa. This leads to superficial invasion, inflammation, and destruction of the mucosa of the small intestine.

Giardiasis may be asymptomatic, although manifestations may develop suddenly or insidiously. Diarrhea is common. It is usually mild, with one or several large, loose stools per day. Diarrhea may be severe, however, with frequent, copious, frothy, malodorous, and greasy stools. Other manifestations include weight loss and weakness; anorexia, nausea, and vomiting; epigastric pain, abdominal cramping and distention, flatulence, and belching. Malabsorption may develop (discussed later in this chapter).

Amebiasis

Amebiasis (amebic dysentery) causes 40,000 to 100,000 deaths annually throughout the world. In the United States it tends to be mild and often asymptomatic.

Amebiasis is caused by the protozoon *Entamoeba histolytica*. Several strains of the protozoon have been identified. Tropical strains tend to be more virulent and pathogenic than those found in temperate climates. Humans are the host for this parasite. It usually is transmitted through food or water contaminated by feces and by person-to-person contact. The parasite enters the intestines, where it may live without causing disease. It may invade the intestinal wall to cause ulceration and inflammation. The cecum, appendix, ascending colon, sigmoid colon, and rectum are most often affected. Ulcers may spread to cause hemorrhage, edema, and mucosal sloughing. The infection may spread via the blood to the liver, lungs, or brain.

Amebiasis is usually asymptomatic. Mild manifestations include abdominal cramps, flatulence, and intermittent diarrhea containing blood and mucus. Severe manifestations of amebic dysentery include frequent watery stools containing blood, mucus, and necrotic tissue; colic, tenesmus, and abdominal tenderness; nausea and vomiting; and fever. The liver may be enlarged and tender to palpation.

Complications are rare, but may include appendicitis, bowel perforation with peritonitis, and fulminating colitis.

Cryptosporidiosis (Coccidiosis)

Cryptosporidiosis causes sporadic mild diarrhea and traveler's diarrhea in all age groups. In people with impaired immune function, such as those with human immunodeficiency virus (HIV) disease, it causes severe diarrhea, malabsorption, and significant weight loss.

TABLE 24–5   Common Protozoal Infections of the Bowel

Disease and Organism	Incubation	Pathogenesis	Manifestations	Management
Giardiasis: *Giardia lamblia*	1 to 3 weeks or more	Trophozoite attaches to mucosa in duodenum and jejunum, causing superficial invasion, inflammation, and tissue destruction.	Diarrhea, mild or severe, daily or intermittent; anorexia, nausea, vomiting; epigastric pain, cramping, distension; flatulence and belching; may be asymptomatic	Metronidazole, quinacrine, furazolidone
Amebiasis: *Entamoeba histolytica*	2 to 4 weeks	Organisms may reside in large intestine without causing disease or can invade colon wall, causing ulceration; may be carried via blood to liver to produce abscess.	Usually asymptomatic; diarrhea may be mild, with few semiformed mucus-containing stools per day, or severe, with 10 to 20 blood-streaked liquid stools per day; abdominal cramps and flatulence; colic, tenesmus, vomiting, tenderness; fatigue, weight loss; prostration and toxicity	Metronidazole and diloxanide furoate or iodoquinol; chloroquine for hepatic abscess
Cryptosporidiosis: *Cryptosporidium*	2 to 10 days	Organisms attach to epithelial surface of small bowel (jejunum), causing villous atrophy and mild inflammatory changes; may secrete enterotoxin.	In immunocompetent clients: Asymptomatic to profuse, watery diarrhea of sudden onset, abdominal cramping; malaise, fever; anorexia, nausea, vomiting. In immunodeficient clients: Profuse watery diarrhea with loss of up to 15 to 20 L per day; severe malabsorption, electrolyte imbalance; weight loss; lymphadenopathy	Self-limiting in immuno-competent clients. For immunodeficient clients: spiramycin, zidovudine (AZT), paromomycin (Humatin), octreotide, eflornithine; fluid and electrolyte replacement; parenteral nutrition as needed

This organism is transmitted by the fecal–oral route. Contaminated water is a frequent source of infection. The organism attaches to bowel epithelium, causing surface damage and inflammation. It does not invade the tissues, but secretes an enterotoxin that causes characteristic watery diarrhea. The disease is self-limited in people with competent immune systems. Watery diarrhea may be accompanied by low-grade fever, nausea, vomiting, abdominal cramps, and general malaise.

Immunocompromised clients develop profuse watery diarrhea with significant fluid and electrolyte losses and severe malabsorption. Lymphadenopathy also may develop.

COLLABORATIVE CARE

Collaborative care includes identifying the causative organism and pharmacologic treatment. Diagnostic testing may include:

- *Stool examination for ova and parasites.* Many protozoa are shed intermittently rather than continuously. Stools are collected sequentially (e.g., every other day for a total of three specimens). Freshly collected stool is examined microscopically to identify protozoa, trophozoites (their immature forms), or their cysts. A laxative may be given prior to the specimen collection to increase protozoal shedding.
- *Indirect hemagglutination assay (IHA),* a blood test to detect antibodies to specific protozoa. This test may not differentiate current from previous infection.

- *Sigmoidoscopy,* to examine bowel mucosa and collect a stool or exudate specimen for examination. In this case, no bowel preparation is performed before the sigmoidoscopy.
- *Duodenal string test (Entero-Test), duodenal aspiration, or duodenal biopsy* when giardiasis is suspected. Duodenal aspirate is stained and examined microscopically for the protozoa. Small bowel biopsy can identify *Cryptosporidium* infection.

Pharmacologic treatment includes both local and systemic antiparasitic drugs, such as iodoquinol (Amebaquine), paromomycin (Humatin), and metronidazole (Flagyl), furazolidone (Furoxone), or albendazole (Albenza). Treatment is usually provided on an outpatient basis. Severe amebic dysentery may require hospitalization for intravenous fluid and electrolyte replacements. Nursing care related to common antiprotozoal drugs is outlined in the box on page 646.

NURSING CARE

Nurses need to teach the public how parasitic diseases are transmitted and how to avoid spreading the infection. Prevention of amebiasis and giardiasis involves:

- Provision of safe water supplies.
- Appropriate disposal of human feces.
- Safe food storage, handling, and preparation.

Medication Administration

Antiprotozoal Agents

LOCAL (GASTROINTESTINAL) AGENTS

Iodoquinol (Yodoxin, Amebaquine)
Paromomycin (Humatin)

These drugs exert a local amebicidal effect in the intestines and are poorly absorbed when administered orally. Local agents have the advantage of provoking fewer side effects than systemically active agents.

Nursing Responsibilities

- Assess for potential contraindications:
  a. Hypersensitivity to the drug or drug class.
  b. Iodoquinol: malnutrition, thyroid disorders; hepatic or renal impairment, optic neuropathy, or hypersensitivity to iodine.
  c. Paromomycin: ulcerative bowel lesions; hypersensitivity to aminoglycoside antibiotics, impaired renal function, intestinal obstruction.
- Observe for adverse effects: anorexia, nausea, vomiting, abdominal cramping, diarrhea, and increased flatulence; report skin rash, visual disturbances, or changes in blood work to primary care provider.

Client and Family Teaching

- Take as prescribed for the full course of therapy.
- Take with food to reduce gastrointestinal effects.
- Keep follow-up appointments as recommended to evaluate the effects of treatment.
- Report adverse effects to the physician.
  a. Any change in vision
  b. Numbness, tingling or pain in extremities
  c. Chills, fever, skin rash or boils
  d. A change in urination or character of urine
  e. Diminished hearing or tinnitus
  f. Weight loss, diarrhea, fatty stools
  g. Candidiasis of the mouth or vagina
- Practice good handwashing, particularly after using the toilet, to prevent spreading the disease to others.

SYSTEMIC AGENTS

Metronidazole (Flagyl, Satric, Metzol, others)
Furazolidone (Furoxone), Albendazole (Albenza)

Clients with symptomatic protozoal infections are generally treated with a systemic antiprotozoal agent. Metronidazole is the most widely used of these antiprotozoal agents and is the drug of choice for treating amebiasis. Furazolidone, available as an elixir, often is used to treat children.

Nursing Responsibilities

- Assess for possible contraindications to therapy:
  a. Hypersensitivity to the prescribed agent or related drugs.
  b. Liver dysfunction or blood dyscrasias
  c. Concurrent use of alcohol or an MAOI
  d. Pregnancy
- Administer as ordered.
  a. Metronidazole may be given orally after meals or as a continuous or intermittent intravenous infusion.
  b. Administer furazolidone and albendazole orally with meals to minimize gastric distress.
- Observe for possible adverse effects; notify the physician if significant. Gastrointestinal effects are common.
  a. Peripheral neuropathy and CNS effects may occur with metronidazole.
  b. Blood dyscrasias may develop with furazolidone or albendazole; monitor CBC and report abnormal results.
  c. Furazolidone can cause hypoglycemia; carefully monitor blood glucose in diabetic clients.
  d. Report abnormal liver function test results.
- Monitor the character and number of stools; obtain specimens as ordered to evaluate the effectiveness of therapy.

Client and Family Teaching

- Take the drug as prescribed for the full duration of the prescription.
- Taking oral preparations after meals helps minimize gastrointestinal side effects. Notify the physician if nausea and vomiting continue.
- Do not use alcohol while taking these drugs. An Antabuse-type response with severe headache, flushing, and vomiting may occur.
- Report adverse effects to the physician, including dizziness and other nervous system changes, sore throats, fatigue, bruising, or infection.
- Candidiasis of the mouth or vagina may occur with metronidazole therapy. Report symptoms to the physician.
- A harmless change in urine color to deep yellow (quinacrine) or rust or brown (metronidazole or chloroquine) may occur while taking these drugs.
- If you are diabetic taking furazolidone, carefully monitor blood glucose levels as hypoglycemia may develop.
- Practice good handwashing, particularly after using the toilet, to prevent transmitting the protozoa to others.

- Adequate handwashing after defecating and before handling food.

Instruct people living in high-risk areas (tropical climates, areas with untreated water supplies) to boil, filter, or treat water supplies with iodine to eliminate protozoal contamination. Instruct them to avoid foods that cannot be peeled or cooked. Teach the manifestations of protozoal infections and where to obtain treatment.

Nursing assessment, diagnoses, and interventions for the client with a protozoal GI infection are similar to those indicated for clients with bacterial or viral infections. *Diarrhea* and *Risk for deficient fluid volume* are priority nursing diagnoses. See previous sections of this chapter for specific nursing interventions related to these diagnoses.

Emphasize the importance of keeping toilet areas clean and maintaining good personal hygiene. Advise the client to avoid rectal contact during sexual activity. Other household members should also have stool specimens examined for parasites. No drug is safe or effective to prevent protozoal infections of the bowel.

THE CLIENT WITH A HELMINTHIC DISORDER

Helminths are parasitic worms, capable of causing infectious diseases in humans. Helminths are subclassified as round worms (nematodes), flukes (trematodes), or tapeworms (cestodes).

PATHOPHYSIOLOGY AND MANIFESTATIONS

Although all helminths can infect humans, the definitive host and intermediate hosts vary with each organism. In nearly all instances of helminthic disorders, the organism enters the body through the gastrointestinal tract in contaminated and inadequately cooked foods. Some of these organisms remain in the intestinal tract; others migrate to infect the liver, lungs, or other structures. Few helminths are common in the United States; Table 24–6 summarizes the most common helminths and their effects.

TABLE 24–6   Selected Helminthic Diseases

	Infection	Host	Area	Pathogenesis	Manifestations
Nematode Infections	Ascariasis	Humans	Worldwide, cosmopolitan; warm, moist climates	Eggs are ingested in fecally contaminated food and drink; motile larvae migrate to lungs and back to small intestine, where they mature to produce more eggs.	Pulmonary: Low-grade fever, cough, blood-tinged sputum, wheezing, dyspnea, substernal chest pain. GI: Ulcerlike epigastric pain, vomiting, abdominal distention
	Enterobiasis (Pinworm infection)	Humans	Worldwide, cosmopolitan	Infect cecum; eggs deposit on perianal skin, organisms may be transmitted to others or reinfect host by oral ingestion.	Nocturnal perianal and perineal pruritus; insomnia, irritability, restlessness
	Hookworm disease	Humans	Tropics and subtropics	Larvae enter through skin or by ingestion and migrate to lungs, up bronchial tree, and down esophagus to mature in upper small bowel, where they attach and suck blood.	Skin: Pruritic dermatitis at site of entry Pulmonary: Dry cough, wheezing, blood-tinged sputum GI: Anorexia, diarrhea, abdominal pain Systemic: Anemia, pallor, cardiac insufficiency
	Trichinosis	Pigs; dogs, cats, rats, many wild animals	Temperate areas where pork is consumed	Larvae are ingested in undercooked meat; adult female burrows into mucosa of small intestine to produce larvae that disseminate via blood and lymphatic system to body tissues and become encysted in striated muscle.	GI: Diarrhea, abdominal cramps, malaise Muscle: Fever; muscle pain, tenderness, edema, and spasm Systemic: Periorbital and facial edema, sweating; photophobia and conjunctivitis; manifestations of inflammation in tissues invaded by larvae
Cestode Infections	Fasciolopsiasis (intestinal fluke) Tapeworm	Humans; other mammals and fish	Worldwide	Organism is ingested by eating uncooked fish or meat containing embryo cysts, by fecal contamination, or by swallowing infected intermediate hosts, such as arthropods, fleas, or lice; head (scolex) of adult worm attaches in upper small intestine, and eggs form in individual segments.	Large tapeworms: Often asymptomatic; infection may cause mild nausea, diarrhea, abdominal pain; anemia, thrombocytopenia, and mild leukopenia Small tapeworms: May be asymptomatic; diarrhea, abdominal pain, anorexia, vomiting, weight loss, and irritability

COLLABORATIVE CARE

The primary means of diagnosing helminthic disorders is examination of the stool for ova and parasites. Enterobiasis is diagnosed by the presence of the parasite's eggs on the perianal skin or on cellulose tape placed over the anus. A CBC may also be ordered. Anemia may be present, particularly with hookworm disease. *Eosinophilia* (an increased percentage of eosinophils in the blood) is common in helminthic disorders. With trichinosis, serum muscle enzymes such as the creatinine kinase (CK) and aspartate aminotransferase (AST) are typically elevated. Serologic testing for antibodies to the worm may also be performed. Blood, duodenal washings, and cerebrospinal fluid (CSF) may be examined for the presence of the trichinosis larvae. Inflamed muscle may be biopsied.

Helminthic infections often are treated with a single oral dose or 3-day course of pyrantel pamoate (Antiminth) or mebendazole (Vermox). Doses may need to be repeated every 2 weeks for clients with heavy infections. These drugs are generally safe, requiring few precautions. Giving the drug after meals minimizes gastrointestinal side effects. Treatment is followed by a stool culture at 2 weeks to evaluate effectiveness. If necessary, an additional course of the drug is prescribed. Other members of the household are generally also treated.

Most clients with trichinosis recover spontaneously without long-term effects. The intestinal phase of the disease is treated with albendazole, taken twice daily for as long as 60 days, or a 13-day course of mebendazole. Hospitalization may be required during the muscle invasion phase of the disease if the infection is severe. Corticosteroids may be used to reduce the inflammation and manage the symptoms.

NURSING CARE

Many helminthic disorders are acquired by consuming food that has been fecally contaminated or contains larvae of the organism. Emphasize the importance of not fertilizing food or grain crops with fecal material, particularly human feces. Teach clients to cook all meats and fish adequately to destroy possible larvae. In general, pickled or salt-preserved meats and fish are no safer than raw. Smoking, another means of preserving fish and meat, may not achieve temperatures high enough to destroy the organisms. Vegetables grown in soil that may be contaminated with eggs or larvae should be peeled or cooked prior to eating.

Emphasize the importance of safe water supplies. Encourage people traveling to areas in which water supplies are questionable to drink only bottled water or carry purification tablets. Work with clients who have private water systems to protect water from fecal contamination by either humans or animals.

Because many clients with these disorders are asymptomatic, nurses need to be alert for histories that indicate risk and subtle manifestations of the disorder.

Use standard precautions to minimize the risk of spreading these infections to other clients. Wear gloves and gowns as necessary to prevent fecal contamination of hands and uniforms. On rare occasions, parasites may be present in the sputum or vomitus, so handle these secretions with care also. Disinfect toilets, toilet seats, and commodes after use. To the client, emphasize the importance of washing hands after using the toilet and before handling food to prevent reinfection.

The client with a helminthic disorder may feel dirty or be ashamed of the disease. Emphasize the prevalence of these disorders, and assure the client that infection can occur despite good health practices when the eggs or larva of the organism are prevalent.

Discuss measures to prevent spread of the disease in the household. Emphasize the importance of hygiene measures including changing bedding, daily cleaning of toilets with disinfectant, and, of course, handwashing.

CHRONIC INFLAMMATORY BOWEL DISEASE

THE CLIENT WITH INFLAMMATORY BOWEL DISEASE

Chronic inflammatory bowel disease (IBD) includes two separate but closely related conditions: ulcerative colitis and Crohn's disease. These conditions have a number of similarities. The etiology of both illnesses is unknown, but both have a geographic distribution and a genetic component. IBD occurs more frequently in the United States and northern European nations than it does in southern Europe and countries in the Southern Hemisphere. IBD is 2 to 4 times more prevalent in Jewish populations of the United States and Europe than it is in non-Jewish Caucasians, African Americans, Hispanics, and Asians (Braunwald et al., 2001). It tends to run in families. Other studies suggest that factors such as an infectious agents and altered immune responses play a role in the development of IBD. Autoimmunity is thought to play a role (see Chapter 9). ⊕ Lifestyle factors (such as smoking) may also affect its development.

The peak incidence of IBD is in young adults between the ages of 15 and 35 years. A second peak occurs between age 60 and 80 (Braunwald et al., 2001). IBD is a chronic and recurrent disease process. Responses to physiologic or psychologic stresses do not cause IBD, but often play a role in exacerbations of the disease.

Despite the similarities, ulcerative colitis and Crohn's disease have distinct differences. Ulcerative colitis primarily affects the large bowel in a continuous pattern, progressing distally to proximally. In Crohn's disease, a patchy pattern of

TABLE 24–7 Characteristics of Ulcerative Colitis and Crohn's Disease

	Characteristic	Ulcerative Colitis	Crohn's Disease
Clinical	Gender	Equal	Equal
	Age at onset	15 to 35 years; secondary peak between 50 and 70 years	10 to 30 years
	Course of disease	Typically chronic and intermittent	Slowly progressive, relapsing
	Diarrhea	5 to 30 stools per day with blood and mucus	Common, usually less severe than colitis, with no obvious blood or mucus in stool
	Abdominal pain	Cramping in left lower quadrant; relieved by defecation	Cramping or steady right lower quadrant or periumbilical pain; tenderness and mass noted in right lower quadrant
	Nutritional deficit	Common; involves anemia, hypoalbuminemia, and weight loss	Common and significant: involves anemia, weight loss, and multiple vitamin and mineral deficits
	Constitutional manifestations	Fever rare; may have associated arthritic, skin, or other organ involvement, such as erythema nodosum or uveitis	Fever, malaise, fatigue; may have some associated conditions plus urinary complications
Pathologic	Depth of involvement	Mucosa and submucosa	Transmural (entire bowel wall)
	Portion of bowel involved	Typically rectum and sigmoid colon; may extend to involve entire large bowel	Any portion of GI tract; terminal ileum and ascending colon involvement predominates
	Distribution	Continuous from rectum	Patchy; skip lesions
	Appearance of mucosa	Granular, dull, hyperemic, friable; disease uniform in affected bowel; pseudopolyps may be seen	Cobblestone appearance, with areas of normal tissue surrounded by ulceration and fissures
Complications	Acute	Toxic megacolon, perforation, massive hemorrhage	Obstruction, fistulization, abscess formation, malabsorption
	Long-term	Colorectal cancer	Colon cancer

involvement is seen, affecting primarily the small intestine. Ulcerative colitis shows mainly mucosal involvement; in Crohn's disease, the submucosal layers of the bowel are affected. A comparison of ulcerative colitis and Crohn's disease is found in Table 24–7. *Multisystem Effects of Inflammatory Bowel Disease* are illustrated on page 650.

ULCERATIVE COLITIS

Ulcerative colitis is a chronic inflammatory bowel disorder that affects the mucosa and submucosa of the colon and rectum. Its annual incidence in the United States is about 11 per 100,000 people (Braunwald et al., 2001).

Chronic intermittent colitis (recurrent ulcerative colitis) is the most common form of the disease. Its onset is insidious, with attacks that last 1 to 3 months occurring at intervals of months to years. Typically, only the distal colon is affected, with few systemic manifestations of the disease. Approximately 15% of people with ulcerative colitis develop *fulminant colitis,* with involvement of the entire colon, severe bloody diarrhea, acute abdominal pain, and fever. Clients with fulminant disease are at high risk for complications.

Physiology Review

The wall of the colon has three layers: the mucosa, the submucosa, and the muscularis externa. The mucosal layer contains an abundance of goblet cells and glands which secrete lubricating mucus to facilitate the movement of feces. The colon wall forms a series of pouches, or *haustra*. These pouches allow the colon to expand and contract. Feces moves through the colon by both peristaltic waves and by segmentation movements that mix the contents of adjacent haustra. As feces moves, water and other substances such as bile salts are reabsorbed.

Pathophysiology

The inflammatory process of ulcerative colitis begins at the rectosigmoid area of the anal canal and progresses proximally. In most clients, the disease is confined to the rectum and sigmoid colon. It may progress to involve the entire colon, stopping at the ileocecal junction.

Ulcerative colitis begins with inflammation at the base of the crypts of Lieberkühn in the distal large intestine and rectum. Microscopic, pinpoint mucosal hemorrhages occur, and crypt abscesses develop (Figure 24–4 ■). These abscesses penetrate the superficial submucosa and spread laterally, leading to necrosis and sloughing of bowel mucosa. Further tissue damage is caused by inflammatory exudates and the release of inflammatory mediators, such as prostaglandins and other cytokines (see Chapter 8 ⊖⊃ for further discussion of the inflammatory process). The mucosa is red and edematous due to vascular congestion, friable (easily broken), and ulcerated. It bleeds easily,

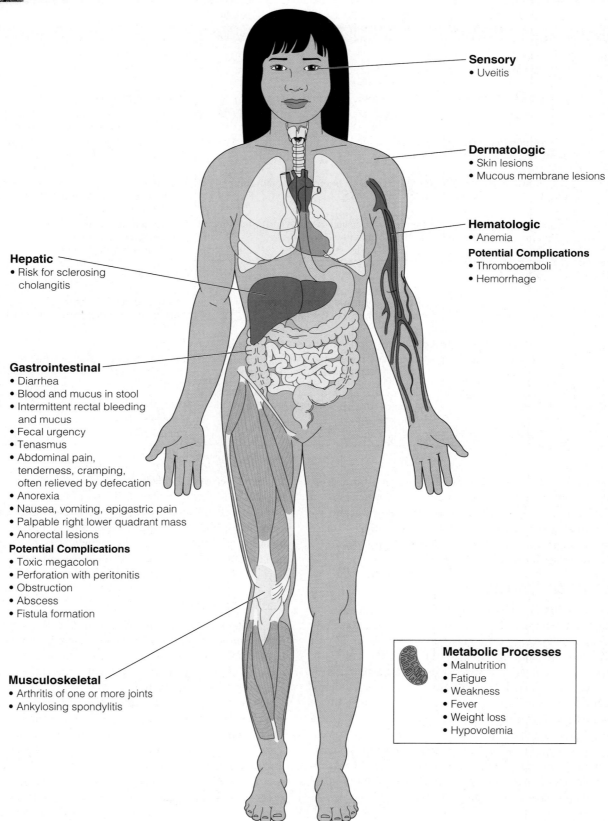

Sensory
• Uveitis

Dermatologic
• Skin lesions
• Mucous membrane lesions

Hematologic
• Anemia
Potential Complications
• Thromboemboli
• Hemorrhage

Hepatic
• Risk for sclerosing cholangitis

Gastrointestinal
• Diarrhea
• Blood and mucus in stool
• Intermittent rectal bleeding and mucus
• Fecal urgency
• Tenasmus
• Abdominal pain, tenderness, cramping, often relieved by defecation
• Anorexia
• Nausea, vomiting, epigastric pain
• Palpable right lower quadrant mass
• Anorectal lesions
Potential Complications
• Toxic megacolon
• Perforation with peritonitis
• Obstruction
• Abscess
• Fistula formation

Musculoskeletal
• Arthritis of one or more joints
• Ankylosing spondylitis

Metabolic Processes
• Malnutrition
• Fatigue
• Weakness
• Fever
• Weight loss
• Hypovolemia

Crypts of
Lieberkuhn

Figure 24–4 ■ Photomicrograph of the mucosa of the large intestine showing the entrances to the crypts of Lieberkühn. The crypts are the focal points for ulcerative colitis.

Source: Photo Researchers, Inc.

and hemorrhage is common. Edema creates a granular appearance. Pseudopolyps, tonguelike projections of bowel mucosa into the lumen, may develop as the epithelial lining of the bowel regenerates. Chronic inflammation leads to atrophy, narrowing, and shortening of the colon, with loss of its normal haustra.

MANIFESTATIONS

Diarrhea is the predominant symptom of ulcerative colitis. Stools contain both blood and mucus. Nocturnal diarrhea may occur. Mild ulcerative colitis is characterized by fewer than five stools per day, intermittent rectal bleeding and mucus, and few constitutional symptoms. Severe ulcerative colitis can lead to more than 6 to 10 bloody stools per day, extensive colon involvement, anemia, hypovolemia, and malnutrition. Rectal inflammation causes fecal urgency and tenesmus. Left lower quadrant cramping relieved by defecation is common. Other systemic manifestations include fatigue, anorexia, and weakness.

Clients with severe disease also may have systemic manifestations such as arthritis involving one or several joints, skin and mucous membrane lesions, or *uveitis* (inflammation of the uvea, the vascular layer of the eye, which may also involve the sclera and cornea). Some clients develop thromboemboli, with blood vessel obstruction due to clots carried from the site of their formation. Sclerosing cholangitis (inflammation and scarring of the bile ducts) may occur (Tierney et al., 2001).

Complications

Acute complications of ulcerative colitis include hemorrhage, toxic megacolon, and colon perforation. Massive hemorrhage may occur with severe attacks of the disease. **Toxic megacolon,** a condition characterized by acute motor paralysis and dilation of the colon to greater than 6 cm, may affect part or all of the colon. The transverse segment of the bowel is most often affected. Toxic megacolon may be triggered by electrolyte imbalances or narcotic administration (Braunwald et al., 2001). Manifestations of toxic megacolon include fever, tachycardia,

hypotension, dehydration, abdominal tenderness and cramping, and a change in the number of stools per day. Perforation is rare, but the risk of this dangerous complication is increased with toxic megacolon. Perforation leads to peritonitis, and has a mortality rate of about 15% (Braunwald et al., 2001).

The risk for colorectal cancer is increased in clients with ulcerative colitis. When the entire colon is involved by ulcerative colitis, the risk is 20 to 30 times greater than for the general public (Porth, 2002). Beginning 8 to 10 years after the diagnosis, yearly colonoscopies with biopsy to detect masses or cell dysplasia are recommended for clients who have extensive ulcerative colitis (Tierney et al., 2001).

CROHN'S DISEASE

Like ulcerative colitis, **Crohn's disease,** also known as regional enteritis, is a chronic, relapsing inflammatory disorder affecting the gastrointestinal tract. The overall incidence of Crohn's disease in the United States is approximately 7 per 100,000 people (Braunwald et al., 2001).

Crohn's disease can affect any portion of the GI tract from the mouth to the anus, but usually affects the terminal ileum and ascending colon. Only the small bowel is involved in about 30% to 40% of clients with Crohn's disease. The disease is limited to the colon only in 15% to 20% of those affected. Both the small and large intestine are involved in the majority (Braunwald et al., 2001).

Pathophysiology

Crohn's disease typically begins as a small inflammatory *aphthoid lesion* (shallow ulcers with a white base and elevated margin, similar to a canker sore) of the mucosa and submucosa of the bowel. These initial lesions may regress, or the inflammatory process can progress to involve all layers of the intestinal wall. Deeper ulcerations, granulomatous lesions, and fissures (knifelike clefts that extend deeply into the bowel wall) develop. The inflammatory process involves the entire bowel wall (transmural).

The lumen of the affected bowel assumes a "cobblestone appearance" as fissures and ulcers surround islands of intact mucosa over edematous submucosa. The inflammatory lesions of Crohn's disease are not continuous; rather, they often occur as "skip" lesions with intervening areas of normal-appearing bowel. Some evidence suggests that despite its normal appearance, the entire bowel is affected by this disorder.

As the disease progresses, fibrotic changes in the bowel wall cause it to thicken and lose flexibility, taking on an appearance that has been likened to a rubber hose. The inflammation, edema, and fibrosis can lead to local obstruction, abscess development, and the formation of fistulas between loops of bowel or bowel and other organs (Figure 24–5 ■). Fistulas between loops of bowel are known as enteroenteric fistulas; those that occur between bowel and bladder are known as enterovesical fistulas; and fistulas that occur between bowel and skin are known as enterocutaneous fistulas. Perineal fistulas are relatively common, originating in the ileum.

Depending on the severity and extent of the disease, malabsorption and malnutrition may develop as the ulcers prevent

Figure 24–5 ■ The progression of Crohn's disease.

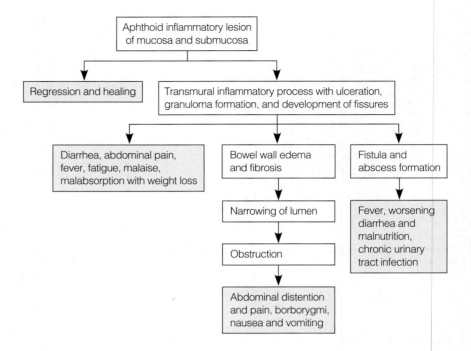

absorption of nutrients. When the jejunum and ileum are affected, the absorption of multiple nutrients may be impaired, including carbohydrates, proteins, fats, vitamins, and folate. Disease in the terminal ileum can lead to vitamin B_{12} malabsorption and bile salt reabsorption. The ulcerations can also lead to protein loss and chronic, slow blood loss with consequent anemia.

MANIFESTATIONS

Because the GI system involvement in Crohn's disease can be so diverse, manifestations may vary among clients. The majority of people with Crohn's disease experience continuous or episodic diarrhea. Stools are liquid or semiformed and typically do not contain blood, although blood may be passed if the colon is involved. Abdominal pain and tenderness is also common. The pain may be located in the right lower quadrant and relieved by defecation. A palpable right lower quadrant mass is often present. Systemic manifestations such as fever, fatigue, malaise, weight loss, and anemia are common. Anorectal lesions such as fissures, ulcers, fistulas, and abscesses also are common and may occur years before intestinal disease is apparent. If the stomach and duodenum are involved, nausea, vomiting, and epigastric pain may occur.

Complications

Certain complications of Crohn's disease (e.g., intestinal obstruction, abscess, and fistula) are so common that they are considered part of the disease process. For many clients, the disease initially presents with one of these complications. Intestinal obstruction is a common complication caused by repeated inflammation and scarring of the bowel that leads to fibrosis and stricture. Obstruction of the bowel lumen causes abdominal distention, cramping pain, and borborygmi. Nausea and vomiting may occur.

Fistulas may be asymptomatic, particularly if they occur between loops of small bowel. When fistulization causes an abscess, chills and fever, a tender abdominal mass, and leukocy-

tosis develop. A fistula between the small bowel and colon may exacerbate diarrhea, weight loss, and malnutrition. When the bladder is involved, recurrent urinary tract infections occur.

Perforation of the bowel is uncommon, but can lead to generalized peritonitis. Massive hemorrhage also is an uncommon complication of Crohn's disease. Long-standing Crohn's disease increases the risk of cancer of the small intestine or colon by 5 to 6 times. This cancer risk, however, is significantly lower than the risk associated with ulcerative colitis.

COLLABORATIVE CARE

Collaborative care for inflammatory bowel disease begins by establishing the diagnosis and the extent and severity of the disease. Treatment is supportive, including medications and dietary measures to decrease inflammation, promote intestinal rest and healing, and reduce intestinal motility. Many clients with IBD require surgery at some point to manage the disease or its complications.

Diagnostic Tests

Diagnostic testing is used to establish the diagnosis of IBD, assess the extent of the disease, and evaluate the effects of the disorder.

- *Sigmoidoscopy* or *colonoscopy* is performed to inspect the bowel mucosa for characteristic changes of IBD: edema, inflammation, mucus and pus, mucosal ulcers or abscesses, and either a continuous or segmental pattern of involvement. Biopsy of bowel mucosa may differentiate ulcerative colitis or Crohn's disease from cancer and other inflammatory bowel disorders. There is a small risk of bowel perforation during these exams, particularly if the disease is severe. Nursing implications for these diagnostic tests are listed in the boxes on pages 619 and 624.

- *Radiologic examination* of the entire gastrointestinal tract includes an upper GI series with small bowel follow-through and a barium enema. These studies can show the characteristic small and large bowel changes of IBD, such as ulcerations, strictures, fistulas, shortening and loss of colon haustra, or complications such as a dilated colon in toxic megacolon. Nursing implications for the client having a barium enema are listed in the box on page 623; see the box on page 628 for nursing implications for a small bowel series.
- *Stool examination* for blood and mucus and *stool cultures* are done to rule out infectious causes of bowel inflammation and diarrhea.
- *CBC with hemoglobin* and *hematocrit* shows anemia from chronic inflammation, blood loss, and malnutrition; and leukocytosis due to inflammation and possible abscess formation. The sedimentation rate is typically elevated during periods of acute inflammation.
- *Serum albumin* may be decreased because of malabsorption, malnutrition, protein loss through intestinal lesions, and chronic inflammation.
- *Folic acid* and *serum levels* of most vitamins, including A, B complex, C, and the fat-soluble vitamins, often are decreased due to malabsorption.

- *Liver function tests* may show elevated liver enzymes (such as ALT, alkaline phosphatase, AST, GGTP, and LDH) and bilirubin levels if sclerosing cholangitis is present.

Medications

The ultimate goal of care is to terminate acute attacks as quickly as possible and reduce the incidence of relapse. Drug therapy plays a key role in achieving this goal. Locally acting and systemic anti-inflammatory drugs are the primary medications used to manage mild to moderate IBD. Drugs to suppress the immune response may be used to treat clients with severe disease.

Sulfasalazine (Azulfidine) is a sulfonamide antibiotic that is poorly absorbed from the gastrointestinal tract and acts topically on the colonic mucosa to inhibit the inflammatory process. The active anti-inflammatory ingredient in sulfasalazine, 5-aminosalicylic acid, also is available in preparations that do not contain sulfa, such as olsalazine and mesalamine. They have the advantage of causing fewer adverse effects than sulfasalazine. Specific preparations, their method of action, and nursing implications for these medications are outlined in the box below and on the following page.

Medication Administration

Inflammatory Bowel Disease

SULFASALAZINE (AZULFIDINE)

Sulfasalazine is an anti-inflammatory drug used for its local effect on the intestinal mucosa in inflammatory bowel disease. The active part of the drug is 5-aminosalicylic acid, which inhibits prostaglandin production in the bowel. Prostaglandin is an important mediator of the inflammatory process; blocking its production reduces inflammation.

Nursing Responsibilities

- Assess for contraindications, including pregnancy or a history of hypersensitivity to sulfonamides or salicylates.
- Assess baseline values for renal function tests (serum creatinine, BUN, urinalysis), liver function tests, and CBC.
- Administer as ordered. Suppositories or retention enemas may be administered at bedtime. Administer oral forms with a full glass of water.
- Have resuscitation equipment available; anaphylactic responses may occur.
- Evaluate for therapeutic response, including reduced number of stools, reduced mucus and blood, and improved stool consistency.
- Monitor for possible adverse responses:
  a. Skin rash, dermatitis, urticaria, or pruritus
  b. Evidence of blood dyscrasias, such as bleeding, easy bruising, fever
  c. Leukopenia, thrombocytopenia, hemolytic anemia, or anagranulocytosis
  d. Changes in urinary output or renal function studies
  e. Evidence of hepatitis or myocarditis

Client and Family Teaching
- Take oral preparations after meals to decrease gastric distress.

- Drink at least 2 quarts of fluid per day to reduce the risk of kidney damage.
- Use sunscreen to prevent burns; this drug increases sensitivity to sun.
- Do not take aspirin, vitamin C, or any other over-the-counter medications containing aspirin or vitamin C without consulting your doctor.
- This medication may interfere with the effectiveness of oral contraceptives; use alternative methods of contraception.
- Notify your doctor if you develop skin rash or hives, sore throat or mouth, bleeding gums, joint pain, easy bruising, or fever.

MESALAMINE (ASACOL ROWASA) AND OLSALAZINE (DIPENTUM)

Mesalamine and olsalazine contain the same active ingredient, 5-aminosalicylic acid, as sulfasalazine, but cause fewer adverse effects. Their mechanism of action is the same as that of sulfasalazine. These drugs are available as suppositories, suspension for enema, or oral tablets.

Nursing Responsibilities
- Assess for possible contraindications such as pregnancy, lactation, or hypersensitivity to these drugs or aspirin.
- Administer as ordered. If more than one dose per day is ordered, space doses evenly over the 24-hour period.
- Evaluate for desired effects (as for sulfasalazine) and potential adverse effects.
  a. Nausea, diarrhea, abdominal cramps, or flatulence
  b. CNS effects including headache, dizziness, insomnia, weakness, or fatigue
  c. Rash or itching
  d. Flulike symptoms, general malaise

(continued on page 654)

Medication Administration

Inflammatory Bowel Disease (continued)

Client and Family Teaching

- Teach the recommended method of administration, including how to insert rectal suppositories or administer a retention enema.
- Shake suspension forms well prior to using.
- Diarrhea is the most common side effect of these drugs. Notify your doctor if adverse effects occur.

CORTICOSTEROIDS

Methylprednisolone   Prednisolone
(Medrol, Solu-Medrol)   (Delta-Cortel)
                           Prednisone

Glucocorticoids are hormones produced by the adrenal cortex. These hormones are necessary for the stress response. Cortisol, the main glucocorticoid, has potent anti-inflammatory effects. Corticosteroids are used to treat acute episodes of IBD. Because of their multiple and significant side effects, they are not used to maintain remission.

Nursing Responsibilities

- Assess for conditions that may be adversely affected by corticosteroid drugs: peptic ulcer disease, glaucoma or cataracts, diabetes, or psychiatric disorders.
- Obtain baseline vital signs and weight; monitor both routinely during therapy. Hypertension and weight gain may result from salt and water retention.
- Monitor for edema.
- Administer as ordered. For daily or alternate-day dosing, administer in the morning, when physiologic glucocorticoid levels are highest, to reduce adrenal cortisone suppression.
- Administer oral preparations with food to decrease gastrointestinal side effects. Antacids or histamine H_2-receptor blocking agents, such as cimetidine (Tagamet), may be prescribed during corticosteroid therapy.

- Monitor for desired effects reduced diarrhea, less blood and mucus in the stool, and less abdominal cramping.
- Monitor for adverse effects:
  a. Increased susceptibility to infection and masking of early signs of infection
  b. Hyperglycemia
  c. Hypokalemia, as manifested by muscle weakness, nausea, vomiting, and cardiac rhythm disturbances
  d. Edema, hypertension, and signs of heart failure
  e. Peptic ulcer formation and possible gastrointestinal hemorrhage (abdominal pain, black or tarry stools, and signs of bleeding)
  f. Changes in mental status, including depression, euphoria, aggression, and behavioral changes
  g. With long-term use, Cushingoid effects, such as abnormal fat deposits in the face (moon faces) and trunk (buffalo hump), muscle wasting and thin extremities, thinning of the skin, and osteoporosis

Client and Family Teaching

- Take as prescribed; do not change the dose or time of day. Do not stop the medication abruptly. The dose will be tapered down gradually when the drug is discontinued.
- Notify the physician if adverse or Cushingoid effects occur.
- Take with food or at mealtimes to decrease the gastrointestinal effects.
- Monitor weight. If a gain of more than 5 pounds is noted notify the physician.
- Moderate salt intake and avoid foods and snacks high in sodium, such as processed meats and potato chips. Increase intake of foods high in potassium, such as fruits, vegetables, and lean meats.
- Carry a card or wear a bracelet or tag at all times identifying corticosteroid use.

For acute exacerbations of IBD, corticosteroids are given to reduce inflammation and induce remission. For ulcerative colitis, the drug may be administered by enema for its local effect and to minimize systemic effects. Hydrocortisone can be administered by enema. Intravenous corticosteroids may be required to treat severe disease; oral preparations are used for less severe manifestations and long-term therapy. Many clients are unable to withdraw from steroid therapy without experiencing relapse and may need chronic low-dose therapy.

Mercaptopurine (6-MP, Purinethol) and other immunosuppressive agents such as azathioprine (Imuran) and cyclosporine (Sandimmune) may be used to treat clients who have not responded to other treatments or who require chronic steroid therapy. These drugs may allow withdrawal from corticosteroids, maintain remission, and facilitate healing. Long-term therapy may be required to produce a beneficial effect. For more information about immunosuppressive drugs, see Chapter 9. ⏎

Newer treatments for IBD employ other immune response modifiers, such as monoclonal antibodies to suppress tumor necrosis factor (TNF, an inflammatory mediator substance),

and natural anti-inflammatory cyctokines such as interleukins (Braunwald et al., 2001).

Although antibiotic therapy generally is not indicated in IBD, metronidazole (Flagyl) has active anti-inflammatory effects. It may be prescribed to help prevent remission after ileal resection in Crohn's disease. See the Medication Administration box on page 646 for the nursing implications for metronidazole. Ciprofloxacin (Cipro) is an alternative to metronidazole.

Antidiarrheal agents, such as loperamide and diphenoxylate, may be given to slow gastrointestinal motility and reduce diarrhea. These drugs are safe for clients with mild, chronic symptoms, but they are not given during acute attacks because they may precipitate toxic dilation of the colon.

Dietary Management

Antigens in the diet may stimulate the immune response in the bowel, exacerbating IBD. As a result, dietary management for inflammatory bowel disease is individualized. Some clients benefit from eliminating all milk and milk products from the diet. Increased dietary fiber may help reduce diarrhea and relieve rectal symptoms, but is contraindicated for clients with intestinal strictures caused by repeated inflammation and scarring.

All food is withheld to promote bowel rest during an acute exacerbation of Crohn's disease. Nutritional status is maintained using enteral or total parenteral nutrition (TPN). See Chapter 20 for more information about enteral feedings and TPN. TPN carries a higher risk of complications than does enteral nutrition. An elemental diet such as Ensure, which contains all essential nutrients in a residue-free formula, may be prescribed. Enteral diets provide essential nutrients to the small intestine to support cell growth, but are not always palatable.

Surgery

Surgical interventions for IBD differ, depending on the primary disease process and the portion of the bowel affected. Generally, surgery is performed only when necessitated by complications of the disease or failure of conservative treatment measures.

Bowel obstruction is the leading indication for surgery in Crohn's disease. Other complications that may require surgical intervention include perforation, internal or external fistula, abscess, and perianal complications. Resection of the affected portion of bowel with an end-to-end anastomosis to preserve as much bowel as possible is the usual treatment. The disease process tends to recur in other areas following removal of affected bowel segments. There is an increased risk of fistula formation following surgery. Bowel strictures may be treated with a strictureplasty. In this procedure, longitudinal incisions are made in the narrowed segment to relieve the stricture while preserving bowel.

Clients with extensive chronic ulcerative colitis may require a **total colectomy** (surgical removal of the colon) to treat the disease itself, for complications such as toxic megacolon, perforation, or hemorrhage, or as a prophylactic measure due to the high colon cancer risk associated with extensive ulcerative colitis. The surgical procedure of choice for extensive ulcerative colitis is a *total colectomy with an ileal pouch-anal anastomosis (IPAA)*. In this procedure, the entire colon and rectum are removed; a pouch is formed from the terminal ileum; and the pouch is brought into the pelvis and anastomosed to the anal canal (Figure 24–6 ■). A temporary or loop ileostomy (described below) is generally performed at the same time and is maintained for 2 to 3 months to allow the anal anastomosis to heal. When the healing is complete, the ileostomy is closed, and the client has 6 to 8 daily bowel movements through the anus.

Advanced age, obesity, or other factors may preclude an IPAA. For these clients, a permanent ileostomy or continent ileostomy may be created.

An intestinal **ostomy** is a surgically created opening between the intestine and the abdominal wall which allows the passage of fecal material. The surface opening is called a **stoma** (Figure 24–7 ■).

The precise name of the ostomy depends on the location of the stoma. An **ileostomy** is an ostomy made in the ileum of the small intestine. In an ileostomy, the colon, rectum, and anus are usually completely removed (*total proctocolectomy with permanent ileostomy*). The anal canal is closed, and the end of the terminal ileum is brought to the body surface through the right abdominal wall to form the stoma. A temporary or *loop ileostomy* may be formed to eliminate feces and allow tissue healing for 2 to 3 months following an IPAA. A loop of ileum is

Figure 24–6 ■ Ileal pouch-anal anastomosis.

Figure 24–7 ■ A healthy-appearing stoma.

Courtesy of Carol Williams, RN, BS, UC Davis Medical Center.

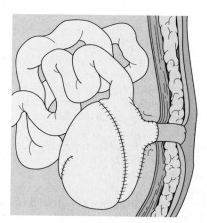

Figure 24–8 ■ Continent (Kock's) ileostomy.

brought to the body surface to form a stoma and allow stool drainage into an external pouch. When the ileostomy is no longer necessary, a second surgery is performed to close the stoma and repair the bowel, restoring fecal elimination through the anus.

In a *continent* (or *Kock's*) *ileostomy,* (Figure 24–8 ■) an intra-abdominal reservoir is constructed and a nipple valve formed (the ileum folded back on itself) from the terminal ileum, before it is brought to the surface of the abdominal wall. Stool collects in the internal pouch; the nipple valve prevents it from leaking through the stoma. A catheter is inserted into the pouch to drain the stool.

Nursing care of the client with an ileostomy is outlined below and on the following page. Procedure 24–1 on page 658 describes how to apply one- and two-piece drainable ostomy pouches.

NURSING CARE OF THE CLIENT HAVING AN ILEOSTOMY

PREOPERATIVE CARE

- Provide routine preoperative care and teaching as outlined in Chapter 7. ∞
- Refer to an enterostomal therapist for marking and teaching about the stoma location, ostomy care, and options for ostomy appliances. *It is important to begin teaching prior to surgery to facilitate learning and acceptance of the ostomy postoperatively.*
- Discuss the availability of a local United Ostomy Association chapter, and provide a referral as necessary or desired. *Local chapters often have members with ostomies who are willing to provide both preoperative and postoperative teaching, listening, and support.*
- Provide preoperative bowel preparation as ordered. *Cathartics, enemas, and preoperative antibiotics are often ordered to reduce the risk of abdominal contamination and infection after surgery.*

POSTOPERATIVE CARE

- Provide routine postoperative care and teaching as outlined in Chapter 7.
- Apply an ostomy pouch over the stoma. (See Procedure 24–1.) *Stool from an ileostomy is expressed continuously or irregularly, and it is liquid in nature; continuous use of a pouch to collect the drainage is therefore necessary.*
- Assess frequently for bleeding, stoma viability, and function. In the early postoperative period, small amounts of blood in the pouch are expected. A healthy stoma appears pink or red and moist as a result of mucus production (Figure 24–7). It should protrude approximately 2 cm from the abdominal wall. *Frequent assessment is particularly important in the initial postoperative period to ensure stoma health and monitor for possible complications. A dusky, brown, black, or white stoma indicates circulatory compromise. Other possible stoma complications include retraction (indentation or loss of the external portion of the stoma) or prolapse (outward telescoping of the stoma, that is, an abnormally long stoma).*
- As the stoma starts to function, empty the pouch, explaining the procedure to the client. Initial drainage is dark green, viscid, and usually odorless. Drainage gradually thickens and becomes yellow-brown. Empty the pouch when it is one-third full. Measure drainage, and include it as output on intake and output records. Rinse the pouch and reapply the clamp. *Emptying the pouch when it is no more than one-third full helps prevent the skin seal from breaking as a result of the weight of the pouch. Because of the potential for excess fluid loss through ileostomy drainage, it is important to include it as fluid output.*
- Assess the peristomal skin. Skin around the stoma should remain clean and pink and free of irritation, rashes, inflammation, or excoriation. *Skin complications may arise from appliance irritation or hypersensitivity, excoriation from a leaking appliance, or* Candida albicans, *a yeast infection.*

- Protect peristomal skin from enzymes and bile salts in the ileostomy effluent. Using a skin barrier on the pouch is essential. Change the pouch if leakage occurs or if the client complains of burning or itching skin. *Enzymes and bile salts normally reabsorbed in the large intestine are irritating to the skin. Excoriation of skin surrounding the stoma impairs the first line of defense against microorganisms and can interfere with the ability to achieve a tight skin seal and prevent pouch leakage.*
- Report the following abnormal assessment findings to the physician:
  a. Allergic or contact dermatitis. *A rash may result from contact with fecal drainage or indicate sensitivity to pouch, paste, tape, or sealant.*
  b. Purulent ulcerated areas surrounding the stoma. *Disruption of the protective barrier of the skin allows bacterial entry.*
  c. A red, bumpy, itchy rash or white-coated area. *This is a manifestation of* Candida albicans, *a yeast infection.*
  d. Bulging around the stoma. *This finding may indicate herniation, caused by loops of intestine protruding through the abdominal wall.*
- Apply protective ointments to the perirectal area of clients with newly functioning ileoanal reservoirs and anastomoses. *This helps protect the skin from the initial stools. As stools thicken and become fewer per day, the client experiences less perirectal irritation.*

CLIENT AND FAMILY TEACHING

- While caring for the ostomy, explain procedures to the client. *Teaching is immediate and ongoing to facilitate acceptance of the ostomy and self-care.*
- Teach to manage the pouch clamp, to empty, rinse, and perform pouch changes. *Self-care is vital to independence and self-esteem.*
- Instruct now to use an electric razor to shave the peristomal hair if necessary. *An electric razor prevents accidental cutting of the stoma with a razor blade.*
- Teach to check the stoma and peristomal skin with each pouch change. *Ongoing assessment is important for optimal health and function of the stoma and surrounding skin. Stripping of tape or excessively frequent pouch removal may cause mechanical trauma to peristomal skin. Chronic skin irritation by ileostomy effluent may lead to* pseudoveracous lesions, *or wartlike nodules.*
- Instruct to report abnormal appearance of the stoma or surrounding skin (as noted previously and below) to the physician:
  a. Narrowing of the stoma lumen. *This indicates stenosis and may interfere with fecal elimination.*
  b. Lacerations or cuts in the stoma. *The stoma contains no nerves, so trauma may occur without pain.*
  c. Separation of the stoma from the abdominal surface. *This potential complication may require surgical repair.*

(continued on page 657)

NURSING CARE OF THE CLIENT HAVING AN ILEOSTOMY (continued)

- Emphasize the importance of adequate fluid and salt intake; the risk for dehydration and hyponatremia is increased particularly during hot weather, when fluid is lost through perspiration as well as ileostomy drainage. Water intake should be sufficient to maintain pale urine and an output of at least 1 quart per day. When exercising in hot weather, the client should consume extra water and salt. High-potassium foods, such as bananas and oranges, may also be recommended. *Loss of the reabsorptive surface of the large bowel increases the amount of water and sodium loss in the stool. If the ileostomy is high (more proximal in the ileum), additional potassium losses may also occur.*
- Discuss signs and symptoms of fluid and electrolyte imbalances:
  a. Extreme thirst
  b. Dry skin and oral mucous membrane
  c. Decreased urine output
  d. Weakness, fatigue
  e. Muscle cramps
  f. Abdominal cramps, nausea, vomiting
  g. Shortness of breath
  h. Orthostatic hypotension (feeling faint when suddenly changing positions)
- Discuss dietary concerns. A low-residue diet is recommended initially (see Table 24–8). Foods that may cause excessive odor or gas are typically avoided as well. *Because food blockage is a potential problem, high-fiber foods are limited, and foods that may cause blockage, such as popcorn, corn, nuts, cucumbers, cel-*

ery, fresh tomatoes, figs, strawberries, blackberries, and caraway seeds are avoided. Symptoms of food blockage include abdominal cramping, swelling of the stoma, and absence of ileostomy output for over 4 to 6 hours.
- Teach self-care measures to relieve food blockage:
  a. Take a warm shower or tub bath. *This can help relax the abdominal muscles.*
  b. Assume a knee-chest position. *The knee-chest position reduces intra-abdominal pressure.*
  c. Drink warm fluids or grape juice if not vomiting. *This provides a mild cathartic effect.*
  d. Massage peristomal area. *Massage may stimulate peristalsis and fecal elimination.*
  e. Remove pouch if the stoma is swollen, and apply a pouch with a larger opening. *If the stoma swells, the pouch may create a mechanical obstruction to output.*
- Notify the physician or enterostomal therapy nurse if:
  a. The above measures fail to relieve the obstruction.
  b. Signs of a partial obstruction persist including high-volume odorous fluid output, abdominal cramps, nausea, and vomiting.
  c. There is no ileostomy output for 4 to 6 hours.
  d. Signs of fluid and electrolyte imbalance occur, such as weakness, dizziness, lightheadedness, or headache.
Should self-care measures not succeed in breaking up a blockage, ileostomy lavage, as *described in Procedure 24–2 may be required.*

TABLE 24–8 Low-Residue Diet

Food Group	Allowed	Avoid
Beverages	Coffee, teas, juices, carbonated beverages; milk limited to 2 cups per day	Alcohol, prune juice
Breads and cereals	Products made from refined flours (white bread, crackers) or finely milled grains (e.g., corn flakes, crisp rice cereal, puffed wheat)	Whole-grain breads, rolls, or cereal; breads or rolls with seeds, nuts, or bran
Desserts	Gelatins, tapioca, plain custards, or puddings; angel-food or sponge cake; ice cream or frozen desserts without fruit or nuts	Any desserts containing dried fruits, nuts, seeds, or coconut; rich pastries, pies
Fruits	Fruit juices and strained fruits; cooked or canned apples, apricots, cherries, peaches, pears; bananas	All other raw or cooked fruits
Meats and other protein sources	Roasted, baked, or broiled tender or ground beef, veal, pork, lamb, poultry, or fish; smooth peanut butter; cottage, cream, American, or mild chedder cheeses in small amounts	Tough or spiced meats and those prepared by frying; highly flavored cheeses; nuts
Potatoes, rice, and pasta	Peeled potatoes; white rice; most pasta products	Potato skins, potato chips, or fried potatoes; brown rice; whole-grain pasta products
Sweets	Sugar, honey, jelly, hard candy and gumdrops, plain chocolates	Jam, marmalade; candy made with seeds, nuts, coconut
Vegetables	Vegetable juices and strained vegetables; cooked or canned vegetables	Raw or whole cooked vegetables
Other	Salt, ground seasonings; cream sauce and plain gravy	Chili sauce, horseradish; popcorn, seeds of any kind; whole spices, olives, vinegar

Procedure 24–1

Changing a One- or Two-Piece Drainable Ostomy Pouch

SUPPLIES

- One-or two-piece pouch
- Skin barrier paste
- Skin prep
- Clamp
- Pouch deodorant
- Measuring guide
- Adhesive remover
- Skin cleanser
- Washcloths
- Plastic bag

Explain the procedure and provide for privacy Follow standard precautions.

PROCEDURE

1. Remove soiled pouch (and the flange if a two-piece pouch) by gently pulling on the pouch or flange and pushing on skin. Use adhesive remover to remove skin barrier paste.
2. Empty pouch, discarding it and the flange (if applicable) in a plastic bag. Save the tail closure clamp. The pouch from a two-piece system may be cleaned out and reused.

3. Cleanse skin and stoma with warm water and skin cleanser or mild soap. Rinse skin and stoma, and pat dry.
4. Note stoma color and peristomal skin condition.
5. If necessary, clip or shave peristomal hair.
6. Use measuring guide or previous pattern to check size of stoma (Figure 24–9A ■).
   a. Presized pouch: check to verify that size is correct.
   b. Cut-to-fit pouch or flange: Trace the correct size of the stoma onto the back of the flange, and cut the opening to match the pattern. The opening should be no more than 1/8 inch larger than stoma.

7. Apply skin prep to skin covered by a wafer, pouch, or tape. Allow to dry.
8. Remove backings from pouch or flange.
9. Apply a bead of skin barrier paste around the stoma base or around the opening of the pouch or flange. Allow the paste to air-dry for 1 to 2 minutes.
10. Center the pouch or flange over the stoma, and press to adhere (Figure 24–9B ■).
11. For a two-piece pouch, snap the pouch onto skin barrier flange.
12. Place deodorizing tablets or a few drops of liquid pouch deodorizer (in some cases, antiseptic mouthwash may be used) in the pouch. Apply the clamp.
13. "Picture frame" the pouch with tape to provide extra security.

Figure 24–9 ■ *A,* A guide for measuring the stoma. *B,* Applying the disposable pouch.

Procedure 24–2

Ileostomy Lavage

SUPPLIES

- Disposable irrigation sleeve
- 60 mL catheter-tipped syringe
- #14 Fr. catheter
- Water-soluble lubricant
- Normal saline for irrigation
- Bedpan
- Clean ostomy pouch

Explain the procedure and provide for privacy. Follow standard precautions.

PROCEDURE

1. Remove the pouch. Apply disposable irrigation sleeve.

2. Clamp the bottom of the sleeve, or place it into the bedpan.
3. Gently examine stoma digitally to break up any mass proximal to stoma and determine direction of the bowel.
4. Lubricate catheter, and insert into stoma until blockage is reached. If the catheter does not reach the blockage after 8 to 10 cm, notify the physician. This may indicate a more proximal obstruction.
5. Instill 30 to 50 mL normal saline.
6. Remove catheter. Allow stoma to drain.
7. Repeat the procedure until the mass is removed.

8. When the blockage is removed, remove the irrigation sleeve.
9. Clean peristomal skin.
10. Apply pouch and clamp.

POSTPROCEDURE

1. Document the procedure, amount of solution used, consistency of results, and the client's tolerance of the procedure.
2. Discuss dietary concerns to help determine cause of blockage.

Complementary Therapies

The chronic nature of inflammatory bowel disease and adverse effects of many prescribed treatments lead many clients with IBD to seek or use complementary therapies. Chiropractic care, megavitamin therapy, dietary supplements, and herbal medi-

cine have been reported as common complementary therapies for IBD (Heuschkel et al., 2002; Verhoef et al., 2002). A study by Langmead et al (2002) concluded that herbal remedies such as slippery elm, fenugreek, devil's claw, Mexican yam, termentil and wei tong ning have antioxidant effects and may provide an effect similar to that of 5-aminosalicylic acid preparations. Many complementary therapies for IBD may interact with prescribed medications; instruct the client to discuss all potential therapies with the primary care provider.

NURSING CARE

Health Promotion

Although inflammatory bowel disease cannot, at this time, be predicted or prevented, effective management may help the client avoid complications of the disease. Stress the importance of complying with the prescribed treatment regimen and promptly reporting manifestations of exacerbations to the physician.

Assessment

Assessment data related to inflammatory bowel disease includes the following subjective and objective data.

- Health history: current manifestations, including onset, duration, severity (number of stools per day, presence of blood or mucus in stool, abdominal pain or cramping, tenesmus); usual diet, ability to maintain weight and nutrition, food intolerances; associated manifestations such as arthragias, fatigue, malaise; current medications; previous treatment and diagnostic tests
- Physical examination: general appearance; weight; vital signs including orthostatic vitals and temperature; abdominal assessment including shape, contour, bowel sounds, palpation for tenderness and masses, presence of stoma or scars

Nursing Diagnoses and Interventions

When planning nursing care for the client with inflammatory bowel disease, it is vital to consider the chronic, recurrent nature of the disorder. Teaching is a major aspect of care. Diarrhea and disturbed body image are significant nursing care problems for the client with IBD. With severe disease, impaired nutrition must be considered a priority problem as well.

Diarrhea

During an acute exacerbation of IBD, diarrhea can be frequent and painful. The frequency of defecation and associated abdominal pain and cramping may interfere with ADLs and increase the risk for fluid volume deficit and impaired skin integrity.

- Record the frequency, amount, and color of stools using a stool chart. Measure and record liquid stool as output. *The severity of diarrhea is an indicator of the severity of the disease and helps determine the need for fluid replacement.*

PRACTICE ALERT *Observe stools for obvious blood and test for occult blood as indicated. Report grossly bloody stools or hematochezia, which may indicate hemorrhage and necessitate emergency surgery.* ■

- Assess vital signs every 4 hours. *Tachycardia, tachypnea, and fever may be indicators of fluid volume deficit.*

- Weigh daily and record. *Rapid weight loss (over days to a week) usually indicates fluid loss, whereas weight loss over weeks to months may indicate malnutrition.*
- Assess for other indications of fluid deficit: warm, dry skin, poor skin turgor, dry shiny mucous membranes, weakness, lethargy, complaints of thirst. *The extent of fluid loss may not be readily evident with diarrhea, particularly if the client uses the bathroom without assistance. Systemic manifestations of fluid volume deficit may be the first indicators of the problem.*
- Maintain bowel rest by keeping NPO or limiting oral intake to elemental feedings as indicated. *Bowel rest during an acute exacerbation of IBD promotes healing and reduces diarrhea and other symptoms.*
- Administer prescribed anti-inflammatory and antidiarrheal medications as indicated. *Anti-inflammatory medications reduce the extent of bowel inflammation and diarrhea. Unless contraindicated, antidiarrheal medications help reduce fluid loss and increase comfort.*

PRACTICE ALERT *When giving antidiarrheal medications to a client with ulcerative colitis, closely observe for manifestations of toxic megacolon: fever, tachycardia, hypotension, dehydration, abdominal pain and cramping, and an abrupt relief of diarrhea.* ■

- Maintain fluid intake by mouth or intravenously as indicated. *The client with IBD requires fluid to replace ongoing losses, as well as fluid to meet the usual daily needs of the body. If an elemental diet or total parenteral nutrition is prescribed, additional fluids may be required to meet fluid intake needs.*
- Provide good skin care. *Fluid deficit and tissue dehydration increase the risk for skin excoriations or breakdown.*
- Assess perianal area for irritation or denuded skin from the diarrhea. Use gentle cleansing agents, such as Periwash or Tucks, or cottonballs saturated with witch hazel. Apply a protective cream, such as zinc oxide–based preparations, to protect skin from the irritating effects of diarrheal stool. *Digestive enzymes in the stool are very corrosive, increasing the risk of skin breakdown where exposed to diarrheal stool.*

Disturbed Body Image

The client with IBD may experience frustration at not being able to control, or even predict, fecal elimination, particularly when the disease is severe. Diarrhea can interfere with the ability to complete tasks, maintain employment or engage in social activities, and even meet basic needs such as eating, sleeping, and sexual activity. Body image can suffer as a result. Treatment of IBD, be it total colectomy with ileal pouch-anal anastomosis, ileostomy, or chronic corticosteroid therapy, also can affect the view of self.

- Accept feelings and perception of self. *Negating or denying the reality of the client's perception impairs trust.*
- Encourage discussion of physical changes and their consequences as they relate to self-concept. *This demonstrates acceptance and provides an opportunity to express the impact of the disease and its treatment on the client's life.*

- Encourage discussion about concerns regarding the effect of the disease or treatment on close personal relationships. *This demonstrates understanding and provides an opportunity for the client to express feelings about the impact of the disease on relationships and significant others.*
- Encourage the client to make choices and decisions regarding care. *This increases the client's sense of control over the disease and his or her future.*
- Discuss possible treatment options and their effects openly and honestly. *Open discussion allows more informed decisions.*
- Involve the client in care, teaching and demonstrating as needed. *This encourages and facilitates independence and decision making.*
- Provide care in an accepting, nonjudgmental manner. *Acceptance of the client despite potential embarrassment about odors or diarrhea enhances self-esteem.*
- Arrange for interaction with other clients or groups of people with IBD or ostomies. *The client may feel that no one who has not experienced a similar problem can understand his or her feelings.*
- Teach coping strategies (odor control, dietary modifications, and so on), and support their use. *This facilitates healthy adaptation to the disease.*

Imbalanced Nutrition: Less Than Body Requirements

Crohn's disease can significantly alter the bowel's ability to absorb nutrients. In both forms of IBD, blood and protein-rich fluid may be lost in diarrheal stools. With malabsorption and continuing nutrient losses, multiple nutrient deficits can develop, affecting growth and development, healing, muscle mass, bone density, and electrolyte balances.

- Monitor laboratory results, including hemoglobin and hematocrit, serum electrolytes, and total serum protein and albumin levels. *These studies provide an indicator of nutritional status.*
- Provide the prescribed diet: high-kcal, high-protein, low-fat diet with restricted milk and milk products if lactose intolerance is present. *Calories and protein are important to replace lost nutrients. Fat restriction helps reduce diarrhea and nutrient loss, particularly when significant portions of the terminal ileum have been resected.*
- Provide parenteral nutrition as necessary if the client is unable to absorb enteral nutrients. *Parenteral nutrition can help reverse nutritional deficits and promote weight gain and healing in the client with acute symptoms.*
- Arrange for dietary consultation. Consider food preferences as allowed. *Providing preferred foods in the prescribed diet increases intake and supports nutritional status.*
- Provide or administer elemental enteral nutrition and supplements as ordered. *Elemental enteral nutritional supplements support healing while providing for bowel rest. They can replace losses and improve nutritional status more rapidly than diet alone.*
- Include family members, the primary food preparer in particular, in teaching and dietary discussions. *Families can reinforce teaching and help the client maintain required restrictions or kcal intake.*

Using NANDA, NIC, and NOC

Chart 24–3 shows links between NANDA nursing diagnoses, NIC, and NOC when caring for the client with inflammatory bowel disease.

Home Care

Inflammatory bowel disease is a chronic condition for which the client needs to provide daily self-management. For this rea-

---

CHART 24–3   LINKS BETWEEN NANDA, NIC, AND NOC

The Client with Inflammatory Bowel Disease

NURSING DIAGNOSES	NURSING INTERVENTIONS	NURSING OUTCOMES
• Acute Pain	• Medication Management	• Comfort Level
• Deficient Fluid Volume	• Fluid Monitoring	• Fluid Balance
	• Fluid/Electrolyte Management	• Hydration
• Diarrhea	• Diarrhea Management	• Symptom Severity
• Imbalanced Nutrition: Less Than Body Requirements	• Nutrition Management	• Nutritional Status
	• Weight Gain Assistance	
• Risk for Impaired Skin Integrity	• Skin Surveillance	• Tissue Integrity: Skin and Mucous Membranes
• Ineffective Coping	• Coping Enhancement	• Coping
	• Decision-Making Support	• Decision Making
	• Emotional Support	• Social Support
	• Family Involvement Promotion	

Note: Data from Nursing Outcomes Classification (NOC) *by M. Johnson & M. Maas (Eds.), 1997, St. Louis: Mosby;* Nursing Diagnoses: Definitions & Classification 2001–2002 *by North American Nursing Diagnosis Association, 2001, Philadelphia: NANDA;* Nursing Interventions Classification (NIC) *by J.C. McCloskey & G. M. Bulechek (Eds.), 2000, St. Louis: Mosby. Reprinted by permission.*

son, teaching is a vital component of care. Teach the client and family about the following topics.

- The type of inflammatory bowel disease affecting the client, including the disease process, short- and long-term effects, the relationship of stress to disease exacerbations, and the manifestations of complications
- Prescribed medications, including drug names, desired effects, schedules for tapering the doses if ordered (as with corticosteroids), and possible side effects or adverse reactions and their management
- The recommended diet and the rationale for any specific restrictions
- Use of nutritional supplements such as Ensure to maintain weight and nutritional status
- Indicators of malabsorption and impaired nutrition; recommendations for self-care and when to seek medical intervention
- If discharged with a central catheter and home parenteral nutrition, written and verbal instructions on catheter care, troubleshooting, and TPN administration (Have the client and a family member demonstrate catheter care and TPN maintenance.)
- The importance of maintaining a fluid intake of at least 2 to 3 quarts per day, increasing fluid intake during warm weather, exercise or strenuous work, and when fever is present
- The increased risk for colorectal cancer and importance of regular bowel exams
- Risks and benefits of various treatment options

If surgery is planned or has been done, include the following topics in home care instructions.

- Ileal pouch-anal anastomosis or ileostomy care as indicated
- Where to obtain ostomy supplies
- Use of nonprescription drugs, such as enteric-coated and timed-release capsules that may not be adequately absorbed before elimination through the ileostomy
- Community and national ostomy support groups (see Box 24–2)

Provide referrals to a dietary consultant or nutritionist, a community health care agency, home care services, and home intravenous care services as indicated. See the Nursing Care Plan on page 662.

BOX 24–2 ■ Resources for Home Care

Local and national resource groups that may be helpful for the client with an ostomy:

- Canadian Foundation for Ileitis and Colitis
  21 St. Clair Avenue E., Suite 301
  Toronto, Ontario M4T 1L9
  CANADA
  416-920-5035
- Crohn's and Colitis Foundation of America
  386 Park Avenue S.
  New York, NY 10016-8804
  800-932-2423
  www.ccfa.org
- United Ostomy Association, Inc.
  36 Executive Park, Suite 120
  Irvine, CA 92714
  800-826-0826
  www.uoa.org

MediaLink | OSTOMY RESOURCES

MALABSORPTION SYNDROMES

Malabsorption is a condition in which the intestinal mucosa ineffectively absorbs nutrients—including carbohydrates, proteins, fats, water, electrolytes, minerals, and vitamins—resulting in their excretion in the stool. Multiple different bowel disorders can lead to malabsorption.

Diseases of the small intestine often cause malabsorption. Other medical and/or surgical conditions can result in malabsorption if they affect digestion or the intestinal mucosa. Primary diseases of the small bowel mucosa, such as sprue, Crohn's disease, and acute infections, can lead to malabsorption. It may also result from *maldigestion,* inadequate preparation of chyme for absorption. For example, major gastric resections, pancreatic disorders with impaired pancreatic enzyme secretion, and biliary disorders that affect bile secretion can impair digestion and absorption of chyme. Selected causes of impaired absorption and digestion are listed in Table 24–9.

Regardless of the cause, malabsorption causes common manifestations resulting from impaired absorption of chyme

TABLE 24–9   Selected Causes of Malabsorption

Cause	Related Factors or Conditions
Impaired absorption	Sprue
	Short bowel syndrome
	Acute enteritis and other bowel infections or infestations
	AIDS-related opportunistic infections and Kaposi's sarcoma
	Celiac disease
	Crohn's disease
	Intestinal ischemia or infarction
	Scleroderma
Impaired digestion	Lactose intolerance
	Gastrectomy
	Chronic pancreatitis, cancer of the pancreas
	Cystic fibrosis
	Biliary obstruction
	Cirrhosis, hepatitis, or liver failure
	Zollinger-Ellison syndrome

Nursing Care Plan
A Client with Ulcerative Colitis

Cortez Lewis is a 42-year-old real estate agent and mother of three school-age children. She has had ulcerative colitis for 18 years and has been treated with prednisone and sulfasalazine. Over the past 4 months she has been having abdominal pain and cramping and frequent bloody diarrhea stools. During the same period, she has lost 20 lb (9 kg), and has had difficulty maintaining her career. She recently developed several lesions of the lower leg identified as erythema nodosum. A recent colonoscopy revealed extensive involvement of the entire colon. On admission, Mrs. Lewis states, "I'm tired of fighting this disease. I am a prisoner in my home because of the diarrhea." She is admitted for a total proctocolectomy and ileal pouch-anal anastomosis.

ASSESSMENT

Janet Wheeler, RN, completes the admission assessment. Mrs. Lewis now weighs 115 lb (52.2 kg). She complains of abdominal cramping, pain, and frequent bloody diarrhea stools. Several reddened lesions are noted on her lower legs. Physical assessment findings include T 98° F (36.6° C), P 72, R 20, and BP 104/72. Skin cool and pale. Abnormal laboratory findings include hemoglobin 7.3 g/dL (normal 11.7 to 15.7 g/dL); hematocrit 23.3% (normal 35% to 47%); WBC 15,580/mm³ (normal 3500 to 11,000/mm³); platelet count 995,000/mm³ (normal 150,000 to 450,000/mm³); serum protein 4.6 g/dL (normal 6 to 8 g/dL); serum albumin 2.4 g/dL (normal 3.5 to 5 g/dL). Preparation for surgery is begun.

DIAGNOSIS

- *Imbalanced nutrition: Less than body requirements* related to impaired absorption
- *Diarrhea* related to inflammation of bowel
- *Risk for deficient fluid volume* related to abnormal fluid loss
- *Risk for impaired tissue integrity* related to drainage from temporary ileostomy
- *Pain* related to surgical intervention
- *Risk for sexual dysfunction* related to temporary ileostomy

EXPECTED OUTCOMES

- Resume prescribed diet within 5 days after surgery.
- Demonstrate normal fecal elimination through the temporary ileostomy.
- Maintain adequate fluid balance.

- Demonstrate appropriate ostomy care prior to discharge.
- Report a tolerable level of discomfort.
- Verbalize feelings about sexuality and acknowledge importance of discussing sexual issues with husband.

PLANNING AND IMPLEMENTATION

- Discuss dietary modifications related to nutritional status and presence of ileostomy. Provide referral to dietitian for diet planning and teaching.
- Teach importance of maintaining a high fluid intake and manifestations of dehydration.
- Teach to empty and change ostomy pouch of choice.
- Teach stoma and peristomal skin assessment with each pouch change.
- Teach food blockage management.
- Refer to local United Ostomy Association.
- Provide list of local medical suppliers for ostomy appliances.

EVALUATION

On discharge, Mrs. Lewis is caring for her ileostomy, demonstrating her ability to empty, rinse, and change the pouch. The ET nurse has provided written and verbal instructions on ileostomy care. Mrs. Lewis verbalizes her understanding of the recommended diet and the need to limit high-fiber food intake and avoid enteric-coated and timed-release medications. The ET nurse has discussed sexual aspects of having an ileostomy and has given Mrs. Lewis a booklet, "Sex and the Female Ostomate," available through the United Ostomy Association. Mrs. Lewis is looking forward to the planned surgery to close the temporary ileostomy.

Critical Thinking in the Nursing Process

1. Why is the client with an ileostomy at risk for dehydration? How can Mrs. Lewis monitor her fluid status at home?
2. Why were Mrs. Lewis's hemoglobin and hematocrit low on admission? If her hemoglobin had been low but her hematocrit normal on admission, what might be the explanation?
3. Outline a teaching plan that could be given to clients for home care of an ileostomy.
4. Develop a care plan for Mrs. Lewis for the nursing diagnosis, *Risk for impaired skin integrity*.

See Evaluating Your Response in Appendix C.

---

and the nutrients it contains (Table 24–10). Predominant GI manifestations include anorexia; abdominal bloating; diarrhea with loose, bulky, foul-smelling stools; and steatorrhea (fatty stools). Weight loss, weakness, general malaise, muscle cramps, bone pain, abnormal bleeding, and anemia are common systemic manifestations of malabsorption. These manifestations result from malnutrition and fluid loss due to poor absorption.

Three common malabsorption disorders in adults are sprue, lactose intolerance, and short bowel syndrome.

THE CLIENT WITH SPRUE

Sprue is a chronic primary disorder of the small intestine in which the absorption of nutrients, particularly fats, is impaired. The severity of the disease depends on the extent of mucosal involvement in the intestine and the duration of the disease. Two major forms of sprue are celiac disease (celiac sprue) and tropical sprue.

TABLE 24–10	Local and Systemic Manifestations of Malabsorption	
Category	Manifestation	Cause
Local (GI)	Diarrhea	Impaired absorption of fluid and electrolytes, leading to excess water in the stool
	Abdominal distention	Gas formation from fermentation of undigested carbohydrates
	Steatorrhea	Impaired fat absorption leading to excess fat in feces
Systemic	Weight loss	Carbohydrate, protein, and fat deficit
	Weakness and malaise	Kcal deficit, anemia, fluid, and electrolyte losses
	Anemia	Vitamin B_{12}, folic acid, and iron deficits
	Bone pain	Calcium and vitamin D deficits
	Muscle cramps, paresthesias	Protein wasting, vitamin B_{12} and electrolyte deficits
	Easy bruising and bleeding	Vitamin K deficit
	Glossitis, cheilosis	Iron, folic acid, and vitamin B_{12} deficits

PHYSIOLOGY REVIEW

Most absorption of nutrients occurs in the small intestine. The mucosa of the small intestine is arranged in microscopic folds, which in turn contain even smaller fingerlike projections called *villi*. The cells of the villi are covered with microscopic hairs, *microvilli*, projecting from the cell membrane. The folds, villi, and microvilli of the intestinal mucosa provide a huge surface area for nutrient absorption. Cells of the intestines are specialized to absorb different nutrients. Readily digested nutrients are absorbed in the proximal intestine; others are absorbed more distally in the intestines. Nutrients are absorbed by the processes of simple diffusion (water and small lipids), facilitated diffusion (water soluble vitamins), and active transport (glucose and amino acids). Once absorbed into the cells of the villi, nutrients enter the blood or lymph for systemic distribution.

PATHOPHYSIOLOGY AND MANIFESTATIONS

Sprue is characterized by flattening of the intestinal mucosa with a loss of villi and microvilli. With the loss of villi, intestinal absorptive surface is lost, and digestive enzyme production, including disaccharidase and particularly lactase, is reduced.

Celiac Sprue

Celiac sprue, also known as *celiac disease* or *nontropical sprue,* is a chronic malabsorption disorder characterized by sensitivity to the gliadin fraction of gluten, a cereal protein. Gluten is found in wheat, rye, barley, and oats. It is also used as a filler in many prepared foods and in medications. The cause

of celiac sprue is unknown; however, genetic, environmental, and immune factors are known to play a role in its development. Caucasians of European descent are most commonly affected (Braunwald et al., 2001). Manifestations of celiac sprue often develop in childhood, but may develop at any age.

In celiac sprue, it appears that the intestinal mucosa is damaged by an immunologic response. Gliadin acts as an antigen (a substance that induces the formation of antibodies that interact specifically with it), prompting the formation of antibodies and immune complexes. These complexes may deposit in the intestinal mucosa, prompting an inflammatory response and loss of villi. Gluten also may directly damage the villi, causing cell loss, inflammation, and edema. The villi shorten and atrophy, resulting in loss of intestinal folds and absorptive surface.

Manifestations of celiac sprue may develop at any age. Local manifestations include abdominal bloating and cramps, diarrhea, and steatorrhea. Systemic manifestations result from the effects of malabsorption and resulting deficiencies. Anemia is common. Clients with celiac disease are often small in stature, and may have delayed maturity. Other signs of nutrient deficiencies include tetany, vitamin deficiencies, muscle wasting, and even rickets (impaired bone development). When gluten is removed from the diet, the manifestations resolve.

Gastrointestinal malignancies and intestinal lymphoma are potential complications of celiac sprue. Other complications include intestinal ulceration and development of refractory sprue, or disease that no longer responds to a gluten-free diet.

Tropical Sprue

Tropical sprue is a chronic disease of unknown cause, although bacterial infection or toxins are thought to contribute. Tropical sprue occurs chiefly in the Caribbean, south India, and southeast Asia. Its onset may be abrupt or insidious. The pathophysiologic changes in bowel mucosa closely resemble those of celiac sprue, although gluten intake has no effect on this condition.

Manifestations of tropical sprue include sore tongue, diarrhea, and weight loss. Initially, diarrhea may be explosive and watery; as the disease progresses, stools become fewer in number and more solid with obvious steatorrhea. Folic acid deficiency is common. Vitamin B_{12} and iron deficiencies may occur, resulting in glossitis; stomatitis; dry, rough skin; and anemia.

COLLABORATIVE CARE

With any malabsorptive disorder, the initial focus of management is to identify the cause. Once this has been determined, specific therapy can be prescribed.

Diagnostic Tests

Laboratory and diagnostic testing are used to make the differential diagnosis for various causes of malabsorption syndromes and to determine the severity of nutrient deficiencies.

- *Fecal fat* is measured to document the presence of steatorrhea. All stool is collected over a 72-hour period. The client is placed on a high-fat (100 g/day) diet for 3 days prior to and during the collection period. No alcohol is to be consumed for 24 hours prior to and during the collection period. The expected result is less than 7 g of fat per 24 hours (Malarkey & McMorrow, 2000). The fat content of stool is increased in many malabsorptive disorders, including celiac and tropical sprue.

- *Serologic testing* for IgA endomysial antibodies, and IgG and IgA antigliadin antibodies is used to diagnose celiac sprue and evaluate compliance with the prescribed gluten-free diet.
- *Serum levels of protein, albumin, cholesterol, electrolytes,* and *iron* may be ordered to evaluate for nutrient deficiencies. The *hemoglobin, hematocrit,* and *RBC indices* are used to evaluate anemia. *Prothrombin time* is increased in vitamin K deficiency.
- *Enteroscopy* uses an extra-long fiberoptic endoscope to visualize and biopsy the upper small intestine. This procedure permits direct examination of intestinal mucosa and collection of a tissue specimen for biopsy. This invasive procedure involves risks, such as perforation, bleeding, and aspiration of gastric contents, but provides valuable diagnostic information about malabsorptive syndromes. Nursing care of the client undergoing an enteroscopy is outlined in Chapter 21.
- *Upper GI series with small bowel follow-through* may be done to evaluate the structures of the upper GI tract. With sprue, the typical "feathery" pattern of barium in the small bowel is lost, and the barium may precipitate and clump. Nursing care of the client undergoing an upper gastrointestinal series with small bowel follow-through is in the Nursing Implications box on page 628.

Medications

Clients with severe nutritional deficits may require vitamin and mineral supplements, as well as iron and folic acid to correct anemia. Vitamin K may be administered parenterally if the prothrombin time is prolonged. In clients whose disease fails to respond to dietary management, corticosteroids may be ordered to suppress the inflammatory response.

Tropical sprue is treated with a combination of folic acid and tetracycline. This regimen is continued for 1 to 2 months. Nutrient deficiencies are treated as for celiac sprue.

Dietary Management

The client with celiac sprue is placed on a gluten-free diet. This treatment is generally successful, as long as the client avoids gluten totally. Gluten is so widely used in prepared foods that this may be no easy task. Consultation with a dietitian and detailed dietary instructions are necessary. Clients need to become aware of hidden sources of gluten and to analyze dietary labels. Common sources of gluten and foods to be avoided are indicated in Table 24–11.

The prescribed diet is also high in calories and protein to correct nutrient deficits. Fat content is restricted to minimize steatorrhea. Initially, the diet usually is restricted in lactose as well to compensate for the loss of lactase-containing microvilli. Foods containing lactose may be reintroduced once remission has occurred (Tierney et al., 2001).

NURSING CARE

Nursing care for the client with sprue focuses on the effects of the disorder on health and nutrition, as well as the client's ability to manage the disease.

Assessment

- Health history: onset, duration, and severity of symptoms; number and character of stools; history of travel to the Caribbean or southeast Asia; previous teaching related to disorder; current treatment and diet
- Physical examination: vital signs; abdominal shape, contour, bowel sounds; manifestations of malnutrition (e.g., anemia, small stature, muscle wasting, signs of other nutrient deficiencies)

TABLE 24–11 Dietary Sources of Gluten		
Food Group	**Contain Gluten**	**May Contain Gluten**
Cereals, grains, and grain products	Bread, crackers, cereal, and pasta containing wheat, rye, or barley grain or flour	Seasoned rice and potato mixes
Beverages	Malt, Postum, Ovaltine, beers, and ales	Commercial chocolate milk, cocoa, and other beverage mixes, such as instant tea mix, dietary supplements
Desserts	Cakes, cookies, and pastries made with wheat, rye, or barley flour	Commercial ice cream and sherbet
Meats and other protein sources		Meat loaf, cold cuts and prepared meats, breaded meats; cheese products; soy protein meat substitutes; commercial egg products
Fruits and vegetables		Commercial seasoned vegetable mixes or vegetables with sauce; canned baked beans; commercial pie fillings
Miscellaneous		Commercial salad dressings and mayonnaise; ketchup and prepared mustard; gravy, white sauce; nondairy creamer; syrups; commercial pickles

Nursing Diagnoses and Interventions

Diarrhea and malnutrition are significant problems for the client with sprue and the priority foci for nursing intervention.

Diarrhea

Steatorrhea and diarrhea typically occur with sprue because fat, water, and other nutrients are poorly absorbed, remaining in the bowel to be eliminated in the stool. Diarrhea can interfere with lifestyle, ADLs, skin integrity, and fluid and electrolyte balance.

- Assess and document the frequency and nature of stools. *Bowel elimination reflects the severity of the disease and efficacy of treatment. With effective treatment, stools become less frequent and more normal in color and appearance.*
- Weigh daily, monitor intake and output, and assess skin turgor and mucous membranes for indications of fluid balance. *Diarrhea increases the risk for hypovolemia and dehydration resulting from excess fluid loss in the stool.*
- Assess and document perianal skin condition. *Frequent defecation can irritate skin and mucous membranes, increasing the risk of breakdown.*
- Promote a liberal fluid intake. *Oral fluids help replace fluid lost through diarrheal stool.*

Imbalanced Nutrition:
Less than Body Requirements

Celiac sprue is a chronic condition. With continuing malabsorption, multiple nutrient deficits may occur, resulting in impaired growth and development, impaired healing, muscle wasting, bone disease, and electrolyte imbalances.

- Maintain accurate dietary intake records. *Assessment of dietary intake provides information about compliance with the prescribed diet as well as the adequacy of nutrient intake.*
- Monitor laboratory results, including hemoglobin and hematocrit, serum electrolytes, total serum protein, and albumin levels. *These studies provide information about nutritional status.*

- Arrange for dietary consultation. Provide for food preferences as allowed. *An individualized diet developed to address the client's food preferences as well as nutrient needs will promote appetite and food intake.*
- Provide the prescribed high-kcal, high-protein, low-fat, gluten-free diet for the client with celiac sprue. Restrict lactose (dairy product) intake as indicated. *Calories and protein are important to replace lost nutrients. Fat restriction helps reduce diarrhea and nutrient loss. Lactose may be restricted during initial treatment, then slowly reintroduced into the diet as the gut heals and its normal structure is restored.*
- Provide parenteral nutrition as ordered if the client is unable to absorb enteral nutrients. *Parenteral nutrition can help reverse nutritional deficits and promote weight gain when symptoms are acute.*
- Administer ordered nutritional supplements. *Nutritional supplements often are necessary to replace losses and restore nutrient levels to normal more rapidly than diet alone can achieve.*
- Include family members, the primary food preparer in particular, in teaching and dietary discussions. *Families can reinforce teaching and help the client maintain required restrictions or kcal intake.*

Using NANDA, NIC, and NOC

Chart 24–4 shows links between NANDA nursing diagnoses, NIC, and NOC for the client with sprue and other malabsorption disorders.

Home Care

Although tropical sprue can be treated with antibiotic and folic acid therapy, the client with celiac sprue has a chronic condition that requires continuing dietary management.

Provide a detailed list of foods that contain gluten and need to be eliminated from the diet, as well as foods that are allowed. Teach the client and family how to identify gluten-containing commercial products by reading labels and lists of ingredients. Encourage purchasing and using a gluten-free cookbook.

CHART 24–4 LINKS BETWEEN NANDA, NIC, AND NOC

The Client with Malabsorption Syndrome

NURSING DIAGNOSES	NURSING INTERVENTIONS	NURSING OUTCOMES
• Imbalanced Nutrition: Less Than Body Requirements	• Nutrition Management • Weight Gain Assistance	• Nutritional Status
• Diarrhea	• Diarrhea Management • Fluid Management	• Bowel Elimination • Symptom Severity • Hydration
• Deficient Knowledge	• Teaching: Prescribed Diet • Teaching: Disease Process	• Knowledge: Diet • Knowledge: Disease Process

Note: Data from Nursing Outcomes Classification (NOC) by M. Johnson & M. Maas (Eds.), 1997, St. Louis: Mosby; Nursing Diagnoses: Definitions & Classification 2001–2002 by North American Nursing Diagnosis Association, 2001, Philadelphia: NANDA; Nursing Interventions Classification (NIC) by J.C. McCloskey & G. M. Bulechek (Eds.), 2000, St. Louis: Mosby. Reprinted by permission.

If corticosteroids have been prescribed, stress the importance of taking the medication as ordered. Emphasize the need to avoid stopping the medication abruptly and to notify all caregivers that a corticosteroid is part of the client's medication regimen. Instruct to frequently monitor weight. A weight gain of 5 lb (2.3 kg) or more in less than a week usually reflects fluid gain, a possible adverse effect of corticosteroids. Other potential effects include decreased resistance to infection, an impaired inflammatory response, and changes in the metabolism of carbohydrates, proteins, and fats.

THE CLIENT WITH LACTASE DEFICIENCY

For carbohydrates to be absorbed from the small intestine, they first must be broken down into simple sugars, or monosaccharides. Lactose is the primary carbohydrate in milk and milk products. It is a disaccharide, requiring the enzyme lactase for digestion and absorption. Lactase deficiency can lead to *lactose intolerance* and symptoms of malabsorption.

Lactase deficiency affects up to 90% of Asians and Native Americans and 70% of African Americans. It also is common among Jewish Americans and Hispanics. Less than 25% of Caucasians are affected (Tierney et al., 2001). Lactase deficiency usually is genetic in origin, but also occurs secondarily to celiac sprue, Crohn's disease, and other disorders affecting the mucosa of the small intestine.

Many people with lactase deficiency are asymptomatic. Small to moderate amounts of milk (one to two 8-ounce glasses) of milk may be well tolerated. Symptoms of lactose intolerance include lower abdominal cramping, pain, and diarrhea following milk ingestion. Undigested lactose ferments in the intestine, forming gases that contribute to bloating and flatus. Lactic and fatty acids produced by this fermentation irritate the bowel, leading to increased motility and abdominal cramping. The undigested lactose draws water into the intestine, which contributes to increased motility and diarrhea. The diarrhea associated with lactose intolerance may be explosive.

COLLABORATIVE CARE

The diagnosis of lactose intolerance usually is based on the history of intolerance to milk and milk products, and a trial of a lactose-free diet. If symptoms resolve when lactose intake is eliminated, the diagnosis of lactose intolerance is confirmed.

The *lactose breath test* is a noninvasive test that may be used to diagnose lactose intolerance. Expired hydrogen gas (H_2) is measured following oral administration of 50 g of lactose. If lactose is digested and absorbed normally, then little change occurs in the amount of exhaled H_2 from fasting to postlactose administration. With lactose intolerance, exhaled H_2 increases following lactose administration as the sugar ferments in the bowel.

For the *lactose tolerance test,* 100 g of lactose solution is orally administered, followed by measurement of blood glu-

cose levels at intervals of 30, 60, and 120 minutes. If lactose is digested and absorbed normally, the blood glucose rises more than 20 mg/dL. The expected blood glucose elevation does not occur in lactose intolerance.

A lactose-free or reduced lactose diet relieves the manifestations of the disorder. Some clients require total elimination of milk and milk products from the diet. Many can tolerate limited amounts of lactose. Milk pretreated with lactase is readily available. Nonprescription lactase enzyme preparations are available to improve milk tolerance. Yogurt containing bacterial lactases may be well tolerated. Calcium supplementation is often recommended, particularly for women on a reduced-lactose or lactose-free diet.

NURSING CARE

Nursing care for the client with lactose intolerance focuses on providing education and support. Discuss sources of lactose: Milk, ice cream, and cottage cheese are high in lactose; aged cheese and yogurt contain much smaller amounts. Potential hidden sources of lactose include sherbets, desserts made from milk and milk chocolate, sauces and gravies, and cream soups. Suggest a trial of lactase-treated milk or lactase enzyme supplements. Emphasize the importance of obtaining nutrients contained in dairy products from other sources. Proteins may be obtained from meats, eggs, legumes, and grains. Other sources of calcium include sardines, oysters, and salmon, as well as plant sources such as beans, cauliflower, rhubarb, and green leafy vegetables.

THE CLIENT WITH SHORT BOWEL SYNDROME

Resection of significant portions of the small intestine may result in a condition known as short bowel syndrome. The severity of the disorder depends on the total amount of bowel resected, as well as the portions of bowel removed. Removal of the proximal portions, including the duodenum, jejunum, and proximal ileum, and distal portion of the ileum are associated with more severe malabsorption and symptoms than resection of midportions of the ileum (Braunwald et al., 2001).

Small bowel may be resected due to tumors, infarction of bowel mucosa, incarcerated hernias, Crohn's disease, trauma, and enteropathy resulting from radiation therapy.

Resection of the small intestine affects the absorption of water, nutrients, vitamins, and minerals. Transit time of ingested foods and fluids is reduced, and digestive processes are impaired. The bowel undergoes an adaptive process in which the remaining villi enlarge and lengthen to increase absorptive surface following resection. For many clients, absorption and bowel function returns to preoperative or near-normal levels. Others have continued significant impairment of digestion and absorption, leading to nutrient deficiencies, weight loss, and diarrhea.

COLLABORATIVE CARE

Laboratory and diagnostic studies are used to evaluate nutrient deficiencies. Total serum proteins and albumin are reduced, as are serum levels of folate, iron, vitamins, minerals, and electrolytes. Anemia and a prolonged prothrombin time (indicative of vitamin K deficiency) may develop.

Management of short bowel syndrome focuses on alleviating symptoms. Clients often simply require frequent, small, high-kcal, high-protein feedings. Multivitamin and mineral supplementation is also frequently necessary. Antidiarrheal medications are used to reduce bowel motility, allowing a greater amount of time for nutrient absorption. Some clients are affected by gastric hypersecretion following bowel resection. For these clients, a proton-pump inhibitor such as omeprazole (Prilosec) may be ordered. Clients with severe manifestations of short bowel syndrome may require total parenteral nutrition.

NURSING CARE

Nursing care for the client with short bowel syndrome focuses on the problems of potential fluid volume deficit, malnutrition, and diarrhea.

Fluid losses are generally greatest in the initial periods following surgery, warranting the closest attention at that time. Frequent assessment of vital signs, intake and output, daily weights, skin turgor, and condition of mucous membranes is vital. It is important to remember that the risk also is high when other abnormal fluid losses occur through, for example, fever, increased respiratory rate, draining wounds, or excess perspiration.

Document nutritional status, including weight, anthropometric measurements, laboratory values, and kcal intake. Provide nutritional supplementation with enteral feedings as needed. Maintain central lines and total parenteral nutrition, using aseptic technique.

For diarrhea, document the number and character of stools. Administer antidiarrheal medications as ordered. If the client is lactose intolerant, limit intake of milk and milk products. Provide good skin care of the perianal region to prevent breakdown from frequent bowel movements. Refer to the discussion of nursing care for the client with sprue for other measures for altered nutrition and diarrhea.

The client and family affected by this condition require extensive education. Because there is no way to cure or replace the lost bowel at this time, the client must manage the disorder on a day-to-day basis. Provide instructions about the recommended diet and medication regimen. Emphasize the importance of maintaining an adequate fluid intake, particularly in hot weather or during strenuous exercise. Teach the client to monitor his or her weight frequently and report changes. Include teaching about possible manifestations of dehydration and nutrient deficiencies that should be reported to the physician. Referring the client to a dietitian or counselor can help the person cope with what may be a lifelong problem.

NEOPLASTIC DISORDERS

Cancer remains the second leading cause of death in the United States, preceded only by heart disease. Although cancer may affect any portion of the digestive tract, the large intestine and rectum are the most common sites. Malignant neoplasms of the lower bowel are the second leading cause of death from cancer (after lung cancer), making this a significant health care concern.

THE CLIENT WITH POLYPS

A **polyp** is a mass of tissue that arises from the bowel wall and protrudes into the lumen. Polyps may develop in any portion of the bowel, but they occur most often in the sigmoid colon and rectum. They vary considerably in size and may be single or multiple. It is estimated that approximately 30% of people over the age of 50 have polyps. Although most polyps are benign, some have the potential to become malignant.

PATHOPHYSIOLOGY AND MANIFESTATIONS

Polyps are identified by their structure and tissue type. Most polyps are adenomas, benign epithelial tumors that are considered premalignant lesions. Less than 1% of polyps become malignant; however, virtually all colorectal cancers arise from adenomatous polyps (Braunwald et al., 2001; Porth, 2002).

Adenomatous polyps represent disruption of the normal process of cell proliferation to replace epithelial cells lining the intestine. Cells are constantly being reproduced to replace those shed as feces moves through the colon. Disruption of the normal process of cell division and maturation can lead to formation of a polyp composed of tightly packed epithelial cells. The cells may appear grossly normal or show signs of dysplasia. Polyps may develop as tubular, villous, or tubulovillous adenomas.

Tubular adenomas (also called *pedunculated* polyps) are more common, accounting for about 65% of benign polyps of the large intestine (Porth, 2002). A tubular adenoma is a globe-like structure attached to the intestinal wall by a thin, stalk-like stem (Figure 24–10 ■). The incidence of this type of polyp increases with age, although it occurs in all age groups and in both sexes. Most are small, 1 cm or less in diameter, although they may be as large as 4 to 5 cm. The malignant potential of these polyps seems to be related to their size. One percent of those under 1 cm in diameter are cancerous, whereas 35% of adenomas larger than 2 cm are cancerous (Porth, 2002).

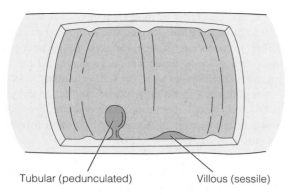

Tubular (pedunculated)   Villous (sessile)

Figure 24–10 ■ Tubular (or pedumculated) and villous (or sessile) polyps.

Villous adenomas (also called *sessile* polyps) have a broad base and an elevated, cauliflower-like surface. They typically develop in the rectosigmoid colon. This type of polyp is often larger than tubular adenomas, usually more than 5 cm. Villous adenomas are less common, accounting for about 10% of colon polyps. They have a higher malignant potential than tubular adenomas, estimated at 25% to 40%. Some adenomatous polyps contain both tubular epithelium and villi and are known as *tubulovillous adenomas.*

Familial polyposis is an uncommon autosomal dominant genetic disorder characterized by hundreds of adenomatous polyps throughout the entire large intestine. Both pedunculated and sessile polyps are seen, usually developing after puberty. Unless treated, the risk of malignancy is almost 100% by age 40 (Braunwald et al., 2001).

Most polyps are asymptomatic, found coincidentally during routine examination or diagnostic testing. Intermittent painless rectal bleeding, bright or dark red, is the most common presenting complaint. A large polyp may cause abdominal cramping, pain, or manifestations of obstruction. Diarrhea and mucous discharge may be associated with a large villous adenoma.

COLLABORATIVE CARE

The diagnosis of intestinal polyps is generally based on diagnostic studies such as sigmoidoscopy or colonoscopy. A rectal polyp may be palpable on digital examination, but further studies are necessary to determine its size and type, the extent of colon involvement, and to assess for malignancy.

- *Colonoscopy* provides the most reliable diagnosis of polyps, allowing visual inspection of the large intestine, biopsy of masses or lesions, and polypectomy. Nursing care of the client undergoing a colonoscopy is outlined in the Nursing Implications box on page 624.

Once identified, polyps are generally removed because of the risk of malignancy. Pedunculated polyps and small villous lesions may be removed during colonoscopy using an electrocautery snare or hot biopsy forceps passed through the scope. This relatively safe procedure has less than a 2% risk of complications such as perforation or hemorrhage. Large villous

adenomas are completely excised and examined histologically for evidence of malignancy. In some cases, the colon segment containing the polyp is resected; a total colectomy with ileorectal anastomosis may be performed for multiple polyps in different anatomic parts of the colon.

Treatment following polypectomy depends on histologic examination of the excised tissue. Because polyps tend to recur, follow-up colonoscopy is recommended in 3 years and then every 5 years if no further polyps are detected. When the polyp is found to be malignant, follow-up care is determined by the tissue type and degree of invasion. See the next section of this chapter.

NURSING CARE

Health Promotion

The incidence of intestinal polyps increases with age. They affect men and women equally. It is believed that an adenomatous polyp requires more than 5 years of growth to become significant in size and malignant potential (Braunwald et al., 2001). Advise all clients to have a screening colonoscopy at age 50 and every 5 years thereafter for early detection of polyps.

Assessment

Polyps are a "silent" disease, with few or no symptoms.

- Health history: rectal bleeding; personal or family history of intestinal polyps or colorectal cancer

Nursing Diagnoses and Interventions

Nursing care for the client with polyps focuses on education and assisting the client through diagnostic testing and polyp removal. Before and after colonoscopy and polypectomy, provide direct care and teaching about the procedure, expected sensations during the procedure, and anticipated postoperative care. Cathartics are prescribed prior to colonoscopy; cleansing enemas also may be ordered. Observe for evidence of fluid and electrolyte imbalance during preoperative preparation. If enemas are ordered, use normal saline (not tap water) to reduce the risk of electrolyte imbalances. Following polypectomy, observe closely for possible complications such as hemorrhage.

The following nursing diagnoses may be appropriate for the client with polyps.

- *Risk for noncompliance* with recommended screening and follow-up, related to lack of understanding
- *Impaired tissue integrity* related to removal of polyps from bowel
- *Risk for deficient fluid volume* related to bowel preparation

Home Care

Include the following topics when teaching for home care.

- The significance of polyps and their relationship to colorectal cancer
- The importance of keeping follow-up appointments and undergoing repeat colonoscopy as ordered: at 3 years following polypectomy, then every 5 years unless additional polyps are found; every 6 months for clients with familial polyposis

- Symptoms to report to the physician, such as diarrhea, pain, rectal bleeding, lightheadedness, or other indications of possible blood loss

Discuss the high risk for colorectal cancer with clients with familial polyposis and their families. Include its genetic transmission: Offspring have a 50% risk of inheriting the disorder. Referral to an enterostomal therapist for discussion about colectomy with ileoanal reservoir may help the client with decisions about treatment options.

THE CLIENT WITH COLORECTAL CANCER

Colorectal cancer, malignancy of the colon or rectum, is the third most common cancer diagnosed in the United States. In the United States, about 148,300 new cases of colorectal cancer were diagnosed in 2002, and over 56,000 people died from this disease (American Cancer Society [ACS], 2002). Earlier diagnosis and improved treatment have improved the survival rate for colorectal cancer. Its incidence, which is nearly equal among men and women, is declining in the United States. Colorectal cancer occurs most frequently after age 50. The incidence continues to rise with increasing age. With early diagnosis and treatment, the 5-year survival rate for colorectal cancer is 90%; however, less than half of colorectal cancers are diagnosed at this early stage. The 5-year survival rate drops to 65% when it has spread locally at the time of diagnosis, and 8% when distant sites are involved (ACS, 2002).

Although the specific cause of colorectal cancer is unknown, a number of risk factors have been identified (Box 24–3). Genetic factors are strongly linked to the risk for colorectal cancer. Up to 25% of people who develop colorectal cancer have a family history of the disease (Braunwald et al., 2001). Persons with familial adenomatous polyposis inevitably will develop colon cancer unless the colon is removed (Tierney et al., 2001). Hereditary nonpolyposis colorectal cancer (also known as Lynch syndrome) is an autosomal dominant disorder that significantly increases the risk for developing colorectal and other cancers. Tumors associated with Lynch syndrome often affect the ascending colon, and tend to occur at an earlier age (Braunwald et al., 2001). Inflammatory bowel disease (ulcerative colitis and Crohn's disease) also increases the risk of colorectal cancer.

Diet plays a role in the development of colorectal cancer. The disease is prevalent in economically prosperous countries where people consume diets high in calories, meat proteins, and fats. This dietary pattern, common in the United States, is thought to increase the population of anaerobic bacteria in the gut. These anaerobes convert bile acids into carcinogens (Braunwald et al., 2001). Diets high in fruits and vegetables, folic acid, and calcium appear to reduce the risk of colorectal cancer. Cereal fiber, once thought to reduce colorectal cancer risk, does not now appear to play a role either way in its development. Other factors that may reduce the risk of colorectal cancer include use of aspirin and other NSAIDs and hormone replacement therapy in post menopausal women (Tierney et al., 2001).

PATHOPHYSIOLOGY

Nearly all colorectal malignancies are adenocarcinomas that begin as adenomatous polyps. Most tumors develop in the rectum and sigmoid colon, although any portion of the colon may be affected (Figure 24–11 ■). The tumor typically grows undetected, producing few symptoms. By the time symptoms occur, the disease may have spread into deeper layers of the bowel tissue and adjacent organs. Colorectal cancer spreads by direct extension to involve the entire bowel circumference, the submucosa, and outer bowel wall layers. Neighboring structures such as the liver, greater curvature of the stomach, duodenum, small intestine, pancreas, spleen, genitourinary tract, and abdominal wall also may be involved by direct extension. Metastasis to regional lymph nodes is the most common form of tumor spread. This is not always an orderly process; distal nodes may contain cancer cells while regional nodes remain normal. Cancerous cells from the primary tumor may also spread by way of the lymphatic system or circulatory system to secondary sites such as the liver, lungs, brain, bones, and kidneys. "Seeding" of the tumor to other areas of the peritoneal cavity can occur when the tumor extends through the serosa or during surgical resection.

BOX 24–3	■ Risk Factors for Colorectal Cancer

- Age over 50 years
- Polyps of the colon and/or rectum
- Family history of colorectal cancer
- Inflammatory bowel disease
- Exposure to radiation
- Diet: high animal fat and kcal intake

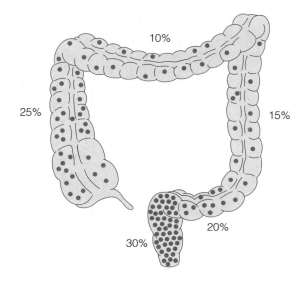

Figure 24–11 ■ The distribution and frequency of cancer of the colon and rectum.

MANIFESTATIONS AND COMPLICATIONS

As noted earlier, bowel cancer often produces no symptoms until it is advanced. Because it grows slowly, 5 to 15 years of growth may occur before symptoms develop. The manifestations depend on its location, type and extent, and complications. Bleeding is often the initial manifestation that prompts clients to seek medical care. Other common early symptoms include a change in bowel habits, either diarrhea or constipation. Pain, anorexia, and weight loss are characteristic in advanced disease. A palpable abdominal or rectal mass may be present. Occasionally the client presents with anemia from occult bleeding.

The primary complications associated with colorectal cancer: (1) bowel obstruction due to narrowing of the bowel lumen by the lesion; (2) perforation of the bowel wall by the tumor, allowing contamination of the peritoneal cavity by bowel contents; and (3) direct extension of the tumor to involve adjacent organs.

Most recurrences of colorectal cancer after tumor removal occur within the first 4 years. The size of the primary tumor does not necessarily relate to long-term survival. The number of involved lymph nodes, penetration of the tumor through the bowel wall, and tumor adherence to adjacent organs are better predictors of the prognosis for the disease (Braunwald et al., 2001).

COLLABORATIVE CARE

The focus of collaborative care for colorectal cancer is early detection and intervention. Colorectal cancer is always treated by surgical resection, with chemotherapy and radiation therapy used as adjuncts.

Screening

The American Cancer Society recommends annual digital rectal examination beginning at age 40, with annual fecal occult blood testing beginning at age 50. Because colorectal tumors bleed in-

termittently, several fecal occult blood specimens typically are collected over a period of several days. Debate exists regarding recommendations for periodic (every 3 to 5 years) flexible sigmoidoscopy or colonoscopy for everyone over age 50.

Diagnostic Tests

- *CBC* is ordered to detect anemia resulting from chronic blood loss and tumor growth.
- *Fecal occult blood* (by guaiac or hemoccult testing) is ordered to detect blood in the feces, because nearly all colorectal cancers bleed intermittently.
- *Carcinoembryonic antigen (CEA)* is a tumor marker that can be detected in the blood of clients with colorectal cancer. CEA levels are used to estimate prognosis, monitor treatment, and detect cancer recurrence. Because this test is not specific for colorectal cancer and does not always detect early-stage cancer, it is not used as a screening measure (Malarkey & McMorrow, 2000).
- *Sigmoidoscopy* or *colonoscopy* is the primary diagnostic test used to detect and visualize tumors. It also allows tissue collection for biopsy. While flexible sigmoidoscopy can detect 50% to 65% of colorectal cancers, many clinicians recommend colonoscopy, endoscopic examination of the entire colon. Tumors typically appear as raised, red, centrally ulcerated, bleeding lesions. (See the boxes on pages 619 and 624 for nursing implications for these tests.)
- *Chest X-ray* is obtained to detect tumor metastasis to the lung.
- *Computed tomography (CT) scan, magnetic resonance imaging (MRI),* or *ultrasonic examination* may be used to assess tumor depth and involvement of other organs by direct extension or metastasis.
- *Tissue biopsy* is obtained at the time of endoscopy to confirm cancerous tissue and evaluate cell differentiation (see Chapter 10). Current staging methods primarily use the TNM system, as outlined in Table 24–12.

TABLE 24–12 The TNM Classification for Colorectal Cancer			
Stage	**Primary Tumor (T)**	**Regional Lymph Nodes (N)**	**Distant Metastasis (M)**
	TX—Primary tumor cannot be assessed TO—No evidence of primary tumor	NX—Regional lymph node cannot be assessed	MX—Presence of distant metastasis cannot be assessed
Stage 0	Tis—Carcinoma in situ	NO—No regional lymph node metastasis	MO—No distant metastasis
Stage I	T1—Tumor invades submucosa T2—Tumor invades muscularis propria		
Stage II	T3—Tumor invades through muscularis propria into subserosa or into non-peritonealized pericolic or perirectal tissues T4—Tumor perforates visceral peritoneum or directly invades other organs or structures		
Stage III	Any T	N1—Metastasis in 1 to 3 pericolic or perirectal lymph nodes N2—Metastasis in 4 or more pericolic or perirectal lymph nodes N3—Metastasis in any lymph node along course of a major named vascular trunk	
Stage IV	Any T	Any N	M1—Distant metastasis

Surgery

Surgical resection of the tumor, adjacent colon, and regional lymph nodes is the treatment of choice for colorectal cancer. Options for surgical treatment vary from destruction of the tumor by laser photocoagulation performed during endoscopy to abdominoperineal resection with permanent colostomy. When possible, the anal sphincter is preserved and colostomy avoided.

Laser photocoagulation uses a very small, intense beam of light to generate heat in tissues toward which it is directed. The heat generated by the laser beam can be used to destroy small tumors. It is also used for palliative surgery of advanced tumors to remove obstruction. Laser photocoagulation can be performed endoscopically and is useful for clients who cannot tolerate major surgery.

Other surgical treatment options for small, localized tumors include local excision and fulguration. These procedures also may be performed during endoscopy, eliminating the need for abdominal surgery. Local excision may be used to remove a disk of rectum containing the tumor in clients with a small, well-differentiated, mobile polypoid lesion. *Fulguration* or electrocoagulation is used to reduce the size of some large tumors for clients who are poor surgical risks. This procedure requires general anesthesia and may need to be repeated at intervals.

Most clients with colorectal cancer undergo surgical resection of the colon with anastomosis of remaining bowel as a curative procedure. The distribution of regional lymph nodes determines the extent of resection as these may contain metastatic lesions. Most tumors of the ascending, transverse, descending, and sigmoid colon can be resected.

Tumors of the rectum usually are treated with an abdominoperineal resection in which the sigmoid colon, rectum, and anus are removed through both abdominal and perineal incisions. A permanent sigmoid colostomy is performed to provide for elimination of feces. Nursing care of the client having bowel surgery is outlined in the box below.

NURSING CARE OF THE CLIENT HAVING BOWEL SURGERY

PREOPERATIVE NURSING CARE

- Provide routine preoperative care for the surgical client as outlined in Chapter 7.
- Arrange for consultation with enterostomal therapy (ET) specialist if appropriate. *The ET nurse is trained to identify and mark an appropriate stoma location, taking into consideration the level of ostomy, skinfolds, and the client's clothing preferences. Initial ostomy care teaching also is provided by the ET nurse during the preoperative visit.*
- Insert a nasogastric tube if ordered. *Although it is often inserted in the surgical suite just prior to surgery, the nasogastric tube may be placed preoperatively to remove secretions and empty stomach contents.*
- Perform bowel preparation procedures as ordered. *Oral and parenteral antibiotics as well as cathartics and enemas may be prescribed preoperatively to clean the bowel and reduce the risk of peritoneal contamination by bowel contents during surgery.*

POSTOPERATIVE NURSING CARE

- Provide routine care for the surgical client (Chapter 7).
- Monitor bowel sounds and degree of abdominal distention. *Surgical manipulation of the bowel disrupts peristalsis, resulting in an initial ileus. Bowel sounds and the passage of flatus indicate a return of peristalsis.*
- Assess the position and patency of the nasogastric tube, connecting it to low suction. If the tube becomes clogged, gently irrigate with sterile normal saline. *A nasogastric or gastrostomy tube is used postoperatively to provide gastrointestinal decompression and facilitate healing of the anastomosis. Ensuring its patency is important for comfort and healing.*
- Assess color, amount, and odor of drainage from surgical drains and the colostomy (if present), noting any changes or the presence of clots or bright bleeding. *Initial drainage may be bright red and then become dark and finally clear or greenish yellow over the first 2 to 3 days. A change in the color, amount or odor of the drainage may indicate a complication such as hemorrhage, intestinal obstruction, or infection.*
- Alert all personnel caring for the client with an abdominoperineal resection to avoid rectal temperatures, suppositories, or other rectal procedures. *These procedures could disrupt the anal suture line, causing bleeding, infection, or impaired healing.*
- Maintain intravenous fluids while nasogastric suction is in place. *The client on nasogastric suction is unable to take oral food and fluids and, moreover, is losing electrolyte-rich fluid through the nasogastric tube. If replacement fluid and electrolytes are not maintained, the client is at risk for dehydration; sodium, potassium, and chloride imbalance; and metabolic alkalosis.*
- Provide antacids, histamine$_2$-receptor antagonists, and antibiotic therapy as ordered. *The above medications may be ordered for the postoperative client, depending on the procedure performed. Antibiotic therapy is a common measure to prevent infection resulting from contamination of the abdominal cavity with gastric contents.*
- Resume oral food and fluids as ordered. Initial feedings may be clear liquids, progressing to full liquids, and then frequent small feedings of regular foods. Monitor bowel sounds and monitor for abdominal distention frequently during this period. *Oral feedings are reintroduced slowly to minimize abdominal distention and trauma to the suture lines.*
- Begin discharge planning and teaching. Consult with a dietitian for instructions and menu planning; reinforce teaching. Teach about potential postoperative complications, such as abdominal abscess, or bowel obstruction, their signs and symptoms, and preventive measures.

Colostomies

Surgical resection of the bowel may be accompanied by a colostomy for diversion of fecal contents. A **colostomy** is an ostomy made in the colon. It may be created if the bowel is obstructed by the tumor, as a temporary measure to promote healing of anastomoses, or as a permanent means of fecal evacuation when the distal colon and rectum are removed. Colostomies take the name of the portion of the colon from which they are formed: ascending colostomy, transverse colostomy, descending colostomy, and sigmoid colostomy (Figure 24–12 ■).

A *sigmoid colostomy* is the most common permanent colostomy performed, particularly for cancer of the rectum. It is usually created during an abdominoperineal resection. This procedure involves the removal of the sigmoid colon, rectum, and anus through abdominal and perineal incisions. The anal canal is closed, and a stoma formed from the proximal sigmoid colon. The stoma usually is located on the lower left quadrant of the abdomen.

When a *double-barrel colostomy* is performed, two separate stomas are created (Figure 24–13 ■). The distal colon is not removed, but bypassed. The proximal stoma, which is functional, diverts feces to the abdominal wall. The distal stoma, also called the mucus fistula, expels mucus from the distal colon. It may be pouched or dressed with a 4 × 4 gauge dressing. A double-barrel colostomy may be created for cases of trauma, tumor, or inflammation, and it may be temporary or permanent.

An emergency procedure used to relieve an intestinal obstruction or perforation is called a *transverse loop colostomy.* During this procedure, a loop of the transverse colon is brought out from the abdominal wall and suspended over a plastic rod or bridge, which prevents the loop from slipping back into the abdominal cavity. The loop stoma may be opened at the time of surgery or a few days later at the client's bedside. The bridge may be removed in 1 to 2 weeks. Transverse loop colostomies are typically temporary.

In a *Hartmann procedure,* a common temporary colostomy procedure, the distal portion of the colon is left in place and is oversewn for closure. A temporary colostomy may be done to

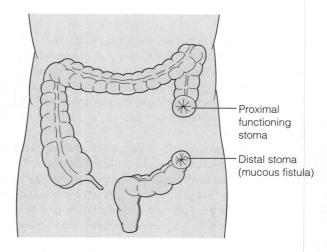

Figure 24–13 ■ A double-barrel colostomy. The proximal stoma is the functioning stoma; the distal stoma expels mucus from the distal colon.

allow bowel rest or healing, such as following tumor resection or inflammation of the bowel. It also may be created following traumatic injury to the colon, such as a gunshot wound. Anastomosis of the severed portions of the colon is delayed because bacterial colonization of the colon would prevent proper healing of the anastomosis. About 3 to 6 months following a temporary colostomy, the colostomy is closed and the colon is reconnected. Clients with temporary colostomies require the same care as clients with permanent colostomies. See the Nursing Care box on page 673.

Radiation Therapy

While radiation therapy is not used as a primary treatment for colon cancer, it is used along with surgical resection for treating rectal tumors. Small rectal cancers may be treated with intracavitary, external, or implantation radiation. Rectal cancer has a high rate of regional recurrence following complete surgical resection, particularly when the tumor has invaded tissues outside the bowel wall or regional lymph nodes. Pre- or postoperative radiation therapy reduces the recurrence of pelvic tumors, although the effect of radiation therapy on long-term survival is less clear. Radiation therapy also is used preoperatively to shrink large rectal tumors enough to permit surgical removal of the tumor (Braunwald et al., 2001).

Chemotherapy

Chemotherapeutic agents, such as intravenous fluorouracil (5-FU) and folinic acid (leucovorin), are also used postoperatively as adjunctive therapy for colorectal cancer. When combined with radiation therapy, chemotherapy reduces the rate of tumor recurrence and prolongs survival for clients with stage II and stage III rectal tumors. The benefit for colon cancers is less clear, but chemotherapy may be used to reduce its spread to the liver and prevent recurrence. Irinotecan (CPT-11) or oxaliplatin also may be used in chemotherapy regimens for colorectal cancer. Further discussion about chemotherapy and nursing implications is included in Chapter 10. ∞

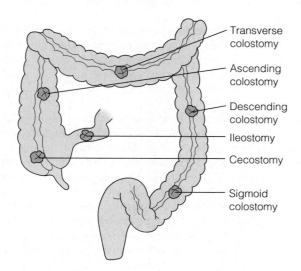

Transverse colostomy

Ascending colostomy

Descending colostomy

Ileostomy

Cecostomy

Sigmoid colostomy

Figure 24–12 ■ Various ostomy levels and sites.

NURSING CARE OF THE CLIENT WITH A COLOSTOMY

- Assess the location of the stoma and the type of colostomy performed. *Stoma location is an indicator of the section of bowel in which it is located and a predictor of the type of fecal drainage to expect.*
- Assess stoma appearance and surrounding skin condition frequently (see the box page 656). *Assessment of stoma and skin condition is particularly important in the early postoperative period, when complications are most likely to occur and most treatable.*
- Position a collection bag or drainable pouch over the stoma. *Initial drainage may contain more mucus and serosanguineous fluid than fecal material. As the bowel starts to resume function, drainage becomes fecal in nature. The consistency of drainage depends on the stoma location in the bowel.*
- If ordered, irrigate the colostomy, instilling water into the colon similar to an enema procedure. *The water stimulates the colon to empty.*
- When a colostomy irrigation is ordered for a client with a double-barrel or loop colostomy, irrigate the proximal stoma. Digital assessment of the bowel direction from the stoma can assist in determining which is the proximal stoma. *The distal bowel carries no fecal contents and does not need irrigation. It may be irrigated for cleansing just prior to reanastomosis.*
- Empty a drainable pouch or replace the colostomy bag as needed or when it is no more than one-third full. *If the pouch is allowed to overfill, its weight may impair the seal and cause leakage.*
- Provide stomal and skin care for the client with a colostomy as for the client with an ileostomy (see the box on page 656). *Good skin and stoma care is important to maintain skin integrity and function as the first line of defense against infection.*
- Use caulking agents, such as Stomahesive or karaya paste, and a skin barrier wafer as needed to maintain a secure ostomy pouch. This may be particularly important for the client with a loop colostomy. *The main challenge for a client with a transverse loop colostomy is to maintain a secure ostomy pouch over the plastic bridge.*
- A small needle hole high on the colostomy pouch will allow flatus to escape. This hole may be closed with a Band-Aid and opened only while the client is in the bathroom for odor control. *Ostomy bags may "balloon" out, disrupting the skin seal, if excess gas collects.*

CLIENT AND FAMILY TEACHING

- Prior to discharge, provide written, verbal, and psychomotor instruction on colostomy care, pouch management, skin care, and irrigation for the client. *Whether the colostomy is temporary or permanent, the client will be responsible for its manage-*

ment. Good understanding of procedures and care enhances the ability to provide self-care, as well as self-esteem and control.
- Allow ample time for the client (and family, if necessary) to practice changing the pouch, either on the client or a model. *Practice of psychomotor skills improves learning and confidence.*
- If an abdominoperineal resection has been performed, emphasize the importance of using no rectal suppositories, rectal temperatures, or enemas. Suggest that the client carry medical identification or a MedicAlert tag or bracelet. *These measures are important to prevent trauma to the tissues when the rectum has been removed.*
- The diet for a client with a colostomy is individualized and may require no alteration from that consumed preoperatively. Dietary teaching should, however, include information on foods that cause stool odor and gas and foods that thicken and loosen stools. Foods that cause these effects on ostomy output are listed below.

Foods That Increase Stool Odor
- Asparagus
- Beans
- Cabbage
- Eggs
- Fish
- Garlic
- Onions
- Some spices

Foods That Increase Intestinal Gas
- Beer
- Broccoli
- Brussels sprouts
- Cabbage
- Carbonated drinks
- Cauliflower
- Corn
- Cucumbers
- Dairy products
- Dried beans
- Peas
- Radishes
- Spinach

Foods That Thicken Stools
- Applesauce
- Bananas
- Bread
- Cheese
- Yogurt
- Pasta
- Pretzels
- Rice
- Tapioca
- Creamy peanut butter

Foods That Loosen Stools
- Chocolate
- Dried beans
- Fried foods
- Greasy foods
- Highly spiced foods
- Leafy green vegetables
- Raw fruits and juices
- Raw vegetables

Foods That Color Stools
- Beets
- Red gelatin

NURSING CARE

Health Promotion

Primary prevention of colorectal cancer is a significant nursing care issue. Teach clients about dietary recommendations provided by the American Cancer Society for the prevention of colorectal cancer. These recommendations include decreasing the amount of fat, refined sugar, and red meats in the diet while

increasing intake of dietary fiber. Foods that contain high amounts of fiber include raw fruits and vegetables, legumes, and whole-grain products.

Stress the importance of regular health examinations, including digital rectal exams. Discuss recommendations for regular hemoccult testing of stool after age 40. Include the importance of seeking medical treatment if blood is noted in or on the stool. Teach clients the warning signs for cancer, including those specific to bowel cancer, such as a change in bowel habits.

Assessment

- Health history: usual bowel patterns and any recent changes; weight loss, fatigue, decreased activity tolerance; presence of blood in the stool; pain with defecation, abdominal discomfort, perineal pain; usual diet; family history of colon cancer, other specific risk factors such as inflammatory bowel disease or colon polyps
- Physical examination: general appearance; weight; abdominal shape, contour; bowel sounds, abdominal tenderness; stool hemoccult or guaiac.

Nursing Diagnoses and Interventions

In planning and implementing care, consider both physical care needs and emotional response to the diagnosis. Because colorectal cancer is often advanced at the time of diagnosis, the prognosis, even with treatment, may be poor. Denial and anger are common. Extensive abdominal surgery and potentially a colostomy may be necessary, and the effects of chemotherapy and radiation therapy can leave the client fatigued and discouraged.

PRACTICE ALERT *If an abdominoperineal resection has been performed, alert all care personnel to avoid rectal temperatures, suppositories, or other procedures that could damage sutures.* ■

Nursing care includes providing emotional support, teaching, and direct care before and after diagnostic procedures and surgery and during adjunctive treatments. Priority nursing diagnoses include *Pain, Imbalanced nutrition,* and *Anticipatory grieving. Risk for sexual dysfunction* should be considered as a priority diagnosis if a colostomy has been created.

Pain

The client with colorectal cancer may experience pain related to preparatory procedures, diagnostic examinations, and surgery. Following an abdominoperineal resection, "phantom" rectal pain related to severing nerves during the wide excision of the rectum may develop. Finally, the primary tumor itself and, potentially, metastatic tumors may impinge on nerves and other organs, causing pain. In the early postoperative period, an epidural infusion or patient-controlled analgesia (PCA) often is used to manage pain. PCA, routine administration of ordered analgesics, or a continuous analgesia delivery (CAD) system also may be used for pain management when the tumor is far enough advanced to preclude surgical resection. See Chapter 4 for more information on caring for clients with pain. ⊙⊙

- Assess frequently for adequate pain relief. Use subjective and objective information, including the location, intensity, and character of the pain, as well as nonverbal signs, such as grimacing; muscle tension; apparent dozing; changes in pulse or blood pressure; rapid, shallow respirations. *The client may assume that pain is to be expected or tolerated or may fear becoming addicted to analgesic medications. Careful questioning and assessment can provide accurate information about pain status, allowing better control of discomfort.*

- Ask client to rate pain using a pain scale. Document the level of pain. *Pain is a subjective experience. Clients perceive and respond to pain differently. Religion and ethnic background may affect the response to pain.*
- Assess analgesic effectiveness 30 minutes after administration. Monitor for pain relief and adverse effects. *The method of delivery, dosage, or medication itself may need to be adjusted to provide adequate pain relief.*
- Assess the incision for inflammation or swelling; assess drainage catheters and tubes for patency. *Poorly controlled pain or pain that changes may be related to organ distention from an obstructed nasogastric tube, urinary catheter, or wound drain, or may indicate an infection.*
- Assess the abdomen for distention, tenderness, and bowel sounds. *Intra-abdominal bleeding, peritonitis, or paralytic ileus can cause pain that may be confused with incisional pain.*
- Administer analgesia prior to an activity or procedure. *Adequate pain relief reduces muscle tension, allowing for more comfortable participation in activities.*
- Assist with adjunctive relief measures, such as positioning, diversional activities, management of environmental stimuli, guided imagery, and teaching relaxation techniques. *These measures enhance the effects of analgesia by reducing muscle tension.*
- Splint incision with a pillow, and teach the client how to self-splint when coughing and deep breathing, *to prevent respiratory complications related to fear of pain.*

Imbalanced Nutrition: Less Than Body Requirements

Bowel preparation for diagnostic procedures and surgery, surgery, radiation therapy, and chemotherapy place the client with colorectal cancer at risk for nutritional deficiencies. Fluid and electrolyte replacement is provided following surgery, along with possible total parenteral nutrition (see Chapter 20). ⊙⊙ Adequate kcal and nutrient intake is necessary for healing after surgery. Additionally, if the tumor is advanced, metabolic needs may be increased and the appetite decreased.

- Assess nutritional status, using data such as height and weight, skinfold measurements, body mass index (BMI) calculation (see Chapter 20), and laboratory data including serum albumin level. Refer to dietitian or nutritionist for dietary management. *The client who is malnourished before beginning aggressive cancer treatment requires more vigorous nutrition management to promote healing.*
- Assess readiness for resumption of oral intake after surgery or procedures using data such as statements of hunger, presence of bowel sounds, passage of flatus, and minimal abdominal distention. *Manipulation of the bowel interrupts peristalsis of the GI tract. It is important to ensure that peristalsis has resumed prior to resumption of oral intake.*
- Monitor and document food and fluid intake. *Documentation helps determine the adequacy of kilocalories and other nutrient intake.*
- Weigh daily. *Weight fluctuation may indicate adequate or inadequate dietary intake.*

- Maintain total parenteral nutrition and central intravenous lines as ordered. *Parenteral nutrition prevents tissue catabolism and promotes healing when food intake is disrupted for more than 2 to 3 days.*
- When oral intake resumes, help the client develop a meal plan that incorporates food preferences and considers the client's schedule and environment. *Consideration of likes, dislikes, and circumstances in meal planning promotes an adequate intake.*

Anticipatory Grieving

When a bowel resection is performed for colorectal cancer, the client needs to adjust to the loss of a major body part as well as to the diagnosis of cancer. Even when the prognosis for recovery is good, many people perceive cancer as fatal. Supporting the client and family during the initial stages of grieving can improve physical recovery as well as psychologic coping and eventual adaptation.

- Work to develop a trusting relationship with the client and family. *This increases the nurse's effectiveness in helping them work through the grieving process.*
- Listen actively, encouraging the client and family to express their fears and concerns. Assist to identify strengths, past experiences, and support systems.
  a. Demonstrate respect for cultural, spiritual, and religious values and beliefs; encourage use of these resources to cope with losses.
  b. Encourage discussion of the potential impact of loss on individual family members, family structure, and family function. Assist family members to share concerns with one another.
  c. Refer to cancer support groups, social services, or counseling as appropriate.
  These resources can be used throughout the grieving process.

Risk for Sexual Dysfunction

Colorectal cancer and ostomy surgery increase the risk for sexual dysfunction, defined as a change in sexual function so that it becomes unsatisfying, unrewarding, inadequate (NANDA, 2001). Physical factors that can lead to sexual dysfunction include disruption of nerves and blood vessels that supply the genitals, radiation therapy, chemotherapy, and other medications prescribed after surgery.

Psychologically, an *ostomate* (client with an ostomy), experiences an altered body image and may develop low self-esteem. The client may feel undesirable and fear rejection. He or she may be concerned about odors or pouch leakage during sexual activity. This emotional stress can also contribute to sexual dysfunction. Self-image changes following an ostomy are addressed in the Nursing Research box below.

- Provide opportunities for the client and family to express feelings about the cancer diagnosis, ostomy, and effects of other treatments. *Encouraging verbalization of feelings about the*

Nursing Research

Evidence-Based Practice for Ostomies

Nurses often identify Disturbed body image as a nursing diagnosis for clients who have ostomy surgery. In a prospective study, researchers studied body image changes in clients with cancer who had an ostomy created (Jenks et al., 1997).

All study participants had primary bowel or bladder cancer and required a temporary or permanent ostomy. The majority of the participants had a permanent incontinent ostomy created. In addition, most participants were treated with chemotherapy, radiation therapy, or a combination of the two. Both quantitative and qualitative measures were used to assess participants' body image preoperatively and at 1 and 6 months postoperatively.

Body image scores were lowest in the preoperative measurement, improving postoperatively and achieving the highest scores at the 6-month measurement. Qualitative data supported cancer and its associated threat of death as the predominant concern of study subjects. At 6 months, at least some participants demonstrated reintegration of body image through qualitative statements.

IMPLICATIONS FOR NURSING

Clients undergoing ostomy surgery for cancer may be more concerned about the effect of the cancer on their lives than the effect of the ostomy. Adaptation to a life-threatening disease and survival are more critical issues for the client and deserve higher priority for nursing care focus. As the threat of the cancer diagnosis is reduced, strategies to improve and reintegrate body image will be more effective. Nurses need to acknowledge and accept the client's feelings and behavior toward the ostomy in the initial postoperative period. Progressive involvement in stoma care is important, as is preventing major leakage accidents. Education is a key strategy to promote body image; as the client acquires new skills, self-concept is enhanced.

Critical Thinking in Client Care

1. It is important for nurses to show acceptance of the client and the ostomy in the initial postoperative period. What behaviors by the nurse will demonstrate acceptance?
2. This study suggested that the client's overriding concern with the cancer diagnosis affected body image in the preoperative period. How might this concern also affect preoperative teaching? What can the nurse do to improve learning during this stressful period?
3. How might the results of a study such as this differ if the study participants were undergoing ostomies to treat inflammatory bowel disease such as ulcerative colitis?

Note. From "The Influence of Ostomy Surgery on Body Image in Patients with Cancer" by J. M. Jenks, K. H. Morin, & N. Tomaselli, November 1997, Applied Nursing Research, 10(4), 174–180.

diagnosis, ostomy, and treatments provides an opportunity to validate that feelings of anger and depression are normal responses to the diagnosis and change in body function.

- Provide consistent colostomy care. *An accepting attitude and consistent care that provides a secure appliance and controls odor and leakage instills a sense of confidence in the client.*
- Encourage expression of sexual concerns. Provide privacy and caregivers who have established trust with the client and family and are comfortable in discussions about sexual concerns. *Sexuality is a very private concern to most people. The client and family are not likely to express their concerns openly unless trust has been established.*
- Reassure the client and significant other that the effect of physical illness and prescribed interventions on sexuality usually is temporary. *The client and partner may misinterpret an initial decrease in libido as evidence that sexual activity will not be possible or resume following recovery.*
- Refer the client and partner to social services or a family counselor for further interventions. *Clients are often discharged from acute care settings well before concerns about sexual activity surface. Ongoing counseling provides a continuing resource.*
- Arrange for a visit from a member of the United Ostomy Association. *People who are living and coping with an ostomy can provide information and support, helping the new ostomate overcome feelings of isolation and rejection.*

Using NANDA, NIC, and NOC

Chart 24–5 shows links between NANDA nursing diagnoses, NIC, and NOC when caring for the client with colorectal cancer.

Home Care

During the diagnostic and preoperative periods, provide instruction about the following topics.

- Tests to be performed and preparatory procedures, including dietary restrictions, laxatives, enemas, and food and fluid restrictions just prior to the procedure
- Recommended postprocedure care and potential adverse effects to report
- Preoperative care, such as intestinal preparation and food and fluid restrictions

If a colostomy is planned, refer to an enterostomal therapist for stoma placement and initial teaching.

Once treatment has been initiated, include the following topics (as appropriate) in teaching for home care.

- Pain management
- Skin care and management of potential adverse effects of radiation therapy and/or chemotherapy (Refer to Chapter 10 for further discussion of teaching needs related to these therapies.) ⬭
- Incision and ostomy care
- Recommended diet
- Follow-up appointments and care

If the tumor is inoperable or a cure is not anticipated, provide information about pain and symptom management. Discuss the hospice philosophy and available services. Provide a referral to a local hospice or home health department.

CHART 24–5 NANDA, NIC, AND NOC LINKAGES

The Client with Colorectal Cancer

NURSING DIAGNOSES	NURSING INTERVENTIONS	NURSING OUTCOMES
• Pain	• Pain Management • Patient-Controlled Analgesia (PCA) Assistance	• Comfort Level • Pain Control • Pain: Disruptive Effects
• Ineffective Health Maintenance	• Ostomy Care • Teaching: Procedure/Treatment	• Bowel Elimination • Self-Care: Toileting
• Imbalanced Nutrition: Less Than Body Requirements	• Nutrition Management • Total Parenteral Nutrition (TPN) Administration	• Nutritional Status • Nutritional Status: Nutrient Intake
• Anticipatory Grieving	• Anticipatory Guidance • Family Support • Support System Enhancement	• Coping • Grief Resolution • Psychosocial Adjustment: Life Change
• Risk for Sexual Dysfunction	• Body Image Enhancement • Sexual Counseling	• Body Image • Self-Esteem

Note: Data from Nursing Outcomes Classification (NOC) by M. Johnson & M. Maas (Eds.), 1997, St. Louis: Mosby; Nursing Diagnoses: Definitions & Classification 2001–2002 by North American Nursing Diagnosis Association, 2001, Philadelphia: NANDA; Nursing Interventions Classification (NIC) by J.C. McCloskey & G. M. Bulechek (Eds.), 2000, St. Louis: Mosby. Reprinted by permission.

Nursing Care Plan
A Client with Colorectal Cancer

William Cunningham is a 65-year-old retired railroad employee, husband, and father of three grown children. For the past 3 months, Mr. Cunningham has noticed small amounts of blood in his stools and occasional mucus. He has a sensation of pressure in the rectum, and notices that his stools are smaller in diameter, about the size of a pencil. After palpating a mass on digital examination of the rectum, the physician orders a colonoscopy. A large sessile lesion is found in the rectum and biopsied. The pathology report shows the lesion to be adenocarcinoma. Mr. Cunningham is scheduled for an abdominoperineal resection and sigmoid colostomy.

ASSESSMENT

Madonna Hart, RN, completes the admission assessment. Mr. Cunningham states that his bowel habits have recently changed, but denies pain or other symptoms. Physical assessment findings include T 98.4 F (36.9° C), P 82, R 18, and BP 118/78. He is 70 inches (178 cm) tall and weighs 185 lb (84 kg). Laboratory findings are normal except for the previous pathology report of adenocarcinoma of rectal lesion.

Mr. Cunningham states, "I really don't want a colostomy, but if that is what it takes to get rid of this, I'm ready to get it over with."

DIAGNOSIS

- *Pain* related to surgical intervention
- *Risk for impaired skin integrity (peristomal)* related to fecal drainage and pouch adhesive
- *Risk for constipation/diarrhea* related to effects of surgery on bowel function
- *Risk for disturbed body image* related to colostomy
- *Risk for sexual dysfunction* related to wide rectal incision, radiation therapy, and colostomy

EXPECTED OUTCOMES

- Report pain within an acceptable range that allows ease of movement and ambulation.

- Perform colostomy care using correct technique.
- Demonstrate willingness to discuss changes in sexual function.
- Wear clothing to enhance physical and emotional self-esteem.

PLANNING AND IMPLEMENTATION

- Provide analgesia as ordered, evaluating its effectiveness.
- Discuss foods that cause odor and gas.
- Teach colostomy care.
- Maintain consistent nursing personnel assignment to facilitate trust.
- Refer to the local United Ostomy Association.
- Provide a list of local medical supply companies for ostomy supplies.
- Provide for privacy when teaching and discussing concerns about ostomy.

EVALUATION

On discharge, Mr. Cunningham is able to empty and rinse out his colostomy pouch. He is changing the pouch and caring for surrounding skin appropriately. Ms. Hart has given him verbal and written instructions on colostomy care. He verbalizes understanding of phantom rectal pain, and the importance of avoiding rectal temperatures and rectal suppositories. He expresses an understanding of the need to avoid heavy lifting, and the importance of follow-up care. Ms. Hart has referred Mr. Cunningham to a home health agency in his community for further questions and follow-up care.

Critical Thinking in the Nursing Process

1. What is the cause of phantom rectal pain?
2. Why is it important to discuss dietary concerns with a client with a colostomy, especially odor- and gas-forming foods?
3. Outline a plan to teach Mr. Cunningham how to irrigate a colostomy.
4. Develop a care plan for Mr. Cunningham for the nursing diagnosis, *Disturbed body image.*

See Evaluating Your Response in Appendix C.

STRUCTURAL AND OBSTRUCTIVE DISORDERS

Any portion of the intestines may be affected by a structural or obstructive disorder. When the structural defect is in the bowel wall, the intestine may be directly affected, as is the case with diverticula. Defects in the abdominal wall may allow intra-abdominal contents (such as loops of bowel) to protrude, indirectly affecting bowel function. Likewise, obstructions may result from disease of the bowel itself or from obstruction of the bowel lumen by an external force.

THE CLIENT WITH A HERNIA

A **hernia** is a defect in the abdominal wall that allows abdominal contents to protrude out of the abdominal cavity. Trauma,

surgery, and increased intra-abdominal pressure caused by such conditions as pregnancy, obesity, weight lifting, or tumors are risk factors for hernia formation.

PATHOPHYSIOLOGY AND MANIFESTATIONS

Hernias are classified by location (Figure 24–14 ■), and may be congenital or acquired. Approximately 80% of hernias occur in the groin (inguinal or femoral hernias). Inguinal hernias often are congenital, caused by improper closure of the tract that develops as the testes descend into the scrotum during fetal development. Groin hernias may be acquired, resulting from weakness of fascia in a region called Hesselbach's area or from dilation of the femoral ring (e.g., during pregnancy and childbirth). Another 10% are ventral or incisional hernias of the

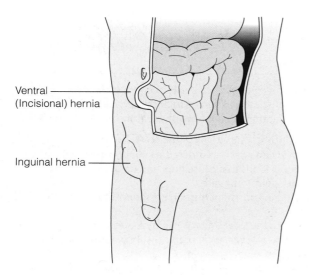

Figure 24–14 ■ An abdominal wall (ventral or incisional) hernia and an inguinal hernia.

abdominal wall. These generally are acquired, caused by weakening of normal abdominal wall musculature. Umbilical hernias also are congenital, and usually are detected in infancy. Hiatal hernias develop in the diaphragm (see Chapter 21).

Abdominal contents (peritoneum, bowel, and other abdominal organs) can protrude through the abdominal wall to form a sac covered by skin and subcutaneous tissues. In most cases, abdominal contents move into the sac when intra-abdominal pressure increases, then return to the abdominal cavity when pressure returns to normal or when manual pressure is placed on the bulging sac. This is known as a *reducible hernia.* The risk for complications is low with a reducible hernia. If the contents of a hernia cannot be returned to the abdominal cavity, it is said to be *incarcerated.* Contents of an incarcerated hernia are trapped, usually by a narrow neck or opening to the hernia. Incarceration increases the risk of complications, including obstruction and strangulation. Obstruction occurs when the lumen of the bowel contained within the hernia becomes occluded, much like the crimping of a hose. A *strangulated hernia* develops when blood supply to bowel and other tissues in the hernia sac is compromised, leading to necrosis. The affected bowel can infarct, leading to perforation with contamination of the peritoneal cavity. Manifestations of a strangulated hernia include severe abdominal pain and distention, nausea, vomiting, tachycardia, and fever.

Inguinal Hernias

Inguinal hernias usually affect males, and may be classified as indirect or direct inguinal hernias. *Indirect inguinal hernias* are caused by improper closure of the tract that develops as the testes descend into the scrotum before birth. A sac of abdominal contents protrudes through the internal inguinal ring into the inguinal canal. It often descends into the scrotum. Although indirect inguinal hernias are congenital defects, they often are not evident until adulthood, when increased intra-abdominal pressure and dilation of the inguinal ring allow abdominal contents to enter the channel.

Direct inguinal hernias are acquired defects that result from weakness of the posterior inguinal wall. Direct inguinal hernias usually affect older adults. *Femoral hernias* are also acquired defects in which a peritoneal sac protrudes through the femoral ring. These hernias usually affect obese or pregnant women.

Inguinal hernias often produce no symptoms and are discovered during routine physical examination. They may cause a lump, swelling, or bulge in the groin, particularly with lifting or straining. An inguinal hernia may cause sharp pain or a dull ache that radiates into the scrotum. A palpable mass may be present in the groin, although it may be felt only with increased intra-abdominal pressure (as occurs during coughing) and invagination of the scrotum toward the inguinal ring.

Umbilical Hernia

Pregnancy and obesity also contribute to the development of umbilical hernias in adults. *Umbilical hernias* may be congenital and evident during infancy, or acquired as the tissue closing the umbilical ring weakens, allowing protrusion of abdominal contents. These hernias are more common in women. Other predisposing factors include multiple pregnancies with prolonged labor, ascites, and large intra-abdominal tumors.

Umbilical hernias tend to enlarge steadily and contain omentum, although they may also contain small or large bowel. The hernia may cause sharp pain on coughing or straining or a dull, aching sensation. Strangulation is a common complication of umbilical hernias.

Incisional or Ventral Hernia

Incisional or *ventral hernias* occur at a previous surgical incision or following abdominal muscle tears. Inadequate healing of the incision or tear can lead to hernia development. Contributing factors include poor wound closure, postoperative infection, age or debility, obesity, inadequate nutrition, and excess incisional stress caused by vigorous coughing.

Ventral hernias are characterized by a bulge at the incisional site, often noted when the client pulls to a sitting position from a lying position. Ventral hernias often are asymptomatic, and the risk of incarceration is low because of the size of the defect.

COLLABORATIVE CARE

The diagnosis of a hernia is made by a physical examination. The client is examined in a supine and sitting or standing position. A bulge may be seen or felt when the client coughs or bears down. No laboratory or diagnostic testing is usually required, unless bowel obstruction or strangulation is suspected.

Surgical repair, or *herniorrhaphy,* is the usual treatment of hernia. Surgery is generally well tolerated by people of all ages and carries a much lower risk than the complications of incarceration, obstruction, and strangulation. Emergency surgery is indicated for a hernia that is incarcerated, painful, or tender. In a herniorrhaphy, the abdominal wall defect is closed by suturing or with wire or mesh over the defect. If incarceration has occurred or strangulation is suspected, the abdomen is explored at the time of surgery and any infarcted bowel resected. Heavy lifting and heavy manual labor are restricted for approximately 3 weeks after surgery.

When surgery is contraindicated, the client may be taught to reduce the hernia by lying down and gently pushing against the mass. A binder or truss may be worn to prevent or control the protrusion. An incarcerated hernia should not be reduced by the client.

NURSING CARE

Assessment

- Health history: manifestations of hernia, such as bulging in the groin or of the abdominal wall when coughing, straining, or moving from lying to sitting; pain (abdominal, groin, or scrotal); history of hernia or abdominal surgery
- Physical examination: observe for bulging of the abdominal wall or around the umbilicus when raising head and shoulders from supine position; wearing gloves, palpate inguinal region for bulges when the client coughs or bears down (Valsalva maneuver).

Nursing Diagnoses and Interventions

Herniorrhaphy is generally an uncomplicated procedure, usually performed as same-day surgery. Preoperative assessment and teaching and immediate postoperative care are the primary nursing care needs. Care is similar to that provided for a client with an appendectomy.

Risk for Ineffective Tissue Perfusion: Gastrointestinal

When providing care for a client with a known hernia, the possibility of obstruction and strangulation must be considered throughout nursing assessments. While nursing interventions may not be able to prevent these complications, rapid identification of the problem allows timely surgical treatment. Prompt treatment may prevent major complications related to infection and peritoneal contamination by bowel contents.

PRACTICE ALERT *Promptly report any acute increase in abdominal, groin, perineal, or scrotal pain. An abrupt increase in the intensity of pain may indicate bowel ischemia due to strangulation.* ■

- Assess bowel sounds and abdominal distention at least every 8 hours. *A change in bowel sounds—either cessation of sounds or an onset of hyperactive, high-pitched sounds—may indicate obstruction. With obstruction, abdominal girth may increase.*
- Notify primary care provider if the hernia becomes painful or tender. *Pain and tenderness may indicate incarceration and increased risk for strangulation.*
- If signs of possible obstruction or strangulation occur, notify the physician. Place client in supine position with the hips elevated and knees slightly bent. Withhold all food and fluids (NPO), and begin preparations for surgery. *This position helps relax abdominal muscles and may facilitate reduction of the hernia. Strangulation or obstruction require immediate surgical intervention.*

Using NANDA, NIC, and NOC

Chart 24–6 shows links between NANDA nursing diagnoses, NIC and NOC for the client having a herniorrhaphy.

Home Care

Include the following topics when teaching clients about hernias and home care.

- Rationale for examining the groin and abdomen for bulges
- The nature of hernia, risk factors, and manifestations
- Surgical intervention for hernia
- How to reduce a hernia if necessary
- The importance of seeking immediate medical intervention for signs of strangulation or obstruction
- The need to notify the physician if upper respiratory infection and cough develops preoperatively (forceful coughing is not recommended postoperatively)
- Postoperative pain management and activity restrictions

THE CLIENT WITH INTESTINAL OBSTRUCTION

Intestinal obstruction is failure of intestinal contents to move through the bowel lumen. Intestinal obstructions may affect either the large or small bowel. The small intestine is more commonly affected; only about 15% of bowel obstructions occur in

---

CHART 24–6 NANDA, NIC, AND NOC LINKAGES

The Client with Herniorrhaphy

NURSING DIAGNOSES	NURSING INTERVENTIONS	NURSING OUTCOMES
• Pain	• Pain Management	• Pain Control
• Risk for Infection	• Incision Site Care	• Wound Healing: Primary Intention
• Urinary Retention	• Urinary Catheterization: Intermittent	• Urinary Elimination

Note: Data from Nursing Outcomes Classification (NOC) by M. Johnson & M. Maas (Eds.), 1997, St. Louis: Mosby; Nursing Diagnoses: Definitions & Classification 2001–2002 by North American Nursing Diagnosis Association, 2001, Philadelphia: NANDA; Nursing Interventions Classification (NIC) by J.C. McCloskey & G. M. Bulechek (Eds.), 2000, St. Louis: Mosby. Reprinted by permission.

the large intestine. Obstruction is the most common reason for small bowel surgery.

PHYSIOLOGY REVIEW

The GI tract contains layers of smooth muscle that contract in rhythmic waves. These waves of contraction, known as *peristalsis,* move along the whole length of the digestive tract to propel contents along the tract. Pacesetter cells in the smooth muscle control the rate of peristalsis.

PATHOPHYSIOLOGY

Intestinal obstructions may be either mechanical or functional in nature. *Mechanical* obstructions may be caused by (1) problems outside the intestine, such as bands of scar tissue or hernias, (2) problems within the intestine, such as tumors or inflammatory bowel disease, or (3) obstruction of the intestinal lumen. The obstruction may be partial or complete. *Functional* obstruction occurs when peristalsis fails to propel intestinal contents although there is no mechanical obstruction. *Adynamic ileus* (also known as *paralytic ileus* or simply *ileus*) is the most common functional obstruction, and probably accounts for most intestinal obstructions altogether (Braunwald et al., 2001). Obstructions are further classified by the portion of intestine affected.

When the intestine is obstructed, gas and fluid accumulate proximal to and within the obstructed segment, distending the bowel. Swallowed air accounts for most of the gas. Ingested fluid, saliva, gastric juice, and pancreatic secretions contribute to accumulated fluid. Water and sodium are drawn into the bowel lumen, contributing to fluid accumulation, distention, and vascular fluid losses.

In some mechanical obstructions, such as a strangulated hernia, blood supply to the affected portion of bowel also is impaired, leading to necrosis and bacterial peritonitis.

Significant bowel distention, vomiting, and third spacing of fluids in the bowel and peritoneal cavity can lead to massive loss of fluids and electrolytes with resulting hypovolemia, hypokalemia, renal insufficiency, and shock.

Small Bowel Obstruction

Adhesions, or bands of scar tissue, and hernias account for 70% to 75% of mechanical small bowel obstructions (Braunwald et al., 2001). In adults, adhesions develop following abdominal surgery or inflammatory processes. Adhesions usually produce a *simple obstruction,* or single blockage in one portion of the intestine (Figure 24-15A ■). The obstruction produced by an incarcerated hernia is a *closed-loop obstruction,* with two different portions of the bowel lumen obstructed (Figure 24-15 B).

Tumors, either intrinsic (of the bowel itself) or extrinsic (of another organ but affecting the bowel because of their size), can progressively occlude the bowel lumen and eventually obstruct it (Figure 24–15C). Other, less common causes of bowel obstruction include intussusception (rare in adults) (Figure 24–15D); volvulus, the rotation of loops of bowel about a fixed point (Figure 24–15E); foreign bodies; stricture; and inflammatory bowel disease.

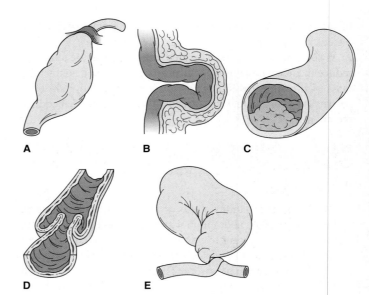

Figure 24–15 ■ Selected causes of mechanical obstruction. *A,* Adhesions; *B,* incarcerated hernia; *C,* tumor; *D,* intussusception; *E,* volvulus.

Both volvulus and an incarcerated hernia can cause a *strangulated obstruction.* In a strangulated obstruction, not only is the lumen of the bowel obstructed, but also the blood supply to the affected portion is compromised.

In a functional obstruction or adynamic ileus, peristalsis stops due to either neurogenic or muscular impairment. The bowel lumen remains patent, but contents are not propelled forward. Temporary ileus commonly follows gastrointestinal surgery. It may also result from tissue anoxia or peritoneal irritation due to hemorrhage, peritonitis, or perforation of an organ. Other conditions that can precipitate paralytic ileus include renal colic, spinal cord injuries, uremia, and electrolyte imbalances, hypokalemia in particular. In addition, the effects of some narcotics, anticholinergic drugs, and antidiarrheal medications such as diphenoxylate can produce a functional obstruction.

MANIFESTATIONS

The manifestations of a small bowel obstruction vary, depending on the level of obstruction and how rapidly it develops. Cramping or colicky abdominal pain that may be intermittent or increasing in intensity is common. Vomiting is common, particularly in high or proximal obstructions, because distention of the lumen stimulates the vomiting center. As bacterial fermentation occurs, vomitus becomes feculent, particularly with a low or distal obstruction. Flatus and feces already present in the lower bowel may be expelled early in the obstructive process, but this expulsion ceases as the obstruction continues.

Early in the course of a mechanical obstruction, borborygmi and high-pitched tinkling bowel sounds are present, as the intestine attempts to propel contents past the obstruction. Visible peristaltic waves may be noted in the distended loops of bowel in thin clients. In the later stages, the bowel becomes silent. With a paralytic ileus, bowel sounds are greatly diminished or absent throughout the process. Abdominal distention is minimal with proximal obstructions, but may be pronounced with distal obstruction and paralytic ileus. The abdomen may be tender to palpation as well.

In addition to abdominal and gastrointestinal manifestations, signs of fluid and electrolyte imbalance develop. Hypovolemia can develop rapidly as extracellular fluid is sequestered in the bowel and vomiting occurs. Although early vital signs may be normal, changes are noted as dehydration and hypovolemia develop. The client becomes tachycardic and tachypneic, and blood pressure falls. Temperature may be elevated. Urine output drops, and signs of hypovolemic shock may be seen.

Complications

Hypovolemia and hypovolemic shock with multiple organ dysfunction is a significant complication of bowel obstruction and can lead to death. Renal insufficiency from hypovolemia can lead to acute renal failure. Pulmonary ventilation may be impaired as abdominal distention elevates the diaphragm and interferes with respiratory processes.

Strangulation associated with incarcerated hernia or volvulus impairs the blood supply to the bowel. Gangrene may rapidly result, causing bleeding into the bowel lumen and peritoneal cavity and eventual perforation. With perforation, bacteria and toxins from the strangulated intestine enter the peritoneum and, potentially, the circulation, resulting in peritonitis and possible septic shock.

The mortality rate in clients with obstruction of the small bowel is approximately 10%. When strangulation occurs, the mortality rate is between 20% and 75% (Braunwald et al., 2001). Delays in surgical intervention contribute to the higher mortality rate, pointing out the necessity of prompt diagnosis and intervention.

Large Bowel Obstruction

Obstruction of the large intestine occurs much less frequently than small bowel obstruction, accounting for approximately 15% of all bowel obstructions in adults. Although any portion of the colon may be affected, obstruction usually occurs in the sigmoid segment. Cancer of the bowel is the most common cause; other causes include volvulus, diverticular disease, inflammatory disorders, and fecal impaction.

If the ileocecal valve between the small and large intestines is competent, distention proximal to the obstruction is limited to the colon itself. This is known as a *closed-loop obstruction*. It can lead to massive colon dilation as the ileum continues to empty gas and fluid into the colon. Increasing pressure within the obstructed colon impairs circulation to the bowel wall. Gangrene and perforation are potential complications. Approximately 15% of clients with large bowel obstruction have an incompetent ileocecal valve, which allows relief of colonic pressure by reflux into the ileum (Braunwald et al., 2001)

Constipation and colicky abdominal pain are usual manifestations of large bowel obstruction. The pain is often deep and cramping; severe, continuous pain may signal bowel ischemia and possible perforation. Vomiting is a late sign, if it occurs at all. The abdomen is distended, with high-pitched, tinkling bowel sounds with rushes and gurgles. On palpation, localized tenderness or a mass may be noted.

COLLABORATIVE CARE

The management of a bowel obstruction focuses on relieving the pressure and obstruction, and providing supportive care. The intestine is decompressed, and fluid and electrolyte balance is restored. Surgery may be necessary to relieve a mechanical obstruction or if strangulation is suspected.

Diagnostic Tests

Radiologic studies (X-rays and CT scan) are used to confirm the diagnosis of bowel obstruction. Laboratory testing is used to evaluate for the presence of infection and fluid and electrolyte imbalances.

- *WBC* often shows mild leukocytosis due to an inflammatory response to changes within the obstructed bowel lumen. With strangulation, leukocytosis is marked.
- *Serum amylase* levels may be elevated, particularly when strangulation is present.
- *Serum osmolality* and *electrolyte levels* are affected by fluid and electrolyte losses from vomiting and fluid sequestering in the bowel lumen. With hypovolemia, the serum osmolality and urine specific gravity increase. Potassium and chloride are lost through vomiting, leading to hypokalemia and hypochloremia.
- *Arterial blood gases* may reveal metabolic alkalosis (pH > 7.45, bicarbonate >26 mEq/L, P_{CO_2} > 45 mmHg) with small bowel obstruction due to loss of hydrochloric acid from the stomach.
- *Abdominal X-ray* often shows distended loops of intestine with fluid and gas in a small bowel obstruction. Free air under the diaphragm indicates a perforation. A distended colon may be visualized with a large bowel obstruction.
- *X-ray* or *CT scan with contrast media* may be required to confirm a mechanical obstruction and assess the completeness of the obstruction. Meglumine diatrizoate (Gastrografin) is often used to provide contrast rather than barium when a bowel obstruction is suspected.

PRACTICE ALERT *Unlike barium, meglumine diatrizoate contains iodine; therefore, it is vital to ask about iodine or seafood hypersensitivity prior to exam.* ■

- *Barium enema* may be used to confirm the diagnosis of large bowel obstruction and determine its location, unless perforation is suspected. See the Nursing Implications box on page 623 for nursing care related to a barium enema.
- *Sigmoidoscopy* or *colonoscopy* may be done to identify the cause when large bowel obstruction occurs. See pages 619 and 624 for nursing care related to these diagnostic studies.

Gastrointestinal Decompression

Most partial small bowel obstructions are successfully treated with gastrointestinal decompression using a nasogastric or long intestinal tube. Functional obstructions respond to treatment with bowel rest and intestinal decompression as well. Intestinal tubes (see Figure 24–3) may be inserted through the nares or via gastrostomy. A balloon or weighted tip draws the tube from the stomach into the intestine and to the area of obstruction via peristalsis. Collected fluid and gas is removed using low suction until persitalsis resumes or the obstruction is relieved.

Surgery

Surgical intervention is required for complete mechanical obstructions as well as for strangulated or incarcerate obstructions of the small intestine. Clients with incomplete mechanical obstruction may also require surgery if the obstruction persists.

Prior to surgery, a nasogastric tube is inserted to relieve vomiting and abdominal distention and to prevent aspiration of intestinal contents. Fluid and electrolyte balance must be restored before surgery as well. Isotonic intravenous fluids, such as normal (physiologic) saline, Ringer's solution, or other balanced electrolyte solutions, are used. Additional electrolytes may be added to the solution to correct low levels. It is particularly important to correct hypokalemia prior to surgery. Acid-base imbalances are also addressed, often using intravenous acidifiers or alkalinizing agents. If strangulation has occurred, the client may require plasma or blood replacement. Intravenous broad-spectrum antibiotics are administered prophylactically (see the section on peritonitis).

A laparotomy usually is performed to allow inspection of the small intestine and removal of infarcted or gangrenous tissue. If the obstruction was caused by adhesions, they are removed or lysed. Obstructing tumors are resected, and foreign bodies are removed. Any bowel that appears to be gangrenous is resected, usually followed by an end-to-end anastomosis of remaining intestine. If a large tumor mass or dense adhesions are found, the area of obstruction may be bypassed by anastomosis of proximal small bowel to small or large intestine distal to the obstruction. Nursing care of the client having bowel surgery is included in the box on page 671.

Obstructions of the large intestine usually necessitate surgery. The primary goal is to relieve colonic distention and prevent perforation; the secondary goal is to remove the obstructing lesion. In some cases, colonoscopy may be used to relieve the distention. If the client's condition prohibits major surgery or the obstructing tumor is advanced, laser photocoagulation may be used to enlarge the bowel lumen. Removal of the obstructing lesion is the preferred treatment. The proximal and distal bowel segments may be anastomosed, or a permanent colostomy or ileostomy may be required. (The previous section on bowel cancer discusses these surgical interventions.)

NURSING CARE

Health Promotion

Teach health promotion activities, such as increasing dietary fiber intake, maintaining a generous fluid intake, and exercising daily to help prevent constipation and possible large bowel obstruction, particularly in the older adult. Stress the importance of complying with dietary restrictions (such as avoiding popcorn) for clients who experience repeated small bowel obstructions.

Assessment

Nurses may be instrumental in the early identification of intestinal obstructions in older adults, the homebound client, or the institutionalized client. Early identification and intervention significantly reduces morbidity from bowel obstruction.

- Health history: complaints of abdominal pain and bloating, constipation; previous history of bowel obstruction or risk factors such as hernia, inflammatory bowel disease, diverticulosis, or previous abdominal surgery; current medications
- Physical examination: vital signs including orthostatic blood pressure and pulse, temperature; skin color, temperature, texture, and turgor; color and moisture of mucous membranes; abdominal shape, contour, bowel sounds, presence of tenderness or masses on palpation

Nursing Diagnoses and Interventions

In clients with a suspected or confirmed bowel obstruction, frequent assessment for complications such as fluid and electrolyte imbalance, acid-base imbalances, hypovolemic shock, perforation, and peritonitis is necessary.

Deficient Fluid Volume

Because of the large collection of fluid in the bowel proximal to an obstruction, the accompanying vomiting, and nasogastric suction, the client with an intestinal obstruction often has a fluid volume deficit. If not corrected promptly, hypovolemic shock, acute renal failure, and multiple organ system dysfunction from poor tissue perfusion may result.

- Monitor vital signs, pulmonary artery pressures, cardiac output (CO), and central venous pressure (CVP) hourly. *A decrease in blood pressure, tachycardia, and tachypnea may indicate hypovolemia. Although invasive, hemodynamic parameters such as pulmonary artery pressures, CO, and CVP allow accurate assessment of fluid volume status.*
- Measure urinary output hourly and nasogastric drainage every 2 to 4 hours. *A urinary output of 30 mL per hour or more usually indicates an adequate glomerular filtration rate (GFR), another indicator of fluid volume. Nasogastric output provides a tool for evaluating fluid replacement needs.*

PRACTICE ALERT *Promptly report urine output less than 30 mL per hour. This often indicates hypovolemia and an increased risk for shock and acute renal failure.* ■

- Maintain intravenous fluids and blood volume expanders as ordered. The amount of fluid administered is calculated to meet ongoing fluid needs and replace previous and current losses. *Restoration and maintenance of blood volume is necessary to maintain cardiac output and tissue and organ perfusion.*
- Measure abdominal girth every 4 to 8 hours. Mark the level of measurement on the abdomen. *A reference mark allows consistent, accurate measurements. An increase in abdominal girth indicates increasing intestinal distention.*

- Notify the physician of changes in status. *Changes in vital signs, pain, and signs of increasing distention can indicate the need for immediate surgical intervention.*

Ineffective Tissue Perfusion: Gastrointestinal

Perfusion of the intestinal wall and mucosa may be impaired by the obstructive process itself (e.g., strangulation or volvulus) or by significant intestinal distention. The goal is to maintain tissue perfusion and promote normal peristalsis and bowel elimination.

- Monitor vital signs hourly. Assess peripheral pulses, skin color, temperature, and capillary refill. *Cardiovascular assessment is vital to detect early signs of hypovolemic shock resulting from sequestering large volumes of fluid in the intestines. Hypovolemia and shock can convert mild bowel ischemia to infarction as the blood supply to the tissue falls.*
- Monitor urine output hourly. Report output of less than 30 mL per hour. *Urine output is a good indicator of the glomerular filtration rate (GFR) and tissue perfusion. The urine output often falls before vital sign changes are apparent in hypovolemia.*
- Monitor temperature at least every 4 hours. *An elevated temperature may be an early indication of sepsis from bowel perforation as a result of gangrene.*
- Frequently assess pain. *A change in the character of pain or a rapid increase in its intensity may signal bowel infarction or perforation.*
- Maintain NPO status until peristalsis resumes. *Enteral food or fluids may increase distention and bowel ischemia. They also are restricted until the possibility of perforation is eliminated.*

Ineffective Breathing Pattern

Significant abdominal distention from a bowel obstruction can cause the diaphragm to flatten, impairing pulmonary ventilation. Following surgery, splinting of abdominal muscles to avoid pain can lead to shallow respirations. These factors, plus the risk of aspiration of gastrointestinal contents during vomiting, place the client at high risk for respiratory complications, particularly with a small bowel obstruction.

- Assess respiratory rate, pattern, and lung sounds at least every 2 to 4 hours. *Tachypnea, shortness of breath, or apparent dyspnea may be early signs of respiratory compromise. Diminished breath sounds, particularly in the bases of the lungs, or crackles indicate poor lung expansion and possible impaired ventilation.*
- Monitor arterial blood gas results for possible effects of altered respiratory status. *Tachypnea may lead to respiratory alkalosis as excess carbon dioxide is eliminated. Conversely, impaired chest expansion can lead to respiratory acidosis because of alveolar hypoventilation.*
- Elevate the head of the bed. *Elevating the head of the bed reduces the work of breathing and improves alveolar ventilation by reducing the pressure of abdominal distention on the diaphragm.*
- Provide a pillow or folded bath blanket to use in splinting the abdomen while coughing postoperatively. *Splinting abdominal muscles and incisions improves the ease and effectiveness of coughing postoperatively.*

- Maintain nasogastric or intestinal tube patency. *Maintaining gastrointestinal suction helps reduce abdominal distention and prevent aspiration associated with vomiting.*
- Encourage use of incentive spirometer or other assistive device hourly. *These devices encourage deep breathing, opening distal airways and preventing atelectasis.*
- Contact respiratory therapy as indicated. *The respiratory therapist may suggest or perform additional measures to maintain effective pulmonary ventilation.*
- Provide good oral care at least every 4 hours. *Dehydration and nasogastric suction dry mucous membranes of the mouth and throat, increasing the risk of bacterial growth. Many respiratory infections result from aspirated organisms.*

Using NANDA, NIC, and NOC

Linkages between NANDA, NIC, and NOC when caring for the client with intestinal obstruction are similar to those for clients with appendicitis or peritonitis. (See Chart 24–2.)

Home Care

Include the following topics when teaching the client with intestinal obstruction in preparation for home care.

- Wound care
- Activity level, return to work, and any other recommended restrictions
- Recommended follow-up care
- Care of temporary colostomy (if appropriate) and planned reanastamosis
- For recurrent obstructions, their cause, early identification of symptoms, and possible preventive measures

THE CLIENT WITH DIVERTICULAR DISEASE

Diverticula are saclike projections of mucosa through the muscular layer of the colon (Figure 24–16 ■). Diverticula may occur anywhere in the gastrointestinal tract, excluding the rectum. The vast majority, however, affect the large intestine, with 90% to 95% occurring in the sigmoid colon.

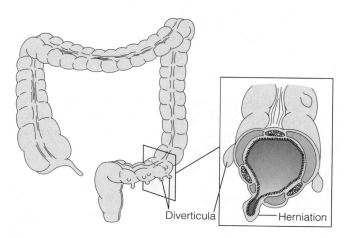

Diverticula   Herniation

Figure 24–16 ■ Diverticula of the colon.

People in the United States, Australia, the United Kingdom, and France have high and increasing incidence rates of diverticular disease. The disease is uncommon in Africa and Asia. Both sexes are equally affected. The incidence of diverticula increases with age: While only 5% of people under age 40 have diverticula, more than 50% of people over age 80 are affected. Millions of people have diverticular disease, but less than one-third of those affected develop symptoms (Tierney et al., 2001).

Cultural factors, diet in particular, are thought to play an important role in the development of diverticula. A diet consisting of highly refined and fiber-deficient foods is believed to be the major factor contributing to the disease. Diverticular disease was essentially unknown before grain milling (which removes two-thirds of the fiber from flour) became prevalent in the early 1900s. Decreased activity levels and postponement of defecation have been suggested as contributing factors. The increasing incidence of diverticula with aging suggests that decreased blood supply or nutrition of the bowel wall may be additional related factors (Bullock & Henze, 2000).

PATHOPHYSIOLOGY AND MANIFESTATIONS

Diverticula form when increased pressure within the bowel lumen causes bowel mucosa to herniate through defects in the colon wall. The circular and longitudinal (teniae coli) muscles often thicken or hypertrophy in the area affected by diverticula. This narrows the bowel lumen, increasing intraluminal pressure. Deficient dietary fiber and a lack of fecal bulk contribute to muscle hypertrophy and narrowing of the bowel. Contraction of the muscles in response to normal stimuli such as meals may occlude the narrowed lumen, further increasing intraluminal pressure. The high pressure causes mucosa to herniate through the muscle wall, forming a diverticulum. Areas where nutrient blood vessels penetrate the circular muscle layer are the most common sites for diverticula formation.

Diverticulosis

Diverticulosis indicates the presence of diverticula. More than two-thirds of clients with diverticulosis are asymptomatic. When manifestations such as episodic pain (usually left-sided), constipation, and diarrhea occur, they often can be attributed to irritable bowel syndrome, which commonly accompanies diverticular disease. (Irritable bowel syndrome is discussed earlier in this chapter.) As the disease progresses, abdominal cramping, narrow stools (decrease in caliber), increased constipation, occult bleeding in the stools, weakness, and fatigue may develop.

Complications of diverticulosis include hemorrhage and diverticulitis. A diverticulum may bleed, whether it is inflamed or not, possibly due to erosion of an adjacent blood vessel by a fecalith in the diverticulum.

Diverticulitis

Diverticulitis is inflammation in and around the diverticular sac. It typically affects only one diverticulum, usually in the sigmoid colon. Undigested food and bacteria collect in the diverticula, forming a hard mass (*fecalith*) that impairs the mucosal blood supply, allowing bacterial invasion. Mucosal ischemia leads to perforation. With microscopic perforation, inflammation is localized. Gross perforation of a diverticulum results in more extensive bacterial contamination and can lead to abscess formation or peritonitis.

Pain is a common manifestation of diverticulitis. It is usually left-sided and may be mild to severe and either steady or cramping. The client may also experience either constipation or increased frequency of defecation. Depending on the location and severity of the inflammation, nausea, vomiting, and a low-grade fever may occur. On examination, the abdomen may be distended, with tenderness and a palpable mass in the left lower quadrant resulting from the inflammatory response.

The older adult may have less specific manifestations, complaining of vague abdominal pain. A palpable mass and signs of a large bowel obstruction may be present.

Complications associated with diverticulitis (in addition to peritonitis and abscess formation) include bowel obstruction, fistula formation, and hemorrhage. Severe or repeated episodes of diverticulitis may lead to scarring and fibrosis of the bowel wall, further narrowing the bowel lumen. This increases the risk for obstruction of the large bowel. Acutely inflamed tissue may adhere to the small bowel, increasing the potential for small bowel obstruction as well. Fistulas may form, usually between the sigmoid colon and the bladder. Urinary tract infection is the usual sign of a colovesical fistula. Fistulas may also perforate into the small intestine, ureter, vagina, perineum, or abdominal wall. Bleeding from perforation of a vessel wall can occur with diverticulitis. Although it may be significant, bleeding usually stops spontaneously.

COLLABORATIVE CARE

Management of diverticular disease varies from no prescribed treatment to surgical resection of affected colon, depending on the severity of the disease and its complications.

Diagnostic Tests

Diagnostic testing is used to identify diverticular disease when the disease is symptomatic or complications develop.

- *WBC count* may show leukocytosis with a left shift (an increased number of immature WBCs) due to inflammation in diverticulitis.
- *Hemoccult* or *guaiac testing* of stool may show the presence of occult blood.
- *Barium enema* may be used to confirm diverticular disease. In addition to illustrating diverticula, X-rays can reveal segmental spasm and muscular thickening with a narrowed bowel lumen. Barium enema is contraindicated in early acute diverticulitis because of the risk of barium leakage into the peritoneal cavity.
- *Abdominal X-ray* films may show free abdominal air associated with diverticulitis and perforation. When there is a risk of perforation, water-soluble contrast media may be used to illustrate an abscess, fistulas, or narrowing of the bowel lumen.

- *CT scan* may be done with or without contrast media to assess inflammation and detect an abscess or fistula.
- *Flexible sigmoidoscopy* or *colonoscopy* may be done to detect diverticulosis, assess for strictures or bleeding, and rule out tumor as the cause of the client's symptoms.

Medications

Systemic broad-spectrum antibiotics effective against usual bowel flora are prescribed to treat acute diverticulitis. Oral antibiotics such as metronidazole (Flagyl) and ciprofloxacin (Cipro) or trimethoprim-sulfamethoxazole (Septra, Bactrim) may be prescribed if symptoms are mild. Severe, acute attacks often necessitate hospitalization and treatment with intravenous fluids and antibiotics effective against anaerobic and gram-negative bacteria. Therapy may include a second-generation cephalosporin such as cefoxitin (Mefoxin), or another antibiotic such as piperacillin-taxobactam (Zosyn) or ticarcillin-clavulanate (Timentin). Antibiotics and their nursing implications are discussed in Chapter 8.

Pentazocine (Talwin) may be prescribed for relief of pain associated with diverticulitis. This analgesic causes less increase in colonic pressure than morphine or meperidine (Demerol).

Although a stool softener such as docusate sodium (Colace) may be prescribed, it is important to note that laxatives (which can further increase intraluminal pressure in the colon) are avoided for the client with diverticular disease.

Dietary Management

Dietary modification is central to the management of diverticular disease. It appears that dietary changes can reduce the risk of complications of diverticulosis. A high-fiber diet is recommended; it increases stool bulk, decreases intraluminal pressures, and may reduce spasm (Table 24–13). Bran is a low-cost fiber supplement that can be added to cereal, soups, salads, or other foods. Commercial bulk-forming products, such as psyllium seed (Metamucil) or methylcellulose also may be recommended. These products are discussed in the Medication Administration box on page 624. The client may be advised to avoid foods with small seeds (such as popcorn, caraway seeds, figs, or berries), which could obstruct diverticula.

TABLE 24–13	Foods Recommended in a High-Fiber, High-Residue Diet
Food Group	**Recommended Foods**
Cereals and grains	Wheat or oat bran; cooked cereals, such as oatmeal; dry cereals, such as bran buds or flakes, corn flakes, shredded wheat; whole-grain breads or crackers; brown rice; popcorn
Fruits	Unpeeled raw apples, peaches, and pears; blackberries, raspberries, strawberries; oranges
Vegetables	Dried beans (navy, kidney, pinto), lima beans; broccoli; peas; corn; squash; raw vegetables, such as carrots, celery, and tomatoes; potatoes (with skins)

Bowel rest is prescribed during an acute episode of diverticulitis. The client initially may be NPO with intravenous fluids and possibly total parenteral nutrition. Feeding is resumed gradually. Initially, a clear liquid diet is prescribed with gradual advancement to a soft, low-roughage diet (i.e., a diet low in insoluble fiber) with daily added psyllium seed to soften stool and increase its bulk. Among the foods the client should avoid are wheat and corn bran, vegetable and fruit skins, nuts, and dry beans. The high-fiber diet is resumed following full recovery.

Surgery

Clients with acute diverticulitis require surgery, usually to treat generalized peritonitis or an abscess that fails to respond to medical treatment. Hemorrhage that recurs or cannot be controlled may also necessitate surgery. Elective surgery may be performed for recurrent episodes of diverticulitis or persistent diverticulitis with continuing pain, tenderness, and a palpable mass.

The affected bowel segment is resected, and if possible an anastomosis of the proximal and distal portions is performed. When an acute infection and diverticulitis are present, a two-stage Hartmann procedure is required. A temporary colostomy is created and anastomosis delayed until the inflammation has subsided. A second surgery is performed 2 to 3 months later to reconnect the bowel and close the temporary colostomy. Refer to the boxes on pages 671 and 673 for nursing care of the client with bowel surgery and a colostomy.

NURSING CARE

Health Promotion

Teaching clients in many different settings about the benefits of a high-fiber diet is important primary prevention for diverticular disease. Nurses working with groups and individuals in the community should emphasize the importance of a high-fiber diet and its benefits in preventing diverticular disease and other disorders. In such facilities as residential or foster care settings, the nurse can work with dietary staff and care providers to increase the amount of fiber in residents' diets, unless this is contraindicated by a preexisting condition.

Assessment

Because most clients with diverticular disease have few or no symptoms, nursing assessment focuses on manifestations of complications.

- Health history: abdominal pain or cramping, chronic constipation or irregular bowel habits; nausea and vomiting; history of diverticular disease or irritable bowel syndrome
- Physical examination: bowel sounds, presence of abdominal tenderness of masses and location; stool for occult blood

Nursing Diagnoses and Interventions

Clients with acute diverticulitis are acutely ill and have multiple nursing care needs. Priority nursing diagnoses include *Impaired tissue integrity, Pain,* and *Anxiety* related to the possibility of a significant complication or possible surgery.

Impaired Tissue Integrity: Gastrointestinal

During an acute attack of diverticulitis, inflammation and mucosal ischemia place the client at risk for perforation and peritonitis. In addition to maintaining bowel rest to reduce the risk of perforation, the nurse monitors for manifestations of perforation and possible sepsis.

- Monitor vital signs including temperature at least every 4 hours. *Tachycardia and tachypnea may be early indications of increased inflammation and resulting fluid shift. Fever greater than 101°F (38.3°C) may indicate increased or spread of inflammation. Note, however, that little temperature elevation may occur in the older client. A change in behavior or increasing lethargy may be subtle indications of infection in the older adult.*
- Assess abdomen every 4 to 8 hours or more often as indicated, including measuring abdominal girth, auscultating bowel sounds, and palpating for tenderness. Promptly report significant changes to the physician. *Increasing abdominal distention, a decrease or change in the quality of bowel sounds, and/or increasing tenderness or guarding may indicate spread of the infectious process or peritonitis.*
- Assess for evidence of lower intestinal bleeding by visual examination and guaiac testing of stools for occult blood. *Perforation of a diverticulum may produce either intestinal or intra-abdominal bleeding and require immediate treatment such as surgery.*
- Maintain intravenous fluids, total parenteral nutrition, and accurate intake and output records. *During acute diverticulitis, oral intake is usually prohibited or restricted. Intravenous fluids are given to maintain fluid and electrolyte balance; total parenteral nutrition is used to maintain nutritional status, facilitating healing and recovery.*

Pain

Pain is a common manifestation of acute diverticulitis. It results from inflammation of the bowel and edema of affected tissues. If surgery is required, postoperative pain is managed with narcotic analgesics.

- Ask the client to rate pain using a pain scale. Document the level of pain, and note any changes in location or character of pain. *The perception and response to pain is individual and is affected by past experiences, culture, ethnic background, and many other factors. A change in the character or intensity of the pain may indicate a complication such as perforation or abscess formation.*
- Administer prescribed analgesic or maintain patient-controlled analgesia (PCA) as ordered. Assess analgesic effectiveness. Avoid administering morphine. Provide adjunctive medications as ordered, and encourage use of adjunctive techniques, such as relaxation, positioning, and distraction. Notify the physician if pain management is inadequate. *If client has not obtained adequate pain relief, further assessment and intervention are required.*
- Maintain bowel rest and total body rest (bed rest with limited activity). *Rest helps reduce inflammation and promote healing, increasing comfort.*
- Reintroduce oral foods and fluids slowly, providing a soft, low-fiber diet with bulk-forming agents. *This allows con-*

tinued healing of the affected bowel while promoting soft, easily expelled stools.

Anxiety

The client with acute diverticulitis faces not only hospitalization, but also potential serious complications such as peritonitis and hemorrhage. Surgery and formation of a temporary colostomy may be necessary. Furthermore, episodes of acute diverticulitis are often recurrent, and the client may fear future problems.

- Assess and document level of anxiety. *Severe anxiety or panic states can interfere with the ability to respond to instructions and assist with care. Low to moderate anxiety levels enhance learning and compliance with prescribed interventions.*
- Demonstrate empathy and awareness of the perceived threat to health. *It is important to recognize and respect the client's feelings and perceptions as reality.*
- Attend to physical care needs. *This provides reassurance that these needs will be met and relieves concerns about them.*
- Spend as much time as possible with the client. *Presence of a caring nurse helps relieve fears of abandonment or that help will not be available if needed. It also enhances trust and provides opportunity for expression of fears or concerns.*
- Assess level of understanding about disease and condition. *This allows misperceptions that may contribute to anxiety to be corrected.*
- Encourage supportive family and friends to remain with the client as much as possible. *This provides a supportive environment for the client and also distracts from physical concerns.*
- Assist the client to identify and use appropriate coping mechanisms. *Coping mechanisms provide immediate relief of anxiety while the client adapts to the situation.*
- Involve the client and family (as appropriate) in care decisions. *This increases the client's sense of control over the situation.*

Using NANDA, NIC, and NOC

Chart 24–7 shows links between NANDA nursing diagnoses, NIC and NOC when caring for the client with diverticulitis.

Home Care

The client with diverticular disease is responsible for its day-to-day management. Discuss the following topics when preparing for home care.

- Prescribed high-fiber diet and the need to maintain the diet for life to reduce the incidence of complications, including ways to increase dietary fiber
- Complications of diverticular disease and its manifestations

Provide a referral to a dietitian for further teaching as indicated.
Prior to discharge of the client with acute diverticulitis, discuss the following:

- Food and fluid limitations, including recommendations for a low-residue diet during the initial period of healing
- Colostomy management (if a temporary colostomy has been created), including where to obtain supplies and dietary management
- Planned procedure to reanastomose the colon and revise the colostomy. Refer to community health care agencies as indicated.

CHART 24–7

NANDA, NIC, AND NOC LINKAGES

The Client with Diverticulitis

NURSING DIAGNOSES	NURSING INTERVENTIONS	NURSING OUTCOMES
• Constipation • Diarrhea • Deficient Knowledge • Pain • Risk for Deficient Fluid Volume	• Nutrition Management • Bowel Management • Diarrhea Management • Teaching: Prescribed Diet • Pain Management • Fluid Management	• Symptom Control • Bowel Elimination • Symptom Severity • Knowledge: Diet • Comfort Level • Fluid Balance

Note: Data from Nursing Outcomes Classification (NOC) by M. Johnson & M. Maas (Eds.), 1997, St. Louis: Mosby; Nursing Diagnoses: Definitions & Classification 2001–2002 by North American Nursing Diagnosis Association, 2001, Philadelphia: NANDA; Nursing Interventions Classification (NIC) by J.C. McCloskey & G. M. Bulechek (Eds.), 2000, St. Louis: Mosby. Reprinted by permission.

Nursing Care Plan
A Client with Diverticulitis

Roseline Ukoha is a 45-year-old married school teacher who has two children. For the past 2 days, she has experienced intermittent abdominal pain and bloating. The pain increased in severity over the past 9 to 10 hours, and she developed nausea, lower back pain, and discomfort radiating into the perineal region. Mrs. Ukoha reports having had no bowel movement for the past 2 days. The emergency department nurse, Jasmine Sarino, RN, completes her admission assessment.

ASSESSMENT

Mrs. Ukoha relates a 10-year history of chronic irritable bowel symptoms, including alternating constipation and diarrhea and intermittent abdominal cramping. She states that she thought these symptoms were due to the stress of teaching middle school, and that they never became severe enough to seek medical advice. When questioned about her diet, she calls it a typical American high-fat, fast-food diet, usually consisting of a sweet roll and coffee for breakfast, a hamburger or sandwich and soft drink for lunch, and a balanced dinner, usually including meat, a vegetable or salad, and potatoes or pasta, "except on pizza night!"

Physical assessment findings include T 101°F (38.3°C), P 92, R 24, and BP 118/70. Abdomen is slightly distended and tender to light palpation. Bowel sounds are diminished. Diagnostic tests include the following abnormal results: WBC 19,900/mm³ (normal 3500 to 11,000/mm³) with increased immature and mature neutrophils on differential; hemoglobin 12.8 g/dL (normal 13.3 to 17.7 g/dL); hematocrit, 37.1% (normal 40% to 52%). Abdominal X-ray films show slight to moderate distention of the large and small bowel with suggestion of possible early ileus. A small amount of free air is noted in the peritoneal cavity.

The diagnosis of probable diverticulitis with diverticular rupture is made, and Mrs. Ukoha is admitted to the medical unit for intravenous fluids, antibiotic therapy, and bowel rest.

DIAGNOSIS

- *Pain* related to inflamed bowel and possible peritonitis
- *Risk for deficient fluid volume* related to inflammation
- *Impaired tissue integrity: Gastrointestinal* related to perforated diverticulum
- *Deficient knowledge* related to disease process and dietary management

EXPECTED OUTCOMES

- Verbalize adequate pain relief.
- Experience no adverse effects of prescribed bed rest.
- Maintain adequate fluid balance while hospitalized, as demonstrated by balanced intake and output, stable weight, good skin turgor and mucous membrane moisture, and laboratory values within the normal range.
- Heal adequately without further evidence of peritonitis.
- Verbalize understanding of the recommended high-fiber diet and the need to increase physical activity and fluid intake to promote optimal bowel function at home.

PLANNING AND IMPLEMENTATION

- Assess comfort status frequently, providing analgesics as needed.
- Maintain intravenous infusion as prescribed.
- Measure intake and output; weigh daily.
- Provide mouth care every 2 to 4 hours until oral intake resumes, then every 4 hours until client assumes self-care.
- Measure temperature every 4 hours.
- Advance diet from clear liquids to low-residue diet when allowed.
- Provide instruction and dietary consultation for high-fiber diet.

EVALUATION

On discharge, Mrs. Ukoha is afebrile, and her abdomen is flat and only slightly tender to palpation. She is taking food and fluids well and has resumed a normal pattern of bowel elimination. She will continue oral antibiotic therapy for another 2 weeks at home. She verbalizes an understanding of the need to continue her low-residue diet for the next week, and maintain a high-fiber diet thereafter. She says she is glad her problem turned out to be diverticulosis instead of cancer as she had feared, and states that she can deal with this now that she knows how.

Critical Thinking in the Nursing Process

1. Why was Mrs. Ukoha hospitalized immediately and placed on intravenous fluids and antibiotics?
2. Mrs. Ukoha reports, "I had a small bowel movement of mucus. Is this normal, or is something wrong?" What would be your response?
3. How did Mrs. Ukoha's previous diet contribute to her diverticular disease and diverticulitis? Did the symptoms of irritable bowel syndrome also contribute? How?
4. Develop a teaching plan to instruct clients with diverticular disease about dietary recommendations.

See Evaluating Your Response in Appendix C.

ANORECTAL DISORDERS

Anorectal lesions include hemorrhoids, a normal condition common to all adults that may become enlarged and painful; anal fissure; anorectal fistulas; anorectal abscess; and pilonidal disease. Fecal incontinence also may be considered an anorectal disorder.

THE CLIENT WITH HEMORRHOIDS

The anus and anal canal contain two superficial venous plexuses with the hemorrhoidal veins. When pressure on these veins is increased or venous return impeded, they can develop *varices,* or varicosities, thus becoming weak and distended. This condition is commonly known as **hemorrhoids,** or piles. When asymptomatic, hemorrhoids are considered to be a normal condition found in all adults.

PATHOPHYSIOLOGY AND MANIFESTATIONS

Hemorrhoids develop when venous return from the anal canal is impaired. Straining to defecate in the sitting or squatting position increases venous pressure and is the most common cause of distended hemorrhoids. Pregnancy increases intra-abdominal pressure, raising venous pressure, and is a second important cause of hemorrhoids. Other factors that may contribute to symptomatic hemorrhoids include prolonged sitting, obesity, chronic constipation, and the low-fiber diet common to Western nations.

Hemorrhoids are classed as either internal or external. *Internal* hemorrhoids affect the venous plexus above the mucocutaneous junction of the anus (Figure 24–17 ■). Internal hemorrhoids rarely cause pain, usually presenting with bleeding. Bleeding from internal hemorrhoids is bright red and unmixed with the stool. It can vary in quantity from streaks on toilet tissue to enough to color the water in the toilet. Recur-

rent bleeding of internal hemorrhoids may be sufficient to cause anemia. Mucus discharge and a feeling of incomplete evacuation of stool also may be manifestations of internal hemorrhoids.

External hemorrhoids affect the inferior hemorrhoidal plexus below the mucocutaneous junction. Bleeding is rare with external hemorrhoids. Anal irritation, a feeling of pressure, and difficulty cleaning the anal region may be manifestations of external hemorrhoids.

As they enlarge, hemorrhoids may prolapse or protrude through the anus. Initially, prolapse occurs only with defecation and the hemorrhoids spontaneously regress back into the anal canal. Eventually, the client may need to manually replace internal hemorrhoids after defecation, or they may become permanently prolapsed and replacement not possible. Symptoms of permanently prolapsed hemorrhoids include mucus discharge and clothing soilage.

"Normal" hemorrhoids are not painful. Pain is associated with ulcerated or thrombosed hemorrhoids, and it can be severe. Prolapsed hemorrhoids may become strangulated as a result of congestion and edema, leading to thrombosis. Hemorrhoidal thrombosis causes extreme pain and may lead to infarction of skin and mucosa overlying the hemorrhoid. Internal hemorrhoids associated with portal hypertension in liver disease may bleed profusely if ruptured. (See Chapter 22 ∞ for further discussion of portal hypertension.)

A *thrombosed external hemorrhoid* is a thrombosis of the subcutaneous external hemorrhoidal veins of the anal canal, rather than a true hemorrhoid. It appears as a painful bluish hematoma beneath the skin and typically occurs following a sudden increase in venous pressure, for example, heavy lifting, coughing, or straining. Pain is significant at onset but gradually subsides. Spontaneous rupture with bleeding may occur. Thrombosed external hemorrhoids resolve spontaneously without intervention.

COLLABORATIVE CARE

Because hemorrhoids are a normal condition, management is conservative unless complications such as permanent prolapse or thrombosis occur.

Hemorrhoids are diagnosed by the client's history and by examination of the anorectal area. External hemorrhoids can be seen on visual inspection, especially if thrombosed. The client is asked to strain (Valsalva's maneuver) during the examination to detect prolapse. Internal hemorrhoids are usually not palpable or tender on digital examination of the rectum. *Anoscopic* examination is used to detect and evaluate internal hemorrhoids. For this exam, a speculum or endoscope is introduced into the anus to provide visual inspection of the tissues. Internal hemorrhoids are vascular structures that protrude into the lumen. Additional diagnostic examinations including testing of stool for occult blood and sigmoidoscopy are performed to rule

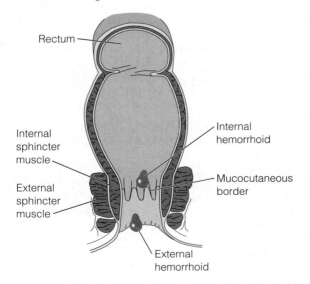

Figure 24–17 ■ The location of internal and external hemorrhoids.

out cancer of the colon or rectum, which may aggravate hemorrhoidal symptoms or produce similar manifestations. If liver disease with portal hypertension is suspected, liver function studies are ordered.

Hemorrhoids that are not permanently prolapsed or acutely thrombosed generally are treated conservatively. A high-fiber diet and increased water intake to increase stool bulk, improve its softness, and reduce straining is effective for most clients with internal or external hemorrhoids. Bulk-forming laxatives such as psyllium seed (Metamucil) or stool softeners such as docusate sodium (Colace) may be prescribed to improve constipation and reduce straining as well. Suppositories and local ointments such as Preparation H or Nupercaine have an anesthetic and astringent effect, reducing discomfort and irritation of surrounding tissues. They have little or no effect on the hemorrhoid itself. Warm sitz baths, bed rest, and local astringent compresses may be recommended to reduce the swelling of edematous prolapsed hemorrhoids after digital reduction.

Hemorrhoids that are permanently prolapsed, are thrombosed, or produce significant symptoms may be treated more aggressively. *Sclerotherapy* involves injecting a chemical irritant into tissues surrounding the hemorrhoid to induce inflammation and eventual fibrosis and scarring. It is used to treat recurrent bleeding and early prolapse of internal hemorrhoids. The treatment produces minimal pain. Enlarged or prolapsing hemorrhoids also may be treated with rubber band ligation. A rubber band is placed snugly around the hemorrhoidal plexus and surrounding mucosa, causing the tissue to necrose and slough within 7 to 10 days. Treatment is limited to one hemorrhoidal complex at a time, so repeat treatments may be necessary. Pain should be minimal if the band is placed appropriately; persistent pain following band ligation may signal an infection. Bleeding can occur as the hemorrhoid sloughs. Other procedures used to treat hemorrhoids include cryosurgery, in which hemorrhoids are necrosed by freezing with a cryoprobe, infrared photocoagulation, or electrocoagulation.

Clients with chronic symptoms, permanent prolapse, chronic bleeding and anemia, or painful thrombosed hemorrhoids may be treated surgically with a *hemorrhoidectomy*. In this procedure, hemorrhoids are surgically excised, leaving normal skin and surrounding tissues. This procedure may use conventional techniques or a laser to remove both internal and external hemorrhoids. Few complications are associated with hemorrhoidectomy.

NURSING CARE

Primary prevention of symptomatic hemorrhoids involves education of clients of all ages. Stress the importance of maintaining an adequate intake of dietary fiber, a liberal fluid intake, and regular exercise to maintain stool bulk, softness, and regularity. Discuss the need to respond to the urge to defecate rather than postponing defecation. Teach appropriate constipation management, including the use of bulk-forming laxatives.

BOX 24–4 ■ Perianal Postoperative Care

ASSESSMENT
- Monitor vital signs every 4 hours for 24 hours.
- Inspect rectal dressing every 2 to 3 hours for 24 hours.
- Monitor urinary output.

PAIN CONTROL
- Assist to position of comfort, usually side-lying.
- Provide analgesics as prescribed.
- Keep fresh ice packs over the rectal dressing as ordered.
- Assist with sitz bath 3 to 4 times per day.
- Provide a flotation pad for use when sitting.

ELIMINATION
- Give stool softeners as prescribed.
- Give an analgesic before the first postoperative bowel movement if possible.
- When tolerated, encourage fluid intake of at least 2000 mL per day.

CLIENT AND FAMILY TEACHING
- Take sitz bath after each bowel movement for 1 to 2 weeks after surgery.
- Drink at least 2 quarts of fluid per day.
- Eat adequate dietary fiber, and exercise moderately.
- Take stool softeners as prescribed.
- Report to the physician the following symptoms: rectal bleeding, continued pain on defecation, fever greater than 101°F (38.3°C), purulent rectal drainage.

Most clients with hemorrhoids are treated in community settings where the primary nursing focus is educational. Discuss the appropriate use of over-the-counter preparations for the relief of minor hemorrhoidal symptoms. If necessary, teach clients how to reduce prolapsed hemorrhoids digitally.

Teach manifestations of possible hemorrhoidal complications, such as chronic bleeding, prolapse, and thrombosis. Stress the need to seek medical evaluation if symptoms persist. Discuss the link between manifestations of hemorrhoids and colorectal cancer, and urge the client to seek medical intervention for persistent, unresolved, or progressive symptoms.

When a hemorrhoidectomy is performed, the client requires more direct nursing intervention. Postoperative care of the client with perianal surgery is outlined in Box 24–4. Anal packing may be in place for the first 24 hours following the procedure. When removed, observe the client closely for bleeding. Pain is a common postoperative problem. Although the operative procedure is minor, postoperative discomfort can be significant because the anal region is richly innervated and muscle spasms may occur. In addition to systemic analgesics, sitz baths usually are ordered. These not only help promote relaxation and reduce discomfort but also clean the anal area. Use of a rubber ring or donut device minimizes pressure on the surgical site while the client sits in the bath.

The client may remain hospitalized until after the first postoperative bowel movement. Stool softeners, adequate fluids, and analgesia before defecation can reduce anxiety and discomfort. Adequate cleaning following defecation, usually with a sitz bath, is vital.

Whether caring for a client with hemorrhoids or a hemorrhoidectomy, consider the following nursing diagnoses.

- *Pain* related to inflamed anal tissues
- *Constipation* related to dietary habits and/or delay of defecation
- *Risk for infection* related to disruption of anal tissue

THE CLIENT WITH AN ANORECTAL LESION

Unlike the rectum, which is relatively insensitive to pain, the anal canal is richly supplied with sensory nerves and highly sensitive to painful stimuli. Lesions of the anorectal area may cause significant pain, particularly with defecation. Infection is a potential complication of anorectal lesions because of contamination by fecal bacteria. The superior boundary of the anal canal (the anorectal juncture or pectinate line) contains 8 to 12 anal crypts where anorectal abscesses or fistulas can form.

Anal Fissure

Anal fissures or ulcers occur when the epithelium of the anal canal over the internal sphincter becomes denuded or abraded. Irritating diarrheal stools and tightening of the anal canal with increased sphincter tension are frequent causes of anal fissures. Other factors that may contribute to their development include childbirth trauma, habitual cathartic use, laceration by a foreign body, and anal intercourse. Chronic inflammation and infection of surrounding tissues accompanies an anal fissure.

Clients with anal fissures typically have periods of exacerbation and remission. Because they occur below the mucocutaneous line, anal fissures are painful. The pain occurs with defecation and may be described as tearing, burning, or cutting. Bright red bleeding is noted with a bowel movement as well. Bleeding is typically minor and noted on toilet tissue. Because of fear of defecation, the client may develop constipation, which further disrupts normal bowel habits and aggravates symptoms.

The diagnosis of anal fissure is made on gentle digital examination of the anal canal and anoscopy using a small anoscope. Treatment is usually conservative, involving dietary changes to increase fiber intake and stool bulk, increased fluid intake and bulk-forming laxatives. A topical agent such as hydrocortisone cream may be prescribed. Surgical intervention with an internal sphincterotomy, an incision into the internal sphincter to increase its diameter, is considered when the fissure does not heal with medical intervention.

Anorectal Abscess

Invasion of the pararectal spaces by pathogenic bacteria can lead to an *anorectal abscess.* Commonly caused by infection that extends from the anal crypt into a pararectal space, the abscess may appear small but often contains a large amount of pus. Multiple pathogens may be present, including *Escherichia coli, Proteus,* streptococci, and staphylococci. Other factors

that may contribute to the development of an anorectal abscess include infection of a hair follicle, sebaceous gland, or sweat gland; and abrasions, fissures, or anal trauma. The incidence of anorectal abscess is higher in men.

Pain is the primary manifestation of an anorectal abscess. Sitting or walking may aggravate the pain, but it is unrelated to defecation. External swelling, redness, heat, and tenderness are apparent on examination. With a deeper abscess, swelling may not be visible, but the abscess is palpable on digital examination.

If the abscess either does not drain spontaneously or is not drained surgically, adjacent anatomic spaces will be affected. Systemic sepsis is also a potential complication.

Incision and drainage (I & D) is the treatment of choice for an anorectal abscess because it rarely resolves with antibiotic therapy alone. This treatment often leads to a persistent fistula, which is surgically closed after the infection has cleared.

Anorectal Fistula

A fistula is a tunnel or tubelike tract with openings at each end. *Anorectal fistulas* have one opening in the anal canal with the other usually found in perianal skin. Most occur spontaneously or as a result of anorectal abscess drainage. Crohn's disease is a predisposing factor to fistula development as well.

The primary manifestation of an anorectal fistula is intermittent or constant drainage or discharge, which may be purulent. This may be accompanied by local itching, tenderness, and pain associated with defecation.

Digital and anoscopic examination with gentle probing of the fistula tract are used to establish the diagnosis. Although some fistulas may heal spontaneously, the treatment of choice is a fistulotomy. The primary opening of the fistula is removed, and the tract is opened to allow it to heal by secondary intention, from the inside outward. If the sphincter is involved, a two-stage operation may be done to preserve the muscle and prevent fecal incontinence.

Pilonidal Disease

The client with *pilonidal disease* has an acute abscess or chronic draining sinus in the sacrococcygeal area. Underlying the abscess or sinus is a cyst with granulation tissue, fibrosis, and, often, hair tufts. This disease usually affects young hirsute (hairy) males and is probably due to hair entrapment in deep tissues of the sacrococcygeal area. Some researchers, however, believe that it is a congenital disorder.

The lesion of pilonidal disease is generally asymptomatic unless it becomes acutely infected. Manifestations of acute inflammation accompany infection, including pain, tenderness, redness, heat, and swelling of the affected area. Purulent discharge may be noted from one or more sinuses or openings in the midline.

The preferred treatment option for pilonidal disease is incision and drainage. The sinus tract and underlying cyst are excised and closed by either primary- or secondary-intention healing. The client may be instructed to remove hair from the area routinely by shaving or using a depilatory to prevent further hair entrapment and recurrence of the problem.

NURSING CARE

Clients with anorectal disorders are often treated in the community, and the primary nursing responsibility is education. Teach the importance of maintaining a high-fiber diet and liberal fluid intake to increase stool bulk and softness and thereby decrease discomfort with defecation. Stress the importance of responding to the urge to defecate to prevent constipation.

Following surgical treatment of any of these disorders, teach the client to keep the perianal region clean and dry. If a dressing is in place, instruct to avoid soiling it with urine or feces during elimination. Following removal of the dressing, teach to clean the area gently with soap and water following a bowel movement. Discuss the use of sitz baths for cleaning and comfort. Suggest taking an analgesic if necessary prior to defecation, but caution that some analgesics may promote constipation. Teach signs and symptoms of infection or other possible complications to report to the physician. If an antibiotic has been prescribed, provide written and verbal instructions about its use, its desired and possible adverse effects, and their management.

 EXPLORE MediaLink

NCLEX review questions, case studies, care plan activities, MediaLink applications, and other interactive resources for this chapter can be found on the Companion Website at www.prenhall.com/lemone.

Click on Chapter 24 to select the activities for this chapter. For animations, video clips, more NCLEX review questions, and an audio glossary, access the Student CD-ROM accompanying this textbook.

TEST YOURSELF

1. A client presents at the urgent care clinic with complaints of diarrhea for the past week. The nurse should first:

   a. Advise the client to abstain from all food intake until the diarrhea subsides
   b. Ask the client to describe the number and character of daily stools
   c. Question the client about possible exposure to an enterotoxin or protozoal infection
   d. Recommend an over-the-counter antidiarrheal preparation such as Pepto-Bismol

2. The nurse caring for a client admitted with possible appendicitis appropriately plans which of the following?

   a. Initiate bowel preparation for a barium enema
   b. Restrict intake to clear liquids
   c. Prepare for possible immediate appendectomy
   d. Insert saline lock for intravenous antibiotic therapy

3. When teaching a client with inflammatory bowel disease about prescribed sulfasalazine, the nurse instructs the client to:

   a. Use a sunscreen while taking the drug
   b. Take the drug on an empty stomach
   c. Limit fluid intake to 1500 mL per day or less
   d. Take vitamin C while on this drug

4. A client reports frequent large, fatty, foul-smelling stools. The nurse recognizes this as:

   a. Hematochezia, a manifestation of GI bleeding
   b. Characteristic of inflammatory bowel disease
   c. A common early manifestation of colorectal cancer
   d. Steatorrhea, a manifestation of malabsorption

5. A client tells the nurse that both his father and grandfather died of colon cancer, and he is worried that he is going to die from "the same horrible disease." Which of the following does the nurse include in her recommendations?

   a. There is no genetic link seen in colon cancer, so his risk is equal to that of people with no family history of the disease
   b. He should plan for annual digital rectal exams and periodic colonoscopy (every 3 to 5 years) for early identification of possible tumors
   c. He should have annual CEA levels drawn to screen for early tumor development
   d. It is imperative that he change his diet immediately, significantly increasing his intake of dietary fiber

See Test Yourself answers in Appendix C.

BIBLIOGRAPHY

Ackley, B.J., & Ladwig, G. B. (2002). *Nursing diagnosis handbook: A guide to planning care* (5th ed.). St. Louis: Mosby.

American Cancer Society. (2002). Cancer reference information: What are the key statistics for colon and rectum cancer? Available http://www.cancer.org

Bailey, C. (2001). Focus. Older patients' experiences of pre-treatment discussions: An analysis of qualitative data from a study of colorectal cancer. *NT Research, 6*(4), 736–746.

Baker, D. (2001). Current surgical management of colorectal cancer. *Nursing Clinics of North America, 36*(3), 579–592.

Ball, E. M. (2000). Ostomy guide, part two. A teaching guide for continent ileostomy. *RN, 63*(12), 35–36, 38, 40.

Bliss, D. Z., Jung, H., Savik, K., Lowry, A., LeMoine, M., Jensen, L., Werner, C., & Schaffer, K. (2001). Supplementation with dietary fiber improves fecal incontinence. *Nursing Research, 50*(4), 203–213.

Braunwald, E., Fauci, A. S., Kasper, D. L., Hauser, S. L., Longo, D. L., & Jameson, J. L. (2001). *Harrison's principles of internal medicine* (15th ed.). New York: McGraw-Hill.

Breeze, J. (2001). Colorectal cancer. *Nursing Times, 97*(11), 39–41.

Bullock, B. A., & Henze, R. L. (2000). *Focus on pathophysiology.* Philadelphia: Lippincott.

Burger, E. T. (2001). Preparing adult patients for international travel. *Nurse Practitioner: American Journal of Primary Health Care, 26*(5), 13–15, 19–25.

Cox, J. A., Rogers, M. A., & Cox, S. D. (2001). Treating benign colon disorders using laparoscopic colectomy. *AORN Journal, 73*(2), 375, 377–380, 382+.

Deglin, J. H., & Vallerand, A. H. (2001). *Davis's drug guide for nurses* (7th ed.). Philadelphia: F.A. Davis.

Dest, V. M. (2000). Oncology today: New horizons. Colorectal cancer. *RN, 63*(3), 53–59.

Erwin-Toth, P. (2001). Caring for a stoma is more than skin deep. *Nursing, 31*(5), 36–40.

Fontaine, K. L. (2000). *Healing practices: Alternative therapies for nursing.* Upper Saddle River, NJ: Prentice Hall Health.

Gallo, J. J., Busby-Whitehead, J., Rabins, P. V., Silliman, R. A., & Murphy, J. B. (Eds.). (1999). *Reichel's care of the elderly: Clinical aspects of aging* (5th ed.). Philadelphia: Lippincott Williams & Wilkins.

Gauf, C. L. (2000). Diagnosing appendicitis across the life span. *Journal of the American Academy of Nurse Practitioners, 12*(4), 129–133.

Heuschkel, R., Afzal, N., Wuerth, A., Zurakowski, D., Leichtner, A., Kemper, K., & Tolia, V. (2002). Complementary medicine use in children and young adults with inflammatory bowel disease. *American Journal of Gastroenterology, 97*(2), 382–388.

Jenks, J. M., Morin, K. H., & Tomaselli, N. (1997). The influence of ostomy surgery on body image in patients with cancer. *Applied Nursing Research, 10*(4), 174–180.

Joachim, G. (2000). Responses of people with inflammatory bowel disease to foods consumed. *Gastroenterology Nursing, 23*(4), 160–167.

Johnson, M., Bulechek, G., Dochterman, J. M., Maas, M., & Moorhead, S. (2001). *Nursing diagnoses, outcomes, & interventions.* St. Louis: Mosby.

Johnson, M., Maas, M., & Moorhead, S. (Eds.). (2000). *Nursing outcomes classification (NOC)* (2nd ed.). St. Louis: Mosby.

Kinney, A. Y., Choi, Y., DeVellis, B., Millikan, R., Kobetz, E., & Sandler, R. S. (2000). Attitudes toward genetic testing in patients with colorectal cancer. *Cancer Practice: A Multidisciplinary Journal of Cancer Care, 8*(4), 178–186.

Kuhn, M. A. (1999). *Complementary therapies for health care providers.* Philadelphia: Lippincott.

Langmead, L., Dawson, C., Hawkins, C., Banna, N., Loo, S., & Rampton, D. S. (2002). Antioxidant effects of herbal therapies used by patients with inflammatory bowel disease: An in vitro study. *Alimentary Pharmacologic Therapy, 16*(2), 197–205.

Lehne, R. A. (2001). *Pharmacology for nursing care* (4th ed.). Philadelphia: Saunders.

Levine, C. D. (1999). Toxic megacolon: Diagnosis and treatment challenges. *AACN Clinical Issues: Advanced Practice in Acute and Critical Care, 10*(4), 492–499.

Lord, L. M., Schaffner, R., DeCross, A. J., & Sax, H. C. (2000). Management of the patient with short bowel syndrome. *AACN Clinical Issues: Advanced Practice in Acute and Critical Care, 11*(4), 604–618.

Malarkey, L.M., & McMorrow, M.E. (2000). *Nurse's manual of laboratory tests and diagnostic procedures* (2nd ed.). Philadelphia: Saunders.

Mason, I. (2001). Inflammatory bowel disease. *Nursing Times, 97*(9), 33–35.

McCloskey, J. C., & Bulechek, G. M. (Eds.) (2000). *Nursing interventions classification (NIC)* (3rd ed.). St. Louis: Mosby.

McConnell, E. A. (2001). Appendicitis: What a pain! *Nursing, 31*(8): 32hn1–3.

_____. (2001). What's behind intestinal obstruction? *Nursing, 31*(10), 58–63.

Meeker, M. H., & Rothrock, J. C. (1999). *Alexander's care of the patient in surgery* (11th ed.). St. Louis: Mosby.

North American Nursing Diagnosis Association. (2001). *NANDA nursing diagnoses: Definitions & classification 2001–2002.* Philadelphia: NANDA.

Olson, S. J., & Zawacki, K. (2000). Hereditary colorectal cancer. *Nursing Clinics of North America, 35*(3), 671–685.

Pontieri-Lewis, V. (2000). Colorectal cancer: Prevention and screening. *MEDSURG Nursing, 9*(1), 9–15, 20.

Porth, C. M. (2002). *Pathophysiology: Concepts of altered health states* (6th ed.). Philadelphia: Lippincott.

Rankin-Box, D. (2000). An alternative approach to bowel disorders. *Nursing Times, 96*(19), NT-plus 24, 26.

Rayhorn, N. (1999). Understanding inflammatory bowel disease. *Nursing, 29*(12), 57–61.

Sercombe, J. (2000). Inflammatory bowel disease and smoking. *Professional Nurse, 15*(7), 439–442.

_____. (2001). Surgical therapy for inflammatory bowel disease. *Nursing Times, 97*(10), 34–36.

Shepherd, M. (2000). Treating diarrhea and constipation. *Nursing Times, 96*(6), NTplus 15–16.

Tierney, L. M., McPhee, S. J., & Papadakis, M. A. (2001). *Current medical diagnosis & treatment* (40th ed.). New York: Lange Medical Books/McGraw-Hill.

Verhoef, M. J., Rapchuk, I., Liew, T., Weir, V., & Hilsden, R. J. (2002). Complementary practitioners' views of treatment for inflammatory bowel disease. *Canadian Journal of Gastroenterology, 16*(2), 95–100.

Whitney, E. N., & Rolfes, S. R. (2002). *Understanding nutrition* (9th ed.). Belmont, CA: Wadsworth.

Wilkinson, J. M. (2000). *Nursing diagnosis handbook with NIC interventions and NOC outcomes* (7th ed.). Upper Saddle River, NJ: Prentice Hall Health.

Wood, M. C., & Ryan, C. T. (2000). Patient resources. Resources on colorectal cancer for patients. *Cancer Practice: A Multidisciplinary Journal of Cancer Care, 8*(6), 308–310.

Young, M. (2000). Caring for patients with coloanal reservoirs for rectal cancer. *MEDSURG Nursing, 9*(4), 193–197.

RESPONSES TO ALTERED URINARY ELIMINATION

Assessing Clients with Urinary System Disorders

MediaLink

www.prenhall.com/lemone
Additional resources for this chapter can be found on the Student CD-ROM accompanying this textbook, and on the Companion Website at www.prenhall.com/lemone. Click on Chapter 25 to select the activities for this chapter.

CD-ROM
- Audio Glossary
- NCLEX Review

Animations
- Urinary System
- Renal Function

Companion Website
- More NCLEX Review
- Functional Health Pattern Assessment
- Case Study
    Renal Calculi
- MediaLink Application
    Kidney Function

LEARNING OUTCOMES

After completing this chapter, you will be able to:

- Review the anatomy and physiology of the urinary system.

- Explain the role of the urinary system in maintaining homeostasis.

- Identify specific topics for consideration during a health history interview of the client with health problems involving the urinary system.

- Describe techniques for assessing the integrity and function of the urinary system.

- Identify abnormal findings that may indicate impairment of the urinary system.

The functions of the renal system are to regulate body fluids, to filter metabolic wastes from the bloodstream, to reabsorb needed substances and water into the bloodstream, and to eliminate metabolic wastes and water as urine. Any alteration in the structure or function of the renal system affects the whole body. In turn, healthy urinary system function depends on the health of other body systems, especially the circulatory, endocrine, and nervous systems.

REVIEW OF ANATOMY AND PHYSIOLOGY

The organs of the urinary system are the paired kidneys, the paired ureters, the urinary bladder, and the urethra (Figure 25–1 ■). Each structure is essential to the total functioning of the urinary system.

The Kidneys

The two kidneys are located outside the peritoneal cavity and on either side of the vertebral column at the levels of T12 through L3. These highly vascular, bean-shaped organs are approximately 4.5 inches (11.4 cm) long and 2.5 inches (6.4 cm) wide. The lateral surface of the kidney is convex; the medial

surface is concave and forms a vertical cleft, the hilum. The ureter, renal artery, renal vein, lymphatic vessels, and nerves enter or exit the kidney at the level of the hilum.

The kidney is supported by three layers of connective tissue: the outer renal fascia, the middle adipose capsule, and the inner renal capsule. The renal fascia, made up of dense connective tissue, surrounds the kidney (and the adrenal gland, a discrete organ that sits on top of each kidney) and anchors it to surrounding structures. The middle adipose capsule is a fatty mass that holds the kidney in place and also cushions it against trauma. The inner renal capsule provides a barrier against infection and helps protect the kidney from trauma.

The functions of the kidney are to:

- Balance solute and water transport.
- Excrete metabolic waste products.
- Conserve nutrients.
- Regulate acid-base balance.
- Secrete hormones to help regulate blood pressure, erythrocyte production, and calcium metabolism.
- Form urine.

Figure 25–1 ■ The urinary system. *A,* Anterior view of the urinary system in a female. *B,* The kidneys are shown in relation to the vertebrae and ribs.

Figure 25–2 ■ Internal anatomy of the kidney.

Capsule

Renal cortex

Renal medulla (pyramid)

Major calyx

Renal column

Minor calyx

Renal artery

Renal vein

Renal pelvis

Ureter

Internally, each kidney has three distinct regions: the cortex, medulla, and pelvis. The outer region, or renal cortex, is light in color and has a granular appearance (Figure 25–2 ■). This region of the kidney contains the glomeruli, small clusters of capillaries. The glomeruli bring blood to and carry waste products from the nephrons, the functional units of the kidney.

The renal medulla, just below the cortex, contains cone-shaped tissue masses called renal pyramids, formed almost entirely of bundles of collecting tubules. Areas of lighter-colored tissue called renal columns are actually extensions of the cortex and serve to separate the pyramids. The collecting tubules that make up the pyramids channel urine into the innermost region, the renal pelvis.

The renal pelvis is continuous with the ureter as it leaves the hilum. Branches of the pelvis known as the major and minor calyces extend toward the medulla and serve to collect urine and empty it into the pelvis. From the pelvis, urine is channeled through the ureter and into the bladder for storage. The walls of the calyces, the renal pelvis, and the ureter contain smooth muscle that moves urine along by peristalsis.

Each kidney contains approximately 1 million nephrons, which process the blood to make urine (Figure 25–3 ■). Each nephron contains a tuft of capillaries called the glomerulus, which is completely surrounded by the glomerular capsule (or Bowman's space). Together, the glomerulus and its surrounding capsule are called the renal corpuscle. The endothelium of the glomerulus allows capillaries to be extremely porous. Thus, large amounts of solute-rich fluid pass from the capillaries into the capsule. This fluid, called the filtrate, is the raw material of urine. Filtrate leaves the capsule and is channeled into the proximal convoluted tubule (PCT) of the nephron. Microvilli on the tubular cells increase the surface area for reabsorption of substances from the filtrate into plasma in the peritubular capillaries. Substances moved by active transport include glucose,

sodium, potassium, amino acids, proteins, and vitamins. About 70% of the water in the filtrate, as well as chloride and bicarbonate, are reabsorbed by passive transport. The filtrate then moves into the U-shaped loop of Henle and is concentrated. The descending limb of the U is relatively thin and freely per-

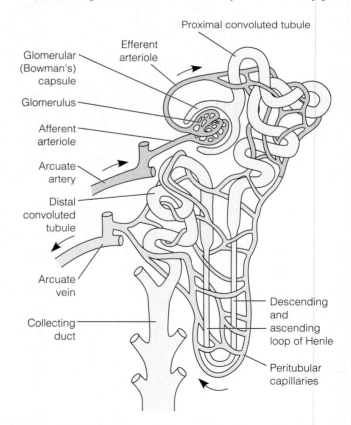

Proximal convoluted tubule

Efferent arteriole

Glomerular (Bowman's) capsule

Glomerulus

Afferent arteriole

Arcuate artery

Distal convoluted tubule

Arcuate vein

Collecting duct

Descending and ascending loop of Henle

Peritubular capillaries

Figure 25–3 ■ The structure of a nephron, showing the glomerulus within the glomerular capsule.

meable to water, whereas the ascending segment is thick and thereby less permeable. The distal convoluted tubule (DCT) receives filtrate from the loop of Henle. Although this segment is structurally similar to the PCT, it lacks microvilli and is more involved with secreting solutes into the filtrate than in reabsorbing substances from it. The collecting duct receives the newly formed urine from many nephrons and channels urine through the minor and major calyces of the renal pelvis and into the ureter.

The Ureters

The ureters are bilateral tubes approximately 10 to 12 inches (25 to 30 cm) long. They transport urine from the kidney to the bladder through peristaltic waves originating in the renal pelvis. The wall of the ureter has three layers: an inner epithelial mucosa, a middle layer of smooth muscle, and an outer layer of fibrous connective tissue.

The Urinary Bladder

The urinary bladder is posterior to the symphysis pubis and serves as a storage site for urine. In males, the bladder lies immediately in front of the rectum; in females, the bladder lies next to the vagina and the uterus. Openings for the ureters and the urethra are inside the bladder: the trigone is the smooth triangular portion of the base of the bladder outlined by these three openings (Figure 25–4 ■).

The layers of the bladder wall (from internal to external) are the epithelial mucosa lining the inside, the connective tissue submucosa, the smooth muscle layer, and the fibrous outer layer. The muscle layer, called the detrusor muscle, consists of fibers arranged in inner and outer longitudinal layers and in a middle circular layer. This arrangement allows the bladder to expand or contract according to the amount of urine it holds.

The size of the bladder varies with the amount of urine it contains. In healthy adults, the bladder holds about 300 to 500 mL of urine before internal pressure rises and signals the need to empty the bladder through **micturition** (also called *urination* or voiding). However, the bladder can hold more than twice that amount if necessary. The bladder has an internal urethral sphincter that relaxes in response to a full bladder and signals the need to urinate. A second external urethral sphincter is formed by skeletal muscle and is under voluntary control.

The Urethra

The urethra is a thin-walled muscular tube that channels urine to the outside of the body. It extends from the base of the bladder to the external urinary meatus. In females, the urethra is approximately 1.5 inches (3 to 5 cm) long, and the urinary meatus is anterior to the vaginal orifice. In males, the urethra is approximately 8 inches (20 cm) long and serves as a channel for semen as well as urine. The prostate gland encircles the urethra at the base of the bladder in males. The male urinary meatus is located at the end of the glans penis.

FORMATION OF URINE

The complex structures of the kidneys process about 180 L (47 gal) of blood-derived fluid each day. Of this amount, only 1% is excreted as urine; the rest is returned to the circulation. (The normal characteristics of urine on laboratory analysis are listed in Table 25–1.) Urine formation is accomplished entirely by the nephron through three processes: glomerular filtration, tubular reabsorption, and tubular secretion (Figure 25–5 ■).

Glomerular Filtration

Glomerular filtration is a passive, nonselective process in which hydrostatic pressure forces fluid and solutes through a membrane. The amount of fluid filtered from the blood into the capsule per minute is called the **glomerular filtration rate (GFR)**. Three factors influence this rate: the total surface area available for filtration, the permeability of the filtration membrane, and the net filtration pressure.

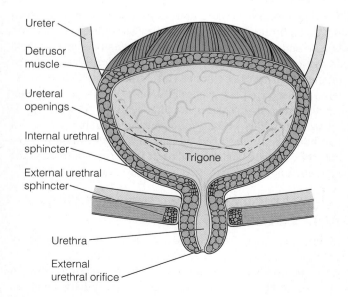

Figure 25–4 ■ Internal view of the urinary bladder and trigone.

TABLE 25–1	Characteristics of Normal Urine
Color	Pale to deep yellow, clear
Odor	Aromatic
Specific gravity	1.001–1.030
pH	4.5–8.0
Protein	Negative to trace
Glucose	Negative
Ketones	Negative
WBCs	0–5/high power field (hpf)
RBCs	0–5/hpf
Casts	Negative to occasional

MediaLink | URINARY SYSTEM ANIMATION

Key

A → Filtration

B → Reabsorption

C → Secretion

Interlobular arteries

Afferent arterioles

Glomerular capillaries

Efferent arterioles

Glomerular capsule

Rest of renal tubule

Peritubular capillaries

To interlobular veins

Urine

A

B

C

Figure 25–5 ■ Schematic view of the three major mechanisms by which the kidneys adjust to the composition of plasma: *A*, glomerular filtration; *B*, tubular reabsorption; and *C*, tubular secretion.

The glomerulus is a far more efficient filter than most capillary beds, because the filtration membrane of the glomerulus is much more permeable to water and solutes than are other capillary membranes. In addition, the glomerular blood pressure is much higher, resulting in higher net filtration pressure.

Net filtration pressure is responsible for the formation of filtrate and is determined by two forces: hydrostatic pressure ("push") and osmotic pressure ("pull"). The glomerular hydrostatic pressure pushes water and solutes across the membrane. This pressure is opposed by the osmotic pressure in the glomerulus (primarily the colloid osmotic pressure of plasma proteins in the glomerular blood) and the capsular hydrostatic pressure exerted by fluids within the glomerular capsule. The difference between these forces determines the net filtration pressure, which is directly proportional to the GFR.

The normal GFR in both kidneys is 120 to 125 mL/min in adults. This rate is held constant under normal conditions by intrinsic controls (or renal autoregulation). The myogenic mechanism, which responds to pressure changes in the renal blood vessels, controls the diameter of the afferent arterioles, thereby achieving autoregulation. An increase in systemic blood pressure causes the renal vessels to constrict, whereas a decline in blood pressure causes the afferent arterioles to dilate. These changes adjust the glomerular hydrostatic pressure and, indirectly, maintain the glomerular filtration rate.

Another intrinsic control of the GFR is the result of the **renin-angiotensin mechanism** at work in the kidneys. Special cells known as the juxtaglomerular apparatus are located in the distal tubules and respond to slow filtrate flow by releasing chemicals that cause intense vasodilation of the afferent arterioles. Conversely, an increase in the flow of filtrate promotes vasoconstriction, decreasing the GFR. A drop in systemic blood pressure often triggers the juxtaglomerular cells to release renin. Renin acts on a plasma globulin, angiotensinogen, to release angiotensin I, which is in turn converted to angiotensin II. As a vasoconstrictor, angiotensin II activates vascular smooth muscle throughout the body, causing systemic blood pressure to rise. Thus, the renin-angiotensin mechanism is a factor in renal autoregulation, even though its main purpose is the control of systemic blood pressure.

Glomerular filtration is also under an extrinsic control mechanism through the sympathetic nervous system. During periods of extreme stress or emergency, sympathetic nervous system stimulation causes strong constriction of the afferent arterioles and inhibits filtrate formation. The sympathetic nervous system also stimulates the juxtaglomerular cells to release renin, increasing systemic blood pressure.

Tubular Reabsorption

Tubular reabsorption is a transepithelial process that begins as the filtrate enters the proximal tubules. In healthy kidneys, virtually all organic nutrients such as glucose and amino acids are reabsorbed. However, the tubules constantly regulate and adjust the rate and degree of water and ion reabsorption in response to hormonal signals. Reabsorption may be active or passive. Substances reclaimed through active tubular reabsorption are usually moving against electrical and/or chemical gradients. These substances, including glucose, amino acids, lactate, vitamins, and most ions, require an ATP-dependent carrier to be transported into the interstitial space. In passive tubular reabsorption, which includes diffusion and osmosis, substances move along their gradient without expenditure of energy.

Tubular Secretion

The final process in urine formation is tubular secretion, which is essentially reabsorption in reverse. Substances such as hydrogen and potassium ions, creatinine, ammonia, and organic acids move from the blood of the peritubular capillaries into the tubules themselves as filtrate. Thus, urine consists of both filtered and secreted substances. Tubular secretion is important for disposing of substances not already in the filtrate, such as medications. This process eliminates undesirable substances that have been reabsorbed by passive processes and rids the body of excessive potassium ions. It is also a vital force in the regulation of blood pH.

MAINTAINING NORMAL COMPOSITION AND VOLUME OF URINE

Maintaining the normal composition and volume of urine involves a countercurrent exchange system. In this system, fluid flows in opposite directions through the parallel tubes of the loop of Henle and the vasa recta, tiny capillaries that run along the loop of Henle. Fluid is exchanged across these parallel membranes in response to a concentration gradient (Figure 25–6 ■). When the filtrate enters the proximal convoluted

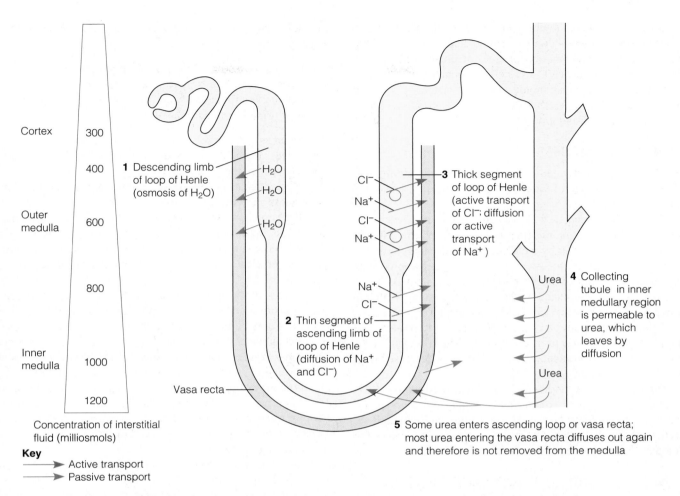

Figure 25–6 ■ The countercurrent exchange system, responsible for establishing and maintaining an osmotic gradient necessary to the composition, volume, and pH of urine.

tubule, its osmolality (at 300 mOsm/kg) is essentially the same as that of the plasma and the interstitial fluid of the renal cortex. Note the following steps in the process.

1. The descending loop of Henle is highly permeable to water and allows chloride and sodium to enter the loop through diffusion. The hyperosmotic interstitium causes water to move out of the descending loop, so that the remaining filtrate becomes increasingly concentrated.
2. The lumen of the ascending loop of Henle is impermeable to water but allows chloride and sodium to move out into the interstitium of the medulla. As a result, the filtrate in the ascending loop becomes hypo-osmotic, and the medullary interstitium becomes hyperosmotic.
3. As the filtrate progresses through the ascending limb of the loop of Henle and enters the distal convoluted tubule, sodium and chloride are removed and water is retained. Thus, the filtrate becomes more dilute.
4. As the filtrate passes through the deep medullary regions, urea (an end product of protein metabolism and, along with water, the main constituent of urine) begins to diffuse out from the collecting tubules into the interstitial space and establishes a concentration gradient to facilitate water movement.

5. Some urea enters the ascending loop of Henle. Urea entering the vasa recta typically diffuses out again.

The dilution or concentration of urine is largely determined by the action of antidiuretic hormone (ADH), which is secreted by the posterior pituitary gland. ADH causes the pores of the collecting tubules to enlarge, so that increased amounts of water move into the interstitial space. As the end result, water is reabsorbed and urine is more highly concentrated. When ADH is not secreted, the filtrate passes through the system without further water reabsorption, so that the urine is more dilute.

Urine is composed, by volume, of about 95% water and 5% solutes. The largest component of urine by weight is urea. Other solutes normally excreted in the urine include sodium, potassium, phosphate, sulfate, creatinine, uric acid, calcium, magnesium, and bicarbonate.

CLEARANCE OF WASTE PRODUCTS

The kidneys excrete water-soluble waste products and other chemicals or substances from the body. This process is called renal plasma clearance, which refers to the ability of the kidneys to clear (cleanse) a given amount of plasma of a particular substance in a given time (usually 1 minute). The kidneys clear 25 to 30 g of urea (a nitrogenous waste product formed in the liver from the breakdown of amino acids) each day. They also clear creatinine (an end product of creatine phosphate, found in skeletal muscle), uric acid (a metabolite of nucleic acid metabolism), and ammonia as well as bacterial toxins and water-soluble drugs. Tests of renal clearance are often used to determine the GFR and glomerular damage.

RENAL HORMONES

Hormones either activated or synthesized by the kidneys include the active form of vitamin D, erythropoietin, and natriuretic hormone.

Vitamin D is necessary for the absorption of calcium and phosphate by the small intestine. In an inactive form, vitamin D enters the body either by dietary intake or through the action of ultraviolet rays on cholesterol in the skin. Activation occurs in two steps, the first in the liver and the second in the kidneys. The renal step is stimulated by parathyroid hormone, which in turn responds to a decreased plasma calcium level.

Erythropoietin stimulates the bone marrow to produce red blood cells in response to tissue hypoxia. The stimulus for the production of erythropoietin by the kidneys is decreased oxygen delivery to kidney cells.

The right atria of the heart releases natriuretic hormone in response to increased volume and stretch, as occurs in increased extracellular volume. This hormone inhibits ADH secretion, so that the collecting tubules are less porous and a large amount of dilute urine is produced.

ASSESSING URINARY SYSTEM FUNCTION

The nurse conducts both a health assessment interview (to collect subjective data) and a physical assessment (to collect objective data) to assess the function of the urinary system.

The Health Assessment Interview

This section provides guidelines for collecting subjective data through a health assessment interview specific to urinary elimination. Problems with urinary elimination may be assessed as part of the total health assessment, or may be part of a focused interview if the client has problems specific to the urinary system.

Current urinary status should include the following data.

- Color, odor, and amount of urine
- Difficulty initiating a stream of urine
- Frequency of urination
- Painful urination (**dysuria**)
- Excessive urination at night (**nocturia**)
- Blood in the urine (**hematuria**)
- Voiding scant amounts of urine (**oliguria**)
- Voiding excessive amounts of urine (**polyuria**)
- Discharge
- Flank pain

If you identify a problem with urinary elimination, analyze its onset, characteristics and course, severity, precipitating and relieving factors, and any associated symptoms, noting the tim-

ing and circumstances. For example, you may ask the following questions.

- Have you noticed any burning when you urinate?
- Do you have difficulty starting to urinate?
- When did you first notice that you were unable to control the loss of urine from your bladder?

Further explore any abnormalities in the client's current urinary status. Focus questions on changes in patterns of urination, changes in the urine, and pain.

Assess changes in patterns of urination by asking the client these questions: How many times a day do you urinate? Do you feel that you empty your bladder each time? How many times do you get up at night to urinate? Do you experience a very strong desire to urinate and feel that you just cannot wait? Have you noticed that you urinate small amounts of dark, strong-smelling urine?

Changes in the urine that should be explored include the presence of blood or a cloudy appearance of the urine. If the client has noticed blood, explore the use of medications (such as anticoagulants or dye-containing drugs) and other bleeding problems. Women may not understand that blood in the toilet after urination is normal during menstruation. Cloudy, foul-smelling urine often indicates infection (**pyuria**); ask the client about temperature elevations, chills, and general malaise. Cloudy urine in men may result from retrograde ejaculation (when semen is discharged into the bladder instead of from the penis) during intercourse.

If the client reports pain, explore its location, duration, and intensity. Kidney pain is experienced in the back and the costovertebral angle (the angle between the lower ribs and adjacent vertebrae) and may spread toward the umbilicus. Renal colic is severe, sharp, stabbing, and excruciating; often it is felt in the flank, bladder, urethra, testes, or ovaries. Bladder and urethral pain is usually dull and continuous but may be experienced as spasms. The client with a distended bladder experiences constant pain increased by any pressure over the bladder.

Information about surgeries or other treatment of previous urinary problems is essential to the health history, as is a family history of altered structure or function. A family history of renal problems may be the first clue to abnormalities in the client's urinary function. Explore information regarding family occurrence of end-stage renal disease, renal calculi, and frequent infections as well as related problems such as hypertension and diabetes mellitus.

Questions about lifestyle, diet, and work history should explore cigarette smoking, exposure to toxic chemicals, usual fluid intake, type of fluid intake, and self-care measures to replace fluids lost during work or physical activity in hot temperatures.

Interview questions and leading statements, categorized by functional health patterns, can be found on the Companion Website.

Physical Assessment

Physical assessment of the urinary system may be performed as part of a total health assessment, as part of an abdominal assessment, or as part of the back examination (for the kidneys).

MediaLink | FUNCTIONAL HEALTH PATTERN ASSESSMENT

For clients with known or suspected problems of this system, assessment requires the techniques of inspection, palpation, percussion, and auscultation. Auscultate immediately after inspection because percussion or palpation may increase bowel motility and interfere with sound transmission during auscultation.

The equipment necessary to assess the urinary system is a urine specimen cup and disposable gloves. At the beginning of the assessment, the client may be sitting or lying supine. Prior to the examination, collect all necessary equipment and explain the techniques to the client to decrease anxiety.

Before beginning the assessment, ask the client to provide you with a clean-catch urine specimen and give the client a specimen cup. Assess the specimen for color, odor, and clarity before you send it to the laboratory.

Because the examination involves exposure of the genital area, give the client a gown and drape the client appropriately to minimize exposure.

Guidelines for percussion and palpation of the kidneys are outlined in the Box 25–1.

BOX 25–1   ■ Guidelines for Physical Assessment of the Kidneys

PERCUSSION OF THE KIDNEYS

Percussion of the kidneys helps assess pain or tenderness. Assist the client to a sitting position, and stand behind the client. For indirect percussion, place the palm of your nondominant hand over the costovertebral angle (see Figure A). Strike this area with the ulnar surface of your dominant hand, curled into a fist (see Figure B). For direct percussion, also strike the area over the costovertebral angle with the ulnar surface of your dominant hand, curled into a fist. Repeat the technique for the other kidney.

You should do percussion of the kidneys with only enough force so the client feels a gentle thud. Percussion is usually done at the end of the assessment.

PALPATION OF THE KIDNEYS

Although the technique of palpation of the kidneys is outlined here, this technique is best performed by an advanced practitioner, because it involves deep palpation. In addition, the kidneys are difficult to palpate.

Assist the client to the supine position and stand at the right side of the client. To palpate the left kidney, reach across the client and place your left hand under the client's left flank with your palm upward. Elevate the left flank with your fingers, displacing the kidney upward. Ask the client to take a deep breath and use the palmer surface of your right hand to palpate the kidney (Figure C). Repeat the technique for the right kidney.

B Percussing the kidney.

12th rib

Costovertebral angle

A Location of the kidneys and the costovertebral angle.

C Palpating the left kidney.

Skin Assessment with Abnormal Findings (✓)

- Inspect the skin and mucous membranes, noting color, turgor, and excretions.
  - ✓ Pallor of the skin and mucous membranes may indicate kidney disease with resultant anemia.
  - ✓ Decreased turgor of the skin may indicate dehydration.
  - ✓ Edema may indicate fluid volume excess.

(Either change in turgor may indicate renal insufficiency with either excess fluid loss or retention.)

  - ✓ An accumulation of uric acid crystals, called *uremic frost*, may be seen on the skin of the client with untreated renal failure.

Abdominal Assessment with Abnormal Findings (✓)

- Inspect the abdomen, noting size, symmetry, masses or lumps, swelling, prominent veins, distention, glistening, or skin tightness.
  - ✓ Enlargements or asymmetry may indicate a hernia or superficial mass.
  - ✓ Prominent veins may indicate renal dysfunction.
  - ✓ Distention, glistening, or skin tightness may be associated with fluid retention.
  - ✓ Ascites is an accumulation of fluid in the peritoneal cavity.

Urinary Meatus Assessment with Abnormal Findings (✓)

(This technique is not part of a routine assessment, but it is an important component in clients with health problems of the urinary system.)

- For the male client: With the client in a sitting or standing position, compress the tip of the glans penis with your gloved hand to open the urinary meatus (Figure 25–7 ■).
- For the female client: With the client in the dorsal lithotomy position, spread the labia with your gloved hand to expose the urinary meatus.
  - ✓ Increased redness, swelling, or discharge may indicate infection or sexually transmitted disease.
  - ✓ Ulceration may indicate a sexually transmitted disease.
  - ✓ In male clients, a deviation of the meatus from the midline may suggest a congenital defect.

Kidney Assessment with Abnormal Findings (✓)

- Auscultate the renal arteries by placing the bell of the stethoscope lightly in the areas of the renal arteries, located in the left and right upper abdominal quadrants.

Figure 25–7 ■ Inspecting the urinary meatus of the male.

  - ✓ Systolic bruits ("whooshing" sounds) may indicate renal artery stenosis.
- Percuss the kidneys for tenderness or pain.
  - ✓ Tenderness and pain on percussion of the costovertebral angle suggest glomerulonephritis or glomerulonephrosis.
- Palpate the kidneys.
  - ✓ A mass or lump may indicate a tumor or cyst.
  - ✓ Tenderness or pain on palpation may suggest an inflammatory process.
  - ✓ A soft kidney that feels spongy may indicate chronic renal disease.
  - ✓ Bilaterally enlarged kidneys may suggest polycystic kidney disease.
  - ✓ Unequal kidney size may indicate hydronephrosis.

Bladder Assessment with Abnormal Findings (✓)

- Percuss the bladder for tone and position.
  - ✓ A dull percussion tone over the bladder of a client who has just urinated may indicate urinary retention.
- Palpate the bladder (over the symphysis pubis and abdomen) for distention.
  - ✓ A distended bladder may be palpated at any point from the symphysis pubis to the umbilicus and is felt as a firm, rounded organ.

EXPLORE MediaLink

NCLEX review questions, case studies, care plan activities, MediaLink applications, and other interactive resources for this chapter can be found on the Companion Website at www.prenhall.com/lemone.

Click on Chapter 25 to select the activities for this chapter. For animations, video clips, more NCLEX review questions, and an audio glossary, access the Student CD-ROM accompanying this textbook.

TEST YOURSELF

1. What substance primarily determines the concentration of urine?

   a. Thyroxine
   b. Renin
   c. Aldosterone
   d. ADH

2. What gland encircles the male urethra at the base of the bladder?

   a. Spleen
   b. Pancreas
   c. Prostate
   d. Adrenal

3. Your client tells you of having to get up to void several times a night. You record this finding as:

   a. Polyuria
   b. Nocturia

   c. Dysuria
   d. Hematuria

4. Before beginning the physical examination of the urinary system, you should ask the client to:

   a. Empty the bladder
   b. Take several deep breaths
   c. Collect a clean-catch urine specimen
   d. Drink several glasses of water

5. Following surgery, your client has not voided for 12 hours. What assessment should you make?

   a. Palpate for bladder distention
   b. Auscultate for bowel sounds
   c. Inspect for edema of the urethra
   d. Percuss for gastric tympany

See Test Yourself answers in Appendix C.

BIBLIOGRAPHY

Bevan, M. (2001). Assessing renal function in older people. *Nursing Older People, 13*(2), 27–28.

Criner, J. (2001). Urinary incontinence in a vulnerable population: Older women. *Seminars in Perioperative Nursing, 10*(1), 33–37.

Edwards, S. (2000). Fluid overload and monitoring indices. *Professional Nurse, 15*(9), 568–572.

Godfrey, K. (1997). Continence: Incontinence in ethnic groups. *Community Nurse, 3*(5), 42.

Gray, M. (2000). Urinary retention. Management in the acute care setting. *American Journal of Nursing, 100*(7), 40–47.

Irwin, B. (2001). Incontinence. *Practice Nurse, 22*(4), 31–32, 43.

Johnson, S. (2000). From incontinence to confidence. *American Journal of Nursing, 100*(2), 69–76.

Kirton, C. (1997). Assessing for bladder distention. *Nursing97, 27*(4), 64.

Lyneham, J. (2001). Physical examination (abdomen, thorax, and lungs): A review. *Australian Journal of Advanced Nursing, 18*(3), 31.

Sheppard, M. (2001). Assessing fluid balance. *Nursing Times, 97* (6 Ntplus), XI–XII.

Weber, J., & Kelley, J. (2002). *Health assessment in nursing.* (2nd ed.). Philadelphia: Lippincott.

Wilson, S., & Giddens, J. (2001). *Health assessment for nursing practice.* St. Louis: Mosby.

Nursing Care of Clients with Urinary Tract Disorders

www.prenhall.com/lemone

Additional resources for this chapter can be found on the Student CD-ROM accompanying this textbook, and on the Companion Website at www.prenhall.com/lemone. Click on Chapter 26 to select the activities for this chapter.

CD-ROM
- Audio Glossary
- NCLEX Review

Companion Website
- More NCLEX Review
- Case Study
  Urinary Tract Infection
- Care Plan Activity
  Urinary Tract Infection
- MediaLink Application
  Urinary Tract Disorders

LEARNING OUTCOMES

After completing this chapter, you will be able to:

- Apply knowledge of the structure and function of the urinary tract to caring for clients with urinary tract disorders.

- Describe the pathophysiology of commonly occurring urinary tract disorders.

- Identify laboratory and diagnostic tests used to diagnose disorders affecting the urinary tract.

- Compare and contrast the manifestations of common urinary tract disorders.

- Discuss the nursing implications of medications prescribed for clients with urinary tract disorders.

- Provide appropriate nursing care for clients having surgery of the urinary tract.

- Use the nursing process as a framework for providing individualized care to clients with urinary tract disorders.

The urinary system includes the kidneys, ureters, urinary bladder, and urethra. This organ system can be affected by a variety of disorders, including congenital malformations, infections, obstructions, trauma, tumors, and neurologic conditions. Any portion of the system—from the kidney through the urethra—can be affected with serious or even life-threatening consequences unless the problem is appropriately diagnosed and treated. Kidney disorders can affect urine production and waste elimination directly, and are discussed in the next chapter. Disorders of the **urinary drainage system** (the kidney pelvis, ureters, bladder, and urethra) may obstruct urine flow or spread to the kidneys, affecting urine production and elimination. The anatomy and physiology and nursing assessment related to the urinary tract is presented in Chapter 25.

When caring for clients with urinary tract disorders, it is important to consider the client's modesty in voiding, possible difficulty in discussing the genitals, embarrassment about being exposed for examination and testing, and fear of changes in body image or function. These psychosocial issues may interfere with the client's willingness to seek help, discuss treatment, and learn about preventive measures.

Nursing interventions for clients with urinary tract disorders are directed toward primary prevention, early detection, and management of the disorder through health teaching and nursing care.

THE CLIENT WITH A URINARY TRACT INFECTION

Bacterial infections of the urinary tract are a common reason for seeking health services, second only to upper respiratory infections. More than 8 million people are treated annually for urinary tract infection (UTI) (Porth, 2002). Community-acquired UTIs are common in young women, and unusual in men under the age of 50.

Most community-acquired UTIs are caused by *Escherichia coli,* a common gram-negative enteral bacteria. About 10% to 15% of symptomatic UTIs are caused by *Staphylococcus saprophyticus,* a gram-positive organism. Catheter-associated UTIs often involve other gram-negative bacteria such as *Proteus, Klebsiella, Seratia,* and *Pseudomonas.*

PHYSIOLOGY REVIEW

The urinary tract is normally sterile above the urethra. Adequate urine volume, a free flow from the kidneys through the urinary meatus, and complete bladder emptying are the most important mechanisms maintaining sterility. Pathogens that enter and contaminate the distal urethra are washed out during voiding. Other defenses for maintaining sterile urine include its normal acidity and bacteriostatic properties of the bladder and urethral cells. The peristaltic activity of the ureters and a competent ureterovesical junction help maintain sterility of the upper urinary tract. As the ureter enters the bladder, its distal portion tunnels between the mucosa and muscle layers of the bladder wall (Figure 26–1 ■). During voiding, increased *intra-*

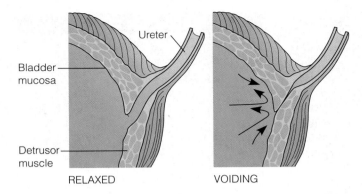

Figure 26–1 ■ A competent ureterovesical junction. Note how increased intravesicular pressure during voiding occludes the distal portion of the ureter, preventing reflux.

vesicular (within the bladder) pressure compresses the ureter, preventing **reflux,** or backflow of urine toward the kidneys. In males, a long urethra and the antibacterial effect of zinc in prostatic fluid also help prevent contamination of this normally sterile environment.

PATHOPHYSIOLOGY AND MANIFESTATIONS

Pathogens usually enter the urinary tract by ascending from the mucous membranes of the perineal area into the lower urinary tract. Bacteria that have colonized the urethra, vagina, or perineal tissues are the usual source of infection (Porth, 2002). From the bladder, bacteria may continue to ascend the urinary tract, eventually infecting the *parenchyma* (functional tissue) of the kidneys (Braunwald et al., 2001). Hematogenous spread of infection to the urinary tract is rare. Infections introduced in this manner are usually associated with previous damage or scarring of the urinary tract. Bacteria introduced into the urinary tract may cause asymptomatic bacteriuria or in an inflammatory response with manifestations of UTI.

Urinary tract infections can be categorized in several ways. Anatomically, UTIs may affect the lower or the upper urinary tract. Lower urinary tract infections include *urethritis,* inflammation of the urethra; *prostatitis,* inflammation of the prostate gland (discussed in Chapter 47); and **cystitis,** inflammation of the urinary bladder. The most common upper urinary tract infection is **pyelonephritis,** inflammation of the kidney and renal pelvis. The infection may involve superficial tissues such as the bladder mucosa, or may invade other tissues such as prostate or renal tissues. Epidemiologically, UTIs are identified as community acquired or nosocomial, associated with catheterization.

Clients can be predisposed to UTI by a variety of factors (Box 26–1). Some risk factors cannot be changed (e.g., aging and the short urethra of the female). In women, sexual activity increases the risk for UTI, as bacteria are introduced into the bladder via the urethra during sexual intercourse. Use of spermicidal compounds with a diaphragm, cervical cap, or condom alters the normal bacterial flora of the vagina and perineal tissues, and further increases the risk for UTI. Some females lack a normally protective mucosal enzyme and have decreased

MediaLink | URINARY TRACT INFECTION CASE STUDY

BOX 26–1 ■ Risk Factors for UTI

FEMALE
- Short, straight urethra
- Proximity of urinary meatus to vagina and anus
- Sexual intercourse
- Use of diaphragm and spermicidal compounds for birth control
- Pregnancy

MALE
- Uncircumsized
- Prostatic hypertrophy
- Rectal intercourse

BOTH
- Aging
- Urinary tract obstruction
- Neurogenic bladder dysfunction
- Vesicoureteral reflux
- Genetic factors
- Catheterization

levels of cervicovaginal antibodies to enterobacteria, further increasing their risk. Prostatic hypertrophy and bacterial prostatitis are risk factors among males. Circumcision appears to have a protective effect. Anal intercourse also is a risk factor for men. Congenital or acquired factors contributing to the risk of infection include urinary tract obstruction by tumors or calculi, structural abnormalities such as strictures, impaired bladder innervation, bowel incontinence, and chronic diseases such as diabetes mellitus. Instrumentation of the urinary tract (e.g., catheterization or cystoscopy) is a major risk factor for UTI. Even when performed under strict aseptic conditions, catheterization can result in bladder infection. The placement of the catheter prevents the flushing action of voiding, and bacteria may ascend to the bladder either through the catheter lumen or via exudate between the urethral mucosa and the catheter.

Older clients have an increased incidence of UTI. The greatest degree of increase is seen in men, as the ratio of female to male UTI in older adults changes from 50:1 to less than 5:1. An increased risk of urinary stasis, chronic disease states (such as diabetes mellitus), and an impaired immune response contribute to the higher incidence of UTI in the older adult. In men, the prostate typically hypertrophies with aging, potentially resulting in urinary retention as the urethra narrows. Prostatic secretions are lessened, diminishing their protective, antibacterial effect. In older women, loss of tissue elasticity and weakening of perineal muscles often contribute to the development of a cystocele or rectocele. Resulting changes in bladder and urethral position increase the risk of incomplete bladder emptying.

Cystitis

Cystitis, inflammation of the urinary bladder, is the most common UTI. The infection tends to remain superficial, involving the bladder mucosa. The mucosa becomes hyperemic (red) and may hemorrhage. The inflammatory response causes pus to form. This process causes the classic manifestations associated with cystitis (see the box below). Typical presenting symptoms of cystitis include **dysuria** (painful or difficult urination), urinary frequency and **urgency** (a sudden, compelling need to urinate), and **nocturia** (voiding two or more times at night). In addition, the urine may have a foul odor and appear cloudy (*pyuria*) or bloody (**hematuria**) because of mucus, excess white cells in the urine, and bleeding of the inflamed bladder wall. Suprapubic pain and tenderness also may be present.

Older clients may not experience the classic symptoms of cystitis. Instead, they often present with nonspecific manifestations such as nocturia, incontinence, confusion, behavior change, lethargy, anorexia, or "just not feeling right." Fever may be present; however, hypothermia also may develop in an older adult.

Cystitis occurs most frequently in adult females, usually because of colonization of the bladder by bacteria normally found in the lower gastrointestinal tract. These bacteria gain entry by ascending the short, straight female urethra. In addition to the risk factors listed in Box 26–1, personal hygiene practices and voluntary urinary retention can contribute to the risk for UTI in women.

Although the bacteriostatic effect of prostatic fluid and a longer urethra provide an effective barrier to bladder infection for adult males, prostatic hypertrophy commonly associated with aging increases the risk of cystitis in elderly males. An enlarged prostate can impede urine flow, leading to incomplete bladder emptying and urinary stasis. Bacteria are not completely flushed with voiding, allowing colonization of the bladder.

Cystitis is usually uncomplicated and readily responds to treatment. When left untreated, the infection can ascend to involve the kidneys. Severe or prolonged infection may lead to sloughing of bladder mucosa and ulcer formation. Chronic cystitis can lead to bladder stones (discussed later in this chapter).

Catheter-Associated UTI

At least 10% to 15% of hospitalized clients with indwelling urinary catheters develop bacteriuria. The longer the catheter remains in place, the greater the risk for infection. Bacteria, including *E. coli, Proteus, Pseudomonas, Klebsiella,* and others, reach the bladder by either migrating through the column of urine within the catheter or by moving up the mucous sheath of the urethra outside the catheter (Braunwald et al., 2001). Bacteria enter the catheter system at the connection between the catheter and drainage system or through the emptying tube of the drainage bag. Colonization of perineal skin by bowel flora is a common source of infection in catheterized women.

Catheter-associated UTIs often are asymptomatic. Gram-negative bacteremia is the most significant complication asso-

Manifestations of Cystitis

• Dysuria	• Pyuria
• Frequency	• Hematuria
• Urgency	• Suprapubic discomfort
• Nocturia	

Nursing Research

Evidence-Based Practice for Intermittent Catheterization

Urinary tract infection is a common complication in clients with spinal cord injury (SCI). Intermittent catheterization has significantly reduced the incidence of UTI in this client population; however, maintaining sterile technique requires using a new kit for each catheterization and may be cost prohibitive. Clean (nonsterile) intermittent catheterization is the method most frequently used to manage neurogenic bladder. The cost of nonsterile intermittent catheterization is significantly lower than that of sterile intermittent catheterization, as the catheter is cleaned and reused for up to 1 week. A study by Prieto-Fingerhut et al. (1997) found that sterile intermittent catheterization resulted in a lower rate of UTI (although the difference was not statistically significant) and reduced costs for antibiotic therapy. While the rate of infection in the nonsterile catheterization group was higher, the cost of catheterization supplies was significantly lower.

IMPLICATIONS FOR NURSING

Several factors should be considered when choosing to use sterile versus nonsterile technique for intermittent catheterization. While the cost of sterile supplies is higher, the incidence of urinary tract infection and the need for antibiotic therapy is reduced by using sterile technique. Other factors that should be considered include the client's immune status and the potential for delaying the client's rehabilitation following SCI during UTI treatment.

Critical Thinking in Client Care

1. Why is intermittent catheterization (using either clean or sterile technique) associated with a lower rate of UTI than that for indwelling catheters?
2. Sterile technique generally is used when catheterizing clients in acute care settings. Would clean technique be appropriate in this situation? Why or why not?

Note. From "A Study Comparing Sterile and Nonsterile Urethral Catheterization in Patients with Spinal Cord Injury" by T. Prieto-Fingerhut, K. Banoveac, and C. M. Lynne, 1997, Rehabilitation Nursing, 22(6), 299–302.

Manifestations of Acute Pyelonephritis

URINARY	SYSTEMIC
• Urinary frequency	• Vomiting
• Dysuria	• Diarrhea
• Pyuria	• Acute fever
• Hematuria	• Shaking chills
• Flank pain	• Malaise
• Costovertebral tenderness	

bacteriuria or cystitis can lead to acute pyelonephritis. Risk factors include pregnancy (because of slowed ureteral peristalsis), urinary tract obstruction, and congenital malformation. Urinary tract trauma, scarring, calculi (stones), kidney disorders such as polycystic or hypertensive kidney disease, and chronic diseases such as diabetes may also contribute to pyelonephritis. *Vesicoureteral reflux,* a condition in which urine moves from the bladder back toward the kidney, is a common risk factor in children who develop pyelonephritis and is also seen in adults when bladder outflow is obstructed.

The infection spreads from the renal pelvis to the renal cortex. The pelvis, calyces, and medulla of the kidney are primarily affected, with white blood cell infiltration and inflammation. The kidney becomes grossly edematous. Localized abscesses may develop on the cortical surface of the kidney (Bullock & Henze, 2000). As with cystitis, *E. coli* is the organism responsible for 85% of the cases of acute pyelonephritis. Other organisms commonly found include *Proteus* and *Klebsiella,* bacteria that normally inhabit the intestinal tract.

The onset of acute pyelonephritis is typically rapid, with chills and fever, malaise, vomiting, flank pain, costovertebral tenderness, urinary frequency, and dysuria (see the Manifestations box above). Symptoms of cystitis also may be present. The older adult may present with a change in behavior, acute confusion, incontinence, or a general deterioration in condition.

Chronic Pyelonephritis

Chronic pyelonephritis involves chronic inflammation and scarring of the tubules and interstitial tissues of the kidney (Bullock & Henze, 2000). It is a common cause of chronic renal failure. It may develop as a result of UTIs or other conditions that damage the kidneys, such as hypertension or vascular conditions, severe vesicoureteral reflux, or obstruction of the urinary tract.

The client with chronic pyelonephritis may be asymptomatic or have mild manifestations such as urinary frequency, dysuria, and flank pain. Hypertension can develop as kidney tissue is destroyed.

COLLABORATIVE CARE

Treatment of UTI focuses on eliminating the causative organism, preventing relapse or reinfection, and identifying and correcting any contributing factors. Drug treatment with antibiotics and urinary anti-infectives is commonly used. In some cases, surgery may be indicated to correct contributing factors.

ciated with these UTIs. Most catheter-associated UTIs resolve quickly when the catheter is removed and a short course of antibiotic is administered. Intermittent catheterization carries a lower risk of infection than does an indwelling catheter, and is preferred for clients who are unable to empty their bladder by voiding (see the Nursing Research box above).

Pyelonephritis

Pyelonephritis is inflammation of the renal pelvis and *parenchyma,* the functional kidney tissue. *Acute pyelonephritis* is a bacterial infection of the kidney; *chronic pyelonephritis* is associated with nonbacterial infections and inflammatory processes that may be metabolic, chemical, or immunologic in origin.

Acute Pyelonephritis

Acute pyelonephritis usually results from an infection that ascends to the kidney from the lower urinary tract. Asymptomatic

Diagnostic Tests

Laboratory testing for UTI includes:

- *Urinalysis* to assess for pyuria, bacteria, and blood cells in the urine. A bacteria count greater than 100,000 (10^5) per milliliter is indicative of infection. Rapid tests for bacteria in the urine include using a *nitrite dipstick* (which turns pink in the presence of bacteria) and the *leukocyte esterase test,* an indirect method of detecting bacteria by identifying lysed or intact white blood cells (WBCs) in the urine.

  Urine should be a midstream clean-catch specimen; if necessary, straight catheterization or "mini-cath," with strict aseptic technique may be used. Catheterization is avoided if possible to reduce the risk of further infection.

- *Gram stain of the urine* may be done to identify the infecting organism by shape and characteristic (Gram positive or negative).
- *Urine culture and sensitivity* tests may be ordered to identify the infecting organism and the most effective antibiotic. Culture requires 24 to 72 hours, so treatment to eliminate the most common organisms often is initiated without culture.
- *WBC with differential* may be done to detect typical changes associated with infection, such as *leukocytosis* (elevated WBC) and increased numbers of neutrophils.

In men and in adult women with recurrent infections or persistent bacteriuria, additional diagnostic testing may be ordered to evaluate for structural abnormalities and other contributing factors.

- *Intravenous pyelography (IVP),* also known as *excretory urography,* is used to evaluate the structure and excretory function of the kidneys, ureters, and bladder. As the kidneys clear an intravenously injected contrast medium from the blood, the size and shape of the kidneys, their calices and pelvises, the ureters, and the bladder can be evaluated, and structural or functional abnormalities, such as vesicoureteral reflux, may be detected.
- *Voiding cystourethrography* involves instilling contrast medium into the bladder, then using X-rays to assess the bladder and urethra when filled and during voiding. This study can detect structural or functional abnormalities of the bladder and urethral strictures. This test has a lower risk of allergic response to the contrast dye than IVP.
- *Cystoscopy,* direct visualization of the urethra and bladder through a cystoscope, may be used to diagnose conditions such as prostatic hypertrophy, urethral strictures, bladder calculi, tumors, polyps or diverticula, and congenital abnormalities. A tissue biopsy may be obtained during the procedure, and other interventions performed (e.g., stone removal or stricture dilation).
- *Manual pelvic* or *prostate examinations* are done to assess for structural changes of the genitourinary tract, such as prostatic enlargement, cystocele, or rectocele.

Nursing implications for these diagnostic procedures are presented in the following box.

Nursing Implications for Diagnostic Tests

The Client with UTI

INTRAVENOUS PYELOGRAPHY (IVP)

Preparation

- Assess knowledge and understanding of procedure, clarifying information as needed.
- Schedule IVP prior to any ordered barium test or gallbladder studies using contrast material.
- Ask about allergy to seafood, iodine, or radiologic contrast dye. Notify physician or radiologist if allergies are known.
- Verify the presence of a signed consent for the procedure.
- Assess renal and fluid status, including serum osmolality, creatinine, and blood urea nitrogen (BUN) levels. Notify the physician of any abnormal values.
- Instruct the client to complete ordered pretest bowel preparation, including prescribed laxative or cathartic (see page 624) the evening before the test, and an enema or suppository the morning of the test. Withhold food for 8 hours prior to the test; clear liquids are allowed.
- Obtain baseline vital signs and record.

After the Test

- Monitor vital signs and urine output.
- Report manifestations of delayed reaction to the contrast media such as dyspnea, tachycardia, itching, hives, or flushing.

Client and Family Teaching

- X-rays and a dye that is rapidly excreted in the urine are used to show the structures of the kidney, ureters, and bladder. The test takes about 30 minutes.
- A laxative and possibly an enema or suppository are used before the test to clear the bowel of feces and gas. Do not eat after the ordered time the evening before the test; you may drink clear fluids such as water, coffee, or tea (without creamer).
- As the dye is injected, you may feel a transient flushing or burning sensation, along with possible nausea and a metallic taste.
- Notify your doctor immediately if you develop a rash, difficulty breathing, rapid heart rate, or hives during or after the test.
- Increase fluid intake after the test is completed.

VOIDING CYSTOURETHROGRAPHY

Preparation

- Assess knowledge and understanding of the procedure, clarifying information as needed.
- Verify the presence of a signed consent for the procedure.
- Ask about allergy to seafood, iodine, or radiologic contrast dye. Notify physician or radiologist if allergies are known. Because the dye is not injected, allergic reactions are rare, and allergy does not contraindicate the examination.
- Instruct to consume only clear liquids the morning of the exam, or as recommended by radiology.
- Insert indwelling catheter if ordered.

Client and Family Teaching

- The bladder is filled with dye solution and X-rays are taken of the filled bladder and of the bladder and urethra during urination.

Nursing Implications for Diagnostic Tests

The Client with UTI *(continued)*

- This procedure causes little or no discomfort and takes approximately 30 to 45 minutes to complete.
- After the procedure, increase your fluid intake to help eliminate the contrast dye and to reduce burning on urination.
- Report signs of infection, such as frequency, urgency, painful urination, cloudy or bloody urine, or malodorous urine.

CYSTOSCOPY

Preparation

- Assess knowledge and understanding of the procedure, clarifying information as needed.
- Verify the presence of a signed consent for the procedure.
- Instruct in pretest preparation as ordered, including prescribed laxatives the evening prior to the test and any ordered food or fluid restrictions.
- Administer sedation and other medications as ordered prior to the test.

Client and Family Teaching

- Cystoscopy is performed in a special cystoscopy room, using local or general anesthesia. You may feel some pressure or a need to urinate as the scope is inserted through the urethra into the bladder. The procedure takes approximately 30 to 45 minutes.
- Do not attempt to stand without assistance immediately after the procedure as you may feel dizzy or faint.
- Burning on urination for a day or two after the procedure is to be expected.
- Immediately notify the physician if your urine remains bloody for more than three voidings after the procedure, or if you develop bright bleeding, low urine output, abdominal or flank pain, chills, or fever.
- Warm sitz baths, analgesic agents, and antispasmodic medications may relieve discomfort after the procedure.
- Increase fluid intake to decrease pain and difficulty voiding and reduce the risk of infection.
- Laxatives may be ordered after the procedure to prevent constipation and straining, which may cause urinary tract bleeding.

Medications

Most uncomplicated infections of the lower urinary tract can be treated with a short course of antibiotic therapy. Upper urinary tract infections, in contrast, usually require longer treatment (2 or more weeks) to eradicate the infecting organism.

Short-course therapy (either a single antibiotic dose or a 3-day course of treatment) reduces treatment cost, increases compliance, and has a lower rate of side effects. Single dose therapy is associated with a higher rate of recurrent infection and continued vaginal colonization with *E. coli*, making a 3-day course of treatment the preferred option for uncomplicated cystitis. Oral trimethoprim-sulfamethoxazole (TMP-SMZ), TMP, or a quinolone antibiotic such as ciprofloxacin (Cipro) or enoxacin (Penetrex) may be ordered.

Men and women with pyelonephritis, urinary tract abnormalities or stones, or a history of previous infections with antibiotic-resistant infections require a 7 to 10 day course of TMP-SMZ, ciprofloxacin, ofloxacin (Floxin), or an alternate antibiotic. The client with severe illness may need hospitalization. Intravenous ciprofloxacin, gentamicin, ceftriaxone (Rocephin), or ampicillin may be prescribed for severe illness or sepsis associated with UTI. See Chapter 8 🔗 for the nursing implications for antibiotic therapy.

The outcome of treatment for UTI is determined by follow-up urinalysis and culture. *Cure,* as evidenced by no pathogens present in the urine, is the desired outcome. When therapy fails to eradicate bacteria in the urine, it is known as *unresolved bacteriuria. Persistent bacteriuria* or *relapse* occurs when a persistent source of infection causes repeated infection after initial cure. *Reinfection* is the development of a new infection with a different pathogen following successful UTI treatment (Tierney et al., 2001).

Clients who experience frequent symptomatic UTIs may be treated with prophylactic antibiotic therapy with a drug such as TMP-SMZ, TMP, or nitrofurantoin (Furadantin, Nitrofan). TMP and nitrofurantoin do not achieve effective plasma concentrations at recommended doses, but do reach effective concentrations in the urine. Nitrofurantoin also may be used to treat UTI in pregnant women. Nursing implications for these urinary anti-infectives and for phenazopyridine (Pyridium), a urinary analgesic, are outlined on page 710.

Antibiotics and urinary anti-infectives are not generally recommended to treat asymptomatic bacteriuria in catheterized clients. The preferred treatment for catheter-associated UTI is removal of the indwelling catheter followed by a 10 to 14 day course of antibiotic therapy to eliminate the infection.

Surgery

Surgery may be indicated for recurrent UTI if diagnostic testing indicates calculi, structural anomalies, or strictures that contribute to the risk of infection. Table 26–1 lists major causes of urinary tract obstruction that may contribute to UTI.

TABLE 26–1	Major Causes of Urinary Tract Obstruction by Location
Location	**Obstructive Process**
Kidney pelvis	Calculi Polycystic kidney disease Infection and scarring
Ureters	Calculi Scarring and stricture Congenital defects or strictures External processes such as pregnancy, tumors, lymph node enlargement
Bladder	Neurogenic bladder Tumors Calculi and other foreign bodies
Urethra	Benign prostatic hypertrophy Tumors Scarring and stricture Trauma

Medication Administration
Urinary Anti-Infectives and Analgesics

URINARY ANTI-INFECTIVES

Nitrofurantoin (Furadantin; Macrodantin)
Trimethoprim (Proloprim, Trimpex)

Urinary anti-infectives are usually used prophylactically to prevent recurrence of UTI in clients with frequent symptomatic infections. Nitrofurantoin also may be used to treat UTI in pregnant women.

Nursing Responsibilities

- Ensure adequate fluid intake (1500 to 2000 mL per day) to maintain a urine output of at least 1500 mL of urine per 24 hours. Do not overhydrate.
- Administer with meals to minimize GI side effects, such as nausea, gastric upset, and abdominal cramping.
- Trimethoprim is contraindicated for use in clients with renal or hepatic impairment; nitrofurantoin is contraindicated for clients with impaired renal function. Report abnormal laboratory values such as elevated creatinine or BUN, bilirubin, alanine aminotransferase (ALT), aspartate aminotransferase (AST), and lactic dehydrogenase (LDH).
- Use with caution in older or chronically ill clients. Monitor closely for adverse effects.
- Do not administer trimethoprim to pregnant women because of possible adverse effects on the fetus.
- Monitor the client taking nitrofurantoin for an acute or chronic pulmonary reaction with manifestations of dyspnea, cough, chills, fever, and chest pain. Discontinue the drug and notify the physician.
- Nitrofurantoin may cause peripheral neuropathy, especially in older clients and adult diabetics. Notify the physician if symptoms develop.
- Nitrofurantoin oral suspension may stain the teeth; have the client rinse the mouth thoroughly after administering.
- Monitor for signs of phenytoin toxicity (sedation, ataxia, and increased blood levels) if trimethoprim is given concurrently. Phenytoin doses may need to be reduced.

Client and Family Teaching

- These drugs are used along with hygiene practices to prevent recurrent UTI. Take as directed, even when no symptoms are present.

- Drink six to eight glasses of water or fluid per day while taking these drugs.
- Take the drug with meals or food to reduce gastric effects; however, avoid milk products because they may interfere with absorption.
- Trimethoprim should not be taken during pregnancy. Contact your physician before attempting to become pregnant.
- Contact your doctor if you develop any of the following: chest pain, difficulty breathing, cough, chills, and fever; numbness and tingling or weakness of the extremities; rash or pruritus (itching).
- If you are taking an oral suspension of nitrofurantoin, rinse your mouth thoroughly after each dose to avoid staining the teeth.
- Nitrofurantoin turns the urine brown. This is not harmful and subsides when the drug is discontinued.
- If you are taking trimethoprim along with phenytoin (Dilantin) or a related anticonvulsant, contact your doctor if you become sedated or begin to stagger.

URINARY ANALGESIC

Phenazopyridine (Pyridium)

Phenazopyridine is a urinary tract analgesic that may be used for symptomatic relief of the pain, burning, frequency, and urgency associated with UTI during the first 24 to 48 hours of therapy. Its use is somewhat controversial, because it does not treat the infection and may delay effective treatment in the client with recurrent UTI who saves a dose or two "for the next time."

Nursing Responsibilities

- Monitor renal function (urine output, weight, serum creatinine, and BUN) during treatment; report changes.
- Stop the drug and contact the physician if sclera or skin become yellow-tinged. This may indicate reduced excretion and toxicity.

Client and Family Teaching

- Take with meals to minimize gastric upset.
- This drug turns urine orange or red. Protect your clothing from staining.
- Promptly contact your doctor if symptoms of UTI recur; do not take phenazopyridine before you seek medical treatment.
- If you notice a yellow tinge to your skin or eyes, stop taking the drug and notify the physician.

Stones, or *calculi*, in the renal pelvis or in the bladder are an irritant and provide a matrix for bacterial colonization. Treatment may include surgical removal of a large calculus from the renal pelvis or cystoscopic removal of bladder calculi. *Percutaneous ultrasonic pyelolithotomy* or *extracorporeal shock wave lithotripsy (ESWL)* (described in the next section of this chapter) may be used instead of surgery to crush and remove stones. (See page 709 for nursing care related to cystoscopy.)

Ureteroplasty, surgical repair of a ureter, may be indicated for structural abnormality or stricture of a ureter. This may be combined with a ureteral reimplantation if vesicoureteral reflux is present. The client returns from these surgeries with an indwelling urinary catheter (Foley or suprapubic) and a **ureteral stent** (a thin catheter inserted into the ureter to provide for urine flow and ureteral support), which remains in place for 3 to 5 days. Care of the client with a ureteral stent is outlined in the box on the next page.

Complementary Therapies

Complementary therapies such as aromatherapy or herbal preparations may be used in conjunction with antibiotics to treat UTI. Adding bergamot, sandalwood, lavender, or juniper oil to bath water helps relieve the discomfort of UTI. Herbal supplements such as saw palmetto have a urinary antiseptic

NURSING CARE OF THE CLIENT WITH A URETERAL STENT

Ureteral stents are used to maintain patency and promote healing of the ureters (see figure below). A stent may be temporary, used during and after a surgical procedure, or it may be used for longer periods in clients with ureteral obstruction due to tumors, strictures, or other causes.

Stents may be positioned during surgery or cystoscopy. They are made of a nontoxic material such as silicone or polyurethane,

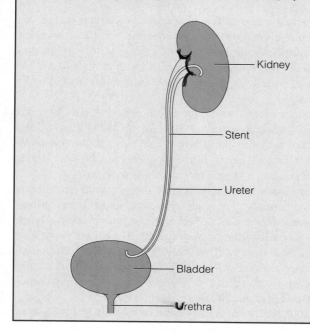

with side drainage holes placed along the length of the stent. Stents are radiopaque for easy radiographic identification. One or both ends of the stent may be pigtail or J-shaped to prevent migration.

- Label all drainage tubes including stents for easy identification. Attach each catheter and stent to a separate closed drainage system. *Careful labeling allows close monitoring of output from all sources and reservoirs. Separate drainage systems minimize the risk of infection.*
- If the stent has been brought to the surface, secure it and maintain its position. *The stent is usually placed in the renal pelvis. It is important to secure it well to prevent trauma to the kidney, inadvertent removal of the stent, and ureter obstruction.*
- Monitor urine output, including color, consistency, and odor. Monitor for signs of infection or bleeding: fever, tachycardia, pain, hematuria, and cloudy or malodorous urine. *The stent facilitates urine flow but may become obstructed because of bleeding, calculi, or sediment. Obstruction may result in hydronephrosis and kidney damage. The stent itself is a foreign body in the urinary tract and can increase the risk of UTI.*
- Maintain fluid intake, encouraging fluids that acidify urine, such as apple and cranberry juice. *The stent can precipitate calculus formation as well as UTI. Increasing fluid intake and acidifying the urine help prevent these complications.*
- For an indwelling stent, stress the need for regular follow-up to monitor for and prevent complications such as UTI and calculi. *The client with an indwelling stent may tend to forget that the stent is in place and become lax in compliance with follow-up and preventive measures.*

effect, and may be beneficial in treating or preventing UTI. Consult a qualified herbologist for recommended doses and appropriate use.

NURSING CARE

Health Promotion

Teach measures to prevent UTI to all clients, particularly to young, sexually active women. Encourage clients to maintain a generous fluid intake of 2.0 to 2.5 quarts per day, increasing intake during hot weather or strenuous activity. Discuss the need to avoid voluntary urinary retention, emptying the bladder every 3 to 4 hours. Instruct women to cleanse the perineal area from front to back after voiding and defecating. Teach to void before and after sexual intercourse to flush out bacteria introduced into the urethra and bladder. Teach measures to maintain the integrity of perineal tissues: Avoid bubble baths, feminine hygiene sprays, and vaginal douches; wear cotton briefs, avoid synthetic materials; if postmenopausal, use hormone replacement therapy or estrogen cream. Unless contraindicated, suggest measures to maintain acid urine: Drink two glasses of cran-

berry juice daily; take ascorbic acid (vitamin C), and avoid excess intake of milk and milk products, other fruit juices, and sodium bicarbonate (baking soda).

Assessment

Focused assessment data for the client with a UTI includes the following:

- Health history: current symptoms, including frequency, urgency, burning on urination, voidings per night; color, clarity, and odor of urine; other manifestations such as lower abdominal, back, or flank pain, nausea or vomiting, fever; duration of symptoms and any treatment attempted; history of previous UTIs and their frequency; possibility of pregnancy and type of birth control used; chronic diseases such as diabetes; current medications and any known allergies
- Physical examination: general health; vital signs including temperature; abdominal shape, contour, tenderness to palpation (especially suprapubic); percuss for costovertebral tenderness (see Box 25–1)

See Chapter 25 ⬡ for complete nursing assessment of the urinary system.

URINARY TRACT INFECTION CARE PLAN

MediaLink

Nursing Diagnoses and Interventions

The client's general health, abilities for self-care, and risk factors that may contribute to UTI are considered when planning and implementing nursing care for the client with a UTI. Priority nursing diagnoses focus on comfort, urinary elimination, and teaching/learning needs.

Pain

Pain is a common manifestation of both lower and upper UTI. Urinary tract pain is caused primarily by distention and increased pressure within the tract. The severity of the pain is related to the rate at which inflammation and distention develop, not their degree.

In cystitis, inflammation causes a sensation of fullness; dull, constant suprapubic pain; and possibly low back pain. The inflamed bladder wall and urethra cause dysuria, pain, and burning on urination. Bladder spasms may develop, causing periodic severe, stabbing discomfort. Pain associated with pyelonephritis is often steady and dull, localized to the outer abdomen or flank region. Urologic disorders rarely cause central abdominal pain.

- Assess pain: timing, quality, intensity, location, duration, and aggravating and alleviating factors. *A change in the nature, location, or intensity of the pain could indicate an extension of the infection or a related but separate problem.*

PRACTICE ALERT *The older adult with a UTI may not complain of dysuria with a UTI. Be alert for other manifestations of UTI such as incontinence, cloudy, or malodorous urine. Inflammatory and immune responses tend to diminish with aging, reducing the irritative symptoms of UTI.* ■

- Teach or provide comfort measures such as warm sitz baths, warm packs or heating pads, balanced rest and activity. Systemic analgesics, urinary analgesics, or antispasmodic medication may be used as ordered. *Warmth relaxes muscles, relieves spasms, and increases local blood supply. Because pain can stimulate a stress response and delay healing, it should be relieved when possible.*
- Increase fluid intake unless contraindicated. *Increased fluid dilutes urine, reducing irritation of the inflamed bladder and urethral mucosa.*

Impaired Urinary Elimination

Inflammation of the bladder and urethral mucosa affects the normal process and patterns of voiding, causing frequency, urgency, and burning on urination, as well as nocturia. Urine may be blood-tinged, cloudy, and malodorous. The client with short- or long-term urinary retention (see the section on urinary retention later in this chapter) requires additional measures to assess for and prevent UTI.

- Monitor (or instruct the client to monitor) color, clarity, and odor of urine. *Urine should return to clear yellow*

within 48 hours, unless drug therapy causes a change in the color of urine. If clarity does not return, further investigation may be necessary.

PRACTICE ALERT *Provide for easy access to a bedpan, urinal, commode, or bathroom. Make sure that lighting is adequate and that pathways are free of obstacles. Frequency, urgency, and nocturia increase the risk of urinary incontinence and of injury due to falls, particularly in the older or debilitated client.* ■

- Instruct to avoid caffeinated drinks, including coffee, tea, and cola; citrus juices, drinks containing artificial sweeteners; and alcoholic beverages. *Caffeine, citrus juices, and artificial sweeteners irritate bladder mucosa and the detrussor muscle, and can increase urgency and bladder spasms.*
- Use strict aseptic technique and a closed urinary drainage system when inserting a straight or indwelling urinary catheter. *Bacteria colonizing the perineal tissues or on the nurse's hands can be introduced into the bladder during catheterization. Aseptic technique reduces this risk.*
- When possible, use intermittent straight catheterization to relieve urinary retention. Remove indwelling urinary catheters as soon as possible. *Using intermittent straight catheterization allows the bladder to fill and completely empty in a more normal manner, maintaining physiologic function. The risk of infection associated with an indwelling catheter is about 3% to 5% per day of catheterization* (Braunwald et al., 2001).
- Maintain the closed urinary drainage system, and use aseptic technique when emptying catheter drainage bag. Maintain gravity flow, preventing reflux of urine into the bladder from the drainage system. *Bacteria can enter the drainage system when its integrity is interrupted (e.g., disconnecting the catheter from the drainage system) or during emptying of the drainage bag. These bacteria can ascend the column of urine to the bladder, causing UTI.*
- Provide perineal care on a regular basis and following defecation. Use antiseptic preparations only as ordered. *Regular cleansing of perineal tissues reduces the risk of colonization by bowel or other bacteria. While antiseptic solutions may be ordered for catheter care, they can dry perineal tissues and reduce normal flora, increasing the risk of colonization by pathogens, and should not routinely be used.*

Ineffective Health Maintenance

The client with a urinary tract infection is at an increased risk for future UTI and needs to understand the disease process, risk factors, measures to prevent recurrent infection, diagnostic procedures, and home care. In addition, once the manifestations of UTI are relieved, motivation to continue the treatment plan declines. Failure to complete the full course of therapy and recommended follow-up can lead to continued bacteriuria and recurrent infections.

- Teach how to obtain a midstream clean-catch urine specimen. *Cleansing of the urinary meatus and perineal area reduces contamination of the specimen by external cells and bacteria. Ninety percent of urethral bacteria are cleared in the first 10 mL of voided urine; a midstream specimen is representative of urine in the bladder.*
- Assess knowledge about the disease process, risk factors, and preventive measures. *The client may have little understanding of UTI, its causes, and contributing factors.*
- Discuss the prescribed treatment plan and the importance of taking all prescribed antibiotics.

PRACTICE ALERT *Symptoms are largely relieved within 24 to 48 hours of starting antibiotic therapy; however, bacteria may remain in the urinary tract. Completing the prescribed regime is important to prevent recurrent infections and resistant bacteria.* ■

- Help the client develop a plan for taking medications, such as taking them with meals (unless contraindicated) or setting out all doses for the day in the morning. *Missed doses of antibiotic can result in subtherapeutic blood levels and reduced effectiveness. Taking medication in association with a regular daily activity such as meals helps clients remember doses.*
- Instruct to keep appointments for follow-up and urine culture. *Follow-up urine culture, often scheduled 7 to 14 days after completion of antibiotic therapy, is vital to ensure complete eradication of bacteria and prevent relapse or recurrence.*
- Teach measures to prevent future UTI (see the preceding Health Promotion section). *Keeping urine dilute and acidic, and voiding regularly flush bacteria out of the bladder and urethra. The proximity of the female urethral meatus to the vagina and anus increases the risk of bacterial contamination, especially during intercourse. Bubble baths, feminine hygiene sprays, synthetic fibers, and douches may dry and irritate perineal tissues, promoting bacterial growth.*

Using NANDA, NIC, and NOC

Chart 26–1 shows links between NANDA nursing diagnosis, NIC and NOC for the client with UTI.

Home Care

Because both upper and lower urinary tract infections are usually managed in the community, teaching is the most important nursing intervention. Provide instruction on the following topics.

- Risk factors for UTI and how to minimize or eliminate these factors through increased fluid intake, regular elimination, and personal hygiene measures
- Early manifestations of UTI and the importance of seeking medical intervention promptly
- Maintaining optimal immune system function by attending to physical and psychosocial stressors, such as lack of adequate rest, poor nutrition, and high levels of emotional stress
- The importance of completing the prescribed treatment and keeping follow-up appointments
- Minimizing the risk of UTI when an indwelling urinary catheter is necessary:
  1. Use alternatives to an indwelling catheter when possible. For urinary incontinence, try scheduled toileting, incontinence pads or diapers, and external catheters if possible. For urinary retention, teach the client or a family member to perform straight catheterization every 3 to 4 hours using clean technique.
  2. Teach care measures such as perineal care, managing and emptying the collection chamber, maintaining a closed system, and bladder irrigation or flushing if ordered when an indwelling catheter is necessary.

CHART 26–1 NANDA, NIC, AND NOC LINKAGES

The Client with UTI

NURSING DIAGNOSES	NURSING INTERVENTIONS	NURSING OUTCOMES
• Pain	• Medication Management	• Comfort Level
• Impaired Urinary Elimination	• Urinary Elimination Management	• Urinary Elimination
• Ineffective Health Maintenance	• Health Education	• Knowledge: Health Behaviors
	• Teaching: Procedure/Treatment	• Knowledge: Treatment Regimen

Note. Data from Nursing Outcomes Classification (NOC) by M. Johnson & M. Maas (Eds.), 1997, St. Louis: Mosby; Nursing Diagnoses: Definitions & Classification 2001–2002 by North American Nursing Diagnosis Association, 2001, Philadelphia: NANDA; Nursing Interventions Classification (NIC) by J.C. McCloskey & G. M. Bulechek (Eds.), 2000, St. Louis: Mosby. Reprinted by permission.

Nursing Care Plan
A Client with Cystitis

Miija Waisanen is a 25-year-old second-year nursing student. She was recently married, and she and her husband live in an apartment near the college she attends. Mrs. Waisanen has never been pregnant, and she is using a diaphragm for birth control. She presents at the local urgent care clinic complaining of low back pain, frequency, urgency, and burning on urination that began the day before.

ASSESSMENT

Patrice Ramiros, RN, admits Mrs. Waisanen to the clinic. Mrs. Waisanen denies having had similar symptoms in the past or ever having been diagnosed with a urinary tract infection. She describes her pain as a constant, dull ache that does not change with movement. She feels the need to urinate almost constantly, but experiences difficulty in starting her stream, and burning pain and cramping when voiding. She reports getting up four times the night before to urinate. She denies painful intercourse and states that her last menstrual period began only 2 weeks ago. Physical examination reveals: BP 112/68; P 90 and regular, afebrile. Suprapubic tenderness noted but no flank or costovertebral angle tenderness. Clean-catch urine specimen shows hematuria, multiple WBCs, and a bacteria count greater than 10^5 per milliliter.

The nurse practitioner prescribes trimethoprim-sulfamethoxazole (TMP-SMZ) 160 mg/800 mg PO bid for 3 days, and aspirin or acetaminophen gr x PO every 4 hours as needed for pain. Mrs. Waisanen is instructed to return to the clinic in 7 days for a follow-up urine culture, or sooner if her symptoms do not improve.

DIAGNOSIS

- *Pain* related to infection and inflammatory process in the urinary tract
- *Impaired urinary elimination* related to inflammation as evidenced by frequency, urgency, nocturia, and dysuria
- *Deficient knowledge* related to lack of information about risk factors for UTI

EXPECTED OUTCOMES

- Report relief of low back pain and burning on urination.
- Regain a normal voiding pattern without frequency, urgency, nocturia, and abnormal urine characteristics.

- Verbalize understanding of the disease process, related risk factors, follow-up instructions, and symptoms of recurrence indicating the need for medical attention.

PLANNING AND IMPLEMENTATION

- Teach comfort measures: warm sitz baths, a heating pad on low heat applied to her lower back or abdomen, rest, increased fluid intake, avoiding caffeinated beverages, and aspirin or acetaminophen as ordered.
- Advise to refrain from sexual intercourse until infection and inflammation have cleared to avoid further irritation of inflamed tissues.
- Discuss the possible relationship between using a diaphragm for birth control and UTI in women.
- Discuss dietary and hygiene practices to prevent UTI, symptoms indicating the need for further intervention, and the risks of undertreatment.

EVALUATION

Six months later, Mrs. Waisanen rotates through the urgent care clinic for her community-based nursing experience. Ms. Ramiros asks how she is doing. Mrs. Waisanen reports that her symptoms and urine cleared within about a day after starting the antibiotic and she has had no further problems. She has seen her women's health care nurse practitioner to change her birth control to oral contraceptives, increased her intake of fluid and vitamin C, and no longer puts off urinating until she "has time to go!"

Critical Thinking in the Nursing Process

1. What physiologic and psychosocial factors put Mrs. Waisanen at risk for developing a UTI?
2. Compare and contrast the benefits and drawbacks to short-course therapy versus conventional therapy for UTI.
3. Why was it appropriate for the nurse practitioner to use short-course therapy with the advice to return if symptoms did not clear?
4. Develop a care plan for Mrs. Waisanen for the nursing diagnosis *Ineffective health maintenance.*

See Evaluating Your Response in Appendix C.

THE CLIENT WITH URINARY CALCULI

Urinary calculi, stones in the urinary tract, are the most common cause of upper urinary tract obstruction (Porth, 2002). The term **lithiasis** means "stone formation"; when the stones form in the kidney, it is known as *nephrolithiasis;* when they form elsewhere in the urinary tract (for example, the bladder), it is called *urolithiasis.* Stones may form and obstruct the urinary tract at any point (Figure 26–2 ■). In the United States and other industrialized countries, renal or kidney stones are the most common.

Urolithiasis affects up to 720,000 people annually in the United States (Tierney et al., 2001). In the United States, the incidence varies by region, with the highest frequency in southern and midwestern states. Males are affected more often than females by a 4:1 ratio (Porth, 2002). Calculi are more common among whites than blacks. Most people affected are in young or middle adulthood.

Although the majority of stones are idiopathic (having no demonstrable cause), a number of risk factors have been identified. The greatest risk factor for stone formation is a prior personal or family history of urinary calculi. A genetic predisposi-

Figure 26–2 ■ Development and location of calculi within the urinary tract.

tion toward the accumulation of certain mineral substances in the urine or a congenital lack of protective factors may explain the familial link. Other identified risk factors include dehydration with resultant increased urine concentration, immobility, and excess dietary intake of calcium, oxalate, or proteins. Gout, hyperparathyroidism, and urinary stasis or repeated infections also contribute to calculus formation.

PHYSIOLOGY REVIEW

Normally, a balance exists in the kidneys between the need to conserve water and eliminate poorly soluble materials such as calcium salts. This balance is affected by factors such as diet,

environmental temperature, and activity. Protective inorganic and organic substances in the urine, such as pyrophosphate, citrate, and glycoproteins, normally inhibit stone formation.

PATHOPHYSIOLOGY

Three factors contribute to urolithiasis: supersaturation, nucleation, and lack of inhibitory substances in the urine.

When the concentration of an insoluble salt in the urine is very high, that is, when the urine is supersaturated, crystals may form. Usually, these crystals disperse and are eliminated because the bonds holding them together are weak. However, a nucleus of crystals may develop stable bonds to form a stone. More often, crystals form around an organic matrix or mucoprotein nucleus to become a stone. The stimulus required to initiate crystallization in supersaturated urine may be minimal. Ingesting a meal high in insoluble salt, or decreased fluid intake as occurs during sleep, allows the concentration to increase to the point where precipitation occurs and stones are formed and grow. When fluid intake is adequate, no stone growth occurs. The acidity or alkalinity of the urine and the presence or absence of calculus-inhibiting compounds also affect lithiasis.

Most (75% to 80%) kidney stones are *calcium stones*, composed of calcium oxalate and/or calcium phosphate. These stones are generally associated with high concentrations of calcium in the blood or urine. *Uric acid stones* develop when the urine concentration of uric acid is high. They are more common in men, and may be associated with gout. Genetic factors contribute to the development of uric acid stones and calcium stones. *Sturvite stones* are associated with UTI caused by urease-producing bacteria such as *Proteus*. These stones can grow to become very large, filling the renal pelvis and calyces. They often are called *staghorn stones* because of their shape. *Cystine stones* are rare, associated with a genetic defect. The types of renal calculi, contributing factors, and recommended dietary modifications are listed in Table 26–2.

TABLE 26–2	Risk Factors and Interventions for Renal Calculi	
Stone Type and Incidence	**Risk Factors**	**Management**
Calcium phosphate and/or oxalate 75%–80%	Hypercalciuria and hypercalcemia: hyperparathyroidism, immobility, bone disease, vitamin D intoxication, multiple myeloma, renal tubular acidosis, prolonged steroid intake Alkaline urine Dehydration Inflammatory bowel disease	Pharmacology: Thiazide diuretics, phosphates, calcium-binding agents Dietary: Limit foods high in calcium and oxalate, increase foods that acidify urine Other: Increase hydration, exercise
Sturvite 15%–20%	UTIs, especially *Proteus* infections	Pharmacology: Antibiotic therapy for UTI Other: Surgical intervention or lithotripsy to remove stone
Uric acid 5%–10%	Gout, increased purine intake, acid urine	Pharmacology: Potassium citrate, allopurinol Dietary: Low purine diet Other: Increase hydration
Cystine (uncommon)	Genetic defect, acid urine	Pharmacology: Penicillamine, sodium bicarbonate Dietary: Sodium restriction Other: Increase hydration

Manifestations of Urinary Calculi

KIDNEY STONES
- Often asymptomatic
- Dull, aching flank pain
- Microscopic hematuria
- Manifestations of UTI

URETERAL STONES
- Renal colic
  - Acute, severe flank pain on affected side
  - Often radiates to suprapubic region, groin, and external genitals
- Nausea, vomiting, pallor, and cool, clammy skin

BLADDER STONES
- May be asymptomatic
- Dull suprapubic pain, possibly associated with exercise or voiding
- Gross or microscopic hematuria
- Manifestations of UTI

Manifestations of Acute and Chronic Hydronephrosis

Acute	Chronic
• Acute, colicky pain; may radiate into groin	• Dull, aching flank pain
• Hematuria, pyuria	• Hematuria, pyuria
• Fever	• Fever
• Nausea, vomiting, abdominal pain	• Palpable flank mass

MANIFESTATIONS

The symptoms caused by urinary calculi vary with their size and location (see the box above). Manifestations develop as a result of obstructed urine flow with resulting distention, and tissue trauma caused by passage of the rough-edged, crystalline stone.

Calculi affecting the kidney calices and pelvis may cause few symptoms. If the stone has gradually or partially obstructed urinary flow, dull, aching flank pain may be present, but renal calculi often are silent, without symptoms. Bladder calculi may cause few symptoms other than dull suprapubic pain with exercise or after voiding.

Renal colic, acute, severe flank pain on the affected side, develops when a stone obstructs the ureter, causing ureteral spasm. The pain of renal colic may radiate to the suprapubic region, groin, and external genitals (the scrotum or labia). The severity of the pain often causes a sympathetic response with associated nausea, vomiting, pallor, and cool, clammy skin.

Manifestations of UTI, including chills and fever, frequency, urgency, and dysuria, may accompany urinary calculi at any level. Trauma to the urinary tract by the calculi may cause gross or microscopic hematuria. Gross hematuria is often the only sign of bladder stones.

Complications

Obstruction

Stones can obstruct the urinary tract at any point from the calyces of the kidney to the distal urethra, impeding the outflow of urine. If the obstruction develops slowly, there may be few or no symptoms, whereas sudden obstruction (e.g., blockage of a ureter by a passing stone) may cause severe manifestations. Urinary tract obstruction can ultimately lead to renal failure. The degree of obstruction, its location, and the duration of impaired urine flow determine the effect on renal function.

Hydronephrosis

The kidneys continue to produce urine, causing increased pressure and distention of the urinary tract behind the obstruction. **Hydronephrosis,** distention of the renal pelvis and calyces, and *hydroureter,* distention of the ureter, are possible results. If the pressure is unrelieved, the collecting tubules, proximal tubules, and glomeruli of the kidney are damaged, causing a gradual loss of renal function.

Acute hydronephrosis typically causes colicky pain on the affected side. The pain may radiate into the groin. Chronic hydronephrosis develops slowly, and may have few manifestations other than dull, aching back or flank pain. When hydronephrosis is significant, a palpable mass may be felt in the flank region. Hematuria and signs of UTI such as pyuria, fever, and discomfort may occur. Gastrointestinal symptoms such as nausea, vomiting, and abdominal pain may accompany hydronephrosis (see the box above).

INFECTION. The urinary stasis associated with partial or complete obstruction increases the risk of urinary tract infection. Either upper or lower UTI may develop.

COLLABORATIVE CARE

Management of urinary calculi focuses on relieving acute symptoms, destroying or removing stones, and preventing further stone formation. Asymptomatic stones (those not causing pain, infection, or obstruction) are treated conservatively.

Diagnostic Tests

Laboratory and diagnostic tests that may be ordered when urinary calculi are suspected include the following:

- *Urinalysis* to assess for hematuria and the possible presence of WBCs and crystal fragments. The urine pH is helpful in identifying the type of stone.
- *Chemical analysis* of any stones passed in the urine determines the type of stone and suggests measures to prevent further stone formation. Retrieving stones or teaching the client to do so is a nursing responsibility. All urine is strained and may be saved. Any visible stones or sediment are sent for analysis.
- *Urine calcium, uric acid,* and *oxalate* measure the amount of these substances excreted over a 24-hour period, and may be assessed to help identify possible causes of lithiasis. Elevated

Nursing Implications for Diagnostic Tests

24-Hour Urine Specimen Collection

Preparation of the Client

- Check for ordered diet or medication regimen modifications during the collection period. Notify appropriate individuals and departments.
- Obtain a specimen container with preservative (if indicated). Label the container with identifying data, test, time started, and time of completion.
- Obtain a clean commode, bedpan, or urine-collection device for the toilet and place it in the room.
- Post notices—on the chart, in the Kardex file, on the door, over the bed, and over the toilet—alerting all personnel to save all urine.
- When collection is to begin, instruct client to completely empty the bladder and discard this urine.
- Save all urine produced during the 24-hour period in a container, refrigerating it or keeping it on ice as indicated.
- When the collection period is to end, have client empty the bladder completely and save this specimen as part of the total. Take the full specimen with requisition to the lab for analysis.
- Chart appropriately.

Client and Family Teaching

- This test requires you to collect all your urine over 24 hours.
- You may have to follow some dietary or medication modifications.
- Urinate (and save your urine) before you move your bowels; do not discard any toilet tissue in the urine container.

calcium levels occur in hyperparathyroidism, Cushing's syndrome, and osteoporosis, all of which may contribute to lithiasis. Uric acid levels may be elevated in clients with gout and those at risk for forming uric acid calculi. Urine oxalate excretion may help to differentiate calcium oxalate from calcium phosphate stones. See the box above for nursing responsibilities for collecting a 24-hour urine specimen.

- *Serum calcium, phosphorus,* and *uric acid* levels may be obtained to help identify factors contributing to calculus formation.
- *KUB* (kidneys, ureters, and bladder) is a flat-plate X-ray of the lower abdomen that requires no special preparation. Calculi may be identified as opacities in the kidneys, ureters, and bladder.
- *Renal ultrasonography* is a noninvasive test that uses reflected sound waves to detect stones and evaluate the kidneys for possible hydronephrosis (see the box that follows).
- *Computed tomography (CT scan)* of the kidney, with or without contrast medium, uses X-rays directed at the kidney from many angles to provide a computer-generated photograph that shows calculi, ureteral obstruction, and other renal disorders.
- *IVP* may be done to visualize the kidneys, ureters, and bladder after injection of a contrast medium. IVP may be done

Nursing Implications for Diagnostic Tests

Urolithiasis

RENAL ULTRASOUND

Preparation of the Client

- No special preparation is indicated; however, barium in the bowel may interfere with results. If both studies are ordered, the renal ultrasound should be scheduled first.

Client and Family Teaching

- This test is noninvasive and does not use radiation. You should feel no discomfort.
- Food, fluids, and ordered medications are not restricted prior to this test.
- The test takes approximately 30 to 60 minutes to complete. During this time, you need to remain relatively still.
- A conductive paste or gel (which may be cold) is applied to your back and flank to allow sound wave transmission. Then a transducer is passed over the skin, producing pictures of the reflected sound waves.

COMPUTED TOMOGRAPHY (CT SCAN) OF THE KIDNEY

Preparation of the Client

- Verify the presence of a signed informed consent.
- Check for allergies to iodine, X-ray contrast dye, and seafood. Inform the radiology department if such an allergy exists.
- Prepare the client as ordered: NPO 4 hours prior to examination; laxatives and/or enemas may be ordered to remove gas, fecal material, or retained barium from the bowel.

Client and Family Teaching

- The test requires 30 to 60 minutes to complete, and you must lie still during the procedure.
- Lie flat on your back during the test while a doughnut-shaped scanner revolves around your body. This can cause a sensation of claustrophobia. The machine emits loud clicking sounds as it rotates.
- The radiology technician is not in the room, but you can communicate through an intercom system at all times.
- If contrast medium is used, you may experience a flushing sensation and nausea as it is injected.

when KUB, renal ultrasonography, and CT scan fail to demonstrate clear evidence of urinary calculi.
- *Cystoscopy* is used to visualize and possibly remove calculi from the urinary bladder and distal ureters.

Medications

An acute episode of renal colic is treated with analgesia and hydration. A narcotic analgesic such as morphine sulfate is given, often intravenously, to relieve pain and reduce ureteral spasm. Indomethacin, a nonsteroidal anti-inflammatory drug (NSAID), given as a suppository, may reduce the amount of narcotic analgesia required for acute renal colic. Oral or intravenous fluids reduce the risk of further stone formation and promote urine output.

After analysis of the calculus, various medications may be ordered to inhibit or prevent further lithiasis. A thiazide diuretic, frequently prescribed for calcium calculi, acts to reduce urinary calcium excretion and is very effective in preventing further stones. Potassium citrate alkalinizes urine (raises the pH), and is often prescribed to prevent stones that tend to form in acidic urine (uric acid, cystine, and some forms of calcium stones). See Table 26–2 for other preparations related to types of stones. Nursing responsibilities focus on teaching the client about the prescribed medication, its importance in preventing further stone formation, and potential adverse effects.

Dietary Management

Diet modifications are often prescribed to change the character of the urine and prevent further lithiasis.

Increased fluid intake of 2.5 to 3.0 L per day is recommended, regardless of stone composition. A fluid intake to ensure the production of approximately 2.0 to 2.5 L of urine a day prevents the stone-forming salts from becoming concentrated enough to precipitate. Fluid intake should be spaced throughout the day and evening. Some authorities recommend that clients drink one to two glasses of water at night to prevent concentration of urine during sleep.

Recommended dietary changes may include reduced intake of the primary substance forming the calculi. For calcium stones, dietary calcium and vitamin D enriched foods are limited. Limiting vitamin D inhibits the absorption of calcium from the GI tract. Calcium stones may be either a calcium phosphate salt, calcium oxalate, or a combination of both; therefore, phosphorus and/or oxalate may also be limited in the diet.

The client with uric acid stones requires a diet low in purines. Organ meats, sardines, and other high-purine foods are eliminated from the diet. Foods with moderate levels of purines, such as red and white meats and some seafoods, may be limited.

In addition to limiting certain foods, the diet may be modified to maintain a urinary pH that does not promote lithiasis. Uric acid and cystine stones tend to form in acid urine. Foods which tend to alkalinize the urine may be recommended. Because alkaline urine promotes formation of calcium stones and urinary tract infections, the diet may be modified to lower the pH of the urine. Foods that affect urinary pH and foods high in various stone components are summarized in Table 26–3.

Surgery

Treatment of existing calculi depends on the location of the stone, the extent of obstruction, renal function, the presence or absence of UTI, and the client's general state of health. In general, the stone is removed if it is causing severe obstruction, infection, unrelieved pain, or serious bleeding (Braunwald et al., 2001).

Lithotripsy, using sound or shock waves to crush a stone, is the preferred treatment for urinary calculi. Several techniques are available. **Extracorporeal shock wave lithotripsy (ESWL)** is a noninvasive technique for fragmenting kidney stones using shock waves generated outside the body. Acoustic shock waves are aimed under fluoroscopic guidance at the stone (Figure 26–3 ■). These shock waves travel through soft tissue without causing damage, but shatter the stone as its

TABLE 26–3	Examples of Food and Fluids for Teaching Clients with Urolithiasis
Foods high in calcium	Beans and lentils, chocolate and cocoa, dried fruits, canned or smoked fish except tuna, flour, milk and milk products
Foods high in oxalate	Asparagus, beer and colas, beets, cabbage, celery, chocolate and cocoa, fruits, green beans, nuts, tea, tomatoes
Purine-rich foods	Goose, organ meats, sardines and herring, venison; moderate in beef, chicken, crab, pork, salmon, veal
Acidifying foods	Cheese, cranberries, eggs, grapes, meat and poultry, plums and prunes, tomatoes, whole grains
Alkalinizing foods	Green vegetables, fruit (except as noted above), legumes, milk and milk products, rhubarb

Figure 26–3 ■ Extracorporeal shock wave lithotripsy. Acoustic shock waves generated by the shock wave generator travel through soft tissue to shatter the urinary stone into fragments, which are then eliminated in the urine.

Courtesy of Dormier Medical Products.

greater density stops their progress. Repeated shock waves pulverize the stone into fragments small enough to be eliminated in the urine. The procedure may require 30 minutes to 2 hours to complete. Intravenous or oral sedation or a transcutaneous electrical nerve stimulator (TENS unit) are used to maintain comfort during the procedure (Meeker & Rothrock, 1999). See the box on the next page for nursing care of the client undergoing a lithotripsy procedure.

Lithotripsy also may be performed using a percutaneous ultrasonic or laser technique. *Percutaneous ultrasonic lithotripsy* uses a nephroscope inserted into the kidney pelvis through a small flank incision (Figure 26–4 ■). The stone is fragmented using a small ultrasonic transducer, and the fragments are re-

NURSING CARE OF THE CLIENT HAVING LITHOTRIPSY

PREOPERATIVE CARE

- Assess knowledge and understanding of the procedure, providing information as needed. *Anxiety is reduced, and recovery is enhanced and hastened when the client is fully prepared for surgery.*
- Follow directions from the radiology department, physician, or anesthetist for withholding food and fluids and for bowel preparation prior to surgery. *Conscious sedation, general anesthesia, or spinal anesthesia may be required, depending on the procedure. Fecal material in the bowel may impede fluoroscopic visualization of the kidney and stone.*

POSTOPERATIVE CARE

- In the initial period, monitor vital signs frequently. *The kidney is highly vascular; therefore, hemorrhage and resulting shock are potential complications of lithotripsy. Bleeding may be internal or retroperitoneal and difficult to detect.*

- Monitor amount, color, and clarity of urine output. *Urine is often bright red initially, but bleeding should diminish within 48 to 72 hours. Cloudy urine may indicate the presence of an infection.*
- Maintain placement and patency of urinary catheters. Anchor ureteral catheters or nephrostomy tubes securely. Irrigate gently if ordered. *A kinked or plugged catheter may result in hydroureter, hydronephrosis, and kidney damage. Decreased urinary output and flank pain are possible symptoms of obstructed urine flow. Excessive force in irrigation may cause trauma and bleeding.*
- Prepare for discharge by teaching care of indwelling catheter, urine-collection device, and incision site (if present). Teach signs and symptoms to report: urine leakage from incision for more than 4 days, symptoms of infection, pain, bright hematuria. *Many clients are discharged with dressings and catheters in place. The client and family need necessary information to provide self-care.*
- Teach measures to reduce the risk of further lithiasis. *Many clients have repeated episodes of lithiasis and renal colic. Prevention of stone formation is important to preserve renal function.*

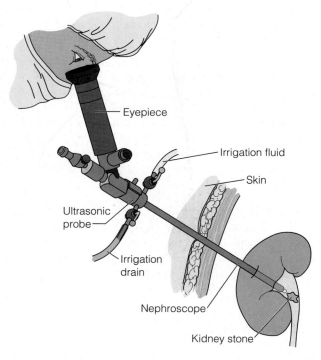

Figure 26–4 ■ Percutaneous ultrasonic lithotripsy. A nephroscope is inserted into the renal pelvis, and ultrasonic waves are used to fragment the stone. The fragments then are removed through the nephroscope.

moved through the nephroscope. *Laser lithotripsy* is an alternative to ultrasonic lithotripsy. Laser beams are used to disintegrate the stone, without damaging soft tissue. A nephroscope or a ureteroscope (passed up the ureter from the bladder during cystoscopy) is used to guide the laser probe into direct contact with the stone (Meeker & Rothrock, 1999).

A double J stent may be inserted into the affected ureter to maintain its patency following ESWL or other lithotripsy pro-

cedures. See the box on page 711 for nursing care of the client with a ureteral stent.

On rare occasions, surgical intervention is necessary to remove a calculus in the renal pelvis or ureter. *Ureterolithotomy* is incision in the affected ureter to remove a calculus. *Pyelolithotomy* is incision into and removal of a stone from the kidney pelvis. A staghorn calculus which invades the calices and renal parenchyma, may require a *nephrolithotomy* for removal. See Chapter 7 ⊖⊃ for care of the surgical client.

Bladder stones may be removed using an instrument passed through a cystoscope to crush the stones. The remaining stone fragments are then irrigated out of the bladder using an acid solution to counteract the alkalinity that precipitated stone formation.

NURSING CARE

Nursing care for the client with urolithiasis is directed at providing for comfort during acute renal colic, assisting with diagnostic procedures, ensuring adequate urinary output, and teaching the client information necessary to prevent future stone formation.

Health Promotion

Discuss the importance of maintaining an adequate fluid intake with all clients. Stress the need to increase fluid intake during warm weather and strenuous exercise or physical labor. Discuss the relationship between weight-bearing activity and retention of calcium in the bones. Encourage all clients to remain as physically active as possible to prevent bone resorption and possible hypercalciuria.

Instruct clients with known gout to maintain a generous fluid intake so as to produce at least 2 L of urine every day. Discuss the risk of lithiasis with clients who have frequent UTIs, and teach measures to reduce the incidence of UTI and the risk for lithiasis.

Assessment

Obtain subjective and objective assessment data specific to urolithiasis.

- Health history: complaints of flank, back, or abdominal pain, radiation, characteristics and timing, aggravating or relieving factors; other symptoms such as nausea and vomiting; possible contributing factors such as dehydration; previous or family history of kidney stones; current or previous treatment measures
- Physical examination: general appearance including position, vital signs; skin color, temperature, moisture, turgor; abdominal, flank, or costovertebral tenderness; amount, color, and characteristics of urine (presence of hematuria, bacteria, pyuria, pH)

Nursing Diagnoses and Interventions

Acute Pain

Pain is the primary outward manifestation of urolithiasis, particularly when a stone lodges within a ureter, causing acute obstruction and distention. Invasive and noninvasive procedures to remove or crush stones also may be painful. Clients undergoing surgery also experience incisional pain.

PRACTICE ALERT *The intensity of renal colic pain can cause a vasovagal response with resulting hypotension and syncope. Always provide for the client's safety.* ■

- Assess pain using a standard pain scale and its characteristics. Administer analgesia as ordered and monitor its effectiveness. *The intensity, type of pain, and its responsiveness to analgesia provide valuable clues as to its cause. Regular administration of prescribed analgesics controls pain more effectively than waiting until pain becomes intolerable. Administering an ordered NSAID on a routine schedule may significantly reduce the need for narcotic analgesia in clients with renal colic.*
- Unless contraindicated, encourage fluid intake and ambulation in the client with renal colic. *Increased fluids and ambulation increase urinary output, facilitating movement of the calculus through the ureter and decreasing pain.*
- Use nonpharmacologic measures such as positioning, moist heat, relaxation techniques, guided imagery, and diversion as adjunctive therapy for pain relief. *Adjunctive pain relief measures can enhance the effectiveness of analgesics and other prescribed treatment.*
- If surgery has been performed, monitor urinary output, catheters, incision, and wound drainage. *Pain may be a symptom of proximal distention due to a blocked catheter. Infection or hematoma at the surgical site can significantly increase perceived pain.*

Impaired Urinary Elimination

Obstruction of the urinary tract is the primary problem associated with urolithiasis. Obstruction can ultimately lead to stasis, infection, or irreversible renal damage.

- Monitor amount and character of urine output. If catheterized, measure output hourly. Document any hematuria, dysuria, frequency, urgency, and pyuria. Strain all urine for stones, saving any recovered stones for laboratory analysis. *The amount of urine output helps determine possible urinary tract obstruction and adequacy of hydration. Hematuria, gross or microscopic, is often associated with calculi and with procedures used to remove stones, such as cystoscopy or lithotripsy. A change in the amount of hematuria may indicate stone passage or a complication. Dysuria, frequency, urgency, and cloudy urine are symptoms of UTI, often associated with urolithiasis. Antibiotic therapy may be required. Analysis of stones recovered from the urine can direct measures to prevent further lithiasis.*

PRACTICE ALERT *A stone that completely obstructs the ureter can lead to hydronephrosis and kidney damage on the affected side. Report symptoms of hydronephrosis such as dull flank pain or aching and changes in renal function studies (BUN and serum creatinine). Because the other kidney continues to function, urine output may not fall significantly with obstruction of one ureter. A rising BUN and serum creatinine may be early signs of renal failure.* ■

- Maintain patency and integrity of all catheter systems. Secure catheters well, label as indicated, and use sterile technique for all ordered irrigations or other procedures. *A kinked or plugged catheter, particularly a ureteral catheter or nephrostomy tube, may damage the urinary system. Labeling catheters can prevent mistakes, such as inappropriate irrigation or clamping. Any catheter increases the risk of infection; aseptic technique in all procedures reduces this risk.*

Deficient Knowledge

The client with urolithiasis has multiple learning needs. These include information about the disease and its possible consequences, any diagnostic or therapeutic procedures performed, and strategies to prevent future lithiasis.

- Assess understanding and previous learning. *Relating information to previously learned material enhances retention and understanding.*
- Present all material in a manner appropriate to knowledge base, developmental and educational level, and current needs. *Learning is an active process that requires the client's participation. Tailoring teaching to the individual increases involvement.*
- Teach about all diagnostic and treatment procedures. *Knowing what to expect reduces anxiety, enhances compliance, and hastens recovery.*
- If the client will be managed in the community, teach to:
  a. Collect and strain all urine, saving any stones.
  b. Report stone passage to the physician and bring the stone in for analysis.
  c. Report any changes in the amount or character of urine output to physician.

When pain can be managed with oral analgesics, urinary stones are managed in the community. The client needs to know how and why to collect the calculus and indicators of complications, such as reduced urine output and cloudy or bloody urine.

- Teach measures to prevent further urolithiasis.
  a. Increase fluid intake to 2500 to 3500 mL per day.
  b. Follow recommended dietary guidelines.
  c. Maintain activity level to prevent urinary stasis and bone resorption.
  d. Take medications as prescribed.

  The risk of recurrent lithiasis is approximately 50%; however, this risk can be reduced by measures to prevent conditions favoring stone formation.

- Teach about the relationship between urinary calculi and UTI, emphasizing preventive measures and the importance of prompt treatment. *Urinary tract infection promotes urolithiasis and thus requires prompt treatment to reduce this risk.*

Using NANDA, NIC, and NOC

Chart 26–2 shows links between NANDA nursing diagnoses, NIC, and NOC for the client with urinary calculi.

Home Care

The client with urinary calculi needs to know how to manage existing stones and what to do to reduce the risk of future stone formation. Discuss the following topics to prepare the client and family for home care.

- Importance of maintaining a fluid intake adequate to produce 2.0 to 2.5 quarts of urine per day
- Prescribed medications, their management, and potential adverse effects
- Dietary recommendations
- Prevention, recognition, and management of UTI
- Any further diagnostic or treatment measures planned

When the client is to be discharged with dressings, a nephrostomy tube, or a catheter, teach the client and family about the following:

- How to change dressings, maintaining aseptic technique
- Assessment of the wound and skin for healing and possible complications such as infection or skin breakdown
- How to manage drainage systems and maintain their patency
- Emptying drainage bags and assessing urine output
- When to contact the physician and recommendations for follow-up care

CHART 26–2   NANDA, NIC, AND NOC LINKAGES

The Client with Urinary Calculi

NURSING DIAGNOSES	NURSING INTERVENTIONS	NURSING OUTCOMES
• Acute Pain	• Pain Management • Analgesic Administration	• Pain Control • Pain: Disruptive Effects
• Impaired Urinary Elimination	• Fluid Management • Specimen Management	• Urinary Elimination
• Deficient Knowledge	• Teaching: Disease Process • Teaching: Procedure/Treatment	• Knowledge: Illness Care • Knowledge: Treatment Regimen

Note. Data from Nursing Outcomes Classification (NOC) by M. Johnson & M. Maas (Eds.), 1997, St. Louis: Mosby; Nursing Diagnoses: Definitions & Classification 2001–2002 by North American Nursing Diagnosis Association, 2001, Philadelphia: NANDA; Nursing Interventions Classification (NIC) by J.C. McCloskey & G. M. Bulechek (Eds.), 2000, St. Louis: Mosby. Reprinted by permission.

Nursing Care Plan
A Client with Urinary Calculi

Richard Leton, age 44, owns a small business. He is admitted to the medical unit from the emergency department after awakening at 4:00 A.M. with severe right-sided pain. His CBC is normal, and urinalysis reveals microscopic hematuria, but no protein or bacteria. A renal ultrasound shows a 4 to 5 mm stone partially obstructing the right ureter.

Stephen Phillips, Mr. Leton's admitting nurse, notes that he is pale, diaphoretic, and very anxious. He complains of nausea and asks for an emesis basin. Mr. Leton received 4 mg of intravenous morphine sulphate shortly after admission to the ED, approxi-

mately 2.5 hours ago. He denies pain at this time, but says, "I'm scared to death that it'll come back—I couldn't even move, it hurt so bad."

ASSESSMENT

Mr. Leton's history reveals no previous episodes of renal calculi. He felt well until the pain awakened him during the night. He admits that he has been working under a deadline to complete a construction project and that he probably has not been drinking

(continued on page 722)

Nursing Care Plan
A Client with Urinary Calculi (continued)

enough fluids "considering how hot it's been." Physical assessment findings include T 100.4°F (38.0°C) PO, P 98, R 24, and BP 160/86. Color is pale to ashen, skin cool and moist. Abdomen firm with moderate tenderness in the right upper outer quadrant. The ED physician orders an IV of 5% dextrose in 1/2 normal saline at 200 mL/hr until nausea relieved, then PO fluids of at least 3000 mL/24 hr; morphine sulfate (MS) 2 to 10 mg IV prn severe pain; indomethacin (Indocin) 50 mg per rectal suppository q8h; promethazine (Phenergan) 25 mg PO or per suppository q6h prn nausea; activity to tolerance; and strain all urine, sending recovered stones for analysis.

DIAGNOSIS

- *Anxiety* related to anticipation of recurrent severe pain
- *Risk for imbalanced nutrition: Less than body requirements,* related to nausea
- *Acute pain* related to partial obstruction of right ureter by calculus
- *Impaired urinary elimination* related to partial obstruction of ureter by calculus
- *Deficient knowledge* related to lack of information about disease process, contributing factors, and management

EXPECTED OUTCOMES

- Demonstrate reduced anxiety by relaxed facial expression, vital signs within his normal range, and ability to rest when not disturbed.
- Consume at least 50% of diet and 100% of ordered fluids without nausea or vomiting.
- Request analgesia as needed at onset of pain; report effective pain relief.
- Maintain urine output of 2500 mL/24 hr with no signs of infection or obstruction (such as increased pain, dysuria, pyuria, or hematuria).
- Relate an understanding of the process of urolithiasis and contributing factors.
- Verbalize dietary, fluid intake, and other measures to reduce risk of future stone formation.

PLANNING AND IMPLEMENTATION

- Reassure that measures to prevent further episodes of renal colic are being implemented, and that medication is available to relieve pain promptly.
- Assess the effectiveness of analgesia and its adverse effects, especially nausea.
- Maintain IV as ordered until oral fluid intake exceeds 200 mL of fluid per hour while awake.
- Measure and strain all urine. Assess urine for color, clarity, and odor.
- Teach about urolithiasis and its risk factors, especially as they relate to Mr. Leton.
- Teach the importance of maintaining a high fluid intake, especially when working outdoors in hot weather; recommended dietary modifications and their rationale; ordered medications and their effects; how to identify and prevent UTI; and symptoms that should be reported to the physician.

EVALUATION

Mr. Leton passed the obstructing stone the evening after admission and is discharged the following day. On discharge, he denies pain or nausea, his urine is clear and pale yellow, and urinalysis is normal. Laboratory analysis shows that the calculus was calcium. Mr. Leton is able to state the importance of continuing a high fluid intake. He verbalizes that he will reduce his intake of calcium-rich foods, such as milk and milk products, and that he will increase his intake of foods to acidify his urine. He is able to list foods to include in his diet. He states, "You'd better believe I'll follow my diet, drink my water, and make sure I don't get an infection. I hope to never feel pain like that again!"

Critical Thinking in the Nursing Process

1. What factors contributed to the onset and timing of Mr. Leton's ureteral colic?
2. What is the rationale for administering indomethacin, an NSAID, to a client with ureteral colic?
3. Why did Mr. Phillips include a nursing intervention to assess for a relationship between Mr. Leton's nausea, his pain, and the ordered analgesic agent?

See Evaluating Your Response in Appendix C.

THE CLIENT WITH A URINARY TRACT TUMOR

A malignancy can develop in any part of the urinary tract; however, 90% develop in the bladder, about 8% develop in the renal pelvis, and only 2% in the ureter or urethra (Braunwald et al., 2001). When diagnosed early, the 5-year survival rate for bladder cancer is 94% (American Cancer Society [ACS], 2002).

An estimated 56,500 new cases of bladder cancer were diagnosed in the United States in 2002, and 12,600 people died as a result of the disease. The incidence of bladder cancer is about 4 times higher in men than it is in women, and about twice as high in whites as it is in blacks (ACS, 2002). Most people who develop bladder cancer are over age 60.

Two major factors are implicated in the development of bladder cancer: the presence of carcinogens in the urine and chronic inflammation or infection of bladder mucosa (See Box 26–2). Cigarette smoking is the primary risk factor for bladder cancer. The risk in smokers is twice that of nonsmokers (ACS, 2002). The chemicals and dyes used in the plastics, rubber, and cable industries; substances in the work environment of textile workers, leather finishers, spray painters, hair dressers, and petroleum workers; and the chronic use of phenacetin-containing analgesic agents also are associated with a higher risk. Additional risk factors for bladder cancer include residence in an urban area, chronic UTIs, and bladder calculi. The parasite *Schistosoma haematocium,* endemic to Egypt and the Sudan, also increases the risk for bladder cancer (Porth, 2002).

PATHOPHYSIOLOGY

Most urinary tract malignancies arise from epithelial tissue. Transitional epithelium lines the entire tract from the renal pelvis through the urethra. Carcinogenic breakdown products of certain chemicals and from cigarette smoke are excreted in the urine and stored in the bladder, possibly causing a local influence on abnormal cell development. Squamous cell carcinoma of the urinary tract occurs less frequently than transitional epithelial cell tumors.

Urinary tract tumors begin as nonspecific cellular alterations that develop into either flat or papillary lesions. These lesions may be either superficial or invasive. About 75% of bladder tumors are papillary lesions (*papillomas*), a polyplike structure attached by a stalk to the bladder mucosa (Figure 26–5 ■). Papillomas are generally superficial, noninvasive tumors that bleed easily and frequently recur (Braunwald et al., 2001). They rarely progress to become invasive, and the prognosis for recovery is good.

Carcinoma in situ (CIS), which occurs less frequently, is a poorly differentiated flat tumor that invades directly and is associated with a poorer prognosis. Bladder tumors are rated by their cell type and grade. Grade I tumors are highly differentiated and rarely progress to become invasive, whereas grade III tumors are poorly differentiated and usually progress (Braunwald et al., 2001). The staging of bladder tumors is outlined in Table 26–4. See Chapter 10 ◯◯ for more information about tumor grading and staging. When metastasis oc-

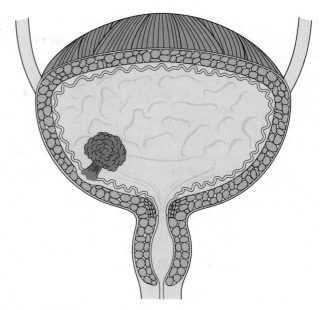

Figure 26–5 ■ A papillary transitional cell carcinoma of the urinary bladder with minimal invasion of the bladder wall.

curs, the pelvic lymph nodes, lungs, bones, and liver are most commonly involved.

MANIFESTATIONS

Painless hematuria is the presenting sign in 75% of urinary tract tumors. Hematuria may be gross or microscopic and is often intermittent, causing delay in seeking treatment (Porth, 2002). Inflammation surrounding the tumor occasionally causes manifestations of a urinary tract infection, including frequency, urgency, and dysuria. Ureteral tumors may cause colicky pain from obstruction. Tumors of the urinary tract typically cause few outward signs and may not be discovered until obstructed urine flow causes flank pain or renal failure.

COLLABORATIVE CARE

Treatment of the client with a tumor of the urinary tract focuses on removal or destruction of the cancerous tissue, prevention of further invasion or metastasis, and maintenance of renal and urinary function.

TABLE 26–4	Bladder Tumor Staging	

Depth of Involvement	TNM (Tumor, Node, Metastasis) Stage	Tumor Involvement
Superficial	T_a	Limited to the bladder mucosa
	T_1	Involvement of the bladder mucosa and submucosal layers
Invasive	T_2	Invasion of superficial muscle of bladder wall
	T_{3a}	Deep muscle invasion
	T_{3b}	Involvement of perivesicular fat
	$T_{3-4}N_+$	Regional (pelvic) lymph node involvement
	$T_{3-4}M_1$	Metastasis to distant lymph nodes or organs

Diagnostic Tests

When a urinary tract tumor is suspected, the following diagnostic tests may be ordered.

- *Urinalysis* is done to evaluate for hematuria. Gross or microscopic hematuria is often the first indicator of a neoplasm in the urinary tract.
- *Urine cytology,* microscopic examination of cells in the urine, is performed to identify abnormal cells (tumor or pretumor cells). Periodic urine cytology is recommended for clients at high risk for bladder cancer or its recurrence due to carcinogen exposure.
- *Ultrasound of the bladder* is a noninvasive test to detect bladder tumors. No dye is required, and the client is not exposed to radiation.
- *Intravenous pyelography* is used to evaluate the structure and function of the kidneys, ureters, and bladder. IVP may reveal a rigid deformity of the bladder wall, obstruction of urine flow at the point of the tumor, or bladder filling or emptying defects.
- *Cystoscopy* and *ureteroscopy* allow direct visualization, assessment, and biopsy of lesions of the urethra, bladder, or ureters using a lighted scope inserted through the urethra. Cystoscopy or ureteroscopy with biopsy allow definitive diagnosis of urinary tract tumors.
- *Computed tomography (CT scan)* or *magnetic resonance imaging (MRI)* are primarily used to evaluate tumor invasion or metastasis.

See the box on pages 708–709 for nursing implications of these diagnostic studies.

Medications

Immunologic or chemotherapeutic agents administered by intravesical instillation (into the bladder) may be used either as the primary treatment for bladder cancer or to prevent recurrence following endoscopic tumor removal. Bacille Calmette-Guérin (BCGLive, TheraCys) is a suspension of attenuated *Mycobacterium bovis* used to treat CIS and recurrent bladder tumors. Instillation into the bladder causes a local inflammatory reaction that eliminates or reduces superficial tumors. Systemic

mycobacterial infection is a rare complication of intravesical BCG therapy that may require antituberculin treatment (Tierney et al., 2001). Other chemotherapeutic agents also may be administered intravesically, including doxorubicin and mitomycin C. Bladder irritation, frequency, dysuria, and contact dermatitis are possible adverse reactions to intravesical chemotherapy.

Radiation Therapy

Radiation is another adjunctive therapy used in the treatment of urinary tumors. Although radiation alone is not curative, it can reduce tumor size prior to surgery and is used as palliative treatment for inoperable tumors and clients who cannot tolerate surgery. Radiation therapy also is used in combination with systemic chemotherapy to improve local and distant relapse rates (Tierney et al., 2001) (see Chapter 10). 🔗

Surgery

A number of surgical procedures, ranging from simple resection of noninvasive tumors to removal of the bladder and surrounding structures, are used to treat urinary tract tumors. Indications for each procedure and specific nursing implications are outlined in Table 26–5.

Transurethral tumor resection may be performed by excision, *fulguration* (destruction of tissue using electric sparks generated by high-frequency current) or *laser photocoagulation* (use of light energy to destroy abnormal tissue). Laser surgery carries the lowest risk of bleeding and perforation of the bladder wall. Following cystoscopic tumor resection, clients are followed at 3-month intervals for tumor recurrence. Recurrences may develop anywhere in the urinary tract, including the renal pelvis, ureter, or urethra (Braunwald et al., 2001).

Cystectomy, surgical removal of the bladder, is necessary to treat invasive cancers. Partial cystectomy may be done to remove a solitary lesion; however, radical cystectomy is the standard treatment for invasive tumors. The bladder and adjacent muscles and tissues are removed. In men, the prostate and seminal vessels are also removed, resulting in impotence. In women, a total hysterectomy and bilateral salpingo-

TABLE 26–5	Surgical Procedures Used to Treat Bladder Tumors	
Procedure	**Indications**	**Nursing Implications**
Transurethral resection of bladder tumor	Diagnose and treat superficial bladder tumors having low rate of recurrence; control bleeding	Maintain continuous bladder irrigation postoperatively; monitor for excessive bleeding; ensure catheter patency. Increase fluids to 2500-3000 mL per day. Give stool softeners to prevent straining.
Partial cystectomy	Resect solitary, isolated tumor at stage B or C not involving trigone	Maintain patency of urethral and/or suprapubic catheter to make sure suture lines are free of pressure; monitor for excess bleeding.
Complete or radical cystectomy	Remove large, invasive tumors; involvement of trigone	Permanent urinary diversion is required. Maintain patency and position of stents; urethral catheter may be in place to drain pelvic cavity.

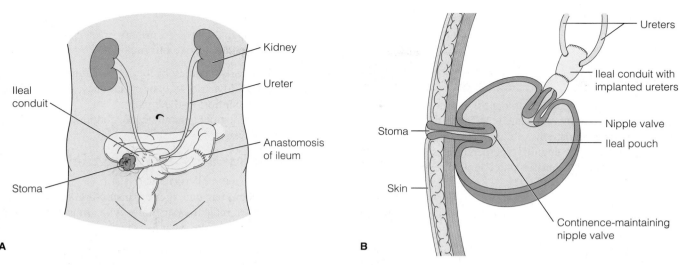

Figure 26–6 ■ Common urinary diversion procedures. *A,* Ileal conduit. A segment of ileum is separated from the small intestine and formed into a tubular pouch with the open end brought to the skin surface to form a stoma. The ureters are connected to the pouch. *B,* A continent urinary diversion. A segment of ileum is separated from the small intestine and formed into a pouch. Nipple valves are formed at each end of the pouch by intussuscepting tissue backward into the reservoir to prevent leakage.

oophorectomy (removal of the uterus, uterine tubes, and ovaries) accompanies the procedure, causing sterility. At the time of surgery, a **urinary diversion** is created to provide for urine collection and drainage. Either an *ileal conduit* (Figure 26–6A■) or a *continent urinary diversion* (Figure 26–6B) is created to collect and drain urine. Table 26–6 describes the most frequently used urinary diversion techniques.

Surgical procedures to remove tumors involving other portions of the urinary tract vary according to the site and stage of the tumor. When the distal ureter is involved, the tumor may be resected and the ureter implanted into the opposite ureter to provide for drainage. A proximal ureteral tumor necessitates removal of the ureter and kidney on the affected side.

TABLE 26–6 Urinary Diversion Procedures

Procedure	Description	Nursing Considerations
Ileal conduit	Portion of ileum is isolated from small intestine, leaving vascular, lymphatic, and neural connections intact; ileum is formed into pouch with open end brought to surface to form a stoma; ureters are inserted into pouch.	Most common urinary diversion. Continuous urine drainage necessitates appliance. Postoperative edema may interfere with urine output. Risk of infection is less than for cutaneous ureterostomy, but potential for reflux is high. Good skin care vital because of constant contact with urine.
Continent internal ileal reservoir or continent ileal bladder conduit (Kock's pouch)	Pouch is created as for ileal conduit but nipple valves are formed by intussuscepting tissue backward into a reservoir to connect pouch to the skin and the ureters to the pouch; filling pressure closes valves, preventing leakage and reflux.	Drainage collection device not necessary. Client must be willing and able to perform clean intermittent self-catheterization every 2 to 4 hours. Continence valve mechanism may fail, requiring surgery for revision.
Indiana continent urinary reservoir	A portion of the terminal ileum, ascending colon, and cecum is isolated from the bowel with vascular and neural connections intact. Reservoir is formed from colon and cecum; portion of the ileum is brought to the surface to form nipple valve and stoma or is attached to urethral stump.	As for Kock's pouch. Client must be able and motivated to manage self-catheterization. Reservoir may absorb urea and electrolytes, resulting in imbalances. Significant portion of bowel is required to form pouch and stoma.
Ileocystoplasty or Camey procedure	Section of the ileum is isolated and formed into U shape. Ureters are implanted in upper portion of the U. Urethra is anastamosed to central section.	Appropriate for men only because urethra is removed with cystectomy in women. Allows client to void by relaxing pelvic muscles and using Valsalva maneuver.

See the box below for nursing care of the client undergoing tumor resection and a urinary diversion.

NURSING CARE

The client who undergoes treatment for a tumor of the urinary tract has many nursing care needs because of alterations in the functional health patterns of elimination, health perception/health management, cognitive/perceptual, self-perception/self-concept, role/relationship, and coping/stress tolerance.

Health Promotion

Encourage all clients not to smoke. Provide referral to smoking cessation programs or clinics for clients who wish to quit smoking. Encourage clients at high risk for developing bladder cancer (see Box 26–2 on page 723) to have periodic examinations, including urinalysis and possible urine cytology.

Assessment

Nursing assessment related to urinary tract cancer includes both subjective and objective information.

- Health history: risk factors; history of hematuria or manifestations of UTI (dysuria, frequency, urgency, pyuria); lower abdominal discomfort or flank pain
- Physical examination: general health; abdominal tenderness; urine for analysis.

Nursing Diagnoses and Interventions

Impaired Urinary Elimination

Whether the client has undergone transurethral resection of a bladder tumor or radical cystectomy with urinary diversion, urinary elimination is altered at least temporarily.

- Monitor urine output from all catheters, stents, and tubes for amount, color, and clarity hourly for the first 24 hours postoperatively, then every 4 to 8 hours. *Decreased urine output*

NURSING CARE OF THE CLIENT HAVING CYSTECTOMY AND URINARY DIVERSION

PREOPERATIVE CARE

- Provide routine preoperative care as outlined in Chapter 7. ⊘
- Assess knowledge of the proposed surgery and its long-term implications, clarifying misunderstandings and discussing concerns. *Clients having surgery for cancer of the urinary tract are trying to cope with diagnosis of cancer and may not fully understand the surgery and its potential effects. Open discussion can facilitate postoperative recovery and adjustment.*
- Begin teaching about postoperative tubes and drains, self-care of stoma, and control of drainage and odor. *Postoperative physiologic and psychologic stressors may interfere with learning. A basic understanding of what to expect in the way of tubes, drains, and procedures reduces stress in the immediate postoperative period. Preoperative teaching can enhance recall and postoperative learning.*
- Assist in identifying stoma site, avoiding folds of skin, bones, scar tissue, and the waistline or belt area. Be sure to consider the client's occupation and style of clothing. The site should be visible to the client and accessible for manipulation. *Stoma placement is a vital component of adjustment and self-care. Care is taken to place the stoma away from areas of constant irritation by clothing or movement. It should be located so that the client can cover and disguise the collecting device, maintain the seal to prevent leakage, and effectively cleanse and maintain the site.*
- Perform bowel-preparation activities as ordered. *Bowel preparation is done to prevent fecal contamination of the peritoneal cavity and to decompress the bowel during surgery.*

POSTOPERATIVE CARE

- Provide routine postoperative care (See Chapter 7).
- Monitor intake and output carefully, assessing urine output every hour for the first 24 hours, then every 4 hours or as ordered. Call the physician if urine output is less than 30 mL per hour. *Tissue edema and bleeding may interfere with urinary output from stoma, catheters, or drains. Maintenance of urine out-*

flow is vital to prevent hydronephrosis and possible renal damage. A urine output of at least 30 mL per hour is necessary for effective renal function.
- Assess color and consistency of urine. Expect pink or bright red urine fading to pink and then clearing by the third postoperative day. Urine may be cloudy due to mucus production by bowel mucosa. *Bright red blood in the urine from a urinary diversion may indicate hemorrhage, necessitating further surgery. Excessive cloudiness or malodorous urine may indicate infection.*
- Assess size, color, and condition of the stoma and surrounding skin every 2 hours for the first 24 hours, then every 4 hours for 48 to 72 hours. Expect the stoma to appear bright red and slightly edematous initially. Slight bleeding during cleansing is normal. *Compromised circulation causes the stoma to appear pale, gray, or cyanotic or blanch when touched. Other complications, such as infection or impaired healing may be evidenced by a change in the appearance of the stoma or incision.*
- Irrigate the ileal diversion catheter with 30 to 60 mL of normal saline every 4 hours or as ordered. *Mucus produced by the bowel wall may accumulate in the newly devised reservoir or obstruct catheters.*
- Monitor serum electrolyte values, acid-base balance, and renal function tests such as BUN and serum creatinine. *Reabsorption of electrolytes from reservoirs created by portions of bowel may result in electrolyte imbalance and metabolic acidosis. Optimal renal function is necessary to maintain a normal state of homeostasis.*
- Teach the client and family about stoma and urinary diversion care, including odor management, skin care, increased fluid intake, pouch application and leakage prevention, self-catheterization for clients with continent reservoirs, and signs of infection and other complications. *The ability to provide self-care is a significant factor in the adjustment to a changed body image. Teaching family members facilitates acceptance and adjustment. The family also needs this knowledge in case illness or disability interferes with the self-care capacity.*

may indicate impaired catheter or drainage system patency. Prompt intervention is necessary to prevent hydronephrosis. A change in color or clarity may indicate a complication such as hemorrhage or infection.

PRACTICE ALERT *Promptly report urine output of less than 30 mL per hour, which may indicate low vascular volume or renal insufficiency. Prompt intervention is vital to restore cardiac output and prevent acute renal failure.* ■

- Label all catheters, stents, and their drainage containers. Maintain separate closed gravity drainage systems for each. *Clear identification of each tube can prevent errors in irrigating and calculating outputs. Separate closed systems minimize the risk and extent of potential bacterial contamination and resultant infection.*

PRACTICE ALERT *Use aseptic techniques and strictly follow guidelines for irrigating catheters. Catheters placed in the kidney pelvis are irrigated using gentle pressure and small amounts of fluid (10 to 15 mL) to avoid damaging renal tissues.* ■

- Secure ureteral catheters and stents with tape; prevent kinking or occlusion; and maintain gravity flow by keeping drainage bag below level of kidneys. *Impaired urine flow can lead to urinary retention and distention of the bladder, a newly created reservoir, or the renal pelvis (hydronephrosis).*
- Encourage fluid intake of 3000 mL per day. *Increased fluid intake maintains a high urinary output, reducing the risk of infection. Dilute urine is less irritating to the skin surrounding the stoma site. Electrolyte reabsorption from reservoirs may increase risk of calculi; high fluid intake and urine output reduce this risk.*

PRACTICE ALERT *Monitor urine output closely for first 24 hours after stents or ureteral catheters are removed. Edema or stricture of ureters may impede output, leading to hydronephrosis and kidney damage.* ■

- Encourage activity to tolerance. *Ambulation promotes drainage of urine from reservoirs and helps prevent calcium loss from bones, which could precipitate calculus formation.*

Risk for Impaired Skin Integrity
The skin surrounding the stoma site of an ileal conduit is at risk for irritation and breakdown. Because urine is acidic and contains high concentrations of electrolytes, it has a corrosive effect on skin. In addition, adhesives and sealants used to prevent pouch leakage may irritate the skin.

- Assess peristomal skin for redness, excoriation, or signs of breakdown. Assess for urine leakage from catheters, stents, or drains. Keep the skin clean and dry. Change wet dressings. *Intact skin is the first line of defense against infection. Impaired skin integrity may lead to local or systemic infection and impaired healing.*

BOX 26–3 ■ **Urinary Stoma Care**

- ■ Gather all supplies: a clean, disposable pouch; liquid skin barrier or barrier ring; 4-by-4 gauze squares; stoma guide; adhesive solvent; clean gloves; and a clean washcloth.
- ■ Assess knowledge, learning needs, and ability and willingness to assist with procedure. Explain the procedure as needed.
- ■ Use standard precautions.
- ■ Remove old pouch, pulling gently away from skin. Warm water or adhesive solvent may be used to loosen the seal if necessary.
- ■ Assess stoma. Normally the stoma is bright red and appears moist. Report a dark purple, black, or very pale stoma to the physician. Slight bleeding with cleansing is normal, especially in the immediate postoperative period.
- ■ Prevent urine flow during cleaning by placing a rolled gauze square or tampon over the stoma opening.
- ■ Cleanse skin around the stoma with soap and water, rinse, and pat or air dry.
- ■ Use the stoma guide to determine correct size for the bag opening and/or protective ring seal. Trim the bag or seal as needed.
- ■ Apply skin barrier; allow to dry.
- ■ Apply the bag with an opening no more than 1 to 2 mm wider than outside of stoma. Allow no wrinkles or creases where the bag contacts the skin.
- ■ Connect bag to the urine-collection device. Dispose of old pouch, used supplies, and gloves appropriately. Wash hands.
- ■ Chart procedure, including stoma appearance and response of the client.

- Ensure gravity drainage of urine collection device or empty bag every 2 hours. *Overfilling of the collection bag may damage the seal, allowing leakage and contact of urine with skin.*
- Change urine collection appliance as needed, removing any mucus from stoma. See Box 26–3 for care of a urinary drainage stoma. *Meticulous care and protection of skin surrounding stoma can maintain integrity and prevent breakdown.*

Disturbed Body Image
A radical cystectomy and urinary diversion affect the client's body image. In most cases, an abdominal stoma is created, requiring either a drainage appliance or regular catheterization of the stoma to drain urine. Removal of the prostate and seminal vesicles or the uterus and ovaries leaves the client sterile. If radiation or chemotherapy is planned as adjunctive therapy, the client may experience hair loss, stomatitis, nausea and vomiting, or other disturbing side effects of therapy.

- Use therapeutic communication techniques, actively listening and responding to the client's and family's concerns. *Clients must know their feelings and concerns are respected and valued. Denial, anger, guilt, bargaining, or depression are common during grieving and normal for a client undergoing a significant change in body image.*
- Recognize and accept behaviors that indicate use of coping mechanisms, encouraging adaptive mechanisms. *The client may initially use defensive coping mechanisms such as denial, minimization, and dissociation from the immediate*

situation to reduce anxiety and maintain psychologic integrity. Adaptive mechanisms include learning as much as possible about the surgery and its effects, practicing procedures, setting realistic goals, and rehearsing various alternative outcomes.

- Encourage looking at, touching, and caring for the stoma and appliance as soon as possible. Allow the client to proceed gradually, providing support and encouragement. *Accepting the stoma as part of the self is vital to adapting to the changed body image and is indicated by a willingness to provide self-care.*

- Discuss concerns about returning to usual activities, perceived relationship changes, and resumption of sexual relations. Provide referral to support group or provide for contact with someone who has successfully adjusted to a urinary diversion. *Clients and families may be reluctant to discuss topics of concern. An atmosphere of openness and acceptance facilitates expression of concerns and anxieties related to the changed body image.*

Risk for Infection

Diagnostic instrumentation procedures, surgical manipulation, and disruption of normal urinary tract defense mechanisms increase the risk of ascending urinary tract infection. When an ileal conduit or artificial bladder is created using bowel tissue, the normal bacteriostatic activity of bladder mucosa is lost. In addition, the peristaltic action of the ureters may be disrupted, and the ureterovesical junction no longer prevents urine reflux. Adjunctive chemotherapy or radiation treatments may impair normal immune function and further increase the risk of infection.

- Maintain separate closed drainage systems, keeping drainage bags lower than the kidney, and prevent loops or kinks in drainage tubing, which impede urine flow. *Although urine is sterile when it leaves the kidney, bacteria grow rapidly in urine. Prevention of urine reflux is essential to preventing UTI.*

- Monitor for signs of infection: elevated temperature, cloudy or foul-smelling urine, hematuria, general malaise, back or abdominal pain, and nausea and vomiting. *Infection undermines*

PRACTICE ALERT *Impaired immune function (due to aging or the effects of chemotherapy) and urine cloudiness (related to the effects of urine on ileal mucosa) can mask usual signs of UTI such as fever and altered urine clarity. Be alert for more generalized manifestations such as increased fatigue and malaise.* ■

the healing process. Early detection and treatment help prevent long-term consequences such as chronic pyelonephritis.

- Teach signs and symptoms of infection and self-care measures to prevent UTI. *The client with a cystectomy and ileal diversion, urostomy, or continent reservoir is at risk of UTI for life because of impaired urinary defense mechanisms. Using clean or aseptic technique in providing care, increasing fluid intake, and using measures to acidify urine minimize this risk to a certain degree but do not eliminate it.*

Using NANDA, NIC, and NOC

Chart 26–3 shows links between NANDA nursing diagnoses, NIC, and NOC for the client with a urinary tract tumor.

Home Care

The need for individual and family teaching for the client who has had surgery to treat a urinary tract tumor is significant. For many clients, surgery means a lifelong change in urinary elimination. Even the client who has undergone transurethral excision of bladder tumors requires follow-up cystoscopy on a regular basis and needs to be alert for signs of tumor recurrence.

The client who has had a urinary diversion needs teaching about care of the stoma and surrounding skin, prevention of urine reflux and infection, signs and symptoms of UTI and renal calculi, and, in some cases, self-catheterization using clean technique.

CHART 26–3 NANDA, NIC, AND NOC LINKAGES

The Client with Bladder Cancer

NURSING DIAGNOSES	NURSING INTERVENTIONS	NURSING OUTCOMES
• Disturbed Body Image	• Coping Enhancement • Grief Work Facilitation	• Body Image • Grief Resolution
• Ineffective Management of Therapeutic Regimen	• Teaching: Procedure/Treatment • Self-Responsibility Facilitation	• Treatment Behavior: Illness or Injury • Knowledge: Treatment Regimen • Participation: Health Care Decisions
• Risk for Impaired Skin Integrity	• Skin Surveillance • Wound Care	• Tissue Integrity: Skin and Mucous Membranes • Wound Healing: Primary Intention
• Sexual Dysfunction	• Teaching: Sexuality	• Sexual Functioning

Note. Data from Nursing Outcomes Classification (NOC) *by M. Johnson & M. Maas (Eds.), 1997, St. Louis: Mosby;* Nursing Diagnoses: Definitions & Classification 2001–2002 *by North American Nursing Diagnosis Association, 2001, Philadelphia: NANDA;* Nursing Interventions Classification (NIC) *by J.C. McCloskey & G. M. Bulechek (Eds.), 2000, St. Louis: Mosby. Reprinted by permission.*

Nursing Care Plan
A Client with a Bladder Tumor

Ben Hussain is a 61-year-old automobile salesman. He is married and has five children, all of whom are grown and living away from home. One week ago, Mr. Hussain became alarmed when his urine became bright red. Even though he had no other symptoms, he called his physician. The physician ordered a urinalysis and urine cytology, revealing gross hematuria and poorly differentiated abnormal cells. Cystoscopy and tissue biopsy confirm a stage C tumor involving the bladder trigone. Mr. Hussain is admitted for a radical cystectomy and continent urinary diversion.

ASSESSMENT

Mr. Hussain's admission history, obtained by Tara Mills, RN, his primary nurse, indicates that he has lost 10 to 15 pounds over the last few months. He smoked two to three packs of cigarettes per day for 40 years, but cut back to a pack a day about a year ago. He says he could not quit smoking entirely. He drinks five to six cups of coffee daily and consumes a moderate amount of alcohol, averaging three to four drinks a day. Mr. Hussain says that he is "a little nervous about surgery and what they're going to find." Ms. Mills notes that he fidgets and talks rapidly throughout their interview. He also expresses concern about how he will handle the pain after surgery, because he has never been hospitalized before his cystoscopy. Physical assessment findings include T 98.2°F (36.7°C) PO, P 84, R 18, and BP 154/86. Examinations of the skin, neuromuscular, and cardiac systems are within normal limits. Scattered expiratory crackles are noted on auscultation of lung fields. Bowel sounds are very active; Mr. Hussain explains that he began taking his bowel-preparation laxative the day before admission. Slight tenderness is noted in the suprapubic region. Mr. Hussain's urine is clear and bright pink. Complete blood count (CBC) and chemistry screening results are within normal limits. Surgery is planned for 9:00 A.M. the following day.

DIAGNOSIS

- *Anxiety* related to undetermined extent of disease and fear of pain
- *Deficient knowledge* related to care and management of continent urinary diversion
- *Impaired urinary elimination* related to cystectomy and urinary diversion
- *Risk for impaired gas exchange* related to smoking history and effects of anesthesia

EXPECTED OUTCOMES

- Verbalize decreased feelings of anxiety.
- Demonstrate appropriate postoperative pain relief through subjective reports of pain severity and objective findings.
- Be able to care for urinary diversion and surrounding skin, prior to discharge.
- Demonstrate self-catheterization of stoma using appropriate technique prior to discharge.
- Maintain normal urine output with acceptable color and clarity and no signs of infection.

- Maintain adequate gas exchange as evidenced by good skin color, O_2 saturation greater than 95%, and clear lung sounds upon auscultation.

PLANNING AND IMPLEMENTATION

- Spend as much time as possible with Mr. Hussain and his family preoperatively, answering questions fully and encouraging expression of fears.
- Provide written and verbal explanations when feasible.
- Administer analgesia on a regular basis for the first 48 to 72 hours. Monitor for objective signs of unrelieved pain.
- Explain all procedures related to stoma and diversion care as they are being performed.
- Encourage Mr. Hussain to look at stoma and touch it when ready.
- Teach stoma and skin care, as well as self-catheterization, emphasizing measures to prevent skin irritation and urinary tract infection.
- Monitor urine output, color, clarity, and consistency every hour for first 24 hours, then every 4 hours for 24 hours, then every 8 hours. Report output of less than 30 mL per hour, bright bleeding, excessively cloudy or malodorous urine.
- Assist with use of incentive spirometer every hour while awake. Ambulate as soon as possible. Assess lung sounds every 4 hours, reporting increased crackles or diminished breath sounds.
- Refer Mr. and Mrs. Hussain to local stoma group on discharge.

EVALUATION

On discharge, Mr. Hussain has performed self-catheterization and stoma and skin care several times. His wife also is able to catheterize the stoma and demonstrate skin care. His urine is pale yellow and slightly cloudy. Mr. Hussain is ambulating independently and using oxycodone (Percocet) twice a day for pain relief. His lungs are clear, and he is very proud of having "survived" 7 days without a cigarette. He says, "Now I'm going to shoot for 7 weeks, then 7 months, then 7 years without a smoke!" A home health referral is made to continue teaching Mr. Hussain to care for his diversion and appliance.

Critical Thinking in the Nursing Process

1. How does cigarette smoking contribute to the increased risk of urinary tract tumors?
2. Suppose Mr. Hussain had become confused, disoriented, and tremorous and had begun to experience visual hallucinations 2 to 3 days postoperatively. What would you suspect the cause to be? What would be the appropriate response?
3. Develop a care plan for Mr. Hussain for the nursing diagnosis, *Risk for sexual dysfunction*.

See Evaluating Your Response in Appendix C.

THE CLIENT WITH URINARY RETENTION

Urinary retention, incomplete emptying of the bladder, can lead to overdistention of the bladder, poor detrusor muscle contractility, and inability to urinate. If the problem persists, hydroureter and hydronephrosis can result.

PHYSIOLOGY REVIEW

Normally, bladder emptying is controlled by the interaction of muscle tone and the autonomic nervous system. The sympathetic nervous system (SNS) relaxes the detrusor muscle, allowing the bladder to fill with urine. The internal sphincter, a continuation of the detrusor muscle, remains closed during filling. Pressures within the bladder remain low during filling, in contrast to high sphincter and urethral pressures. Voluntary muscles of the external sphincter and pelvic floor help maintain these high pressures. When the bladder contains 150 to 300 mL of urine, signals from stretch receptors in the bladder wall are transmitted to the spinal cord and cerebral cortex. Reflexive bladder emptying can be consciously inhibited. During *micturition* (bladder emptying), parasympathetic stimulation causes the detrusor muscle of the bladder fundus to contract, opening the internal sphincter. The external sphincter then relaxes, allowing urine to flow out.

PATHOPHYSIOLOGY

Either mechanical obstruction of the bladder outlet or a functional problem can cause urinary retention. *Benign prostatic hypertrophy (BPH)* is a common cause; difficulty initiating and maintaining urine flow is often the presenting complaint in men with BPH. Acute inflammation associated with infection or trauma of the bladder, urethra, or vulvovaginal tissues may also interfere with micturition. Scarring due to repeated urinary tract infection can lead to urethral stricture and a mechanical obstruction. Bladder calculi may also obstruct the urethral opening from the bladder.

Surgery, particularly abdominal or pelvic surgery, may disrupt detrusor muscle function, leading to urine retention. Drugs also may interfere with its function. Anticholinergic medications such as atropine, glycopyrrolate (Robinul), propantheline bromide (Pro-Banthine), scopolamine hydrochloride (Transderm-Scop), and others can lead to acute urinary retention and bladder distention. Many other drug groups have anticholinergic side effects and may cause urinary retention. Among these are antianxiety agents such as diazepam (Valium), antidepressant and tricyclic drugs such as imipramine (Tofranil), antiparkinsonian drugs, antipsychotic agents, and some sedative/hypnotic drugs. In addition, antihistamines common in over-the-counter cough, cold, allergy, and sleep-promoting drugs have anticholinergic effects and may interfere with bladder emptying. Diphenhydramine (Benadryl) is an example of a nonprescription antihistamine.

Voluntary urinary retention (particularly common among nurses!) may lead to overfilling of the bladder and a loss of detrusor muscle tone.

The client with urinary retention is unable to empty the bladder completely. Overflow voiding or incontinence may occur, with 25 to 50 mL of urine eliminated at frequent intervals. Assessment reveals a firm, distended bladder that may be displaced to one side of midline. Percussion of the lower abdomen reveals a dull tone, reflective of fluid in the bladder.

COLLABORATIVE CARE

Mechanical obstructions are treated by removing or repairing the obstruction when possible. Resection of the prostate gland may be done for urinary retention related to BPH. Bladder calculi are removed, and measures to prevent their formation are instituted.

An indwelling urinary catheter or intermittent straight catheterization can prevent urinary retention and overdistention of the bladder. Cholinergic medications such as bethanechol chloride (Urecholine), which promote detrusor muscle contraction and bladder emptying, may be used. A medication with no anticholinergic side effects may be substituted when urinary retention is related to drug therapy.

NURSING CARE

Health promotion measures to prevent urinary retention include monitoring urine output in at-risk clients and evaluating drug regimens for medications known to interfere with detrusor muscle function. Pay particular attention to elimination when these drugs are ordered (or used by) a client with BPH or other mechanical obstruction of urine flow.

Impaired Urinary Elimination

Nursing measures to promote urination include placing the client in normal voiding position and providing for privacy. Additional measures include running water, placing the client's hands in warm water, pouring warm water over the perineum, or taking a warm sitz bath.

In acute urinary retention, catheterization may be necessary to relieve bladder distention and prevent hydronephrosis. Use a relatively small catheter (16 Fr. for a man, 14 Fr. for a woman). A coudé-tipped catheter is passed more easily in the older man with an enlarged prostate. Using 2% lidocaine gel (10 mL injected into the male urethra or lubrication of the catheter with the gel for a woman) reduces discomfort during catheterization and promotes pelvic muscle relaxation (Gray, 2000b). Carefully observe the client as the distended bladder drains.

PRACTICE ALERT *Some clients may experience a vasovagal response, becoming pale, sweaty, and hypotensive if the bladder is rapidly drained. Draining urine in 500 mL increments, clamping the catheter for 5 to 10 minutes between increments, may prevent this response. Hematuria also may occur with rapid bladder decompression. Promptly notify the physician if hematuria develops (Gray, 2000b).* ■

Home care for the client with urinary retention varies, depending on the cause. Some clients may be taught intermittent self-catheterization. Instruct all clients who have experienced urinary retention to avoid over-the-counter drugs that affect micturition, especially those with an anticholinergic effect (allergy and cold medications, many nonprescription sleep aids). Other home care measures include double-voiding (urinate, remain on the toilet for 2 to 5 minutes, then urinate again), scheduled voiding, or, when other measures fail, an indwelling catheter. When an indwelling catheter is necessary, teach the client and family to use clean technique when changing from overnight bag to leg bag, and to promptly report signs of UTI to the primary care provider.

THE CLIENT WITH NEUROGENIC BLADDER

The neurologic connections influencing bladder filling, the perception of fullness and the need to void, and bladder emptying are complex. Disruption of the central or peripheral nervous systems may interfere with normal mechanisms, causing **neurogenic bladder.**

PATHOPHYSIOLOGY

As noted in the physiology section of urinary retention, bladder filling and emptying is controlled by the central nervous system (CNS). This neurologic control can be disrupted at any level: the cerebral cortex (voluntary impulses); the micturition center of the midbrain; the spinal cord tracts; or the peripheral nerves of the bladder itself.

Spastic Bladder Dysfunction

A simple reflex arc exists between the bladder and the spinal cord at levels S2 through S4. The stimulus of more than 400 mL of urine in the bladder causes reflex contraction of the detrusor muscle and bladder emptying unless voluntary control (cerebral input) is used to suppress it. Disruption of CNS transmission above the sacral spinal cord segment typically leads to *spastic neurogenic bladder.* Both sensory and voluntary control of urination are interrupted partially or totally, while the sacral reflex arc remains intact. The stimuli generated by bladder filling cause frequent spontaneous detrusor muscle contraction and involuntary bladder emptying. Spinal cord injury above the sacral segment is the most common cause of a spastic bladder. Other causes include stoke, multiple sclerosis, and other CNS lesions (Porth, 2002).

Flaccid Bladder Dysfunction

Damage to the sacral spinal cord at the level of the reflex arc, the cauda equina, or the sacral nerve roots causes loss of detrusor muscle tone and a *flaccid neurogenic bladder.* The perception of bladder fullness is lost, and the bladder becomes overdistended, with weak and ineffective detrusor muscle contractions. Flaccid neurogenic bladder is seen with myelomeningocele and during the spinal shock phase of a spinal cord injury above the sacral region. During the spinal shock phase, all reflex activity below the level of spinal cord injury is suppressed.

Peripheral neuropathies may also cause bladder atony and overfilling. Either sensory or motor pathways (or both) may be disrupted, leading to incomplete bladder emptying and large residual volumes after voiding (Porth, 2002). Diabetes mellitus is the most common cause of peripheral bladder neuropathy. Other causes include multiple sclerosis, chronic alcoholism, and prolonged overdistention of the bladder.

COLLABORATIVE CARE

Management of neurogenic bladder focuses on maintaining continence and avoiding complications associated with overfilling or incomplete emptying of the bladder. Because self-care is the goal, teaching is a primary intervention for the health care team.

Diagnostic Tests

The following diagnostic tests may be ordered for the client with a neurogenic bladder.

- *Urine culture* to detect possible urinary tract infection related to impaired bladder function.
- *Urinalysis* and *serum BUN* and *creatinine* to evaluate renal function. Ascending infection or hydronephrosis resulting from bladder overfilling and vesicoureteral reflux can damage the kidneys. Impaired renal function may lead to blood cells or protein in the urine, and elevated BUN and creatinine levels.
- *Postvoid catheterization* to measure residual urine. After voiding, the bladder normally contains less than 50 mL of urine. Amounts greater than 50 mL may indicate ineffective detrusor muscle contractions, common in neurogenic bladder.
- *Cystometrography* to evaluate bladder filling and the detrusor muscle tone and function.

Medications

Medications may be prescribed to increase or decrease the contractility of the detrusor muscle, increase or decrease the tone of the internal sphincter, or to relax the external urethral sphincter.

Bethanechol, a cholinergic drug, stimulates detrusor muscle contraction in flaccid neurogenic bladder. It is generally used to manage short-term urinary retention (e.g., following surgery or childbirth). It may used in combination with bladder-training techniques to promote complete emptying of a neurogenic bladder. Anticholinesterase drugs such as neostigmine (Prostigmin) and pyridostigmine (Mestinon) also may be used to increase detrusor muscle tone.

Anticholinergic drugs (parasympathetic blockers) relax the detrusor muscle and contract the internal sphincter, increasing bladder capacity in clients with spastic bladder dysfunction. Oxybutynin (Ditropan) and tolterodine (Detrol) inhibit the muscarinic effects of acetylcholine on smooth muscle, reducing detrusor muscle spasticity and promoting bladder filling. Other anticholinergic drugs also may be used, including propantheline (Pro-Banthine) or flavoxate (Urispas). Dry mouth, blurred vision, and constipation are potential adverse effects of anticholinergic medications. See the Medication Administration box on page 732 for drugs used to modify detrusor muscle activity.

Medication Administration
The Client with Neurogenic Bladder

CHOLINERGIC DRUGS TO STIMULATE MICTURITION

Bethanechol chloride (Urocholine)

Bethanechol stimulates the parasympathetic nervous system, increasing detrusor muscle tone and producing a contraction strong enough to initiate micturition. It is used primarily to treat acute postoperative and postpartum urinary retention.

Nursing Responsibilities

- Assess for contraindications, including hypersensitivity, hyperthyroidism, peptic ulcer disease, asthma, significant bradycardia or hypotension, coronary heart disease, epilepsy, and parkinsonism.
- Do not give to clients who have had recent gastrointestinal or bladder surgery or those with possible gastrointestinal or urinary tract obstruction.
- Give oral forms on an empty stomach to reduce the risk of nausea and vomiting.
- Administer parenteral bethanechol subcutaneously. Keep atropine, the antidote for bethanechol overdose or toxicity, available.
- Observe for desired effect within 30 to 60 minutes after oral administration, 5 to 15 minutes after injection.
- Assess for adverse effects such as malaise, headache, abdominal cramping, nausea, hypotension with reflex tachycardia, wheezing, and dyspnea.

Client and Family Teaching

- Take the medication 1 hour before or 2 hours after meals.
- Use caution when rising from a recumbent or sitting position; you may feel dizzy or lightheaded.

ANTICHOLINERGIC DRUGS TO TREAT SPASTIC BLADDER

Oxybutynin (Ditropan)
Tolterodine (Detrol)
Propantheline bromide (Pro-Banthine)
Flavoxate hydrochloride (Urispas)

Anticholinergic drugs inhibit the response to acetylcholine, relaxing the detrusor muscle and increasing internal sphincter tone. The combination of detrusor relaxation and internal sphincter contraction increases the bladder capacity of clients with spastic or hyperreflexive neurogenic bladder. Of these medications, tolterodine has the most specific effects on the detrusor muscle with fewer anticholinergic side effects.

Nursing Responsibilities

- Assess for contraindications, such as glaucoma, gastrointestinal or urinary tract obstruction, severe ulcerative colitis or toxic megacolon, unstable cardiovascular status, or myasthenia gravis.
- Observe for the desired effect of increased bladder capacity with decreased incontinence and spasm.
- Monitor for possible interaction with other drugs such as narcotic analgesics, antidysrhythmic medications, antihistamines, antidepressants, or psychoactive drugs.
- Monitor heart rate and blood pressure, especially when given to clients with known cardiovascular disease.
- Assess for adverse effects such as urinary hesitancy or retention, dysrhythmias, mental status changes, and gastrointestinal disturbances.

Client and Family Teaching

- Promptly report eye pain, rapid heart beat, difficulty breathing, rash or hives, or changes in mental function to your primary care provider.
- These drugs may cause drowsiness or blurred vision. Use caution when driving, operating machinery, or performing other tasks requiring mental acuity.
- Hard candies help relieve dry mouth associated with these drugs.
- Do not use alcohol or nonprescription antihistamines while taking these drugs.

Treatments

Dietary

Dietary measures to reduce the risk for UTI and urinary calculi may be suggested for the client with neurogenic bladder. A moderate to high fluid intake and a diet that acidifies the urine are helpful. Cranberry juice is recommended to maintain urine acidity. See Table 26–3 for additional foods to include or avoid in the diet to help prevent UTI and urolithiasis. The timing of fluid intake may be regulated to promote continence.

Bladder Retraining

Clients with spastic neurogenic bladder may use measures to stimulate reflex voiding, allowing scheduled toileting. Techniques include using trigger points, for example, stroking or pinching the abdomen, inner thigh, or glans penis. Pulling pubic hairs, tapping the suprapubic region, or inserting a gloved finger into the rectum and gently stretching the anal sphincter can also stimulate urination.

The *Credé's method* (applying pressure to the suprapubic region with the fingers of one or both hands), manual pressure on the abdomen, and the Valsalva maneuver (bearing down while holding one's breath) promote bladder emptying for the client with a spastic or flaccid bladder.

PRACTICE ALERT *Increasing lower abdominal and bladder pressure with the Credé's method can stimulate autonomic dysreflexia in some clients with spinal cord injuries. Autonomic dysreflexia is a medical emergency in which the blood pressure rises rapidly due to SNS stimulation. ■*

See Chapter 41 for a discussion of autonomic dysreflexia.

The client with a flaccid bladder may require catheterization to completely empty the bladder. An indwelling catheter may be used initially, but intermittent catheterization is preferred. Clean intermittent self-catheterization is performed every 3 to 4 hours to prevent overdistention of the bladder (see Procedure 41–1). 🔗

Surgery

Surgery may be required when urination cannot be effectively managed using more conservative measures. *Rhizotomy,* or destruction of the nerve supply to the detrusor muscle or the external sphincter, may be used for clients with hyperreflexia or spasticity. Urinary diversion is another surgical technique used when conservative management fails. Implantation of an artificial sphincter may be useful for some clients with neurogenic bladder. See Table 26–6 for urinary diversion techniques and page 726 nursing care of the client undergoing a urinary diversion.

NURSING CARE

Nursing care of the client with a neurogenic bladder is directed toward promoting urinary drainage and continence, preventing complications, and teaching the client and family self-care techniques.

Assessment

Nursing assessment for neurogenic bladder includes obtaining a complete nursing history, focusing on information related to CNS or spinal cord injury or disease, as well as disorders that affect the peripheral nervous system (e.g., diabetes). Ask about measures used to stimulate or control urination. Inspect and palpate the lower abdomen and suprapubic region for tenderness or bladder distention. Percuss the suprapubic region for a dull percussion tone indicative of a full bladder. Dullness up to the level of the umbilicus indicates at least 500 mL of urine in the bladder (Gray, 2000). Assess urine for color, clarity, and odor. Collect a specimen for analysis as indicated.

Nursing Diagnoses and Interventions

Although each client has individual nursing care needs, examples of nursing diagnoses appropriate for the client with a neurogenic bladder include the following:

- *Impaired urinary elimination* related to impaired bladder innervation
- *Self-Care deficit: Toileting* related to neurologic injury
- *Risk for impaired skin integrity* related to urinary incontinence
- *Risk for infection* related to impaired urination reflex

Home Care

Include the following in teaching for the client with neurogenic bladder and family members.

- Measures to stimulate reflex voiding and promote bladder emptying
- Use of prescribed medications, including desired and adverse effects, and interactions with other drugs
- Manifestations of UTI or urolithiasis, and measures to reduce the risk of these complications

THE CLIENT WITH URINARY INCONTINENCE

The most common manifestation of impaired bladder control is **urinary incontinence,** or involuntary urination. Incontinence can have significant impact, leading to physical problems such as skin breakdown, infection, and rashes. Psychosocial consequences include embarrassment, isolation and withdrawal, feelings of worthlessness and helplessness, and depression.

Approximately 13 million people in the United States have some degree of urinary incontinence. The estimated cost of managing incontinence is $10 billion yearly. Urinary incontinence is especially common among older clients (see the box below). Up to 30% of older women living in the community experience urinary incontinence. In long-term care, foster care, and homebound populations, the incidence is about 50% (Gallo et al., 1999; Tierney et al., 2001). The actual prevalence of urinary incontinence is nearly impossible to determine. Embarrassment and the availability of products to protect clothing and prevent detection contribute to clients' not seeking evaluation of and treatment for incontinence.

Nursing Care of the Older Adult

MINIMIZING THE RISK FOR UTI AND UI

Older adults have a higher incidence of two common urinary tract disorders: urinary tract infection (UTI) and urinary incontinence (UI).

URINARY TRACT INFECTION

Aging affects normal protective mechanisms to prevent UTI. The pH of urine increases with aging, allowing bacteria to grow and multiply more readily. Glucosuria, more common in older adults due to the higher incidence of diabetes, facilitates bacterial growth. Incomplete bladder emptying and urinary retention are more common due to problems such as prostatic hypertrophy in men, bladder prolapse in women, and neurogenic bladder in both sexes. Changes in vaginal pH in women and decreased prostatic secretions in men may also contribute to an increased incidence of UTI.

While many UTIs in older adults are asymptomatic and self-limited, infections can lead to bacteremia, sepsis, and shock. Manifestations of UTI in the elderly include dysuria, urgency, frequency, incontinence, occasional hematuria, and confusion. Symptoms such as fever, chills, and flank pain and tenderness may be absent. Dementia may make diagnosis more difficult.

URINARY INCONTINENCE

Urinary incontinence, the involuntary loss of urine, is a common problem in older adults. While incontinence should never be considered a *normal* consequence of aging, age-related changes contribute to its development. Bladder capacity tends to decline with

(continued on page 734)

Nursing Care of the Older Adult

MINIMIZING THE RISK FOR UTI AND UI (continued)

age and involuntary bladder muscle contractions are more common. In women, decreased estrogen levels and pelvic muscle relaxation decrease bladder outlet and urethral resistance pressures. Decreased estrogen also causes atrophic vaginitis and urethritis, with manifestations of dysuria and urgency. Other risk factors for UI in older adults include impaired mobility and chronic degenerative diseases, impaired cognition, medications, low fluid intake, diabetes, and stroke.

Assessing for Home Care

Assessment for urinary problems in the older adult focuses on risk factors, the extent and manifestations of the disorder, and contributing factors. Using clear language, ask about problems with urine loss, its frequency, and any contributing factors. Inquire about frequency, urgency, and burning on urination. Identify current medications and the time of day each is taken. Assess patterns of fluid intake and output. Assess the abdomen for evidence of bladder distention or tenderness. Perform a mental status examination if indicated.

Assess the home environment (whether in the community or a residential living facility) for possible barriers to urinary elimination:

- Inadequate lighting, particularly at night
- Narrow doorways that may interfere with access to the toilet
- Inadequate toilet facilities
- The need for mobility aids such as safety bars, a raised toilet seat, or a bedside commode

Teaching for Home Care

Discuss the following points to help prevent UTI and UI in the older adult.

- Maintain a generous fluid intake. Reduce or eliminate fluid intake after the evening meal to reduce nocturia.

- Wear comfortable clothing that is easy to remove for toileting.
- Maintain good hygiene, but do not bathe more often than necessary; frequent bathing and feminine hygiene sprays or douches may dry perineal tissues, increasing the risk of UTI or UI.
- Perform pelvic muscle exercises (Kegel exercises) several times a day to increase perineal muscle tone.
- Reduce consumption of caffeine-containing beverages (coffee, tea, colas), citrus juices, and artificially sweetened beverages containing Nutra-Sweet.
- Use behavioral techniques such as scheduled toileting, habit training, and bladder training to reduce the frequency of incontinence. *Scheduled toileting* is toileting at regular intervals (e.g., every 2 to 4 hours). *Habit training* is toileting the client on a schedule that corresponds with the normal pattern. *Bladder training* gradually increases the bladder capacity by increasing the intervals between voidings and resisting the urge to void.
- See your primary care provider regularly for a pelvic or prostate exam.
- For women, discuss possible benefits and risks of hormone replacement therapy, physical therapy, or surgery to treat incontinence.
- Report a change in urine color, odor, or clarity or symptoms such as burning, frequency, or urgency to your primary care provider.

Resources for Home Care

National Association for Continence
P.O. Box 8310
Spartanburg, SC 29305-8310
864-579-7900
Website: http://www.nafc.org

PATHOPHYSIOLOGY

Urinary continence requires a bladder able to expand and contract and sphincters that can maintain a urethral pressure higher than that in the bladder. Incontinence results when the pressure within the urinary bladder exceeds urethral resistance, allowing urine to escape. Any condition causing higher than normal bladder pressures or reduced urethral resistance can potentially result in incontinence. Relaxation of the pelvic musculature, disruption of cerebral and nervous system control, and disturbances of the bladder and its musculature are common contributing factors.

Incontinence may be an acute, self-limited disorder, or it may be chronic. The causes may be congenital or acquired, reversible or irreversible. Congenital disorders associated with incontinence include *epispadias* (absence of the upper wall of the urethra), and *meningomyelocele* (a neural tube defect in which a portion of the spinal cord and its surrounding meninges protrude through the vertebral column). Central nervous system or spinal cord trauma, stroke, and chronic neurologic disorders such as multiple sclerosis and Parkinson's disease are examples of acquired, irreversible causes of incontinence. Reversible causes include acute con-

fusion, medications such as diuretics or sedatives, prostatic enlargement, vaginal and urethral atrophy, UTI, and fecal impaction.

Incontinence is commonly categorized as stress incontinence, urge incontinence (also known as overactive bladder), overflow incontinence, and functional incontinence. Table 26–7 summarizes each type with its physiologic cause and associated factors. *Mixed incontinence,* with elements of both stress and urge incontinence, is common. *Total incontinence* is loss of all voluntary control over urination, with urine loss occurring without stimulus and in all positions.

Incontinence is associated with an increased risk for falls, fractures, pressure ulcers, urinary tract infection, and depression. It contributes to the stress of caregivers, and may be a factor in institutionalizing the client.

COLLABORATIVE CARE

Urinary incontinence management is directed at identifying and correcting the cause if possible. If the underlying disorder cannot be corrected, techniques to manage urine output can often be taught.

TABLE 26-7   Types of Urinary Incontinence

	Description	Pathophysiology	Contributing Factors
Stress	Loss of urine associated with increased intra-abdominal pressure during sneezing, coughing, lifting. Quantity of urine lost is usually small.	Relaxation of pelvic musculature and weakness of urethra and surrounding muscles and tissues leads to decreased urethral resistance	• Multiple pregnancies • Decreased estrogen levels • Short urethra, change in angle between bladder and urethra • Abdominal wall weakness • Prostate surgery • Increased intra-abdominal pressure due to tumor, ascites, obesity
Urge	Involuntary loss of urine associated with a strong urge to void	Hypertonic or overactive detrusor muscle leads to increased pressure within bladder and inability to inhibit voiding	• Neurologic disorders such as stroke, Parkinson's disease, multiple sclerosis; peripheral nervous system disorders • Detrusor muscle overactivity associated with bladder outlet obstruction, aging, or disorders such as diabetes
Overflow	Inability to empty bladder, resulting in overdistention and frequent loss of small amounts of urine	Outlet obstruction or lack of normal detrusor activity leads to overfilling of bladder and increased pressure	• Spinal cord injuries below S2 • Diabetic neuropathy • Prostatic hypertrophy • Fecal impaction • Drugs, especially those with anticholinergic effect
Functional	Incontinence resulting from physical, environmental, or psycho-social causes	Ability to respond to the need to urinate is impaired	• Confusion or dementia • Physical disability or impaired mobility • Diuretic therapy or sedation • Depression • Regression

Evaluation for incontinence begins with a complete history, including the duration, frequency, volume, and associated circumstances of urine loss. A voiding diary (Figure 26–7 ■) is often used to collect detailed information. The history also includes information about chronic or acute illnesses, previous surgeries, and current medication use, both prescription and over the counter.

Physical assessment includes abdominal, rectal, and pelvic assessment as well as evaluation of mental and neurologic status, mobility, and dexterity. Findings often associated with incontinence in women include weak abdominal and pelvic muscle tone, cystocele or urethrocele, and atrophic vaginitis. In men, an enlarged prostate gland is the physical finding most commonly associated with incontinence.

See page 736 for a research model for diagnosing urge incontinence using specific client assessment data.

Diagnostic Tests

- *Urinalysis* and *urine culture* using a clean-catch specimen are done to rule out infection and other acute causes of incontinence.
- *Postvoiding residual (PVR) volume* is measured to determine how completely the bladder empties with voiding. Less than 50 mL PVR is expected; when 100 mL or more is obtained, further testing is indicated.
- *Cystometrography* is used to assess neuromuscular function of the bladder by evaluating detrusor muscle function, pressure within the bladder, and the filling pattern of the blad-

der. The client describes sensations and any urge to void as sterile water or saline is instilled into the bladder. Normally, the urge to void is perceived at 150 to 450 mL, and the bladder feels full at 300 to 500 mL. Bladder pressure and volume are recorded on a graph. When the bladder is full, the client voids, and intravesical pressure is noted during voiding.

- *Uroflowmetry* is a noninvasive test used to evaluate voiding patterns. The uroflowmeter, contained in a funnel, measures the rate of urine flow, the continuous flow time, and the total voiding time.
- *Intravenous pyelography* may be ordered to evaluate structure and function of the upper and lower urinary tract.
- *Cystoscopy* or *ultrasonography* may be ordered to identify structural disorders contributing to incontinence, such as an enlarged prostate or a tumor.

Nursing implications for the specialized studies for urinary incontinence are outlined in the box on page 736.

Medications

Both stress and urge incontinence may improve with drug treatment.

Drugs that contract the smooth muscles of the bladder neck may reduce episodes of mild stress incontinence. Phenylpropanolamine (Acutrim, Allerest, Contac, others), a commonly used decongestant and nonprescription diet aid, is an effective preparation. Adverse effects such as hypertension, palpitations, and nervousness may limit its use.

Your Daily Voiding Diary   Date _____

This diary will help you and your health care team identify factors causing bladder control problems. Choose a 24-hour period when you can record your fluid intake (type and amount), urine output and episodes of urine leakage, any strong urge to void just prior to leaking, and your activity when leak episodes occur. The line below illustrates how to use your diary.

Time	Fluid Intake Amount	Type	Urine Output			Leaks			Urge Yes / No	Activity
7 am	2 cups	coffee	sm	(med)	lg	(sm)	med	lg	Yes	walking
			sm	med	lg	sm	med	lg		
			sm	med	lg	sm	med	lg		
			sm	med	lg	sm	med	lg		
			sm	med	lg	sm	med	lg		
			sm	med	lg	sm	med	lg		
			sm	med	lg	sm	med	lg		
			sm	med	lg	sm	med	lg		
			sm	med	lg	sm	med	lg		
			sm	med	lg	sm	med	lg		
			sm	med	lg	sm	med	lg		
			sm	med	lg	sm	med	lg		
			sm	med	lg	sm	med	lg		
			sm	med	lg	sm	med	lg		
			sm	med	lg	sm	med	lg		
			sm	med	lg	sm	med	lg		
			sm	med	lg	sm	med	lg		

I used ___ pads today.   I used ___ diapers today.

Questions to ask my health care team: _____
_____
_____

Figure 26–7 ■ A sample voiding diary.

Source: Adapted: from Your Daily Bladder Diary, *National Kidney and Urologic Diseases Information Center, National Institute of Diabetes and Digestive and Kidney Disease (NIDDK), National Institutes of Health.*

Nursing Implications for Diagnostic Tests

Urinary Incontinence

POSTVOIDING RESIDUAL VOLUME

Preparation of the Client

- Instruct the client to notify the nurse when the urge to void (urinate) is felt.
- Have client void into a collection device. Instruct to empty bladder as completely as possible. Provide for privacy to avoid "shy-bladder" syndrome.
- Immediately after voiding, catheterize using aseptic technique and a straight catheter. Drain bladder completely of residual urine.
- Record time; amount voided; amount obtained on catheterization; color, clarity, and odor of urine; and any other significant data.

Client and Family Teaching

- This test is used to determine how completely you empty your bladder with voiding.
- Residual urine (urine left in the bladder after urination) increases the risks of urinary infection and incontinence.

- This test poses a slight risk of infection. Report symptoms of frequency, urgency, pain on urination, nocturia, and cloudy, bloody, or malodorous urine.

CYSTOMETROGRAM (CMG)

Preparation of the Client

- Verify a signed consent for the test.
- Check for UTI as indicated by urinalysis or manifestations; infection may interfere with test results.
- No food or fluid restriction is required for this test.

Client and Family Teaching

- This test evaluates bladder capacity, and the motor (contraction) and sensory functions of the bladder.
- You will be given privacy during the procedure and will not be unnecessarily exposed.
- Do not strain to void during the test; straining may invalidate the results

(continued on page 737)

Nursing Implications for Diagnostic Tests

Urinary Incontinence *(continued)*

- You will be asked to describe sensations as the bladder is filled, including the first urge to void, the sensation of being unable to delay urination any longer, and others such as pain, sweating, or nausea.
- The test requires about 45 minutes to complete.
- Report persistent hematuria or signs of infection to the physician.
- A warm tub or sitz bath may help to relieve discomfort after testing.

UROFLOWMETRY
Preparation of the Client
- Withhold medications that may interfere with test results.

Client and Family Teaching
- This is a rapid, simple test to measure the volume of urine voided per second.
- Privacy is provided during testing. Male clients void while standing; females, while sitting.
- You will urinate into a funnel.
- Drugs affecting bladder and sphincter tone, movement during testing, and straining during voiding may invalidate test results.
- Increase your fluid intake and do not urinate for several hours prior to the test to ensure a full bladder and a strong urge to void during testing.
- No discomfort or risk is associated with this test.

When incontinence is associated with postmenopausal atrophic vaginitis, estrogen therapy may be effective. Both systemic estrogens and local creams are used.

Clients with urge incontinence may be treated with preparations that increase bladder capacity. The primary drugs used to inhibit detrusor muscle contractions and increase bladder capacity include oxybutinin (Ditropan), an anticholinergic drug, and tolterodine (Detrol), a more specific antimuscarinic agent. These drugs can be taken once or twice a day, and have fewer side effects than less specific anticholinergic drugs. Drugs with anticholinergic effects are contraindicated for the client with acute glaucoma. Urinary retention is a potential side effect that must be considered when these drugs are used (see the Medication Administration box on page 732).

Surgery

Surgery may be used to treat stress incontinence associated with cystocele or urethrocele and overflow incontinence associated with an enlarged prostate gland.

Suspension of the bladder neck, a technique that brings the angle between the bladder and urethra closer to normal, is effective in treating stress incontinence associated with urethrocele in 80% to 95% of clients. A laparoscopic, vaginal, or abdominal approach may be used to perform this surgery. Care of the client with a bladder neck suspension is outlined in the Nursing Care box on page 738.

Prostatectomy, using either the transurethral or suprapubic approach, is indicated for the client who is experiencing

---

Nursing Research

Evidence-Based Practice for Urinary Incontinence

While an accurate diagnosis of stress urinary incontinence often is made based on clinical data, motor urge incontinence has been more difficult to accurately diagnose without urodynamic testing. This presents difficulty for nurses and nurse practitioners planning care for incontinent clients when urologic testing is not feasible or readily available. A model developed by Gray, McClain, Peruggia, Patrie, and Steers (2001) may be useful to address this problem in cognitively intact adults. By comparing client data with urolodynamic testing results, this team of researchers identified factors predictive of motor urge incontinence. These factors included age, gender, and three key symptoms: diurnal frequency (urinating more often than every 2 hours while awake), nocturia (awakening with urge to urinate more than once per night if under age 65, twice per night if over age 65), and urge incontinence (urine loss associated with a strong desire to urinate). The presence of all three symptoms was more than 92% predictive of motor urge incontinence in study participants of all ages (range 18 to 89; median 61) and both genders.

Implications for Nursing
Asking specific questions about urinary tract symptoms can facilitate accurate identification of the nursing diagnosis, *Urge urinary*

incontinence. Accurate diagnosis is vital to planning and implementing appropriate care measures, and achieving the desired outcome of continence. Successful treatment promotes self-esteem and provides positive reinforcement for continuing planned strategies.

Critical Thinking in Client Care
1. What nursing care measures and client teaching will you provide for the client with stress incontinence that may not be appropriate or necessary for the client with urge incontinence? For the client with urge incontinence but not stress incontinence?
2. Identify circumstances in which it may not be possible or feasible to have the client undergo urodynamic testing to differentiate stress, urge, or mixed (stress and urge) incontinence.
3. The clients in this study lived independently in the community and were cognitively intact. Can the data in this study be generalized to clients residing in a long-term care facility? Can the results be applied to all types of incontinence? Why or why not?

Note. From "A Model for Predicting Motor Urge Urinary Incontinence" by M. Gray et al., 2001, Nursing Research, 50(2), p. 116–122.

NURSING CARE OF THE CLIENT HAVING A BLADDER NECK SUSPENSION

PREOPERATIVE CARE

- Provide routine preoperative care and teaching as outlined in Chapter 7. ∞
- Discuss the need to avoid straining and the Valsalva maneuver postoperatively. Suggest measures such as increasing fluid and fiber intake and using a stool softener to prevent postoperative constipation. *Straining and increased abdominal pressure during the Valsalva maneuver may place excessive stress on suture lines and interfere with healing.*

POSTOPERATIVE CARE

- Provide routine postoperative care as outlined in Chapter 7.
- Monitor urine output, including quantity, color, and clarity. Expect urine to be pink initially, gradually clearing. *Bright red urine, excessive vaginal drainage, or incisional bleeding may indi-*

cate hemorrhage. Instrumentation of the urinary tract increases the potential for UTI; cloudy urine may be an early sign.
- Maintain stability and patency of suprapubic and/or urethral catheters. Secure catheters in position. *Maintaining bladder decompression eliminates pressure on suture lines. Preventing movement or pulling on catheters reduces the risk for resultant pressure on surgical incisions.*
- Carefully monitor urine output after catheter removal. *Difficulty voiding is common following catheter removal. Early intervention to prevent bladder distention is important to prevent pressure on suture lines.*
- If the urethral or suprapubic catheter will remain in place on discharge, teach proper care to the client and family members as needed. *Appropriate self-care and early recognition of problems reduce the risk for significant complications.*

---

overflow incontinence as a result of an enlarged prostate gland and urethral obstruction. Care of the client with a prostatectomy is outlined in Chapter 47. ∞

Other surgical procedures of potential benefit in the treatment of incontinence include implantation of an artificial sphincter, formation of a urethral sling to elevate and compress the urethra, and augmentation of the bladder with bowel segments to increase bladder capacity.

Complementary Therapies

Biofeedback and relaxation techniques may help reduce episodes of urinary incontinence. Biofeedback uses electronic monitors to teach conscious control over physiologic responses of which the individual is not normally aware. Developing awareness of perceptible information allows the client to gain voluntary control over urination. Biofeedback is widely used to manage urinary incontinence.

NURSING CARE

Health Promotion

Although urinary incontinence rarely causes serious physical effects, it frequently has significant psychosocial effects, and can lead to lowered self-esteem, social isolation, and even institutionalization. Get the word out—inform all clients that UI is not a normal consequence of aging and that treatments are available. To reduce the incidence of UI, teach all women to perform pelvic floor exercises (Box 26–4) to improve perineal muscle tone. Advise women to seek advice from their women's health care or primary care practitioner about using topical or systemic hormone therapy during menopause to maintain perineal tissue integrity. Advise older men to have routine prostate examinations to prevent urethral obstruction and overflow incontinence.

BOX 26–4 ■ Pelvic Floor (Kegel) Exercises

- Identify the pelvic muscles with these techniques:
  a. Stop the flow of urine during voiding and hold for a few seconds.
  b. Tighten the muscles at the vaginal entrance around a gloved finger or tampon.
  c. Tighten the muscles around the anus as though resisting defecation.
- Perform exercises by tightening pelvic muscles, holding for 10 seconds, and relaxing for 10 to 15 seconds. Continue the sequence (tighten, hold, relax) for 10 repetitions.
- Keep abdominal muscles and breathing relaxed while performing exercises.
- Initially, exercises should be performed twice per day, working up to four times a day.
- Encourage exercising at a specific time each day or in conjunction with another daily activity (such as bathing or watching the news). Establish a routine because these exercises should be continued for life.
- Assistive devices, such as vaginal cones and biofeedback, may be useful for clients who have difficulty identifying appropriate muscle groups.

Assessment

Nursing assessment for the client with urinary incontinence includes both subjective and objective data.

- Health history: voiding diary; frequency of incontinent episodes, amount of urine loss and activities associated with incontinence; methods used to deal with incontinence; use of Kegel exercises or medications; any chronic diseases, related surgeries, etc.; effects of incontinence on usual activities, including social activities
- Physical examination: physical and mental status, including any physical limitations or impaired cognition; inspect, palpate, and percuss abdomen for bladder distention; inspect perineal tissues for redness, irritation, or tissue breakdown;

observe for bulging of bladder into vagina when bearing down; assess pelvic muscle tone as indicated

Nursing Diagnoses and Interventions

In planning nursing care, consider the client's mental status, mobility, and motivation. Behavioral techniques can be effective, but require long-term commitment and the physical and mental capability to use them.

Nursing care and modification of routines can restore continence fully or partially even in the institutionalized client. Scheduled toileting, bladder training, and prompted voiding combined with positive reinforcement such as praise can reduce the need for diapers, incontinence pads, and indwelling catheters.

Urinary Incontinence: Stress and/or Urge

Exercises to strengthen pelvic floor muscles, dietary modifications, and bladder training programs often are effective to restore and maintain continence.

- Instruct to keep a voiding diary, recording the time and amount of all fluid intake and urinary output, status at the time of voiding (dry or wet) and on arising from sleep, and activities. *Voiding diaries provide valuable information for identifying the type of incontinence and possible measures to reduce or eliminate incontinent episodes.*
- Teach pelvic floor muscle exercises (Box 26–4). Instruct to consciously tighten pelvic muscles when the need to void is perceived and to relax the abdomen while walking to the bathroom. *Improved pelvic muscle strength helps retain urine and prevent stress incontinence by increasing urethral pressure. Exercises also decrease abnormal detrusor muscle contractions, decreasing pressure within the bladder.*

> **PRACTICE ALERT**   *Do not advise clients who have difficulty emptying the bladder completely to stop urine flow while voiding to identify pelvic floor muscles. Repeated interruption of micturition can interfere with complete bladder emptying and increase the risk for UTI.* ∎

- Using the client's voiding diary, suggest dietary and fluid intake modifications to reduce stress and urge incontinence. Include limiting caffeine, alcohol, citrus juice, and artificial sweetener consumption; limiting fluid intake to no less than 1.5 to 2.0 L per day; and limiting evening fluid intake. *Caffeine, alcohol, and citrus juices are bladder irritants and tend to promote detrusor instability, increasing the risk of urge incontinence. Artificial sweeteners may also irritate the bladder. Fluid intake of 1.5 to 2.0 L per day is adequate to maintain health for most clients; excess fluid may increase stress incontinence if bathroom facilities are not readily available.*

> **PRACTICE ALERT**   *Limiting total fluid intake to less than 1.5 to 2.0 L per day is not recommended for clients with urinary incontinence. Inadequate fluid increases urine concentration, leading to bladder wall irritation and possibly increasing problems of urge incontinence.* ∎

Self-Care Deficit: Toileting

Functional incontinence may be the predominant problem in an institutionalized older adult. Limited mobility, impaired vision, dementia, lack of access to facilities and privacy, and tight staffing patterns increase the risk for incontinence in previously continent residents. The primary problem in functional incontinence is an outside factor that interferes with the ability to respond normally to the urge to void. An immobilized client may wet the bed if a call light is not within reach; a client with Alzheimer's disease may perceive the urge to void but be unable to interpret its meaning or respond by seeking a bathroom. For these clients, self-care deficit in toileting is a primary problem.

- Assess physical and mental abilities and limitations, usual voiding pattern, and ability to assist with toileting. *A thorough assessment allows planned interventions to address specific needs and promote independence.*
- Provide assistive devices as needed to facilitate independence, such as raised toilet seats, grab bars, a bedside commode, or night lights. *Fostering independence in toileting bolsters self-concept and maintains a positive body image.*
- Plan a toileting schedule based on the client's normal elimination patterns to achieve approximately 300 mL of urine output with each voiding. *Allowing the bladder to fill to a point at which the urge to void is experienced and then emptying it completely helps maintain normal bladder capacity and bacteriostatic functions.*
- Position for ease of voiding—sitting for females, standing for males—and provide privacy. *Normal positioning, usual toileting facilities, and privacy enhance the ability to void on schedule and empty the bladder completely.*
- Adjust fluid intake so that the majority of fluids are consumed during times of day when the client is most able to remain continent. Unless fluids are restricted, maintain a fluid intake of at least 1.5 to 2.0 L per day. *An adequate fluid intake is vital to promote hydration and urinary function. Overly concentrated urine can irritate the bladder, increasing incontinence.*
- Assist with clothing that is easily removed (e.g., elastic-waisted pants or loose dresses). Velcro and zipper fasteners may be easier to use than snaps and buttons. *Clothing that is difficult to remove can increase the risk of incontinence in the client with mobility problems or impaired dexterity.*

Social Isolation

Urinary incontinence increases the risk for social isolation due to embarrassment, fear of not having ready access to a bathroom, body odor, or other factors. Social isolation, in turn, can increase problems of incontinence, because normal cues and relationships are lost, and the need to remain dry is less strongly felt.

- Assess reasons for and extent of social isolation. Verify the degree of social isolation with the client or significant other. *Do not assume that social isolation is only related to urinary incontinence. Other problems frequently associated with aging (such as a hearing deficit) may be primary or contributing factors.*

- Refer client for urologic examination and incontinence evaluation. *Clients who assume that urinary incontinence is a normal part of the aging may not be aware of treatment options.*
- Explore alternative coping strategies with client, significant other, staff, and other health team members. *Protective pads or shields, good perineal hygiene, scheduled voiding, and clothing that does not interfere with toileting can enhance continence.*

Using NANDA, NIC, and NOC

Chart 26–4 shows links between NANDA nursing diagnoses, NIC and NOC when caring for the client with urinary incontinence.

Home Care

Because urinary incontinence is a contributing factor in the institutionalization of many older people, client and family teaching can have a significant impact on maintaining independence and residence in the community. Address possible causes of incontinence and appropriate treatment measures. Refer for urologic examination if not already completed. Discuss fluid intake management, perineal care, and products for clothing protection.

CHART 26–4 NANDA, NIC, AND NOC LINKAGES

The Client with Urinary Retention or Incontinence

NURSING DIAGNOSES	NURSING INTERVENTIONS	NURSING OUTCOMES
• Urinary Retention	• Urinary Bladder Training • Urinary Catheterization: Intermittent • Urinary Retention Care	• Urinary Continence • Urinary Elimination
• Functional Urinary Incontinence	• Prompted Voiding • Urinary Habit Training • Urinary Elimination Management	• Urinary Continence • Urinary Elimination • Tissue Integrity: Skin & Mucous Membranes
• Stress Urinary Incontinence	• Pelvic Muscle Exercise • Urinary Incontinence Care • Weight Management	• Urinary Continence
• Urge Urinary Incontinence	• Fluid Management • Medication Management	• Urinary Continence

Note. Data from Nursing Outcomes Classification (NOC) *by M. Johnson & M. Maas (Eds.), 1997, St. Louis: Mosby;* Nursing Diagnoses: Definitions & Classification 2001–2002 *by North American Nursing Diagnosis Association, 2001, Philadelphia: NANDA;* Nursing Interventions Classification (NIC) *by J.C. McCloskey & G. M. Bulechek (Eds.), 2000, St. Louis: Mosby. Reprinted by permission.*

Nursing Care Plan
A Client with Urinary Incontinence

Anna Giovanni, a 76-year-old retired teacher, has been widowed for 10 years and lives alone. Mrs. Giovanni's eldest daughter expresses concern that her mother seems increasingly reluctant to leave her apartment to visit friends and family. She reports a strong odor of urine throughout her mother's apartment and that her mother's bed is often wet. She expresses worry about needing to place her mother in a nursing home if she cannot continue to live independently.

ASSESSMENT

Jane Oberle, RN, a nurse practitioner, examines Mrs. Giovanni who admits that she has problems with urine leakage when laughing and coughing, and a strong urge to void on hearing the sound of running water. At night, her urge to void is so strong that she often cannot reach the bathroom in time. Mrs. Giovanni denies a history of UTIs, neurologic disorders, or difficulty with her bowels. She had a hysterectomy at age 52 and was on hormone replace-

ment therapy for about 10 years afterward. She is taking digoxin 0.125 mg daily, furosemide 40 mg twice daily, and potassium chloride 20 mEq 3 times daily for mild heart failure.

Physical assessment reveals a moderate cystourethrocele and atrophy of vaginal and vulvar tissues. Moderate perineal dermatitis is noted. Pelvic floor strength is weak. Urinalysis is within normal limits, and postvoiding residual urine is 5 mL.

Analysis of Mrs. Giovanni's voiding diary shows moderate consumption of tea and juices throughout the day, nine daytime voidings and four night voidings with an average volume of about 250 mL per void. She notices urine leakage most often in the late afternoon and at night. Ms. Oberle identifies a diagnoses of stress incontinence with an urgency component and decides to try a conservative approach before referring Mrs. Giovanni for further testing and possible cystourethrocele repair. She prescribes estrogen cream, tolterodine (Detrol), and a barrier cream to treat Mrs. Giovanni's vulvitis.

Nursing Care Plan

A Client with Urinary Incontinence *(continued)*

DIAGNOSIS

- *Stress urinary incontinence* related to weak pelvic floor musculature and tissue atrophy
- *Urge urinary incontinence* related to excess intake of caffeine and citrus juices
- *Impaired skin integrity* related to constant contact of urine with perineal tissues
- *Ineffective coping* related to inability to control urine leakage

EXPECTED OUTCOMES

- Remain dry between voidings and at night.
- Demonstrate improved perineal muscle strength.
- Regain and maintain perineal skin integrity.
- Return to her previous level of social activity.

PLANNING AND IMPLEMENTATION

- Teach how to identify pelvic floor muscles and how to perform Kegel exercises.
- Suggest drinking decaffeinated tea and noncitrus fruit juices (grape, apple, and cranberry).
- Encourage to minimize fluid intake after evening meal.
- Change afternoon dose of furosemide from 9:00 P.M. to 3:00 P.M.
- Instruct to void by the clock, gradually increasing intervals from every 45 to 60 minutes to every 2 to 2.5 hours. Advise to maintain shorter voiding intervals for 2 to 3 hours after furosemide doses.
- Teach to cleanse perineal area, wiping front to back, after each voiding or incident of urine leakage.
- Introduce commercial products available for clothing and furniture protection, encouraging experimentation to identify the most helpful product(s).
- Provide a commode for bedside at night and adequate lighting to prevent injury.
- Schedule follow-up visits and evaluations to reinforce teaching.

EVALUATION

Three months after her initial visit, Mrs. Giovanni states that she is doing very well, experiencing occasional leakage of small amounts of urine, primarily when sneezing, coughing, or laughing. She finds a minipad adequate for protection and is often able to remain dry all day. She has had no further problems with enuresis since changing her evening furosemide dose to late afternoon and limiting her fluids after dinner. She can make it to the bathroom and no longer needs the bedside commode. Her perineal tissue is intact, and she demonstrates improved muscle strength. Anna's daughter says her mother is beginning to resume her normal social activities, and that she is no longer worried about her mother's ability to care for herself independently.

Critical Thinking in the Nursing Process

1. What factors in Mrs. Giovanni's past medical history and current medication regimen contributed to her nighttime incontinence?
2. What is the rationale for including an intervention to teach Mrs. Giovanni about perineal cleansing as part of her care plan?
3. Develop a care plan for Mrs. Giovanni for the nursing diagnosis, *Situational low self-esteem* related to urinary incontinence.

See Evaluating Your Response in Appendix C.

 ## EXPLORE MediaLink

NCLEX review questions, case studies, care plan activities, MediaLink applications, and other interactive resources for this chapter can be found on the Companion Website at www.prenhall.com/lemone.

Click on Chapter 26 to select the activities for this chapter. For animations, video clips, more NCLEX review questions, and an audio glossary, access the Student CD-ROM accompanying this textbook.

TEST YOURSELF

1. A 23-year-old woman presents to the urgency clinic with symptoms of a urinary tract infection. The nursing history reveals that the client was treated 3 months previously for a UTI. Additional questions the nurse should ask include

   a. Did you complete your antibiotic prescription for your first UTI?

   b. What form of birth control are you using?
   c. Does your partner have similar symptoms?
   d. How much fluid do you drink each day?

2. Recognizing the risk for urolithiasis in the immobilized client, the nurse appropriately plans to:
   a. Administer a calcium supplement
   b. Regularly monitor urine pH
   c. Maintain an indwelling urinary catheter
   d. Increased fluid intake to 3,000 mL per day

3. The nurse teaching a group of community members about wellness and disease prevention includes which of the following as a measure to reduce the risk for bladder cancer?
   a. Do not start smoking; if you smoke, stop
   b. Avoid using hair dyes and pesticides in the home
   c. Limit your intake of coffee and other caffeinated beverages
   d. Empty your bladder every two hours

4. The nurse evaluates her teaching as effective when the client with a newly created continent ileal diversion is able to:
   a. Demonstrate care for the collection device
   b. State the importance of promptly reporting cloudy urine to the physician
   c. Demonstrate self catheterization of the stoma
   d. Identify factors contributing to his risk for bladder cancer

5. The nurse identifies which of the following as a high priority goal for a client with stress incontinence?
   a. Can identify products for protecting clothing and furniture
   b. States chronic and benign nature of the disorder
   c. Performs pelvic floor muscle exercises as taught at least twice a day
   d. Limits intake of beverages containing caffeine and artificial sweeteners

See Test Yourself answers in Appendix C.

BIBLIOGRAPHY

Ackley, B. J., & Ladwig, G. B. (2002). *Nursing diagnosis handbook: A guide to planning care* (5th ed.). St. Louis: Mosby.

Ahya, S. N., Flood, K., & Paranjothi, S. (Eds.). (2001). *The Washington manual of medical therapeutics* (30th ed.). Philadelphia: Lippincott Williams & Wilkins.

American Cancer Society. (2002). *Cancer facts and figures 2002.* Atlanta: Author.

Bardsley, A. (1999). Assessment of incontinence. *Elder Care, 11*(9), 36–39.

Baxter, A. (1999). Bladder cancer: Its diagnosis and treatment. *Nursing Times, 95*(41), 42–44.

Braunwald, E., Fauci, A. S., Kasper, D. L., Hauser, S. L., Longo, D. L., & Jameson, J. L. (2001). *Harrison's principles of internal medicine* (15th ed.). New York: McGraw-Hill.

Bullock, B. A., & Henze, R. L. (2000). *Focus on pathophysiology.* Philadelphia: Lippincott.

Fontaine, K. L. (2000). *Healing practices: Alternative therapies for nursing.* Upper Saddle River, NJ: Prentice Hall Health.

Gallo, J. J., Busby-Whitehead, J., Rabins, P. V., Silliman, R. A., & Murphy, J. B. (Eds.). (1999). *Reichel's care of the elderly: Clinical aspects of aging* (5th ed.). Philadelphia: Lippincott Williams & Wilkins.

Gray, M. (2000a). Urinary retention: Management in the acute care setting. Part 1. *American Journal of Nursing, 100*(7), 40–47.

——————. (2000b). Urinary retention: Management in the acute care setting. Part 2. *American Journal of Nursing, 100*(8), 36–43.

Gray, M., McClain, R., Peruggia, M., Patrie, J., & Steers, W. D. (2001). A model for predicting motor urge urinary incontinence. *Nursing Research, 50*(2), 116–122.

Hanchett, M. (2002). Techniques for stabilizing urinary catheters. *American Journal of Nursing, 102*(3), 44–48.

Johnson, M., Bulechek, G., Dochterman, J. M., Maas, M., & Moorhead, S. (2001). *Nursing diagnoses, outcomes, & interventions.* St. Louis: Mosby.

Johnson, M., Maas, M., & Moorhead, S. (Eds.). (2000). *Nursing outcomes classification (NOC)* (2nd ed.). St. Louis: Mosby.

Johnson, S. T. (2000). From incontinence to confidence. *American Journal of Nursing, 100*(2), 69–70, 72–75.

Lekan-Rutledge, D. (2000). Diffusion of innovation. A model for implementation of prompted voiding in long-term care settings. *Journal of Gerontology Nursing, 26*(4), 25–33.

Lyons, S. S., & Specht, J. K. (2000). Prompted voiding protocol for individuals with urinary incontinence. *Journal of Gerontology Nursing, 26*(6), 5–13.

Malarkey, L.M., & McMorrow, M.E. (2000). *Nurse's manual of laboratory tests and diagnostic procedures* (2nd ed.). Philadelphia: Saunders.

Maloney, C., & Cafiero, M. R. (1999). Urinary incontinence. Noninvasive treatment options. *Advance for Nurse Practitioners, 7*(6), 36–42.

McCloskey, J. C., & Bulechek, G. M. (Eds.) (2000). *Nursing interventions classification (NIC)* (3rd ed.). St. Louis: Mosby.

McConnell, E. A. (2001). Myths & facts … about kidney stones. *Nursing, 31*(1), 73.

Meeker, M. H., & Rothrock, J. C. (1999). *Alexander's care of the patient in surgery* (11th ed.). St. Louis: Mosby.

National Kidney and Urologic Diseases Information Clearinghouse. (1998). Urinary incontinence in women. National Institute of Diabetes and Digestive and Kidney Diseases (NIDDK), National Institutes of Health. Available www.niddk.nih.gov/health/urolog/pubs/uiwomen/uiwomen.htm

Nicolle, L. E. (2001). Urinary tract infections in long-term care facilities. *Infections Control & Hospital Epidemiology, 22*(3), 167–175.

North American Nursing Diagnosis Association. (2001). *NANDA nursing diagnoses: Definitions & classification 2001–2002.* Philadelphia: NANDA.

Porth, C. M. (2002). *Pathophysiology: Concepts of altered health states* (6th ed.). Philadelphia: Lippincott.

Prieto-Fingerhut, T., Banovac, K., & Lynne, C. M. (1997). A study comparing sterile and nonsterile urethral catheterization in patients with spinal cord injury. *Rehabilitation Nursing, 22*(6), 299–302.

Ratliff, C. R., & Donovan, A. M. (2001). Frequency of peristomal complications. *Ostomy & Wound Management, 47*(8), 26–29.

Springhouse. (1999). *Nurse's handbook of alternative & complementary therapies.* Springhouse, PA: Author.

Suchinski, G. A., Piano, M. R., Rosenberg, N., & Zerwic, J. J. (1999). Treating urinary tract infections in the elderly. *Dimensions of Critical Care Nursing, 18*(1), 21–27.

Tierney, L. M., McPhee, S. J., & Papadakis, M. A. (2001). *Current medical diagnosis & treatment* (40th ed.). New York: Lange Medical Books/McGraw-Hill.

Vinsnes, A. G., Harkless, G. E., Haltbakk, J., Bohm, J., & Hunskaar, S. (2001). Healthcare personnel's attitudes towards patients with urinary incontinence. *Journal of Clinical Nursing, 10*(4), 455–462.

Young. J. (2000). Action stat. Kidney stone. *Nursing, 30*(7), 33.

Nursing Care of Clients with Kidney Disorders

LEARNING OUTCOMES

After completing this chapter, you will be able to:

- Relate the pathophysiology of common kidney disorders to normal renal physiology (see Chapter 25).

- Relate manifestations of kidney disease to the pathophysiology of the disorder.

- Discuss diagnostic studies used to identify disorders of the kidneys.

- Discuss the nursing implications for medications used to treat clients with kidney disorders.

- Identify specific dietary modifications ordered for clients with kidney disorders.

- Compare and contrast dialysis procedures used to manage acute and chronic renal failure.

- Discuss nursing care of the client undergoing dialysis.

- Provide appropriate nursing care for the client who has had kidney surgery or a renal transplant.

- Use the nursing process to plan and provide individualized care to clients with renal disorders.

MediaLink

www.prenhall.com/lemone

Additional resources for this chapter can be found on the Student CD-ROM accompanying this textbook, and on the Companion Website at www.prenhall.com/lemone. Click on Chapter 27 to select the activities for this chapter.

CD-ROM
- Audio Glossary
- NCLEX Review

Animation
- Furosemide

Companion Website
- More NCLEX Review
- Case Study
    Acute Glomerulonephritis
- Care Plan Activity
    Acute Glomerulonephritis
- MediaLink Application
    Kidney Disorders

The internal environment of the body normally remains in a relatively constant or *homeostatic* state. The kidneys help maintain homeostasis by regulating the composition and volume of extracellular fluid. They excrete excess water and solutes and also can conserve water and solutes when deficits occur. In addition, the kidneys help regulate acid-base balance and they excrete metabolic wastes. Regulation of blood pressure is also a key function of the kidneys.

Both primary kidney disorders (such as glomerulonephritis) and systemic diseases (such as diabetes mellitus) can affect renal function. In North America, more than 20 million people are affected by kidney and urinary tract diseases. Every year, approximately 1 in every 1000 people in the United States develops end-stage renal disease (ESRD), the final phase of chronic renal failure in which little or no kidney function remains. Chronic renal disease accounts for about 80,000 deaths per year and is a major cause of lost work time and wages. Ironically, the increased prevalence of chronic renal disease in recent years is partially related to the success of dialysis and transplantation.

AGE-RELATED CHANGES IN KIDNEY FUNCTION

Glomeruli in the renal cortex (see Chapter 25 ⊂⊃ for a review of normal kidney structure and function) are lost with aging, reducing kidney mass. Because of the large functional reserve of the kidneys, however, renal function remains adequate unless additional stressors affect the renal system. The **glomerular filtration rate (GFR),** the amount of filtrate made by the kidneys per minute, declines due to age-related factors affecting the renovascular system (such as arteriosclerosis, decreased renal vascularity, and decreased cardiac output). By age 80, the GFR may be less than half of what it was at age 30.

Age-related changes in renal function have significant implications. The kidneys are less able to concentrate urine and compensate for increased or decreased salt intake. When combined with diminished effectiveness of antidiuretic hormone (ADH) and a reduced thirst response, both common in aging, this decreased ability to concentrate urine increases the risk for dehydration. Potassium excretion may be decreased because of lower aldosterone levels. As a result, fluid and electrolyte imbalances are more common and potentially critical in the older client.

Decreased GFR in the older adult also reduces the clearance of drugs excreted through the kidneys. This reduced clearance prolongs the half-life of drugs and may necessitate lower drug doses and longer dosing intervals. Common medications affected by decreased GFR include:

- Cardiac drugs: digoxin, procainamide
- Antibiotics: aminoglycosides, tetracyclines, cephalosporins
- Histamine H_2 antagonists: cimetidine
- Antidiabetic agents: chlorpropamide

When caring for older adults, it is especially important to monitor drugs that are toxic to the renal tubules. Radiologic dyes and aminoglycoside, tetracycline, and the cephalosporin antibiotics are part of this group.

Age-related changes in renal function and related nursing implications are summarized in Table 27–1.

THE CLIENT WITH A CONGENITAL KIDNEY MALFORMATION

Congenital kidney disorders can affect the form and/or function of the kidney. Functional congenital kidney disorders are usually identified in childhood or adolescence. If function is not affected, congenital malformations may be detected only coincidentally. Malformations include agenesis, hypoplasia, alterations in kidney position, and horseshoe kidney.

Agenesis, absence of the kidney, and *hypoplasia,* underdevelopment of the kidney, typically affect only one of these paired organs. Renal function remains normal unless the unaffected kidney is compromised. Abnormal kidney position af-

TABLE 27–1 Nursing Implications of Age-Related Changes in Kidney Function		
Functional Change	**Effect**	**Implications**
Decreased glomerular filtration rate (GFR)	Decreased clearance of drugs excreted primarily through the kidneys increases drug half-life and blood levels, and risk of drug toxicity.	Monitor carefully for signs of toxicity, especially when administering digoxin, aminoglycoside antibiotics, tetracycline, vancomycin, chlorpropamide, procainamide, cimetidine, and cephalosporin antibiotics.
Decreased number of functional nephrons; lower levels of aldosterone; increased resistance to ADH	Decreased ability to conserve water and sodium; impaired potassium excretion; and decreased hydrogen ion excretion, resulting in reduced ability to compensate for acidosis.	Monitor for dehydration and hyponatremia; maintain fluid intake of 1500 to 2500 mL/day unless contraindicated; monitor for hyperkalemia, especially if taking a potassium-sparing diuretic, heparin, angiotensin-converting enzyme (ACE) inhibitor, beta-blocker, or NSAID; increased risk for acidosis.
Reduced numbers of functional nephrons	Decreased renal reserve with increased risk of failure.	Avoid giving nephrotoxic drugs if possible; monitor urine output and blood chemistries for early signs of renal failure.

fects the ureters and urine flow, potentially leading to urinary stasis, increased risk of urinary tract infection (UTI), and lithiasis, or stone formation (see Chapter 26).

One in every 500 to 1000 people has *horseshoe kidney,* making it one of the most common renal malformations (Porth, 2002). Failure of the embryonic kidneys to ascend normally can result in a single, horseshoe-shaped organ. The two kidneys are fused at either the upper or lower pole (usually the lower). This malformation does not typically affect renal function; however, because the ureters cross the fused poles, there is an increased risk for *hydronephrosis,* or distention of the renal pelvis and calyces with urine (see Chapter 26). Recurrent UTI and renal calculi are also common in clients with horseshoe kidney.

Renal ultrasonography and intravenous pyelography are used to diagnose horseshoe kidney. Correction of the abnormality is rarely necessary, although surgical resection of the isthmus (connection between the kidneys) may be done to relieve ureteral obstruction or allow access to the abdominal aorta, which lies behind it.

Nursing care for clients with horseshoe kidney or other congenital malformations is primarily educational. Because abnormal kidney shape or position increases the risk of infection and stone formation, teach the client to maintain a fluid intake of at least 2500 mL per day. Emphasize the importance of avoiding dehydration by increasing fluids during hot weather and strenuous exercise. Teach hygiene practices such as perineal cleansing and voiding before and after intercourse to help prevent UTI. Teach the early manifestations of UTI and instruct to seek treatment promptly to prevent infection of the kidney. See Chapter 26.

THE CLIENT WITH POLYCYSTIC KIDNEY DISEASE

Polycystic kidney disease, a hereditary disease characterized by cyst formation and massive kidney enlargement, affects both children and adults. This disease has two forms: The autosomal dominant form affects adults; the autosomal recessive form is present at birth (Bullock & Henze, 2000; Porth, 2002). Autosomal recessive polycystic kidney disease is rare. It usually is diagnosed prenatally or in infancy. Renal failure generally develops during childhood, necessitating kidney transplant or dialysis. Autosomal dominant polycystic kidney disease is relatively common, affecting 1 in every 300 to 1000 people and accounting for approximately 10% of clients with ESRD in the United States (Braunwald et al., 2001). This section focuses on autosomal dominant polycystic kidney disease, the more common, adult form of the disorder.

PATHOPHYSIOLOGY

Renal cysts are fluid-filled sacs affecting the nephron, the functional unit of the kidneys. They develop in the tubular epithelium of the nephron, filling with straw-colored glomerular filtrate. The cysts may range in size from microscopic to several centimeters in diameter and affect the renal cortex and

Figure 27–1 ■ A polycystic kidney. The functional tissue of the kidneys is gradually destroyed and replaced with fluid-filled cysts.

Source: A. Glauberman/Photo Researchers, Inc.

medulla of both kidneys. As the cysts fill, enlarge, and multiply, the kidneys also enlarge. Renal blood vessels and nephrons are compressed and obstructed, and functional tissue destroyed (Figure 27–1 ■). The renal parenchyma atrophies and becomes fibrotic and scarred (Braunwald et al., 2001).

People affected by polycystic kidney disease often develop cysts elsewhere in the body, including the liver, spleen, pancreas, and other organs. Up to 10% of people affected experience subarachnoid hemorrhage from a type of congenital intracranial aneurysm. People with polycystic kidney disease also have an increased incidence of incompetent or "floppy" cardiac valves.

MANIFESTATIONS

Polycystic kidney disease is slowly progressive. Symptoms usually develop by age 40 to 50. Common manifestations include flank pain, microscopic or gross **hematuria** (blood in the urine), **proteinuria** (proteins in the urine), and *polyuria* and *nocturia,* as the concentrating ability of the kidney is impaired. Urinary tract infection and renal calculi are common, as cysts interfere with normal urine drainage. Most clients develop hypertension from disruption of renal vessels. The kidneys become palpable, enlarged, and knobby. Symptoms of renal insufficiency and chronic renal failure typically develop by age 60 to 70.

COLLABORATIVE CARE

Diagnostic tests used to determine the extent of polycystic kidney disease include the following:

- *Renal ultrasonography* is the diagnostic procedure of choice for polycystic kidney disease. Reflected sound waves are used to assess kidney size and to identify, locate, and differentiate renal masses such as cysts, tumors, and calculi. (See the box on page 717 for the nursing implications for renal ultrasound.)
- *Intravenous pyelography (IVP),* a radiologic examination, is used to evaluate the structure and excretory function of the

kidneys, ureters, and bladder. An intravenously injected contrast medium illuminates kidney size and shape, the calyces and pelvis, the ureters, and the bladder as it is cleared from the blood. Cysts can be detected and sized, and the extent of kidney involvement determined. (See the Nursing Implications box on page 708 for an IVP.)

- *Computed tomography (CT scan)* of the kidney uses X-rays passed through the kidneys at many angles to create a detailed picture of renal tissue densities and composition. CT may be done with or without contrast media. Kidney CT is used to detect and differentiate renal masses such as cystic disease or tumors. (See the Nursing Implications box on page 717.)

Management of adult polycystic kidney disease is largely supportive. Care is taken to avoid further renal damage by nephrotoxic substances, UTI, obstruction, or hypertension. A fluid intake of 2000 to 2500 mL per day is encouraged to help prevent UTI and lithiasis. Hypertension associated with polycystic disease is generally controlled using angiotensin-converting enzyme (ACE) inhibitors or other antihypertensive agents (see Chapter 33). Ultimately, dialysis or renal transplantation is required. Clients with polycystic kidney disease are typically good candidates for transplantation because of the absence of associated systemic disease.

NURSING CARE

For those with adult polycystic kidney disease, an autosomal dominant disorder, discuss genetic counseling and screening of family members for evidence of the disease. This is particularly important if renal transplantation is contemplated and family members are potential donors. Consider the following nursing diagnoses when planning care for the client with polycystic kidney disease.

- *Excess fluid volume* related to impaired renal function
- *Anticipatory grieving* related to potential loss of kidney function
- *Deficient knowledge* regarding measures to help preserve kidney function
- *Risk for ineffective coping* related to potential genetic transmission of the disorder to offspring

Teach the client with polycystic kidney disease about the disease, its genetic nature, and usual course. Discuss measures to maintain optimal renal function. Instruct to maintain a fluid intake of at least 2500 mL per day. Include additional information about preventing UTI (such as hygiene measures) and early manifestations of UTI. Stress the importance of seeking treatment to prevent further kidney damage. Advise to avoid drugs that are potentially toxic to the kidneys and to check with primary care provider before taking any new drug.

THE CLIENT WITH A GLOMERULAR DISORDER

Disorders and diseases involving the glomerulus are the leading cause of chronic renal failure in the United States. They are the underlying disease process for half of those people needing dialysis and result in 12,000 deaths per year.

Glomerular disorders may be either primary, involving mainly the kidney, or secondary to a multisystem disease or hereditary condition. Primary glomerular disease is often immunologic or idiopathic in origin. Diabetes mellitus, systemic lupus erythematosus (SLE), and Goodpasture's syndrome are frequently implicated in secondary glomerular disorders.

PHYSIOLOGY REVIEW

The glomerulus is a tuft of capillaries surrounded by a thin, double-walled capsule (Bowman's capsule). (See Figure 25–3) About 20% of the resting cardiac output flows through the glomeruli of the kidneys, forming approximately 180 L of plasma ultrafiltrate. More than 99% of this filtrate is reabsorbed in the renal tubules. The rate of glomerular filtration (GFR) is controlled by opposing forces: The pressure and amount of blood flowing through the glomeruli promote filtration, and the pressure in Bowman's capsule and colloid osmotic pressure of the blood oppose it. The total surface area of glomerular capillaries also affects the GFR. The glomerular capillary membrane has three layers: the capillary endothelial layer, the basement membrane, and the capsule epithelial layer. Water and the smallest solutes (such as electrolytes) pass freely across this membrane, while larger molecules (such as plasma proteins) are retained in the blood.

PATHOPHYSIOLOGY

Glomerular disease affects both the structure and function of the glomerulus, disrupting glomerular filtration. The capillary membrane becomes more permeable to plasma proteins and blood cells. This increased permeability in the glomerulus causes the manifestations common to glomerular disorders: hematuria, proteinuria, and edema. The GFR falls, leading to **azotemia** (increased blood levels of nitrogenous waste products), and hypertension. Glomerular involvement may be diffuse, involving all glomeruli, or focal, involving some glomeruli while others remain essentially normal.

Both hematuria and proteinuria are caused by glomerular capillary membrane damage, which allows blood cells and proteins to escape from the blood into the glomerular filtrate. Hematuria may be either gross or microscopic. Proteinuria is considered to be the most important indicator of glomerular injury, because it increases progressively with increased glomerular damage. Loss of plasma proteins leads to *hypoalbuminemia* (low serum albumin levels), which in turn reduces the plasma oncotic pressure (osmotic pressure created by plasma proteins), leading to edema.

As plasma proteins are lost, the forces opposing filtration diminish, and the amount of filtrate increases. The increased flow of filtrate stimulates the renin-angiotensin-aldosterone mechanism (see Chapter 25), producing vasoconstriction and a fall in GFR. Increased aldosterone production causes salt and water retention which further contribute to edema. As the GFR falls, filtration and elimination of nitrogenous wastes, including urea, decreases, causing azotemia. **Oliguria,** urine output of less than 400 mL in 24 hours, may result from the decreased GFR. Hypertension results from fluid retention and disruption of the renin-angiotensin system, a key regulator of blood pressure.

The major primary glomerular disorders include acute glomerulonephritis, rapidly progressive glomerulonephritis, chronic glomerulonephritis, and nephrotic syndrome. Diabetic nephropathy and lupus nephritis are the most common secondary forms of glomerular disease.

Acute Glomerulonephritis

Glomerulonephritis is inflammation of the glomerular capillary membrane. Acute glomerulonephritis can result from systemic diseases or primary glomerular diseases, but acute poststreptococcal glomerulonephritis (also known as acute proliferative glomerulonephritis) is the most common form. Infection of the pharynx or skin with group A β-hemolytic streptococcus is the usual initiating event for this disorder. Staphylococcal or viral infections, such as hepatitis B, mumps, or varicella (chickenpox), can lead to a similar postinfectious acute glomerulonephritis (Porth, 2002). This primarily childhood disease also can affect adults.

In acute glomerulonephritis, circulating antigen-antibody immune complexes formed during the primary infection become trapped in the glomerular membrane, leading to an inflammatory response. The complement system is activated, and vasoactive substances and inflammatory mediators are released. Endothelial cells proliferate, and the glomerular membrane swells and becomes permeable to plasma proteins and blood cells (Figure 27–2 ■). Renal involvement is diffuse, spread throughout the kidneys.

MANIFESTATIONS AND COMPLICATIONS

Acute glomerulonephritis is characterized by an abrupt onset of hematuria, proteinuria, salt and water retention, and evidence of azotemia occurring 10 to 14 days after the initial infection. The urine often appears brown or cola-colored. Salt and water retention increase extracellular fluid volume, leading to hypertension and edema. The edema is primarily noted in the face, particularly around the eyes (*periorbital* edema). Dependent edema, affecting the hands and upper extremities in particular, may also be noted. Other manifestations may include fatigue, anorexia, nausea and vomiting, and headache (see the box below).

The older adult may have less apparent symptoms. Nausea, malaise, arthralgias, and proteinuria are common manifestations; hypertension and edema are seen less often. Pulmonary infiltrates may occur early in the disorder, often due to worsening of a preexisting condition such as heart failure.

The prognosis for adults with acute glomerulonephritis is less favorable than it is for children. The symptoms may resolve spontaneously within 10 to 14 days. Full recovery is usual in children, whereas 60% or more affected adults recover completely. The remainder have persistent symptoms, and some have permanent kidney damage (Porth, 2002).

Rapidly Progressive Glomerulonephritis

Rapidly progressive glomerulonephritis (RPGN) is characterized by manifestations of severe glomerular injury without a specific, identifiable cause. This type of glomerulonephritis often progresses to renal failure within months. It may be idiopathic (primary), or secondary to a systemic disorder such as SLE or Goodpasture's syndrome. It affects people of all ages.

In RPGN, glomerular cells proliferate and, together with macrophages, form crescent-shaped lesions that obliterate Bowman's space (Porth, 2002). Glomerular damage is diffuse, leading to a rapid, progressive decline in renal function. Irreversible renal failure often develops over weeks to months (Braunwald et al., 2001; Bullock & Henze, 2000).

Clients with RPGN typically present with complaints of weakness, nausea, and vomiting. Some may relate a history of a flulike illness preceding the onset of the glomerulonephritis. Other symptoms include oliguria and abdominal or flank pain. Moderate hypertension may develop. On urinalysis, hematuria and massive proteinuria are noted.

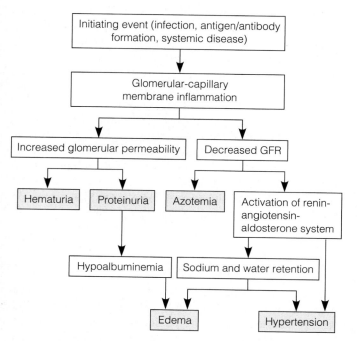

Figure 27–2 ■ The pathogenesis of glomerulonephritis.

Manifestations of Acute Glomerulonephritis

- Hematuria, cola-colored urine
- Proteinuria
- Salt and water retention
- Edema, periorbital and facial, dependent
- Hypertension
- Azotemia
- Fatigue
- Anorexia, nausea, and vomiting
- Headache

Goodpasture's Syndrome

Goodpasture's syndrome is a rare autoimmune disorder of unknown etiology. It is characterized by formation of antibodies to the glomerular basement membrane. These antibodies also may bind to alveolar basement membranes, damaging alveoli and causing pulmonary hemorrhage. Goodpasture's syndrome usually affects young men between 18 and 35, although it can occur at any age and affect women as well.

Although the glomeruli may be nearly normal in appearance and function in Goodpasture's syndrome, extensive cell proliferation and crescent formation characteristic of rapidly progressive glomerulonephritis are more common. Renal manifestations include hematuria, proteinuria, and edema. Rapid progression to renal failure may occur. Alveolar membrane damage can lead to mild or life-threatening pulmonary hemorrhage. Cough, shortness of breath, and hemoptysis (bloody sputum) are early respiratory manifestations.

Chronic Glomerulonephritis

Chronic glomerulonephritis is typically the end stage of other glomerular disorders such as RPGN, lupus nephritis, or diabetic nephropathy. In many cases, however, no previous glomerular disease has been identified.

Slow, progressive destruction of the glomeruli and a gradual decline in renal function are characteristic of chronic glomerulonephritis. The kidneys decrease in size symmetrically, and their surfaces become granular or roughened. Eventually, entire nephrons are lost.

Symptoms develop insidiously, and the disease is often not recognized until signs of renal failure develop. Chronic glomerulonephritis may also be diagnosed when hypertension and impaired renal function are found coincidentally during a routine physical examination or treatment for an unrelated disorder. Viral or bacterial infectious diseases can exacerbate the disorder, prompting its diagnosis.

The course of chronic glomerulonephritis varies, with years to decades between the diagnosis and the development of end-stage renal failure.

Nephrotic Syndrome

Nephrotic syndrome is a group of clinical findings as opposed to a specific disorder. It is characterized by massive proteinuria, hypoalbuminemia, hyperlipidemia, and edema. A number of disorders can affect the glomerular capillary membrane, changing its porosity and allowing plasma proteins to escape into the urine. *Minimal change disease (MCD)* is the most common cause of nephrotic syndrome in children and accounts for 20% of adults with nephrotic syndrome (Braunwald et al., 2001). In MCD, the size and form of glomeruli appear normal by light microscopy. The prognosis for MCD is good. In adults, *membranous glomerulonephropathy* is the most common cause of idiopathic nephrotic syndrome. The glomerular basement membrane thickens, although no inflammation is present. This form of nephrotic syndrome also occurs with some systemic diseases such as SLE and hepatitis B, and with drugs such as gold or penicillamine. *Focal sclerosis,* in which scarring (sclerosis) of glomeruli occurs, and *membran-*

Figure 27–3 ■ Severe edema characteristic of nephrotic syndrome.

Source: Science Photo Library/Library Researcher, Inc.

oproliferative glomerulonephritis, caused by thickening and proliferation of glomerular basement membrane cells, are additional forms of nephrotic syndrome.

With plasma protein loss in the urine and resulting hypoalbuminemia, the oncotic pressure of the plasma falls. Fluid shifts from the vascular compartment to interstitial spaces, causing the edema characteristic of nephrotic syndrome. Salt and water retention, possibly due to activation of the renin-angiotensin system, contribute to the edema. Edema may be severe, affecting the face and periorbital area as well as dependent tissues (Figure 27–3 ■).

Loss of plasma proteins stimulates the liver to increase albumin production and lipoprotein synthesis. As a result, serum triglyceride and low-density lipoprotein (LDL) levels increase, as do urine lipids (*lipiduria*). Hyperlipidemia increases the risk for atherosclerosis in clients with nephrotic syndrome.

Thromboemboli (mobilized blood clots) are a relatively common complication of nephrotic syndrome. Loss of clotting and anticlotting factors along with plasma proteins are thought to disrupt the coagulation system, increasing the risk for renal vein thrombosis, deep vein thrombosis, and pulmonary embolism. Renal vein thrombosis can cause flank or groin pain on one or both sides, gross hematuria, and a reduced GFR (Porth, 2002).

Nephrotic syndrome usually resolves without long-term effects in children. The prognosis for adults is less optimistic. Less than 50% of adults recover completely. Many have persistent proteinuria and may develop progressive renal impairment. As many as 30% of adults with nephrotic syndrome develop end-stage renal failure.

Diabetic Nephropathy

Diabetic nephropathy, kidney disease common in the later stages of diabetes mellitus (DM), is the leading cause of end-stage renal disease in North America. Thirty percent of clients with type 1 DM and about 20% of type 2 diabetic clients develop nephropathy. ESRD resulting from diabetic nephropathy is seen more frequently in blacks with type 2 DM, and in whites with type 1 DM (Braunwald et al., 2001).

Initial evidence of microproteinuria indicating renal damage is typically seen within 10 to 15 years after the onset of diabetes. Overt proteinuria and nephropathy generally develop within 15 to 20 years of the initial diagnosis.

The characteristic lesion of diabetic nephropathy is glomerulosclerosis and thickening of the glomerular basement membrane. Arteriosclerosis, a common feature of long-term diabetes and hypertension, contributes to the disease, as do nephritis and tubular lesions. Pyelonephritis, inflammation of the kidney, is also implicated in the development of diabetic nephropathy. A further discussion is found in Chapter 18.

Lupus Nephritis

Systemic lupus erythematosus (SLE) is an inflammatory autoimmune disorder affecting the connective tissue of the body. Between 40% and 85% of clients with SLE develop manifestations of nephritis (Braunwald et al., 2001). Immune complexes that form within the glomerular capillary wall are the usual trigger for glomerular injury in SLE. Manifestations of lupus nephritis range from microscopic hematuria to massive proteinuria. Its progession may be slow and chronic or *fulminant,* with a sudden onset and the rapid development of renal failure. Most clients with minimal or mild lesions survive for at least 10 years. Improved management of the underlying disease, immunotherapy, dialysis, and renal transplantation have significantly improved the prognosis in recent years.

COLLABORATIVE CARE

Management of all types of glomerulonephritis, acute and chronic, primary and secondary, focuses on identifying the underlying disease process and preserving kidney function. In most glomerular disorders, there is no specific treatment to achieve a cure. Treatment goals are to maintain renal function, prevent complications, and support the healing process.

Diagnostic Tests

Laboratory and diagnostic testing are valuable to identify the cause of glomerulonephritis and evaluate kidney function.

The following studies may be ordered to help identify the underlying cause or etiology.

- *Throat or skin cultures* detect infection by group A β-hemolytic streptococci. Although poststreptococcal glomerulonephritis typically follows the acute infection by 1 to 2 weeks, treatment to eradicate any remaining organisms is initiated to minimize antibody production.
- *Antistreptolysin O (ASO) titer* and other tests detect streptococcal *exoenzymes* (bacterial enzymes that stimulate the immune response in acute poststreptococcal glomerulonephritis). Other titers such as antistreptokinase (ASK) or antideoxyribonuclease B (ADNAase B) may be obtained as well.
- *Erythrocyte sedimentation rate (ESR)* is a general indicator of inflammatory response. It may be elevated in acute poststreptococcal glomerulonephritis and in lupus nephritis.

- *KUB* (kidney, ureter, bladder) *abdominal X-ray* may be done to evaluate kidney size and rule out other causes of the client's manifestations. The kidneys may be enlarged in acute glomerulonephritis, whereas bilateral small kidneys are typical of late chronic glomerulonephritis.
- *Kidney scan,* a nuclear medicine procedure, allows visualization of the kidney after intravenous administration of a radioisotope. In glomerular diseases, the uptake and excretion of the radioactive material are delayed.
- *Biopsy,* microscopic examination of kidney tissue, is the most reliable diagnostic procedure for glomerular disorders. Biopsy helps determine the type of glomerulonephritis, the prognosis, and appropriate treatment. Renal biopsy is usually done percutaneously, by inserting a biopsy needle through the skin into the kidney to obtain a tissue sample. Open biopsy, which requires surgery, may also be done.

See the box on page 750 for the nursing implications for diagnostic tests used to evaluate glomerular disorders.

The following studies are used to evaluate kidney function:

- *Blood urea nitrogen (BUN)* measures urea nitrogen, the end product of protein metabolism. It is created by the breakdown and metabolism of both dietary and body proteins. Urea is eliminated from the body by filtration in the glomerulus; minimal amounts are reabsorbed in the renal tubules. Glomerular diseases interfere with filtration and elimination of urea nitrogen, causing blood levels to rise. Increased protein catabolism (destruction), which may occur with GI bleeding or tissue breakdown, can also raise the BUN. Normal BUN values are listed in Table 27–2. Levels up to 50 mg/dL or 17.7 mmol/L indicate mild azotemia, and levels higher than 100 mg/dL or 35.7 mmol/L indicate severe renal impairment.
- *Serum creatinine* measures the amount of creatinine in the blood. Creatinine is also a metabolic by-product, produced in relatively constant amounts by skeletal muscles. It is excreted entirely by the kidneys, making the serum creatinine a good indicator of kidney function. Normal values (see Table 27–2) are lower in the older adult because of decreased muscle mass. Levels greater than 4 mg/dL indicate serious impairment of renal function.
- *Urine creatinine* also is an indicator of renal function and the GFR. Urine creatinine levels decrease when renal function is impaired as it is not effectively eliminated from the body.
- *Creatinine clearance* is a specific indicator of renal function used to evaluate the GFR. The *clearance,* or amount of blood cleared of creatinine in 1 minute, depends on the amount and pressure of blood being filtered and the filtering ability of the glomeruli. Levels normally decline with aging as the GFR decreases in the older adult. Disorders such as glomerulonephritis affect glomerular filtration, decreasing the creatinine clearance.
- *Serum electrolytes* are evaluated because impaired kidney function alters their excretion. Monitoring serum electrolytes is particularly important to prevent complications associated with imbalances.

Nursing Implications for Diagnostic Tests

Glomerular Disease

CREATININE CLEARANCE

Preparation of the Client

- Obtain a 24-hour urine specimen container without preservative.
- Instruct to begin the specimen collection at the designated time by voiding and discarding this initial specimen. Collect all urine voided for the next 24 hours, emptying the bladder at the end of the collection time and saving the specimen. Do not discard toilet paper in the specimen container.
- Instruct to void and save the specimen prior to defecating to prevent contamination or loss of urine.
- Refrigerate or keep the urine specimen on ice during the collection period.
- Post signs in the client's room and bathroom indicating the hours of urine collection to prevent inadvertent discarding of the urine.
- Collect or have laboratory personnel collect a venous blood sample during the 24-hour urine collection period.
- Note the client's name, age, weight, and height on the laboratory requisition.

Client and Family Teaching

- Generally, no special diet is required during the test.
- Follow instructions for 24-hour specimen collection if the test is being done on an outpatient basis.

KIDNEY SCAN (RENAL SCAN)

Preparation of the Client

- Informed consent is required. Provide teaching and answer questions as needed.
- Make sure that the client is well hydrated prior to the procedure. Provide two to three glasses of water before the procedure if indicated.
- Obtain weight (used to calculate the amount of radioisotope to be injected).
- Have void prior to the procedure.
- After the procedure, increase fluid intake to promote excretion of the radioisotope.
- No special radioactivity precautions are indicated; instruct to flush the toilet immediately after voiding and to wash hands thoroughly.
- Because of the slight potential for harm to a developing fetus, pregnant personnel should not be assigned to care for clients during the first 24 hours after this procedure.

Client and Family Teaching

- Increase fluid intake before and after the renal scan.
- No special diet or other preparation is required.
- The test takes 1 to 4 hours.
- No anesthesia is required, and you will experience no pain or discomfort other than that associated with remaining still for a period of time.

RENAL BIOPSY

Preparation of the Client

- Informed consent is required for a kidney biopsy. Answer questions and provide additional information as needed.
- Maintain npo status from midnight before the procedure.
- Note hemoglobin and hematocrit prior to the procedure.
- If the procedure is to be performed at the bedside, obtain biopsy tray and other necessary supplies.
- Following procedure, apply a pressure dressing and position supine to help maintain pressure on the biopsy site.
- Monitor closely for bleeding during the first 24 hours after the procedure:
  a. Check vital signs frequently. Notify the physician of tachycardia, hypotension, or other signs of shock.
  b. Monitor biopsy site for bleeding.
  c. Check hemoglobin and hematocrit, comparing with pre-procedure values.
  d. Observe for and report complaints of flank or back pain, shoulder pain (caused by diaphragmatic irritation if hemorrhage occurs), pallor, lightheadedness.
  e. Monitor urine output for quantity and hematuria. Initial hematuria should clear within 24 hours.
- Monitor for other potential complications such as inadvertent penetration of the liver or bowel. Report abdominal pain, guarding, and decreased bowel sounds.
- Encourage fluids during the initial postprocedure period.

Client and Family Teaching

- Local anesthesia is used at the injection site. The procedure may be uncomfortable but should not be painful.
- When the needle is inserted, you will be instructed not to breathe to prevent kidney motion.
- The entire procedure takes approximately 10 minutes.
- Avoid coughing during the first 24 hours after the procedure. Strenuous activity such as heavy lifting may be prohibited for approximately 2 weeks after the procedure.
- Report any signs and symptoms of complications, such as hemorrhage or urinary tract infection, to the physician.

- *Urinalysis* often shows red blood cells and proteins in the urine of clients with a glomerular disorder. These substances, normally too large to enter glomerular filtrate, escape due to increased porosity of glomerular capillaries in glomerular disorders. A 24-hour urine specimen is used to determine the amount of protein in the urine.

Medications

Although no drugs are available to cure glomerular disorders, medications are used to treat underlying disorders, reduce inflammation, and manage the symptoms.

Antibiotics are prescribed for the client with poststreptococcal glomerulonephritis to eradicate any remaining bacteria,

TABLE 27–2	Changes in Laboratory Values Associated with Kidney Disease	
Test	**Normal Value**	**Value in Renal Disease**
Blood urea nitrogen (BUN)	5–20 mg/dL Slightly higher in older adult	20–50 mg/dL or higher
Creatinine, serum	Female: 0.5–1.1 mg/dL Male: 0.6–1.2 mg/dL Slightly lower in older adult	Elevated; levels >4 mg/dL indicate severe impairment of renal function
Creatinine clearance	Female: 88–128 mL/min Male: 97–137 mL/min Values decline in older adult	Reduced renal reserve: 32.5–90.0 mL/min Renal insufficiency: 6.5–32.5 mL/min Renal failure: <6.5 mL/min
Serum albumin	3.2–5 g/dL; 3.2–4.8 g/dL in older adult	Decreased in nephrotic syndrome
Serum electrolytes	Potassium: 3.5–5.0 mEq/L Sodium: 136–145 mEq/L Calcium: 4.5–5.5 mEq/L or 8.2–10.5 mg/dL Phosphorus: 3.0–4.5 mg/dL	Increased in renal insufficiency Decreased in nephrotic syndrome Decreased in renal failure Increased in renal failure
Red blood cell count	Female: 4.0–5.5 million/mm³ Male: 4.5–6.2 million/mm³	Decreased in chronic renal failure
Urine creatinine	Female: 600–1800 mg/24 hours Male: 800–2000 mg/24 hours	Decreased in disorders of impaired renal function
Urine protein	Resting: 50–80 mg/24 hours Ambulatory: <150–250 mg/24 hours	Increased in disorders of impaired renal function
Urine red blood cells	<2–3/HPF; no RBC casts	Present in glomerular disorders

removing the stimulus for antibody production. Nephrotoxic antibiotics, such as the aminoglycoside antibiotics, streptomycin, and some cephalosporins, are avoided.

Aggressive immunosuppressive therapy is used to treat acute inflammatory processes such as rapidly progressive glomerulonephritis, Goodpasture's syndrome, and exacerbations of SLE. When begun early, immunosuppressive therapy significantly reduces the risk of end-stage renal disease and renal failure. Prednisone, a glucocorticoid, is prescribed in relatively large doses of 1 mg per kilogram of body weight per day (e.g., a 160-pound man would receive 70 to 75 mg per day). Other immunosuppressive agents such as cyclophosphamide (Cytoxan) or azathioprine (Imuran) are prescribed in conjunction with corticosteroids. Corticosteroid use in poststreptococcal glomerulonephritis may actually worsen the condition, so is avoided.

Oral glucocorticoids such as prednisone also are used in high doses to induce remission of nephrotic syndrome. When glucocorticoids alone are ineffective, other immunosuppressive agents such as cyclophosphamide or chlorambucil (Leukeran) may be used to induce or maintain remission. See Chapter 9 ⟳ for more information about corticosteroids and other immunosuppressive drugs.

ACE inhibitors may be ordered to reduce protein loss associated with nephrotic syndrome. These drugs reduce proteinuria and slow the progression of renal failure. They have a protective effect on the kidney in clients with diabetic nephropathy. Nonsteroidal anti-inflammatory drugs (NSAIDs) also reduce proteinuria in some clients, but can increase salt and water retention (Braunwald et al., 2001).

Antihypertensives may be prescribed to maintain the blood pressure within normal levels. Blood pressure management is important because systemic and renal hypertension are associated with a poorer prognosis in clients with glomerular disorders.

Treatments

Bed rest may be ordered during the acute phase of poststreptococcal glomerulonephritis. When the edema of nephrotic syndrome is significant or the client is hypertensive, sodium intake may be restricted to 1 to 2 g per day. Dietary protein may be restricted if azotemia is present. When proteins are restricted, those included in the diet should be complete or high-value proteins. Complete proteins supply the essential amino acids required for growth and tissue maintenance. Complete and incomplete proteins are compared in Table 27–3.

Plasma exchange therapy (**plasmapheresis**), a procedure to remove damaging antibodies from the plasma, is used in

TABLE 27–3	Complete and Incomplete Protein Sources	
	Complete Proteins	**Incomplete Proteins**
Definition	Provide all essential amino acids needed for growth and tissue maintenance	Lack one or more essential amino acids or contain inadequate proportions
Examples	Milk, eggs, cheese, meats, poultry, fish, and soy	Vegetables, breads, cereals and grains, legumes, seeds, and nuts

conjunction with immunosuppressive therapy to treat RPGN and Goodpasture's syndrome. Plasma and glomerular-damaging antibodies are removed using a blood cell separator. The red blood cells are then returned to the client along with albumin or human plasma to replace the plasma removed. This procedure is usually done in a series of treatments. It is not without risk, and informed consent is required. Potential complications of plasma exchange therapy include those associated with intravenous catheters, fluid volume shifts, and altered coagulation.

Renal failure resulting from a glomerular disorder may necessitate dialysis to restore fluid and electrolyte balance and remove waste products from the body. Dialysis procedures and related nursing care are explained in the acute renal failure section later in this chapter.

NURSING CARE

Health Promotion

Discuss the importance of effectively treating streptococcal infections in all age groups to help reduce the risk for acute glomerulonephritis. Stress the importance of completing the full course of antibiotic therapy to eradicate the infecting bacteria. Teach clients with diabetes mellitus and SLE about potential renal effects of their disease. Discuss measures to reduce the risk of associated nephritis, such as effectively managing the disease, treating hypertension, and avoiding drugs and substances that are potentially toxic to the kidneys.

Assessment

Review Chapter 25 ⊖⊃ for complete assessment of the renal and urinary systems. Focused assessment data related to glomerular disorders includes the following:

- Health history: complaints of facial or peripheral edema or weight gain, fatigue, nausea and vomiting, headache, general malaise, abdominal or flank pain; cough or shortness of breath; changes in amount, color, or character of urine (e.g., frothy urine); history of skin or pharyngeal streptococcal infection, diabetes, SLE, or kidney disease; current medications
- Physical examination: General appearance; vital signs; weight; presence of periorbital, facial, or peripheral edema; skin for lesions, infection; inspect throat, obtain culture as indicated; urine specimen for color, character, odor

Nursing Diagnoses and Interventions

Nursing care is supportive and educational. Monitoring renal function and fluid volume status are key components of care, as is protecting the client from infection. Both manifestations of glomerular disorders and their treatment can interfere with a client's ability to maintain usual roles and responsibilities.

Excess Fluid Volume

Excess fluid volume and resulting edema are common manifestations of glomerular disorders. When proteins are lost in the urine, the oncotic pressure of plasma falls, and fluid shifts into the interstitial spaces. The body responds to this fluid shift by retaining sodium and water to maintain intravascular volume, leading to excess fluid volume.

- Monitor vital signs, including blood pressure, apical pulse, respirations, and breath sounds, at least every 4 hours. Report significant changes. *Excess fluid increases the cardiac workload and the blood pressure. Tachycardia may result. Associated electrolyte imbalances can cause dysrhythmias. Increased pulmonary vascular pressure can lead to pulmonary edema, tachypnea, dyspnea, and crackles (rales) in the lungs.*
- Record intake and output every 4 to 8 hours, or more frequently as indicated. *Accurate intake and output records help determine fluid volume status.*

PRACTICE ALERT *Weigh daily, using consistent technique (time of day, scale, and clothing). Accurate daily weights are the best indicator of approximate fluid balance (Wise et al., 2000).* ■

- Monitor serum electrolytes, hemoglobin and hematocrit, BUN, and creatinine. *Glomerular disorders affect fluid balance and may alter electrolyte balance as well, potentially leading to complications such as cardiac dysrhythmias (see Chapter 5). ⊖⊃ Increased intravascular volume can result in low hemoglobin and hematocrit values. BUN and creatinine provide information about renal function.*
- Maintain fluid restriction as ordered. Offer ice chips (in limited and measured amounts) and frequent mouth care to relieve thirst. With the client, develop a fluid intake schedule. *Fluids may be restricted to reduce fluid overload, edema, and hypertension. Ice chips and frequent mouth care moisten mucous membranes and help relieve thirst while maintaining oral tissue integrity. Including the client in planning fluid intake promotes a sense of control and understanding of the treatment regimen.*

PRACTICE ALERT *Carefully monitor and regulate intravenous infusions; include fluid used to dilute IV medications as intake. Significant "hidden" fluid intake can occur with intravenous medication administration.* ■

- Arrange dietary consultation regarding sodium or protein-restricted diets. *Including the client and dietitian in planning allows individualization of the diet to client preferences. The glomerular disorder may reduce appetite; considering food preferences can help maintain adequate nutrition.*
- Monitor for desired and adverse effects of prescribed medications. *Diuretic therapy helps reduce excess fluid volume; however, glomerular disorders can affect the client's response to treatment. In addition, diuretics can exacerbate electrolyte imbalances and muscle weakness often associated with glomerular disorders.*
- Provide frequent position changes and good skin care. *Perfusion may be altered by tissue edema, increasing the risk of breakdown.*

Fatigue

Fatigue is a common manifestation of glomerular disorders. Anemia, loss of plasma proteins, headache, anorexia, and nausea compound this fatigue. The ability to maintain usual physical and mental activities may be impaired.

- Document energy level. *As glomerular function improves, fatigue begins to resolve, and energy increases.*
- Schedule activities and procedures to provide adequate rest and energy conservation. Prevent unnecessary fatigue. *Adequate rest and energy conservation reduce fatigue and improve the client's ability to tolerate and cope with required treatments and activities.*
- Assist with ADLs as needed. *The goal is to conserve limited energy reserves.*
- Discuss the relationship between fatigue and the disease process with client and family. *Understanding the nature of the disease and associated fatigue helps the client and family cope with reduced energy and comply with prescribed rest.*
- Reduce energy demands with frequent, small meals and short periods of activity. Limit the number of visitors and visit length. *Small, frequent meals reduce the energy needed for eating and digestion. Limiting visitors and visit length helps conserve energy. In addition, nurses can assist the fatigued client who may be reluctant to ask visitors to leave.*

Ineffective Protection

The effects of both the glomerular disorder and treatment with anti-inflammatory and cytotoxic drugs can depress the immune system, increasing the risk for infection. The anti-inflammatory effect of corticosteroids may also mask early manifestations of infection.

PRACTICE ALERT *Monitor vital signs, temperature, and mental status every 4 hours. An elevated temperature may indicate infection; anti-inflammatory drugs may moderate this response, however. Tachycardia, increasing lethargy, or confusion may be the initial signs of infection.* ∎

- Assess frequently for other signs of infection such as purulent wound drainage, productive cough, adventitious breath sounds, and red or inflamed lesions. Monitor for manifestations of UTI, such as dysuria, frequency and urgency, and cloudy, foul-smelling urine. *Early identification and treatment of infection is important to prevent systemic complications in the susceptible client.*
- Monitor CBC, focusing on the WBC and differential. *An elevated WBC and increased numbers of immature WBCs in the blood (left shift) may be early indicators of infection.*
- Use good handwashing technique. Protect from cross-infection by providing a private room and restricting ill visitors. *Clients with decreased resistance to infection need increased protection.*
- Avoid or minimize invasive procedures. *Maintaining the protective skin barrier is especially important for the client with altered immune status.*
- If catheterization is required, use sterile intermittent straight catheterization or maintain a closed drainage system for an indwelling catheter. Prevent urine reflux from the drainage system to the bladder or the bladder to the kidneys by ensuring a patent, gravity system. *The urinary tract is a frequent entry point for infection, particularly in the hospitalized or institutionalized client. Maintaining strict asepsis during catheterization is vital. Intermittent catheterization is associated with a lower risk of UTI than an indwelling catheter.*
- Provide a nutritionally sound diet with complete proteins. *A well-balanced, nutritionally sound diet is important to maintain nutritional status and support immune function.*
- Teach measures to prevent infection. *Care often is provided in the home, requiring the client and family to use appropriate infection control measures.*

Ineffective Role Performance

The manifestations and treatment of glomerular disorders can affect the ability to maintain usual roles and activities. Fatigue and muscle weakness may limit physical and social activities. Bed rest or activity limitations may be ordered to minimize the degree of proteinuria. If azotemia is present, malaise, nausea, and mental status changes can interfere with role function. Facial and periorbital edema affect the client's self-esteem and may lead to isolation.

- Establish a strong therapeutic relationship. *It is important to gain the client's trust and confidence.*
- Encourage self-care and participation in decision making. *Increased autonomy helps restore self-confidence and reduce powerlessness.*
- Provide for time for verbalization of thoughts and feelings; listen actively, acknowledging and accepting fears and concerns. *Adequate time and active listening encourage expression of concerns and the affect of the disease or treatments on daily life. This helps the client deal with the illness, its treatment, and associated losses.*
- Support coping skills, helping the client identify personal strengths. *This support helps the client gain confidence.*
- When possible, enlist the support of family, other clients, and friends. *These people can provide physical, psychologic, emotional, and social support.*
- Discuss the effect of the disease and treatments on roles and relationships, helping identify potential changes in roles, relationships, and lifestyle. Help the client and family develop a plan for alternative behaviors and relationships, encouraging the client to maintain usual roles to the extent possible. *Developing a plan helps reduce the strain of role changes and maintain a sense of dignity and control.*
- Provide accurate and optimistic information about the disorder and its short- and long-term effects. *The client and family need accurate information to plan for the future.*
- Evaluate the need for additional support and social services for the client and family. Provide referrals as indicated. *Depending on client and family strengths, the severity of the disorder, and its treatment and prognosis, ongoing social support services may be necessary to facilitate coping and adaptation.*

Using NANDA, NIC, and NOC

Chart 27–1 shows links between NANDA nursing diagnoses, NIC, and NOC when caring for the client with a glomerular disorder.

CHART 27–1 NANDA, NIC, AND NOC LINKAGES

The Client with a Glomerular Disorder

NURSING DIAGNOSES	NURSING INTERVENTIONS	NURSING OUTCOMES
• Excess Fluid Volume	• Fluid Management • Fluid Monitoring	• Fluid Balance
• Fatigue • Imbalanced Nutrition: Less than Body Requirements • Ineffective Role Performance	• Energy Management • Nutrition Management • Nutrition Monitoring • Coping Enhancement	• Energy Conservation • Nutritional Status: Nutrient Intake • Coping • Psychosocial Adjustment: Life Change

Note. Data from Nursing Outcomes Classification (NOC) by M. Johnson & M. Maas (Eds.), 1997, St. Louis: Mosby; Nursing Diagnoses: Definitions & Classification 2001–2002 by North American Nursing Diagnosis Association, 2001, Philadelphia: NANDA; Nursing Interventions Classification (NIC) by J.C. McCloskey & G. M. Bulechek (Eds.), 2000, St. Louis: Mosby. Reprinted by permission.

Home Care

Glomerular disorders may be self-limited or progressive. In either case, the course is lengthy, ranging from months to years. Self-management is essential. Provide instructions for the client and family, including the following topics.

• Information about the disease and the prognosis

• Prescribed treatment, including activity and diet restrictions; the use and potential effects, both beneficial and adverse, of all medications
• Risks, manifestations, prevention, and management of complications such as edema and infection
• Signs, symptoms, and implications of improving or declining renal function
• Measures to prevent further kidney damage, such as nephrotoxic drugs to avoid

Nursing Care Plan
A Client with Acute Glomerulonephritis

Jung-Lin Chang is a 23-year-old graduate student in biology. He presents at the university health center, with brown and foamy urine. The physician there admits him to the infirmary and orders a throat culture, ASO titer, CBC, BUN, serum creatinine, and urinalysis.

ASSESSMENT
Connie King, the nurse admitting Mr. Chang, notes that his history is essentially negative for past kidney or urinary problems. He relates having had a "pretty bad" sore throat a couple of weeks before admission. However, it was during midterms, so he took a few antibiotics he had from a previous bout of strep throat, increased his fluids, and did not see a doctor. The sore throat resolved, and he felt well until noticing the change in his urine. He admits that his eyes seemed a little puffy, but he thought this was due to lack of sleep and fatigue. He has eaten little the past 2 days, but was not alarmed because his food intake is irregular most of the time.

Physical assessment findings include: T 98.8° F (37.1° C) PO, P 98, R 18, and BP 136/90. Weight 165 pounds (75 kg), up from his normal of 160 (72.5 kg). Moderate periorbital edema and edema of hands and fingers noted.

Throat culture is negative, but the ASO titer is high. CBC essentially normal. BUN 42 mg/dL, serum creatinine 2.1 mg/dL. Urinalysis reveals the presence of protein, red blood cells, and RBC casts. A subsequent 24-hour urine protein analysis shows 1025 mg of protein (normal 30 to 150 mg/24 hours).

The physician diagnoses acute poststreptococcal glomerulonephritis and places Mr. Chang on bed rest with bathroom privileges. He orders fluid restriction (1200 mL/day) and a restricted sodium and protein diet.

DIAGNOSIS
• *Excess fluid volume* related to plasma protein deficit and sodium and water retention
• *Risk for imbalanced nutrition: Less than body requirements* related to anorexia
• *Anxiety* related to prescribed activity restriction
• *Risk for ineffective therapeutic regimen management* related to lack of information about glomerulonephritis and treatment

EXPECTED OUTCOMES
• Maintain blood pressure within normal limits.
• Return to usual weight with no evidence of edema.
• Consume adequate calories following prescribed dietary limitations.
• Verbalize reduced anxiety regarding ability to continue studies.
• Demonstrate an understanding of acute glomerulonephritis and prescribed treatment regimen.

PLANNING AND IMPLEMENTATION
• Vital signs every 4 hours; notify physician of significant changes.
• Weigh daily; intake and output every 8 hours.
• Schedule fluids allowing 650 mL on day shift, 450 mL on evening shift, and 100 mL on night shift.

Nursing Care Plan
A Client with Acute Glomerulonephritis (continued)

- Arrange dietary consultation to plan a diet that includes preferred foods as allowed.
- Provide small meals with high-carbohydrate between-meal snacks.
- Encourage Mr. Chang to talk about his condition and its potential effects.
- Assist with problem solving and exploring options for maintaining studies.
- Enlist friends and family to listen and provide support.
- Teach Mr. Chang and his family about acute glomerulonephritis and prescribed treatment.
- Instruct in appropriate antibiotic use.

EVALUATION

Mr. Chang is released from the infirmary after 4 days. He decides to return to his parents' home for the 6 to 12 weeks of convalescence prescribed by his doctor. Mr. Chang's renal function gradually returns to normal with no further azotemia and minimal proteinuria after 4 months. He verbalizes understanding of the relationship

between the strep throat, his inappropriate use of antibiotics, and the glomerulonephritis. He says, "I may not always remember to take every pill on time in the future, but I sure won't save them for the next time again!"

Critical Thinking in the Nursing Process

1. How did Mr. Chang's use of "a few" previously prescribed antibiotics to treat his sore throat affect his risk for developing poststreptococcal glomerulonephritis?
2. What additional risk factors did Mr. Chang have for developing glomerulonephritis?
3. The initial manifestations of acute poststreptococcal glomerulonephritis and rapidly progressive glomerulonephritis are very similar. What diagnostic test would the physician use to make the differential diagnosis? Develop a plan of care for a client undergoing this examination.

See Evaluating Your Response in Appendix C.

THE CLIENT WITH A VASCULAR KIDNEY DISORDER

Renal function is dependent on an adequate supply of blood. Blood supports renal cell metabolism and is vital to kidney function, the nephron in particular. The kidney can regulate fluid, electrolyte, and acid-base balance and serve as a major organ of excretion only when its blood supply is sufficient. Vascular disorders, therefore, can have a significant impact on renal function.

HYPERTENSION

Hypertension, sustained elevation of the systemic blood pressure, can result from or cause kidney disease.

Prolonged hypertension damages the walls of arterioles and accelerates the process of atherosclerosis. This damage primarily affects the heart, brain, kidneys, eyes, and major blood vessels. In the kidney, arteriosclerotic lesions develop in the *afferent* (leading into) and *efferent* (going out of) arterioles and the glomerular capillaries. The glomerular filtration rate declines and tubular function is affected, resulting in proteinuria and microscopic hematuria. Approximately 10% of deaths attributed to hypertension result from renal failure (Braunwald et al., 2001).

Malignant hypertension is a rapidly progressive form of hypertension that may develop in clients with untreated primary hypertension. The diastolic pressure is in excess of 120 mmHg and may be as high as 150 to 170 mmHg. Malignant hypertension affects less than 1% of hypertensive clients; it is more common in African Americans than in people of European ancestry. Untreated, malignant hypertension causes a rapid decline in renal function due to vessel changes, renal ischemia, and infarction.

Approximately 5% to 10% of hypertensive clients have *secondary hypertension,* which is actually a manifestation of

an underlying disease. Renal vascular disease and diseases of the renal parenchyma, such as diabetic nephropathy, are commonly associated with secondary hypertension.

Management of hypertension to maintain the blood pressure within normal limits is vital to prevent kidney damage. When hypertension is secondary to kidney disease, adequate blood pressure control can slow the decline in renal function. Hypertension and its management is discussed in depth in Chapter 33. ⊘

RENAL ARTERY OCCLUSION

Renal arteries can be occluded by either a primary process affecting the renal vessels or by emboli, clots, or other foreign material. Risk factors for *acute renal artery thrombosis* (formation of a blood clot in the renal artery) include severe abdominal trauma, vessel trauma from surgery or angiography, aortic or renal artery aneurysms, and severe aortic or renal artery atherosclerosis. Emboli from the left side of the heart can travel via the aorta to occlude the renal artery. Emboli may form as a result of atrial fibrillation (irregular and uncoordinated electrical activity of the atria), following myocardial infarction, as vegetative growths on heart valves associated with bacterial endocarditis, or from fatty plaque in the aorta.

Renal arterial occlusion may be asymptomatic when the occlusion develops slowly and the affected vessels are small. Acute occlusion leading to ischemia and infarction typically causes sudden, severe localized flank pain, nausea and vomiting, fever, and hypertension. Hematuria and oliguria may occur. In the older client, the new onset of hypertension or worsening of previously controlled hypertension may signal renal artery thrombosis.

Laboratory studies reveal leukocytosis (elevated WBC), and elevated renal enzyme levels, including aspartate transaminase (AST) and lactic dehydrogenase (LDH). These enzymes, normally present in renal cells, are released into the circulation when cells necrose and die. With bilateral arterial occlusion and infarction, renal function deteriorates rapidly, leading to acute renal failure (Braunwald et al., 2001).

Surgery to restore blood flow to the affected kidney may be indicated for acute occlusion. Management usually is more conservative, using anticoagulant therapy, hypertension control, and supportive treatment.

RENAL VEIN OCCLUSION

A thrombus (clot) formed in a renal vein can occlude the vessel. The cause of the thrombus often is unclear. In adults, renal vein thrombosis usually occurs with nephrotic syndrome. Other predisposing factors include pregnancy, oral contraceptive use, and certain malignancies.

Gradual or acute deterioration of renal function may be the only manifestation of renal vein occlusion. If the thrombus breaks loose, it can become a pulmonary embolism. The definitive diagnosis is made by visualizing the thrombus through renal venography.

Thrombolytic drugs such as streptokinase or tPA may be given to dissolve or break up the thrombus. Anticoagulant therapy also is used to prevent further clotting and pulmonary emboli. Renal function often improves with treatment.

RENAL ARTERY STENOSIS

Renal artery stenosis (narrowing) causes 2% to 5% of all cases of hypertension (Braunwald et al., 2001). It can affect one or both kidneys.

Atherosclerosis with gradual occlusion of the renal artery lumen by plaque is the primary cause of renal artery stenosis in men. In younger women, the most common cause is fibromuscular dysplasia, structural abnormalities involving the intimal, medial, or adventitial layers of the arterial wall.

Renal artery stenosis is suspected when hypertension develops before age 30 or after age 50 with no prior history of high blood pressure. An epigastric bruit (murmur) and other manifestations of vascular insufficiency may also be present. The affected kidney appears small and atrophied on renal ultrasound. The captopril test for renin activity and renal angiography are used to confirm the diagnosis. Clients with renovascular hypertension show higher levels of renin activity following administration of captopril, an ACE inhibitor drug (see Chapter 33) than clients with essential or primary hypertension (Braunwald et al., 2001). Renal angiography uses radiologic contrast dye injected into the renal arteries to allow visualization of renal blood vessels.

The preferred treatment for renal artery stenosis is dilation of the stenotic vessel by percutaneous transluminal angioplasty. In this procedure, a balloon-tipped catheter is inserted via the femoral artery and aorta to dilate the renal artery. It relieves symptoms immediately in 90% of clients with fibromuscular dysplasia. One year after treatment, 60% remain symptom-free. Some clients require a bypass graft of the renal artery. A section of saphenous vein or hypogastric artery is grafted from the aorta to the renal artery beyond the stenosis.

The blood pressure may not return to normal following treatment, but is more easily managed using medications.

THE CLIENT WITH KIDNEY TRAUMA

The kidneys are relatively well protected by the rib cage and back muscles, but trauma due to blunt force or penetrating injury may inflict damage. Many renal injuries heal uneventfully, but prompt diagnosis and immediate treatment can be life-saving in the event of major damage.

PATHOPHYSIOLOGY AND MANIFESTATIONS

Blunt force is the most common cause of kidney injury. Falls, motor vehicle accidents, and sports injuries can damage the kidney. The injury may be minor, causing a contusion or small hematoma, or more serious, resulting in laceration or other damage. The kidney may fragment or "shatter," causing significant blood loss and urine extravasation. Tearing of the renal artery or vein may cause rapid hemorrhage, with shock and possible death.

Gunshot wounds, knife wounds, impalement injuries, and fractured ribs can penetrate the kidney. Minor penetrating injuries may lacerate the capsule or renal cortex. Major injuries include laceration or destruction of renal parenchyma or the vascular supply. Renal artery, renal vein, and renal pelvis lacerations are critical injuries.

The primary manifestations of kidney trauma are hematuria (gross or microscopic), flank or abdominal pain, and oliguria or anuria. There may be localized swelling, tenderness, or ecchymoses in the flank region. Retroperitoneal bleeding from the kidney may cause Turner's sign, a bluish discoloration of the flank. Signs of shock may be present, including hypotension, tachycardia, tachypnea, cool and pale skin, and an altered level of consciousness.

COLLABORATIVE CARE

Hemoglobin and hematocrit levels fall in significant renal injury with hemorrhage. Hematuria is typically noted on urinalysis. AST levels rise within 12 hours of significant renal trauma. Renal ultrasonography is used to diagnose bleeding and kidney damage. A CT scan and IVP to visualize renal structures may be done to establish a definitive diagnosis. Renal arteriography is used when major injury is suspected and surgery is anticipated.

Treatment of minor kidney injuries is generally conservative, including bed rest and observation. In these injuries, bleeding is typically minor and self-limiting. With major or critical trauma, immediate treatment focuses on controlling hemorrhage and treating or preventing shock. Surgery or percutaneous arterial embolization during angiography may be required to stop the bleeding. Major lacerations may require surgical repair, partial nephrectomy, or total **nephrectomy** (removal) of the affected kidney.

NURSING CARE

Nursing care for the client who has experienced renal trauma focuses on timely and accurate assessment and appropriate intervention to preserve life and prevent complications. Obtain a urine specimen for analysis when kidney trauma is suspected. Monitor level of consciousness, vital signs, skin color and temperature, and urine output for possible signs of shock. See Chapter 6 ⊘⊘ for additional nursing care measures for the client who has had a traumatic injury or who develops shock.

THE CLIENT WITH A RENAL TUMOR

Renal tumors may be either benign or malignant, primary or metastatic. Benign renal tumors are infrequent and are often found only on autopsy. Primary renal malignancies account for about 2% of adult cancers and approximately 12,000 deaths per year. Most primary renal tumors arise from renal cells; a primary tumor also may develop in the renal pelvis, although less frequently. Metastatic lesions to the kidney are associated with lung and breast cancer, melanoma, and malignant lymphoma.

Males are affected by renal cancer more than females by a 2:1 ratio. The highest incidence is seen in people over the age of 55 years. Smoking and obesity are risk factors; chronic irritation associated with renal calculi may also contribute. Some renal cancers are associated with genetic factors. Clients with end-stage renal disease also may develop renal cancer.

PATHOPHYSIOLOGY AND MANIFESTATIONS

Most (85% to 95%) primary renal tumors are renal cell carcinomas (Braunwald et al., 2001; Porth, 2002). These tumors arise from tubular epithelium and can occur anywhere in the kidney. The tumor, which can range in size up to several centimeters, has clearly defined margins and contains areas of ischemia, necrosis, and hemorrhage. Renal tumors tend to invade the renal vein, and often have metastasized when first identified. Metastasis tend to occur in the lungs, bone, lymph nodes, liver, and brain (Bullock & Henze, 2000).

Renal tumors are often silent, with few manifestations. The classic triad of symptoms, gross hematuria, flank pain, and a palpable abdominal mass, is seen in only about 10% of people with renal cell carcinoma. Hematuria, often microscopic, is the most consistent symptom. Systemic manifestations include fever without infection, fatigue, and weight loss. See the box above.

The tumor may produce hormones or hormonelike substances, including parathyroid hormone, prostaglandins, prolactin, renin, gonadotropins, and glucocorticoids. These substances produce *paraneoplastic syndromes,* with additional manifestations such as hypercalcemia, hypertension, and hyperglycemia. The progression of renal cell carcinomas varies from prolonged periods of stable disease to very aggressive. Table 27–4 outlines the staging and prognosis for renal cell cancers.

Manifestations of Renal Tumors

- Microscopic or gross hematuria
- Flank pain
- Palpable abdominal mass
- Fever
- Fatigue
- Weight loss
- Anemia or polycythemia

COLLABORATIVE CARE

Hematuria is often the only initial manifestation of renal cancer; its presence indicates a need for further diagnostic studies, including:

- *Renal ultrasonography* to detect renal masses and differentiate cystic kidney disease from renal carcinoma.
- *CT scan* to determine tumor density, local extension of the tumor, and regional lymph node or vascular involvement.
- *IVP* and *MRI* may be done to evaluate renal structure and function.
- *Renal angiography, aortography,* and *inferior venacavography* may be used to evaluate the extent of vascular involvement prior to surgery.
- *Chest X-ray, bone scan, and liver function studies* to identify potential metastases.

Radical nephrectomy is the treatment of choice for kidney tumors. In a radical nephrectomy, the adrenal gland, upper ureter, fat and fascia surrounding the kidney, as well as the entire kidney,

TABLE 27–4 Renal Cell Cancer Staging

Stage	Extent of Tumor	Prognosis
I	Confined to the kidney capsule	66% 5-year survival
II	Invasion through the capsule but confined to local fascia	64% 5-year survival
III	Regional lymph node, ipsilateral renal vein, or inferior vena cava involvement	42% 5-year survival
IV	Locally invasive or distant metastases	11% or less 5-year survival

Note. Adapted from Harrison's Principles of Internal Medicine *(15th ed.) by E. Braunwald et al. (Eds.), 2001, New York: McGraw-Hill.*

NURSING CARE OF THE CLIENT HAVING A NEPHRECTOMY

PREOPERATIVE CARE

- Provide routine preoperative care as outlined in Chapter 7. ⊝⊚
- Report abnormal laboratory values to the surgeon. *Bacteriuria, blood coagulation abnormalities, or other significant abnormal values may affect surgery and postoperative care.*
- Discuss operative and postoperative expectations as indicated, including the location of the incision (Figure 27–4) and anticipated tubes, stents, and drains. *Preoperative teaching about postoperative expectations reduces anxiety for the client and family during the early postoperative period.*

POSTOPERATIVE CARE

- Provide routine postoperative care as described in Chapter 7.
- Frequently assess urine color, amount, and character, noting any hematuria, pyuria, or sediment. Promptly report oliguria or anuria, as well as changes in urine color or clarity. *Preserving function of the remaining kidney is critical; frequent assessment allows early intervention for potential problems.*
- Note the placement, status, and drainage from ureteral catheters, stents, nephrostomy tubes, or drains. Label each clearly. Maintain gravity drainage; irrigate only as ordered. *Maintaining drainage tube patency is vital to prevent potential hydronephrosis. Bright bleeding or unexpected drainage may indicate a surgical complication.*
- Support the grieving process and adjustment to the loss of a kidney. *Loss of a major organ leads to a body image change and grief response. When renal cancer is the underlying diagnosis, the client may also grieve the loss of health and potential loss of life.*

- Provide the following home care instructions for the client and family.
  a. The importance of protecting the remaining kidney by preventing UTI, renal calculi, and trauma. See Chapter 26 for measures to prevent UTI and calculi. *Damage to the remaining kidney by UTI, renal calculi, or trauma can lead to renal failure.*
  b. Maintain a fluid intake of 2000 to 2500 mL per day. *This important measure helps prevent dehydration and maintain good urine flow.*
  c. Gradually increase exercise to tolerance, avoiding heavy lifting for a year after surgery. Participation in contact sports is not recommended to reduce the risk of injury to the remaining kidney. *Lifting is avoided to allow full tissue healing. Trauma to the remaining kidney could seriously jeopardize renal function.*
  d. Care of the incision and any remaining drainage tubes, catheters, or stents. *This routine postoperative instruction is vital to prepare the client for self-care and prevent complications.*
  e. Report signs and symptoms to the physician, including manifestations of UTI (dysuria, frequency, urgency, nocturia, cloudy, malodorous urine) or systemic infection (fever, general malaise, fatigue), redness, swelling, pain, or drainage from the incision or any catheter or drain tube site. *Prompt treatment of postoperative infection is vital to allow continued healing and prevent compromise of the remaining kidney.*

---

are removed. Regional lymph nodes may also be resected. Although nephrectomy can be done using a laparoscopic approach, laparotomy primarily is used for radical nephrectomy. Nursing care for the client having a nephrectomy is summarized above.

No effective treatment is available for advanced renal carcinoma with metastases. Biologic therapies such as interferon α or interleukin-2 have been used, but rarely achieve a durable effect. No chemotherapy drug consistently causes tumor regression in more than 20% of clients (Braunwald et al., 2001).

NURSING CARE

Nursing Diagnoses and Interventions

Nursing care for the client with renal cancer focuses on needs related to the cancer diagnosis and to the surgical intervention. Postoperative pain may be significant and the risk for respiratory complications is high. The remaining kidney must be protected from damage to preserve renal function. Psychologically, the client may grieve the loss of a major organ and the diagnosis of cancer.

Pain

The size and location of the incision used for a radical nephrectomy (Figure 27–4 ■) make pain management a challenge. Intercostal blocks, patient-controlled analgesia (PCA), or routine analgesic administration can effectively relieve the discomfort. Nursing care focuses on assessing pain relief, providing supportive measures to enhance analgesia, and ensuring that pain or the fear of pain does not lead to respiratory complications.

- Assess frequently for adequate pain relief. Use a standard pain scale and nonverbal signs such as grimacing, tense body position, apparent dozing, elevated pulse, change of blood pressure, or rapid, shallow respirations. Notify the physician of inadequate pain relief. *The client may assume that pain is to be expected or may fear becoming addicted to analgesics. Careful questioning and assessment allow effective pain management. Responses to analgesics are individual, and the prescribed dose may need to be adjusted.*
- Assess the incision for inflammation or swelling and drainage catheters and tubes for patency. *An obstructed catheter can lead to hydronephrosis, hematoma, or abscess, increasing incisional pain.*

PRACTICE ALERT
Assess for abdominal distention, tenderness, and bowel sounds. Intra-abdominal bleeding, peritonitis, or paralytic ileus can cause pain that may be confused with incisional pain. ■

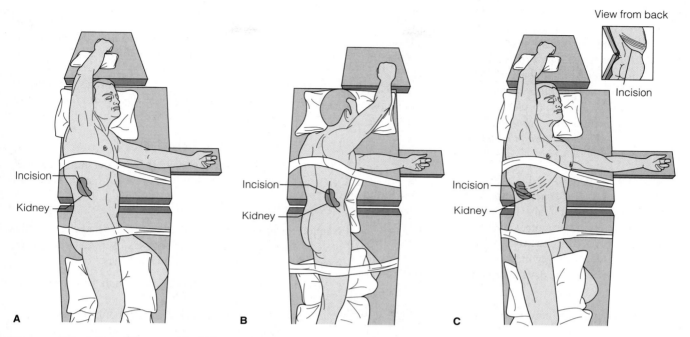

Figure 27—4 ■ Incisions used for kidney surgery. *A*, Flank. *B*, Lumbar. *C*, Thoracoabdominal.

• Use adjunctive pain relief measures such as positioning, diversional activities, management of environmental stimuli, guided imagery, and relaxation techniques. *These can enhance the effects of analgesia.*

Ineffective Breathing Pattern

The location of the incision combined with respiratory depressant effects of narcotic analgesics increases the risk for respiratory complications in the client who has had a nephrectomy.

• Position to promote respiratory excursion, using semi-Fowler's position and side-lying positions as allowed and tolerated. *Lung expansion is improved in semi-Fowler's and Fowler's positions.*

> **PRACTICE ALERT** *Assess respiratory status frequently, including rate and depth, cough, breath sounds, oxygen saturation, and temperature. Pneumothorax on the operative side is common. Early identification and intervention can prevent major respiratory complications.* ■

• Change position frequently, ambulate as soon as possible. *These measures promote lung expansion and the movement of mucus out of airways.*
• Encourage frequent (every 1 to 2 hours) deep breathing, spirometer use, and coughing. Assist to splint the incision. *These measures promote alveolar ventilation, gas exchange, and airway clearance.*

Risk for Impaired Urinary Elimination

Surgery involving the urinary tract increases the risk for altered renal function and urine elimination. In addition, removal of one kidney dictates extra caution to maintain renal circulation, a sterile urinary tract, and free urine flow.

• Monitor vital signs, CVP, and urine output every 1 to 2 hours initially, then every 4 hours. *Hypovolemia due to hemorrhage, diuresis, or fluid sequestering (third spacing) reduces blood flow to the kidney and increases the risk of renal ischemia with possible acute tubular necrosis and acute renal failure.*
• Frequently assess the amount and nature of drainage on surgical dressings and from drainage tubes, stents, and catheters. Measure and record output from each drain or catheter separately. *Frequent and accurate assessment of drainage helps to identify excess bleeding, abnormal fluid loss, infection, or other potential surgical complications.*

> **PRACTICE ALERT** *Prevent kinking, twisting, or tension on drains and tubes. Do not clamp. Irrigate carefully and only with a physician's order. Notify the physician immediately if any tube becomes dislodged. It is vital to maintain the patency of drains, particularly any affecting the remaining kidney, to prevent excess pressure of hydronephrosis.* ■

• Maintain fluid intake with intravenous fluids until oral intake is resumed. Encourage an intake of 2000 to 2500 mL per day as soon as the client tolerates oral liquids. *A liberal fluid intake prevents dehydration, helps to dilute any nephrotoxic substances, and promotes good urinary output.*
• Use strict aseptic technique in caring for all urinary catheters, tubes, stents, drains, and incisions. *Asepsis is vital to prevent infection and possible compromise of the remaining kidney.*

- Following catheter removal, assess frequently for urinary retention. Notify the physician if the client is unable to void within 4 to 6 hours or if manifestations of retention (distended bladder, discomfort, urinary dribbling) develop. *Maintenance of urine output is vital to prevent stasis and possible complications such as infection and hydronephrosis.*
- Monitor laboratory results, including urinalysis, BUN, serum creatinine, and serum electrolytes. Report abnormal findings to the physician. *Abnormal values may indicate early acute renal failure; prompt intervention is necessary to preserve renal function.*

Anticipatory Grieving

The client having a radical nephrectomy for renal cancer not only loses a major organ but also has to adjust to the diagnosis of cancer. Although the prognosis for recovery may be good, many people perceive cancer as always fatal. Providing support for the client and family during the initial stages of grieving can improve physical recovery, psychologic coping, and eventual adaptation.

- Work to develop a trusting relationship with the client and family. *Trust increases the nurse's effectiveness in helping them work through the process of grieving.*
- Listen actively, encouraging the client and family to express fears and concerns. *As they begin to express their concerns, client and family can begin to deal more effectively with them.*
- Assist the client and family to identify strengths, past experiences, and support systems. *These resources can be employed in working through the grieving process.*
- Demonstrate respect for cultural, spiritual, and religious values and beliefs; encourage use of these resources to cope with losses. *Value and belief systems can provide a structure and form for dealing with the grieving process.*

- Encourage discussion of the potential impact of loss on the client and the family structure and function. Assist family members to share concerns with one another. *Sharing of fears and concerns among family members promotes involvement and support of the entire family unit so that the individual is not left to cope alone.*
- Refer to cancer support groups, social services, or counseling as appropriate. *Support groups and counseling services provide additional resources for coping.*

Using NANDA, NIC, and NOC

Chart 27–2 shows links between NANDA nursing diagnoses, NIC, and NOC when caring for the client with renal cancer.

Home Care

If renal cancer was detected at an early stage and cure is anticipated, teaching for home care focuses on protecting the remaining kidney. Include the following topics.

- Measures to prevent infection, renal calculi, hydronephrosis, and trauma
  a. Maintain a fluid intake of 2000 to 2500 mL per day, increasing the amount during hot weather or strenuous exercise.
  b. Urinate when the urge is perceived, and before and after sexual intercourse.
  c. Properly clean the perineal area.
  d. Manifestations of UTI, and the importance of early and appropriate evaluation and intervention.
  e. If the client is an older adult male, manifestations of prostatic hypertrophy, a major cause of urinary tract obstruction, and the importance of routine screening examinations.
  f. Avoid contact sports such as football or hockey; use measures to prevent motor vehicle accidents and falls, which could damage the kidney.

CHART 27–2 NANDA, NIC, AND NOC LINKAGES

The Client with Renal Cancer

NURSING DIAGNOSES	NURSING INTERVENTIONS	NURSING OUTCOMES
• Acute Pain	• Medication Management • Patient-Controlled Analgesia (PCA) Assistance	• Pain: Disruptive Effects • Pain Level
• Ineffective Breathing Pattern	• Cough Enhancement • Positioning • Respiratory Monitoring	• Respiratory Status: Airway Patency • Respiratory Status: Ventilation
• Risk for Impaired Urinary Elimination • Anticipatory Grieving	• Urinary Elimination Management • Coping Enhancement • Grief Work Facilitation	• Urinary Elimination • Coping • Grief Resolution

Note. Data from Nursing Outcomes Classification (NOC) by M. Johnson & M. Maas (Eds.), 1997, St. Louis: Mosby; Nursing Diagnoses: Definitions & Classification 2001–2002 by North American Nursing Diagnosis Association, 2001, Philadelphia: NANDA; Nursing Interventions Classification (NIC) by J.C. McCloskey & G. M. Bulechek (Eds.), 2000, St. Louis: Mosby. Reprinted by permission.

RENAL FAILURE

Renal failure is a condition in which the kidneys are unable to remove accumulated metabolites from the blood, leading to altered fluid, electrolyte, and acid-base balance. The cause may be a primary kidney disorder, or renal failure may be secondary to a systemic disease or other urologic defects. Renal failure may be either acute or chronic. **Acute renal failure** has an abrupt onset and with prompt intervention is often reversible. **Chronic renal failure** is a silent disease, developing slowly and insidiously, with few symptoms until the kidneys are severely damaged and unable to meet the excretory needs of the body. Both forms of renal failure are characterized by azotemia, increased levels of nitrogenous wastes in the blood.

Renal failure is common and costly. In 1999, approximately 89,000 new clients began receiving treatment for **end-stage renal disease (ESRD)**. Annually, more than 243,000 clients with ESRD undergo dialysis, about 13,500 have kidney transplants, and another 53,000 are awaiting kidney transplants. The annual cost of ESRD treatment (in 1999 dollars) is $17.87 billion. The cost is also measured in lives and lifestyle. The 5-year survival rate for clients undergoing dialysis is 31.3 % (National Kidney and Urologic Diseases Information Clearinghouse [NKUDIC], 2001). Although many clients report satisfaction with their quality of life, often clients on dialysis are unable to work, and the family structure may disintegrate under the strain of treatment.

THE CLIENT WITH ACUTE RENAL FAILURE

Acute renal failure (ARF) is a rapid decline in renal function with azotemia and fluid and electrolyte imbalances. Approximately 5% of all hospitalized clients develop ARF; the incidence jumps to as much as 30% in critical and special care units (Braunwald et al., 2001). The mortality rate for ARF in seriously ill clients is up to 88%. This high death rate is probably more related to the populations affected by ARF—older clients and the critically ill—than to the disorder itself (Porth, 2002).

Major trauma or surgery, infection, hemorrhage, severe heart failure, severe liver disease, and lower urinary tract obstruction are risk factors for ARF. Drugs and radiologic contrast media that are toxic to the kidney (*nephrotoxic*) also increase the risk for ARF. Older adults develop ARF more frequently due to their higher incidence of serious illness, hypotension, major surgeries, diagnostic procedures, and treatment with nephrotoxic drugs. The older adult also may have some degree of preexisting renal insufficiency associated with aging.

The most common causes of acute renal failure are ischemia and nephrotoxins. The kidney is particularly vulnerable to both because of the amount of blood that passes through it. A fall in blood pressure or volume can cause ischemia of kidney tissues. Nephrotoxins in the blood damage renal tissue directly.

PHYSIOLOGY REVIEW

The functional unit of the kidneys, the nephron (Figure 25–3), produces urine through three processes: glomerular filtration, tubular reabsorption, and tubular secretion. In the *glomerulus,* a filtrate of water and small solutes is formed. The solute concentration of this filtrate is equal to that of plasma, with the exception of large molecules such as plasma proteins and blood cells. The glomerular filtration rate (GFR), the amount of filtrate formed per minute, is affected by blood volume and pressure, the autonomic nervous system, and other factors. From the glomerulus, the filtrate flows into the *tubules,* where its composition is changed by the processes of *tubular reabsorption* and *tubular secretion.* Most water and many filtered solutes such as electrolytes and glucose are reabsorbed. Metabolic waste products such as urea, hydrogen ion, ammonia, and some creatinine are secreted into the tubule for elimination. By the time urine exits the collecting duct into the renal pelvis, 99% of the filtrate has been reabsorbed.

PATHOPHYSIOLOGY

The causes of acute renal failure are commonly categorized as prerenal, intrarenal, and postrenal. Prerenal causes account for 55% to 60% of ARF, intrarenal for 35% to 40%, and postrenal for less than 5%. Table 27–5 summarizes the causes of acute renal failure.

Prerenal ARF

Prerenal causes of ARF affect renal blood flow and perfusion. Any condition that significantly decreases vascular volume, cardiac output, or systemic vascular resistance can affect renal blood flow. The kidneys normally receive 20% to 25% of the cardiac output to maintain the GFR. A drop in renal blood flow to less than 20% of normal causes ischemic changes in kidney tissue and a fall in GFR. If renal perfusion is rapidly restored, these changes are reversible. Continued ischemia can lead to tubular cell necrosis and significant nephron damage (Porth, 2002). Intrarenal ARF may result.

Intrarenal ARF

Intrarenal failure is characterized by acute damage to the renal parenchyma and nephrons. Intrarenal causes include diseases of the kidney itself and acute tubular necrosis, the most common intrarenal cause of ARF.

In acute glomerulonephritis, glomerular inflammation can reduce renal blood flow and cause ARF. Vascular disorders affecting the kidney, such as vasculitis (inflammation of the blood vessels), malignant hypertension, and arterial or venous occlusion, can damage nephrons sufficiently to result in acute renal failure.

Acute Tubular Necrosis

Nephrons are especially susceptible to injury from ischemia or exposure to nephrotoxins. **Acute tubular necrosis (ATN),**

TABLE 27-5 Causes of Acute Renal Failure

	Cause	Examples
Prerenal	Hypovolemia	Hemorrhage, dehydration, excess fluid loss from GI tract, burns, wounds
	Low cardiac output	Heart failure, cardiogenic shock
	Altered vascular resistance	Sepsis, anaphylaxis, vasoactive drugs
Intrarenal	Glomerular / microvascular injury	Glomerulonephritis, DIC, vasculitis, hypertension, toxemia of pregnancy, hemolytic uremic syndrome
	Acute tubular necrosis	Ischemia due to conditions associated with prerenal failure; toxins such as drugs, heavy metals; hemolysis, rhabdomyolysis (muscle cell breakdown)
	Interstitial nephritis	Acute pyelonephritis, toxins, metabolic imbalances, idiopathic
Postrenal	Ureteral obstruction	Calculi, cancer, external compression
	Urethral obstruction	Prostatic enlargement, calculi, cancer, stricture, blood clot

destruction of tubular epithelial cells, causes an abrupt and progressive decline of renal function. Prolonged ischemia is the primary cause of ATN. When ischemia and nephrotoxin exposure occur concurrently, the risk for ATN and tubular dysfunction is especially high. See *Pathophysiology Illustrated* on the next page for the pathogenesis of acute renal failure due to ATN. Risk factors for ischemic ATN include major surgery, severe hypovolemia, sepsis, trauma, and burns. The impact of ischemia resulting from vasodilation and fluid loss in sepsis, trauma, and burns often is compounded by toxins released by bacteria or from damaged tissue.

Ischemia lasting more than 2 hours causes severe and irreversible damage to kidney tubules with patchy cellular necrosis and sloughing. The GFR is significantly reduced as a result of (1) ischemia, (2) activation of the renin-angiotensin system, and (3) tubular obstruction by cellular debris, which raises the pressure in the glomerular capsule.

Common nephrotoxins associated with ATN include the aminoglycoside antibiotics and radiologic contrast media. Many other drugs (e.g., nonsteroidal anti-inflammatory drugs and some chemotherapy drugs), heavy metals such as mercury and gold, and some common chemicals such as ethylene glycol (antifreeze) are also potentially toxic to the renal tubule. The risk for ATN is higher when nephrotoxic drugs are given to older clients or clients with preexisting renal insufficiency, and when used in combination with other nephrotoxins. Dehydration increases the risk by increasing the toxin concentration in nephrons.

Nephrotoxins destroy tubular cells by both direct and indirect effects. As tubular cells are damaged and lost through necrosis and sloughing, the tubule becomes more permeable. This increased permeability results in filtrate reabsorption, further reducing the ability of the nephron to eliminate wastes.

Rhabdomyolysis may cause up to 25% of all cases of ARF (Wallace, 2001). It is caused by release of excess myoglobin from injured skeletal muscles. Myoglobin is a protein that acts as the oxygen reservoir for muscle fibers, much as hemoglobin does for the blood. Muscle trauma, strenuous exercise, hyperthermia or hypothermia, drug overdose, infection, and other factors can precipitate rhabdomyolysis. The myoglobin clogs renal tubules causing ischemic injury, and contains an iron pig-

ment that directly damages the tubules. *Hemolysis,* red blood cell destruction, releases hemoglobin into the circulation, with much the same effect as rhabdomyolysis.

Postrenal ARF

Obstructive causes of acute renal failure are classified as postrenal. Any condition that prevents urine excretion can lead to postrenal ARF. Benign prostatic hypertrophy is the most common precipitating factor. Others include renal or urinary tract calculi and tumors. See Chapter 25 for further discussion of urinary tract obstruction.

COURSE AND MANIFESTATIONS

The course of acute renal failure typically includes three phases: initiation, maintenance, and recovery.

Initiation Phase

The *initiation phase* may last hours to days. It begins with the initiating event (e.g., hemorrhage) and ends when tubular injury occurs. If ARF is recognized and the initiating event is effectively treated during this phase, the prognosis is good. The initiation phase of ARF has few manifestations; in fact, it is often identified only when manifestations of the maintenance phase develop.

Maintenance Phase

The *maintenance phase* of ARF is characterized by a significant fall in GFR and tubular necrosis. Oliguria may develop, although many clients continue to produce normal or near normal amounts of urine (nonoliguric ARF). Even though urine may be produced, the kidney cannot efficiently eliminate metabolic wastes, water, electrolytes, and acids from the body during the maintenance phase of ARF. Azotemia, fluid retention, electrolyte imbalances, and metabolic acidosis develop. These abnormalities are more severe in the oliguric client than in the nonoliguric one, leading to a poorer prognosis with oliguria.

During the maintenance phase, salt and water retention cause edema, increasing the risk for heart failure and pulmonary edema. Impaired potassium excretion leads to hyperkalemia.

Intrarenal (or intrinsic) causes of acute renal failure have the greatest effect on renal function because the functional unit of the kidney, the nephron, is damaged. The course of intrinsic renal failure often is longer, and recovery is prolonged. Acute tubular necrosis (ATN) accounts for 75% of intrinsic acute renal failure. In ATN, tubular epithelial cells are destroyed by either ischemic or toxic injury.

1. Severe hypotension, hypovolemia, and shock lead to ischemia of tubular epithelium. Renal tubular cells are very sensitive to anoxia. Cellular ATP is depleted, calcium accumulates within the cells, and free radicals damage cell membranes. Ischemia causes patchy necrosis and rupture of the basement membrane in the proximal convoluted tubule and ascending limb of the loop of Henle (Figure A).

2. Nephrotoxins include some drugs (the aminoglycoside antibiotics, in particular), radiologic dyes, pesticides, and heavy metals. Hemoglobin (e.g., released by hemolysis resulting from transfusion reaction) and myoglobin (released by muscle cells due to trauma, extreme exercise, hypo- or hyperthermia) also are nephrotoxic. Nephrotoxins damage tubular cells by their direct effects on the cell itself, or by indirect effect (e.g., vasoconstriction and ischemia). Nephrotoxic damage primarily affects the proximal tubule in a uniform pattern. It frequently is less severe than ischemic damage (Figure B).

3. Injured tubular cells release intracellular debris, which combines with proteins within the tubules to form casts. These casts, together with sloughed necrotic cells occlude the tubular lumen, increasing tubular pressure and disrupting the flow of glomerular filtrate. Glomerular filtration slows. The increased pressure pushes filtrate out of the damaged tubule into interstitial tissues (backleak). Renal blood flow and glomerular filtration may be further reduced by intrarenal angiotensin II release and vasoconstriction (Figure C).

4. Impaired tubular function affects the ability to eliminate salt, water, and metabolic waste products. As a result, oliguria, hyperkalemia, azotemia, and metabolic acidosis develop, causing the manifestations of acute renal failure.

763

When the serum potassium level is greater than 6.0 to 6.5 mEq/L, manifestations of its effect on neuromuscular function develop. These include muscle weakness, nausea and diarrhea, electrocardiographic changes, and possible cardiac arrest. Other electrolyte imbalances include hyperphosphatemia and hypocalcemia. Metabolic acidosis results from impaired hydrogen ion elimination by the kidneys.

Anemia develops after several days of ARF due to suppressed erythropoietin secretion by the kidneys. Immune function may be impaired, increasing the risk for infection. Other manifestations of the maintenance phase include:

- Edema and hypertension due to salt and water retention.
- Confusion, disorientation, agitation or lethargy, hyperreflexia, and possible seizures or coma due to azotemia, electrolyte and acid-base imbalances.
- Anorexia, nausea, vomiting, and decreased or absent bowel sounds.
- Uremic syndrome if ARF is prolonged (see the section on chronic renal failure that follows).

Recovery Phase

The recovery phase of ARF is characterized by a process of tubule cell repair and regeneration and gradual return of the GFR to normal or pre-ARF levels. Diuresis may occur as the nephrons and GFR recover, and retained salt, water, and solutes are excreted. Serum creatinine, BUN, potassium, and phosphate levels remain high and may continue to rise in spite of increasing urine output. Renal function improves rapidly during the first 5 to 25 days of the recovery phase, and continues to improve for up to 1 year.

COLLABORATIVE CARE

Preventing acute renal failure is a goal in caring for all clients, especially those in high-risk groups. Maintaining an adequate vascular volume, cardiac output, and blood pressure is vital to preserve kidney perfusion. Nephrotoxic drugs are avoided if possible. When a nephrotoxic drug or substance must be used, the risk of ARF can be reduced by using the minimum effective dose, maintaining hydration, and eliminating other known nephrotoxins from the medication regimen.

Treatment goals for acute renal failure are to (1) identify and correct the underlying cause, (2) prevent additional kidney damage, (3) restore the urine output and kidney function, and (4) compensate for renal impairment until kidney function is restored. Fluid and electrolyte balance is a key component in managing ARF.

The client's history and physical assessment can provide clues about the initiating event for ARF. Impaired perfusion for as few as 30 minutes may cause significant renal ischemia.

Diagnostic Tests

Diagnostic tests are used to identify the cause of acute renal failure and monitor its effects on homeostasis.

- *Urinalysis* often shows the following abnormal findings in acute renal failure.

  a. A fixed specific gravity of 1.010 (equal to the specific gravity of plasma) as the tubules are unable to concentrate the filtrate
  b. Proteinuria if glomerular damage is the cause of ARF
  c. The presence of red blood cells (due to glomerular dysfunction), white blood cells (related to inflammation), and renal tubular epithelial cells (indicating ATN)
  d. Cell casts, which are protein and cellular debris molded in the shape of the tubular lumen (In ARF, RBC, WBC, and renal tubular epithelial casts may be present. Brownish pigmented casts and positive tests for occult blood indicate hemoglobinuria or myoglobinuria.)

- *Serum creatinine* and *BUN* are used to evaluate renal function. In ARF, serum creatinine levels increase rapidly, within 24 to 48 hours of the onset. Creatinine levels generally peak within 5 to 10 days. Creatinine and BUN levels tend to increase more slowly when urine output is maintained. The onset of recovery is marked by a halt in the rise of the serum creatinine and BUN.

- *Serum electrolytes* are monitored to evaluate the fluid and electrolyte status. The serum potassium rises at a moderate rate and is often used to indicate the need for dialysis. Hyponatremia is common, due to the water excess associated with ARF.

- *Arterial blood gases* often show a metabolic acidosis due to the kidneys' inability to adequately eliminate metabolic wastes and hydrogen ions (see Chapter 5).

- *Complete blood count* shows reduced RBCs, moderate anemia, and a low hematocrit. ARF affects erythropoietin secretion and RBC production. Iron and folate absorption may also be impaired, further contributing to anemia.

Laboratory findings associated with kidney disease are summarized in Table 27–2.

- *Renal ultrasonography* is used to identify obstructive causes of renal failure, and to differentiate acute renal failure from end-stage chronic renal failure. In ARF, the kidneys may be enlarged, whereas they typically appear small and shrunken in chronic renal failure. (See page 717 for nursing care of the client having a renal ultrasound or CT scan.)

- *Computed tomography (CT)* scan also may be done to evaluate kidney size and identify possible obstructions.

- *Intravenous pyelography (IVP), retrograde pyelography,* or *antegrade pyelography* may also be used to evaluate kidney structure and function. Radiologic contrast media are used with extreme caution because of their potential nephrotoxicity. Retrograde pyelography, in which contrast dye is injected into the ureters, and antegrade pyelography, in which the contrast medium is injected percutaneously into the renal pelvis, are preferred because they have fewer nephrotoxic effects than IVP. (See the Nursing Implications box on page 708.)

- *Renal biopsy* may be necessary to differentiate between acute and chronic renal failure (see the Nursing Implications box for diagnostic tests on page 750)

Medications

The primary focus in drug management for acute renal failure is to restore and maintain renal perfusion and to eliminate drugs that are nephrotoxic from the treatment regimen.

Intravenous fluids and blood volume expanders are given as needed to restore renal perfusion. Dopamine (Intropin), administered in low doses by intravenous infusion, increases renal blood flow. Dopamine is a sympathetic neurotransmitter that improves cardiac output and dilates blood vessels of the mesentery and kidneys when given in low therapeutic doses.

If restoration of renal blood flow does not improve urinary output, a potent loop diuretic such as furosemide (Lasix) or an osmotic diuretic such as mannitol may be given with intravenous fluids. The purpose is twofold. First, if nephrotoxins are present, the combination of fluids and potent diuretics may, in effect, "wash out" the nephrons, reducing toxin concentration. Second, establishing urine output may prevent oliguria, and reduce the degree of azotemia and fluid and electrolyte imbalances. Furosemide also may be used to manage salt and water retention associated with ARF.

Aggressive hypertension management limits renal injury when ARF is associated with disorders such as toxemia and pregnancy-induced hypertension. ACE inhibitors or other antihypertensive medications are used to control arterial pressures.

All drugs that are either directly nephrotoxic or that may interfere with renal perfusion (such as potent vasoconstrictors) are discontinued. NSAIDs, nephrotoxic antibiotics, and other potentially harmful drugs are avoided throughout the course of acute renal failure.

The client in acute renal failure has an increased risk of gastrointestinal bleeding, probably related to the stress response and impaired platelet function. Regular doses of antacids, histamine H_2-receptor antagonists (e.g., famotidine or ranitidine), or a proton-pump inhibitor such as omeprazole (Prilosec) are often ordered to prevent GI hemorrhage.

Hyperkalemia may require active intervention as well as restricted potassium intake. Serum levels of greater than 6.5 mEq/L are treated to prevent cardiac effects of hyperkalemia. With significant hyperkalemia, calcium chloride, bicarbonate, and insulin and glucose may be given intravenously to reduce serum potassium levels by moving potassium into the cells. A potassium-binding exchange resin such as sodium polystyrene sulfonate (Kayexalate, SPS Suspension) may be given orally or by enema. This agent removes potassium from the body by exchanging sodium for potassium, primarily in the large intestine. When given orally, it is often combined with sorbitol to prevent constipation. Rectally, it is instilled as a retention enema, allowed to remain in the bowel for approximately 30 to 60 minutes, and then irrigated out using a tap-water enema.

Aluminum hydroxide (AlternaGEL, Amphojel, Nephrox), an antacid, is used to control hyperphosphatemia in renal failure. It binds with phosphates in the GI tract, which are then excreted in the feces.

Because many drugs are eliminated from the body by the kidney, drug dosages may need to be adjusted. Doses within the usual range can lead to potentially toxic blood levels, because their elimination is slowed and half-life prolonged. Nursing implications for medications commonly prescribed for the client in ARF are summarized in the box below.

Medication Administration

The Client with Acute Renal Failure

LOOP DIURETICS
Bumetanide (Bumex)
Ethacrynic acid (Edecrin)
Furosemide (Lasix)
Torsemide (Demadex)

The loop diuretics, named for their primary site of action in the loop of Henle, are *high-ceiling diuretics:* The response increases with increasing doses. These are highly effective diuretics used in early ARF to reestablish urine flow and convert oliguric renal failure to nonoliguric renal failure. Loop diuretics may be given with intravenous dopamine to promote renal blood flow. In ATN due to a nephrotoxin, loop diuretics are used to clear the toxin from the nephrons more rapidly. Loop diuretics cause potassium wasting, which is generally not a concern in ARF because renal failure impairs normal potassium elimination.

Nursing Responsibilities
- Assess weight and vital signs for baseline data.
- Monitor intake and output, daily weight (or more frequently as ordered), vital signs, skin turgor, and other indicators of fluid volume status frequently.
- Assess for orthostatic hypotension as these potent diuretics can lead to hypovolemia.
- Monitor laboratory results, especially serum electrolyte, glucose, BUN, and creatinine levels.

- Administer by mouth or, if ordered, by intravenous injection:
  a. Furosemide undiluted at a rate of no more than 20 mg per minute
  b. Ethacrynic acid 50 mg diluted with 50 mL of normal saline at a rate of no more than 10 mg per minute
  c. Bumetanide undiluted over at least 1 minute or diluted in lactated Ringer's solution, normal saline, or 5% dextrose in water for infusion
  d. Torsemide undiluted over at least 2 minutes.
- Assess response. Urine output typically increases within 10 minutes after intravenous administration.
- Monitor hearing and for complaints such as tinnitus. High doses of loop diuretics increase the risk of ototoxicity especially with ethacrynic acid. These effects may be reversible if detected early and the drug is discontinued.
- Avoid administering concurrently with other ototoxic agents, such as aminoglycoside antibiotics and cisplatin.

Client and Family Teaching
- Unless contraindicated, maintain a fluid intake of 2 to 3 quarts per day.
- Rise slowly from lying or sitting positions, because a fall in blood pressure may cause lightheadedness.

(continued on page 766)

MediaLink | FUROSEMIDE ANIMATION

Medication Administration

The Client with Acute Renal Failure (continued)

- Take in the morning and, if ordered twice a day, late afternoon to avoid sleep disturbance.
- Take with food or milk to prevent gastric distress.
- Nonsteroidal anti-inflammatory drugs (NSAIDs) interfere with the effectiveness of loop diuretics and should be avoided.

OSMOTIC DIURETICS
Mannitol (Osmitrol, Isotol)
Urea (Ureaphil)

The osmotic diuretics act by increasing the osmotic draw in the blood and urine. In the blood, the effect is to pull extracellular water into the vascular system, increasing the GFR. These substances are then freely filtered in the glomerulus and increase the osmotic draw of the urine, inhibiting water reabsorption. The effect is to increase urine volume and flow. In addition, osmotic diuretics dilute waste products in the urine, decreasing the risk of renal damage due to excess concentrations.

Nursing Responsibilities
- Assess urine output. Osmotic diuretics are used in early renal failure to maintain urine output but are contraindicated in anuria. A test dose may be administered; urine output of 30 mL per hour following the test dose shows an adequate response.
- Do not give these diuretics to clients who have heart failure, or who are severely dehydrated. They increase vascular volume and may worsen heart failure. These drugs are not effective unless extracellular volume is adequate.
- Administer mannitol intravenously, diluting before use if indicated. Check solution for crystallization. Dissolve crystals by warming the solution slightly. Infuse 15% to 25% mannitol solutions through a filter over 30 to 90 minutes.
- Administer urea intravenously, diluting in 100 mL of 5% or 10% dextrose in water for every 30 g of urea. Administer no faster than 4 mL per minute through a filter.
- Monitor vital signs, breath sounds, and urinary output.
- Discontinue the drug if signs of heart failure or pulmonary edema develop or if renal function continues to decline.

Client and Family Teaching
- Report shortness of breath, headache, chest pain, or dizziness immediately.

ELECTROLYTES AND ELECTROLYTE MODIFIERS
Calcium chloride
Calcium gluconate
Sodium bicarbonate
Sodium polystyrene sulfonate (Kayexalate)

Calcium chloride or gluconate and sodium bicarbonate are administered intravenously in the initial management of hyperkalemia. Calcium is also administered to correct hypocalcemia and reduce hyperphosphatemia (calcium and phosphate have a reciprocal relationship in the body; as the level of one rises, the level of the other falls). Sodium bicarbonate helps correct acidosis and move potassium back into the intracellular space. Sodium polystyrene sulfonate is not used to replace an electrolyte, but to remove excess potassium from the body by exchanging sodium for potassium in the large intestine.

Nursing Responsibilities
- Assess serum electrolyte levels prior to and during therapy. Report rapid shifts or adverse responses to the physician.
- Administer as appropriate:
  a. Intravenous calcium choride at less than 1 mL per minute; intravenous calcium gluconate at 0.5 mL per minute. Inject into a large vein through a small-bore needle; avoid infiltration because extravasation of intravenous solution will cause tissue necrosis.
  b. Intravenous sodium bicarbonate infusion over 4 to 8 hours; oral tablets as prescribed.
  c. Sodium polystyrene sulfonate as an oral solution mixed with sorbitol to prevent constipation, or as a retention enema mixed with warm water. Leave in the bowel for 30 to 60 minutes, irrigate using a small tap-water enema.
- Monitor for adverse reactions, such as dysrhythmias, electrolyte imbalances, and metabolic alkalosis.

Client and Family Teaching
- Intravenous calcium may make you lightheaded; remain in bed for at least 30 minutes after administration.
- Chew sodium bicarbonate tablets and follow with 8 ounces of water. Do not take with milk.
- Retain the sodium polystyrene sulfonate enema as long as possible.

Fluid Management

Once vascular volume and renal perfusion are restored, fluid intake is usually restricted. The allowed daily fluid intake is calculated by allowing 500 mL for insensible losses (respiration, perspiration, bowel losses) and adding the amount excreted as urine (or lost in vomitus) during the previous 24 hours. For example, if a client with ARF excretes 325 mL of urine in 24 hours, the client is allowed a fluid intake (including oral and intravenous fluids) of 825 mL for the next 24 hours. Fluid balance is carefully monitored, using accurate weight measurements and the serum sodium as the primary indicators.

Dietary Management

Renal insufficiency and the underlying disease process increase the rate of *catabolism* (the breakdown of body proteins) and decrease the rate of *anabolism* (body tissue repair). The client with ARF needs adequate nutrients and calories to prevent catabolism. Proteins are limited to 0.6 g per kilogram of body weight per day to minimize the degree of azotemia. Dietary proteins should be of high biologic value (rich in essential amino acids). Carbohydrates are increased to maintain adequate calorie intake and provide a protein-sparing effect.

Parenteral nutrition providing amino acids, concentrated carbohydrates, and fats may be instituted when the client cannot consume an adequate diet (e.g., due to nausea, vomiting, or underlying critical illness). The disadvantages of parenteral nutrition in the client with ARF are the high volume of fluid required and the risk for infection through the venous line.

Dialysis

Manifestations of uremia, severe fluid overload, hyperkalemia, or metabolic acidosis in a client with renal failure indicate a need to replace renal function. **Dialysis** is the diffusion of solute molecules across a semipermeable membrane from an area of higher solute concentration to one of lower concentration. It is used to remove excess fluid and metabolic waste products in renal failure. Early use of dialysis can reduce the rate of complications. Dialysis may also be used to rapidly remove nephrotoxins in acute tubular necrosis. While dialysis compensates for lost renal elimination functions, it does not replace lost erythropoietin production. Anemia is a continuing problem for the client receiving dialysis.

In dialysis, blood is separated from a dialysis solution (**dialysate**) by a semipermeable membrane. Either **hemodialysis,** a procedure in which blood passes through a semipermeable membrane filter outside the body, or **peritoneal dialysis,** which uses the peritoneum surrounding the abdominal cavity as the dialyzing membrane, may be used for the client with ARF. **Continuous renal replacement therapy (CRRT),** in which blood is continuously circulated through a highly porous hemofilter from artery to vein or vein to vein, is a newer form of dialysis that may be used to treat ARF.

Hemodialysis

Hemodialysis uses the principles of diffusion and ultrafiltration to remove electrolytes, waste products, and excess water from the body. Blood is taken from the client via a vascular access and pumped to the dialyzer (Figure 27–5 ■). The porous membranes of the dialyzer unit allow small molecules such as water, glucose, and electrolytes to pass through, but block larger molecules such as serum proteins and blood cells. The dialysate, a solution of approximately the same composition and temperature as normal extracellular fluid, passes along the other side of the membrane. Small solute molecules move freely across the membrane by diffusion. The direction of movement for any substance is determined by the concentrations of that substance in the blood and the dialysate. Electrolytes and waste products such as urea and creatinine diffuse from the blood into the dialysate. If it is necessary to add something to the blood, such as calcium to replace depleted stores,

Figure 27–5 ■ A hemodialysis system.

it can be added to the dialysate to diffuse into the blood. Excess water is removed by creating a higher hydrostatic pressure of the blood moving through the dialyzer than of the dialysate, which flows in the opposite direction. This process is known as **ultrafiltration.**

Initially, clients with ARF typically undergo daily hemodialysis, then three to four sessions per week as indicated. Hemodialysis is not used if the client is hemodynamically unstable (e.g., with hypotension or low cardiac output). Following are complications associated with hemodialysis.

- Hypotension, the most frequent complication during hemodialysis, is related to changes in serum osmolality, rapid removal of fluid from the vascular compartment, vasodilation, and other factors.
- Bleeding is related to altered platelet function associated with uremia and the use of heparin during dialysis.
- Infection (local or systemic) is related to WBC damage and immune system suppression. *Staphylococcus aureus* septicemia is commonly associated with contamination of the vascular access site. Clients on chronic hemodialysis have higher rates of hepatitis B, hepatitis C, cytomegalovirus, and HIV infection than the general population.

See the box below for nursing care for the client undergoing hemodialysis.

Continuous Renal Replacement Therapy

Clients with acute renal failure may be unable to tolerate hemodialysis and rapid fluid removal if their cardiovascular status is unstable (e.g., due to trauma, major surgery, heart failure). Continuous renal replacement therapy (CRRT), which allows more gradual fluid and solute removal, often is used for these clients. In CRRT, blood is continuously circulated from an artery to a vein or a vein to a vein through a highly porous hemofilter for a period of 12 or more hours. Excess water and solutes such as electrolyes, urea, creatinine, uric acid, and glucose drain into a collection device. Fluid may be replaced with normal saline or a balanced electrolyte solution as needed during CRRT (Figure 27–6 ■). This

NURSING CARE OF THE CLIENT UNDERGOING HEMODIALYSIS

PREDIALYSIS CARE

- Assess vital signs, including orthostatic blood pressures (lying, sitting, and standing), apical pulse, respirations, and lung sounds. *These data provide baseline information to help evaluate the effects of hemodialysis. Hypertension may indicate excess fluid volume. The client who is hypotensive may not tolerate rapid fluid volume changes during dialysis. Abnormal heart sounds (e.g., a gallop or murmur) and changes in heart rate or rhythm may indicate excess fluid volume or electrolyte imbalance. Fluid overload may also cause dyspnea, tachypnea, and rales or crackles in the lungs.*
- Record weight. *Weight changes are an effective indicator of fluid volume.*
- Assess vascular access site for a palpable pulsation or vibration and an audible bruit and for inflammation. *Infection and thrombus formation are the most common problems affecting the access site in hemodialysis clients.*
- Alert all personnel to avoid using the extremity with the vascular access site (or the nondominant arm, if long-term access has not been established) for blood pressures or venipuncture. *These procedures may damage vessels and lead to failure of the AV fistula.*

POSTDIALYSIS CARE

- Assess and document vital signs, weight, and vascular access site condition. *Rapid fluid and solute removal during dialysis may lead to orthostatic hypotension, cardiopulmonary changes, and weight loss.*
- Monitor BUN, serum creatinine, serum electrolyte, and hematocrit levels between dialysis treatments. *These values help determine the effectiveness of the treatment, the need for fluid and diet restrictions, and the timing of future dialysis sessions. The anemia associated with renal failure does not improve with*

dialysis, and iron and folate supplements or periodic blood transfusions may be needed.
- Assess for dialysis disequilibrium syndrome, with headache, nausea and vomiting, altered level of consciousness; and hypertension. *Rapid changes in BUN, pH, and electrolyte levels during dialysis may lead to cerebral edema and increased intracranial pressure.*
- Assess for other adverse responses to dialysis, such as dehydration, nausea and vomiting, muscle cramps, or seizure activity. Treat as ordered. *Excess fluid removal and rapid changes in electrolyte balance can cause fluid deficit, nausea, vomiting, and seizure activity.*
- Assess for bleeding at the access site or elsewhere. Use standard precautions at all times. *Renal failure and heparinization during dialysis increase the risk for bleeding. Frequent exposure to blood and blood products increase the risk for hepatitis B or C or other bloodborne diseases.*
- If a transfusion is given during dialysis, monitor for possible transfusion reaction (e.g., chills and fever; dyspnea; chest, back, or arm pain; and urticaria or itching). *Clients in renal failure may receive multiple transfusions, increasing the risk of transfusion reaction. Close monitoring during and after the transfusion is important to identify early signs of a reaction.*
- Provide psychologic support and listen actively. Address concerns and accept responses such as anger, depression, and noncompliance. Reinforce client and family strengths in coping with renal failure and hemodialysis. *Grieving is a normal response to loss of organ function. The client may feel hopeless or helpless and resent dependence on a machine. The nurse can help the client and family work through these responses and focus on positive aspects of living.*
- Refer to social services and counseling as indicated. *Clients with renal failure may need additional support services to help them adapt to and live with their disease.*

Figure 27–6 ■ Continuous arteriovenous hemofiltration (CAVH).

slower process helps maintain hemodynamic stability and avoid complications associated with rapid changes in ECF composition. The most common CRRT techniques are outlined in Table 27–6.

CRRT is typically performed in an intensive care unit or specialized nephrology unit. Both arterial and venous lines are required for some types of CRRT; for others, a double-lumen venous catheter is used. Strict aseptic technique is vital in caring for vascular access sites to reduce the risk of infection.

Vascular Access

Acute or temporary vascular access for hemodialysis or CRRT usually is gained by inserting a double-lumen catheter into the subclavian, jugular, or femoral vein. The double-lumen catheter has a central partition separating the blood withdrawal side of the catheter from the return side. Blood is drawn into the catheter through small openings in the proximal portion of the catheter, and returned to the circulation through an opening in the distal end of the catheter to avoid withdrawing the blood that has just been dialyzed.

For longer-term vascular access, an *arteriovenous (AV) fistula* (Figure 27–7 ■) is created. In preparation for fistula formation, the nondominant arm is not used for venipuncture or blood pressure measurement during renal failure. The fistula is created by surgical anastomosis of an artery and vein, usually the radial artery and cephalic vein. It takes about a month for the fistula to mature so that it can be used for taking and replacing blood during dialysis. A functional AV fistula has a palpable pulsation and a bruit on auscultation. Venipunctures and blood pressures are avoided on the arm with the fistula.

In chronic renal failure, an *arteriovenous graft* is most often used for vascular access. The graft, a tube made of Gortex, is surgically implanted and connects the artery and the vein. Blood flows through the graft from the artery to the vein. Occasionally, an *external AV shunt* connecting a peripheral artery with a peripheral vein is used for vascular access.

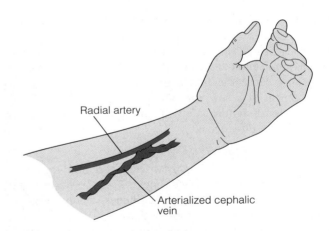

Figure 27–7 ■ An arteriovenous fistula.

TABLE 27–6 Continuous Renal Replacement Therapies		
Type	**Indications**	**Description**
Continuous arteriovenous hemofiltration (CAVH)	Remove fluid and some solutes	Arterial blood circulates through a hemofilter, then returns to client through venous line; ultrafiltrate collects in a drainage bag.
Continuous arteriovenous hemodialysis (CAVHD)	Remove fluid and waste products	Arterial blood circulates through a hemofilter surrounded by dialysate, then returns to client through venous line; ultrafiltrate collects in a drainage bag.
Continuous venovenous hemodialysis (CVVHD)	Remove fluid and waste products	Venous blood circulates through a hemofilter surrounded by dialysate, then returns to client through double-lumen venous catheter; ultrafiltrate collects in a drainage bag.

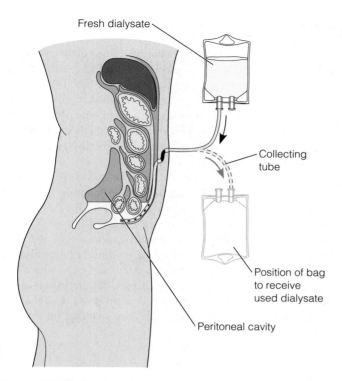
Fresh dialysate

Collecting tube

Position of bag to receive used dialysate

Peritoneal cavity

Figure 27–8 ■ Peritoneal dialysis.

Localized AV fistula, graft, or shunt problems can occur. Infection and clotting or thrombosis are the most common shunt problems. Aneurysms may also develop. Both infection and thrombosis can lead to systemic manifestations such as septicemia and embolization. These local complications may cause the fistula or graft to fail, necessitating development of a new site. The psychologic impact of AV fistula or graft failure is significant, often causing depression and low self-esteem.

Peritoneal Dialysis

In peritoneal dialysis, the highly vascular peritoneal membrane serves as the dialyzing surface (Figure 27–8 ■). Warmed sterile dialysate is instilled into the peritoneal cavity through a catheter inserted into the peritoneal cavity. Metabolic waste products and excess electrolytes diffuse into the dialysate while it remains in the abdomen. Water movement is controlled using dextrose as an osmotic agent to draw it into the dialysate. The fluid is then drained by gravity out of the peritoneal cavity into a sterile bag. This process of dialysate infusion, dwell time of the solution in the abdomen, and drainage is repeated at prescribed intervals.

Because excess fluid and solutes are removed more gradually in peritoneal dialysis, it poses less risk for the unstable client; however, this slower rate of metabolite removal can be a disadvantage in ARF. Peritoneal dialysis increases the risk for developing peritonitis. It is contraindicated for clients who have had recent abdominal surgery, significant lung disease, or peritonitis. See the box on the following page for nursing care for the client having peritoneal dialysis.

NURSING CARE

Health Promotion

Acute renal failure often can be prevented by measures that maintain fluid volume and cardiac output and reduce the risk of exposure to nephrotoxins. Carefully monitor critically ill, postoperative, and other at-risk clients for early signs of hypovolemia (low urine output, altered mental status, changes in vital signs, skin color or temperature). Promptly report a fall in urine output to less than 30 mL per hour and other evidence of decreased cardiac output. Maintain intravenous fluids as ordered. Alert the physician if the client is receiving more than one nephrotoxic drug or if a nephrotoxic drug is ordered for a dehydrated client. Closely observe clients receiving blood or blood cells for early signs of transfusion reaction and intervene appropriately.

Assessment

Both subjective and objective data are useful when assessing the client with acute renal failure.

- Health history: complaints of anorexia, nausea, weight gain, or edema; recent exposure to a nephrotoxin such as an aminoglycoside antibiotic or radiologic procedure using an injected contrast medium; previous transfusion reaction; chronic diseases such as diabetes, heart failure, or kidney disease
- Physical examination: vital signs including temperature; urine output (amount, color, clarity, specific gravity, presence of blood cells or protein); weight; skin color, peripheral pulses; presence of edema (periorbial or dependent); lung sounds, heart sounds, and bowel tones

See page 772 for assessment of the older adult with ARF.

Nursing Diagnoses and Interventions

The client with acute renal failure has numerous nursing care needs related not only to the renal failure but also to the underlying condition that precipitated it. Priority nursing care needs relate to fluid volume alterations, appetite and nutrition, and teaching/learning.

Excess Fluid Volume

In acute renal failure, the kidneys often cannot excrete adequate urine to maintain a normal extracellular fluid balance. Fluid retention is greater in oliguric renal failure than in nonoliguric failure. Rapid weight gain and edema indicate fluid retention. In addition, heart failure and pulmonary edema may develop. In the older adult or severely debilitated client, fluid retention can present a significant management problem.

- Maintain hourly intake and output records. *Accurate intake and output records help guide therapy, especially fluid restrictions.*
- Weigh daily or more frequently, as ordered. Use standard technique (same scale, clothing, or coverings) to ensure accuracy. *Rapid weight changes are an accurate indicator of fluid volume status, particularly in the oliguric client.*
- Assess vital signs at least every 4 hours. *Hypertension, tachycardia, and tachypnea may indicate excess fluid volume.*

NURSING CARE OF THE CLIENT UNDERGOING PERITONEAL DIALYSIS

PREDIALYSIS CARE

- Document vital signs including temperature, orthostatic blood pressures (lying, sitting, and standing), apical pulse, respirations, and lung sounds. *These baseline data help assess fluid volume status and tolerance of the dialysis procedure. Hypertension, abnormal heart or lung sounds, or dyspnea may indicate excess fluid volume. Poor respiratory function may affect the ability to tolerate peritoneal dialysis. Temperature measurement is vital, because infection is the most common complication of peritoneal dialysis.*
- Weigh daily or between dialysis runs as indicated. *Weight is an accurate indicator of fluid volume status.*
- Note BUN, serum electrolyte, creatinine, pH, and hematocrit levels prior to peritoneal dialysis and periodically during the procedure. *These values are used to assess the efficacy of treatment.*
- Measure and record abdominal girth. *Increasing abdominal girth may indicate retained dialysate, excess fluid volume, or early peritonitis.*
- Maintain fluid and dietary restrictions as ordered. *Fluid and diet restrictions help reduce hypervolemia and control azotemia.*
- Have the client empty the bladder prior to catheter insertion. *Emptying the bladder reduces the risk of inadvertent puncture.*
- Warm the prescribed dialysate solution to body temperature (98.6°F or 37°C) using a warm water bath or heating pad on low setting. *Dialysate is warmed to prevent hypothermia.*
- Explain all procedures and expected sensations. *Knowledge helps reduce anxiety and elicit cooperation.*

INTRADIALYSIS CARE

- Use strict aseptic technique during the dialysis procedure and when caring for the peritoneal catheter. *Peritonitis is a common complication of peritoneal dialysis; sterile technique reduces the risk.*
- Add prescribed medications to the dialysate; prime the tubing with solution and connect it to the peritoneal catheter, taping connections securely and avoiding kinks. *This allows dialysate to flow freely into the abdominal cavity and prevents leaking or contamination.*
- Instill dialysate into the abdominal cavity over a period of approximately 10 minutes. Clamp tubing and allow the dialysate to remain in the abdomen for the prescribed dwell time. Keep drainage tubing clamped at all times during instillation and dwell time. *Dialysate should flow freely into the abdomen if the peritoneal catheter is patent. Dialysis, the exchange of solutes and water between the blood and dialysate, occurs across the peritoneal membrane during the dwell time.*

- During instillation and dwell time, observe closely for signs of respiratory distress, such as dyspnea, tachypnea, or crackles. Place in Fowler's or semi-Fowler's position and slow the rate of instillation slightly to relieve respiratory distress if it develops. *Respiratory compromise may result from overly rapid filling or overfilling of the abdomen or from a diaphragmatic defect that allows fluid to enter the thoracic cavity.*
- After prescribed dwell time, open drainage tubing clamps and allow dialysate to drain by gravity into a sterile container. Note the clarity, color, and odor of returned dialysate. *Blood or feces in the dialysate may indicate organ or bowel perforation; cloudy or malodorous dialysate may indicate an infection.*
- Accurately record amount and type of dialysate instilled (including any added medications), dwell time, and amount and character of the drainage. *When more dialysate drains than has been instilled, excess fluid has been lost (output). If less dialysate is returned than has been instilled, a fluid gain has occurred (intake).*
- Monitor BUN, serum electrolyte, and creatinine levels. *These values are used to assess the effectiveness of dialysis.*
- Troubleshoot for possible problems during dialysis.
  a. Slow dialysate instillation. Increase the height of the container and reposition the client. Check tubing and catheter for kinks. Check abdominal dressing for wetness, indicating leakage around the catheter. *Slow dialysate flow may be related to a partially obstructed tube or catheter.*
  b. Excess dwell time. *Prolonged dwell time may lead to water depletion or hyperglycemia.*
  c. Poor dialysate drainage. Lower the drainage container, reposition, check for tubing kinks. Check abdominal dressing. *Tubing or catheter obstruction can also interfere with dialysate drainage.*

POSTDIALYSIS CARE

- Assess vital signs, including temperature. *Comparison of pre- and postdialysis vital signs helps identify beneficial and adverse effects of the procedure.*
- Time meals to correspond with dialysis outflow. *Scheduling meals while the abdomen is empty of dialysate enhances intake and reduces nausea.*
- Teach the client and family about the procedure. *The client may elect to use peritoneal dialysis at home to manage end-stage renal disease and prevent uremia.*

PRACTICE ALERT *Frequently assess breath and heart sounds, neck veins for distention, and back and extremities for edema. Report abnormal findings. Adventitious breath sounds (crackles), abnormal heart sounds such as an S3 or S4 gallop, distended neck veins, and peripheral edema may indicate hypervolemia, heart failure, or pulmonary edema.* ■

- If not contraindicated, place in semi-Fowler's position, *to enhance cardiac and respiratory function.*
- Report abnormal serum electrolyte values and manifestations of electrolyte imbalance. The client with ARF is at particular risk for the following electrolyte imbalances:
  a. *Hyperkalemia* due to impaired potassium excretion. Manifestations include irritability, nausea, diarrhea,

KIDNEY DISORDERS

MediaLink

Nursing Care of the Older Adult

RENAL FAILURE

Structural and functional changes occur in the aging kidney. Structurally, the number of nephrons decreases. The glomerular filtration rate (GFR) decreases, resulting in decreased renal clearance of drugs. Urine concentrating ability decreases, and the kidney is less able to conserve sodium. Renal compensation for acid-base imbalances takes longer. Despite these changes, the kidney retains its ability to regulate fluid and electrolyte homeostasis remarkably well unless additional stresses are added. Any additional stressors such as hypotension, exposure to nephrotoxic drugs, or an inflammatory process such as glomerulonephritis may precipitate renal failure in the older adult.

The manifestations of renal failure often are missed in aging clients (e.g., edema may be attributed to heart failure or high blood pressure to preexisting hypertension). Serum creatinine levels may rise slowly. Because older adults have less muscle mass, they produce less creatinine, a by-product of muscle cell metabolism. Likewise, the BUN may remain within normal limits.

The same measures are used to treat renal failure in older adults as in younger people. Hemodialysis, peritoneal dialysis, and renal transplantation are appropriate if necessary. Treatment options (including conservative treatment or no treatment) and their potential benefits and ramifications should be clearly explained.

Assessing for Home Care

A number of factors should be considered in assessing the older adult's ability to manage treatment such as dialysis at home:

- Does the client have reasonable access to a dialysis center or outpatient unit? Is transportation available?

- Would home hemodialysis be appropriate? Is a caregiver available to be trained to manage dialysis? Does the client's home have appropriate electrical and plumbing fixtures?
- Would continuous ambulatory peritoneal dialysis be appropriate? Does the client have the manual dexterity, will, and cognitive ability to manage dialysis infusions? If not, would intermittent peritoneal dialysis using a dialyzing machine be more appropriate?
- Are family members or other support persons available to provide assistance to the client as needed?

Resources for Home Care
The following resources may be useful for clients with kidney disease.

- American Association of Kidney Patients
  3505 E. Frontage Rd., Suite 315
  Tampa, FL 33607
  800-749-2257
  www.aakp.org
- American Kidney Fund
  6110 Executive Blvd., Suite 1010
  Rockville, MD 20852
  800-638-8299
  www.akfinc.org
- National Kidney Foundation
  30 E. 33rd Street, Suite 1100
  New York, NY 10016
  800-622-9010
  www.kidney.org

---

abdominal cramping, cardiac dysrhythmias, and ECG changes.
  b. *Hyponatremia* due to water retention. Manifestations include nausea, vomiting, and headache, with possible CNS manifestations of lethargy, confusion, seizures, and coma.
  c. *Hyperphosphatemia* due to decreased phosphate excretion. Manifestations include hyperreflexia, paresthesias, and possible tetany.
ARF impairs electrolyte and water excretion, causing multiple electrolyte imbalances.
- Restrict fluids as ordered. Provide frequent mouth care and encourage using hard candies to decrease thirst. If ice chips are allowed, include the water content (approximately one-half of the total volume) as intake. *Fluids are restricted to minimize fluid retention and complications of fluid volume excess.*
- Administer medications with meals. *Giving oral medications with meals minimizes ingestion of excess fluids.*
- Turn frequently and provide good skin care. *Edema decreases tissue perfusion and increases the risk of skin breakdown, especially in the older or debilitated client.*

Imbalanced Nutrition: Less Than Body Requirements
Anorexia and nausea associated with renal failure often interfere with food intake and nutrition. In addition, the disease

process leading to ARF may contribute to increased nutritional needs for healing and decreased food intake.

- Monitor and record food intake, including the amount and type of food consumed. *A detailed intake record helps guide decisions about nutritional status and necessary supplements.*
- Weigh daily. *Weight changes over time (days to weeks) reflect nutritional status, while rapid weight changes are more reflective of fluid volume status. In ARF, weight may remain stable or increase due to fluid retention even though tissue mass is being lost.*
- Arrange for dietary consultation to plan meals within prescribed limitations that consider the client's food preferences. *Diets restricted in protein, salt, and potassium can be unpalatable; including preferred foods as allowed increases intake.*
- Engage the client in planning daily menus. *Participation in meal planning increases the client's sense of control and autonomy.*
- Allow family members to prepare meals within dietary restrictions. Encourage family members to eat with the client. *Familiar foods and social interaction encourage eating and increase enjoyment of meals.*
- Provide frequent, small meals or between-meal snacks. *These measures promote food intake in the fatigued or anorectic client.*

- Administer antiemetics as ordered and provide mouth care prior to meals. *Nausea and a metallic taste in the mouth, common manifestations of uremia, can decrease food intake.*
- Administer parenteral nutrition as ordered if the client is unable to eat or tolerate enteral nutrition. *Preventing or slowing tissue catabolism is important for the client with ARF.*

PRACTICE ALERT *Intravenous lines and parenteral nutrition solutions can increase the risk for infection. Monitor sites carefully for signs of infection or inflammation.* ■

Deficient Knowledge

The client with ARF has multiple learning needs. These include information about ARF, diagnostic and laboratory studies, management strategies, and implications for the recovery period.

- Assess anxiety level and ability to comprehend instruction. Tailor information and presentation to developmental level and physical, mental, and emotional status. *The client with ARF may be critically ill or have uremic effects that hinder learning. During the initial stages of ARF it may be necessary to limit information to immediate concerns.*
- Assess knowledge and understanding. *To enhance understanding and retention, relate information presented to previous learning.*
- Teach about diagnostic tests and therapeutic procedures. *Teaching reduces anxiety and improves understanding and cooperation.*
- Discuss dietary and fluid restrictions. *These measures may be continued after discharge.*
- If the client is discharged prior to the recovery phase of ARF, teach the signs and symptoms of complications, such as fluid volume excess or deficit, heart failure, and electrolyte imbalances. *As kidney function returns, urine output increases, but the concentrating ability of the nephrons and electrolyte*

excretion remain impaired. This impaired function increases the risk of excess fluid loss, possible dehydration, orthostatic hypotension, and electrolyte imbalance.
- Teach how to monitor weight, blood pressure, and pulse. *These are important means of assessing fluid status.*
- Instruct to avoid nephrotoxic drugs and chemicals for up to 1 year following an episode of ARF. *During recovery, nephrons are vulnerable to damage by nephrotoxins such as NSAIDs, some antibiotics, radiologic contrast media, and heavy metals. Because alcohol can increase the nephrotoxicity of some materials, discourage alcohol ingestion.*

Using NANDA, NIC, and NOC

Chart 27–3 shows links between NANDA nursing diagnoses, NIC, and NOC for the client with ARF.

Home Care

Often the client is critically ill when ARF develops. Critical illness and the resulting state of client and family crisis can impair learning and retention of information. Include family members in teaching during the initial stages to promote understanding of what is happening and the reasons for specific treatment measures. Inclusion of the family reduces their anxiety, and provides a valuable resource for reinforcing client teaching about care after discharge.

Client teaching needs for home care include:

- Avoiding exposure to nephrotoxins, particularly those in over-the-counter products.
- Preventing infection and other major stressors that can slow healing.
- Monitoring weight, blood pressure, and pulse.
- Manifestations of relapse.
- Continuing dietary restrictions.
- Knowing when to contact the physician.

CHART 27–3 NANDA, NIC, AND NOC LINKAGES

The Client with Acute Renal Failure

NURSING DIAGNOSES	NURSING INTERVENTIONS	NURSING OUTCOMES
• Anxiety	• Active Listening • Anxiety Reduction	• Anxiety Control • Coping
• Decreased Cardiac Output	• Hemodynamic Regulation • Shock Management	• Cardiac Pump Effectiveness
• Excess Fluid Volume	• Fluid Management • Fluid / Electrolyte Management	• Electrolyte and Acid-Base Balance • Fluid Balance
• Imbalanced Nutrition: Less than Body Requirements	• Enteral Tube Feeding • Nutrition Management • Nutrition Monitoring	• Nutritional Status: Food and Fluid Intake
• Impaired Urinary Elimination	• Urinary Elimination Management	• Urinary Elimination

Note. Data from Nursing Outcomes Classification (NOC) by M. Johnson & M. Maas (Eds.), 1997, St. Louis: Mosby; Nursing Diagnoses: Definitions & Classification 2001–2002 by North American Nursing Diagnosis Association, 2001, Philadelphia: NANDA; Nursing Interventions Classification (NIC) by J.C. McCloskey & G. M. Bulechek (Eds.), 2000, St. Louis: Mosby. Reprinted by permission.

Nursing Care Plan
A Client with Acute Renal Failure

Judy Devak is driving home late one evening when she loses control of her car trying to avoid hitting a deer in the road. Her car strikes a tree and rolls into a deep ditch beside the road, out of sight of passing cars. The wreek is not discovered until 2 hours later. On arrival at the accident scene, the paramedics find Ms. Devak hypotensive: BP 90/60, P 120, and R 24. She is alert and in severe pain, with a fractured right femur. After immobilizing Ms. Devak's neck and back and extricating her from the car, they apply a traction splint to her leg and transport her to the local hospital.

ASSESSMENT

Katie Leaper, RN, obtains a nursing history on Ms. Devak's admission to the intensive care unit. Ms. Devak indicates that she has been healthy, having experienced only minor illnesses and chickenpox as a child. She has never been hospitalized, and knows of no allergies to medications. Ms. Devak is not currently taking prescription or nonprescription drugs. Physical assessment findings include T 97.4° F (36.3° C) PO, P 100, R 18, and BP 124/68. Skin pale, cool, and dry, with multiple scrapes, minor abrasions, and bruises on face and extremities. A linear bruise is noted on her chest and abdomen from the seat belt. Lung sounds clear, heart tones normal, and abdomen tender but soft to palpation. Right leg alignment maintained with skeletal traction. One unit of whole blood was infused prior to ICU admission, a second unit is currently infusing. An indwelling urinary catheter and a nasogastric tube are in place.

During the first few hours after admission, Ms. Leaper notes that Ms. Devak's hourly output has dropped from 55 mL to 45 mL to 28 mL of clear yellow urine. The physician orders a 500 mL intravenous fluid challenge, STAT urinalysis, BUN, and serum creatinine. The fluid challenge elicits only a slight increase in urine output. Urinalysis results show a specific gravity of 1.010 and the presence of WBCs, red and white cell casts, and tubular epithelial cells in the sediment. Ms. Devak's BUN is 28 mg/dL; her serum creatinine, 1.5 mg/dL. The physician diagnoses probable acute renal failure and orders a nephrology consultation. In addition, the physician orders aluminum hydroxide, 10 mL every 2 hours per nasogastric tube, and ranitidine 50 mg intravenously every 8 hours.

DIAGNOSIS

- *Acute pain* related to injuries sustained in accident
- *Anxiety* related to being in the intensive care unit
- *Risk for excess fluid volume* related to impaired renal function
- *Impaired physical mobility* related to skeletal traction
- *Ineffective protection* related to injuries and invasive procedures

EXPECTED OUTCOMES

- Report adequate pain control.
- Verbalize reduced anxiety.
- Maintain stable weight and vital signs within normal range.

- Maintain skin integrity.
- Use the trapeze appropriately to adjust position in bed while maintaining body alignment.
- Remain free of infection, bleeding, or respiratory distress.

PLANNING AND IMPLEMENTATION

- Maintain patient-controlled analgesia.
- Assess frequently for pain control and response to analgesia.
- Encourage expression of thoughts, feelings, and fears about condition and placement in ICU.
- Document vital signs and heart and lung sounds at least every 4 hours.
- Weigh every 12 hours.
- Document hourly intake and output.
- Restrict fluids as ordered, including diluent for all intravenous medications as intake.
- Assist with mouth care every 3 to 4 hours; allow frequent rinsing of mouth and ice chips as allowed.
- Assist with position changes at least every 2 hours; teach use of the overhead trapeze.
- Monitor frequently for signs of infection, bleeding, or respiratory distress.

EVALUATION

After just over 3 days of oliguria, Ms. Devak's urine output increases. By the end of the fourth day she is excreting 60 to 80 mL/hour of urine. Although her BUN, serum creatinine, and potassium levels remain high, they never reach a critical point, and dialysis is not required. She is transferred from the ICU on the fifth day after admission. When Ms. Devak is able to begin eating, she is placed on a low-potassium diet, restricted to 50 g of protein. Her renal function gradually improves. By discharge, results of her renal function studies, including BUN and serum creatinine, are nearly normal. Ms. Devak verbalizes an understanding of the need to avoid nephrotoxins such as NSAIDs until allowed by her physician.

Critical Thinking in the Nursing Process

1. What was the most likely specific precipitating factor for Ms. Devak's acute renal failure? Did anything else contribute to her risk?
2. Why did the physician prescribe aluminum hydroxide and ranitidine? Consider both the acute renal failure and Ms. Devak's placement in the intensive care unit.
3. Ms. Devak is at risk for respiratory distress related to potential fluid volume excess. How does her fractured femur further contribute to risk for respiratory distress?
4. Develop a care plan for Ms. Devak for the nursing diagnosis, *Diversional activity deficit.*

See Evaluating Your Response in Appendix C.

THE CLIENT WITH CHRONIC RENAL FAILURE

Although the kidneys usually recover from acute injury, many chronic conditions can lead to progressive renal tissue destruction and loss of function. Nephron units are lost and renal mass decreases, with progressive deterioration of glomerular filtration, tubular secretion, and reabsorption. This process of chronic renal failure (CRF) may progress slowly for many years without being recognized. Eventually, the kidneys are unable to excrete metabolic wastes and regulate fluid and electrolyte balance adequately, a condition known as end-stage renal disease (ESRD), the final stage of CRF.

The incidence of ESRD is increasing, particularly in older adults. In 1999, more than 89,000 people started treatment for ESRD for a total of about 424,000 people undergoing ESRD treatment (NKUDIC, 2001). Native Americans have the highest incidence of ESRD, followed by African Americans, Asians and European Americans (United States Renal Data System [USRDS], 2001).

Conditions causing CRF typically involve diffuse, bilateral disease of the kidneys with progressive destruction and scarring of the entire nephron. As indicated in Figure 27–9 ■, diabetes is the leading cause of ESRD in all population groups in the United States. Hypertension closely follows diabetes as a major cause of ESRD (USRDS, 2001).

PATHOPHYSIOLOGY AND MANIFESTATIONS

The pathophysiology of CRF involves a gradual loss of entire nephron units. In the early stages, as nephrons are destroyed, remaining functional nephrons hypertrophy. Glomerular capillary flow and pressure increase in these nephrons, and more solute particles are filtered to compensate for lost renal mass. This increased demand predisposes the remaining nephrons to glomerular sclerosis (scarring), resulting in their eventual destruction. This process of continued loss of nephron function may continue even after the initial disease process has resolved (Braunwald et al., 2001). Table 27–7 outlines common pathologic processes leading to nephron destruction and ESRD.

The course of CRF is variable, progressing over a period of months to many years. In the early stage, known as *decreased renal reserve*, unaffected nephrons compensate for the lost nephrons. The glomerular filtration rate (GFR) is about 50% of normal, and the client is asymptomatic with normal BUN and serum creatinine levels. As the disease progresses and the GFR falls to 20% to 50% of normal, azotemia and some manifestations of *renal insufficiency* may be seen. Any further insult to the kidneys at this stage (such as infection, dehydration, exposure to nephrotoxins, or urinary tract obstruction) can further reduce function and precipitate the onset of *renal failure* or overt uremia. This stage is characterized by a GFR of less than 20% of

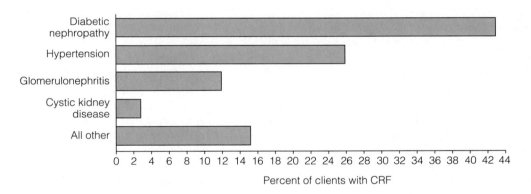

Figure 27–9 ■ The most common causes of chronic renal failure (USRDS, 2001).

TABLE 27–7 Pathophysiology of Chronic Renal Failure

Cause	Examples
Diabetic nephropathy	Changes in the glomerular basement membrane, chronic pyelonephritis, and ischemia lead to sclerosis of the glomerulus and gradual destruction of the nephron
Hypertensive nephrosclerosis	Long-standing hypertension leads to renal arteriosclerosis and ischemia resulting in glomerular destruction and tubular atrophy
Chronic glomerulonephritis	Bilateral inflammatory process of the glomeruli leading to ischemia, nephron loss, and shrinkage of the kidney
Chronic pyelonephritis	Chronic infection commonly associated with an obstructive or neurologic process and vesicoureteral reflux leading to reflux nephropathy (renal scarring, atrophy, and dilated calyces)
Polycystic kidney disease	Multiple bilateral cysts gradually destroy normal renal tissue by compression
Systemic lupus erythematosus	Basement membrane damage by circulating immune complexes leading to focal, local, or diffuse glomerulonephritis

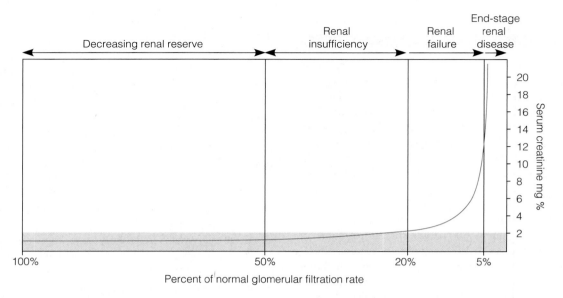

Figure 27-10 ■ The relationship of renal function to BUN and serum creatinine values through the course of chronic renal failure.

normal. The serum creatinine and BUN levels rise sharply (Figure 27-10 ■), the client becomes oliguric, and manifestations of uremia are seen. In ESRD, the final stage of CRF, the GFR is less than 5% of normal and renal replacement therapy is necessary to sustain life (Braunwald et al., 2001; Porth, 2002). Table 27-8 summarizes the stages of chronic renal failure.

Chronic renal failure often is not identified until its final, uremic stage is reached. **Uremia,** which literally means "urine in the blood," refers to the syndrome or group of symptoms associated with ESRD. In uremia, fluid and electrolyte balance is altered, the regulatory and endocrine functions of the kidney are impaired, and accumulated metabolic waste products affect essentially every other organ system (Braunwald et al., 2001; Porth 2002).

Early manifestations of uremia include nausea, apathy, weakness, and fatigue, symptoms that are dismissed as a viral infection or influenza. As the condition progresses, frequent vomiting, increasing weakness, lethargy, and confusion develop (Porth, 2002). The *Multisystem Effects of Uremia* are illustrated on the next page.

Fluid and Electrolyte Effects

Loss of functional kidney tissue impairs its ability to regulate fluid, electrolyte, and acid-base balance. In the early stages of

CRF, impaired filtration and reabsorption lead to proteinuria, hematuria, and decreased urine concentrating ability. Salt and water are poorly conserved, and risk for dehydration increases. Polyuria, nocturia, and a fixed specific gravity of 1.008 to 1.012 are common (Porth, 2002). As the GFR decreases and renal function deteriorates further, sodium and water retention are common, necessitating salt and water restrictions.

Hyperkalemia develops as renal failure progresses. Manifestations of hyperkalemia, such as muscle weakness, paresthesias, and ECG changes, are not usually seen until the GFR is less than 5 mL/min. Phosphate excretion is also impaired, leading to hyperphosphatemia and hypocalcemia. Reduced calcium absorption due to impaired vitamin D activation also contributes to hypocalcemia. Hypermagnesemia develops with advancing renal failure; magnesium-containing antacids are avoided for this reason.

As renal failure advances, hydrogen-ion excretion and buffer production are impaired, leading to metabolic acidosis. Respiratory rate and depth increase (Kussmaul's respirations) to compensate for metabolic acidosis. Although metabolic acidosis is often asymptomatic, other possible manifestations include general malaise, weakness, headache, nausea and vomiting, and abdominal pain (see Chapter 5). ⬡

TABLE 27-8 Stages of Chronic Renal Failure		
Stage	**Glomerular Filtration Rate**	**Manifestations**
Decreased renal reserve	Approximately 50% of normal	None; normal BUN and creatinine
Renal insufficiency	20% to 50% of normal	Polyuria with low, fixed specific gravity; azotemia; anemia; hypertension
Renal failure	<20% of normal	Increasing azotemia; edema, metabolic acidosis, hypercalcemia; possible uremia
End-stage renal disease	<5% of normal	Kidney atrophy and fibrosis; overt uremia

Multisystem Effects of Uremia

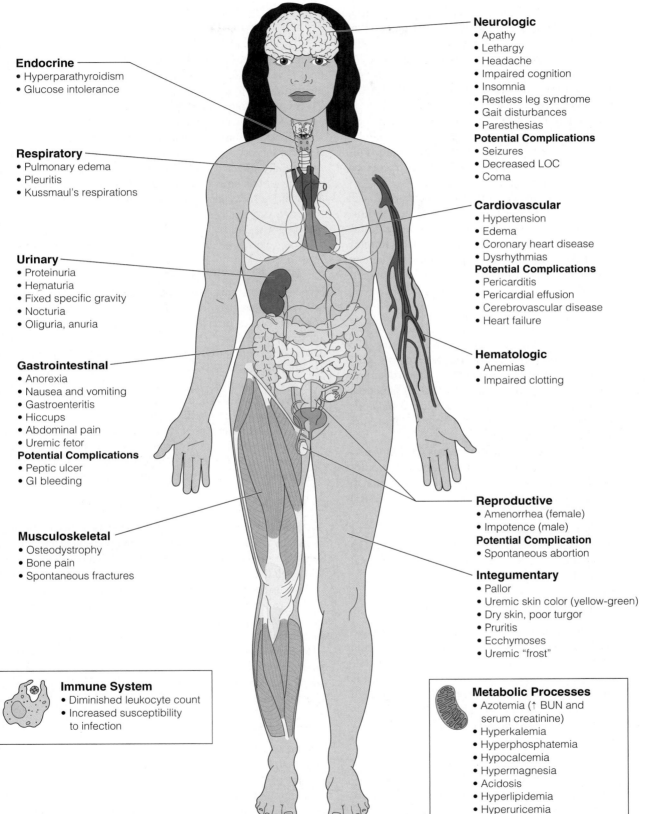

Endocrine
- Hyperparathyroidism
- Glucose intolerance

Respiratory
- Pulmonary edema
- Pleuritis
- Kussmaul's respirations

Urinary
- Proteinuria
- Hematuria
- Fixed specific gravity
- Nocturia
- Oliguria, anuria

Gastrointestinal
- Anorexia
- Nausea and vomiting
- Gastroenteritis
- Hiccups
- Abdominal pain
- Uremic fetor
Potential Complications
- Peptic ulcer
- GI bleeding

Musculoskeletal
- Osteodystrophy
- Bone pain
- Spontaneous fractures

Immune System
- Diminished leukocyte count
- Increased susceptibility to infection

Neurologic
- Apathy
- Lethargy
- Headache
- Impaired cognition
- Insomnia
- Restless leg syndrome
- Gait disturbances
- Paresthesias
Potential Complications
- Seizures
- Decreased LOC
- Coma

Cardiovascular
- Hypertension
- Edema
- Coronary heart disease
- Dysrhythmias
Potential Complications
- Pericarditis
- Pericardial effusion
- Cerebrovascular disease
- Heart failure

Hematologic
- Anemias
- Impaired clotting

Reproductive
- Amenorrhea (female)
- Impotence (male)
Potential Complication
- Spontaneous abortion

Integumentary
- Pallor
- Uremic skin color (yellow-green)
- Dry skin, poor turgor
- Pruritis
- Ecchymoses
- Uremic "frost"

Metabolic Processes
- Azotemia (↑ BUN and serum creatinine)
- Hyperkalemia
- Hyperphosphatemia
- Hypocalcemia
- Hypermagnesia
- Acidosis
- Hyperlipidemia
- Hyperuricemia
- Malnutrition

Cardiovascular Effects

Cardiovascular disease is a common cause of death in ESRD, and results from accelerated atherosclerosis. Hypertension, hyperlipidemia, and glucose intolerance all contribute to the process. Cerebral and peripheral vascular manifestations of atherosclerosis are also seen.

Systemic hypertension is a common complication of ESRD. Hypertension results from excess fluid volume; increased rennin-angiotensin activity, increased peripheral vascular resistance, and decreased prostaglandins. Increased extracellular fluid volume also can lead to edema and heart failure. Pulmonary edema may result from heart failure and increased permeability of the alveolar capillary membrane.

Retained metabolic toxins can irritate the pericardial sac, causing an inflammatory response and signs of pericarditis. *Cardiac tamponade,* a potential complication of pericarditis, occurs when inflammatory fluid in the pericardial sac interferes with ventricular filling and cardiac output. Once a common complication of uremia, pericarditis is less common when dialysis is initiated early.

Hematologic Effects

Anemia is common in uremia, caused by multiple factors. The kidneys produce erythropoietin, a hormone that controls RBC production. In renal failure, erythropoietin production declines. Retained metabolic toxins further suppress RBC production, and contribute to a shortened RBC life span. Nutritional deficiencies (iron and folate) and increased risk for blood loss from the GI tract also contribute to anemia.

Anemia contributes to manifestations such as fatigue, weakness, depression, and impaired cognition. It also affects cardiovascular function, and may be a major contributing factor to coronary heart disease and heart failure associated with ESRD (Porth, 2002).

Renal failure impairs platelet function, increasing the risk of bleeding disorders such as epistaxis and GI bleeding. The mechanism of impaired platelet function associated with renal failure is poorly understood.

Immune System Effects

Uremia increases the risk for infection. High levels of urea and retained metabolic wastes impair all aspects of inflammation and immune function. The WBC declines, humoral and cell-mediated immunity are impaired, and phagocyte function is defective. Both the acute inflammatory response and delayed hypersensitivity responses are affected (Porth, 2002). Fever is suppressed, often delaying the diagnosis of infection.

Gastrointestinal Effects

Anorexia, nausea, and vomiting are the most common early symptoms of uremia. Hiccups also are commonly experienced. Gastroenteritis is frequent. Ulcerations may affect any level of the GI tract and contribute to an increased risk of GI bleeding. Peptic ulcer disease is particularly common in uremic clients. *Uremic fetor,* a urinelike breath odor often associated with a metallic taste in the mouth, may develop. Uremic fetor can further contribute to anorexia.

Neurologic Effects

Uremia alters both central and peripheral nervous system function. CNS manifestations occur early and include changes in mentation, difficulty concentrating, fatigue, and insomnia. Psychotic symptoms, seizures, and coma are associated with advanced uremic encephalopathy.

Peripheral neuropathy is also common in advanced uremia. Both the sensory and motor tracts are involved. The lower limbs are initially affected. "Restless leg syndrome," sensations of crawling or creeping, prickling, or itching of the lower legs with frequent leg movement, increases during rest. Paresthesias and sensory loss typically occur in a "stocking-glove" pattern. As uremia progresses, motor function is also impaired, causing muscle weakness, decreased deep tendon reflexes, and gait disturbances.

Musculoskeletal Effects

Hyperphosphatemia and hypocalcemia associated with uremia stimulates parathyroid hormone secretion. Parathyroid hormone causes increased calcium resorption from bone. In addition, osteoblast (bone-forming) and osteoclast (bone-destructing) cell activity is affected. This bone resorption and remodeling, combined with decreased vitamin D synthesis and decreased calcium absorption from the GI tract, leads to *renal osteodystrophy,* also known as renal rickets. Osteodystrophy is characterized by *osteomalacia,* softening of the bones, and *osteoporosis,* decreased bone mass. Bone cysts may develop. Manifestations of osteodystrophy include bone tenderness, pain, and muscle weakness. The client is at increased risk for spontaneous fractures (Porth, 2002).

Endocrine and Metabolic Effects

Accumulated waste products of protein metabolism are a primary factor involved in the effects and manifestations of uremia. Serum creatinine and BUN levels are significantly elevated. Uric acid levels are increased, contributing to an increased risk of gout.

Tissues become resistant to the effects of insulin in uremia, leading to glucose intolerance. High blood triglyceride levels and lower than normal high-density lipoprotein (HDL) levels contribute to the accelerated atherosclerotic process.

Reproductive function is affected. Pregnancies are rarely carried to term, and menstrual irregularities are common. Reduced testosterone levels, low sperm counts, and impotence affect the male client with ESRD.

Dermatologic Effects

Anemia and retained pigmented metabolites cause pallor and a yellowish hue to the skin in uremia. Dry skin with poor turgor, a result of dehydration and sweat gland atrophy, is common. Bruising and excoriations are frequently seen. Metabolic wastes not eliminated by the kidneys may be deposited in the skin, contributing to itching or pruritus. In advanced uremia, high levels of urea in the sweat may result in *uremic frost,* crystallized deposits of urea on the skin.

COLLABORATIVE CARE

Early management of CRF focuses on eliminating factors that may further decrease renal function and measures to slow the progression of the disease to ESRD. Additional treatment goals are to:

- Maintain nutritional status while minimizing the accumulation of toxic waste products and manifestations of uremia.
- Identify and treat complications of CRF.
- Prepare for renal replacement therapies such as dialysis or renal transplant.

Diagnostic Tests

Diagnostic testing is used both to identify CRF and to monitor kidney function. A number of tests may be performed to determine the underlying renal disorder. Once the diagnosis is established, renal function is monitored primarily through blood levels of metabolic wastes and electrolytes.

- *Urinalysis* is done to measure urine specific gravity and detect abnormal urine components. In CRF, the specific gravity may be fixed at approximately 1.010, equivalent to that of plasma. This fixed specific gravity is due to impaired tubular secretion, reabsorption, and urine concentrating ability. Abnormal proteins, blood cells, and cellular casts may also be noted in the urine.
- *Urine culture* is ordered to identify any urinary tract infection that may hasten the progress of CRF.
- *BUN* and *serum creatinine* are obtained to evaluate kidney function in eliminating nitrogenous waste products. Levels of both are monitored to assess the progress of renal failure. A BUN of 20 to 50 mg/dL signals mild azotemia; levels greater than 100 mg/dL indicate severe renal impairment. Uremic symptoms are seen when the BUN is around 200 mg/dL or higher. Serum creatinine levels of greater than 4 mg/dL indicate serious renal impairment.
- *Creatinine clearance* evaluates the GFR and renal function. In early CRF (renal insufficiency), the GFR is more than 20% of normal and the creatinine clearance 25 mL/min or greater. As the disease progresses and the stage of renal failure is reached, the GFR is reduced to less than 20% of normal and the creatinine clearance to 10 to 30 mL/min. In ESRD, the GFR is less than 5% of normal and the creatinine clearance is 5 to 10 mL/min or less. Nursing implications for creatinine clearance are outlined in the box on page 750.
- *Serum electrolytes* are monitored throughout the course of CRF. The serum sodium may be within normal limits or low because of water retention. Potassium levels are elevated but usually remain below 6.5 mEq/L. Serum phosphate is elevated, and the calcium level is decreased. Metabolic acidosis is identified by a low pH, low CO_2, and low bicarbonate levels.
- *CBC* reveals moderately severe anemia with a hematocrit of 20% to 30% and a low hemoglobin. The number of red blood cells and platelets is reduced.
- *Renal ultrasonography* is done to evaluate kidney size. In CRF, kidney size decreases as nephrons are destroyed and kidney mass is reduced. Preparation of the client and nursing implications for renal ultrasonography are outlined in the box on page 717.
- *Kidney biopsy* may be done to identify the underlying disease process if this is unclear. It is also used to differentiate acute from chronic failure. Kidney biopsy may be performed in surgery or done percutaneously using needle biopsy. The box on page 750 outlines nursing care for a client having a renal biopsy.

Medications

Chronic renal failure affects both the pharmacokinetic and pharmacodynamic effects of drug therapy. Most medications are excreted primarily by the kidney. The half-life and plasma levels of many drugs increase in chronic renal failure. Drug absorption may be decreased when phosphate-binding agents are administered concurrently. Proteinuria can significantly reduce plasma protein levels, leading to manifestations of toxicity when highly protein-bound drugs are given. In addition, any potentially nephrotoxic agent is avoided or used with extreme caution. Drugs such as meperidine, metformin (Glucophage), and other oral hypoglycemic agents eliminated by the kidney are avoided entirely (Braunwald et al., 2001).

Diuretics such as furosemide or other loop diuretics may be prescribed to reduce extracellular fluid volume and edema. Diuretic therapy also can reduce hypertension and cause potassium wasting, lowering serum potassium levels. Other antihypertensive agents are used to maintain the blood pressure within normal levels, slow the progress of renal failure, and prevent complications of coronary heart disease and cerebral vascular disease. Angiotensin-converting enzyme (ACE) inhibitors are preferred, although any class of antihypertensive agent may be prescribed (see Chapter 33).

Other drugs may be used to manage electrolyte imbalances and acidosis. Sodium bicarbonate or calcium carbonate may be used to correct mild acidosis. Oral phosphorus binding agents such as calcium carbonate or calcium acetate are given to lower serum phosphate levels and normalize serum calcium levels. Aluminum hydroxide may be used in acute treatment of hyperphosphatemia. Its use is limited to short term by complications such as encephalopathy and osteodystrophy associated with long-term administration of aluminum-containing preparations (Tierney et al., 2001). Vitamin D supplements may be given to improve calcium absorption.

If the serum potassium rises to dangerously high levels, a combination of bicarbonate, insulin, and glucose may be given intravenously to promote potassium movement into the cells. Sodium polystyrene sulfonate (Kayexalate), a potassium-ion exchange resin, can be given either orally or rectally (as an enema).

Folic acid and iron supplements are given to combat anemia associated with chronic renal failure. A multiple vitamin preparation is also often prescribed, because anorexia, nausea, and dietary restrictions may limit nutrient intake.

Dietary and Fluid Management

As renal function declines, the elimination of water, solutes, and metabolic wastes is impaired. Accumulation of these wastes in the body leads to uremic symptoms. Instituted early in the course of CRF, dietary modifications can slow the progress of nephron destruction, reduce uremic symptoms, and help prevent complications.

Unlike carbohydrates and fats, the body is unable to store excess proteins. Unused dietary proteins are degraded into urea and other nitrogenous wastes, which are then eliminated by the kidneys. Protein-rich foods also contain inorganic ions such as hydrogen ion, phosphate, and sulfites that are eliminated by the kidneys. Research has shown that restricting dietary protein intake slows the progression of CRF and reduces uremic symptoms (Braunwald et al., 2001). A daily protein intake of 0.6 g/kg of body weight, or approximately 40 g/day for an average male client, provides the amino acids necessary for tissue repair. Proteins should be of high biologic value, rich in the essential amino acids. Carbohydrate intake is increased to maintain energy requirements and provide approximately 35 kcal/kg per day.

Water and sodium intake is regulated to maintain the extracellular fluid volume at normal levels. Water intake of 1 to 2 L per day is generally recommended to maintain water balance. Sodium is restricted to 2 g per day initially. More stringent water and sodium restrictions may be necessary as renal failure progresses. The client is instructed to monitor weight daily and report any weight gain in excess of 5 pounds over a 2-day period.

When the GFR falls to less than 10 to 20 mL/min, potassium and phosphorus intake is also restricted. Potassium intake is limited to less than 60 to 70 mEq/day (normal intake is about 100 mEq/day) (Tierney et al., 2001). The client is cautioned to avoid using salt substitutes, which typically contain high levels of potassium chloride. Foods high in phosphorus include eggs, dairy products, and meat.

Renal Replacement Therapies

When pharmacologic and dietary management strategies are no longer effective to maintain fluid and electrolyte balance and prevent uremia, dialysis or kidney transplantation is considered.

A number of considerations affect the choice of long-term treatment. Hemodialysis and peritoneal dialysis each have advantages and disadvantages. Establishing vascular access for hemodialysis may take several months. Planning ahead to develop the access before dialysis is necessary can ease the transition to dialysis. Established access is not a consideration for peritoneal dialysis. The peritoneal catheter can be placed and treatment initiated as soon as it is indicated. When dialysis treatments will be performed at home, initiating instruction before it is required can result in more effective learning. If a family member will serve as a dialysis helper, training begins prior to the onset of uremia.

If transplantation is considered, tissue typing and identification of potential living related donors can be done prior to the onset of ESRD. To make an informed decision, both the client and the potential donor need to understand the risks, benefits, and options available. If the decision for transplant is made early, dialysis can potentially be avoided. The client's age, concurrent health problems, donor availability, and personal preference influence the choice of renal replacement therapy.

Dialysis

Approximately 80% of all people being treated for ESRD in the United States are receiving dialysis at an average maintenance cost of about $35,000 per year (USRDS, 2001). For the client who is not a candidate for renal transplantation or who has had a transplant failure, dialysis is life sustaining.

The most common therapies for ESRD in the United States are hemodialysis performed in a dialysis center, followed by peritoneal dialysis and kidney transplant (NKUDIC, 2001). Both hemodialysis and peritoneal dialysis can be done in the home, but few clients use home hemodialysis. Of the two, peritoneal dialysis is typically the choice for at-home treatment. As the morbidity and mortality for each are comparable, factors such as the desire and ability to manage home care, employment, and availability of a dialysis center become the primary factors influencing the choice of hemodialysis or peritoneal dialysis.

Clients on long-term dialysis have a higher risk for complications and death than the general population. Many have other severe diseases along with ESRD. Infection and cardiovascular disease are common causes of illness and death. The 1-year survival rate for clients receiving dialysis is more than 78%; long-term survival, however, falls to 31% at 5 years and less than 9% at 10 years (NKUDIC, 2001).

The decision to initiate dialysis is not easy. Like insulin therapy for the diabetic, dialysis manages the symptoms of ESRD but does not cure it. Dialysis is a constant factor of life, requiring thinking and planning ahead at all times. Clients on dialysis may not be able to maintain a job. Families often fall apart with the day-to-day stress. Even with dialysis, the client may have constant flulike symptoms, never feeling truly well. Clients on hemodialysis may feel powerless because of their dependence on others for treatment. On the other hand, home peritoneal dialysis places a continuing burden on the client to maintain treatment. In the end, the client may choose to discontinue treatment, preferring death over continued dialysis.

Hemodialysis for ESRD typically is done three times a week for a total of 9 to 12 hours. The amount of dialysis needed (or *dialysis dose*) is individually determined by factors such as body size and residual renal function, dietary intake, and concurrent illness. Hypotension and muscle cramps are common complications during hemodialysis treatments. Infection and vascular access problems are common long-term complications of hemodialysis. Cardiovascular disease is the leading cause of death for clients receiving hemodialysis. The death rate from cardiovascular disease is higher in clients on hemodialysis than those on peritoneal dialysis or who have had a kidney transplant for reasons that are unclear (Braunwald et al., 2001). See the previous section on ARF and the box on page 768 for more information about hemodialysis and related nursing care.

Peritoneal dialysis is currently used by less than 10% of people who require long-term dialysis in the United States. In Canada and Europe, 35% to 45% of clients with ESRD are treated with peritoneal dialysis. In third-world countries, peritoneal dialysis is used to treat the majority of clients with ESRD.

Continuous ambulatory peritoneal dialysis (CAPD) is the most common form of peritoneal dialysis used. Dialysate (2 L) is instilled into the peritoneal cavity, and the catheter is sealed. The client can then continue normal daily activities, emptying the peritoneal cavity and replacing the dialysate every 4 to 6 hours. No special equipment is needed. A variation of CAPD is *continuous cyclic peritoneal dialysis (CCPD)*, which uses a delivery device during nighttime hours and a continuous dwell during the day. CAPD can be performed anywhere, and CCPD allows for home treatment at night, leaving the client free during the day.

Peritoneal dialysis has several advantages over hemodialysis. Heparinization and vascular complications associated with an AV fistula are avoided. The clearance of metabolic wastes is slower but more continuous, avoiding rapid fluctuations in extracellular fluid composition and associated symptoms. More liberal intake of fluids and nutrients is often allowed for the client on CAPD. While glucose absorbed from dialysate can increase blood glucose levels in the diabetic, regular insulin can be added to the infusion to manage hyperglycemia. The client on peritoneal dialysis is better able to self-manage the treatment regimen, reducing feelings of helplessness.

The major disadvantages of peritoneal dialysis include less effective metabolite elimination and risk of infection (peritonitis). Peritoneal dialysis may not be effective for large clients with no residual kidney function. Serum triglyceride levels increase with peritoneal dialysis. Finally, the presence of an indwelling peritoneal catheter may cause a body image disturbance. See the previous section of this chapter and the box on page 771 for more information about and nursing care for the client undergoing peritoneal dialysis.

Kidney Transplant

Kidney transplant has become the treatment of choice for many clients with ESRD. Kidneys are the solid organ most commonly transplanted, and to date kidney transplantation is the most successful of transplantation procedures. The first kidney transplant was performed in 1954; the donor and recipient were identical twins. Kidney transplant as a treatment for ESRD is limited primarily by availability of organs. In 2001, more than 15,000 people received a kidney transplant; however, there currently are more than 52,000 awaiting a transplant (United Network of Organ Sharing [UNOS], 2002b).

Kidney transplant improves both survival and quality of life for the client with ESRD. The client on dialysis has a 62.8% probability of surviving after 2 years of dialysis; the transplant recipient has a greater than 91.5% probability of survival after 2 years. At 5 years, the difference is even greater: 31.3% for dialysis compared with 80.4% for transplant (NKUDIC, 2001). The transplant client is no longer tethered to a dialysis catheter, machine, or center. Dietary and fluid restrictions are reduced, and the body image is more "whole."

Most transplanted kidneys are obtained from cadavers; however, transplants from living donors are increasing. In 2001, of transplanted kidneys, 37.4% came from living donors, most of whom were related to the recipient (UNOS, 2002c). With both cadaver and living donor transplants, a close match between blood and tissue type is desired. Human leukocyte antigens (HLA) are compared between the donor and recipient; six antigens in common is considered to be a "perfect" match. The success of well-matched living-donor transplants is better than for cadaver organ transplants, with a 1-year graft survival of 94% compared to 89% for cadaver transplants (NKUDIC, 2001). Close tissue matching probably accounts for the better outcome with living donors. People with normal kidneys who are in good physical health may donate a kidney. Predonation counseling is vital: Nephrectomy is major surgery and involves a risk of trauma or disease damaging the remaining kidney in the future. If the transplant fails, the psychologic impact on the donor can be significant. Nursing care of the client having a nephrectomy is summarized in the box on page 758.

Cadaver kidneys are obtained from people who meet the criteria for brain death, are less than 65 years old, and are free of systemic disease, malignancy, or infection, including HIV and hepatitis B or C. Kidneys are removed after brain death has been determined, and are preserved by hypothermia or a technique called continuous hypothermic pulsatile perfusion. A kidney preserved by hypothermia is transplanted within 24 to 48 hours. Continuous pulsatile perfusion allows up to 3 days before transplantation. The system used to allocate cadaver kidneys for transplantation is outlined in Box 27–1.

BOX 27–1 ■ How Cadaver Kidneys Are Allocated for Transplant

The scarcity of organs for transplant raises questions about how cadaver kidneys are allocated—who receives a kidney and who does not. Past inequities in the allocation process (e.g., more men than women, more Caucasians than people of color, more rich than poor, and more young than old) led to the development of the United Network for Organ Sharing (UNOS) in 1986. UNOS has policies for organ distribution, including kidneys, hearts, livers, and other transplanted organs.

UNOS maintains national, regional, and local lists of clients awaiting transplants. When an organ becomes available, donor information is entered into the UNOS computer. The computer then runs a match program, generating a list of clients ranked by criteria such as blood and tissue type, organ size, and medical urgency of the client. Factors such as time on the waiting list and distance between the donor and the transplant center also are considered. A candidate with a perfect match (six human leukocyte antigens in common) and compatible blood type gets priority for the kidney, regardless of region or geographic area. Otherwise, the list of clients in the local area is checked first, then the regional list of clients awaiting transplant. If no match is found in the region, the organ becomes available to clients nationwide.

The UNOS allocation system, standardized fees, and Medicare coverage for transplantation have done much to ensure equitable access to available kidneys. Still, controversy exists. Clients with resources for travel may register in several different regions for an organ. Up to 10% of clients receiving a transplant in any center may be foreign nationals competing with U.S. citizens for scarce organ resources. A transplant center can accept or reject a candidate for transplant who has lost a kidney because of noncompliance.

As long as the demand for kidneys exceeds the supply of donor organs, it is likely that controversy will exist regarding their allocation. Nurses can help by identifying potential donors and contacting the transplant coordinator. In addition, nurses can inform the public about organ donation and allocation system, and encourage donation.

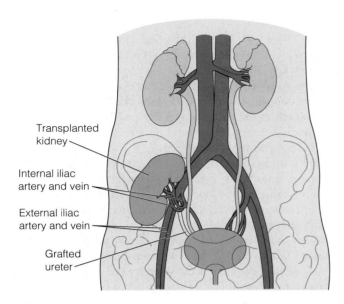

Figure 27–11 ■ Placement of a transplanted kidney in the iliac fossa with anastomosis to the hypogastric artery, iliac vein, and bladder.

The donor kidney is placed in the lower abdominal cavity of the recipient, and the renal artery, vein, and ureter are anastomosed (Figure 27–11 ■). The renal artery of the donor kidney is connected to the hypogastric artery, and the renal vein to the iliac vein. The ureter is connected to one of the recipient's ureters or directly to the bladder, using a tunnel technique to prevent reflux. Nursing care for the client having a kidney transplant is outlined in the box on the next page.

Unless the donor and recipient are identical twins, the grafted organ stimulates an immune response to reject the transplanted organ. Immunosuppressive drugs minimize this response. Azathioprine or mycophenolate mofetil are commonly used, often in combination with prednisone, a corticosteroid. Cyclosporine, a potent immunosuppressive, also may be used. These drugs suppress a portion of the immune system and the inflammatory response, increasing the risk for infections and cancers with long-term therapy. The nursing implications of immunosuppressive therapy are outlined in Chapter 9. ⊙

Glucocorticoids such as prednisone and methylprednisolone are used for both maintenance immunosuppression and to treat acute rejection episodes. Side effects of long-term corticosteroid use include impaired wound healing, emotional disturbances, osteoporosis, and cushingoid effects on glucose, protein, and fat metabolism.

Azathioprine inhibits both cellular and humoral immunity. Because this drug is rapidly metabolized by the liver, the dose may not need to be altered in the presence of renal failure. Bone marrow suppression, abnormalities of liver function, and alopecia are the primary significant adverse effects for azathioprine. The action of mycophenolate mofetil is similar to that of azathioprine. Its advantages are minimal bone marrow suppression and increased potency in preventing or reversing rejection of the transplanted organ (Braunwald et al., 2001).

Cyclosporine primarily affects cellular immunity, the helper T cells in particular. Among its many adverse effects, which include hepatotoxicity and hirsutism, nephrotoxicity is a primary concern for the kidney transplant client.

Even with immunosuppressive therapy, the transplanted kidney can be rejected at any time. Either acute or chronic rejection may develop. *Acute rejection* develops within months of the transplant. It is caused by a cellular immune response with T-lymphocyte proliferation (Porth, 2002). Few manifestations may be apparent other than a rise in serum creatinine and possible oliguria. Methylprednisolone, a glucocorticoid, and OKT3 monoclonal antibody (see Chapter 9) are used to manage acute rejection episodes. OKT3 can cause severe systemic reactions, including chills, fever, hypotension, headache, and possible pulmonary edema (Braunwald et al., 2001). *Chronic rejection,* which may develop months to years following the transplant, is a major cause of graft loss. Both humoral and cellular immune responses are involved in chronic rejection. It does not respond to increased immunosuppression. The presenting manifestations of chronic rejection—progressive azotemia, proteinuria, and hypertension—are those of progressive renal failure.

Hypertension is a possible complication of kidney transplant, resulting from graft rejection, renal artery stenosis, or renal vasoconstriction. Clients may develop glomerular lesions and manifestations of nephrosis. Hypertension and altered blood lipids (increased LDLs and decreased HDLs) increase the risk of death from myocardial infarction and stroke following transplant (Braunwald et al., 2001).

Long-term immunosuppression has adverse effects as well. Infection is a continuing threat. Bacterial and viral infections may develop, as well as fungal infections of the blood, lungs, and central nervous system. Tumors are also common, with carcinoma in situ of the cervix, lymphomas, and skin cancers most prevalent. The risk of congenital anomalies is increased in infants whose mothers have undergone immunosuppressive therapy. Corticosteroid use may lead to bone problems, gastrointestinal disorders such as peptic ulcer disease, and cataract formation.

NURSING CARE

Health Promotion

Measures to reduce the risk of CRF focus on preventing kidney disease and appropriately managing diabetes and hypertension. Promote early and effective treatment of all infections, particularly skin and pharyngeal infections caused by streptococcal bacteria. Discuss measures to reduce the risk for urinary tract infections, and stress the importance of prompt treatment to eradicate the infecting organism. Discuss the relationship between diabetes, hypertension, and kidney disease. Emphasize that maintaining blood glucose levels and the blood pressure within the recommended ranges reduces the risk of adverse effects on the kidneys. Ensure that all clients with less than optimal renal function are well hydrated, particularly when a nephrotoxic drug is prescribed or anticipated.

NURSING CARE OF THE CLIENT HAVING A KIDNEY TRANSPLANT

PREOPERATIVE CARE

- Provide routine preoperative care as outlined in Chapter 7. ∞
- Assess knowledge and feelings about the procedure, answering questions and clarifying information as needed. Listen and address concerns about surgery, the source of the donor organ, and possible complications. *Addressing concerns and reducing preoperative anxiety improve postoperative recovery.*
- Continue dialysis as ordered. *Continued renal replacement therapy is necessary to manage fluid and electrolyte balance and prevent uremia prior to surgery.*
- Administer immunosuppressive drugs as ordered before surgery. *Immunosuppression is initiated before transplantation to prevent immediate graft rejection.*

POSTOPERATIVE CARE

- Provide routine postoperative care as outlined in Chapter 7.
- Maintain urinary catheter patency and a closed system. *Catheter patency is vital to keep the bladder decompressed and prevent pressure on suture lines. A closed drainage system minimizes the risk for urinary tract infection.*
- Measure urine output every 30 to 60 minutes initially. *Careful assessment of urine output helps determine fluid balance and transplant function. Acute tubular necrosis (ATN) is a common early complication, usually due to tissue ischemia during the period between removal of the kidney from the donor and transplantation. Oliguria is an early sign.*
- Monitor vital signs and hemodynamic pressures closely. *Diuresis may occur immediately, resulting in hypovolemia, low cardiac output, and impaired perfusion of the transplanted kidney.*
- Maintain fluid replacement, generally calculated to replace urine output over the previous 30 or 60 minutes, milliliter for milliliter. *Fluid replacement is vital to maintain vascular volume and tissue perfusion.*
- Administer diuretics as ordered. *Loop and/or osmotic diuretics such as furosemide or mannitol may be used to promote postoperative diuresis.*
- Remove the catheter within 2 to 3 days or as ordered. Encourage to void every 1 to 2 hours and assess frequently for signs of urinary retention following catheter removal. *The bladder may have atrophied prior to surgery, reducing its capacity. Urinary retention places stress on suture lines and increases the risk of infection.*
- Monitor serum electrolytes and renal function tests. *These tests are used to monitor graft function and fluid and electrolyte status. Electrolyte imbalances may develop as the transplanted kidney begins to function and diuresis occurs. Elevated serum creatinine and BUN levels may be early signs of rejection or graft failure.*

- Monitor for possible complications:
  a. *Hemorrhage* from an arterial or venous anastomosis can be either acute or insidious. Indicators include swelling at the operative site, increased abdominal girth, and signs of shock, including changes in vital signs and level of consciousness. *Hemorrhage is a surgical emergency, requiring prompt recognition and treatment to preserve the graft.*
  b. *Ureteral anastomosis failure* causes urine leakage into the peritoneal cavity. It may be marked by decreased urine output with abdominal swelling and tenderness. *Failure of the ureteral anastomosis requires surgical intervention.*
  c. *Renal artery thrombosis* is characterized by an abrupt onset of hypertension and reduced GFR. *Renal artery thrombosis can result in transplant failure.*
  d. *Infection* due to immunosuppression is an immediate and continuing risk. The inflammatory response is blunted, and infection may not significantly elevate the temperature. Monitor for signs such as change in level of consciousness, cloudy or malodorous urine, or purulent drainage from the incision. *Prevention and prompt treatment of infections is particularly important in the immunosuppressed client.*
- Include the following in predischarge teaching for the client and family:
  a. The use and effects of prescribed medications, including antihypertensive medications, immunosuppressive agents, prophylactic antibiotics, and others as ordered.
  b. Monitoring vital signs (including temperature) and weight.
  c. Manifestations of organ rejection, such as swelling and tenderness over the graft site, fever, joint aching, weight gain, and decreased urinary output. Stress the importance of promptly reporting signs and symptoms to the physician.
  d. Ordered or recommended dietary restrictions such as restricted carbohydrate and sodium intake, and increased protein intake.
  e. Measures to prevent infection, such as avoiding crowds and obviously ill individuals.
  The client and family will manage care after discharge, and therefore need a good understanding of what to expect, how to monitor graft status, and measures to reduce the adverse effects of medications.
- Provide psychologic support, address concerns, and provide information as needed. *The client knows that transplant success is not guaranteed. In addition, the client has often been managing a chronic disease independently and is used to having a degree of control. Providing information and allowing the client to retain control relieves anxiety and improves recovery.*

Finally, encourage the client with ESRD to investigate options for early transplantation to avoid long-term dialysis.

Assessment

Both subjective and objective data are used to assess the client with CRF.

- Health history: complaints of anorexia, nausea, weight gain, or edema; current treatment (if any), including type and frequency of dialysis or previous kidney transplant; chronic diseases such as diabetes, heart failure, or kidney disease
- Physical examination: mental status; vital signs including temperature, heart and lung sounds, and peripheral pulses;

urine output (if any); weight; skin color, moisture, condition; presence of edema (periorbial or dependent); bowel tones; presence and location of an AV fistula, shunt, or graft, or peritoneal catheter

See the box on page 772 for assessment of the older adult with ESRD.

Nursing Diagnoses and Interventions

Whether the client with ESRD is facing long-term dialysis or renal transplantation, a number of nursing care needs can be identified. This section focuses on nursing care related to impaired renal function, nutritional deficits due to dietary restrictions and nausea, increased risk for infection, and changes in body image.

Impaired Tissue Perfusion: Renal

Capillaries are an integral part of the nephron. As nephrons are destroyed, kidney perfusion progressively declines. As renal perfusion and nephron function falls, the kidney is less able to maintain fluid and electrolyte balance and eliminate waste products from the body.

- Monitor intake and output, vital signs including orthostatic blood pressures, and weight. *These provide important data to identify changes in fluid volume.*

PRACTICE ALERT *Weight changes are a more accurate indicator of fluid volume status in the oliguric or anuric client than intake and output measurements.* ■

- Restrict fluids as ordered. *As renal function declines, the ability to eliminate excess fluid is impaired.*
- Monitor respiratory status, including lung sounds, every 4 to 8 hours. *Fluid volume overload may lead to heart failure and possible pulmonary edema.*
- Monitor BUN, serum creatinine, pH, electrolytes, and CBC. Report significant changes. *As renal function declines, progressive azotemia with increasing BUN and serum creatinine is seen. Metabolic acidosis develops as the kidney is unable to eliminate hydrogen ions and conserve bicarbonate. Hyponatremia, hyperkalemia, hyperphosphatemia, and hypocalcemia are associated with renal failure. The RBC count, hemoglobin, and hematocrit decline due to deficient erythropoietin to stimulate cell production in the bone marrow. An acute fall in hemoglobin and hematocrit may indicate GI bleeding, a risk in clients with ESRD.*
- Report manifestations of electrolyte imbalances, such as cardiac dysrhythmias and other ECG changes, muscle tremors and possible tetany, and Kussmaul's respirations. *Manifestations of electrolyte imbalance may indicate the need for intervention.*
- Administer medications to treat electrolyte imbalances as ordered. *Medications may be prescribed to help maintain electrolyte and acid-base balance and prevent adverse effects of imbalances.*

PRACTICE ALERT *Monitor carefully for desired and adverse effects of all medications. Impaired renal function affects drug elimination and increases the risk for toxic effects.* ■

- Administer antihypertensive medications as ordered. *Hypertension management is an important factor in slowing the progression of CRF.*
- Time activities and procedures to allow rest periods. *The anemia associated with CRF may cause significant fatigue and activity intolerance.*

Imbalanced Nutrition: Less Than Body Requirements

Anorexia, nausea, and vomiting are common manifestations of ESRD and uremia. The client often has a metallic taste and bad breath, which also diminish appetite. A diet restricted in protein and sodium will compound these problems. Food intake may be insufficient to meet metabolic needs. Catabolism, the breakdown of body proteins to meet energy needs, exacerbates azotemia and uremia.

- Monitor food and nutrient intake as well as episodes of vomiting. *Careful monitoring helps determine the adequacy of intake.*
- Weigh daily before breakfast. *This provides the most accurate measurement. Remember that a gain of 2 pounds or more over a 24-hour period is more likely to reflect fluid retention than a gain in body mass.*
- Administer antiemetic agents 30 to 60 minutes before eating. *Antiemetics reduce nausea and the risk of vomiting with food intake.*
- Assist with mouth care prior to meals and at bedtime. *Mouth care improves taste, stimulates the appetite, and maintains the integrity of oral mucous membranes.*
- Serve small meals and provide between-meal snacks. *Small meals are less likely to prompt nausea and help improve food intake.*
- Arrange for a dietary consultation. Provide preferred foods to the extent possible, and involve the client in planning daily menus. Encourage family members to bring food as dietary restrictions allow. *Providing preferred foods within restrictions promotes intake.*
- Monitor nutritional status by tracking weight, laboratory values such as serum albumin and BUN, and anthropometric measurements (see Chapters 19 ⃝ and 20). *Indicators of impaired nutrition develop gradually and may be subtle. Careful assessment is important.*
- Administer parenteral nutrition as prescribed. Routinely monitor blood glucose levels, and use strict aseptic technique when handling the solution and venous access site. *Parenteral nutrition may be necessary to prevent catabolism and increasing azotemia. Hyperglycemia and infection are risks associated with parenteral nutrition (see Chapter 20). Immune system suppression associated with renal failure further increases the risk for infection.*

Risk for Infection

Chronic renal failure affects the immune system and leukocyte function, increasing susceptibility to infection. Invasive devices required for hemodialysis or peritoneal dialysis add to this risk. The client who has had a kidney transplant remains on immunosuppressive therapy for life, further depressing the immune system and increasing the risk for infection.

- Use standard precautions and good handwashing technique at all times. *Handwashing is a primary means of preventing the transfer of organisms. Clients who are on hemodialysis or who have had multiple blood transfusions to treat anemia have an increased risk for hepatitis B, hepatitis C, and HIV infection.*

PRACTICE ALERT *Use strict aseptic technique when managing ports, catheters, and incisions, to reduce the risk of introducing infectious organisms when immune responses are impaired.* ■

- Monitor temperature and vital signs at least every 4 hours. *A low-grade fever or increased pulse rate may indicate an infection in the immunosuppressed client.*
- Monitor WBC count and differential. *Increased WBCs may indicate a bacterial infection; decreased WBCs may indicate viral infection. A shift in the differential showing more immature WBCs (bands) in circulation is another indicator of infection.*
- Culture urine, peritoneal dialysis fluid, and other drainage as indicated. *Culture is done to verify the presence of pathogens.*

PRACTICE ALERT *Monitor clarity of dialysate return. Dialysate should return clear in the client undergoing peritoneal dialysis. Cloudy dialysate may indicate peritonitis, the most common complication of peritoneal dialysis, and should be reported and cultured.* ■

- Provide good respiratory hygiene including position changes, coughing, and deep breathing. *These measures improve clearance of respiratory secretions, reducing the risk for infection.*
- Restrict visits from obviously ill people. Teach the client and family about the risk for infection and measures to reduce the spread of infection. *The client's resistance to infection is impaired, necessitating extra caution in preventing unnecessary exposures.*

Disturbed Body Image

Chronic disease and impaired kidney function can affect the client's body image. Hemodialysis requires an arteriovenous fistula or shunt; a permanent peritoneal catheter is required for peritoneal dialysis. While kidney transplant can restore an image of wholeness, a visible scar remains and the organ may be perceived as "foreign."

- Involve the client in care, including meal planning, dialysis, and catheter, port, or incision care to the extent possible. *Involvement improves acceptance and stimulates discussion about the effect of the disease and treatment measures on the client's life.* See the Nursing Research box below.
- Encourage expression of feelings and concerns, accepting perceptions and feelings without criticism. *Self-expression enhances the client's self-worth and acceptance.*
- Include the client in decision making and encourage self-care. *Increased autonomy enhances the client's sense of control, independence, and self-worth.*
- Support positive gains, but do not support denial. *The client may have difficulty accepting the renal failure, but adaptation to the loss is important.*
- Help the client develop and achieve realistic goals. *Realistic goals allow the client to see progress.*
- Provide positive reinforcement and feedback. *These measures support growth and adaptation.*
- Reinforce effective coping strategies. *Reinforcement helps the client develop positive versus negative strategies for coping.*
- Facilitate contact with a support group or other community members affected by renal failure. *The client benefits by*

Nursing Research

Evidence-Based Practice For the Client on Hemodialysis

In a study of clients undergoing hemodialysis for CRF, researchers in Sweden looked at suffering on three levels: related to sickness and treatment, related to care provided, and related to the client's unique life experience and existence (Hagren, Pettersen, Severinsson, Lutzen, & Clyne, 2001). The study included 15 clients between age 50 and 86.

The researchers identified dependence on the hemodialysis machine and dependence on caregivers as the primary sources of suffering in these clients. This dependence and the loss of freedom associated with hemodialysis affected marital and family relationships and social lives of the sufferers. Accepting dependence on the hemodialysis machine and being seen as an individual by caregivers, thus promoting autonomy, relieved clients' suffering.

IMPLICATIONS FOR NURSING

Treating all clients with ESRD holistically, respecting their individual and unique characteristics and experience, is vital to promote acceptance and autonomy. Listen carefully, responding to each person's concerns. Discuss the effects of the disease and its treatment on the client's life, marital and family relationships, and socialization. Suggest strategies to maintain independence and provide relief for caregivers. When appropriate, discuss alternatives to hemodialysis for treating ESRD, such as kidney transplant or peritoneal dialysis. Peritoneal dialysis may be managed independently by the client, reducing dependence on others and time spent in treatment.

Critical Thinking

1. Identify assessment tools and data you could use to evaluate degree of suffering in the client receiving long-term hemodialysis.
2. In addition to the above, what interventions can you, as the nurse, implement to promote autonomy and acceptance of hemodialysis in the client with ESRD?
3. Develop a teaching plan for families and significant others to help them promote acceptance and autonomy in the client undergoing long-term hemodialysis.

CHART 27–4 NANDA, NIC, AND NOC LINKAGES

The Client with End-Stage Renal Disease

NURSING DIAGNOSES	NURSING INTERVENTIONS	NURSING OUTCOMES
• Chronic Sorrow	• Coping Enhancement • Mood Mangement	• Acceptance: Health Status • Depression Control
• Excess Fluid Volume	• Fluid Management • Fluid / Electrolyte Management	• Electrolyte and Acid-Base Balance • Fluid Balance
• Fatigue	• Energy Management • Environmental Management	• Activity Tolerance • Energy Conservation
• Nausea	• Nausea Management • Nutritional Monitoring	• Nutritional Status: Food and Fluid Intake
• Risk for Infection	• Infection Protection • Wound Care	• Infection Status

Note. Data from Nursing Outcomes Classification (NOC) by M. Johnson & M. Maas (Eds.), 1997, St. Louis: Mosby; Nursing Diagnoses: Definitions & Classification 2001–2002 by North American Nursing Diagnosis Association, 2001, Philadelphia: NANDA; Nursing Interventions Classification (NIC) by J.C. McCloskey & G. M. Bulechek (Eds.), 2000, St. Louis: Mosby. Reprinted by permission.

providing and receiving support in a group of people going through similar circumstances.
- Refer for mental health counseling as indicated or desired. *Counseling can help the client develop effective coping and adaptation strategies.*

Using NANDA, NIC, and NOC

Chart 27–4 shows links between NANDA nursing diagnoses, NIC, and NOC when caring for the client with ESRD.

Home Care

Chronic renal failure and ESRD are long-term processes that require client management. No matter what treatment option is chosen (hemodialysis, peritoneal dialysis, or renal transplantation), day-to-day management falls to the client and family. Teaching for home care includes the following topics.

- Nature of the kidney disease and renal failure, including expected progression and effects
- Monitoring weight, vital signs, and temperature

- Prescribed dietary and fluid restrictions (Involve the client, a dietitian, and the family member usually responsible for cooking. Include strategies to manage nausea and relieve thirst within allowed fluid limits.)
- How to assess and protect a fistula or shunt for hemodialysis (or the extremity to be used if one is anticipated)
- Peritoneal catheter care and the procedure for peritoneal dialysis as indicated (Include a family member or significant other, in case the client is unable to perform the procedure independently at some time.)
- Following kidney transplant, prescribed medications, adverse effects and their management, infection prevention, graft protection, and manifestations of organ rejection

Refer to a dietitian for diet planning and counseling. If home hemodialysis is planned, refer the designated dialysis helper for formal training. Both the National Kidney Foundation and the American Association of Kidney Patients may be able to provide support and educational materials for the client with ESRD (see the box on page 772). Local and state chapters of these organizations can provide additional support.

Nursing Care Plan
A Client with End-Stage Renal Disease

Walter Cohen, 45 years old, is the print shop manager at a local community college. He has been a type 1 diabetic since the age of 20, and was diagnosed with diabetic nephropathy 10 years ago. Despite blood pressure control with antihypertensive medications and frequent blood glucose monitoring with insulin coverage, he developed overt proteinuria 5 years ago and has now progressed to end-stage renal disease. He enters the nephrology unit for temporary he-

modialysis to relieve uremic symptoms. While there, a CAPD catheter will be inserted. Mr. Cohen's desire to continue working is the primary factor in his choice of CAPD over hemodialysis.

ASSESSMENT

Richard Gonzalez, Mr. Cohen's care manager, obtains a nursing assessment. Mr. Cohen states that his diabetes has always been difficult to control. He has had numerous hypoglycemic episodes and

Nursing Care Plan

A Client with End-Stage Renal Disease (continued)

has been hospitalized "four or five times" for ketoacidosis. Recently he has developed symptoms of peripheral neuropathy and increasing retinopathy. He attributed his lack of appetite, nausea, vomiting, and fatigue over the past month to "a touch of the flu." His weight remained stable, so he did not worry about not eating much.

Physical assessment findings include T 97.8°F (36.5°C) PO, P 96, R 20, and BP 178/100. Skin cool and dry, with minor excoriations on forearms and lower legs. Breath odor fetid. Scattered fine rales noted in bilateral lung bases. Soft S_3 gallop noted at cardiac apex. Bilateral pitting edema of lower extremities to just below the knees; fingers and hands also edematous. Abdominal assessment essentially normal, with hypoactive bowel sounds. Urinalysis shows a specific gravity of 1.011, gross proteinuria, and multiple cell casts. CBC results: RBC 2.9 mill/mm³; hemoglobin 9.4 g/dL; hematocrit 28%. Blood chemistry abnormalities include BUN 198 mg/dL; creatinine 18.5 mg/dL; sodium 125 mEq/L; potassium 5.7 mEq/L; calcium 7.1 mg/dL; phosphate 6.8 mg/dL. A temporary jugular venous catheter will be placed for hemodialysis the next day, followed by peritoneal catheter insertion later in the week.

DIAGNOSIS

- *Excess fluid volume* related to failure of kidneys to eliminate excess body fluid
- *Imbalanced nutrition: Less than body requirements* related to effects of uremia
- *Impaired skin integrity of lower extremities* related to dry skin and itching
- *Risk for infection* related to invasive catheters and impaired immune function

EXPECTED OUTCOMES

- Adhere to the prescribed fluid restriction of 750 mL per day.
- Demonstrate reduced extracellular fluid volume by weight loss, decreased peripheral edema, clear lung sounds, and normal heart sounds.
- Consume and retain 100% of prescribed diet, including snacks.
- Demonstrate healing of lower extremity skin lesions.
- Remain free of infection.
- Demonstrate appropriate peritoneal catheter care and CAPD.

PLANNING AND IMPLEMENTATION

- Space fluids, allowing 400 mL from 0700 to 1500, 200 mL from 1500 to 2300, and 100 mL from 2300 to 0700.
- Provide mouth care at least every 4 hours and before every meal.

- Keep sugarless hard candy and ice chips at the bedside; include ice consumed as fluid intake.
- Weigh daily before breakfast; monitor vital signs, and heart and lung sounds every 4 hours.
- Document intake and output every 4 hours.
- Arrange dietary consultation for menu planning.
- Administer prescribed antiemetic 1 hour before meals.
- Monitor food intake, noting percentage and types of food consumed.
- Clean lesions on lower extremities every 8 hours and assess healing.
- Teach CAPD procedure and peritoneal catheter care.
- Assist to identify strengths and needs in health regimen management.

EVALUATION

Mr. Cohen was hospitalized for 2 weeks, undergoing four hemodialysis sessions to reduce uremic symptoms. An arteriovenous fistula has been created in his left arm in case he should need hemodialysis in the future. He begins peritoneal dialysis the second week, and by discharge he is able to manage the catheter care and dialysis runs with the help of his wife. His heart and lung sounds are normal, and he has minimal peripheral edema on discharge. The excoriations on his legs have healed. His temperature is normal, and no evidence of infection is noted. Mr. Cohen remains anorectic and slightly nauseated, but is eating most of his prescribed diet and snacks. He has lost 10 pounds with excess fluid removal by dialysis, but his weight remains stable during the second week. Mr. Cohen and his wife have been introduced to another client who has been on CAPD for several years and promises to help them with problem solving.

Critical Thinking in the Nursing Process

1. How does diabetes mellitus damage the kidneys and lead to ESRD? Why is this more significant for a client with type 1 diabetes than for someone with type 2 diabetes (see Chapter 18)?
2. Why do high levels of urea in the blood often cause changes in cognition and mental status? What manifestations of encephalopathy would you expect to see?
3. How might Mr. Cohen's insulin dosage and diet need to be changed with the institution of peritoneal dialysis? Why?
4. Develop a care plan for the nursing diagnosis, *Disturbed body image*.

See Evaluating Your Response in Appendix C.

EXPLORE MediaLink

NCLEX review questions, case studies, care plan activities, MediaLink applications, and other interactive resources for this chapter can be found on the Companion Website at www.prenhall.com/lemone.

Click on Chapter 27 to select the activities for this chapter. For animations, video clips, more NCLEX review questions, and an audio glossary, access the Student CD-ROM accompanying this textbook.

TEST YOURSELF

1. In obtaining a nursing history from a 22-year-old client admitted with a diagnosis of acute glomerulonephritis, the nurse specifically asks the client about a recent history of which of the following?

   a. Urinary tract infection
   b. Strep throat
   c. X-ray using contrast media
   d. Illicit drug use

2. Appropriate postoperative nursing interventions for the client who has had a partial or total nephrectomy include:

   a. Connecting all catheters and drains to a single collection device
   b. Routine irrigation of all catheters with sterile normal saline
   c. Administering cough suppressant medication as needed
   d. Labeling and securing all catheters, tubes, and drains

3. Important nursing interventions to prevent acute renal failure in the critically ill client include:

   a. Maintaining fluid volume and cardiac output
   b. Avoiding all potentially nephrotoxic drugs

   c. Administering antihypertensive drugs
   d. Assessing for a history of diabetes or systemic lupus erythematosus

4. The nurse evaluates her teaching as effective when the client recovering from acute renal failure states that he will:

   a. Limit his fluid intake to 1500 mL or less per day
   b. Consume only vegetable proteins
   c. Avoid taking drugs that may be nephrotoxic
   d. Self-catheterize for residual urine at least once a week

5. An appropriate goal of nursing care for a client with end-stage renal disease is the client will be able to:

   a. Identify a live-in caregiver
   b. State the advantages and disadvantages of hemodialysis, peritoneal dialysis, and kidney transplant as renal replacement therapies
   c. Demonstrate the ability to independently perform hemodialysis in the home
   d. Relate the hospice philosophy and identify indicators of the need for hospice care

See Test Yourself answers in Appendix C.

BIBLIOGRAPHY

Ackley, B.J., & Ladwig, G. B. (2002). *Nursing diagnosis handbook: A guide to planning care* (5th ed.). St. Louis: Mosby.

American Cancer Society. (2002). *Cancer facts and figures 2002.* Atlanta: Author.

Bartucci, M. R. (1999). Kidney transplantation: State of the art. *AACN Clinical Issues: Advanced Practice in Acute and Critical Care, 10*(2), 153–163.

Braunwald, E., Fauci, A. S., Kasper, D. L., Hauser, S. L., Longo, D. L., & Jameson, J. L. (2001). *Harrison's principles of internal medicine* (15th ed.). New York: McGraw-Hill.

Bullock, B. A., & Henze, R. L. (2000). *Focus on pathophysiology.* Philadelphia: Lippincott.

Deglin, J. H., & Vallerand, A. H. (2001). *Davis's drug guide for nurses* (7th ed.). Philadelphia: F.A. Davis.

Fontaine, K. L. (2000). *Healing practices: Alternative therapies for nursing.* Upper Saddle River, NJ: Prentice Hall Health.

Fox, H. L., & Swann, D. (2001). Goodpasture syndrome: Pathophysiology, diagnosis, and management. *Nephrology Nursing Journal, 28*(3), 305–312.

Gallo, J. J., Busby-Whitehead, J., Rabins, P. V., Silliman, R. A., & Murphy, J. B. (Eds.). (1999). *Reichel's care of the elderly: Clinical aspects of aging* (5th ed.). Philadelphia: Lippincott Williams & Wilkins.

Hagren, B., Pettersen, I. M., Severinsson, E., Lutzen, K., & Clyne, N. (2001). The haemodialysis machine as a lifeline: Experiences of suffering from end-stage renal disease. *Journal of Advanced Nursing, 34*(2), 196–202.

Hayes, D. D. (2000). Caring for your patient with a permanent hemodialysis access. *Nursing, 30*(3), 41–46.

Johnson, M., Bulechek, G., Dochterman, J. M., Maas, M., & Moorhead, S. (2001). *Nursing diagnoses, outcomes, & interventions.* St. Louis: Mosby.

Johnson, M., Maas, M., & Moorhead, S. (Eds.). (2000). *Nursing outcomes classification (NOC)* (2nd ed.). St. Louis: Mosby.

King, B. (2000). Meds and the dialysis patient. *RN, 63*(7), 54–59.

Kostadaras, A. (2001). Erythropoietin for the anemia of chronic renal failure. *Home Health Care Consultant, 8*(7), 27–31.

Lang, M. M., & Towers, C. (2001). Identifying poststreptococcal glomerulonephritis. *Nurse Practitioner: American Journal of Primary Health Care, 26*(8), 34, 37–38, 40–42+.

Lehne, R. A. (2001). *Pharmacology for nursing care* (4th ed.). Philadelphia: Saunders.

Little, C. (2000). Renovascular hypertension. *American Journal of Nursing, 100*(2), 46–51.

Mackenzie, D. L. (1999). When *E. coli* turns deadly. *RN, 62*(7), 28–31.

Malarkey, L.M., & McMorrow, M.E. (2000). *Nurse's manual of laboratory tests and diagnostic procedures* (2nd ed.). Philadelphia: Saunders.

Mallick, N., & El Marasi, A. (1999). Chronic renal failure. *Care of the Critically Ill, 15*(3), 80, 82–84.

McCann, K., & Boore, J. R. (2000). Fatigue in persons with renal failure who require maintenance haemodialysis. *Journal of Advanced Nursing, 32*(5), 1132–1142.

McCloskey, J. C., & Bulechek, G. M. (Eds.) (2000). *Nursing interventions classification (NIC)* (3rd ed.). St. Louis: Mosby.

Meeker, M. H., & Rothrock, J. C. (1999). *Alexander's care of the patient in surgery* (11th ed.). St. Louis: Mosby.

Meister, J., & Reddy, K. (2002). Rhabdomyolysis: An overview. *American Journal of Nursing, 102*(2), 75, 77, 79.

Myhre, M. J. (2000). Herbal remedies, nephropathies, and renal disease. *Nephrology Nursing Journal, 27*(5), 473–480.

National Kidney and Urologic Diseases Information Clearinghouse. (2001). *Kidney and urologic disease statistics for the United States.* NIH Publication No. 02-3895. Available www.niddk.nih.gov/health/kidney/pubs/kustats

North American Nursing Diagnosis Association. (2001). *NANDA Nursing diagnoses: Definitions & classification 2001–2002.* Philadelphia: NANDA.

Porth, C. M. (2002). *Pathophysiology: Concepts of altered health states* (6th ed.). Philadelphia: Lippincott.

Ross, C. A. (2000). Emergency. Dialysis disequilibrium syndrome. *American Journal of Nursing, 100*(2), 53–54.

Schmelzer, M., & Stam, M. A. (2000). A hidden menace: Hemolytic uremic syndrome. *American Journal of Nursing, 100*(11), 26–32.

Seaton-Mills, D. (1999). Acute renal failure: Causes and considerations in the critically ill patient. *Nursing in Critical Care, 4*(6), 293–297.

Sprauve, D. (2000). Understanding chronic renal failure. *Nursing, 30*(4), Hosp Nurs 32hn12, 32hn14.

Tierney, L. M., McPhee, S. J., & Papadakis, M. A. (2001). *Current medical diagnosis & treatment* (40th ed.). New York: Lange Medical Books/McGraw-Hill.

United Network for Organ Sharing. (2002a). *All about UNOS.* Available www.unos.org/Newsroom/allabout_main.htm

———. (2002b). *Critical data. U. S. facts about transplantation.* Available www.unos.org/Newsroom/critdata_main.htm

———. (2002c). *Living donation outpaces cadaveric in 2001.* Available www.unos.org/Newsroom/archive_story_20020426_2001donornumbers.htm

Urden, L. D., Stacy, K. M., & Lough, M. E. (2002). *Thelan's critical care nursing: Diagnosis and management* (4th ed.). St. Louis: Mosby.

U. S. Renal Data System. (2001). *USRDS 2001 annual data report: Atlas of end-stage renal disease in the United States.* Bethesda, MD: National Institute of Diabetes and Digestive and Kidney Diseases (NIDDK).

Welch, J. L., & Davis, J. (2000). Self-care strategies to reduce fluid intake and control thirst in hemodialysis patients. *Nephrology Nursing Journal, 27*(4), 393–395.

Whitney, E. N., & Rolfes, S. R. (2002). *Understanding nutrition* (9th ed.). Belmont, CA: Wadsworth.

Wise, L. C., Mersch, J., Racioppi, J., Crosier, J., & Thompson, C. (2000). Evaluating the reliability and utility of cumulative intake and output. *Journal of Nursing Care Quality, 14*(3), 37–42.

Wallace, L. S. (2001). Rhabdomyolysis: A case study *Medsurg Nursing, 10*(3), 113–120.

Standard Precautions

Standard precautions are designed to reduce the risk of transmission of microorganisms from both recognized and unrecognized sources of infection. They are the primary strategies for preventing nosocomial infections within institutions, and are important to protect health care workers as well. Standard precautions apply to (1) blood; (2) all body fluids, secretions, and excretions except sweat, regardless of whether or not they contain visible blood; (3) nonintact skin; and (4) mucous membranes. Standard precautions are applied to all clients receiving care in hospitals, regardless of their diagnosis or presumed infection status. These precautions are specifically designed for hospitals; however, they also may be implemented in extended and long-term care facilities, and to a more limited extent in providing home care or in other community-based care settings.

HANDWASHING

- Wash your hands (a) after touching blood, body fluids, secretions, excretions, and contaminated items, whether or not gloves are worn; (b) immediately after removing gloves, even if gloves appear to be intact; (c) between contacts with clients; and (d) when otherwise indicated to prevent transfer of organisms to other clients. You may need to wash your hands between tasks and procedures on the same client to prevent cross-contaminating different body sites.

- Use soap and warm water for handwashing when hands are visibly dirty or contaminated with blood or other body fluids.

- If hands are not visibly soiled, use an alcohol-based hand rub for routinely decontaminating hands in all other situations.

GLOVES

- Wear clean, nonsterile gloves when touching blood, body fluids, secretions, excretions, and contaminated items.

- Put on clean gloves just before touching mucous membranes and nonintact skin.

- Change your gloves between tasks and procedures on the same client after contacting material that may contain a high concentration of microorganisms.

- Wear gloves for all invasive procedures such as performing venipuncture or other vascular or surgical procedures.

- Wear gloves if you have cuts, scratches, or other breaks in the skin.

- Remove gloves promptly after use, before touching noncontaminated items and surfaces, and before going to another client; wash hands immediately after removing gloves.

MASK, EYE PROTECTION, FACE SHIELD

Wear a mask and eye protection or a face shield to protect mucous membranes of your eyes, nose, and mouth during procedures and client care activities that are likely to generate splashes or sprays of blood, body fluids, secretions, or excretions.

GOWN

Wear a gown (clean, disposable) to protect your skin and prevent soiling of clothing during procedures and client care activities that are likely to generate splashes or sprays of blood, body fluids, secretions, or excretions. Remove soiled gowns promptly, washing your hands immediately after gown removal.

EQUIPMENT

Handle used client care equipment that is soiled with blood, body fluids, secretions, and excretions in a way that prevents exposing your skin and mucous membranes, contaminating your clothing, and transferring microorganisms to other clients or environments. Ensure that reusable equipment is cleaned and appropriately reprocessed before using for the care of another client.

ENVIRONMENTAL CONTROL

Follow hospital procedures for routine care, cleaning, and disinfecting environmental surfaces, beds, bed rails, bedside equipment, and other frequently touched surfaces.

LINEN

Handle and transport linens soiled with blood, body fluids, secretions, and excretions in a manner that prevents exposing your skin and mucous membranes, contaminating your clothing, and transferring microorganisms to other clients and environments. Place soiled linen in leakage-resistant bags at the location where it is used.

OCCUPATIONAL HEALTH AND BLOODBORNE PATHOGENS

- Take care to prevent injuries when using needles, scalpels, and other sharps; when handling sharp instruments after

Sources. Centers for Disease Control and Prevention (2002). Guidelines for hand hygiene in health-care settings: Recommendations of the Healthcare Infection Control Practices Advisory Committee and the HICPAC/SHEA/APIC/IDSA Hand Hygiene Taskforce. *MMWR, 51*(RR-16), 1–56; Hospital Infection Control Practices Advisory Committee (1997). Part II. Recommendations for isolation precautions in hospitals. Atlanta: Public Health Service, U.S. Department of Health and Human Services, Centers for Disease Control and Prevention.

procedures; when cleaning used instruments; and when disposing of used needles.

- Never recap used needles, manipulate them using both hands, or handle them in a manner that directs the point of a needle toward any part of your body. If it is necessary to protect the needle prior to disposal, use a one-handed "scoop" technique or mechanical device to hold the needle sheath.

- Do not remove used needles from disposable syringes by hand; do not bend, break, or otherwise manipulate used needles by hand.

- Place used disposable syringes and needles, scalpel blades, and other sharp items in appropriate puncture-resistant containers located as close as practical to the area in which the items were used.

- Place reusable syringes and needles in a puncture-resistant container for transport to the reprocessing area.

- Use mouthpieces, resuscitation bags, or other ventilation devices as an alternative to mouth-to-mouth resuscitation methods whenever possible.

CLIENT PLACEMENT

Place clients who contaminate the environment or who do not (or are not expected to) assist in maintaining appropriate hygiene or environmental control (e.g., an ambulatory, confused client with fecal incontinence) in a private room.

2003–2004 NANDA-Approved Nursing Diagnoses

Activity Intolerance
Activity Intolerance, Risk for
Adaptive Capacity: Intracranial, Decreased
Adjustment, Impaired
Airway Clearance, Ineffective
Anxiety
Anxiety, Death
Aspiration, Risk for
Attachment, Parent/Infant/Child, Risk for Impaired
Body Image, Disturbed
Body Temperature: Imbalanced, Risk for
Bowel Incontinence
Breastfeeding, Effective
Breastfeeding, Ineffective
Breastfeeding, Interrupted
Breathing Pattern, Ineffective
Cardiac Output, Decreased
Caregiver Role Strain
Caregiver Role Strain, Risk for
Communication, Readiness for Enhanced
Communication: Verbal, Impaired
Confusion, Acute
Confusion, Chronic
Constipation
Constipation, Perceived
Constipation, Risk for
Coping: Community, Ineffective
Coping: Community, Readiness for Enhanced
Coping, Defensive
Coping: Family, Compromised
Coping: Family, Disabled
Coping: Family, Readiness for Enhanced
Coping (Individual), Readiness for Enhanced
Coping, Ineffective
Decisional Conflict (Specify)
Denial, Ineffective
Dentition, Impaired
Development: Delayed, Risk for
Diarrhea
Disuse Syndrome, Risk for
Diversional Activity, Deficient
Dysreflexia, Autonomic
Dysreflexia, Autonomic, Risk for
Energy Field, Disturbed
Environmental Interpretation Syndrome, Impaired
Failure to Thrive, Adult
Falls, Risk for
Family Processes, Dysfunctional: Alcoholism
Family Processes, Interrupted
Family Processes, Readiness for Enhanced
Fatigue
Fear
Fluid Balance, Readiness for Enhanced
Fluid Volume, Deficient
Fluid Volume, Deficient, Risk for
Fluid Volume, Excess
Fluid Volume, Imbalanced, Risk for
Gas Exchange, Impaired
Grieving, Anticipatory
Grieving, Dysfunctional
Growth, Disproportionate, Risk for
Growth and Development, Delayed

Health Maintenance, Ineffective
Health-Seeking Behaviors (Specify)
Home Maintenance, Impaired
Hopelessness
Hyperthermia
Hypothermia
Identity: Personal, Disturbed
Infant Behavior, Disorganized
Infant Behavior: Disorganized, Risk for
Infant Behavior: Organized, Readiness for Enhanced
Infant Feeding Pattern, Ineffective
Infection, Risk for
Injury, Risk for
Knowledge, Deficient (Specify)
Knowledge (Specify), Readiness for Enhanced
Latex Allergy Response
Latex Allergy Response, Risk for
Loneliness, Risk for
Memory, Impaired
Mobility: Bed, Impaired
Mobility: Physical, Impaired
Mobility: Wheelchair, Impaired
Nausea
Neurovascular Dysfunction: Peripheral, Risk for
Noncompliance (Specify)
Nutrition, Imbalanced: Less than Body Requirements
Nutrition, Imbalanced: More than Body Requirements
Nutrition, Imbalanced: More than Body Requirements, Risk for
Nutrition, Readiness for Enhanced
Oral Mucous Membrane, Impaired
Pain, Acute
Pain, Chronic
Parenting, Impaired
Parenting, Readiness for Enhanced
Parenting, Risk for Impaired
Perioperative Positioning Injury, Risk for
Poisoning, Risk for
Posttrauma Syndrome
Posttrauma Syndrome, Risk for
Powerlessness
Powerlessness, Risk for
Protection, Ineffective
Rape-Trauma Syndrome
Rape-Trauma Syndrome: Compound Reaction
Rape-Trauma Syndrome: Silent Reaction
Relocation Stress Syndrome
Relocation Stress Syndrome, Risk for
Role Conflict, Parental
Role Performance, Ineffective
Self-Care Deficit: Bathing/Hygiene
Self-Care Deficit: Dressing/Grooming
Self-Care Deficit: Feeding
Self-Care Deficit: Toileting
Self-Concept, Readiness for Enhanced
Self-Esteem, Chronic Low
Self-Esteem, Situational Low
Self-Esteem, Risk for Situational Low
Self-Mutilation

Self-Mutilation, Risk for
Sensory Perception, Disturbed (Specify: Visual, Auditory, Kinesthetic, Gustatory, Tactile, Olfactory)
Sexual Dysfunction
Sexuality Patterns, Ineffective
Skin Integrity, Impaired
Skin Integrity, Risk for Impaired
Sleep Deprivation
Sleep Pattern Disturbed
Sleep, Readiness for Enhanced
Social Interaction, Impaired
Social Isolation
Sorrow, Chronic
Spiritual Distress
Spiritual Distress, Risk for
Spiritual Well-Being, Readiness for Enhanced
Spontaneous Ventilation, Impaired
Sudden Infant Death Syndrome, Risk for
Suffocation, Risk for
Suicide, Risk for
Surgical Recovery, Delayed
Swallowing, Impaired
Therapeutic Regimen Management: Community, Ineffective
Therapeutic Regimen Management, Effective
Therapeutic Regimen Management: Family, Ineffective
Therapeutic Regimen Management, Ineffective
Therapeutic Regimen Management, Readiness for Enhanced
Thermoregulation, Ineffective
Thought Processes, Disturbed
Tissue Integrity, Impaired
Tissue Perfusion, Ineffective (Specify: Renal, Cerebral, Cardiopulmonary, Gastrointestinal, Peripheral)
Transfer Ability, Impaired
Trauma, Risk for
Unilateral Neglect
Urinary Elimination, Impaired
Urinary Elimination, Readiness for Enhanced
Urinary Incontinence, Functional
Urinary Incontinence, Reflex
Urinary Incontinence, Stress
Urinary Incontinence, Total
Urinary Incontinence, Urge
Urinary Incontinence, Risk for Urge
Urinary Retention
Ventilatory Weaning Response, Dysfunctional
Violence: Other-Directed, Risk for
Violence: Self-Directed, Risk for
Walking, Impaired
Wandering

Source. NANDA Nursing Diagnoses: Definitions and Classification, 2003–2004. Philadelphia: North American Nursing Diagnosis Association. Used with permission.

APPENDIX C

Evaluate Your Response and Test Yourself Answers

Answers to Test Yourself

Chapter 1: The Medical-Surgical Nurse
1. D 2. A 3. B 4. C 5. C

Chapter 2: The Adult Client in Health and Illness 1. D 2. A 3. B 4. B 5. B

Chapter 3: Community-Based and Home Care of the Adult Client 1. B 2. D 3. C 4. A 5. B

Chapter 4: Nursing Care of Clients in Pain 1. B 2. A 3. B 4. D 5. C

Chapter 5: Nursing Care of Clients with Altered Fluid, Electrolyte, or Acid-Base Balance 1. A 2. D 3. B 4. D 5. A

Chapter 6: Nursing Care of Clients Experiencing Trauma and Shock 1. D 2. A 3. B 4. C 5. B

Chapter 7: Nursing Care of Clients Having Surgery 1. B 2. D 3. C 4. B 5. D

Chapter 8: Nursing Care of Clients with Infection 1. C 2. B 3. D 4. A 5. B

Chapter 9: Nursing Care of Clients with Altered Immunity 1. D 2. A 3. C 4. D 5. B

Chapter 10: Nursing Care of Clients with Cancer 1. C 2. A 3. C 4. B 5. C

Chapter 11: Nursing Care of Clients Experiencing Loss, Grief, and Death 1. C 2. D 3. B 4. A 5. C

Chapter 12: Nursing Care of Clients with Problems of Substance Abuse 1. B 2. A 3. D 4. C 5. B

Chapter 13: Assessing Clients with Integumentary Disorders 1. B 2. C 3. A 4. D 5. D

Chapter 14: Nursing Care of Clients with Integumentary Disorders 1. C 2. B 3. D 4. A 5. B

Chapter 15: Nursing Care of Clients with Burns 1. A 2. C 3. D 4. B 5. C

Chapter 16: Assessing Clients with Endocrine Disorders 1. D 2. A 3. C 4. B 5. B

Chapter 17: Nursing Care of Clients with Endocrine Disorders 1. A 2. C 3. C 4. D 5. B

Chapter 18: Nursing Care of Clients with Diabetes Mellitus 1. A 2. C 3. D 4. C 5. C

Chapter 19: Assessing Clients with Nutritional and Gastrointestinal Disorders 1. A 2. C 3. D 4. A 5. D

Chapter 20: Nursing Care of Clients with Nutritional Disorders 1. C 2. B 3. A 4. C 5. D

Chapter 21: Nursing Care of Clients with Upper Gastrointestinal Disorders 1. D 2. B 3. A 4. D 5. C

Chapter 22: Nursing Care of Clients with Gallbladder, Liver, and Pancreatic Disorders 1. A 2. C 3. D 4. B 5. C

Chapter 23: Assessing Clients with Bowel Elimination Disorders 1. D 2. A 3. D 4. D 5. C

Chapter 24: Nursing Care of Clients with Bowel Disorders 1. B 2. C 3. A 4. D 5. B

Chapter 25: Assessing Clients with Urinary System Disorders 1. D 2. C 3. B 4. C 5. A

Chapter 26: Nursing Care of Clients with Urinary Tract Disorders 1. B 2. D 3. A 4. C 5. C

Chapter 27: Nursing Care of Clients with Kidney Disorders 1. B 2. D 3. A 4. C 5. B

Chapter 28: Assessing Clients with Cardiac Disorders 1. C 2. D 3. C 4. A 5. B

Chapter 29: Nursing Care of Clients with Coronary Heart Disease 1. C 2. B 3. D 4. A 5. B

Chapter 30: Nursing Care of Clients with Cardiac Disorders 1. A 2. C 3. B 4. D 5. C

Chapter 31: Assessing Clients with Hematologic, Peripheral Vascular, and Lymphatic Disorders 1. D 2. A 3. B 4. C 5. A

Chapter 32: Nursing Care of Clients with Hematologic Disorders 1. C 2. D 3. A 4. B 5. A

Chapter 33: Nursing Care of Clients with Peripheral Vascular and Lymphatic Disorders 1. C 2. A 3. D 4. B 5. A

Chapter 34: Assessing Clients with Respiratory Disorders 1. D 2. C 3. B 4. D 5. C

Chapter 35: Nursing Care of Clients with Upper Respiratory Disorders 1. B 2. D 3. C 4. A 5. C

Chapter 36: Nursing Care of Clients with Lower Respiratory Disorders 1. D 2. B 3. A 4. C 5. D

Chapter 37: Assessing Clients with Musculoskeletal Disorders 1. C 2. A 3. B 4. D 5. A

Chapter 38: Nursing Care of Clients with Musculoskeletal Trauma 1. B 2. C 3. C 4. A 5. D

Chapter 39: Nursing Care of Clients with Musculoskeletal Disorders 1. B 2. D 3. D 4. A 5. C

Chapter 40: Assessing Clients with Neurologic Disorders 1. D 2. C 3. B 4. A 5. B

Chapter 41: Nursing Care of Clients with Cerebrovascular and Spinal Cord Disorders 1. B 2. D 3. C 4. A 5. B

Chapter 42: Nursing Care of Clients with Intracranial Disorders 1. D 2. B 3. B 4. A 5. C

Chapter 43: Nursing Care of Clients with Neurologic Disorders 1. C 2. A 3. B 4. D 5. B

Chapter 44: Assessing Clients with Eye or Ear Disorders 1. B 2. C 3. A 4. D 5. C

Chapter 45: Nursing Care of Clients with Eye and Ear Disorders 1. B 2. D 3. C 4. A 5. D

Chapter 46: Assessing Clients with Reproductive System Disorders 1. C 2. D 3. A 4. C 5. B

Chapter 47: Nursing Care of Men with Reproductive System Disorders 1. D 2. A 3. B 4. B 5. C

Chapter 48: Nursing Care of Women with Reproductive System Disorders 1. B 2. A 3. B 4. D 5. C

Chapter 49: Nursing Care of Clients with Sexually Transmitted Infections 1. B 2. A 3. D 4. A 5. C

Evaluate Your Response: Cues for Critical Thinking Questions

Chapter 4: Nursing Care of Clients in Pain

A Client with Chronic Pain

1. Review the factors that affect an individual's response to pain. What have you observed in your own family and friends, as well as clients for whom you have cared?

2. Reflect on the benefits and disadvantages of each alternative. Make your decision based on knowledge about pain and about medications for pain.

3. What factors in Ms. Akers's illness and treatment increase her risk for constipation? What would you include in the plan specific to fluid intake and diet?

Chapter 5: Nursing Care of Clients with Altered Fluid, Electrolyte, or Acid-Base Balance

A Client with Fluid Volume Excess

1. Review the homeostatic mechanisms that control fluid balance and cardiac output. Which mechanisms are employed in this situation?

2. Review the anatomy and physiology of the respiratory system, including cardiopulmonary blood flow. Think about the effects of the upper abdominal organs on respiratory function as well.

3. Use therapeutic communication techniques: What is behind the client's statement? How can you facilitate Mrs. Rainwater's involvement in care decisions?

4. Review the actions and precautions for diuretic therapy. Think about what the client needs to know in terms of timing, possible adverse effects, and other information about diuretic therapy.

A Client with Hypokalemia

1. Review the physiologic effects of potassium, especially its intracellular and neuromuscular effects.

2. Review the potential sites and causes of excess potassium loss.

3. Think about the effects of diuretics on potassium balance and the effects of hypokalemia on digitalis therapy. What is the primary indication for digitalis therapy and how does this contribute to the interaction of these three factors?

4. Review the section in Chapter 24 on constipation and its management. ⊕

A Client with Hyperkalemia

1. Review the causes and manifestations of hyperkalemia.

2. What are the potential effects of hyperkalemia on cardiac conduction? At what level of hyperkalemia are these likely to be seen?

3. Review collaborative treatment measures to rapidly reduce potassium levels. Why would these be used with a K+ of 8.5?

4. Think about the effects of anxiety on learning as you develop a plan to provide teaching to avoid future episodes of hyperkalemia. As you develop your plan, remember the potential long-term effects of chronic renal failure.

A Client with Acute Respiratory Acidosis

1. Review normal gas exchange across the alveolar-capillary membrane and the processes that drive this exchange. Then review the role that carbon dioxide plays as a potential acid.

2. Describe the effect of acidosis on mental function.

3. Consider risk factors for choking: alcohol consumption, taking large bites of food, inadequate chewing, and so forth.

Chapter 6: Nursing Care of Clients Experiencing Trauma and Shock

A Client with Multiple Injuries

1. The definition of *Deficient fluid volume* is decreased intravascular, interstitial, and/or intracellular fluid. Which of Mrs. Souza's vital signs would support this definition? What other assessments could you make that would further support this diagnosis?

2. Consider the physiology of cellular metabolism. How long do brain cells live without oxygen? What happens if circulation is improved but the airway is blocked?

3. What can cause restlessness? Consider comfort, elimination, oxygenation, emotional status, and immobility.

4. List the multiple possibilities for entry of pathogens into the human body. Would age and physical condition increase the risk? What about transmission from health care personnel?

A Client with Septic Shock

1. Review the pharmacologic effects of vasopressors. Consider the pathologic basis for septic shock and how these medications may be effective.

2. Review the content on respiratory acidosis in Chapter 5. ⊕ What do these findings tell you? What is present in Ms. Huang's physical status that would cause these manifestations?

3. Review the content about colloidal intravenous solutions in the chapter. What would you expect them to do when they are administered? How does this correlate to cardiac output? How do you assess increased circulatory volume?

Chapter 7: Nursing Care of Clients Having Surgery

A Client Having Surgery

1. Safety concerns include ambulating and not tripping over scatter rugs or clutter. See information in Chapter 3 on safety in the home. ⊕

2. Medications used to prevent an occurrence such as infection are called prophylactic medications. Her risks for infection are from the surgical wound and microvascular circulation in bone. Teach her to take the complete course of antibiotics prescribed and the possible side effects of the antibiotic. Encourage her to notify the physician if side effects or adverse events occur.

3. When blood stops flowing, it clots. Her immobility is a concern and puts her at risk for thrombosis and emboli. She has a risk for bleeding secondary to the anticoagulant and should inform any health care providers such as dentists that she is taking the anticoagulant.

4. Consider the risk for osteoporosis in addition to the degenerative changes Mrs. Overbeck experienced. She will need calcium sources and vitamin D.

Chapter 8: Nursing Care of Clients with Infection

A Client with Acquired Immunity

1. Review the adult immunizations listed in Table 8–8. ⊕ Consider the geographical area in which the client lives. For example, clients living in areas at risk for Lyme disease should check with their physician about the new Lyme disease vaccine.

2. Review the concept of acquired immunity and the discussion of immunization in this chapter. What affect could nonimmunized persons have on their family and community?

3. Identify possible systemic and local reactions associated with immunizations. List manifestations that the client should report to the primary caregiver.

Chapter 9: Nursing Care of Clients with Altered Immunity

A Client with HIV Infection

1. Considering Ms. Lu's age, how effective is her immune system? How could lifestyle factors affect immune status?

2. At this stage of Ms. Lu's diagnosis, would you expect the physician to order a viral load test? Why or why not?

3. You have been asked to discuss AIDS and safe sex practices to a group of high school freshmen. What information would you present to them?

4. What resources could you provide to Ms. Lu and her fiancé regarding their desire to have a child?

Chapter 10: Nursing Care of Clients with Cancer

1. Review content on altered nutrition in Chapter 20 and the content in this chapter on the nursing diagnosis Altered Nutrition: Less than Body Requirements. Make a list of diagnostic tests for malnutrition with normal values.

2. Consider the type of cancers Mr. Casey has been diagnosed as having. Where in the body do these malignancies commonly metastasize? What would cause the pain?

3. Review a pharmacology book for medications that increase appetite and make a list of those appropriate to Mr. Casey.

4. Sepsis is discussed in Chapter 6. ⌨ Review the content in that chapter on septic shock and outline manifestations. Develop a plan of care for Mr. Casey that is structured by priority of nursing diagnoses.

Chapter 11: Nursing Care of Clients Experiencing Loss, Grief, and Death

A Client Experiencing Loss and Grief

1. Review the physical manifestations of grief described in the chapter and compare and contrast those with the ones verbalized by Mrs. Rogers.

2. Consider the benefits of including Mrs. Rogers's daughter in a meeting of the staff. What type of questions would be most useful in making the daughter feel a part of the plan of care? Why would a statement such as, "Why don't you do more for your mother," be inappropriate?

3. Consider the losses Mrs. Rogers has experienced. Review the material in the chapter on responses to loss. Think about the reasons you would not say, "Oh, you have a lot to live for." Think of two or three questions or statements that would help you assess the reason why Mrs. Rogers said this to you.

Chapter 12: Nursing Care of Clients with Problems of Substance Abuse

1. Consider the interactions of prescribed or over-the-counter medications with alcohol. What if the client has not taken prescribed medications because of chronic alcoholism?

2. Review the effects of Anatbuse. Make a list of possible interactions and side effects.

3. *Imbalanced nutrition: Less than body requirements* is an appropriate nursing diagnosis when a client does not have sufficient nutritional intake to meet metabolic needs. What in Mr. Russell's history and physical assessment supports this diagnosis? What nutritional information should you provide?

Chapter 14: Nursing Care of Clients with Integumentary Disorders

A Client with Herpes Zoster

1. Consider environmental, economic, and language barriers. What agencies in your own city or state exist to provide help? What can you do other than make referrals? If you do make a referral, to whom would it be?

2. Review skin assessment guidelines in Chapter 13. ⌨ How would you determine that the lesions had not improved? What manifestations would indicate secondary infection of the lesions? What would you do next if the lesions are still very painful and have not improved?

3. *Ineffective role performance* is defined as patterns of behavior and self-expression that do not match the environmental context, norms, and expectations. Related factors include inadequate or inappropriate linkage with the health care system and poverty. Based on this information, what interventions would you use? How would you evaluate the effectiveness of your interventions?

A Client with Malignant Melanoma

1. List reasons why people do not seek health care. Do you believe nurses can effect change? If so, what community activities would be most effective?

2. Consider attitudes toward the possibility of future illnesses. How would this affect your plan? What do you believe would be most effective in teaching this age group?

3. Think about what you know about taking prescribed antibiotics as well as the side effects of antibiotic therapy. What would you suggest that Mr. Sanders do?

4. *Powerlessness* is the perception that one's own actions will not significantly affect an outcome. Is this a common response to the diagnosis of cancer? Consider types of communications and interventions that would allow greater decision making for Mr. Sanders.

Chapter 15: Nursing Care of Clients with Burns

A Client with a Major Burn

1. Review the effects of the major burn wound on the renal and gastrointestinal systems. What assessments would indicate effective fluid resuscitation?

2. What type of burns did Mr. Howard have on his arms? Consider the effect of compression on the peripheral vascular system. What assessments would you make to identify this complication?

3. Consider the type of pain the client has. What do you think might happen if the narcotics were given by other routes, such as oral or intramuscularly?

4. Review the effects of a major burn. Consider the damage to cell wall integrity and capillary beds. What effect does the shift of proteins and sodium have on intravascular volume?

Chapter 17: Nursing Care of Clients with Endocrine Disorders

A Client with Graves' Disease

1. What effect does increased TH have on metabolism and cardiac rate and stroke volume? How does this effect compare to that of sympathetic stimulation?

2. Consider the effect of elevating any body part, such as elevating your leg above heart level for a sprained ankle. How does this affect venous return?

3. You will need to consider Mrs. Manuel from both a medical and a surgical perspective. How would you teach her to care for her incision? With removal of most of the thyroid gland, what symptoms would you be sure she knew about? What should she do if these occur?

A Client with Hypothyroidism

1. Make a list of changes in body systems with aging and with decreased TH levels. How would you determine what assessment findings were abnormal?

2. Consider the effects of the following factors: weakness, fatigue, problems with memory. What would you recommend she do in her home to increase her safety?

3. Prepare a list of manifestations of hyperthyroidism. Be sure they are in terms a client would understand.

A Client with Cushing's Syndrome

1. Review Ms. Domico's lab results and compare them to normal results. What altered the findings in her case?

2. How many ways can you think of to assess fluid balance? Consider weight, I&O, and skin. What other assessments provide information?

3. Review Box 17–3. ⊝⊙ How does fatigue differ from "just being tired"? Would increasing hours of sleep be an intervention you would include? Why or why not?

A Client with Addison's Disease

1. Review the functions of the hormones of the adrenal cortex in Chapter 16. ⊝⊙ Consider the effects of stress, and formulate your response with rationale.

2. Review content on fluid imbalance in Chapter 5. ⊝⊙ Make a list of assessments you might make that would indicate severe dehydration. What is the pathophysiology of fluid loss in the client with Addison's disease?

3. Review content on sodium and potassium in Chapter 5 ⊝⊙ and make a list of foods you would suggest Mr. Sardoff eat.

Chapter 18: Nursing Care of Clients with Diabetes Mellitus

A Client with Type 1 Diabetes

1. How do the increased urinary output and increased osmolarity of the blood plasma affect the fluid status of the body? What is the response of the body to decreased intravascular volume?

2. Consider the effects of nicotine on blood vessels. How would these effects, when combined with the pathologic effects of long-standing hyperglycemia, affect blood vessel walls?

3. Review the information about chronic illness in Chapter 2. ⊝⊙ *Powerlessness* is a perceived lack of control over a situation and/or one's ability to significantly affect an outcome. What types of statements by a client would help you make this nursing diagnosis?

4. Compare and contrast the developmental needs and tasks of the young adult and the older adult (see Chapter 2 ⊝⊙). Consider the teaching materials that might have to be adapted to physical changes in the older adult.

Chapter 20: Nursing Care of Clients with Nutritional Disorders

A Client with Obesity

1. Review the physiology of cholesterol formation in the body and the factors that affect this process.

2. Consider developmental stages and teaching strategies for adult learners.

3. Think about individual factors, family and support group influences, and cultural factors that may affect recommended weight loss and exercise strategies.

A Client with Malnutrition

1. Review the physiology of albumin and cholesterol formation in the body.

2. Review Mrs. Chow's diet and compare it to the food pyramid or recommendations for food intake to formulate your response.

3. Consider cultural influences and the client's preferred foods as you plan a diet that is high in calories and protein.

Chapter 21: Nursing Care of Clients with Upper Gastrointestinal Disorders

A Client with Oral Cancer

1. Review the major risk factors for oral cancer and identify the populations most likely to have these risk factors.

2. Work with your classmates to plan (and implement) an education program, considering the developmental/teaching needs of this group of young people.

3. Think about the possible causes for Mr. Chavez's refusal to talk (remember that assessment is the first step of the nursing process). How will you identify factors contributing to his behavior?

A Client with Peptic Ulcer Disease

1. Review the physiology of the gastric mucosal barrier and the pathogenesis of peptic ulcer disease, and the effect of *H. pylori* infection on these processes.

2. Review physiologic responses to stress in your physiology or nursing fundamentals text; compare and apply this information with the physiology of the gastric mucosal barrier and the pathophysiology of ulcer development.

3. Consider Mr. O'Donnell's occupation and schedule, as well as the prescribed medications and when each should be taken.

4. Using journal and text resources as well as your classmates, identify as many stress reduction techniques as possible. Then sort your list into those which could be used while working, and identify ways to effectively teach each technique.

A Client with Gastric Cancer

1. Review the healing process and the normal physiology of the stomach as you formulate your answer to this question.

2. Consider the surgery, immediate postoperative care, and what the client and family should expect in developing your teaching plan.

3. Review Chapter 10 ∞ and nursing care related to chemotherapy.

4. Again, review Chapter 10 ∞ for nursing care measures for clients with cancer; also review Chapter 20 ∞ for strategies to prevent and manage malnutrition.

Chapter 22: Nursing Care of Clients with Gallbladder, Liver, and Pancreatic Disorders

A Client with Cholelithiasis

1. Review the composition of gallstones, as well as the physiology of gallbladder function and bile. Research and discuss dietary practices of the Chickasaw tribe (or of Native Americans).

2. Review Chapter 7 ∞ for care related to a laparotomy (incision into the abdomen).

3. As you develop your plan, consider Mrs. Red Wing's culture, job, and family obligations.

A Client with Hepatitis A

1. In your plan, consider the transmission and pathophysiology of hepatitis A. Review developmental considerations when teaching clients to adapt your teaching to Mr. Johns's level.

2. Review Table 22–2, ∞ as well as the pathophysiology of hepatitis.

3. Review Tables 22–2 and 22–3, ∞ as well as standard precautions.

4. In your plan, consider the living situation (group home), the developmental level of the residents, and the resident care

managers (largely unskilled). Work with your study or clinical group to develop this plan.

A Client with Alcoholic Cirrhosis

1. Review the anatomy and physiology of the liver and its circulation, as well as the pathophysiology of cirrhosis and its complications.

2. Consult your nutrition textbook as needed for foods that are high in calories but low in protein and sodium. When planning for limited protein intake, be sure to include high-quality proteins and limit intake of lower-quality proteins such as legumes.

3. Review the pathophysiology of hepatic encephalopathy and the ∞ medication box on page 591 to develop your responses to this question.

4. Review therapeutic communication skills; consult your nursing diagnosis and care planning text book as you develop this care plan.

A Client with Acute Pancreatitis

1. Review Chapter 12 for assessment data indicative of alcohol withdrawal.

2. Review both the pathophysiology of acute pancreatitis and the acute inflammatory process.

3. Consult your nutrition textbook or the American Dietetic Association web site: www.eatright.org

4. Consult your nursing care planning textbook to develop this care plan.

Chapter 24: Nursing Care of Clients with Bowel Disorders

A Client with Acute Appendicitis

1. Review the acute inflammatory response to an infectious process and the role WBCs play in the immune response. ∞

2. Review Chapter 7. Consider factors such as incision size, abdominal muscle disruption, and manipulation of the bowel in developing your response.

3. Consider points such as pain management, resumption of activities, incision care, and potential complications in developing your teaching plan. Consider the client's education

and developmental stage as well.

4. Review the effects of anxiety on recovery and learning. Identify nursing measures to reduce situational anxiety.

A Client with Ulcerative Colitis

1. Review normal functions of the small and large intestine. Review the usual location of an ileostomy. Review fluid volume deficit in Chapter 5 for manifestations and assessment data.

2. Think about the effect of chronic blood loss and review the effect of malnutrition on the hemoglobin and hematocrit.

3. Review the home care section of inflammatory bowel disease for teaching points to include.

4. Review nursing care for the client with diarrhea, as well as the procedure for ileostomy care.

A Client with Colorectal Cancer

1. Review peripheral innervation and impulse transmission in your anatomy and physiology textbook; think about how nerves in the rectal region are disrupted in an abdominoperineal resection. Also review the phantom ∞ pain phenomenon in Chapter 4.

2. Compare elimination through a colostomy with "normal" bowel elimination through the anus. How do they differ in terms of the passage of flatus? ∞

3. Review Procedure 24–1 and ∞ the nursing care box on page 672. Also review the procedure for administering an enema in your fundamentals or skills textbook.

4. Review this nursing diagnosis in your nursing diagnosis or nursing care planning handbook; be sure to individualize your plan to Mr. Cunningham's situation and needs.

A Client with Diverticulitis

1. Review Mrs. Ukoha's presenting symptoms and laboratory data. Then review the collaborative care section related to diverticulitis.

2. Consider how long Mrs. Ukoha may have been on bowel rest (NPO) prior to having a bowel movement, and the manifestations of diverticular disease.

3. Review the risk factors for and pathophysiology of diverticular disease and diverticulitis.

4. Consult your nutrition textbook and see Table 24–13 ⊕ to develop your teaching plan.

Chapter 26: Nursing Care of Clients with Urinary Tract Disorders

A Client with Cystitis

1. Consider risk factors for UTI as well as factors affecting Mrs. Waisanen's immune function.

2. Consider the indications for short-course antibiotic therapy and the indications for conventional therapy. Think about factors such as cost, compliance, and the risk for adverse effects, as well as how antibiotics work to eradicate bacteria.

3. Identify why *Ineffective health maintenance* may be an appropriate nursing diagnosis for Mrs. Waisanen and the individual factors contributing to this diagnosis as you plan care.

A Client with Urinary Calculi

1. Review the risk factors for urinary lithiasis.

2/3. Using the medications section of collaborative care for the client with urinary calculi in Chapter 26 ⊕ as well as Chapter 4, ⊕ and your pharmacology textbook or drug handbook, review analgesia for the client with renal colic and the intended and adverse effects of the drugs given to Mr. Leton.

A Client with a Bladder Tumor

1. Review the physiology of the bladder and the risk factors for urinary tract tumors.

2. Review Mr. Hussain's health history for possible contributing factors.

3. See Chapter 12 ⊕ for nursing care of clients with problems of substance abuse.

4. Use your nursing care planning and nursing diagnoses textbooks to identify possible outcomes and interventions for *Sexual dysfunction*.

A Client with Urinary Incontinence

1. Review the desired and adverse effects of the prescribed medications.

2. Review the effects of menopause and estrogen deficiency on perineal tissues.

3. Review Mrs. Giovanni's physical examination findings and risk factors for UTI.

4. Identify factors that may contribute to *Situational low self-esteem* in Mrs. Giovanni and nursing measures to address this diagnosis.

Chapter 27: Nursing Care of Clients with Kidney Disorders

A Client with Acute Glomerulonephritis

1. Review Chapter 8 ⊕ and the use of antibiotics to treat infection.

2. Review Mr. Chang's history and the risk factors for acute glomerulonephritis.

3. Review the diagnostic tests used to differentiate different forms of glomerulonephritis on page 750. ⊕

A Client with Acute Renal Failure

1. Review common causes and the pathophysiology of acute renal failure.

2. Review the sections on peptic ulcer disease and stress gastritis in Chapter 21. ⊕

3. Consider the position requirements to maintain body and bone alignment in skeletal traction (Chapter 38). ⊕

A Client with End-Stage Renal Disease

1. Review the usual onset, pathophysiology, and long-term effects of type 1 and type 2 diabetes (Chapter 18). ⊕

2. Consider the effects of urea and ammonia (both neurologic toxins) on brain function.

3. Review the manifestations of uremia.

4. Consider the composition of the dialysate and its possible effect on blood glucose control.

Chapter 29: Nursing Care of Clients with Coronary Heart Disease

A Client with Coronary Artery Bypass Surgery

1. Identify Mr. Clements's modifiable risk factors as you develop your plan. What barriers might need to be overcome to implement strategies to reduce his risk factors?

2. What strategies can you use to overcome denial without creating hostility or impairing the client-nurse relationship?

3. Consider traditional family roles as well as those roles that are unique to these individuals. Identify measures you can use to enlist the spouse's support.

4. Think about therapeutic communications as you formulate your response. Will your age or gender potentially affect your ability to respond effectively to these concerns? Would referral to another health care provider be appropriate?

A Client with Acute Myocardial Infarction

1. Review immediate treatment measures for MI. Are other means available for reestablishing coronary artery perfusion? If you are in a rural area without immediate access to a cardiac catheterization lab, how will this affect your response?

2. Review the section of this chapter on dysrhythmias and their treatment. Research protocols for treating frequent PVCs in the post-MI client at your clinical facility.

3. Review the goals of cardiac rehabilitation and Mrs. Williams's individual risk factors as you develop your teaching plan.

4. Consider the value of using a therapeutic response to Mrs. Williams's statement concerning smoking. Also consider the risks associated with cigarette smoke. How can you respond without supporting Mrs. Williams's desire to smoke and without precipitating anger or resistance? Review Chapter 12. ⊕

A Client with Supraventricular Tachycardia

1. Review the effects of sympathetic and parasympathetic nervous system stimulation on cardiac function.

2. Review the section on supraventricular tachycardias, as well as the antidysrhythmic medications for other treatment options.

3. Use your pharmacology textbook as you develop your teaching plan.

Chapter 30: Nursing Care of Clients with Cardiac Disorders

A Client with Heart Failure

1. Review the prescribed medications and their interactions. Do not forget to consider Mr. Jackson's age in assessing his risk for toxicity and interactions.
2. Review therapeutic communications skills and the use of open-ended statements to evaluate the underlying message of Mr. Jackson's statement.
3. Review exercise recommendations for the client with heart failure (page 885) as well as cardiac rehabilitation principles (Chapter 29).
4. Review the rationale for aspirin therapy in the client with CHD and its effects on platelets and clotting as you formulate your response.
5. Review Chapter 41 for causes of CVA and the section of Chapter 29 on atrial fibrillation.

A Client with Mitral Valve Prolapse

1. Review the pathophysiology and manifestations of MVP, as well as the general treatment measures for valve disorders.
2. Think about the effects of progressive conditioning on cardiac function.
3. Consider the anxiety associated with heart conditions and with a potentially progressive disorder that could affect childbearing and other life activities, as well as ultimately necessitate surgery.
4. Review the manifestations of MVP and of mitral regurgitation.

Chapter 32: Nursing Care of Clients with Hematologic Disorders

A Client with Anemia

1. Consider the effects of Mrs. Matthews's rapid weight loss on fluid balance, as well as the effects of tissue hypoxia on cardiac output.
2. Refer to Box 32–6 and your nutrition text. Be sure to consider Mrs. Matthews's age in designing your menu.
3. Consider factors such as Mrs. Matthews's recent dietary history, the folic acid content of foods, and other pertinent factors in the history and physical assessment
4. In addition to general factors to consider for the older adult (don't forget transportation among other factors), also consider the possible effect of Mrs. Matthews's recent loss and the grieving process.

A Client with Hemophilia

1. Review the pathophysiology of hemophilia and its effect on the clotting process.
2. Consider both the ABCs and Maslow's hierarchy of needs as you respond to this question.
3. Think about the genetic transmission of hemophilia. How might Mr. Cruise's hemophila affect any children that he has? Grandchildren?
4. Review your nursing fundamentals book, nursing skills book, and intravenous therapy text to develop your teaching plan. Also consider previous learning and developmental levels.
5. Consult your nursing care planning text. Consider why this might be an appropriate nursing diagnosis for Mr. Cruise.

A Client with Leukemia

1. Review the physiology of white blood cells, and the immune and inflammatory responses.
2. Think about the risks created by hospitalization in terms of exposure to infection and invasive procedures.
3. Think about the effect of inability to perform self care on self-esteem, self-confidence, and perception of power and control.
4. Use information provided in the nursing care and home care sections of this chapter as well as in Chapter 8.
5. Use your nursing care planning and fundamentals texts to develop your care plan.

A Client with Hodgkin's disease

1. Review Chapter 10 and the effects of chemotherapy and radiation on cancerous cells. Think about the advantages of combining these two therapies in terms of short and long-term desired and adverse effects.
2. Consider the primary and potential risks for infection in community settings as you design your teaching plan. What teaching strategies will you use for a young adult with Mr. Quito's education and experience?
3. Review theories of development and the developmental tasks for the young adult.
4. Use your nursing fundamentals and nursing care planning texts for reference in developing your care plan.

Chapter 33: Nursing Care of Clients with Peripheral Vascular and Lymphatic Disorders

A Client with Hypertension

1. Review Mrs. Spezia's assessment data and the risk factors for primary hypertension.
2. Review the pathophysiology of primary hypertension and of obesity (Chapter 20), as well as the relationship between hypertension and coronary heart disease.
3. Think about resources that are available in your community for homeless people. Talk to community health and social service agencies to identify additional resources.
4. Again, review Mrs. Spezia's assessment data, the pathophysiology of hypertension, and the long-term effects of stress.
5. Use your nursing care planning and nursing diagnosis textbooks to help develop your care plan.

A Client with Peripheral Atherosclerosis

1. Review treatments for peripheral atherosclerosis, as well as lifestyle measures for preventing and treating atherosclerosis and coronary heart disease (Chapter 29).
2. Compare the pathophysiology of peripheral atherosclerosis, intermittent claudication, and coronary heart disease (Chapter 29) to identify similarities and differences.
3. Review the actions of beta blockers and their role in angina prophylaxis.
4. Use your nursing care planning and nutrition textbooks to help develop your care plan.

A Client with Deep Vein Thrombosis

1. Review the pathophysiologic processes of venous thrombosis and inflammation as you develop your answer.

2. Think about questions you could ask for further information as well as potential resources for Mrs. Hipps.

3. Consider assessment data to evaluate Mrs. Hipps's limitations and resources, as well as community resources to help meet her needs.

4. Use your nursing diagnosis and care planning textbooks to develop your plan of care.

Chapter 35: Nursing Care of Clients with Upper Respiratory Disorders

A Client with Peritonsillar Abscess

1/2. Review the manifestations of upper respiratory infections and management of these disorders.

3. Think about the primary uses of the nose, mouth, and pharynx as you consider nursing diagnoses related to upper respiratory disorders.

A Client with Nasal Fracture

1. Consider other measures to restore the client's sense of control over the situation. Consider the potentially traumatic effects of suction on the mucous membranes as well as possible infection control risks.

2. Review the implications and potential dangers of CSF leakage to help you develop your care plan.

3. Think about the benefits and drawbacks of immediate and delayed rhinoplasty.

A Client with Total Laryngectomy

1. Review the options for speech rehabilitation. If available, practice using a speech generator. Practice esophageal speech.

2. Use your nursing care planning and nursing diagnoses handbook to develop your care plan. Consider Mr. Tom's age, occupation, and marital status in your plan of care.

3. Review Chapter 7 ⊖⊃ for surgical nursing care interventions, as well as your nursing fundamentals textbook for wound care strategies.

4. Consider measures to promote airway clearance and ventilation of all lung fields.

Chapter 36: Nursing Care of Clients with Lower Respiratory Disorders

A Client with Pneumonia

1. Review Mrs. O'Neal's assessment data and compare her history with identified risk factors for pneumonia.

2. Review normal immune and inflammatory responses and the role of white blood cells in these processes.

3. Review Chapter 9 ⊖⊃ and altered immune responses for the physiology and effects of anaphylactic shock.

4. Use your nursing care planning and nursing diagnosis textbooks to help develop your care plan.

A Client with Tuberculosis

1. Consider available resources for mentally ill clients, as well as community and public health resources. Consider measures to ensure compliance with the prescribed treatment.

2. Contact your local public health department, the discharge planner for your unit, or the social services department in your clinical facility to help identify available resources.

3. Use your nursing fundamentals text, the nursing care section under Pneumonia, and your nursing diagnosis or care planning handbook as you develop your care plan.

A Client with COPD

1. Review the processes by which cigarette smoke inflicts damage on lung tissue. Use your pediatric and pathophysiology texts for additional information.

2. Review the physiology of the respiratory drive, as well as the effects of chronic elevated carbon dioxide levels in the blood.

3. Review the manifestations of COPD and its complications as well as the section of this chapter on respiratory failure.

4. Use your nursing diagnosis handbook to help identify appropriate goals and interventions for this nursing diagnosis.

A Client with Lung Cancer

1. Review Chapter 10 ⊖⊃ and use your pharmacology text to research the effects of these drugs and the rationale for combination chemotherapy.

2. Use Chapter 10 ⊖⊃ and your pharmacology text to identify probable side effects of this treatment regimen. Then use your nursing care planning book to identify appropriate nursing diagnoses and interventions.

3. Review the pathophysiology and collaborative care sections for lung cancer to develop your response to this question.

A Client with ARDS

1. As you respond to this question, consider additional treatment measures for ARDS and respiratory failure. Also consider the potential long-term consequences and complications of intubation and mechanical ventilation. Discuss strategies for communicating with Ms. Adamson's family and supporting coping and decision-making by Ms. Adamson and her family in an instance such as this.

2. Think about the precipitating factors for ARDS and the factors that may precipitate respiratory failure in a client with COPD. Consider the probable overall respiratory and general health status of the individual affected by each of these conditions.

3. Review the precipitating factors for ARDS and discuss strategies to prevent them.

4. Use your nursing care planning book to identify appropriate goals and nursing interventions for this nursing diagnosis.

Chapter 38: Nursing Care of Clients with Musculoskeletal Trauma

A Client with a Hip Fracture

1. Consider Mrs. Carbolito's age and the fact that she is postmenopausal. What effect does estrogen have on bone health? What might have increased her risk for falls?

2. Review the principles of traction application. What purpose does it

serve prior to surgery? What words could you use that she would understand? Think about the effects of trauma, pain, and suddenly finding oneself in a strange environment on listening and understanding verbal communications.

3. List how each of these manifestations would affect skin integrity, food intake, and bone healing.

A Client with a Below-the-Knee Amputation

1. Design a sequential plan for Mr. Rocke's self-care of the stump. Consider his readiness to learn and the complexity of the care. Is there a risk in letting him assume total responsibility from the beginning? Why or why not?

2. List the factors used to describe Mr. Rocke. How do these affect his ability or willingness to follow up with medical care? What community agencies are available where you live or go to school that would be good sources of assistance and support for Mr. Rocke?

3. Review the information about exercise. How would Mr. Rocke's choice not to do exercises affect his ability to use a prosthesis to walk?

Chapter 39: Nursing Care of Clients with Musculoskeletal Disorders

A Client with Osteoporosis

1. Review the effects of nicotine and caffeine on blood circulation to bones. What effect does alcohol play in bone loss?

2. Review foods that increase blood cholesterol levels. What is considered a normal cholesterol level? You may need to read content in Chapter 29. ⬤ Knowing the client needs calcium, what type of dairy products would you recommend?

3. List activities for the client who is not able to be ambulatory. How many of the activities on your list would help prevent osteoporosis?

4. *Risk for trauma* is defined as an increased risk for accidental tissue injury, such as a fracture. What

interventions would you teach Mrs. Bauer to reduce this risk?

A Client with Osteoarthritis

1. Review information about serum creatinine and BUN in a laboratory studies textbook or on the web. What medications is Mr. Cerulli taking that may be affecting these findings? Consider what teaching is necessary related to these findings.

2. What assessments are significant for confusion? If necessary, review content related to confusion. Review Mr. Cerulli's history in the case study and determine factors that may have contributed to his risk for confusion before, during, and after surgery.

3. *Acute confusion* is defined as an abrupt onset of a cluster of global, transient changes and disturbances in attention, cognition, psychomotor activity, level of consciousness, and/or sleep/wake cycle. What assessments could you make to support this diagnosis for Mr. Cerulli? What interventions might you design for this diagnosis?

A Client with Rheumatoid Arthritis

1. Think about the role differences in a 42-year-old woman and a 72-year-old woman. On the other hand, consider the effects of a chronic illness that may have been present for 30 years. Would your plan differ? Why or why not?

2. List the possible disabilities that may be caused by rheumatoid arthritis. How do you believe these would affect Mrs. James? What agencies in your community are available for support of people with this type of illness? Where would you go for literature to give Mrs. James?

3. *Ineffective role performance* is defined as behaviors and expressions that do not match norms or expectations. Do you believe this is an appropriate nursing diagnosis for Mrs. James? Why or why not? What interventions could be implemented for this diagnosis?

Chapter 41: Nursing Care of Clients with Cerebrovascular and Spinal Cord Disorders

A Client with a Stroke

1. What subjective manifestations does the client with hypertension have? (Review content in Chapter 33.) ⬤

2. How does increased blood pressure affect the walls of blood vessels in the cerebral circulation?

3. Consider referral to community resources as a volunteer tutor for adult literacy, gardening, and/or woodworking. Tutoring college students is another option.

4. Use statements that will encourage Mr. Boren to talk about his arm and how he feels about being unable to use it.

A Client with a SCI

1. What are the developmental tasks of a 19-year-old? How does the inability to meet these tasks affect emotional responses?

2. Think about questions that explore Mr. Valdez's fears in relation to sexuality. Practice questions and statements with friends until you are not embarrassed to ask them.

3. Consider how your own values and beliefs may differ from those of a client.

4. What baseline assessments and information are necessary before developing a plan for urinary elimination needs? Why would self-catheterization be an option? What are the risks of long-term Foley catheterization?

A Client with an Intervertebral Disk

1. What emergency management of any possible spinal cord injury is necessary, and why?

2. Consider social and economic needs. What types of community and health care resources are available for a young single mother?

3. What type of clothing would be most useful for Mrs. Ivans? In what sequence should she dress? What about shoes?

Chapter 42: Nursing Care of Clients with Intracranial Disorders

A Client with a Migraine Headache

1. Review the content in the chapter on migraine headaches. List questions that you would ask specific to onset, length, manifestations, stages, pain, diet, and factors associated with the headache onset.

2. Consider foods that are high in sodium. What would you suggest if Ms. Friedman eats fast foods at least five times a week? Review the food pyramid in Chapter 2 ⊙⊙ and outline a weekly meal plan for Ms. Friedman.

3. Discuss with members of your class those factors that interfere with their normal sleep patterns. What suggestions might you give Ms. Friedman to help her improve her sleep? Why is this important?

A Client with a Seizure Disorder

1. List the teaching topics you would include for Ms. Carlson. Consider how her needs (e.g., for safety) would differ if she lived alone.

2. Describe statements you could use to help Ms. Carlson understand not only the dangers but also the legal issues involved. What if Ms. Carlson does not recognize these concerns?

3. What type of questions could you ask Ms. Carlson to determine why she feels this way? Would you personally find it embarrassing? How can you facilitate Ms. Carlson's understanding for this recommendation?

A Client with Subdural Hematoma

1. Review the manifestations of the types of intracranial hematomas. What assessments are specific to a subdural hematoma? Why is it important to know this?

2. What are some other interventions that might be used? How could family help? What if no family members are available?

3. Acute confusion is a sudden onset of changes in attention, cognition, psychomotor activity, level of consciousness, and/or sleep/wake cycle. What would you determine as priority nursing diagnoses and interventions for Mr. Lee?

A Client with Bacterial Meningitis

1. List the environmental stimuli in the hospital setting. How could these be decreased? What effect do these stimuli have on cognition and behavior that is altered by an intracranial infection?

2. Think about how you would feel if Mr. Cook tried to hit you. How would you respond to him? To whom would you report this?

3. Why would Mr. Cook have pain? How would pain be manifested during the initial treatment period for Mr. Cook? Is it important to consider the respiratory effects of narcotics for him? Defend your answer.

A Client with a Brain Tumor

1. Review content in the chapter on increased intracranial pressure and intracranial surgery. List collaborative and nursing interventions to decrease increased intracranial pressure.

2. What do these manifestations indicate? What would be your priority assessment? Who would you notify?

3. Practice the use of therapeutic communications and what response you would make.

4. Consider the reasons Ms. Lange feels powerless. What nursing interventions might decrease this feeling?

Chapter 43: Nursing Care of Clients with Neurologic Disorders

A Client with AD

1. Think about what information you would need and how you would collect it. Consider such factors as the age of family members, educational level of family members, and stage of the client's AD. What else would you need to know?

2. Review the suggested activities in this section of the chapter. What others can you think of or have you seen used successfully? Osteoarthritis often results in joint stiffness and pain as well as problems with mobility. Would this affect your interventions? If so, how could they be adapted?

3. Consider the type of foods that might be prepared, the timing of meals, and interventions that might be used to decrease agitation before or during meals.

A Client with MS

1. Outline a typical day's activities for Mr. McMurphy that would provide a balance between activity and rest. What assessments would you make to evaluate the effectiveness of this plan?

2. Consider how respiratory infections are spread. Why is Mr. McMurphy at increased risk?

3. The definition of *Risk for injury* is that one is at risk as a result of environmental conditions interacting with the person's adaptive and defensive resources. What factors in this client's history and physical status would support this diagnosis? What interventions would you include in the care plan and why?

A Client with Parkinson's Disease

1. Consider the adaptations that might be made to clothing and shoes. What adaptive devices might be useful?

2. What information would you need to know before you develop your interventions? Include that from Mr. Avneil and what might be available in the community and the long-term care facility.

3. *Chronic sorrow* is a recurring pattern of sadness in response to continual loss. Consider the type of communications you would need to use with Mr. Avneil to identify his degree of sorrow. What other assessment might provide cues to support this diagnosis (think about eating and sleeping)? How might an activity such as reminiscence help?

A Client with Myasthenia Gravis

1. Review the pathophysiology of myasthenia gravis. What is the action of Tensilon?

2. Consider teaching topics for Mrs. Avis that would assist her in conserving energy while preparing meals. List suggestions to conserve energy while eating.

3. *Ineffective role performance* is the state in which behaviors and self-expression do not match such factors as norms and expectations. What changes occur as a result of this illness? What do you think Mrs. Avis expects of herself? What are some interventions you could implement to facilitate acceptance of the change she is experiencing?

Chapter 45: Nursing Care of Clients with Eye and Ear Disorders

A Client with Glaucoma and Cataracts

1. What is the pathophysiology of glaucoma? How does a cataract affect glaucoma?

2. Consider the effects of cortico-steroids on glaucoma. If Mrs. Rainey is to administer several medications at home, identify specific teaching guidelines for her.

3. Consider referral for home health visits. Think about the effect of transferring her for a brief admission to an assisted-living facility.

Chapter 47: Nursing Care of Men with Reproductive System Disorders

A Man with Prostate Cancer

1. Why would Mr. Turner be at risk for altered skin integrity? Outline the interventions you would include on his teaching plan that would promote skin integrity as he cares for himself at home.

2. *Noncompliance* is defined as behaviors that do not coincide with the therapeutic plan agreed upon by the person and the health care professional. Do you think Mr. Turner fully understood his treatment and agreed with his follow-up care? What could be done in the preoperative phase of Mr. Turner's care to better ensure his understanding and desire to have continued medical care?

3. What assessments indicate that Mr. Turner does or does not have bladder distention? Would you report this? If so, to whom?

Chapter 48: Nursing Care of Women with Reproductive System Disorders

A Woman with Endometriosis

1. What is the relationship between Mrs. Hall's manifestations and a decreased RBC count? Review the information in Chapter 32 ∞ and list assessments you would make to identify anemia.

2. List nonthreatening questions you would use to begin the discussion. How might it help to ask these questions at the beginning of the interview? Then list questions that you might use to collect data about the couple's sexual history. Would you be embarrassed to ask them? If so, how might this in turn affect their responses?

3. *Situational low self-esteem* is the state in which a person develops a negative perception of self-worth in response to a current situation. What information in Mrs. Hall's history might provide data to support this nursing diagnosis?

A Woman with Cervical Cancer

1. Review the risk factors for cervical cancer. Consider what might differ for a young woman and an older woman.

2. Review the information in Chapter 10 ∞ on radiation as a treatment for cancer. What interventions would be appropriate for Ms. Gillam?

3. Based on your review of the information on radiation, explain how radiation might cause fatigue. How does fatigue differ from being tired? What interventions would you include in a plan of care for this nursing diagnosis?

A Woman with Breast Cancer

1. Review the information in the chapter on the genetic factors that pose a risk for developing breast cancer. How could you explain this in terms understandable by Mrs. Clemments and her daughters?

2. List the different types of mastectomies. Consider the implications of the differences, and how this would affect your nursing care.

3. Review the information on chemotherapy in Chapter 10. ∞ List the types of chemotherapy and its common side effects. Consider the classifications of medications that are used to treat these side effects.

4. What factors in the treatment of Mrs. Clemments treatment might disrupt the amount and quality of her sleep? What interventions might be used to improve her sleep pattern?

Chapter 49: Nursing Care of Clients with Sexually Transmitted Infections

A Client with Gonorrhea

1. What manifestations does Ms. Cirit have that are typical of the disease? Would you make other assessments? If so, what are they?

2. Review the discussion of HIV in Chapter 9. ∞ Do you believe it is true that infection with gonorrhea may increase the risk of HIV? If so, how would you explain this to Ms. Cirit?

3. *Impaired social interaction* is a state of aloneness or rejection experienced by an individual that is perceived as negative. What assessments of Ms. Cirit might support this diagnosis? What interventions and expected outcomes would you develop?

A Client with Syphilis

1. Describe the assessments you would expect to find in a man with early syphilis.

2. Consider topics such as number of sex partners, patterns of sexual activity, and use of safe sex practices. What other topics should be explored? How can you ask these questions without being embarrassed or embarrassing the client?

3. List possible statements you might make. Do you believe this is a nursing responsibility? If you do not feel comfortable with this topic, what could you do?

CREDITS

All photographs/illustrations not credited on page, under or adjacent to the piece, or not credited below, were photographed/rendered on assignment and are property of Pearson Education/Prentice Hall Health.

Illustrations:

Figure 28–3	Todd A. Buck
Figure 28–7	Todd A. Buck
Figure 34–1	Todd A. Buck
Figure 19–1	Todd A. Buck
Figure 12–2	Todd A. Buck
Figure 44–1	Todd A. Buck
Figure 37–1	Todd A. Buck
Figure 37–4	Todd A. Buck
Figure 44–11	Todd A. Buck

INDEX

SINGLE PC LICENSE AGREEMENT AND LIMITED WARRANTY